Mar... son, 1982

Date Booster dates	Date Booster dates	Date Booster dates	Date Booster dates
Date Booster dates	Date Booster dates	Date Booster dates	Date Booster dates
Date	Date	Date	Date
Date	Date	Date	Date
Date Booster dates	Date Booster dates	Date Booster dates	Date Booster dates

THE MACMILLAN GUIDE TO

FAMILY HEALTH

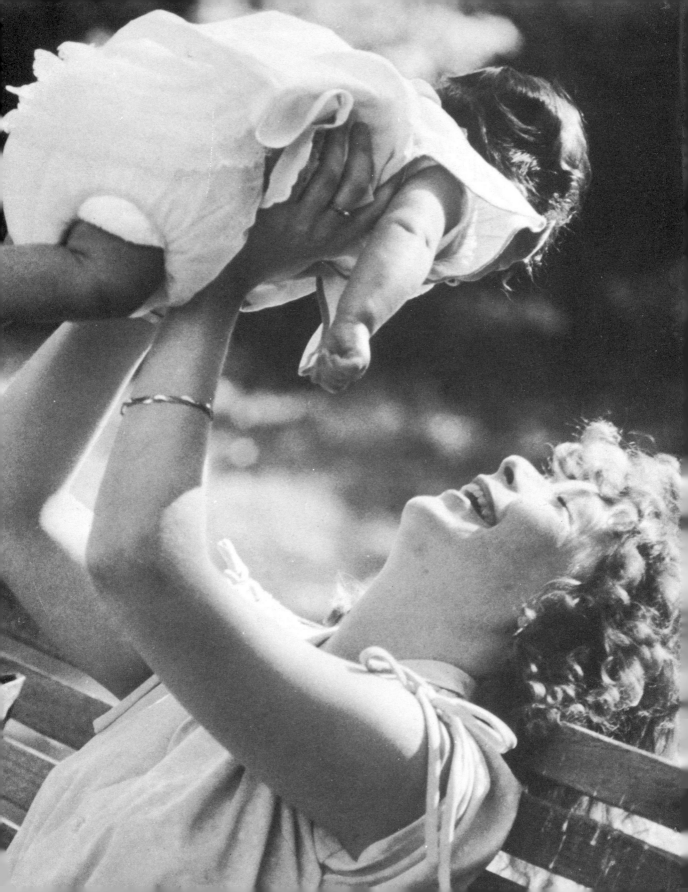

THE MACMILLAN GUIDE TO

FAMILY HEALTH

Editor-in-Chief
Dr Tony Smith MA BM BCh

BOOK CLUB ASSOCIATES
LONDON

Typesetting
Vantage Photosetting Co Ltd

Reproduction
Aero Offset Reproductions Ltd

Printed by
New Interlitho Spa, Milan

Foreword

Whenever you fall ill, whether with a trivial head cold or a life-threatening cancer, you want to know as much as possible about the disease. In the past 20 years medicine has lost much of its aura of secrecy; you can now expect to be told what is wrong with you, what can be done about it, and what the possible outcome may be. Yet at a hospital clinic or even in your own doctor's surgery you may be too anxious or embarrassed to ask all these questions – and if you manage to ask them, the answers may be so complex that you cannot understand them or can remember only parts.

The first aim of the Macmillan Guide to Family Health is, then, to fill the gaps and provide comprehensive answers to basic questions about common and important diseases – to tell you what, in an ideal world, your own doctor would tell you. During preparation of the Guide we have drawn on the experience of both medical specialists and general practitioners so as to balance specialist expertise with the priorities given by family doctors to common and recurrent illnesses.

Secondly, the Guide encourages medical self-reliance. Day-to-day illnesses and accidents usually need no professional treatment – and some may need no treatment at all. Here, the Guide offers the unique aid of self-diagnosis symptom charts. These charts take common symptoms such as headache, vomiting, or pain in a joint and help you to decide whether you can rely on self-treatment or whether you need medical attention. Next, to help you gain the confidence to look after yourself, the Guide explains what happens in minor disorders and what can be done to relieve symptoms. On occasions when medical help is needed for a particular symptom or disorder, the warning signs and degree of urgency are clearly spelt out.

The third – and in some ways most important – aim of the Guide is to help you improve your life style. Contemporary medicine is giving greater emphasis to prevention, and the Guide provides practical advice on diet, exercise, and the essentials of preventive medicine such as immunization against infections. The diseases most likely to strike down people in the prime of life – strokes, heart attacks, and cancers – are at least partly attributable to "self-inflicted" factors such as overeating, over-indulgence in alcohol and tobacco, lack of exercise, and psychological stresses and conflicts.

The technological achievements of medical science mean that doctors can do more than ever before to restore health by replacing or repairing worn-out or damaged joints and heart valves and even transplanting kidneys and other organs. These are, however, treatments of last resort. Each of us is largely responsible for his or her own body, and throughout the Guide we emphasize that the key to a long, healthy life lies in maintenance and prevention rather than in repeated repairs.

Dr Tony Smith
MA BM BCh

Contents

Part IV
Caring for the sick

ADVISERS

Prof H J Gamble
*Professor of Neuroanatomy, St Thomas's
Hospital Medical School, London*

Dr D Haslam MRCGP DRCOG
*General Practitioner, Ramsey,
Cambridgeshire*

Mr S P B Percival MB FRCS
*Consultant Ophthalmic Surgeon,
Scarborough Hospital Group,
Yorkshire*

Dr J L Scheuer
*Senior Lecturer in Anatomy,
St Thomas's Hospital Medical School,
London*

Dr R Turner MB FRCGP
*General Practitioner,
Bexley, Kent*

Dr D J Williams MRCP MRCGP
*Consultant, Accident and Emergency Department,
The Middlesex Hospital, London*

EDITORIAL TEAM

Project editor	Stephen Parker
Project art editor	Patrick Nugent
Text editors	Donald Berwick
	Anthony Whitehorn
Editors	Cathy Meeus
	Lindy Newton
Editorial assistant	Starry Schor
Designers	Julia Goodman
	Bob Gordon
	Julia Harris
	Helen Sampy
Project advisers	Dr Alex Armstrong MBBS
	Dr Helen Dziemidko MBBS
	Elizabeth Fenwick
Managing editor	Jackie Douglas
Art director	Roger Bristow

How to use this book

The Macmillan Guide to Family Health is designed for use in both sickness and health, and the contents of its four parts (The healthy body; Symptoms and self-diagnosis; Diseases, disorders, and other problems; and Caring for the sick) are closely related. The following suggestions should help you take full advantage of the services the book offers to you and your family. (For a complete *Contents* list see the previous two pages.)

Questionnaires to tell you how healthy you are
Begin by checking the current state of your health and the possible effects of life style – including eating and drinking habits – upon future well-being. The questionnaires around which the first part of the book is built will tell you much about yourself (see, for example, *How good is your general health?* on p.13). They also lead you, where appropriate, into relevant sections of Part I, where you will find information and advice about steps you can take to improve your chances for lasting health. And, for a better understanding of all aspects of health and illness, Part I contains a detailed colour *Atlas of the body* (p.49), which you can consult for the name and position of almost any organ in the body.

Have you a current problem?
The major portion of the book is concerned with diagnosis and disease, and here the emphasis is on problem-solving. The best way for you to use this material depends on where your problem lies. The *Self-diagnosis symptom charts* (p.66) in Part II provide a unique method of finding out what a particular symptom (or symptoms) may signify.

The symptom charts have been specifically compiled for people who do not know what is wrong with them – or whether, in fact, anything *is* wrong – but whose bodies are behaving in any one of 99 rather odd ways. The "odd" way may be an ache or pain, a swelling, or difficulty in breathing, swallowing, or sleeping. Look up the symptom that is troubling you in the special *Chart-finder* (p.68), turn to the correct symptom chart, and follow through. (The introduction to Part II gives you thorough instructions for finding the relevant symptom chart for your problem and using it to advantage.) The chart may suggest that your immediate problem is not serious enough to require the services of a doctor, or it may indicate the need for medical help either immediately or within a few days. In most cases you will be referred to another portion of the book in order to gather more information on your tentative self-diagnosis. You may, as one possibility, be directed to a colour photograph in the section containing *Visual aids to diagnosis* (p.233). More often, you will be referred to a Part III article dealing with the disease or disorder that seems likely to have caused your problem.

Diseases and disorders

If you are already seeing a doctor about a specific disorder and would like to know more about it – perhaps just to find out whether your condition is fairly common among people of your age and sex – you can look it up in the general index and turn directly to the relevant article in Part III. In other cases, you may be referred to an article from one of the self-diagnosis symptom charts in Part II. Another alternative is referral from the first part of the book, where you may have learned that an aspect of your current life style is putting your health at risk from a particular disease.

Every article in Part III is organized in such a way as to anticipate questions and answer them frankly in, as far as possible, non-technical language. The facts about any disorder tend to arrange themselves logically around answers to five basic questions:

What are the symptoms?
How common is the problem?
What are the risks?
What should be done?
What is the treatment?

In certain cases additional questions – what, for instance, are the long-term prospects for recovery? – arise, and such questions are asked and answered where appropriate. Illnesses that are too trivial or rare to warrant extensive discussion are covered in a few sentences.

The first three questions are self-explanatory. A word about the last two, however: "What should be done?" involves both what you yourself should do (whether, say, you should see your doctor right away or simply spend a few days in bed) and what you can expect the doctor to do in order to make a firm diagnosis of your condition. Note, too, that in the "What is the treatment?" category specific drugs are not generally identified. The reason for this is that while it is possible to specify the type of drug generally prescribed for a given disorder, the choice of particular drugs within the type is too great to be summarized in a short article. (For more about drugs, see below.)

Most articles in Part III deal with health problems common to both sexes and all ages; but there are also groups of articles concentrating on matters of chief concern to particular segments of the population: men, women, couples, infants and children, adolescents, and the elderly. In addition, there is a series of articles concerned with problems of pregnancy and childbirth.

Caring for the sick

In the last part of the Guide – Part IV – you will find advice on general problems of health care that everyone must face from time to time. The articles cover both professional medical care and self-care procedures, and may be read as tracing the progress of a typical illness from the GP's surgery to the hospital bed, to convalescence at home. From this structure emerges useful information about choosing a family doctor, various medical specialities, hospital services, and problems involved in caring for the sick at home. There are also suggestions about matters seldom spoken about, such as practical ways of coping with terminal illness, death, and funeral arrangements.

Drugs

The *Drug index* (p.778) provides information on the uses of various drugs, the way they are administered, and their possible side-effects. Most drugs commonly in use in Britain are included under trade and chemical names.

Words you may not understand

In reading about medical matters you are certain to come across occasional words or phrases that are either unfamiliar or used in a peculiarly medical sense. Most such words are italicized where appropriate in the following pages; and italicized terms, along with many others, are clearly defined in the *Glossary* (p.788).

First aid for accidents and emergencies

If at any time you need to take first-aid action in order to safeguard your health or the health of others, turn to the quick-reference section *Accidents and emergencies* (p.801). In addition to providing information on life-saving measures for potentially fatal emergencies, these pages also give practical instructions for treating minor, everyday problems such as blisters and grazes.

The Macmillan Guide to Family Health has been prepared after careful consideration by the Editor-in-Chief and the Contributors, and represents an understanding of medical knowledge at the date of publication. However, diagnosis and the application of medical knowledge to treatment *depend on the particular circumstances that are applicable to each individual, and readers are therefore urged always to consult a qualified physician. It is hoped that this book will enable the reader to work with a physician in a more constructive and better informed way.*

Part I

The healthy body

Introduction
Keeping physically fit
Keeping mentally fit
The effects of stress
Eating and drinking sensibly
The dangers of alcohol
The dangers of smoking
Safety and environmental health
Early warning signs of possible serious illness
Atlas of the body

The healthy body

Introduction

Are you in good health? It may be several years since you last saw your doctor or were ill enough to stay in bed for a week, but of course that is no guarantee of future good health. Physical and mental breakdowns are common in middle age. Many such breakdowns are due to years of unhealthy living and are therefore avoidable.

Unless you are one of the relatively few really health-conscious individuals, your current life style is almost certainly less healthy than it should be. Now is the time to modify it. You will benefit, first of all, by lowering the risks of preventable illness. And as you become increasingly fit, you will feel better all round and will find that you are more capable of enjoying life. Certain basic guidelines for healthy living are simple, and medical research shows convincingly that they improve your chances for a long, healthy life. These guidelines are set out below, as the five basic rules for healthy living.

If you follow the guidelines, you will retain your health and vigour, and you will increase your life expectancy. Even if you are middle-aged and overweight, and last took

exercise when you were a teenager, you can move gradually into a healthier living pattern. First, you should check on the present state of your health and the soundness of various aspects of your current life style. The series of questionnaires in this part of the book will help you to evaluate your fitness. And the articles accompanying each questionnaire should serve as a guide to staying healthy.

Certain aspects of life style, behaviour, and recent medical history are especially important in assessing the current state of your health. The questionnaire *How good is your general health?* on the opposite page identifies the most significant factors, as indicated in many recent medical studies. Try this questionnaire first, using it as a starting point for your new health programme.

Our society's current emphasis on diet, exercise, and other aspects of life style is not just an accumulation of fashionable fads. The major diseases of middle age are serious – often fatal – yet are more easily prevented than cured. There is no mystery about what to do. Your life is largely in your hands.

Five basic rules for healthy living

1 If you smoke, give it up. **Now!** There is no longer any doubt about the link between smoking tobacco and the development of serious illnesses such as lung cancer and some forms of heart disease.

2 If you drink alcohol, drink in moderation – no more than an average of two pints of beer (*or* four small measures of spirits *or* four glasses of wine) each day.

3 Take some strenuous exercise at least twice, and preferably three times, each week.

4 Eat sensibly. You need a balanced diet with plenty of fruit and vegetables, but go easy on cream, butter, fatty foods, sugar, cakes, and other sweet things.

5 Do not let yourself get overweight. If you are already obese (see the *Weight chart*, p.28), go on a reducing diet until you are healthily slim.

The health questionnaires

The questionnaires in Part I of this book have been compiled mainly for the use of adults; but most of the questions are applicable to any age group. You will find them helpful as a starting point in evaluating your physical and mental well-being and that of all members of your family. Evaluation is only the first step, however. Where possible, you should go on to take further steps to improve your chances of avoiding illness by reading and acting on the information and advice in the articles that accompany each of the questionnaires.

Two of the questionnaires – those dealing with drinking alcohol and smoking – may not concern you directly. However, they may concern others in your family who can test themselves, and who should read the relevant articles. Emphasize the need for answering honestly. If you cheat on the questions, the only person you are cheating is yourself.

How good is your general health?

Answer YES or NO to the following questions

1 Are you within desirable weight limits for your height (see the *Weight chart,* p.28)?

YES☐ NO☐

2 When walking briskly with people of your own age group, can you match their pace and carry on casual conversation without becoming short of breath?

YES☐ NO☐

3 Can you walk up 3 flights of stairs (each comprising around 15 or 20 steps) without having to pause for breath?

YES☐ NO☐

4 Do you take exercise vigorous enough to make you breathless and sweaty at least 3 times a week?

YES☐ NO☐

5 Do you ordinarily sleep soundly *and* wake up feeling energetic and ready for the day ahead?

YES☐ NO☐

6 At the end of a working day do you usually feel energetic enough to go out and enjoy a social evening?

YES☐ NO☐

7 Do you drink, on average, less than 2 pints of beer (or 4 measures of spirits or 4 glasses of wine) a day?

YES☐ NO☐

8 Are you – and have you been for at least the last 15 years – a non-smoker?

YES☐ NO☐

9 Can you eat more or less what you like without forethought (i.e. without worrying about possible unpleasant after-effects of foods such as cucumbers or onions)?

YES☐ NO☐

10 Do you seldom (less than once a week) take patent medicine or home remedies for a problem such as headache, constipation, or indigestion?

YES☐ NO☐

EVALUATION
If you can answer YES to all the above questions, you are at this moment in good health. More than a total of 3 NO answers suggests the need for serious consideration of some sort of change in life style. In the latter event you should try the more detailed questionnaires in the following pages, and adopt any helpful advice in the accompanying articles that may apply in your case. In addition, all readers will do well to examine the list of symptoms included under *Early warning signs of possible serious illness* (p.48).

Keeping physically fit

It is no accident that the words "fit" and "healthy" are often linked. Level of physical fitness reflects the state of a person's general health; and your body's fitness is largely determined by the amount of physical work that you do. Physical work includes all movements – even such routine activities as walking, eating, sitting, and breathing – but most important from the standpoint of fitness is the quantity and quality of vigorous exercise you take. In these pages you will find an explanation of why exercise can improve your health, well-being, and life expectancy, along with some tips on how to become physically fit by devising your own exercise programme. As a starting point, assess your current level of fitness by means of the *step test* recommended below.

How fit are you?

The step test is designed to assess the efficiency of heart, lungs, and muscles in response to a set amount of exercise. The result gives an indication of almost anyone's general level of fitness.

Note: If you answered NO to question 3 in the questionnaire entitled *How good is your general health?* (p.13), you should *not* attempt this test; see your doctor first.

Before you try the step test . . .
This exercise separates the very unfit from those of average or just-below-average fitness: Walk steadily up 3 flights of stairs (each comprising 15 to 20 steps). Do you have to pause for breath, or are you so breathless when you reach the top that you cannot talk normally? If you answer YES, you are very unfit and should consult your doctor before attempting to get fitter.

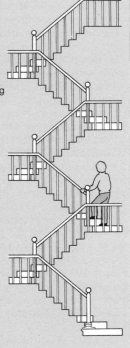

The step test
Choose a bottom stair – or any fixed platform – about 200mm (8in) high. Step on to it with one foot, bring up the other, and then step back down on to the floor (below left). Repeat the up-and-down process at a rate of 24 times a minute for 3 minutes. (A test run will help you get the rhythm right.)
WARNING: Do not continue the exercise if you begin to feel unpleasantly out of breath, dizzy, nauseated, or in any way uncomfortable.
   Stop after 3 minutes and wait for exactly 1 minute. Then check your heartbeat rate by counting your pulse over the next 15 seconds, and this will enable you to read off your fitness rating on the table below.

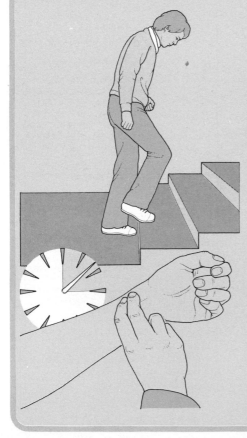

Pulse (heartbeats) counted in 15 seconds				Fitness rating
MEN		WOMEN		
Under 45 years	Over 45 years	Under 45 years	Over 45 years	
Below 18	Below 19	Below 20	Below 21	Excellent
18 to 20	19 to 21	20 to 22	21 to 23	Good
21 to 25	22 to 26	23 to 28	24 to 29	Average
Above 25	Above 26	Above 28	Above 29	Poor

Why exercise is good for you

In the context of physical fitness, "exercise" refers to any activity involving a fairly high degree of physical movement that makes you breathless and sweaty if you do it vigorously. Digging in the garden or washing the car can be just as much "exercise" as a game of soccer or an hour's hard cycling, provided it is done vigorously enough.

There is a sound physiological reason why physical activity is good for you. Any work that muscles do increases their need for oxygen. During physical exercise you must breathe more deeply to get more oxygen into your lungs, and your heart (which is itself almost all muscle) must beat harder and faster to pump blood to the muscles. Heart disease accounts for almost a third of all deaths and a high proportion of serious illness in the industrial West. So an efficient, resilient heart – not to mention strong lungs – means you are less likely to have major health problems. One British survey has shown that middle-aged people with desk jobs who do not exercise in their spare time are twice as susceptible to heart attacks as are comparable people who exercise regularly.

The more you work your muscles, and the larger the number of muscles and joints that you use, the greater the physical gain. The most beneficial kind of exercise is "dynamic" (jogging, say, or swimming). Dynamic exercise strengthens the heart, lungs, and body muscles when it makes you breathless and sweaty. It also keeps joints supple, thus guarding against the early onset of disorders such as osteoarthritis. The alternative "static" exercise (such as weightlifting), which builds specific muscles to excessive degrees, does little to improve your heart and lungs, and little to improve general fitness.

Lack of exercise can contribute to development of various disorders. Anyone whom illness or injury has forced to lie in bed for a time will know how weak their muscles become. The same disuse also affects the bones and can damage organs such as the kidneys. And unexercised, weak muscles put extra strain on other structures such as joints and ligaments by overloading them.

The physical benefits of dynamic exercise are unarguable. There are psychological benefits, too. Many people sleep better after exercise, wake more refreshed, and are more alert and better able to concentrate than they were when unfit. And exercise helps, to some extent, to keep you healthily slim. To sum up, exercise of the right sort should make you feel better, live longer, and have less illness.

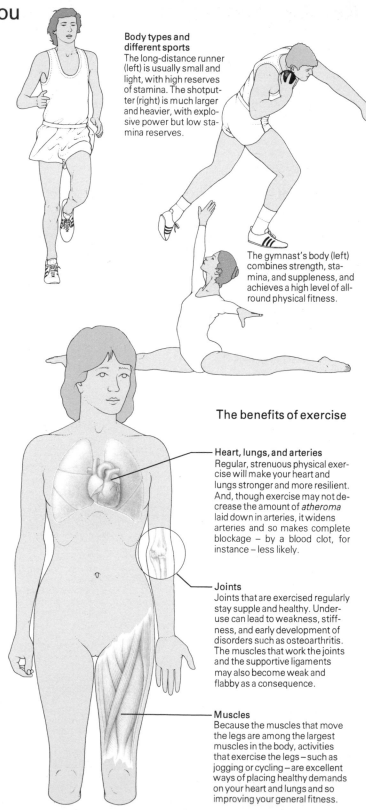

Body types and different sports
The long-distance runner (left) is usually small and light, with high reserves of stamina. The shotputter (right) is much larger and heavier, with explosive power but low stamina reserves.

The gymnast's body (left) combines strength, stamina, and suppleness, and achieves a high level of all-round physical fitness.

The benefits of exercise

Heart, lungs, and arteries
Regular, strenuous physical exercise will make your heart and lungs stronger and more resilient. And, though exercise may not decrease the amount of *atheroma* laid down in arteries, it widens arteries and so makes complete blockage – by a blood clot, for instance – less likely.

Joints
Joints that are exercised regularly stay supple and healthy. Underuse can lead to weakness, stiffness, and early development of disorders such as osteoarthritis. The muscles that work the joints and the supportive ligaments may also become weak and flabby as a consequence.

Muscles
Because the muscles that move the legs are among the largest muscles in the body, activities that exercise the legs – such as jogging or cycling – are excellent ways of placing healthy demands on your heart and lungs and so improving your general fitness.

The essentials of a good exercise programme

The right sort of exercise for you is exercise that will benefit *your* body in its current state of fitness. The following recommendations are based on three pieces of advice that apply to everyone who wants to embark on a successful exercise programme.

1. Have at least two, and preferably three, exercise sessions every week, preferably at regular intervals and stated times. Make each session 20 minutes or longer, with little or no pause for rest. Choose a level of activity high enough to make you breathless, sweaty, and aware of your heart beating – but not so violent that you become dizzy or nauseated, or risk straining muscles or joints. It is always advisable to do warm-up exercises before the main exercise session.

2. You must choose forms of exercise that you enjoy and that you can fit into your schedule. If you dislike sports, energetic gardening and do-it-yourself work around the house are good, purposeful ways of keeping active. Cycling or brisk walking to and from your place of work can easily be fitted into everyday routines. The important thing is not to do whatever you set out to do grudgingly.

3. Do not attempt to get fit too rapidly. Start gently, exercising just hard enough to become aware of mild strain, and heighten your efforts gradually over the course of the first four weeks. If you start a new sport, beware of over-competitiveness. If you take up a potentially very strenuous game such as squash, try to improve on your last performance rather than on your opponent's.

A final note of warning. If you belong to one of the following categories, ask your doctor for advice before you take up any sort of strenuous activity:

- People over 60 years of age, or those over 45 who have had little or no hard exercise since early adulthood.
- Heavy smokers (anyone who smokes more than 20 cigarettes a day).
- People who are seriously overweight (see the *Weight chart* on p.28).
- People under treatment or supervision for a long-term health problem such as high blood pressure, heart disease, diabetes, or kidney disease.
- People with a rating of "poor" according to the fitness test described in *How fit are you?* on p.14.

Warm-up exercises

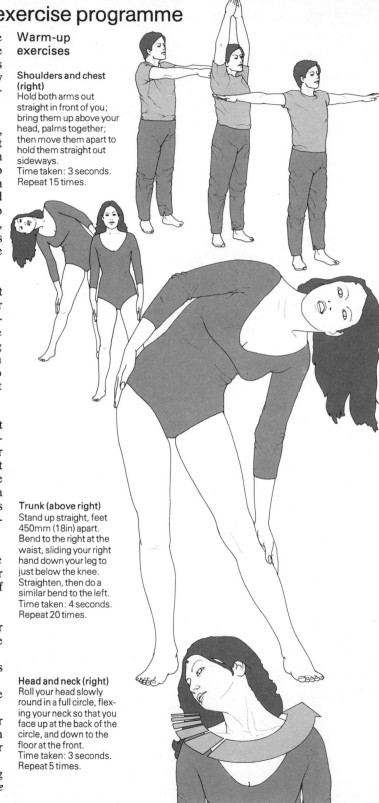

Shoulders and chest (right)
Hold both arms out straight in front of you; bring them up above your head, palms together; then move them apart to hold them straight out sideways.
Time taken: 3 seconds.
Repeat 15 times.

Trunk (above right)
Stand up straight, feet 450mm (18in) apart. Bend to the right at the waist, sliding your right hand down your leg to just below the knee. Straighten, then do a similar bend to the left.
Time taken: 4 seconds.
Repeat 20 times.

Head and neck (right)
Roll your head slowly round in a full circle, flexing your neck so that you face up at the back of the circle, and down to the floor at the front.
Time taken: 3 seconds.
Repeat 5 times.

Hips and trunk
Right: Stand up straight, bend forwards at the waist, and bring one leg up to touch face with knee; then straighten. Repeat for other leg. Time taken: 4 seconds. Repeat 10 times.
Below: Hold arms out sideways, with feet slightly apart. Slowly swing arms and upper body to face right, then swing round to face left. Time taken: 2 seconds. Repeat 20 times.

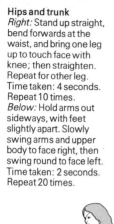

Arms and shoulders using weights
Lie on your back on a firm surface, gripping equal weights in either hand. Keeping arms straight, bring hands together above head. Slowly lower arms back to floor. Time taken: 2 seconds. Repeat 15 times.

Exercise bicycle (below)
A static exercise bicycle is a very useful all-weather fitness machine. Measure each day's performance against your previous performance, and aim for a steady week-by-week improvement. Adjust the braking mechanism on the bicycle as you gradually increase your fitness level.

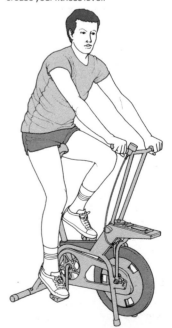

Fitness values of selected common activities
Included in this table are a number of common sports and everyday physical activities, and the fitness benefits they can be expected to provide. At best, such a table can be only an approximate guide. Ratings are based on a level of strenuousness likely to be maintained by ordinary, non-professional participants in each of the various activities. Do not interpret the evaluations as applicable to someone, for example, who is either cycling lazily through flat country lanes or is competing in the Tour de France.

Key to chart symbols

*	Negligible
**	Fair
***	Good
****	Excellent

Activity	Calories consumed in 20 minutes of activity	Value in improving health of heart and lungs	Value in improving suppleness of joints	Value in improving muscle power
Easy walking	60	*	*	*
Housework	90	*	**	**
Light gardening (weeding, etc.)	90	*	**	**
Golf (flat course)	90	*	**	*
Brisk walking	100	**	*	**
Badminton	115	**	***	**
Horse riding	115	**	***	**
Gymnastics	140	**	****	**
Heavy gardening (digging, etc.)	140	**	***	****
Easy jogging	160	***	*	**
Tennis	160	***	***	**
Disco dancing	160	***	****	*
Ice skating	160	***	***	**
Skiing (downhill)	160	***	***	**
Hockey	180	***	***	**
Rowing	180	****	**	****
Soccer	180	***	***	***
Rugby	180	***	***	****
Squash	200	***	***	**
Brisk jogging	210	****	**	**
Bicycling	220	****	**	***
Swimming	240	****	****	****

Keeping mentally fit

As indicated in the section of this book that deals with *mental and emotional problems* (p.294), most of us, though on a fairly even keel for most of the time, undergo occasional periods of great stress. Bereavement, financial difficulties, ill-health, and worry are all part of the fabric of living but it is when several stressful factors occur together that mental health may suffer. Although such stresses do not literally cause mental (and physical) disease, they can play an important part in making you more susceptible to disease (see *Are you under too much stress?* on p.23). So, since you cannot avoid stress, you will do well to study the following pages that advise you how you can develop an attitude of mind which will protect your mental (and physical) health. Some people, unable to cope when subjected to extreme stress, collapse into mental illness. To withstand the tensions of difficult periods everyone needs a generally healthy frame of mind as well as a healthy body. Are *you* fit enough to avoid breaking down under any emotional strains that may unexpectedly occur? The questionnaire entitled *How is your mental health?* (below) will help in assessing the current state of your mental well-being and resilience.

How is your mental health?

Answer YES or NO to the following questions

1 Are you sleeping badly?
YES ☐ NO ☐

2 Do you feel generally tired and lacking in energy?
YES ☐ NO ☐

3 Do you find it hard to concentrate on something, even when you intensely want to do so?
YES ☐ NO ☐

4 Are you so discontented with your job that you suspect you are no longer doing it as well as you should?
YES ☐ NO ☐

5 Do you have few or no interests and activities other than your work?
YES ☐ NO ☐

6 Do you usually try to avoid meeting new people because of the strain of having to think of something to say to them?
YES ☐ NO ☐

7 Do you find it difficult to get along with people?
YES ☐ NO ☐

8 Do trivial setbacks and inconveniences make you irritable or bad-tempered even when you *know* they are trivial?
YES ☐ NO ☐

9 Do you feel really close to nobody, not even members of your immediate family?
YES ☐ NO ☐

10 Do you view life as a continual uphill struggle?
YES ☐ NO ☐

11 Do you tend not to bother too much with your personal appearance?
YES ☐ NO ☐

12 Do you often have headaches?
YES ☐ NO ☐

13 When you think about the future, do you become extremely depressed?
YES ☐ NO ☐

EVALUATION
If you answer YES to no more than 2 questions, you need not worry about your mental fitness. YES answers to 3 or more questions suggest that you should study the following articles, and perhaps accept some of the advice they offer. This is especially important if external events are already producing a stressful period in your life. To estimate the likely impact of current external events upon your mental reserves, see the questionnaire *Are you under too much stress?* on p.23.

How to relieve tension

Some people manage to be easy-going and relaxed no matter what the stresses and pressures on them. For others, even a small problem becomes a major disaster, a source of constant worry or anger. If you are in this latter group, try to remember that strong emotions affect the body physically by releasing the hormone adrenaline into the bloodstream. Adrenaline increases breathing and heartbeat rates, makes the stomach queasy and the muscles tense, and raises blood pressure. If continually repeated, such bodily reactions can become increasingly harmful – especially to people with heart disease, but also to people who are physically sound. The

procedures recommended below and on the next page should serve as aids to dissipate any tension that has built up.

Muscle-relaxation exercises

In most areas of Britain, yoga classes, partly subsidized by the local authority, teach (among other things) muscle relaxation. If you cannot join one of these, however, try practising the following simple exercises on your own; they can help almost anybody to unwind. Be sure to do them regularly, not just when you feel you either *must* relax or burst. A gradually acquired ability to relax will stand you in good stead when trouble comes.

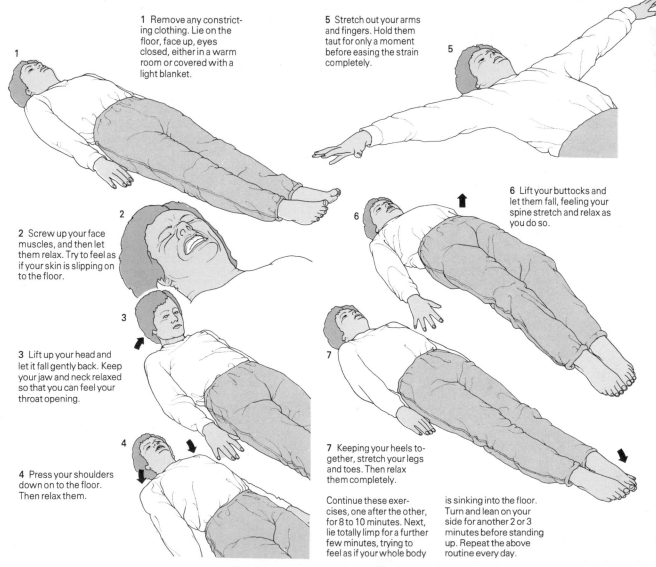

1 Remove any constricting clothing. Lie on the floor, face up, eyes closed, either in a warm room or covered with a light blanket.

2 Screw up your face muscles, and then let them relax. Try to feel as if your skin is slipping on to the floor.

3 Lift up your head and let it fall gently back. Keep your jaw and neck relaxed so that you can feel your throat opening.

4 Press your shoulders down on to the floor. Then relax them.

5 Stretch out your arms and fingers. Hold them taut for only a moment before easing the strain completely.

6 Lift your buttocks and let them fall, feeling your spine stretch and relax as you do so.

7 Keeping your heels together, stretch your legs and toes. Then relax them completely.

Continue these exercises, one after the other, for 8 to 10 minutes. Next, lie totally limp for a further few minutes, trying to feel as if your whole body is sinking into the floor. Turn and lean on your side for another 2 or 3 minutes before standing up. Repeat the above routine every day.

Breathing exercises

Deep breathing is helpful at all times, and a habit of taking deep rather than shallow breaths is one of the strongest weapons against the onset of tension. To develop the habit, sit or lie in a comfortable position, and breathe deeply and slowly, timing the breaths so that you take half as many as usual during the course of one minute. Continue this rhythmic activity for five minutes (but stop if you begin to feel dizzy). Do the exercise twice a day, every day. And if at other times you begin to feel a build-up of tension, make a point of slowing your breathing to the exercise rate for a few minutes; the almost inevitable and immediately noticeable result will be some easing of mental strain. You will gain the full benefit of this deep breathing if you also remember to let your shoulders relax completely at the same time.

Meditation

There are many meditation techniques, all of which have the same goal: to achieve tranquillity by emptying the mind of distracting thoughts and worries.

A number of organizations teach meditation methods. You need not take a course or join a group, though. Most people are capable of acquiring the meditation habit on their own. If you want to learn to meditate, try the following method:

1. With your eyes closed and your back straight, sit in an upright but comfortable chair in a quiet room.

2. Choose a word or phrase that has no emotional overtones for you ("oak", say, or "bring"). Without moving your lips, repeat the word silently to yourself, giving your full attention to the word as a word, not to its meaning. If any thought or image enters your mind, do not actively try to banish it, but do not follow it; instead, fasten your attention on the unspoken sound of the chosen word.

3. Do this steadily for five minutes twice a day for a week – or until you have become adept at emptying your mind of all thoughts for an extended period. Then gradually increase the meditation period until you can manage about 20 minutes at each session.

Some people find it easier to focus their attention on something visual – a wall pattern or a candle, for example – rather than a word. The important thing is to banish thought (and, incidentally, worry) by means of non-emotive concentration.

How to get a good night's sleep

The "average" person has between seven and eight hours of sleep in an "average" day. But, in fact, sleep requirements differ widely. If you always wake up after only five to six hours and find it impossible to drop off again, do not worry; this is probably as much sleep as you need. And there is generally no cause for concern if you seldom have an unbroken night's rest. Many people tend not only to over-estimate their need for sleep but to under-estimate the amount they get during a restless night. Research into sleep-time behaviour and electrical brain waves indicates that few people lying in bed and trying to sleep through the night really get "hardly a wink" of sleep.

A few days – or even a fairly regular diet – of skimpy sleep will do you no harm as long as you remain energetic and healthily alert during waking hours. If, however, you feel over-tired or too tense to relax into sleep when you go to bed, try some of the following eight suggestions. If you continue to suffer from some form of insomnia and it appears to be

How to cope with a crisis

No matter how healthy your normal state of mind and body, it is likely that throughout the course of your life you will not escape an occasional crisis brought on by stress. At any such time the best way to remain on an even keel is to adopt the following attitudes and modes of behaviour:

1 Concentrate on things as they are *now*. Do not increase your mental burdens by brooding about the past. Think about future events only in so far as you can help to shape them; do not worry about a future that you cannot control.

2 Consider your problems one at a time. Reacting to an accumulation of stresses as if they were an interrelated single threat often results in an inability to take positive action. Carried to an extreme, this can lead to serious mental illness.

3 Talk things over with your close relations and friends. Do not complain or burden them with your troubles, but seek – and listen to – their opinions and advice.

affecting your daily routine, consult your doctor. Though prolonged spells of sleeplessness may not themselves damage health, insomnia is sometimes a warning symptom of a mental illness such as *anxiety* (p.300) or *depression* (p.297). (For other possible causes of difficulty in sleeping see *Self-diagnosis symptom chart 4.*)

1. Do not take work to bed with you. If you like to read in bed, read nothing remotely concerned with your job or other matters that may be bothersome.

2. Have at least some physical exercise during the day so that your body feels tired enough to crave rest at bedtime. It often helps to take a short, gentle stroll in the open air an hour or so before going to bed.

3. Try not to go to bed within three hours of having a full meal; a full stomach is not conducive to sleep. A warm, milky drink or even a small whisky at bedtime, however, may make you sleepy.

4. A warm bath – *not* a brisk shower – just before bedtime may help you relax.

5. Although an emotional upset or violent exercise just before going to bed is likely to retard sleep, satisfactory sexual intercourse is apt to have a sedative effect.

6. Make sure that you are neither too hot nor too cold. Most people sleep best in a room temperature of 16 to 18°C (60 to 65°F).

7. Use the relaxation techniques described in the preceding pages.

8. If all else fails, get out of bed and stay up for the rest of the night rather than turning and tossing restlessly. In fact, you may break the cycle of insomnia by making a point of staying up all night just once .

Sleep patterns
The diagram below shows how the brain's activity changes during a night's sleep. Periods of "REM" (Rapid Eye Movement) sleep – during which dreams are thought to occur – alternate with sessions of deep sleep. As morning approaches, sleep becomes gradually more shallow until you awaken

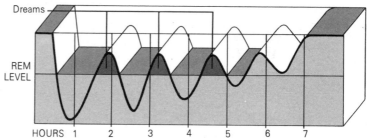

4 Having decided what you want to do about a problem that you *can* influence, act promptly and firmly. Positive action is bound to be healthier than passive brooding.

5 Occupy yourself and your mind as much as possible. Any social activity – cards, sports, theatres, discussion groups – is preferable to solitude at times of great emotional strain.

6 Do not nurse grudges or blame other people for your current trouble. Even if you have been wronged in some way, a constant sense of frustrated hostility will accomplish nothing except further damage to your mental health.

7 Make a point of devoting some time every day to physical relaxation that temporarily frees your mind from its preoccupations. If you go for a walk, for instance, it is much better to concentrate on what you see around you instead of on your problems.

8 Apart from being more sociable and more physically active than usual, it is especially important to stick as nearly as you can to your daily routine. At times of crisis a familiar pattern of regular meals and chores done at specified hours can encourage a sense of security by forcing order upon apparent chaos.

9 So as not to take your cares to bed with you, try not to think about them after 8pm. You will sleep better if you manage to wind down a few hours before going to bed. And if you wake during the night, you are more likely to be relaxed enough to go back to sleep if you were not occupied with problem-solving when you first dropped off.

10 Learn to recognize a crisis, and never be too proud to admit that you are overwhelmed by anxiety and can no longer manage on your own. Consult a doctor sooner rather than later. Alternatively (or in addition), ask for help from an organization such as the *Samaritans* (p.768), which will assist anyone in mental distress. It may surprise you to find that, once you put your problems and fears into words, they no longer seem insurmountable.

The effects of stress

Any substantial change in your routine – including changes for the better as well as changes for the worse – will make demands on your mental and emotional resources. Researchers have shown that as stresses accumulate for an individual, he or she becomes increasingly susceptible to physical illness, mental and emotional problems, and even accidental injuries. Shown here are the parts of the body most susceptible to stress-related diseases – though the exact cause-and-effect process is often unclear.

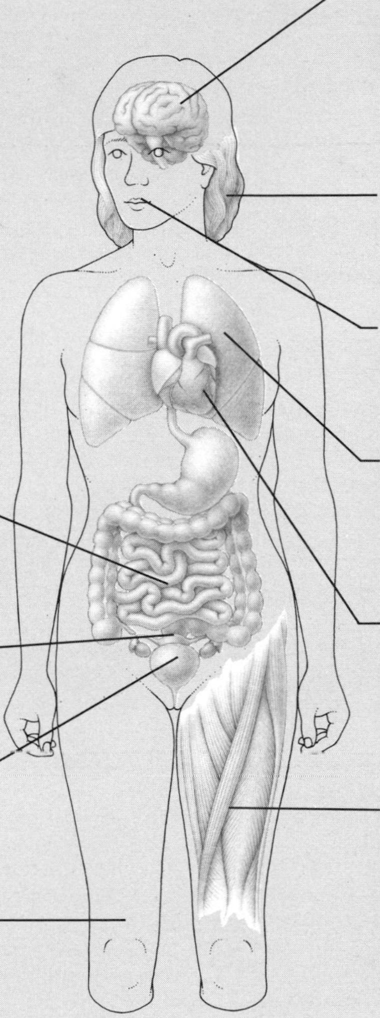

Brain
Many mental and emotional problems – among them anxiety, depression, and schizophrenia – may be precipitated by stress.

Hair
Some forms of baldness – among them alopecia areata – are linked to high levels of stress.

Mouth
Mouth problems such as aphthous (mouth) ulcers and lichen planus often seem to crop up when the individual is under stress.

Lungs
Asthmatics often find that their condition worsens when they are subjected to high levels of mental or emotional stress.

Heart
Attacks of angina and disturbances of heart rate and rhythm often occur at the same time as, or follow closely upon, a period of stress.

Muscles
Various minor muscular twitches and "nervous tics" become more noticeable when the individual is under stress, and the muscular tremor of Parkinson's disease is also more marked at such times.

Digestive tract
Diseases of the digestive tract that may be either caused or exacerbated by stress include gastritis, stomach and duodenal ulcers, ulcerative colitis, and irritable colon.

Reproductive organs
Stress-related problems in this part of the body include amenorrhoea in women, and impotence and premature ejaculation in men.

Bladder
The bladders of many women (and some men) react to stress by becoming "irritable".

Skin
Some people suffer outbreaks of skin disorders such as eczema and psoriasis when subjected to abnormal stress.

Pulse rate during the day
The graph on the right shows how a typical person's pulse rate varies through an ordinary day. Each peak, whether brought on by physical or mental stress, places increased demands on heart, blood vessels, and other body organs. In some cases, such as playing an evening game of squash, the increase in pulse rate is linked to healthy physical exercise. In other cases – such as a confrontation with a superior at work – pent-up emotional conflicts are probably having unhealthy effects on the body.

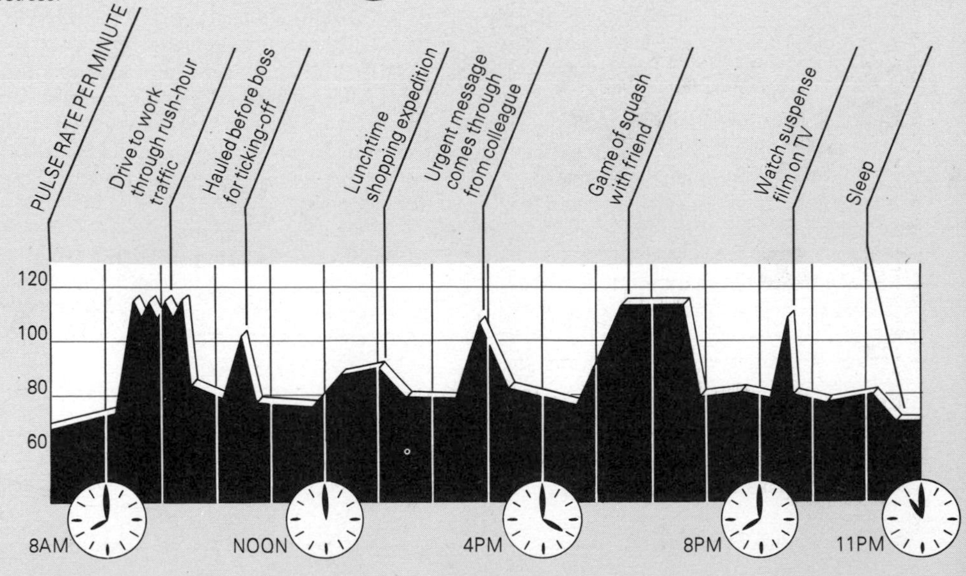

PULSE RATE PER MINUTE

Drive to work through rush-hour traffic

Hauled before boss for ticking-off

Lunchtime shopping expedition

Urgent message comes through from colleague

Game of squash with friend

Watch suspense film on TV

Sleep

120

100

80

60

8AM   NOON   4PM   8PM   11PM

Are you under too much stress?

To assess the current level of stress in your life, answer the following questions, adding up the number of points indicated for each YES answer.

Note: The words "wife" and "husband" apply to any partner, providing the relationship is close and has lasted for some time.

During the past six months

1 Has your wife or husband died?
20 points

2 Have you become divorced or separated from your partner?
15 points

3 Has a close relation (other than husband or wife) died?
13 points

4 Have you been in hospital because of injury or illness?
11 points

5 Have you married, or effected a reconciliation with your husband or wife after a separation?
10 points

6 Have you discovered you are soon to become a parent?
9 points

7 Has there been a major change, whether for better or worse, in the health of a close member of your family?
9 points

8 Have you recently lost your job or retired?
9 points

9 Are you experiencing any sexual difficulties?
8 points

10 Has a new member been born or married into your intimate family circle?
8 points

11 Has a close friend died?
8 points

12 Have your finances got markedly better or worse?
8 points

13 Have you changed your job?
8 points

14 Has any of your children moved out of the family home or started or finished school?
6 points

15 Is trouble with in-laws causing tension within your family?
6 points

16 Is there anyone at home or at work whom you dislike strongly?
6 points

17 Do you frequently suffer from premenstrual tension?
6 points

18 Have you had a resounding personal success, such as rapid promotion at work?
6 points

19 Have you experienced "jet lag" at least twice?
6 points

20 Has there been a major domestic upheaval such as moving house or having an extension built onto your house (though not including a change in family relationships)?
5 points

21 Have you had problems at work that may be putting your job at risk?
5 points

22 Have you taken on a substantial debt or mortgage?
3 points

23 Have you had a minor brush with the law, such as being prosecuted for a traffic offence or failure to have a TV licence?
2 points

EVALUATION
The higher your total score, the more stressful your life. As a general guide, a score of under 30 suggests that you are unlikely to suffer stress-related illness or accidental injury now or in the near future. If your score amounts to 60 or more, the pressures on you are greater than normal. This means you are at risk from one or more stress-related problems, as detailed on the opposite page.

Eating and drinking sensibly

If you have a balanced diet – if, in other words, you do not eat too much of one or two kinds of foods, missing out on essential elements contained in other foods – you are obeying the first rule of sensible eating. Most people in the industrial West do this almost without thinking. Too many of us, however, disobey the second rule: Do not eat more than you need. All other factors being equal, a balanced but *just adequate* diet is the best guarantee of good health.

The following articles explain which foods contain which nutrients and how you can maintain a balanced diet that keeps your body working *well* rather than working merely adequately.

Are you eating and drinking sensibly?

This questionnaire tests the common sense of your current eating and drinking habits. (For a questionnaire dealing specifically with the consumption of alcohol see *Are you drinking too much alcohol?* on p.32.)

Answer YES or NO to the following questions

1 Is your weight within the normal range for your height (see the *Weight chart* on p.28)?
YES ☐ NO ☐

2 Do you generally have 2 or 3 medium-sized meals a day rather than occasional snacks and one big meal?
YES ☐ NO ☐

3 Do you make a point of setting aside specific times for leisurely meals, instead of eating hastily while carrying on with your other activities?
YES ☐ NO ☐

4 Do you use *polyunsaturated* cooking oil and low-fat margarine rather than butter or lard for cooking?
YES ☐ NO ☐

5 Do you eat fried foods sparingly, limiting yourself to no more than 3 or 4 helpings of fried food a week?
YES ☐ NO ☐

6 Do you eat no more than 4 eggs a week?
YES ☐ NO ☐

7 Do you drink, on average, less than 0.5 litre (¾ pint) of milk every day?
YES ☐ NO ☐

8 Do you have a generous portion of at least 2 high-fibre foods every day?
YES ☐ NO ☐

9 Do you often choose to eat fish or white meat – for instance, plaice or chicken – rather than red or fatty meats such as beef or pork?
YES ☐ NO ☐

10 For between-meal snacks and desserts do you eat fresh fruit rather than cakes, sweets, and biscuits?
YES ☐ NO ☐

11 Do you avoid lavish use of salty foods, such as pickles and chutneys?
YES ☐ NO ☐

12 Do you always taste foods before salting them?
YES ☐ NO ☐

13 Do you take tea or coffee without sugar, and do you rarely take sweet soft drinks in general?
YES ☐ NO ☐

14 Do you limit your intake of coffee to 5 cups a day?
YES ☐ NO ☐

EVALUATION
The more YES answers, the healthier your diet and the more sensible your eating habits. The following pages explain why. If you give more than three NO answers, you should examine and alter your eating habits.

The components of a healthy diet

A sound diet contains adequate quantities of six groups of substances: proteins, carbohydrates, and fats, all of which are calorific (that is, energy-productive); and *fibre* (roughage), vitamins, and minerals, which, though essential, are not in themselves calorific. In addition, of course, we need water, without which life is impossible. A human being deprived of both food and drink cannot usually survive for longer than four or five days; life can continue for up to two months on fluid alone.

To understand the part each of these dietary components plays in keeping our bodies healthy, see the accompanying summaries.

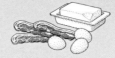

Fats

Fats (technically known as *lipids*) are found in plants – olives and peanuts are examples – as well as in animals. Fats provide energy, and minute quantities are also used for growth and repair. In addition, they make food more palatable and filling. Excess fat is laid down in the body as fatty tissue which, though it may have some insulating properties, can cause serious health problems (see *Obesity*, p.492).

Depending on chemical composition, fats are either *saturated* or *unsaturated* – a distinction that matters to non-experts chiefly in that saturated fats tend to increase the amount of *cholesterol* (p.27) in the blood. Animal fats – especially in milk, butter, cheese, and meat – are mostly highly saturated, and an excess intake of such foods is at least partly responsible for the development of *atheroma*, which causes *atherosclerosis* (p.372). The fat in fish, chicken or turkey, and most vegetable oils is largely unsaturated; in chicken and turkey most of it is in the skin, which need not be eaten. From the standpoint of health the best fats are those, such as sunflower, safflower, corn, or soya-bean oil, that are known as *polyunsaturated*.

Vitamins and minerals

Vitamins are chemicals, usually complex ones, most of which your body cannot make for itself but which it requires in order to function well. There are many types of vitamin, but anyone who eats a reasonably balanced diet is virtually certain to get them all (for fuller information see *Vitamins*, p.494).

The minerals needed in a healthy diet are mostly metals and salts such as iron, phosphorus, calcium, and sodium chloride (table salt). Like vitamins, they are needed only in minute quantities, and you are unlikely to suffer from mineral deficiency if you have a fairly well-balanced diet. In the case of salt, however, too much can be bad for you, especially if you suffer from *high blood pressure* (p.382). Even when food seems rather tasteless, it is probably wise not to add extra salt, and not to eat too much chutney or pickle, which has a relatively high salt content.

Proteins

Proteins are the chemical compounds that form the basis of the structural framework of living matter. We need a regular daily intake of protein for the repair, replacement, and growth of body tissues. Animal proteins (meat, fish, eggs, cheese) can provide a high percentage of our essential intake in exactly the form our bodies need. A wider variety of vegetable proteins (most abundantly found in peas, beans, and other pulses, but also present in grains and so in bread) is necessary for the human body – and lack of variety can cause strict vegetarians to suffer from malnutrition. Protein adds taste and interest to meals. It is satisfying, yet not bulky. If you eat more than your body tissues require, the excess provides extra energy or is converted to fat and stored.

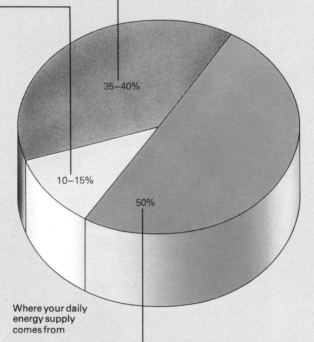

35–40%

10–15%

50%

Where your daily energy supply comes from

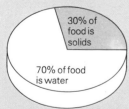

30% of food is solids

70% of food is water

Water

Your body is approximately half water. You lose around 2 litres (up to 4 pints) every day in breathed-out moisture, urine, faeces, and sweat. The lost fluid must be replaced, but about 70 per cent of most foods is water; so you do not actually need to drink 2 litres of fluid in order to replace lost amounts.

Carbohydrates

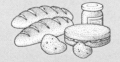

These are chemicals containing carbon, hydrogen, and oxygen. All the foods that we think of as being either "starchy" or "sugary" contain a high proportion of carbohydrates – sugar, bread, biscuits, pasta, potatoes, and cereals, for example. These foods are good sources of energy, and some are useful because they contribute other elements of a balanced diet. Wholemeal bread and potatoes contain fibre, for instance; cereals contain protein; and bread is a good, reliable source of iron.

Sugar, however, is not a valuable dietary ingredient even though it is a quick producer of energy. Most overweight people are fat because they take in too many calories, usually in the form of sugar or high-sugar foods. Moreover, it encourages tooth decay. Nor is it by any means an essential source of energy since other, more nutritionally useful carbohydrates, and proteins and fats, can all be burned to produce energy. In a reducing diet a lack of sugar will force the body to use up stored fat for energy without depriving it of the essential components of a healthy diet.

Fibre (roughage)

The human digestive tract is unable to digest fibre (plant materials such as cellulose and pectin, which are particularly abundant in unrefined flour and cereals, fruit, leafy vegetables, and pulses such as lentils). Fibre is, nonetheless, of great importance to our diet. Not only does it provide bulk to help the large intestine work efficiently in carrying away body wastes, but it may also furnish protection against diverticular disease and cancer of the colon or rectum. Some doctors believe that because fibre affects the way the body uses fats, a high-fibre diet may even help to reduce the development of *atheroma* by lowering the levels of fats (including the level of cholesterol) in the blood.

What is a balanced diet?

Failure to eat sensibly does not stem from eating the "sensibly" foods, but from eating too much of one particular ingredient or not enough of another. If you consume a variety of foodstuffs – and most people do so automatically – you are unlikely to lack the essential nutrients. On the other hand, if you subsist on a restricted selection of foods, your health will suffer accordingly.

Surplus energy from too much fatty or sugar-containing food is stored in the body as fat and can become a serious health problem (see *Obesity*, p.492). A balanced diet gives you all the nutrients and energy you need – but no more. Here are some pointers to help you maintain a balanced diet:

1. Eat meat no more than once a day. Fish and poultry are less fattening than red meat, sausages, and processed meats.

2. Bake or grill food rather than frying it. If you do fry, use *polyunsaturated* oils (such as corn oil) rather than butter, dripping, or lard.

3. Cut down on dairy products, especially fatty foods such as cream, butter, cream cheese, ice cream, and milk – no more than 0.5 litre (¾ pint) of milk each day. Yoghurt, cottage cheese, *unsaturated* margarines, and skimmed milk are better for you.

4. Get your daily quota of *fibre* by eating plenty of leafy vegetables and fruit; eat them raw or lightly cooked because prolonged cooking destroys essential vitamins. Another good source of fibre is potato skin. (Note that a food does *not* have to have a tough or stringy texture in order to contain fibre.)

5. Do not eat more than a total of four eggs a week. Though low in saturated fats, eggs have a very high *cholesterol* content.

6. For dessert or a snack choose fresh fruit rather than sweets, pastries, or puddings.

Finally, remember that most "rules" concerning good and bad eating counsel a policy of perfection. But if you feel fit, take regular exercise, and are not overweight or gaining too much weight, do not worry about the details of what you eat or ponder over recurrent newspaper and TV reports of the latest findings about "good" and "bad" foods. Your diet, so long as it roughly fits the guidelines laid out in these pages, is probably quite all right as it is.

A balanced day's eating

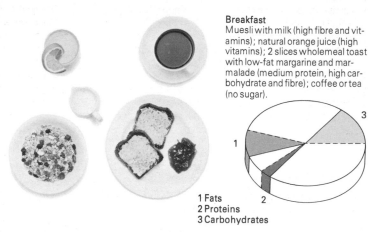

Breakfast
Muesli with milk (high fibre and vitamins); natural orange juice (high vitamins); 2 slices wholemeal toast with low-fat margarine and marmalade (medium protein, high carbohydrate and fibre); coffee or tea (no sugar).

1 Fats
2 Proteins
3 Carbohydrates

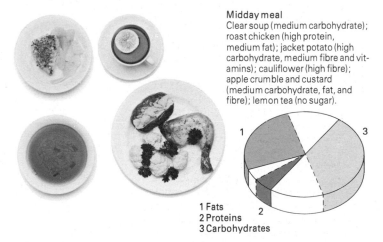

Midday meal
Clear soup (medium carbohydrate); roast chicken (high protein, medium fat); jacket potato (high carbohydrate, medium fibre and vitamins); cauliflower (high fibre); apple crumble and custard (medium carbohydrate, fat, and fibre); lemon tea (no sugar).

1 Fats
2 Proteins
3 Carbohydrates

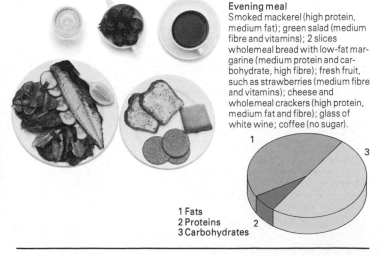

Evening meal
Smoked mackerel (high protein, medium fat); green salad (medium fibre and vitamins); 2 slices wholemeal bread with low-fat margarine (medium protein and carbohydrate, high fibre); fresh fruit, such as strawberries (medium fibre and vitamins); cheese and wholemeal crackers (high protein, medium fat and fibre); glass of white wine; coffee (no sugar).

1 Fats
2 Proteins
3 Carbohydrates

Cholesterol

Cholesterol, a *steroid* chemical, is present in certain foods, mainly – though not exclusively – fatty foods. Small amounts of cholesterol are essential for making and maintaining nerve cells and for synthesizing natural hormones. But you do not have to eat cholesterol-rich foods such as fatty meat and dairy products in order to have your daily quota of the chemical; your liver can utilize other foods for manufacturing all the cholesterol you need. If you were to cut all cholesterol-rich food out of your diet, you would lower the cholesterol content of your blood by only about 15 per cent. That 15 per cent, however, might make all the difference between the healthy functioning of your system and the development of a life-threatening disorder. High cholesterol levels in the blood almost certainly lead to a narrowing of the arteries as a result of the formation of large deposits of *atheroma* in arteries (see *Atherosclerosis*, p.372). So if you include only small quantities of *saturated* foods and other high-cholesterol foods – eggs, for instance – in your diet, you will lower your blood-cholesterol level by an appreciable percentage, with a proportionate lowering of the risk of atherosclerosis.

Counting calories

A calorie is a measurement of energy. If you burn a piece of coal, you can measure the resultant energy (released as heat) in calories. Similarly, your body burns a given quantity of food to release a certain number of calories. Three basic dietary components – proteins, carbohydrates, and fats – produce varying amounts of energy. Weight-for-weight, protein-rich foods have fewer calories than carbohydrate-rich foods, and both are far less calorific than fats.

Note that "calorie" spelled with a small c specifies a relatively small unit of energy. A Calorie (with a big C) is equal to 1,000 calories (with a small c). Most articles about diet (including those in this book) speak in terms of large Calories rather than small calories. Thus when we say that there are 10 Calories in a few lettuce leaves, we mean that the lettuce contains 10,000 calories. The number of Calories you need depends largely on how physically active you are (some examples of average daily requirements are shown on the right). You will probably gain weight if you have a few hundred Calories more than your average requirements – unless you move on to a job that involves more physical exertion or take up an activity that burns up more Calories. And if you are in the later stages of pregnancy or a breast-feeding mother, you may need up to an extra 800 Calories each day to feed your growing baby.

A few people are able to eat more than their daily energy (calorie) requirement without putting on weight. The reason for this is that their bodies are somehow able to burn up the extra calories without putting the excess energy to specific use. As you get older, you may find that it becomes harder to keep your weight down even when your calorific intake remains theoretically "correct" (see *Age and increasing weight*, p.29). So your ability to gain or lose weight depends – partly, at least – on other, less measurable factors than calories alone.

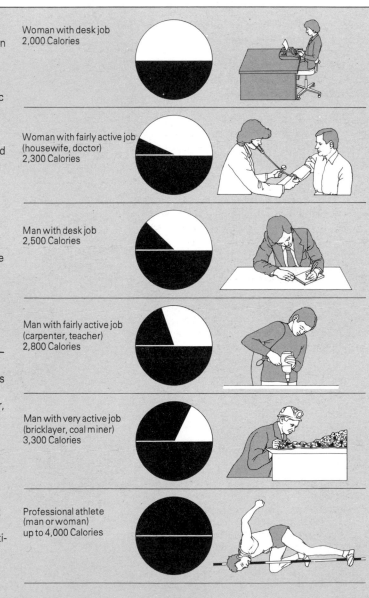

Woman with desk job
2,000 Calories

Woman with fairly active job
(housewife, doctor)
2,300 Calories

Man with desk job
2,500 Calories

Man with fairly active job
(carpenter, teacher)
2,800 Calories

Man with very active job
(bricklayer, coal miner)
3,300 Calories

Professional athlete
(man or woman)
up to 4,000 Calories

How to lose weight

Fat ordinarily accounts for about 10 to 20 per cent of the weight of an adult male, and 25 per cent of the weight of a female. Any more than this is unnecessary and unhealthy. The *weight chart* below shows "desirable" weight for someone of your height. Ideally, your weight should remain roughly constant after the age of 25. Most people do gain a little as they grow older, reaching their heaviest at about 50, but there is no obvious physiological reason for this; it is usually due to a combination of a less active life style and an over-adequate diet (see *Age and increasing weight*, opposite).

If you come into the "overweight" category on the weight chart, you should study the article on *obesity* (p.492). If you are not convinced that you are unhealthily fat, take a critical look at yourself naked in front of a full-length mirror, and jump up and down. If you are seriously overweight, accumulated fat will shake noticeably. Are you still unconvinced? Try pinching a fold of skin from your stomach, just above your navel. If the fold is more than about 25mm (1in) thick, adjust your diet now!

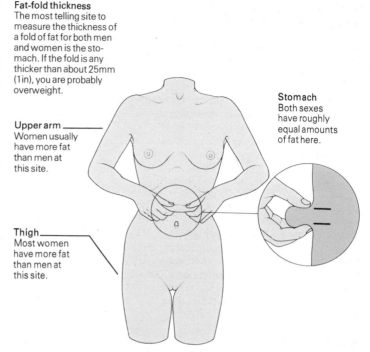

Fat-fold thickness
The most telling site to measure the thickness of a fold of fat for both men and women is the stomach. If the fold is any thicker than about 25mm (1in), you are probably overweight.

Upper arm
Women usually have more fat than men at this site.

Thigh
Most women have more fat than men at this site.

Stomach
Both sexes have roughly equal amounts of fat here.

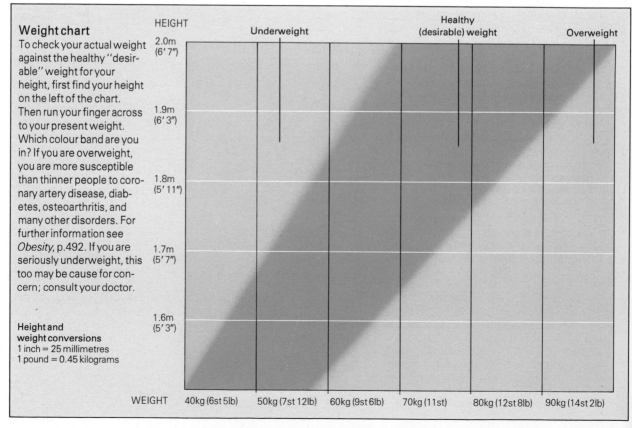

Weight chart
To check your actual weight against the healthy "desirable" weight for your height, first find your height on the left of the chart. Then run your finger across to your present weight. Which colour band are you in? If you are overweight, you are more susceptible than thinner people to coronary artery disease, diabetes, osteoarthritis, and many other disorders. For further information see *Obesity*, p.492. If you are seriously underweight, this too may be cause for concern; consult your doctor.

Height and weight conversions
1 inch = 25 millimetres
1 pound = 0.45 kilograms

HEIGHT

2.0m (6' 7")
1.9m (6' 3")
1.8m (5' 11")
1.7m (5' 7")
1.6m (5' 3")

Underweight　　Healthy (desirable) weight　　Overweight

WEIGHT　40kg (6st 5lb)　50kg (7st 12lb)　60kg (9st 6lb)　70kg (11st)　80kg (12st 8lb)　90kg (14st 2lb)

The step-by-step diet

This diet is not designed to bring swift, dramatic results. It is suitable for people who simply want to remain healthily slim as well as for those who want to lose weight. The aim is to help you lose weight slowly but steadily, modifying your diet so that once you have reached your desirable weight, you can keep it constant.

Fattening foods and drinks are those that, weight for weight, are the most calorific and yet have the least nutritional value. The "step-by-step" reducing diet is based on the principle that the surest way to lose weight is to limit your intake of such things while eating virtually all you want of non-fattening foods *that you like.* Foods listed in group 1, which are mainly sweet or rich in fats, add relatively little bulk to your diet. Those in group 2, though still fattening if eaten in quantity, provide more bulk and contain more of the essential ingredients of a nourishing diet. Group 3 gives a selection of foods that contain comparatively few calories, yet provide hunger-satisfying bulk along with useful nutrients. Proceed as follows:

Step 1 Cut out (or cut down on) all foods listed in group 1. In addition, limit your daily intake of alcoholic beverages to no more than 1 pint of beer (or the equivalent in wine or spirits – see *How much alcohol is there in your favourite drink?* on p.35). Eat normal portions of any food from groups 2 and 3. If you feel hungry at any time, have something from group 3 rather than group 2.

Step 2 If you have not begun to lose weight after two weeks, stop having all group 1 foods that you have continued to eat, and cut down on your consumption of alcohol. Halve your helpings of group 2 foods. Eat as much as you want of group 3 foods.

Step 3 If you still fail to lose weight after a further two weeks, halve your helpings of group 3 foods, and eat as little as you can of the things listed in group 2.

This programme permits you to enjoy varied, flexible, and pleasant meals while on your reducing diet. When you have reached your desirable weight, you can either painlessly remain on the same regime or gradually modify it. If you find yourself putting on weight again, you should then be able to pinpoint offending foods and cut back on them. But remember that it is important to base your choice of diet on foods you like; otherwise you may not stick to the programme.

MEAT	VEGETABLES	DAIRY FOODS	FISH	OTHER
Group 1 foods				
Visible fat on any meat Bacon Duck, goose Sausages, salami Patés		Butter, lard Cream Ice cream (including water-ices)		Thick gravies or sauces Fried foods Sugar, sweets, chocolates Cakes, pies, other pastries, biscuits Puddings, custards Tinned fruits in heavy syrup Dried fruits Nuts Jams, honey, syrups
Group 2 foods				
Lean beef, lamb, pork	Beans Lentils	Eggs Cheeses (other than cottage cheese) Milk	Oily fish such as herrings, mackerel, sardines, and tuna	Pasta Rice Thick soups Bread and crispbreads Cereals (unsweetened) Margarine Polyunsaturated vegetable oils Beef- or yeast-extract drinks
Group 3 foods				
Poultry (not including the skin) other than duck or goose Tongue, liver, kidney, sweetbreads, etc.	Potatoes Vegetables (raw or lightly cooked) Clear or vegetable-only soups	Skimmed milk Yoghurt Cottage cheese	Non-oily fish such as cod, haddock, and whiting Shellfish such as prawns, crabs, and cockles	Bran Fresh fruit Unsweetened fruit juice

Age and increasing weight

As the human body ages, it seems to need less energy – partly because it becomes less active, and partly for other reasons not yet clear. But many old people do not reduce their food intake to correspond with their decreasing energy requirements. In addition, some people drink more alcohol than they did when young, and alcoholic drinks contain calories (energy) in abundance. The overall result is an "energy surplus" which manifests itself as increasing deposits of fatty flesh as old age approaches. The grey area in the accompanying graph shows how the excess energy intake mounts up, as many older people discover when they become obese.

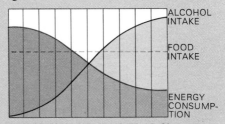

AGE 15 20 25 30 35 40 45 50 55 60

ALCOHOL INTAKE

FOOD INTAKE

ENERGY CONSUMPTION

Mealtimes

If you lead a busy life and are short of time, you may find that you are eating a full meal only about once a day. From the standpoint of health this is bad practice; you would be treating your body with more consideration if you had several small meals instead of a single big one. A given amount of food is used more efficiently by the body if it is spaced throughout the day rather than eaten at one sitting. People who have large, infrequent meals tend to gain more weight and to have a higher level of fat in the blood than do those who eat smaller quantities (but the same total) at regular intervals. Frequent small meals also help prevent digestive ulcers. And because they play a part in keeping blood sugar at a fairly constant level, they prevent hunger from making you tired and irritable. Many people who feel edgy with no evident cause are simply hungry without knowing it.

Sit down and relax at mealtimes. If you eat absent-mindedly while doing something else, whether working or watching television, you are likely to eat more than you realize. Take time to savour your food, too; time aids the digestive process. And finish off each meal with fruit such as an apple – or, better still, a piece of cheese – rather than sweet puddings. (Apples are not quite as good as cheese; they are slightly acidic and contain sugar, and bits of the fruit tend to get stuck between the teeth; all of this predisposes you to dental decay.) Finally, always be sure to clean your teeth thoroughly after eating.

Caffeine

Caffeine, the drug found in coffee, tea, cocoa, and certain soft drinks such as cola, stimulates your central nervous system and makes you feel more energetic. It also acts as a *diuretic*. Although the effects of the drug vary from person to person, 1 or 2 cups of either tea or coffee will generally be enough to produce the stimulant effect. Very large doses of caffeine – 1,000mg (1g, about $\frac{1}{30}$ oz) or more – can lead to restlessness, sleeplessness, trembling, palpitations, and diarrhoea. Such symptoms are apt to occur in people who drink more than 5 or so cups of strong black coffee in a single day. An average-sized cup of coffee contains around 100 mg of caffeine. Weak, milky, or instant coffee contains less caffeine; there is much less in tea and cocoa, and even less in cola beverages. You should try to keep your average consumption below 5 cups of coffee daily.

Although habitual tea or coffee drinkers may become emotionally dependent on the drug, actual addiction (physical dependence, with withdrawal symptoms) does not seem to occur (see *Drug addiction*, p.305). Emotional dependence is unlikely to become a major health problem. Still, it is worth remembering that there are no vitamins or minerals in coffee, tea, or cola. Fruit juice is better all round.

Food hygiene

Badly prepared, cooked, or stored food is a health hazard because of the risk of poisoning. Keep your food clean and free of microbes by following these 10 pieces of advice:

1 Store food in clean, covered containers. To discourage microbial infection keep foods either refrigerated or piping hot.

2 Minimize the need to re-heat left-overs or pre-prepared foods. If you must re-heat something, make sure it is thoroughly cooked before serving it.

3 Make sure you and your family always wash your hands – *not* in the kitchen sink – after using the toilet and before handling food.

4 Cover cuts and sores on your hands with a clean, waterproof dressing, or wear impermeable gloves, when preparing food.

5 Clean working surfaces with hot soapy water before placing unwrapped food on them.

6 Rinse dishes before actually washing them. Use hot soapy water and *clean* dish-cloths for washing. Rinse off soap with hot water, and never dry with a soiled tea-towel.

7 Always keep lids on waste bins; empty and clean them regularly.

8 Do not keep cream cakes, custards, and other milky foods, even if refrigerated, for longer than about 48 hours.

9 Buy pre-cooked foods such as sausage rolls, pork pies, and cold meats only from a busy store with a fast turnover. Take careful note of "sell-by" dates on the containers.

10 Cook poultry thoroughly, especially if you are cooking a pre-frozen bird.

Calorie index

The table below provides a ready method of estimating your daily Calorie intake, as an aid to slimming. Simply look up each food you eat, note down the number of Calories it contains, and total the Calories for a day's meals.

For information on how many Calories you are likely to need for your level of physical activity, see the box on *Counting calories*, p.27. And for detailed advice on how to slim, consult the article on *obesity*, p.492.

Food or drink	Amount and how cooked (raw unless stated)	Calories	Food or drink	Amount and how cooked (raw unless stated)	Calories
Almonds	25g (2 heaped tbs)	150	Honey	5g (tsp)	15
Apple	120g (small)	40	Ice cream	60g (average scoop)	100
Apple pie	240g (average portion)	620	Jam	5g (tsp)	15
Apricots	100g (4 halves, tinned)	100	Kipper	150g (fillet, steamed)	290
Asparagus	150g (6 spears, boiled)	15	Lamb	100g (chop, grilled)	350
Avocado	120g (½ pear)	250	Leeks	100g (4 heaped tbs, boiled)	25
Bacon (middle-cut)	50g (2 rashers, fried)	225	Lemon	100g (average)	20
Banana	150g (average)	65	Lentils	50g (2 heaped tbs, boiled)	50
Beans (baked)	100g (4 tbs, canned)	60	Lettuce	5g (leaf)	5
Beans (runner)	100g (4 tbs, boiled)	20	Mackerel	200g (small, fried)	380
Beef (lean)	100g (4 thin slices, roast)	400	Margarine	5g (pat)	35
Beef (steak)	240g (average, fried)	500	Melon	200g (slice)	25
Beef (steak)	240g (average, grilled)	440	Milk (skimmed)	200ml (glass)	70
Beer	280ml (½ pint)	90	Milk (whole)	200ml (glass)	130
Bran	10g (heaped tbs)	15	Mushrooms	25g (large)	5
Brandy	20ml (single measure)	65	Oats (rolled)	25g (heaped tbs)	105
Bread (white)	25g (small slice)	60	Onions	150g (medium)	40
Bread (wholemeal)	25g (small slice)	60	Orange	150g (medium)	60
Butter	5g (pat)	35	Orange juice (fresh)	200ml (glass)	60
Cabbage	100g (4 heaped tbs, boiled)	15	Orange squash	200ml (glass, diluted)	60
Carrots	100g (4 heaped tbs, boiled)	20	Parsnips	100g (4 heaped tbs, boiled)	65
Cauliflower	100g (4 heaped tbs, boiled)	10	Pasta	25g (heaped tbs)	30
Celery	25g (50mm/2in stick)	2	Paté	25g (25mm/1in cube)	90
Cheese (cheddar)	25g (25mm/1in cube)	100	Peanuts	50g (average packet, roasted)	300
Cheese (cottage)	120g (small carton)	100	Pear	150g (average)	50
Cheesecake	100g (small portion)	400	Peas (fresh)	100g (4 heaped tbs, boiled)	55
Chestnuts	25g (5, roast)	40	Peas (processed)	100g (4 heaped tbs, cooked)	100
Chicken	100g (drumstick, grilled)	140	Pepper (green)	100g (small)	15
Chocolate (milk)	50g (average bar)	250	Pineapple	100g (slice)	50
Chocolate (plain)	50g (average bar)	250	Plaice	150g (fillet, fried)	350
Chocolate cake	100g (small portion)	300	Pork	150g (cutlet, grilled)	300
Cocoa (milk and sugar)	170ml (cup)	155	Porridge	100g (made with water)	45
Cod	200g (fillet, steamed)	170	Potato	100g (medium, boiled)	80
Coffee (black, no sugar)	170ml (cup)	4	Potato	100g (medium, chipped)	300
Cooking oil	25g (tbs)	225	Raspberries	100g (4 heaped tbs)	25
Crab	100g (small, dressed)	100	Rice	25g (heaped tbs, boiled)	35
Cream (double)	25g (tbs)	125	Rice pudding	200g (average portion)	240
Cream (single)	25g (tbs)	55	Salad cream	25g (tbs)	80
Crisps	25g (small packet)	140	Salami	25g (4 slices)	130
Croissant	75g (average)	260	Salmon	100g (canned)	150
Cucumber	50g (25mm/1in slice)	5	Salmon (fresh)	100g (cutlet, steamed)	185
Digestive biscuit	15g (average)	70	Sausage (pork)	25g (small, grilled)	55
Doughnut	100g (average)	400	Shrimps	100g (10, peeled)	95
Drink, soft	200ml (glass)	40	Spinach	100g (4 tbs, boiled)	35
Duck	120g (breast, roast)	380	Sprouts	100g (10, boiled)	20
Egg (white)	25g (medium)	15	Sugar (white)	5g (tsp)	25
Egg (whole)	50g (medium, boiled)	75	Sweetcorn	100g (4 tbs, boiled)	80
Egg (yolk)	25g (medium)	60	Tea (milk, no sugar)	170ml (cup)	20
Flour (white)	25g (heaped tbs)	85	Tomato	25g (small)	5
Fruit cake	100g (small portion)	330	Treacle	25g (tbs)	60
Gooseberries	150g (portion, stewed)	20	Trout	240g (small, fried)	300
Grapes	25g (5)	10	Turkey	100g (2 slices, roast)	150
Haddock	200g (fillet, steamed)	160	Veal	150g (escalope, fried)	300
Ham	90g (3 slices, boiled)	230	Vinegar	25g (tbs)	1
Hamburger	180g (large, grilled)	450	Wine	140ml (glass)	75
Hazelnuts	25g (2tbs heaped)	100	Yoghurt (low fat, fruit)	150g (small carton)	130
Herring	150g (fillet, fried)	330	Yoghurt (low fat, plain)	150g (small carton)	75

Notes: 100g (about 3¾oz) is an average-sized portion; tbs = tablespoonful; tsp = teaspoonful.

The dangers of alcohol

What is generally called "social" or "occasional" drinking is a harmless pleasure that millions of us indulge in. Moderate drinking, whether of beer, wine, or spirits, is not generally harmful to health; but it can evolve almost imperceptibly into excessive, damaging consumption of alcohol. We should never lose sight of the fact that alcohol is a drug; and any drug consumed in excess, or at the wrong time, becomes harmful. Your answers to the questions below will help determine whether you are – or are in danger of becoming – dependent on alcohol. The next few pages look at the harm that over-consumption of alcohol can cause to your body and mind. (For alcohol addiction see *Alcoholism*, p.304.)

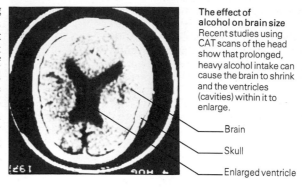

The effect of alcohol on brain size Recent studies using CAT scans of the head show that prolonged, heavy alcohol intake can cause the brain to shrink and the ventricles (cavities) within it to enlarge.

— Brain

— Skull

— Enlarged ventricle

Are you drinking too much alcohol?

Answer YES or NO to the following questions

1 When you have an empty glass at a party, do you always actively look for a refill instead of waiting to be offered one?

YES ☐ NO ☐

2 If given the chance, do you frequently pour out a more generous drink for yourself than seems to be the "going" amount for others?

YES ☐ NO ☐

3 Do you often have a drink or two when you are alone, either at home or in a pub or bar?

YES ☐ NO ☐

4 Is your drinking ever the direct cause of a family quarrel, or do quarrels often seem to occur – if only by coincidence – when you have had a drink or two?

YES ☐ NO ☐

5 Do you feel that you *must* have a drink at a specific time every day – right after work, for instance?

YES ☐ NO ☐

6 When worried or under unusual stress, do you almost automatically take a stiff drink to "settle your nerves"?

YES ☐ NO ☐

7 Are you untruthful about how much you have had to drink when questioned on the subject?

YES ☐ NO ☐

8 Does drinking ever cause you to take time off work, or to miss scheduled meetings or appointments?

YES ☐ NO ☐

9 Do you feel physically deprived if you cannot have at least one drink every day?

YES ☐ NO ☐

10 Do you sometimes crave a drink in the morning?

YES ☐ NO ☐

11 Do you sometimes have "mornings after" when you cannot remember what happened the night before?

YES ☐ NO ☐

EVALUATION
You will do well to regard a YES answer to any one of the above questions as a warning sign; do not increase your consumption of alcohol. Two YES answers suggest that you may already be becoming dependent on drink. Three or more YES answers indicate that you may have a serious drinking problem, which is apt to worsen unless you come to grips with it.

The effects of alcohol

The main effect of alcohol – and a major reason why most people enjoy moderate drinking – is a gradual dulling of the reactions of the brain and nerves. One or two drinks act as a tranquillizer or relaxant. Even in small quantities alcohol is *not* a stimulant, as many people believe. None the less, there is sometimes an agreeable loss of inhibitions, and this may lead to an occasional creative action that might otherwise not have surfaced. Temporarily, too, alcohol can make some drinkers feel – if not actually show themselves to be – unusually alert and witty.

Alcohol is also a *vasodilator*; the rush of blood into the skin from widened blood vessels can make warmth seem to flow into a chilled body. In addition, it is a *diuretic*, causing increased water loss (as heavier and more frequent urination) from the body.

Heavy drinking causes the level of sugar in the blood to fall rapidly. This may lead, a few

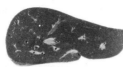
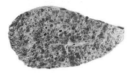

The effects of alcohol on the liver
A slice of healthy liver (upper photograph) shows a smooth, even texture. A slice of cirrhotic liver (lower photograph) reveals diseased tissue riddled with nonfunctioning scar tissue.

hours after a drinking session, to *hypoglycaemia* (p.522), in which the drinker feels weak, dizzy, confused, and abnormally hungry. (If this happens to you, drink something sweet or take a glucose tablet.) Drinking also tends to increase sexual desire while decreasing a man's ability to maintain an erection – possibly because the drug dulls the nerves that control erection and ejaculation. Some of the major alcohol-related diseases are discussed in the box below.

Although alcoholic drinks contain plenty of calories in the form of carbohydrates, they have no other nutritional value. This is why overweight heavy drinkers often develop symptoms of nutritional deficiency (see the article on *Vitamins*, p.494).

Finally, regular heavy drinking leads almost inevitably to problems at work, with your family, and with the law. Alcohol is an important factor in roughly one-third of all road accidents. If you drink and drive, you risk serious injury to yourself and others.

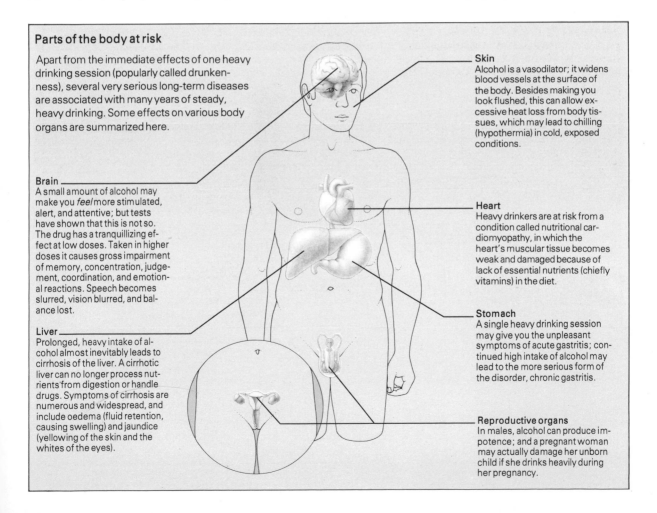

Parts of the body at risk

Apart from the immediate effects of one heavy drinking session (popularly called drunkenness), several very serious long-term diseases are associated with many years of steady, heavy drinking. Some effects on various body organs are summarized here.

Brain
A small amount of alcohol may make you *feel* more stimulated, alert, and attentive; but tests have shown that this is not so. The drug has a tranquillizing effect at low doses. Taken in higher doses it causes gross impairment of memory, concentration, judgement, coordination, and emotional reactions. Speech becomes slurred, vision blurred, and balance lost.

Liver
Prolonged, heavy intake of alcohol almost inevitably leads to cirrhosis of the liver. A cirrhotic liver can no longer process nutrients from digestion or handle drugs. Symptoms of cirrhosis are numerous and widespread, and include oedema (fluid retention, causing swelling) and jaundice (yellowing of the skin and the whites of the eyes).

Skin
Alcohol is a vasodilator; it widens blood vessels at the surface of the body. Besides making you look flushed, this can allow excessive heat loss from body tissues, which may lead to chilling (hypothermia) in cold, exposed conditions.

Heart
Heavy drinkers are at risk from a condition called nutritional cardiomyopathy, in which the heart's muscular tissue becomes weak and damaged because of lack of essential nutrients (chiefly vitamins) in the diet.

Stomach
A single heavy drinking session may give you the unpleasant symptoms of acute gastritis; continued high intake of alcohol may lead to the more serious form of the disorder, chronic gastritis.

Reproductive organs
In males, alcohol can produce impotence; and a pregnant woman may actually damage her unborn child if she drinks heavily during her pregnancy.

How much is too much?

The real question is: how much is too much *for you*? The effect that alcohol has on the body and mind depends on its concentration in the blood. The drug is absorbed into the blood from the digestive system and remains in the blood until broken down by the liver or excreted in the urine. The rate at which the alcohol level in the blood falls is fairly constant. It follows that, whatever the circumstances and however long it may take for you to be affected, once you have reached a certain blood-alcohol peak it will take the drug the same length of time to leave your system as it takes to leave the system of someone else who is affected more slowly or more quickly than you. However, the rate at which the alcohol level in the blood rises is variable, according to the circumstances. So if you want to prevent the amount of alcohol in your blood from rising to a precarious peak, do your drinking with these factors in mind:

Body size: Because there is more blood in a large person than in a small person, the concentration of alcohol in the big person's blood tends to rise more slowly and to reach lower levels overall when identical amounts of alcohol are consumed.

Eating while drinking: Food in the stomach and intestines slows the rate at which alcohol is absorbed into the bloodstream. Thus, if you eat while drinking (or "line your stomach" with food before going to a party), you stand less chance of swiftly reaching a dangerously high blood-alcohol level.

Type of drink and speed of drinking: The more slowly you drink, the less drastic the effects. If you drink whisky, the high alcohol content produces a high concentration of alcohol in your blood more quickly than would beer. If you gulp down a measure of whisky, the alcohol is swiftly absorbed into your system. If you slowly sip a pint of beer, much of the alcoholic content may have been dissipated by the time you have finished it.

Physical tolerance: Regular doses of alcohol induce a gradual "acclimatization" to a substantial quantity in the blood; the brain gets "used to" being bathed in alcohol. As a result, if you have drunk heavily for years, you may be able to look normal and behave in an apparently normal fashion even though your blood level would make a less hardened drinker seem markedly drunk. Appearances are, however, deceptive. Habitual drinkers may talk plausibly and coherently, but their ability to drive a car will still be impaired if their blood alcohol exceeds a certain level.

An unfortunate result of increased tolerance is that you can become dependent on a concentration of alcohol in your blood. Moreover, you gradually need greater and greater amounts of the drug to give you whatever effects you require from drinking. In some people such dependence degenerates into addiction (see *Alcoholism*, p.304).

A further point to remember when drinking is that the level of alcohol in the blood is cumulative (see *The cumulative effects of a day's drinking*, below).

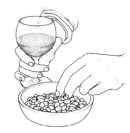

Eating while drinking Consuming food – even titbits at a party – helps to slow the rate of alcohol absorption, so that the level in the blood rises more slowly and peaks at a lower level than if the digestive tract remained empty of food.

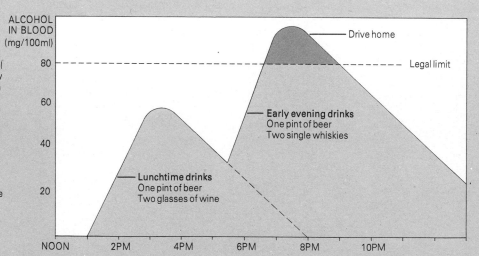

The cumulative effects of a day's drinking

If you have a drink or two at lunchtime, your alcohol level may be safely below the legal limit for driving a car (see the graph, right). But it takes several hours for the body to eliminate even that small amount of alcohol. So another drink or two later on will add to the concentration remaining from your earlier session, and the total may then exceed the safe driving limit.

ALCOHOL IN BLOOD (mg/100ml)

Drive home

Legal limit

80

60

Early evening drinks
One pint of beer
Two single whiskies

40

Lunchtime drinks
One pint of beer
Two glasses of wine

20

NOON   2PM   4PM   6PM   8PM   10PM

How much alcohol is there in your favourite drink?

In its pure form, alcohol is a colourless liquid too strong for the mouth and stomach to tolerate undiluted. There are many types of alcohol, but the type present in varying proportions in alcoholic drinks is known as ethyl alcohol or ethanol. (Another common type is what chemists call methyl alcohol – often spoken of as wood alcohol because it may be distilled from wood – and this is a dangerous poison that should not be drunk.) Shown below is a rundown of the approximate alcoholic content of various kinds of drink. This will give you a rough guide to estimating your actual intake of alcohol during any drinking session.

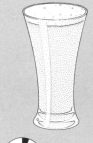 **=** 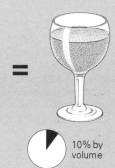 **=** 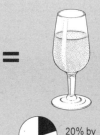 **=**

 5% by volume

10% by volume

 20% by volume

40% by volume

Beer
Most beers, lagers, and ales contain about 5 per cent by volume of alcohol. Some so-called "real ales" are stronger and may contain up to 8 or 9 per cent.

Wine
Typical table wines contain about 10 to 13 per cent by volume of alcohol. The alcoholic content of a wine is not necessarily related to its taste or bouquet; a "powerful, full-bodied" vintage may be less alcoholic than a "light, fragrant" wine.

Fortified wine
A wine such as sherry, port, or vermouth is "fortified" by the addition of extra quantities of alcohol. Such wines may contain up to 20 per cent by volume.

Spirits
Whisky, gin, vodka, brandy, and other "hard" drinks, including most liqueurs, contain about 40 percent by volume of alcohol.

Equivalent sizes
The size of the glass in which each of the various types of drink is conventionally served will obviously determine the total quantity of alcohol in normal drinks at parties or in a pub. So although there is a much smaller proportion of alcohol in beer than in, say, sherry, a single glass of beer is ordinarily many times the size of a single glass of sherry. The following equivalents are based on typical sizes of drinks served in British pubs: The alcoholic content of one half-pint of beer *equals* one glass of wine *equals* one glass of sherry *equals* one measure of whisky.

How alcohol levels are measured

The most accurate method of assessing the amount of alcohol drunk is to measure the concentration of alcohol in the blood. This is expressed as milligrams (mg) of alcohol per 100 millilitres (ml) of blood. A syringe is used to take the blood sample from an arm vein.

There are two other widely used techniques. One involves the analysis of a sample of urine; the other (the "breath test") measures the amount of alcohol in expired air. Because these are both indirect methods, neither is as reliable as the direct analysis of blood. In Britain the legal limit for drivers is set at 80mg alcohol per 100 ml blood.

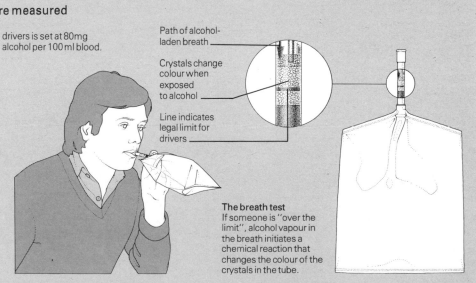

Path of alcohol-laden breath

Crystals change colour when exposed to alcohol

Line indicates legal limit for drivers

The breath test
If someone is "over the limit", alcohol vapour in the breath initiates a chemical reaction that changes the colour of the crystals in the tube.

How to cut down on your drinking

If you average as much as 2½ to 3 pints a day of beer, or the equivalent in wine or spirits, you may be jeopardizing your health. This, then, is the time to start limiting your intake of alcohol. It is not hard to do. The first and most important step is to *want* to cut down. Even if you feel your health is fine at the moment, you should consider the future. (If you want to but find you cannot, accept the probability that drink is becoming a serious problem for you, and you should seek guidance from an organization such as *Alcoholics Anonymous*. See p.768 for further information.) On the opposite page are suggestions on how to cut down without entirely forgoing the pleasures of social drinking.

Effects of alcohol at rising levels

Using results obtained from blood tests, and after observing the behaviour of representative samples of people with alcohol in their blood, medical researchers have produced the following guide to the likely effects of various alcoholic levels on an average individual. For the purposes of the guide it is assumed that stated quantities are drunk by a person weighing about 70kg (11 stones). If you weigh less than this, you should modify the amount you drink accordingly.

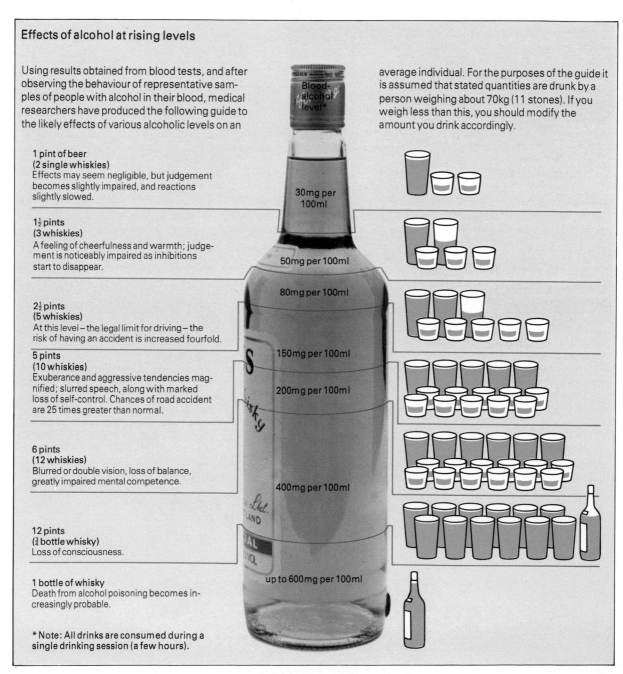

Blood-alcohol level*

1 pint of beer (2 single whiskies)
Effects may seem negligible, but judgement becomes slightly impaired, and reactions slightly slowed.

30mg per 100ml

1½ pints (3 whiskies)
A feeling of cheerfulness and warmth; judgement is noticeably impaired as inhibitions start to disappear.

50mg per 100ml

80mg per 100ml

2½ pints (5 whiskies)
At this level – the legal limit for driving – the risk of having an accident is increased fourfold.

150mg per 100ml

5 pints (10 whiskies)
Exuberance and aggressive tendencies magnified; slurred speech, along with marked loss of self-control. Chances of road accident are 25 times greater than normal.

200mg per 100ml

6 pints (12 whiskies)
Blurred or double vision, loss of balance, greatly impaired mental competence.

400mg per 100ml

12 pints (¾ bottle whisky)
Loss of consciousness.

up to 600mg per 100ml

1 bottle of whisky
Death from alcohol poisoning becomes increasingly probable.

* Note: All drinks are consumed during a single drinking session (a few hours).

Set yourself reasonable limits

Decide not to exceed a certain number of drinks on a given occasion, and stick to your decision. An average of no more than two beers or four measures of whisky a day is a safe limit. You have proved to yourself that you can control your drinking if you set such a target regularly and never exceed it.

Learn to say no

Only too often many of us have "just one more" because others in the group are having another drink or because someone puts pressure upon us, not because we really want a drink. When you reach the sensible limit you have set yourself, politely but firmly refuse to exceed it. If you are being the generous host, pour yourself a glass of water or fruit juice; nobody will notice the difference.

Drink slowly

Never gulp down a drink. Choose your drinks for their flavour, not their "kick", and savour the taste of each sip.

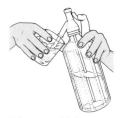

Dilute your drinks
Adding non-alcoholic liquid mixers to strong drinks is a useful way of slowing down your alcohol intake.

Dilute your drinks

If you prefer spirits to beer, try having long drinks. Instead of downing your gin or whisky neat – or nearly so, as in cocktails – have it diluted with tonic, water, or soda water in a tall glass. That way, you can enjoy the flavour as well as the act of drinking, but it will take longer to finish each drink; and you can dally over three or four comparatively weak drinks for a whole evening.

Do not drink on your own

Make a point of confining your drinking to social gatherings. It is sometimes hard to resist the urge to pour oneself a relaxing drink at the end of a hard day, but many formerly heavy drinkers have found that a cup of tea or a soft drink satisfies the need as well as a whisky or gin did, and that the alcoholic drink was just a habit. What really helps you to unwind – even with no drink at all – is a comfortable chair, loosened clothing, and perhaps a soothing gramophone record, television programme, or a good book to read.

Hangovers and alcohol folklore

Hangovers

How bad you feel after an evening's drinking depends partly on your constitution, which you cannot greatly modify, but also on what and how much you have drunk. Most alcoholic drinks contain substances called congeners that are added for colour and flavour. It is the different congeners in different drinks that combine with the amount of alcohol to give a drinking bout its "hangover potential". Brandy, bourbon, and red wines produce the worst hangovers. Gin and vodka contain few congeners and are therefore least likely to cause hangover. With all drinks, smoking seems to contribute towards making the hangover worse.

When prevention fails, rest is the best cure. Because alcohol is a *diuretic* drug, causing an increased rate of output of urine, you should try to compensate for the loss of body fluid by drinking as much water as you can after a drinking spree. And if you have a bad headache, take paracetamol rather than aspirin (the latter will further irritate an already irritated stomach).

Alcohol folklore

There are a number of traditional beliefs associated with drinking, and many people tend to take their truth for granted. Personal experience may have "proved" to you that the following familiar statements are true. But is there medical evidence for their validity? Read on!

1 "It is risky to mix your drinks (for instance, to have beer after whisky, or wine after gin)." There is no evidence that mixing drinks will do more long-term damage to the system than sticking to one type. It seems true, though, that a hangover is more likely when you mix drinks.

2 "Drinking black coffee sobers you up." This is only partly true. Any fluid you take helps to counteract the diuretic effect of alcohol, and a mild stimulant such as coffee (which contains *caffeine* – see p.30) may compensate for the depressant effect of alcohol. But *no* drug can speed the rate at which alcohol is removed from the bloodstream.

3 "A hair of the dog that bit you eases a hangover." If you pour yourself a drink on the morning after a spree, it may make you feel better for two reasons. First, the additional fluid helps to reverse the *dehydrating* effect of alcohol, which is a contributing cause of hangover. Secondly, the characteristic headache of a hangover may be due in part to the sudden change in concentration of alcohol bathing the brain, and a morning-after drink can add just enough alcohol to make the change more gradual. But if you find that you are frequently forced to rely on this method of curing your hangovers, the hangovers themselves are probably withdrawal symptoms of alcohol addiction. This is clear warning that you have a drink problem and should seek help.

4 "The best medicine for a badly chilled body is a stiff drink." Because alcohol is a *vasodilator*, a comfortable feeling of warmth does follow the rush of blood into the surface tissues of the body. But this diversion of blood from vital inner organs actually increases the risk of chilling and *hypothermia* (p.723).

The dangers of smoking

Two out of five people who smoke 20 or more cigarettes a day die before 65; this is twice the proportion for non-smokers. Cigarettes are responsible for about 50,000 needlessly early deaths in Britain every year. If you are a regular smoker, you are probably losing around five and a half minutes of life expectation for each cigarette smoked. Yet, despite the vast medical evidence supporting such statistics, and the publicity given to them, most heavy smokers continue to smoke. And thousands of adolescents every year begin to smoke occasionally, on the assumption that "everybody does". Research indicates that about 85 per cent of these occasional smokers eventually become regular, full-time smokers.

The following pages catalogue the health problems associated with smoking, discuss the dangerous substances in tobacco, and suggest ways to break the habit.

How much is smoking affecting your health?

Smoking in any form is harmful, but the extent of the damage tobacco does to your body depends on several factors: whether you smoke mainly pipes, cigars, or cigarettes; the amount of smoke that you regularly take into your lungs; and the length of time you have been smoking. The numerical weight assigned to each YES answer in the questionnaire below reflects the hazard to health presented by that particular facet of smoking.

If you used to be a smoker but have given up, your chances of suffering from a tobacco-related disease diminish with each successive year. For an indication of where you now stand see *How your chances improve*, p.41.

Score the number of points indicated for each YES answer

1 Do you smoke a pipe?
2 points

2 On average, do you smoke:
a) 1 to 4 cigars a day?
2 points
b) 5 to 9 cigars a day?
4 points
c) over 10 cigars a day?
7 points

3 On average, do you smoke:
a) 1 to 9 cigarettes a day?
10 points
b) 10 to 19 cigarettes a day?
15 points
c) 20 to 39 cigarettes a day?
18 points
d) over 40 cigarettes a day?
24 points

4 Have you been a regular smoker for:
a) less than 15 years?
2 points
b) 15 to 25 years?
7 points
c) 25 to 35 years?
9 points
d) more than 35 years?
13 points

5 If you smoke cigarettes, are they mostly "high tar" ones?
4 points

6 Do you smoke your cigarette or cigar right down to the butt?
7 points

7 Regardless of what or how much you smoke, do you generally inhale (breathe tobacco smoke into your lungs)?
10 points

EVALUATION
There is slight reason for concern if your total score in response to the above questions is under 10 points. Note, however, that if you smoke cigarettes you cannot possibly score less than 10. (For a discussion of why cigarette smoking is the most harmful form see *Cigarettes vs cigars and pipes*, p.40.) A score between 10 and 25 indicates that you are seriously jeopardizing your chances for health and long life. And remember that if you are relatively young and do not "kick" the habit, your score will rise swiftly as time passes. If you already score over 25 points, you are in an extremely high-risk category. Remember, though, that however high your score, it is always worth giving up smoking. Your chances of suffering from a smoking-associated disease begin to diminish as soon as you stop.

Smoking can seriously damage your health

Tobacco smoke contains 3 dangerous chemicals: tar, nicotine, and carbon monoxide. Tar is a mixture of several substances which condense into a sticky, syrup-like substance in the lungs. Nicotine is an addictive drug that is absorbed from the lungs and acts mainly on the nervous system. And carbon monoxide lessens the ability of red blood cells to carry oxygen throughout the body.

Consider the average smoker – someone who gets through 15 to 20 cigarettes a day. Compared with non-smokers he or she is: 14 times more likely to die from cancer of the lung, throat, or mouth; 4 times more likely to die from cancer of the oesophagus; twice as likely to die from cancer of the bladder; and twice as likely to die from a heart attack. In addition, cigarettes are a principal cause of chronic bronchitis and emphysema; and chronic lung disease itself increases the risks of pneumonia and heart failure. Smoking also increases the health risks of high blood pressure.

The usually minor risks of the contraceptive pill are greater among women smokers. A pregnant woman who smokes 15 to 20 cigarettes a day is twice as likely as a non-smoker to have a miscarriage, and more likely to have a premature – and therefore vulnerable – baby. In the immediate post-natal period the mortality rate of babies born to women who smoke is almost 30 per cent higher than the rate for babies born to non-smokers. Furthermore, "passive smoking" – breathing in air contaminated by smoke from other people's tobacco – has recently been shown to increase the risk of lung cancer in non-smokers.

Some brands of cigarette contain less tar and nicotine than others, but there is no such thing as an entirely "safe" cigarette. Neither does switching to "mild" cigarettes always help. Habitually heavy smokers merely adapt their smoking habits to the switch by taking longer puffs, lighting up more often, and inhaling more deeply.

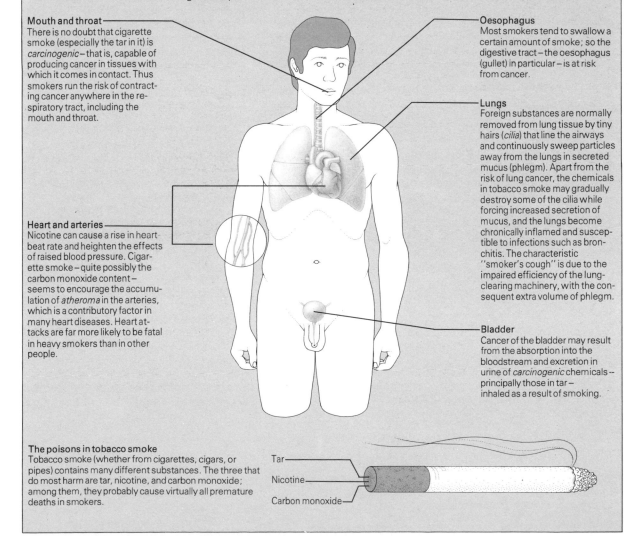

Mouth and throat
There is no doubt that cigarette smoke (especially the tar in it) is *carcinogenic* – that is, capable of producing cancer in tissues with which it comes in contact. Thus smokers run the risk of contracting cancer anywhere in the respiratory tract, including the mouth and throat.

Oesophagus
Most smokers tend to swallow a certain amount of smoke; so the digestive tract – the oesophagus (gullet) in particular – is at risk from cancer.

Lungs
Foreign substances are normally removed from lung tissue by tiny hairs (*cilia*) that line the airways and continuously sweep particles away from the lungs in secreted mucus (phlegm). Apart from the risk of lung cancer, the chemicals in tobacco smoke may gradually destroy some of the cilia while forcing increased secretion of mucus, and the lungs become chronically inflamed and susceptible to infections such as bronchitis. The characteristic "smoker's cough" is due to the impaired efficiency of the lung-clearing machinery, with the consequent extra volume of phlegm.

Heart and arteries
Nicotine can cause a rise in heartbeat rate and heighten the effects of raised blood pressure. Cigarette smoke – quite possibly the carbon monoxide content – seems to encourage the accumulation of *atheroma* in the arteries, which is a contributory factor in many heart diseases. Heart attacks are far more likely to be fatal in heavy smokers than in other people.

Bladder
Cancer of the bladder may result from the absorption into the bloodstream and excretion in urine of *carcinogenic* chemicals – principally those in tar – inhaled as a result of smoking.

The poisons in tobacco smoke
Tobacco smoke (whether from cigarettes, cigars, or pipes) contains many different substances. The three that do most harm are tar, nicotine, and carbon monoxide; among them, they probably cause virtually all premature deaths in smokers.

Tar
Nicotine
Carbon monoxide

Why do smokers smoke?

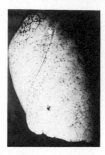

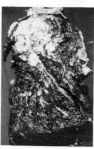

Consider these two pictures. Top: a normal human lung. Bottom: a lung in the advanced stage of cancer.

Most smokers regret their inability to stop, although some are only too ready to blame their hacking cough on a persistent summer cold, or high blood pressure on the stresses of daily life. Such smokers are unable to face up to the fact that their real problem is smoking. The proportion of cigarette smokers in Britain has dropped from 51 per cent in 1956 to around 40 per cent today. Even so, 2 individuals in every 5 are needlessly risking their lives and the health of others by acquiring a habit that is known to be harmful.

Most smokers begin in adolescence, when the possibilities of ill health and death appear too remote to be real. The teenager lights up occasionally because his or her friends do. Cigarettes have become a symbol of swaggering maturity, and also a "prop", a support against outward signs of shyness or awkwardness in social situations. The progression from an occasional cigarette without inhaling to heavy smoking usually occurs so gradually that young people never quite realize when they have finally been "hooked".

If you are a smoker and have adolescent or pre-adolescent children, you can at least set them a good example by stopping now. But remember that adolescents are by nature rebels, and that moralizing or preaching is likely to be counter-productive. Put the facts in their hands – for one thing, that the annual cost to a typical British wage-earner of 20-odd cigarettes a day is about a month's pay – and leave the rest up to their own good sense.

Warning to parents

If you smoke you are, of course, damaging your own health; but you are probably also damaging the health of your children. Tobacco smoke in the air of your household is being inhaled by your children (so-called "passive smoking"). It is an established fact that children whose parents smoke suffer more from diseases of the respiratory tract, such as bronchitis and pneumonia, than do the children of non-smokers.

How to stop smoking

Almost all health risks associated with smoking decrease as soon as you give up, no matter how long you have smoked. Your chances of having a heart attack, for example, fall rapidly when you stop. After five non-smoking years the risk of premature death from smoking-related diseases is almost halved. After 15 years the risk has all but disappeared (see *How your chances improve*, opposite).

Cigarettes vs cigars and pipes

Though the smoke from a cigar or pipe contains a higher concentration of both tar and nicotine than does cigarette smoke, even a few cigarettes a day pose a greater risk to health than would a number of cigars or pipefuls. This may be because, while it is extremely difficult to smoke cigarettes without inhaling, it is difficult to inhale cigar or pipe smoke voluntarily. Cigarette smokers tend to inhale actively, deeply, and constantly. But, because of the very harshness of the smoke from burning cigar or pipe tobacco, it is almost impossible to breathe it directly into healthy lungs.

However, simply switching to a pipe from cigarettes is likely to increase your risk instead of lessening it. This is because you have become accustomed to inhaling and may find yourself retaining the habit without wanting to – and you will now be inhaling even more harmful smoke than before.

Research among smokers indicates that while nearly 4 out of 5 want to stop, only about a quarter of those who try manage to do so. However, many of the smokers who fail to give up are those who are not willing to put up with the inconvenience and withdrawal symptoms that giving up smoking almost inevitably entails. A method such as hypnotism, group therapy, or acupuncture may help. If you want to stop and have been unable to succeed on your own, get in touch with a branch of *Action on Smoking and Health* (known as *ASH* – see p.768), which will probably have some suggestions for supportive outside help in your area.

Most smokers who really want to stop can, in fact, do it by themselves. The following step-by-step procedure has proved effective for thousands of ex-smokers:

Step 1: Analyse your smoking habits. Prepare a 24-hour chart of every cigarette you normally smoke, along with the times when you almost automatically light up – with every cup of coffee or after every meal, for example, or as you begin the day's work. Give yourself two or three weeks in which to study when and why you "need" cigarettes, so that you actually pay attention to every puff you

If you really cannot stop smoking
Are you unable to stop smoking cigarettes no matter how hard you try? If so, you can at least lessen the health risks by adopting the following measures:

1 Choose a low-tar brand of cigarette.

2 Smoke fewer cigarettes.

3 Take fewer puffs per cigarette, and smoke it only halfway down its length.

4 When you are not puffing, keep the cigarette out of your mouth.

5 Do your best not to breathe smoke into your lungs.

6 Be wary of changing to cigars or a pipe. If you do switch, try as hard as you can *never* to inhale.

have. This increasing concern with the act of smoking is a good way to prepare for the task of giving up the habit.

Step 2: Make up your mind that there can be no turning back. List all the reasons why you want to stop, including a run-down of the good things that will happen when you have stopped (for instance, a keener palate, no more morning cough, etc.). Be absolutely convinced that the effort is worth making before you make it.

Step 3: Name the day, circle it on your calendar, and give up totally on that day. This is the most successful and, in the long run, least harrowing way to break the smoking habit. It helps if family or close friends can act together, giving up on the same date and sustaining one another through the difficult early days; or if you choose a time when your usual routine is being broken for another reason (for example, just as you go on holiday). Some smokers have found that it helps to make a great show of stopping by announcing it to the world at large – which makes it a matter of pride for them not to succumb to temptation in a weak moment.

Step 4: Feel free to use any device you can as a cigarette substitute during the difficult early days. It may help to chew gum or use some of the anti-smoking tablets that can be bought over the counter. If your hand seems empty without a cigarette between your fingers, hold a pencil or pen. In addition, practise one of the relaxation exercises recommended elsewhere in this book (see *How to relieve tension,* p.19) in order to counteract the tensions that smoking used to unwind for you. And it often helps to give up – temporarily, at least – some of the activities that you associate with smoking. For instance, if you habitually smoked while having a drink at the neighbourhood pub, stay away from that pub for a while. Avoid situations that encourage smoking; for example, ride only in the non-smoking carriages of trains.

Step 5: Enjoy not smoking! Do not forget that you are saving several pounds a week. Give yourself a positive reward by putting the unspent money into a fund for buying something you could not otherwise afford.

Step 6: During the difficult weeks eat as much as you want, and do not worry about putting on weight. Your appetite is almost certain to increase, and when you are feeling tense and restless (the natural result of trying to overcome an addictive habit) you may often be impelled to nibble at something; so you will probably put on a few pounds. Remember that the first four weeks are the hardest. You can expect to lose your intense craving for tobacco after about eight weeks, and you will then be free to concentrate on eating more sparingly if necessary.

How your chances improve

When you stop smoking, you automatically reduce your chances of dying from a smoking-related disease. The longer you abstain, the less likely you are to succumb, until after about 15 years of non-smoking your chances of early death are just about the same as those of a lifelong non-smoker. Moreover, the length of time you smoked makes little difference to this general trend; so it is *always* worth giving up. The graph (right) shows how the average smoker's chances of dying from lung cancer (compared to those of a non-smoker) decrease from the time he or she stops smoking. This tendency, though less marked than for lung cancer, applies to all illnesses associated with smoking.

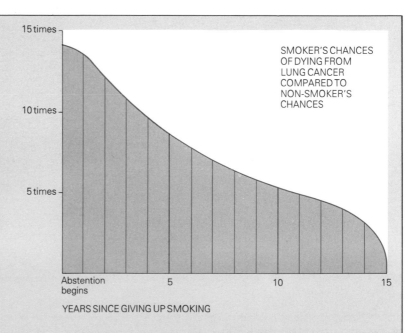

SMOKER'S CHANCES OF DYING FROM LUNG CANCER COMPARED TO NON-SMOKER'S CHANCES

YEARS SINCE GIVING UP SMOKING

Safety and environmental health

Accidents account for around 3 per cent of deaths in Britain and other Western countries – a figure that could be considerably reduced if all of us paid more attention to basic safety precautions. Health-consciousness must also include safety-consciousness.

The work that you do may expose you to a particular set of hazards. Provided you – and your employers – take reasonable precautions, though, your chances of suffering from an occupational disease such as a lung or skin disorder can be kept to a minimum. As for possible risks from the environment – air, water, and so on – most of them are small in comparison with the innumerable other risks of just being alive. For a fuller discussion of *occupational and environmental risks* turn to p.45.

Chief causes of accidental death

The statistics in this table (abstracted from "The Facts about Accidents", a report prepared by the Royal Society for Prevention of Accidents) are rounded-off figures for a recent year in Britain. Note that they apply to death only. Statistics for major and minor non-fatal injuries are less reliable than fatality figures, but probably for every death there are up to 500 corresponding accidents that are not fatal but cause major or minor injury.

As the table indicates, there are several major causes of accidental death, but susceptibility to certain kinds of accident is greater for some age groups than for others. The most dangerous place for virtually everybody is in or near traffic – as a driver, passenger, cyclist, or pedestrian. Accidents account for over half of *all* deaths of people aged 15 to 24, and more than three-quarters of these accidents happen on the road. The next most common cause of accidental deaths among people from 15 to 44 is poisoning, often due to a suspected overdose of drugs. In many such cases, when suicide is suspected but not proved, the death is officially registered as "accidental".

The riskiest room in the house appears to be the kitchen, especially for children. The category "Choking and suffocation" includes principally fatalities caused by choking on insufficiently chewed lumps of food or on vomit, and by suffocation from breathing into plastic bags. Fire also tends to start in kitchens. So the kitchen is a sensible place in which to keep both a *home first-aid kit* (p.816) and a small fire extinguisher or fire blanket.

Age group	Annual number of deaths from all causes per 100,000 people	Percentage of deaths resulting from accidents	Chief cause of accidental death (as percentage of total)	Commonest other causes (in order of frequency)
Under 1	140	3%	Choking and suffocation (70%)	Falls; fire; road accidents.
1–4	55	28%	Road accidents (37%)	Fire; drowning; choking and suffocation.
5–9	30	38%	Road accidents (57%)	Drowning; fire; falls.
10–14	25	37%	Road accidents (53%)	Drowning; choking and suffocation; falls.
15–24	65	55%	Road accidents (76%)	Poisoning; falls; drowning.
25–44	120	17%	Road accidents (53%)	Poisoning; falls; choking and suffocation.
45–64	1,000	3%	Road accidents (44%)	Falls; poisoning; fire.
Over 64	6,000	2%	Falls (61%)	Road accidents; fire; poisoning.

Are you doing enough to prevent accidents?

Death from accidents is high in the mortality tables (just below circulatory and respiratory diseases and cancers). The accompanying questions are designed to test how well you protect yourself and your family from accidental injury. The first group of questions concentrates on guarding against possible hazards in and around the home. The second group deals with safety measures that should be taken against accidents that might happen to you or your family on the road, whether in a vehicle or as pedestrians. The third and last group is mainly concerned with safety on holiday, when unfamiliar surroundings and activities present special hazards.

Basic safety in the home

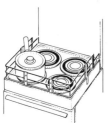

Always make sure that open fires are guarded.

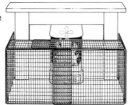

Always place pan handles facing inwards, and use a hob guard if possible.

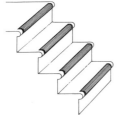

Always ensure stair carpets are secure, and use tread grips if you can.

Group 1   Safety in the home
Answer YES or NO to the following questions

1 If you have a garden, is it fenced and gated so that children cannot run straight from the house into a road?
YES ☐   NO ☐

2 Do all open fires – wood, gas, coal, or electric – have secure guards around them?
YES ☐   NO ☐

3 When cooking, do you guard against accidental tipping by positioning pan handles so that they do not extend outwards?
YES ☐   NO ☐

4 Do you have a hob guard on your cooker?
YES ☐   NO ☐

5 Are you careful never to leave small children unsupervised in the kitchen or bathroom?
YES ☐   NO ☐

6 Are your children's nightclothes and soft toys labelled as being made of non-inflammable materials?
YES ☐   NO ☐

7 Are medicines in your house kept in a secure place, out of children's reach?
YES ☐   NO ☐

8 Are you careful never to store drugs or dangerous chemicals (bleach, paint-stripper, etc.) within children's reach or in unlabelled or wrongly labelled containers?
YES ☐   NO ☐

9 Do you make sure that members of the family do not keep pills by their beds?
YES ☐   NO ☐

10 Do you make a point of preventing young children from playing with objects small enough to be swallowed?
YES ☐   NO ☐

11 Do you keep plastic bags away from your children?
YES ☐   NO ☐

12 Are your carpets firmly fixed, with no ragged spots or edges, and are loose rugs placed in such a way as to minimize the risks of sliding or tripping?
YES ☐   NO ☐

13 Are your stairways, hallways, and other passages well lit (brightly enough, say, for reading a newspaper)?
YES ☐   NO ☐

14 Is it a rule in your house that nothing is left sitting about on the stairs?
YES ☐   NO ☐

15 If you spill or drop something that might be slippery on the floor, do you always clean it up right away?
YES ☐   NO ☐

16 Do you keep non-slip mats both in and alongside the bath or shower?
YES ☐   NO ☐

(Continued overleaf)

Group 2 Safety on the road   Answer YES or NO to the following questions

17 Have you taught your children exactly how, when, and where to cross streets safely?

YES ☐ NO ☐

18 Have your children been taught the basic rules of the road for use when cycling?

YES ☐ NO ☐

19 Do you inspect your family's cycles regularly to see that they are in good repair, their lights are working, and they are the right size for each rider?

YES ☐ NO ☐

20 When walking in streets or open roads at twilight or in the dark, do all members of your family carry a light, or wear something noticeable, such as a white or luminous jacket?

YES ☐ NO ☐

21 Are you always careful to drink less than the legal limit of alcohol if you are going to drive a car soon afterwards? (For legal limits see *How much is too much?* on p.34.)

YES ☐ NO ☐

22 Do you avoid driving when you feel unusually tired or ill, or if you are taking drugs (such as antihistamines) that are known to impair alertness?

YES ☐ NO ☐

23 Do you have your car fully serviced – including lights, tyres, windscreen washer and wiper, brakes, and steering – either every 10,000km (6,000 miles) or at least every 6 months?

YES ☐ NO ☐

24 Do you check at least once a week to make sure that your car windows, lights, mirrors, and reflectors are clean?

YES ☐ NO ☐

25 When driving, do you always try to keep a gap of at least a metre (yard) for each mile-per-hour of speed between your car and the one in front?

YES ☐ NO ☐

26 Do you always make sure that you and all passengers in your car use available seat belts?

YES ☐ NO ☐

27 If you carry dogs or other pets in your car, are they securely separated from the driver by a net or fence?

YES ☐ NO ☐

Group 3 Safety on holiday   Answer YES or NO to the following questions

28 Are all members of your family able to swim, or in the process of learning how to swim?

YES ☐ NO ☐

29 In a boat, does everyone always wear a life-jacket?

YES ☐ NO ☐

30 Do you find out about local tides and currents before bathing in strange waters?

YES ☐ NO ☐

31 If you do any hill walking, hiking, or climbing, do you always go prepared with the right clothing and equipment?

YES ☐ NO ☐

32 When going on an excursion lasting for a day or longer, do you tell someone what your route is and when you expect to be back?

YES ☐ NO ☐

33 Do you and your family take full safety precautions and have the proper equipment and clothing when you engage in possibly dangerous sports?

YES ☐ NO ☐

34 Before taking up a new and potentially dangerous activity such as hang-gliding, do you make sure you get proper tuition from an instructor?

YES ☐ NO ☐

35 When you are about to go abroad, do you always ask your doctor to advise you about necessary vaccinations and – for travel in the tropics – preventive drugs?

YES ☐ NO ☐

EVALUATION
A NO answer to any of the above questions indicates that you are not doing all you should to minimize the risk of accidents. You can – and ought to – take all the protective steps suggested in the questions. For a discussion of some less obvious risks, which may or may not be preventable in your case, see *Occupational and environmental risks* (opposite). (For advice on *accidental falls*, to which the elderly are particularly susceptible, see p.719.)

Occupational and environmental risks

Occupational hazards

Most people tend to live not far from where they happened to be born and to "fall into" their jobs rather than make an active choice. Moreover, it is almost as hard to predict the physical and mental effects of most occupations or dwelling areas as it is to foresee a car crash or a fire. The links between certain kinds of work and specific ailments are sometimes ill-defined. The high rate of alcoholism among bartenders, actors, and writers does not make it inevitable that people who work in public houses, theatres, or newspaper offices will become addicted to drink *because* of their jobs – but it does make it more likely.

In other cases, direct causal links between occupation and disease are more obvious. This is particularly true of respiratory-system disorders resulting from years of exposure to certain chemicals or dusty substances. Examples are pneumoconiosis and related "dust diseases" (such as asbestosis and silicosis) to which miners, stone masons, quarry workers, asbestos handlers, and people who smelt or grind aluminium, iron, and similar metals are susceptible. Less obvious are complaints such as farmer's lung which sometimes affect people who work on the land. Anthrax is an infection that sometimes attacks dock workers or air-cargo handlers who come into contact with contaminated pelts or other animal products. Craftsmen who grind or polish metal are especially susceptible to eye injuries. The prolonged handling of vibrating machinery can lead to Raynaud's disease. And, of course, there is always the clear-cut risk of accidental injury in manual labour, whether skilled or unskilled. Probably the most hazardous of all jobs is deep-sea diving; the risk of death as a direct result of carrying out maintenance of off-shore oil-drilling equipment is very high indeed.

(Continued overleaf)

Air-filter mask

Eye protectors

Ear protectors

Reinforced footwear

Protective headgear

Heavy gloves

Safety at work and in the home

In Britain there is much legislation requiring safe working conditions for employees, especially where machinery is concerned. It is only sensible to apply such guidelines and install safety equipment in the home, particularly as more and more people take to using power tools for gardening and house and car maintenance. The 6 examples given here suggest ways of protecting yourself from injury or illness while using potentially dangerous items. Never leave safety guards off power tools, and make sure you read and follow instruction leaflets carefully.

Are you at risk?

No list of potential hazards can cover the whole ground. For one thing, there are always new industries creating new types of work that may lead to disorders of the body or mind. Then, too, unsuspected links between certain jobs and diseases may still be discovered. There is recent evidence, for instance, that workers exposed to certain chemicals used in the industrial manufacture of polyvinyl chloride (PVC) are susceptible to cancer of the liver. In fact, virtually any job has its health risks; even if safely seated at a desk all day, you are more likely than others to develop coronary artery disease. In general, though, you are most at risk of a specific job-linked disorder if your occupation:
– Exposes your respiratory system to chemicals, floating particles, or gas.
– Exposes your skin to a chemical (especially in concentrated form).
– Exposes your ears to loud noise.
– Exposes you to machinery of any sort.

What should be done?

Nowadays most of the obvious occupational hazards are recognized and publicized, and employers are legally required to take steps to safeguard health and minimize accidents. If your job is even slightly risky, be sure you understand why (your employer or trade-union representative should have leaflets or other information on the subject). Then make sure you take all recommended safety precautions and wear approved protective clothing. Use the ear plugs or muffs provided if you work with noisy machinery, to protect your ears from occupational deafness; never trust to luck instead of wearing a hard hat on a construction site; and so on.

If you are concerned about the adequacy of health-protection measures at your place of work, do not hesitate to broach the subject to someone in authority. A representative of your employer or trade union is the obvious person to see. Otherwise, get in touch with the nearest branch of the *Health and Safety Executive* (a government agency – see your local telephone directory for the address of your nearest branch, or p.768 for the address of the head office). Remember that a major characteristic of job-linked illnesses other than those caused by direct injury is that early symptoms are hardly noticeable but develop relentlessly over months or years. Take precautions *now* to safeguard your future health.

Environmental hazards

The air and water of modern Britain, no matter where you live, are free of serious health risks. As a result of anti-air-pollution laws, the industrial smoke that once caused many cases of bronchitis and emphysema is now largely under control. The greatest modern sources of air pollution are the carbon monoxide and lead in motor-vehicle exhaust fumes, but the risks are probably smaller than some environmentalists maintain. It is less risky, for example, to work in heavy traffic than it is to smoke cigarettes.

True, lead is a powerful poison; workers exposed to high concentrations of the metal may develop damage to their kidneys or nerves. But there is no clear evidence that the concentration of airborne lead is great enough anywhere in Britain to damage health. (There is, however, a possible danger from lead in certain old-fashioned domestic water supplies; see below.)

The safety of the water we drink is even more certain than that of the air we breathe. Statistics show that people who live in soft-water areas are slightly more susceptible to heart disease and that women are slightly more likely to give birth to children with *congenital* malformations than those in hard-water areas. The difference is too small, though, to warrant drastic action such as moving to a theoretically "safer" part of the country (and people living in hard-water areas should not soften drinking water). A relatively greater – though still small – risk comes from the lead that sometimes lines old-fashioned water storage tanks and pipes. If you live in an old house in a soft-water region, you should check your tanks and pipes and replace any that are lead-lined. There is no evidence that anything else in the water supply – chlorine, fluoride, or even traces of agricultural chemicals – can seriously damage health.

So, except for those people who, doctors believe, are particularly susceptible to risks from environmental hazards, there is virtually no reason for most people to "escape" environmental risks by moving house or installing so-called water purifiers. Changing locations is advisable chiefly for sufferers from *chronic bronchitis* (p.354), who do better in warm, dry climates if they can afford to leave Britain. Some sufferers from lung diseases such as emphysema, however, are advised against moving to a high-altitude area, because the low oxygen content of air at such altitudes can cause shortness of breath and difficulty in sleeping. And if you choose to move to a sunny area, remember that heavy doses of sunlight can cause skin cancer in light-skinned people; do not over-expose bare skin to the strong sun.

The facts about cancer

One reason why the *early warning signs of possible serious illness* listed on p.48 should not be ignored is that many of them suggest the possibility of cancer. Since fear of the unknown is far worse than fear of the known, here for your information are some of the basic facts about this most dreaded of diseases:

To begin with, cancer is not a single disease. It is the name of a group of diseases in which body cells multiply and spread uncontrollably. This can happen in virtually any part of the body; and except in blood cancers (such as leukaemia), the unchecked spread of cells develops into a *malignant* tumour, which generally keeps growing and is likely to invade neighbouring tissues, with potentially fatal consequences. (Other, non-cancerous, tumours are known as *benign* because, although they may grow, their cells do not spread.) A cancer that occurs in bone or muscle tissue is technically termed a *sarcoma*. One occurring in the skin, a gland, or the lining of an organ such as the lung, liver, bladder, or brain is a *carcinoma*. But doctors also use many other words as labels for specific types of cancer. Of the 550 or so physical disorders reviewed in this book, approximately 50 deal with some kind of malignant growth.

What causes cancer?

Medical scientists have identified many of the causes of cancer – smoking causes lung cancer, for example – and they believe that around 80 per cent of all cancers are due to contamination of the environment by chemicals termed *carcinogens*. But exactly how the carcinogens cause cells to become malignant is still not known. Among possible carcinogens are industrial substances like asbestos, tar, and chromium, and nuclear radiation. But even some of the things you eat and drink may make you more or less susceptible to malignancy. And although there is no evidence that cancer is contagious or can be inherited, it does seem to be prevalent in some families. The implication is that your home environment and diet may well affect your susceptibility to malignant tumours. For this reason most doctors advise their patients not only to give up smoking and heavy drinking, but to eat certain foods – animal fats in particular – sparingly.

What are the chances for cure?

Many cancers – those of the cervix, rectum, and skin, for instance – can be detected early; and if treated promptly, before malignant cells have spread far, they can often be completely cured. Once cells have spread (*metastasized*) from the primary growth, however, and have formed secondary growths in other parts of the body, the chances for cure become slim. This is why early detection is so important – and why medical people are constantly working to develop new techniques for discovering malignancy in its very early stages. Fortunately, progress is being made all the time, and there are now successful screening tests for early detection of several kinds of bowel and bladder cancer as well as cancer of the cervix and breast. Moreover, painless diagnostic procedures such as *ultrasound* and *radio-isotope scanning* have largely replaced the often unpleasant investigative techniques of a few years ago.

Cancer is still a killer, of course. It accounts for about 1 in every 8 deaths of people under 35 (even so, that is less than the ratio of deaths from road accidents), and 1 in every 4 deaths of those aged 45 or more. Although those figures may be disturbing, the general outlook is improving. In recent years the rate of cure in treating many forms of cancer has been steadily increasing, as the following examples show:

● Early surgical removal of a cancer of the cervix now has an almost 100 per cent rate of cure.
● Drug treatment of cancer of the lymph glands has a cure rate of over 80 per cent.
● Surgical removal of skin or bowel cancer now has a cure rate of more than 50 per cent.
● In acute lymphoblastic leukaemia, which used to be considered a hopeless childhood disease, modern drugs have accomplished a cure rate of nearly 50 per cent.

So never give way to the assumption that cancer is incurable. Instead, be alert for early symptoms, and see your doctor promptly if any develop.

The 5 most common cancer sites in men
1 Lung
2 Prostate
3 Large intestine
4 Urinary tract
5 Blood (leukaemias) and lymph (lymphomas)

The 5 most common cancer sites in women
1 Breast
2 Large intestine
3 Uterus
4 Lung
5 Blood (leukaemias) and lymph (lymphomas)

Early warning signs of possible serious illness

Many serious illnesses begin with apparently minor or localized symptoms which, if recognized early, can alert you to action in time for the disease to be cured or controlled. In most cases, of course, nothing is seriously wrong. Even so, if you experience any of the following symptoms, you should consult the relevant self-diagnosis symptom chart in Part II of this book; you should also consult your doctor without delay.

1	Rapid loss of weight – more than about 4kg (10lb) in 10 weeks – without apparent cause.		**13**	Persistent bluish tinge to the lips, insides of eyelids, or nail beds.
2	A sore, scab, or ulcer, either in the mouth or on the body, that fails to heal within a period of about 3 weeks.		**14**	Extreme shortness of breath for no apparent reason.
3	A skin blemish or mole that begins to bleed or itch, or that changes colour, size, or shape in middle age.		**15**	Vomiting of blood or a substance that resembles coffee grounds.
			16	Persistent indigestion or abdominal pain.
4	Severe headaches that develop for no obvious reason.		**17**	A marked change in normal bowel habits – for example, alternating attacks of diarrhoea and constipation.
5	Sudden attacks of vomiting, without preceding nausea.		**18**	Faeces that look black and tarry.
6	Fainting spells for no apparent reason.		**19**	Rectal bleeding.
7	Visual problems such as seeing "haloes" around lights, or intermittently blurred vision, especially in dim light.		**20**	Unusually cloudy, pink, red, or smoky-looking urine.
8	Increasing difficulty swallowing.		**21**	In men: some discomfort or difficulty when passing urine.
9	Hoarseness that lasts without apparent cause for a week or more.		**22**	In men: discharge from the tip of the penis.
10	A "smoker's" cough or any other nagging cough that has been getting worse.		**23**	In women: a lump (or unusual thickening) in a breast; or any alteration in breast shape (flattening, bulging, or puckering of skin).
11	Blood in coughed-up sputum.		**24**	In women: bleeding or unusual discharge from a nipple.
12	Constantly swollen ankles.		**25**	In women: vaginal bleeding or "spotting" that occurs between periods or at any time after the menopause.

Atlas of the body

Introduction

Until the Middle Ages, medicine was based almost entirely on the teaching of the Ancient Greek physicians Hippocrates and Galen. Their advice on the treatment of common illnesses and injuries was soundly based on practical experience, but they had little understanding of the structure and functioning of the human body. Medieval medicine was still rooted in such concepts as the "four humours" – blood, phlegm, yellow bile, and black bile.

The science of medicine began in the 16th century with the careful dissection and detailed study of corpses by the Italian artist and inventor Leonardo da Vinci. In 1543 the Belgian scientist Andreas Vesalius produced the first comprehensive anatomical textbook, *de humani corporis fabrica* ("The Structure of the Human Body"). Vesalius was able to correct many of the misconceptions in the teachings of the Ancients, and he laid the foundations for modern anatomy (the structure of the body) and physiology (the functioning of the body). The next major landmark came in 1628 when the English physician William Harvey explained for the first time the true nature of how blood circulates around the body.

The twin studies of anatomy and physiology have developed steadily since Harvey's day. They have provided the essential foundations for the scientific study of diseases by pathologists and microbiologists and their treatment by drugs and surgery. But the pace of discovery has accelerated with the recent development of new techniques for studying the body – for example, *CAT scans, ultrasound scans, radio-isotope scans*, and *endoscopy*.

This section of the book deals with the anatomy of the body. It illustrates the major divisions of the body's structure and shows how new techniques have helped us to visualize the structures of internal organs. (Descriptions of how the various parts and systems of the body function are given in the section introductions in Part III.)

Historical beliefs about the body
Until the 16th century, religious and other constraints prevented dissection of corpses – whether healthy or diseased – to study how the human body is put together. As a result, there grew up a number of beliefs about anatomy and physiology that we now know are misconceptions. They seem to us surprising and bizarre; but it is likely that in another hundred years some of the beliefs held today will be exposed in the same way.

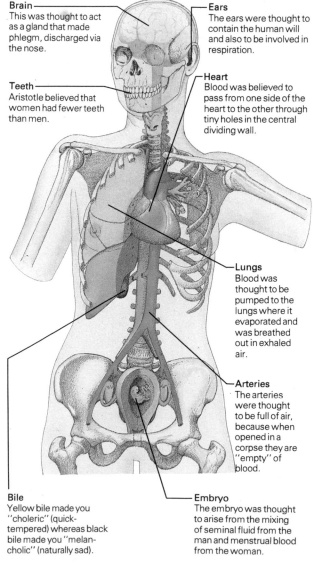

Brain
This was thought to act as a gland that made phlegm, discharged via the nose.

Teeth
Aristotle believed that women had fewer teeth than men.

Ears
The ears were thought to contain the human will and also to be involved in respiration.

Heart
Blood was believed to pass from one side of the heart to the other through tiny holes in the central dividing wall.

Lungs
Blood was thought to be pumped to the lungs where it evaporated and was breathed out in exhaled air.

Arteries
The arteries were thought to be full of air, because when opened in a corpse they are "empty" of blood.

Bile
Yellow bile made you "choleric" (quick-tempered) whereas black bile made you "melancholic" (naturally sad).

Embryo
The embryo was thought to arise from the mixing of seminal fluid from the man and menstrual blood from the woman.

The skeleton

The average human skeleton has 206 bones. There are 32 in each arm, 31 in each leg, 29 in the skull, 26 in the spine, and 25 in the chest. In some skeletons the number of bones varies slightly from the norm – for example, you may have a few extra bones in your hands or feet, or one or more bones may be missing.

The separate bones of the skeleton are connected by joints. There are several types of joint. Fixed joints (*sutures*) hold the bones firmly together, as in the skull. Partly movable joints allow some flexibility, as in the bones of the spine. And freely movable joints provide great flexibility in several planes of movement, as at the shoulder.

The male and female skeletons differ very little. One difference is that male bones are generally slightly larger and heavier than their female counterparts. Also, the cavity in the male pelvis, surrounded by the hip bones and sacrum, is narrower than that of the female pelvis, through which the baby's head and body have to pass during childbirth.

Ossification (bone formation)

In the early months before birth, very little of the skeleton contains actual bone. Most of the bones that eventually form are, in fact, made of cartilage. As the child grows, the cartilage turns into true bone – a process known as "ossification". The areas of ossification appear at set times during the growth of a healthy child. On an X-ray the only areas that show up are those formed of bone (cartilage is pretty much invisible); therefore, it is easy to detect ossification on an X-ray. The series of X-ray photographs below shows how the ankle and foot "bones" of a child gradually appear and grow to replace the "invisible" cartilage until, by the mid-teens, the bones have assumed their mature, adult shape.

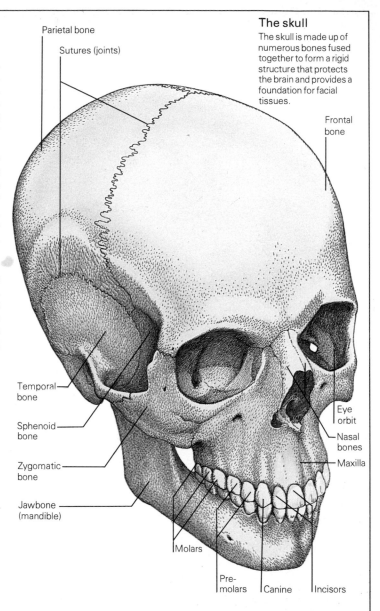

Parietal bone
Sutures (joints)

The skull

The skull is made up of numerous bones fused together to form a rigid structure that protects the brain and provides a foundation for facial tissues.

Frontal bone

Temporal bone
Sphenoid bone
Zygomatic bone
Jawbone (mandible)
Molars
Pre-molars
Canine
Incisors
Maxilla
Nasal bones
Eye orbit

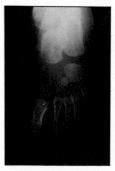

1 year

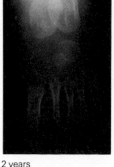

2 years

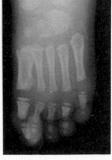

4 years

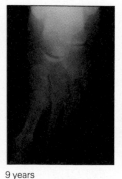

9 years

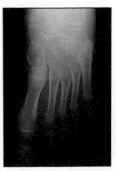

15 years

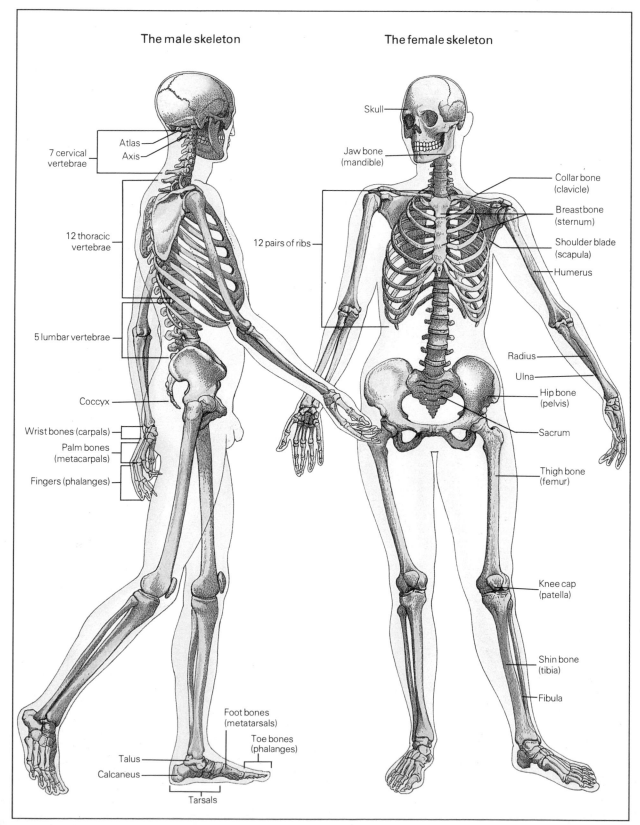

The male skeleton

The female skeleton

7 cervical vertebrae

Atlas

Axis

12 thoracic vertebrae

5 lumbar vertebrae

Coccyx

Wrist bones (carpals)

Palm bones (metacarpals)

Fingers (phalanges)

Skull

Jaw bone (mandible)

12 pairs of ribs

Collar bone (clavicle)

Breastbone (sternum)

Shoulder blade (scapula)

Humerus

Radius

Ulna

Hip bone (pelvis)

Sacrum

Thigh bone (femur)

Knee cap (patella)

Shin bone (tibia)

Fibula

Foot bones (metatarsals)

Toe bones (phalanges)

Talus

Calcaneus

Tarsals

The muscles

There are well over 600 named muscles in the normal body. Each muscle is made up of bundles of closely interlocking muscle fibres, which vary in length from a few millimetres – as in the muscles that move the eyeball – to about 300mm (1ft) – as in the buttock muscles. Some of these fibres contract and relax very quickly; others are designed for the long-term contraction required to maintain body posture.

Each end of a skeletal muscle is attached to a bone (except in the case of a few muscles in the face, which are attached to skin or other tissue), either directly or by means of a tendon. The tendon may be long and tapering or a flat sheet of tissue. Besides the skeletal muscles shown here, there are many other muscles in the body; the heart, for instance, and the digestive-tract walls contain large quantities of muscular tissue.

The muscles of the head and neck (right)

These produce the various movements associated with eating and with positioning of the head. In addition, they are responsible for the vast range of facial expressions that we use to communicate our moods and emotions to others.

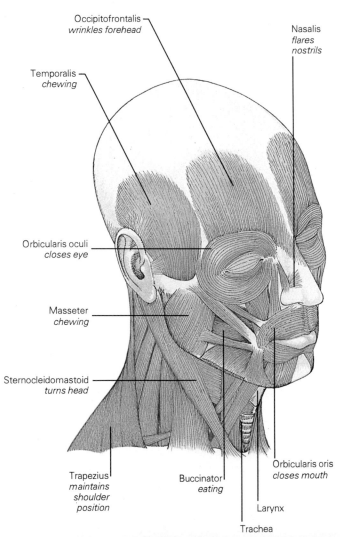

Occipitofrontalis
wrinkles forehead

Nasalis
flares nostrils

Temporalis
chewing

Orbicularis oculi
closes eye

Masseter
chewing

Sternocleidomastoid
turns head

Trapezius
maintains shoulder position

Buccinator
eating

Orbicularis oris
closes mouth

Larynx

Trachea

Muscle biopsies

A muscle biopsy is laboratory examination of a small sample of muscle tissue for signs of disease. The photographs shown here are of very thin slices of healthy muscle, magnified 8,000 times. Each fibre is made of many tiny dark stripes (myosin molecules) and light stripes (actin molecules). In a relaxed muscle (right) the stripes overlap only slightly; in a contracted muscle (far right) they slide over each other, so shortening the length of the muscle.

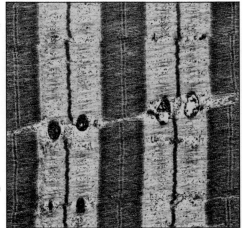

Relaxed muscle fibre

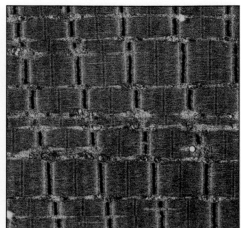

Contracted muscle fibre

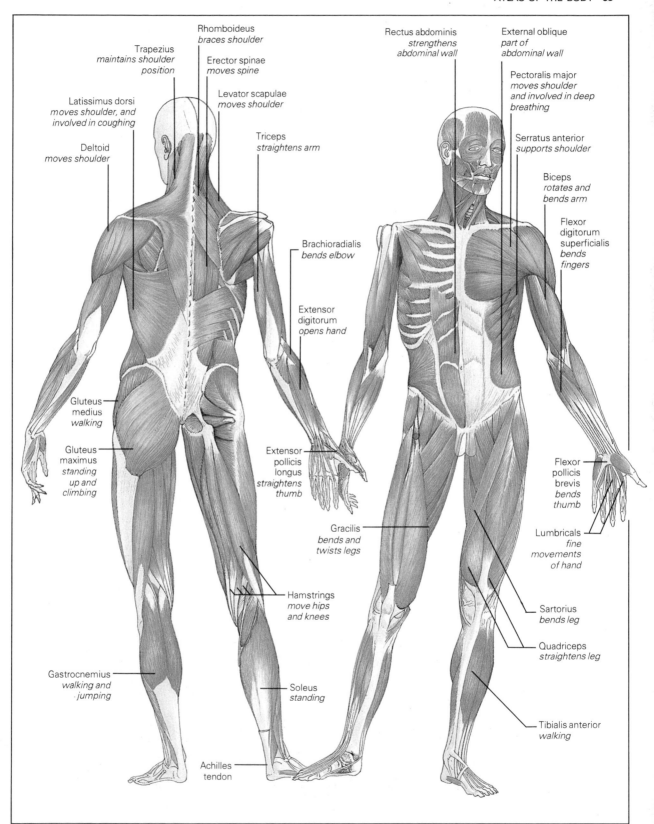

Trapezius
maintains shoulder position

Rhomboideus
braces shoulder

Erector spinae
moves spine

Levator scapulae
moves shoulder

Latissimus dorsi
moves shoulder, and involved in coughing

Deltoid
moves shoulder

Triceps
straightens arm

Rectus abdominis
strengthens abdominal wall

External oblique
part of abdominal wall

Pectoralis major
moves shoulder and involved in deep breathing

Serratus anterior
supports shoulder

Biceps
rotates and bends arm

Flexor digitorum superficialis
bends fingers

Brachioradialis
bends elbow

Extensor digitorum
opens hand

Gluteus medius
walking

Gluteus maximus
standing up and climbing

Extensor pollicis longus
straightens thumb

Gracilis
bends and twists legs

Flexor pollicis brevis
bends thumb

Lumbricals
fine movements of hand

Hamstrings
move hips and knees

Sartorius
bends leg

Quadriceps
straightens leg

Gastrocnemius
walking and jumping

Soleus
standing

Tibialis anterior
walking

Achilles tendon

The brain and nerves

Lying well protected within the rigid, bony box formed by the skull bones is the brain. The main components of the brain are the two cerebral hemispheres, the cerebellum, and the brain stem.

The cerebral hemispheres comprise nearly 90 per cent of brain tissue. Each hemisphere is about 150mm (6in) from front to back, and together they are 110mm (4½in) across. They are made up of intricate folds of nerve tissues whose total surface area is about the same as that of a large sheet of newspaper.

The cerebellum, which is concerned with muscular coordination, lies beneath the rear part of the cerebral hemispheres. It also consists of nerve cells and is divided into two hemispheres.

The brain stem, which is about 75mm (3in) long, contains the nerve centres that control breathing, blood pressure, and other vital yet "automatic" functions; it connects the rest of the brain with the spinal cord.

The brain is a hollow organ. Within it are four interconnected cavities, called ventricles, filled with a fluid called cerebro-spinal fluid. The ventricles are connected to the long, thin cavity that runs down the middle of the spinal cord and which is also filled with cerebro-spinal fluid.

The cranial nerves (below)
There are 12 pairs of cranial nerves that run from the underside of the brain to various organs and parts of the body. Some of the more important nerves carry information from the main sense organs – for example, the optic nerves transmit visual information from the eyes to the brain, where it is coordinated and interpreted.

Nerve junctions
Shown below are 2 small parts of the nervous system – the brachial plexus (upper diagram) in the lower neck, and the sacral plexus (lower diagram) in the lower back. These junctions illustrate the tremendous complexity of the nervous system as a whole.

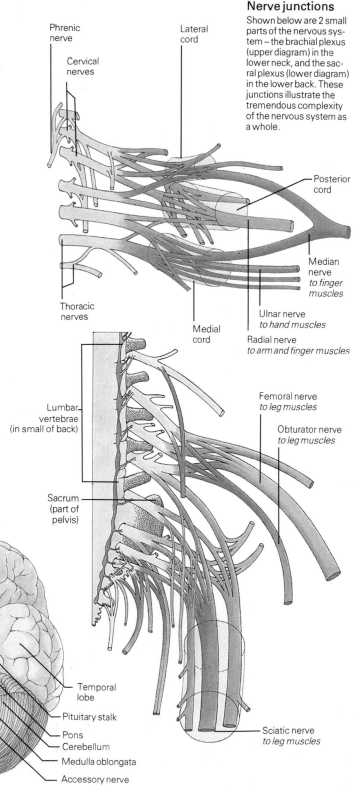

Phrenic nerve

Cervical nerves

Lateral cord

Posterior cord

Median nerve
to finger muscles

Thoracic nerves

Medial cord

Ulnar nerve
to hand muscles

Radial nerve
to arm and finger muscles

Lumbar vertebrae (in small of back)

Femoral nerve
to leg muscles

Obturator nerve
to leg muscles

Sacrum (part of pelvis)

Sciatic nerve
to leg muscles

Frontal lobe

Olfactory nerve

Optic nerve

Oculomotor nerve

Trochlear nerve

Abducent nerve

Trigeminal nerve

Facial nerve

Auditory nerve

Glossopharyngeal nerve

Vagus nerve

Hypoglossal nerve

Temporal lobe

Pituitary stalk

Pons

Cerebellum

Medulla oblongata

Accessory nerve

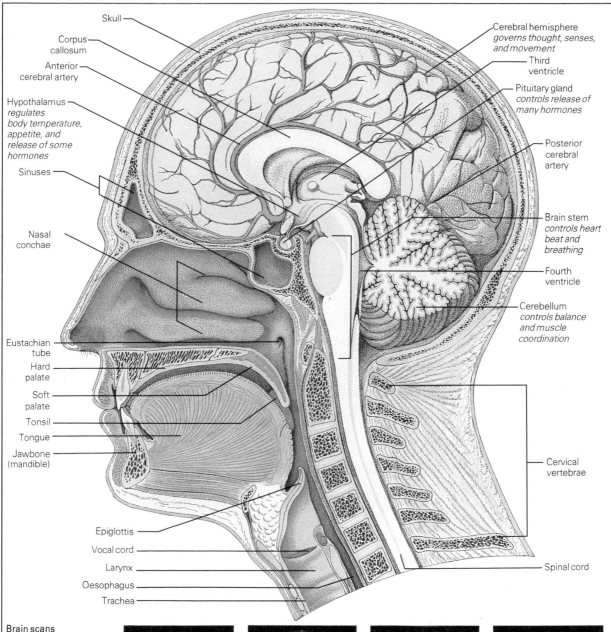

Skull

Corpus callosum

Anterior cerebral artery

Hypothalamus *regulates body temperature, appetite, and release of some hormones*

Sinuses

Nasal conchae

Eustachian tube

Hard palate

Soft palate

Tonsil

Tongue

Jawbone (mandible)

Epiglottis

Vocal cord

Larynx

Oesophagus

Trachea

Cerebral hemisphere *governs thought, senses, and movement*

Third ventricle

Pituitary gland *controls release of many hormones*

Posterior cerebral artery

Brain stem *controls heart beat and breathing*

Fourth ventricle

Cerebellum *controls balance and muscle coordination*

Cervical vertebrae

Spinal cord

Brain scans
These CAT scans are derived from a series of X-ray pictures taken as a camera moves around the head. A computer integrates this information into pictures of horizontal ''slices'' through the head. The darker areas are less dense tissues; the light parts are dense tissues such as the skull bones (see also the body scans on p.58).

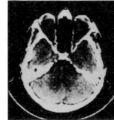

At eye level the skull and nasal bones and the bones of the eye sockets are clearly visible.

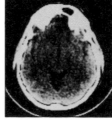

At eyebrow level an air-filled asymmetrical sinus appears as a well-defined dark patch.

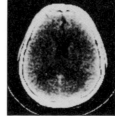

At mid-forehead level the dark, fluid-filled cavities (ventricles) within the brain can be seen.

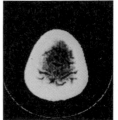

At hair-line level the convolutions on the surface of the brain begin to come into view.

The heart, lungs, and blood vessels

The heart is a cone-shaped organ, made almost entirely of muscle, about the size of your clenched fist. It lies roughly in the centre of the chest; two-thirds of it is to the left of the breast bone, the other third to the right.

The lungs, which are also cone-shaped, lie on either side of the heart. The left lung is slightly smaller than the right one, to accommodate the heart. Between them, the lungs contain about 300 million tiny air sacs (alveoli), whose combined surface area equals that of a tennis court. The tops of the lungs come right up to the collar line, at the base of the neck. When you breathe in deeply, the bases of the lungs extend to the depth of the tenth pair of ribs; when you breathe out, they retract to the level of the eighth pair of ribs.

Bronchogram of the lungs
A small amount of liquid visible on X-rays is trickled down the throat into the lungs, and outlines the branching pattern of the trachea and bronchi (airways).

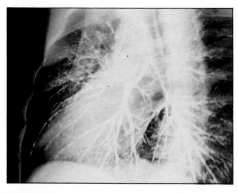

Endoscopic picture of the lungs
The inside of the lungs can be viewed directly by a bronchoscope, a type of endoscope. This picture shows the trachea dividing into the two main bronchi (see also the pictures on p.60).

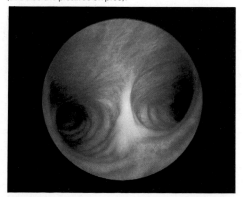

The circulatory system

The circulatory system carries blood to and from every part of the body. Arteries carry blood away from the heart; veins return blood to the heart.

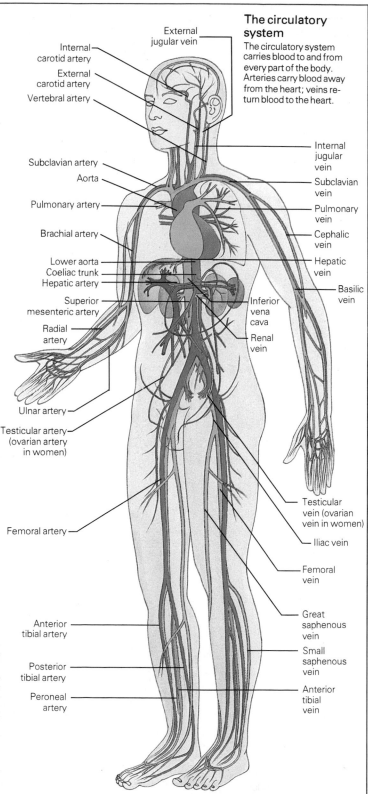

External jugular vein
Internal carotid artery
External carotid artery
Vertebral artery
Subclavian artery
Aorta
Pulmonary artery
Brachial artery
Lower aorta
Coeliac trunk
Hepatic artery
Superior mesenteric artery
Radial artery
Ulnar artery
Testicular artery (ovarian artery in women)
Femoral artery
Anterior tibial artery
Posterior tibial artery
Peroneal artery

Internal jugular vein
Subclavian vein
Pulmonary vein
Cephalic vein
Hepatic vein
Basilic vein
Inferior vena cava
Renal vein
Testicular vein (ovarian vein in women)
Iliac vein
Femoral vein
Great saphenous vein
Small saphenous vein
Anterior tibial vein

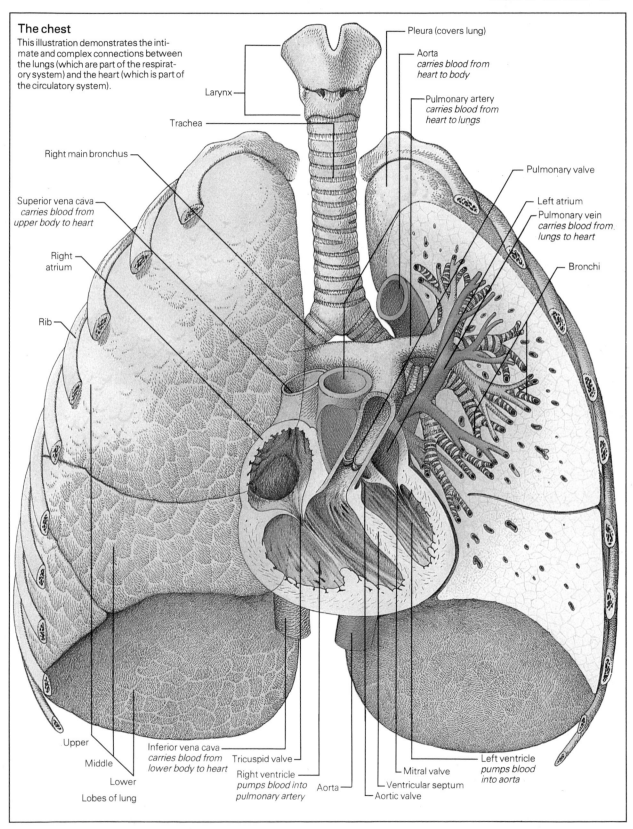

The chest

This illustration demonstrates the intimate and complex connections between the lungs (which are part of the respiratory system) and the heart (which is part of the circulatory system).

Larynx

Trachea

Right main bronchus

Superior vena cava
carries blood from upper body to heart

Right atrium

Rib

Pleura (covers lung)

Aorta
carries blood from heart to body

Pulmonary artery
carries blood from heart to lungs

Pulmonary valve

Left atrium

Pulmonary vein
carries blood from lungs to heart

Bronchi

Upper

Middle

Lower

Lobes of lung

Inferior vena cava
carries blood from lower body to heart

Tricuspid valve

Right ventricle
pumps blood into pulmonary artery

Aorta

Mitral valve

Ventricular septum

Aortic valve

Left ventricle
pumps blood into aorta

The torso

The upper part of the torso is the chest, which contains the heart and lungs (see also the previous page). The chest is separated from the lower part of the torso – the abdomen – by the diaphragm, a dome-shaped sheet of muscle. The edge of the diaphragm is attached to the bottom of the ribcage but, because of its domed shape, its middle reaches to only 25mm (1in) below the level of the nipples.

Packed into the abdomen are the organs of the digestive and urinary systems. The lower part of the abdomen, cradled within the hip bone, is often called the pelvis. In the female, the pelvis contains the reproductive organs.

Body scans
Pictures of horizontal "slices" through the body can be taken by the CAT scanner (see also the brain scans on p.55). The denser the tissue, the lighter it appears on the scan.

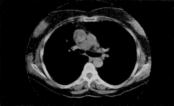

At mid-chest level, the palest areas are the backbone and ribs, the heart appears slightly darker, and the air-filled lungs black.

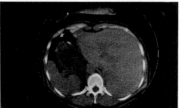

At a level just below the breastbone, the large light area on the right is the liver and the similar, smaller area to the left is the spleen; the darker patch is the stomach.

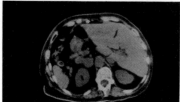

Just above the navel, the liver shows up as a large light area to the right. The light circles on either side of the backbone are the kidneys; the patchy areas are loops of intestine.

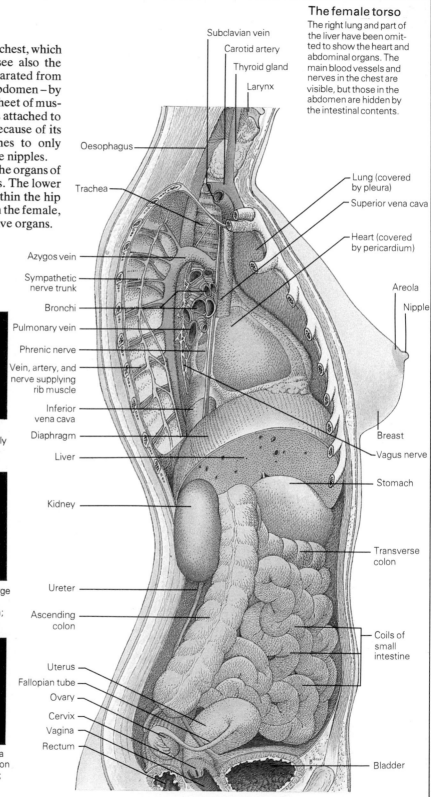

The female torso
The right lung and part of the liver have been omitted to show the heart and abdominal organs. The main blood vessels and nerves in the chest are visible, but those in the abdomen are hidden by the intestinal contents.

Subclavian vein
Carotid artery
Thyroid gland
Larynx
Oesophagus
Trachea
Azygos vein
Sympathetic nerve trunk
Bronchi
Pulmonary vein
Phrenic nerve
Vein, artery, and nerve supplying rib muscle
Inferior vena cava
Diaphragm
Liver
Kidney
Ureter
Ascending colon
Uterus
Fallopian tube
Ovary
Cervix
Vagina
Rectum
Lung (covered by pleura)
Superior vena cava
Heart (covered by pericardium)
Areola
Nipple
Breast
Vagus nerve
Stomach
Transverse colon
Coils of small intestine
Bladder

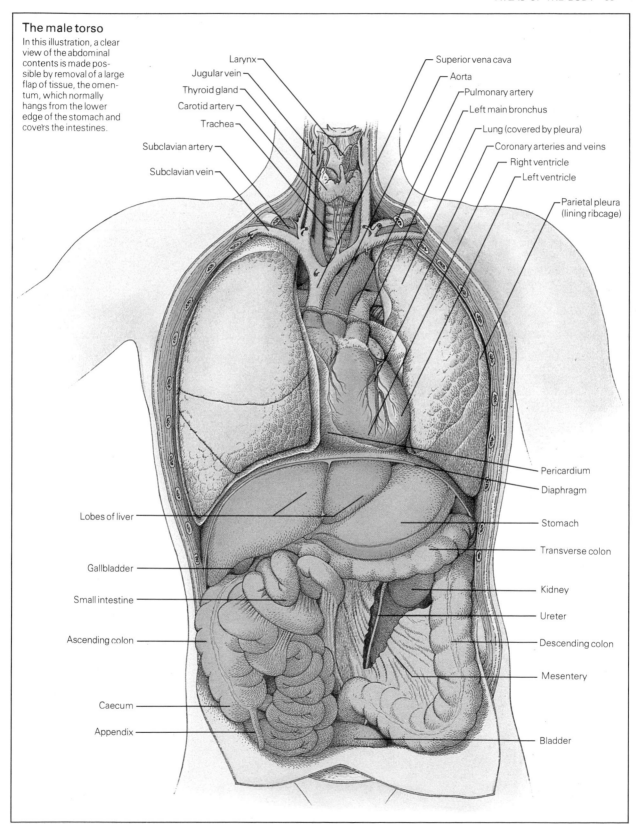

The male torso

In this illustration, a clear view of the abdominal contents is made possible by removal of a large flap of tissue, the omentum, which normally hangs from the lower edge of the stomach and covers the intestines.

Larynx

Jugular vein

Thyroid gland

Carotid artery

Trachea

Subclavian artery

Subclavian vein

Superior vena cava

Aorta

Pulmonary artery

Left main bronchus

Lung (covered by pleura)

Coronary arteries and veins

Right ventricle

Left ventricle

Parietal pleura (lining ribcage)

Pericardium

Diaphragm

Lobes of liver

Stomach

Transverse colon

Gallbladder

Kidney

Small intestine

Ureter

Ascending colon

Descending colon

Mesentery

Caecum

Appendix

Bladder

The digestive organs

The digestive tract is basically one long tube extending from the mouth to the anus. Food passes from the mouth down the oesophagus, a tube about 250mm (10in) long, to the stomach, which holds about 1.5 litres (2½ pints) when fairly full. After the stomach comes the duodenum, a C-shaped tube about the same length as the oesophagus. Small ducts carry digestive juices from the liver and pancreas into the duodenum. The next section of the tract is about 5m (about 16ft) of coiled small intestine, followed by 1.5m (about 5ft) of large intestine which leads into the rectum and, finally, the anus.

The lengths of the various portions of digestive tract vary markedly from person to person. They also vary depending on whether the tissues are alive or not; after death, the muscles in the digestive-tract walls lose their tone and relax, and the tract becomes appreciably longer.

Endoscopy
Modern endoscopes (long, flexible tubes that transmit visual images) can reach and view virtually all parts of the digestive tract. Most regions of the tract are normally flattened and contain murky semi-liquids. So, to obtain a clear view, air is pumped down the endoscope into the tract to hold its walls apart while the photograph is being taken. Below left is a photograph of the stomach lining with its shiny, ridged surface. Below right is the lining of the duodenum. It has a smooth interior on which an abnormality – an ulcer, for instance – would be clearly visible. (See also the picture on p.56.)

The digestive system
The digestive system comprises the digestive tract – the tube from mouth to anus – plus 2 organs, the liver and pancreas, that manufacture digestive juices.

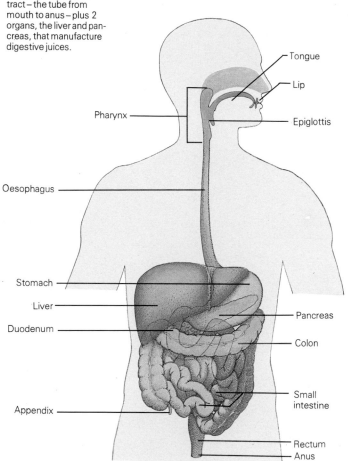

Tongue
Lip
Pharynx
Epiglottis
Oesophagus
Stomach
Liver
Duodenum
Pancreas
Colon
Appendix
Small intestine
Rectum
Anus

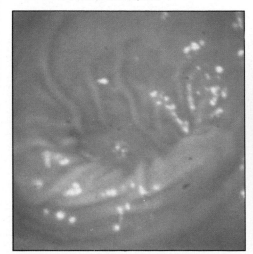

Endoscopic view of stomach

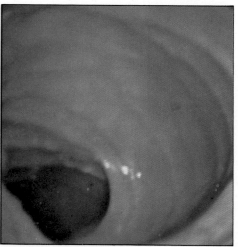

Endoscopic view of duodenum

The abdominal digestive organs

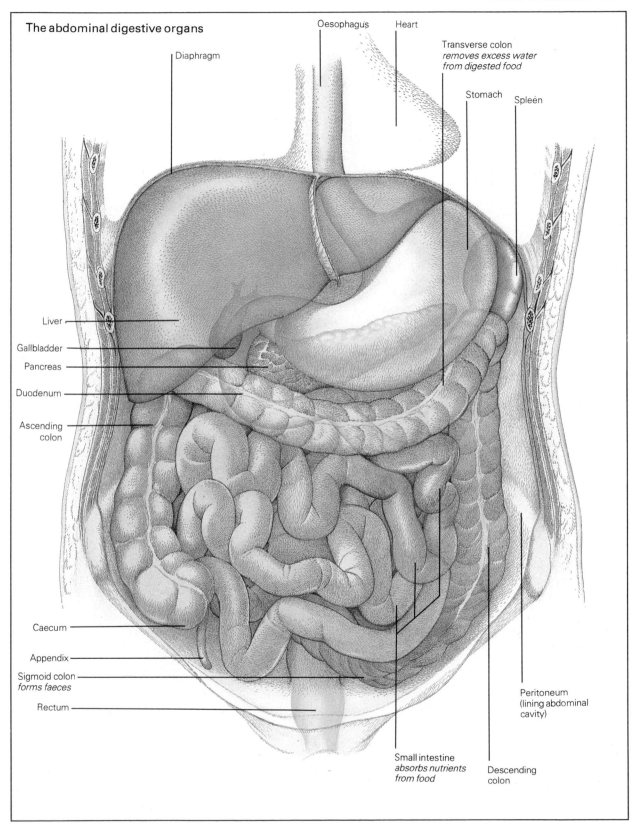

Oesophagus

Heart

Diaphragm

Transverse colon
*removes excess water
from digested food*

Stomach

Spleen

Liver

Gallbladder

Pancreas

Duodenum

Ascending
colon

Caecum

Appendix

Sigmoid colon
forms faeces

Rectum

Peritoneum
(lining abdominal
cavity)

Small intestine
*absorbs nutrients
from food*

Descending
colon

The organs of the lower abdomen

The lower abdominal organs are concerned principally with removal of wastes, in the form of urine and faeces, and with reproduction (see below). The bladder stores urine from the kidneys. It is a muscular sac about 75mm (3in) in diameter when full. The urine is passed to the outside along a tube called the urethra, which in the male is 250mm (about 10in) long but in the female only 25mm (approximately 1in) long. The lower abdominal organs are sometimes called the pelvic organs because they are situated within the cup-shaped hip bone, the pelvis.

The male reproductive organs
In addition to the visible male genitalia (the 2 testes in their pouch, the scrotum, and the penis), there are glands and ducts inside the abdomen; these internal organs are the prostate gland, the 2 seminal vesicles, and the 2 tubes each called the vas deferens.

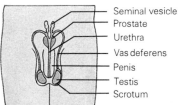

Seminal vesicle
Prostate
Urethra
Vas deferens
Penis
Testis
Scrotum

The female reproductive organs
The female genital organs are all situated within the abdomen, except for the vagina, which leads from the abdominal area to the external genitals, the vulva. Inside the abdomen are the 2 ovaries connected by the 2 fallopian tubes to the uterus (commonly called the womb).

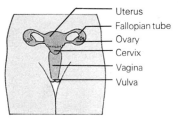

Uterus
Fallopian tube
Ovary
Cervix
Vagina
Vulva

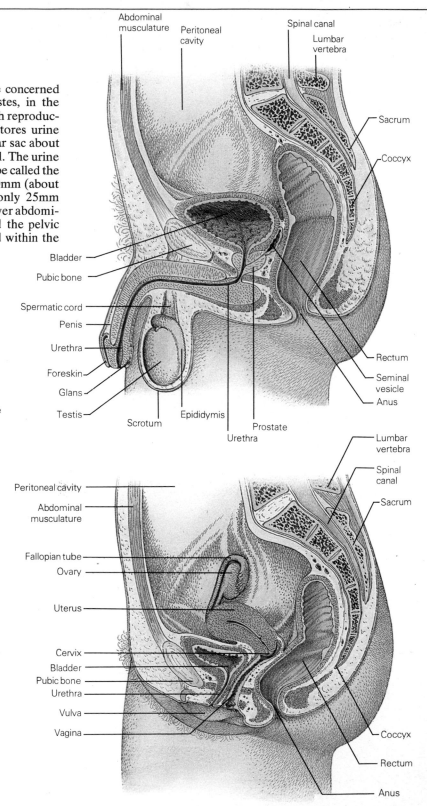

Abdominal musculature
Peritoneal cavity
Spinal canal
Lumbar vertebra
Sacrum
Coccyx
Bladder
Pubic bone
Spermatic cord
Penis
Urethra
Foreskin
Glans
Testis
Scrotum
Epididymis
Prostate
Urethra
Rectum
Seminal vesicle
Anus

Lumbar vertebra
Spinal canal
Sacrum
Peritoneal cavity
Abdominal musculature
Fallopian tube
Ovary
Uterus
Cervix
Bladder
Pubic bone
Urethra
Vulva
Vagina
Coccyx
Rectum
Anus

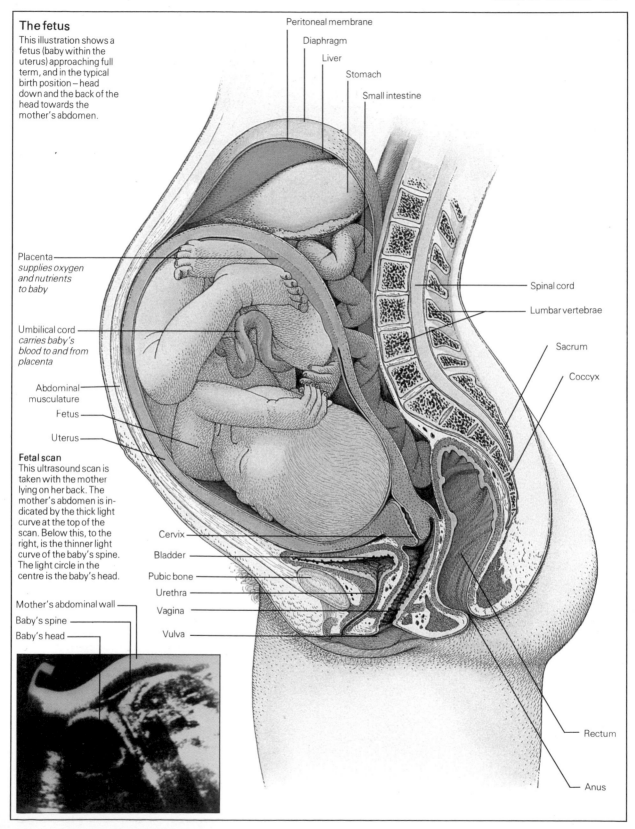

The fetus

This illustration shows a fetus (baby within the uterus) approaching full term, and in the typical birth position – head down and the back of the head towards the mother's abdomen.

Peritoneal membrane

Diaphragm

Liver

Stomach

Small intestine

Placenta
supplies oxygen and nutrients to baby

Umbilical cord
carries baby's blood to and from placenta

Abdominal musculature

Fetus

Uterus

Spinal cord

Lumbar vertebrae

Sacrum

Coccyx

Fetal scan

This ultrasound scan is taken with the mother lying on her back. The mother's abdomen is indicated by the thick light curve at the top of the scan. Below this, to the right, is the thinner light curve of the baby's spine. The light circle in the centre is the baby's head.

Cervix

Bladder

Pubic bone

Urethra

Vagina

Vulva

Mother's abdominal wall

Baby's spine

Baby's head

Rectum

Anus

The special sense organs

The two senses that provide most information about the world around us are sight and hearing. The eyes and ears are delicate and sensitive structures of great complexity, but they lie well protected inside shaped cavities within the skull bones. The eye is "directional" in that six separate muscles swivel it to look at objects in various locations, and this directional information is passed to the brain. The human ear does not have this ability, though many animals are able to pinpoint the direction a sound comes from by moving the external ear (pinna).

Ophthalmoscope view of the retina
The pale disc is the optic disc, where all the nerves come together and leave the eye on their way to the brain. Arteries can be seen radiating from the disc to supply the retina and other structures in the eye with blood.

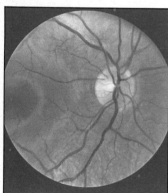

The ear
The outer-ear canal, which is about 20mm ($\frac{3}{4}$in) long, leads through the skull bone to the middle and inner ear. Connecting the middle ear to the back of the throat is another tube about 40mm (approximately 1$\frac{1}{2}$in) long, the eustachian tube. Besides enabling us to hear, the ear also contains the semicircular canals which enable us to keep our balance.

The eye
The eyeball is about 25mm (1in) in diameter. The socket for it in the skull bone is appreciably larger, to allow room for the pairs of muscles that move the eye.

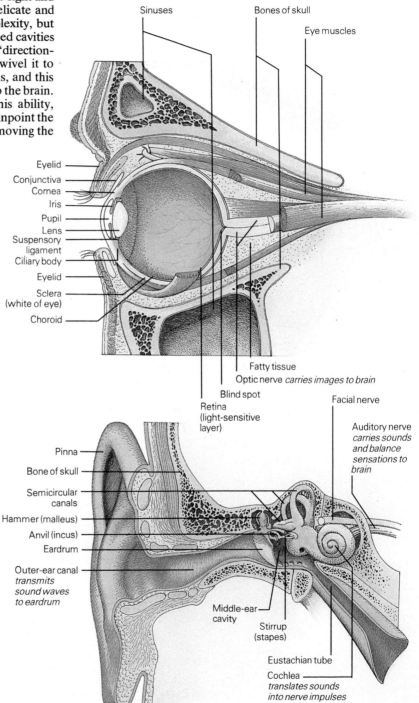

Sinuses

Bones of skull

Eye muscles

Eyelid
Conjunctiva
Cornea
Iris
Pupil
Lens
Suspensory ligament
Ciliary body
Eyelid
Sclera (white of eye)
Choroid

Fatty tissue
Optic nerve *carries images to brain*
Blind spot
Retina (light-sensitive layer)

Pinna
Bone of skull
Semicircular canals
Hammer (malleus)
Anvil (incus)
Eardrum
Outer-ear canal *transmits sound waves to eardrum*

Facial nerve

Auditory nerve *carries sounds and balance sensations to brain*

Middle-ear cavity
Stirrup (stapes)
Eustachian tube
Cochlea *translates sounds into nerve impulses*

Part II

Symptoms and self-diagnosis

Self-diagnosis symptom charts
Visual aids to diagnosis

Self-diagnosis symptom charts

How to use the charts

Each of the self-diagnosis symptom charts in this section is aimed at helping you to track down the possible significance of a particular symptom, either on its own or combined with other symptoms. Every chart takes a common symptom as its starting point, from which you are led by a series of questions and answers to a logical conclusion. The end point you reach will probably refer you elsewhere in this book, and may also tell you to seek professional help (whether routinely or urgently). First find the chart you want by consulting the *Chart-finder* (p.68), which gives you the appropriate *chart number*. Then, after turning to the chart itself, check its relevance by noting the *definition* and *chart group*.

As shown on the two samples on these pages, each chart consists of a series of simple YES or NO *questions*. Always begin at the first question, and follow through to the

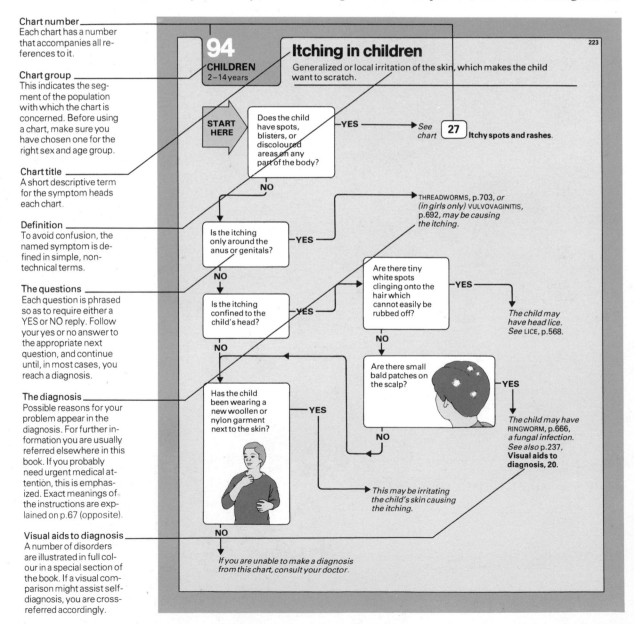

Chart number
Each chart has a number that accompanies all references to it.

Chart group
This indicates the segment of the population with which the chart is concerned. Before using a chart, make sure you have chosen one for the right sex and age group.

Chart title
A short descriptive term for the symptom heads each chart.

Definition
To avoid confusion, the named symptom is defined in simple, non-technical terms.

The questions
Each question is phrased so as to require either a YES or NO reply. Follow your yes or no answer to the appropriate next question, and continue until, in most cases, you reach a diagnosis.

The diagnosis
Possible reasons for your problem appear in the diagnosis. For further information you are usually referred elsewhere in this book. If you probably need urgent medical attention, this is emphasized. Exact meanings of the instructions are explained on p.67 (opposite).

Visual aids to diagnosis
A number of disorders are illustrated in full colour in a special section of the book. If a visual comparison might assist self-diagnosis, you are cross-referred accordingly.

94
CHILDREN
2–14 years

Itching in children
Generalized or local irritation of the skin, which makes the child want to scratch.

223

START HERE

Does the child have spots, blisters, or discoloured areas on any part of the body? — **YES** → *See chart* **27** Itchy spots and rashes.

NO

Is the itching only around the anus or genitals? — **YES** → THREADWORMS, p.703, *or (in girls only)* VULVOVAGINITIS, p.692, *may be causing the itching.*

NO

Is the itching confined to the child's head? — **YES** → Are there tiny white spots clinging onto the hair which cannot easily be rubbed off? — **YES** → *The child may have head lice. See* LICE, p.568.

NO

NO → Are there small bald patches on the scalp? — **YES** → *The child may have* RINGWORM, p.666, *a fungal infection. See also* p.237, **Visual aids to diagnosis, 20.**

NO

Has the child been wearing a new woollen or nylon garment next to the skin? — **YES** → *This may be irritating the child's skin causing the itching.*

NO

If you are unable to make a diagnosis from this chart, consult your doctor.

diagnosis that fits your case. Here you will usually find one – or sometimes more than one – likely explanation of your problem, along with *instructions* on what steps to take. Except in urgent cases, be sure to follow through all cross-references, or you may miss out on further advice. **Important:** Remember that the charts give only tentative diagnoses. For firm diagnosis and treatment always consult your doctor.

What the instructions mean

Call your doctor now!
Seek medical advice within a few hours at the most. Either telephone your doctor for an urgent house call, or go straight to the surgery. If your doctor is unavailable, telephone or visit your local hospital casualty department.

**EMERGENCY
Get medical help now!**
The problem may be life-threatening and needs immediate attention. If you fail to reach your own doctor within minutes, dial 999 and ask for an ambulance; or take the sufferer to the nearest hospital casualty department if he or she can be moved safely.

Consult your doctor.
Do not delay!
Get medical advice within a day or two. Ask your doctor's receptionist for an appointment by tomorrow, or the next day at the latest.

If your problem is not identified as one requiring swift attention, you can assume that an urgent consultation is not vital. Turn to the page(s) indicated for further information and advice.

First aid
Wherever first-aid measures are applicable, a cross-reference to the appropriate page is provided along with a distinctive, easily-spotted symbol: ✚

Boxed information
Some charts contain boxes giving important additional information – either self-help advice or, more often, warnings about possibly dangerous symptoms. Whenever there is a possibility of cancer this is described under **Cancer watch**.

---

134 | **39**
GENERAL all ages

Coughing up blood
Coughing up phlegm that is coloured or streaked bright red or rusty brown, or that is pink and frothy.

START HERE → Is your temperature 39°C (102°F) or above? —**YES**→ **Call your doctor now!** *These symptoms suggest that you may have* PNEUMONIA, p.359, *especially if your phlegm is rusty brown.*

NO

Are you short of breath even though you have not been exercising? —**YES**→ Is your phlegm pink and frothy? —**YES**→ **EMERGENCY Get medical help now!** *You may have a build-up of fluid in the lungs.* See PULMONARY OEDEMA, p.368.

NO / **NO**

Have you recently had an operation, or been confined to bed by an injury or prolonged illness? —**YES**→ **EMERGENCY Get medical help now!** *You may have a blood clot in the lung.* See PULMONARY EMBOLISM, p.406.

NO

Has a cold or bout of flu within the past month left you with a persistent cough? —**YES**→ *Consult your doctor. Coughing may have ruptured a small blood vessel.*

NO

Have you had a cough for many weeks or months? —**YES**→ *Consult your doctor.* **Do not delay!** *These symptoms indicate the possibility of* LUNG CANCER, p.366, *or* TUBERCULOSIS, p.563.

NO

If you are unable to make a diagnosis from this chart, consult your doctor without further delay.

Cancer watch
Coughing up blood may be a sign of lung cancer if you have had a cough for many weeks or months. This diagnosis is particularly likely if you are a smoker.

Consult your doctor without delay!

How to find the chart you need

The special *Chart-finder* index (below) directs you to the number of the chart that deals with your problem. To find the chart you want, follow these steps:

1. Single out your major problem; if you are suffering from two or more symptoms (high fever, a cough, and runny nose, say) select the one that troubles you most.

2. Find the symptom in the chart-finder. For your convenience the charts are indexed according to a variety of key words. Irregular vaginal bleeding, for instance, is listed in three places – under B, I, and V.

3. If you cannot find your main symptom in the chart-finder, look for a chart dealing with a secondary symptom if you have one.

4. When you have found the correct chart, turn to the chart number (*not* page number) indicated and proceed with your self-diagnosis. For a full explanation of how to use the charts see p.66.

CHART-FINDER

1

Feeling under the weather

A vague, generalized feeling of being unwell.

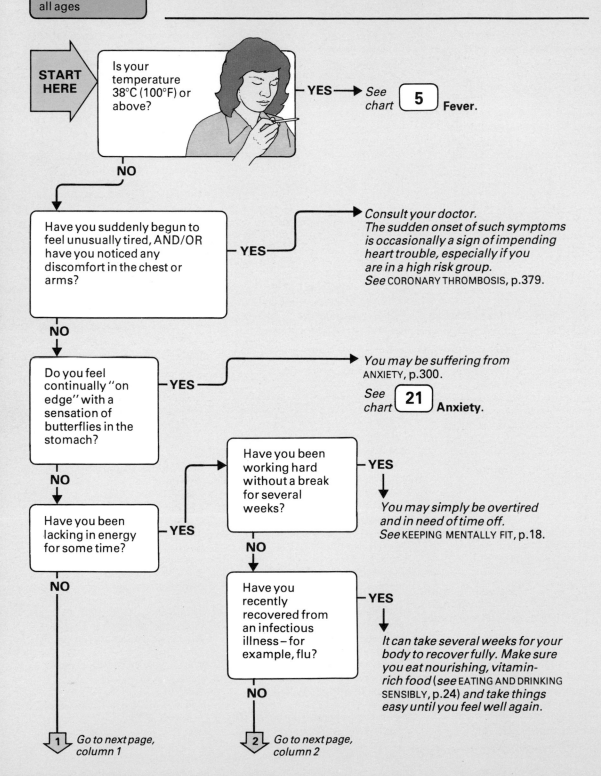

START HERE

Is your temperature 38°C (100°F) or above?

YES → *See chart* **5** **Fever.**

NO

Have you suddenly begun to feel unusually tired, AND/OR have you noticed any discomfort in the chest or arms?

YES → *Consult your doctor.*
The sudden onset of such symptoms is occasionally a sign of impending heart trouble, especially if you are in a high risk group.
See CORONARY THROMBOSIS, p.379.

NO

Do you feel continually "on edge" with a sensation of butterflies in the stomach?

YES → *You may be suffering from* ANXIETY, p.300.
See chart **21** **Anxiety.**

NO

Have you been lacking in energy for some time?

YES → Have you been working hard without a break for several weeks?

YES ↓
You may simply be overtired and in need of time off.
See KEEPING MENTALLY FIT, p.18.

NO

Have you recently recovered from an infectious illness – for example, flu?

YES ↓
It can take several weeks for your body to recover fully. Make sure you eat nourishing, vitamin-rich food (see EATING AND DRINKING SENSIBLY, p.24) *and take things easy until you feel well again.*

NO

NO

1 *Go to next page, column 1*

2 *Go to next page, column 2*

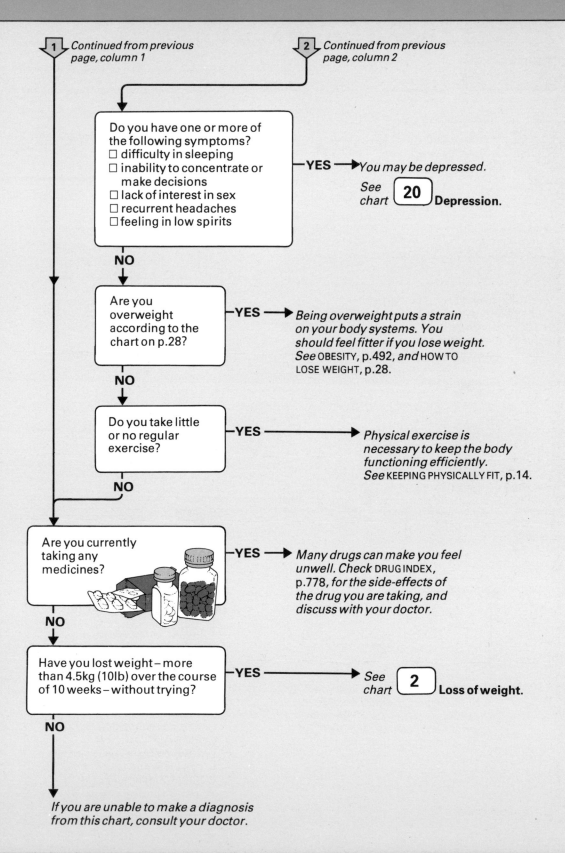

1 *Continued from previous page, column 1*

2 *Continued from previous page, column 2*

Do you have one or more of the following symptoms?
- ☐ difficulty in sleeping
- ☐ inability to concentrate or make decisions
- ☐ lack of interest in sex
- ☐ recurrent headaches
- ☐ feeling in low spirits

YES → *You may be depressed.*

See chart **20** **Depression.**

NO

Are you overweight according to the chart on p.28?

YES → *Being overweight puts a strain on your body systems. You should feel fitter if you lose weight. See* OBESITY, p.492, *and* HOW TO LOSE WEIGHT, p.28.

NO

Do you take little or no regular exercise?

YES → *Physical exercise is necessary to keep the body functioning efficiently. See* KEEPING PHYSICALLY FIT, p.14.

NO

Are you currently taking any medicines?

YES → *Many drugs can make you feel unwell. Check* DRUG INDEX, p.778, *for the side-effects of the drug you are taking, and discuss with your doctor.*

NO

Have you lost weight – more than 4.5kg (10lb) over the course of 10 weeks – without trying?

YES → *See chart* **2** **Loss of weight.**

NO

If you are unable to make a diagnosis from this chart, consult your doctor.

Loss of weight

Loss of 4.5kg (10lb) or more, over a period of 10 weeks or less, without a deliberate change in eating habits.

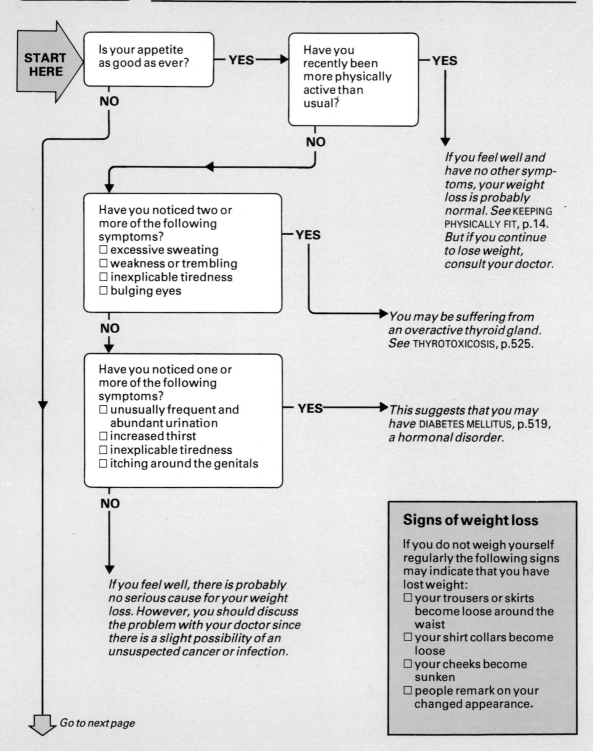

START HERE

Is your appetite as good as ever?

YES → **Have you recently been more physically active than usual?**

YES →

If you feel well and have no other symptoms, your weight loss is probably normal. See KEEPING PHYSICALLY FIT, p.14. *But if you continue to lose weight, consult your doctor.*

NO

NO

Have you noticed two or more of the following symptoms?
☐ excessive sweating
☐ weakness or trembling
☐ inexplicable tiredness
☐ bulging eyes

YES →

You may be suffering from an overactive thyroid gland. See THYROTOXICOSIS, p.525.

NO

Have you noticed one or more of the following symptoms?
☐ unusually frequent and abundant urination
☐ increased thirst
☐ inexplicable tiredness
☐ itching around the genitals

YES →

This suggests that you may have DIABETES MELLITUS, p.519, *a hormonal disorder.*

NO

If you feel well, there is probably no serious cause for your weight loss. However, you should discuss the problem with your doctor since there is a slight possibility of an unsuspected cancer or infection.

Signs of weight loss

If you do not weigh yourself regularly the following signs may indicate that you have lost weight:
☐ your trousers or skirts become loose around the waist
☐ your shirt collars become loose
☐ your cheeks become sunken
☐ people remark on your changed appearance.

⇩ *Go to next page*

Continued from previous page

Have you been having recurrent bouts of diarrhoea?

YES → Are your faeces unusually pale, bulky, and difficult to flush away?

YES →

NO ↓ (from diarrhoea box)

NO ↓ (from faeces box)

You may have faulty digestion. See MALABSORPTION, p.475.

Have you been constipated AND/OR have you noticed blood in your faeces?

YES →

NO ↓

Consult your doctor.
Do not delay!
You may have inflammation of the small intestine (see CROHN'S DISEASE, p.473), *but there is a slight chance of* CANCER OF THE LARGE INTESTINE, p.481.

Have you been re-current attacks of upper abdominal pain?

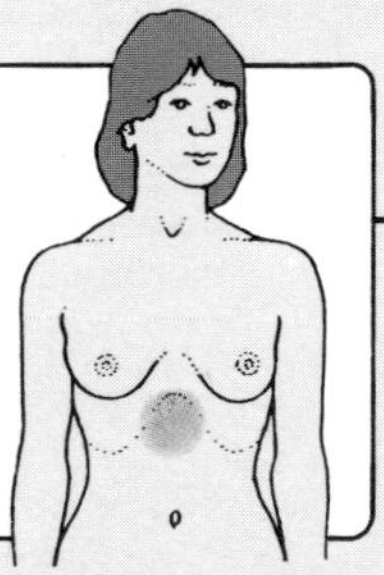

YES →

Consult your doctor.
Do not delay!
You may have a STOMACH ULCER, p.465, *but there is also a possibility of* CANCER OF THE STOMACH, p.466.

NO ↓

Consult your doctor.
Do not delay!
You may have a chronic infection such as TUBERCULOSIS, p.563.

Have you noticed two or more of the following symptoms?
☐ night sweats
☐ recurrent raised temperature
☐ general feeling of ill health
☐ persistent cough
☐ blood in phlegm

YES →

NO ↓

If you are unable to make a diagnosis from this chart, consult your doctor.

Cancer watch

There is a possibility of cancer if weight loss and loss of appetite are combined with abdominal pain OR a change in bowel habit.

Consult your doctor without delay!

3

GENERAL
all ages

Overweight

The chart on p.28 indicates the optimum weight for your height. If you are heavier than this, you are overweight and endangering your health.

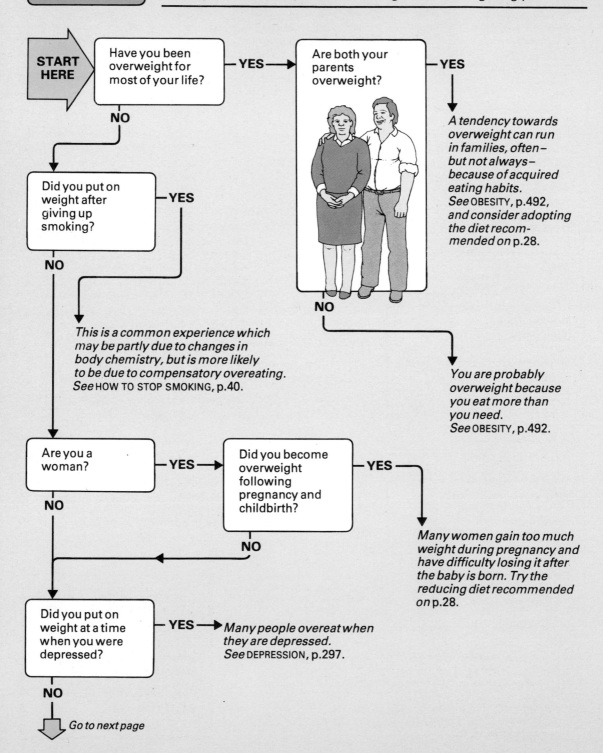

START HERE → Have you been overweight for most of your life? — **YES** → Are both your parents overweight? — **YES**

NO

A tendency towards overweight can run in families, often – but not always – because of acquired eating habits. See OBESITY, p.492, and consider adopting the diet recommended on p.28.

Did you put on weight after giving up smoking? — **YES**

NO

This is a common experience which may be partly due to changes in body chemistry, but is more likely to be due to compensatory overeating. See HOW TO STOP SMOKING, p.40.

NO

You are probably overweight because you eat more than you need. See OBESITY, p.492.

Are you a woman? — **YES** → Did you become overweight following pregnancy and childbirth? — **YES**

NO

NO

Many women gain too much weight during pregnancy and have difficulty losing it after the baby is born. Try the reducing diet recommended on p.28.

Did you put on weight at a time when you were depressed? — **YES** → *Many people overeat when they are depressed. See DEPRESSION, p.297.*

NO

Go to next page

⬇ *Continued from previous page*

Did the weight gain follow a change from a physically strenuous job to sedentary work?

YES → *In your former job you probably needed more calories than you do now. You should adjust your eating habits accordingly.* See COUNTING CALORIES, p.27.

NO

Have you noticed any of the following symptoms since you began to put on weight?
☐ feeling the cold more than you used to
☐ thinning or brittle hair
☐ dry skin

YES → *You may be suffering from an underactive thyroid gland.* See HYPOTHYROIDISM, p.526.

NO

Have you been taking steroid drugs for a problem such as asthma or rheumatoid arthritis?

YES → *Such drugs can cause weight gain. Check* DRUG INDEX, p.778, *for the side-effects of the drug you are taking, and discuss with your doctor.*

NO

Are you over 40?

YES → *Weight gain as you grow older may be a result of such factors as a decline in the amount of exercise you take and changes in the rate that your body burns up food.* See AGE AND INCREASING WEIGHT, p.29.

NO

If you are unable to make a diagnosis from this chart, your excess weight is probably due only to overeating. If after a month of following the recommended reducing diet, you fail to lose weight, consult your doctor.

Losing excess weight

Whatever the cause of your weight gain, following the balanced reducing diet described on p.28 will help you achieve and maintain a healthy weight.

Difficulty in sleeping

Frequent difficulty in falling asleep or staying asleep during the night (often called insomnia).

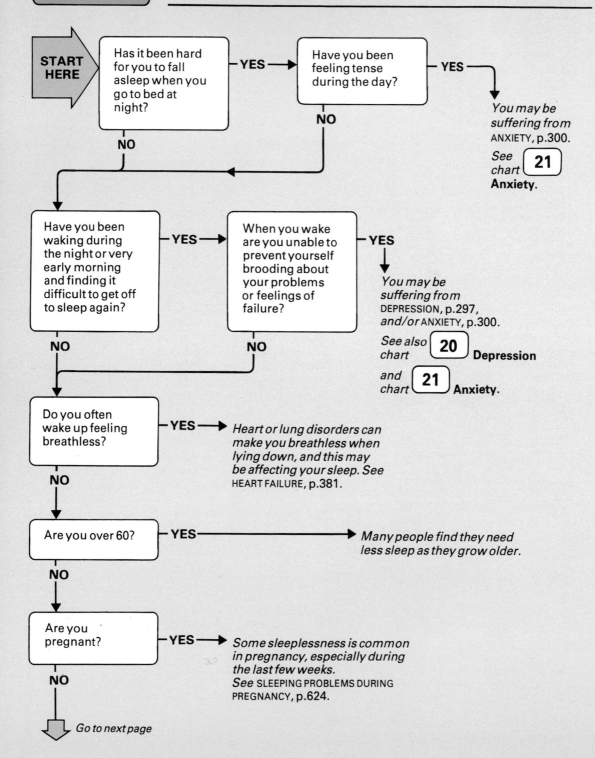

START HERE → Has it been hard for you to fall asleep when you go to bed at night? — **YES** → Have you been feeling tense during the day? — **YES** →

You may be suffering from ANXIETY, p.300.

See chart **21** **Anxiety**.

NO

Have you been waking during the night or very early morning and finding it difficult to get off to sleep again? — **YES** → When you wake are you unable to prevent yourself brooding about your problems or feelings of failure? — **YES** →

You may be suffering from DEPRESSION, p.297, *and/or* ANXIETY, p.300.

See also chart **20** **Depression**

and chart **21** **Anxiety**.

NO   **NO**

Do you often wake up feeling breathless? — **YES** →

Heart or lung disorders can make you breathless when lying down, and this may be affecting your sleep. See HEART FAILURE, p.381.

NO

Are you over 60? — **YES** →

Many people find they need less sleep as they grow older.

NO

Are you pregnant? — **YES** →

Some sleeplessness is common in pregnancy, especially during the last few weeks.
See SLEEPING PROBLEMS DURING PREGNANCY, p.624.

NO

⇩ *Go to next page*

Continued from previous page

On nights when you have difficulty in sleeping, have you drunk more tea or coffee than usual?

YES → The caffeine in tea and coffee is a stimulant and is likely to be the cause of your problem. Try to avoid these drinks in the late afternoon and evening. If you still have trouble sleeping, try cutting out tea and coffee altogether. See CAFFEINE, p.30.

NO ↓

On nights when you have difficulty in sleeping, have you eaten a late, heavy meal, or drunk a lot of alcohol?

YES → These are common causes of difficulty in sleeping. Try eating your evening meals earlier and/or reducing your alcohol intake.

NO ↓

Have you recently stopped taking sleeping pills or tranquillizers?

YES → It can take several weeks for your sleeping pattern to return to normal after using these drugs.

NO ↓

Do you have a sedentary job and do you take little physical exercise on most days?

YES → Your body may not be sufficiently tired to allow you to sleep easily. Try taking some exercise in the fresh air before bedtime. See WHY EXERCISE IS GOOD FOR YOU, p.15.

NO ↓

If you are unable to make a diagnosis from this chart, and self-help suggestions do not work, consult your doctor.

Self-help

If you have difficulty in sleeping for any reason, try the following self-help measures:
☐ reduce your consumption of tea, coffee, and alcohol
☐ avoid large, late evening meals
☐ take a walk in the fresh air before bedtime
☐ have a hot, milky drink before going to bed.

For additional advice, see HOW TO GET A GOOD NIGHT'S SLEEP, p.20.

5

GENERAL
over 14 years

Fever

Temperature of about 38°C (100°F) or above.
For children see chart 90, **Fever in infants**, or chart 91, **Fever in children**.

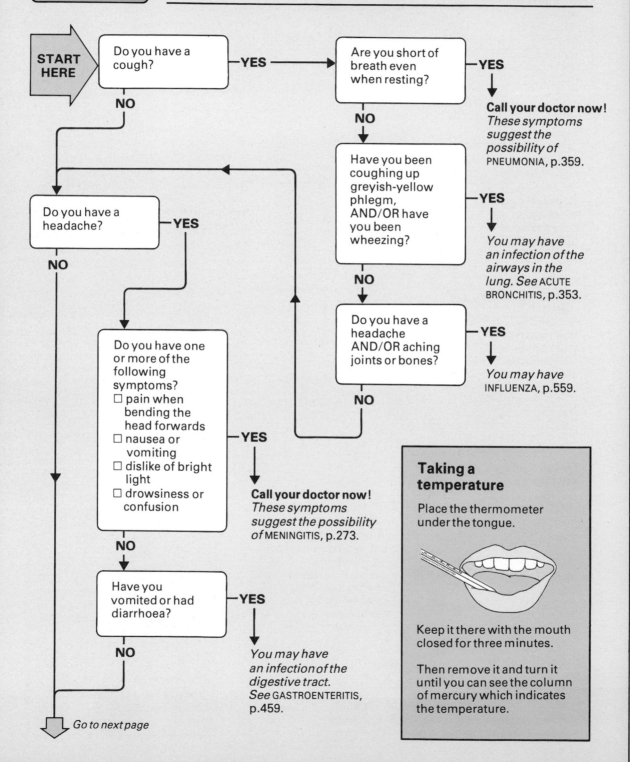

START HERE

Do you have a cough? — **YES** →

Are you short of breath even when resting? — **YES** →

Call your doctor now! *These symptoms suggest the possibility of* PNEUMONIA, p.359.

NO ↓ (cough)

NO ↓ (short of breath)

Have you been coughing up greyish-yellow phlegm, AND/OR have you been wheezing? — **YES** →

You may have an infection of the airways in the lung. See ACUTE BRONCHITIS, p.353.

NO ↓

Do you have a headache? — **YES** →

Do you have a headache AND/OR aching joints or bones? — **YES** →

You may have INFLUENZA, p.559.

NO ↓

Do you have one or more of the following symptoms?
☐ pain when bending the head forwards
☐ nausea or vomiting
☐ dislike of bright light
☐ drowsiness or confusion

— **YES** →

Call your doctor now! *These symptoms suggest the possibility of* MENINGITIS, p.273.

NO ↓

Have you vomited or had diarrhoea? — **YES** →

You may have an infection of the digestive tract. See GASTROENTERITIS, p.459.

NO ↓

⬇ *Go to next page*

Taking a temperature

Place the thermometer under the tongue.

Keep it there with the mouth closed for three minutes.

Then remove it and turn it until you can see the column of mercury which indicates the temperature.

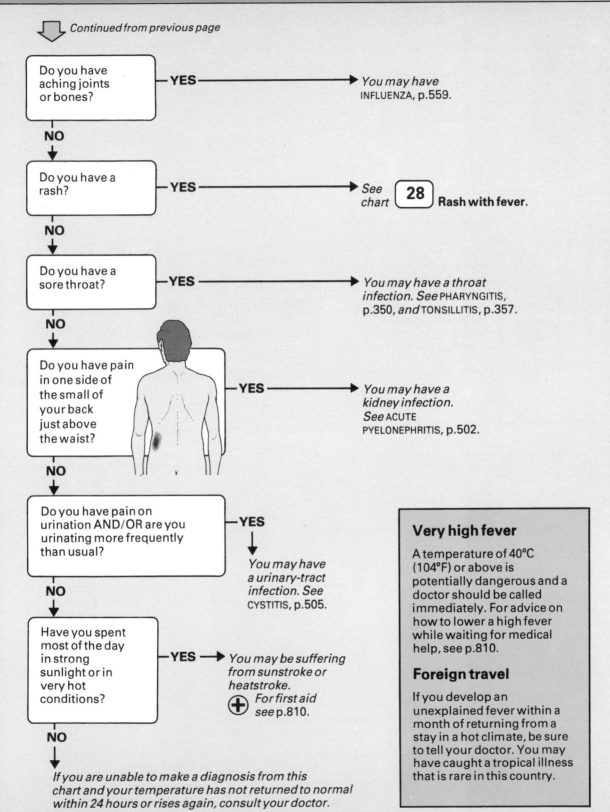

Continued from previous page

Do you have aching joints or bones? — **YES** → *You may have* INFLUENZA, p.559.

NO

Do you have a rash? — **YES** → *See* chart **28** **Rash with fever**.

NO

Do you have a sore throat? — **YES** → *You may have a throat infection. See* PHARYNGITIS, p.350, *and* TONSILLITIS, p.357.

NO

Do you have pain in one side of the small of your back just above the waist? — **YES** → *You may have a kidney infection. See* ACUTE PYELONEPHRITIS, p.502.

NO

Do you have pain on urination AND/OR are you urinating more frequently than usual? — **YES** → *You may have a urinary-tract infection. See* CYSTITIS, p.505.

NO

Have you spent most of the day in strong sunlight or in very hot conditions? — **YES** → *You may be suffering from sunstroke or heatstroke.* ✚ *For first aid see* p.810.

NO

If you are unable to make a diagnosis from this chart and your temperature has not returned to normal within 24 hours or rises again, consult your doctor.

Very high fever

A temperature of 40°C (104°F) or above is potentially dangerous and a doctor should be called immediately. For advice on how to lower a high fever while waiting for medical help, see p.810.

Foreign travel

If you develop an unexplained fever within a month of returning from a stay in a hot climate, be sure to tell your doctor. You may have caught a tropical illness that is rare in this country.

Excessive sweating

Sweating that occurs other than in hot conditions or during or just after exercise.

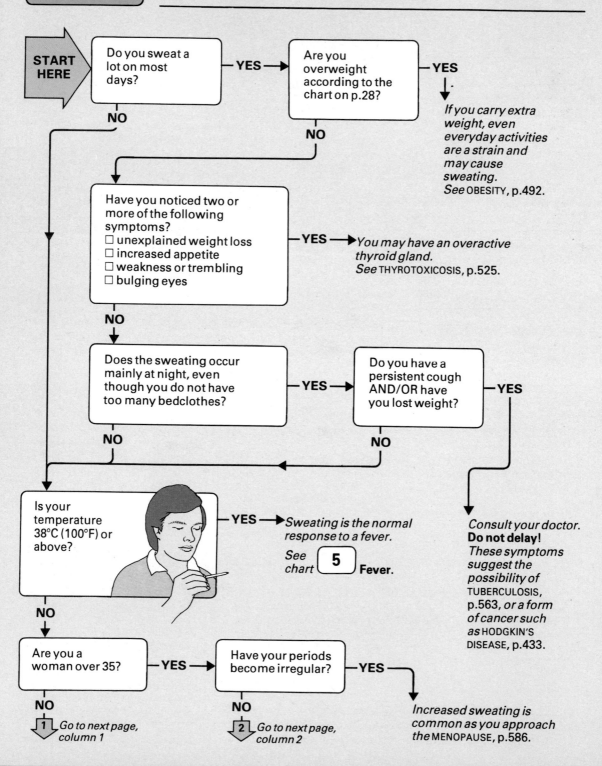

START HERE → Do you sweat a lot on most days?
- **YES** → Are you overweight according to the chart on p.28?
  - **YES** → *If you carry extra weight, even everyday activities are a strain and may cause sweating.* See OBESITY, p.492.
  - **NO** ↓

Have you noticed two or more of the following symptoms?
- ☐ unexplained weight loss
- ☐ increased appetite
- ☐ weakness or trembling
- ☐ bulging eyes
- **YES** → *You may have an overactive thyroid gland.* See THYROTOXICOSIS, p.525.
- **NO** ↓

Does the sweating occur mainly at night, even though you do not have too many bedclothes?
- **YES** → Do you have a persistent cough AND/OR have you lost weight?
  - **YES** → *Consult your doctor.* **Do not delay!** *These symptoms suggest the possibility of* TUBERCULOSIS, p.563, *or a form of cancer such as* HODGKIN'S DISEASE, p.433.
  - **NO** ↓
- **NO** ↓

Is your temperature 38°C (100°F) or above?
- **YES** → *Sweating is the normal response to a fever.* See chart **5** Fever.
- **NO** ↓

Are you a woman over 35?
- **YES** → Have your periods become irregular?
  - **YES** → *Increased sweating is common as you approach the* MENOPAUSE, p.586.
  - **NO** → **2** Go to next page, column 2
- **NO** → **1** Go to next page, column 1

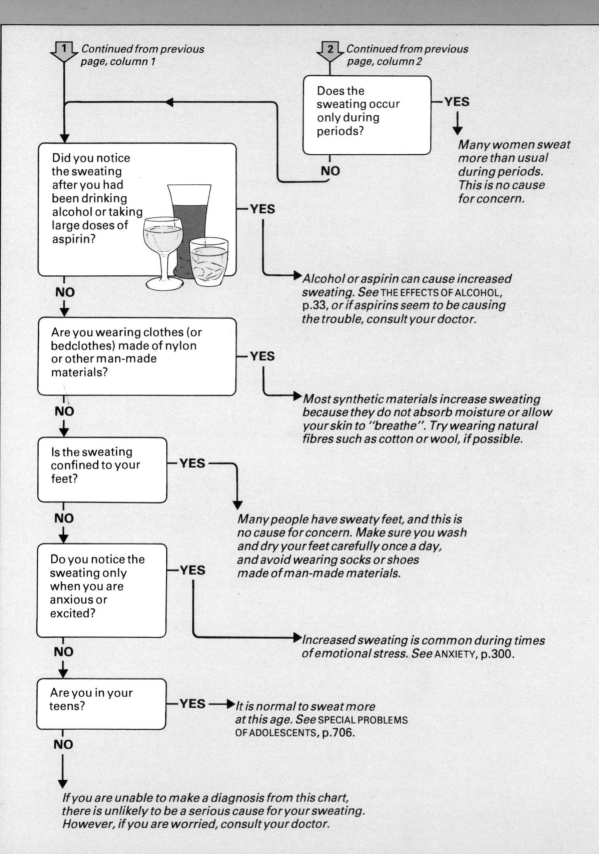

1 Continued from previous page, column 1

2 Continued from previous page, column 2

Does the sweating occur only during periods?

YES → Many women sweat more than usual during periods. This is no cause for concern.

NO

Did you notice the sweating after you had been drinking alcohol or taking large doses of aspirin?

YES → Alcohol or aspirin can cause increased sweating. See THE EFFECTS OF ALCOHOL, p.33, or if aspirins seem to be causing the trouble, consult your doctor.

NO

Are you wearing clothes (or bedclothes) made of nylon or other man-made materials?

YES → Most synthetic materials increase sweating because they do not absorb moisture or allow your skin to "breathe". Try wearing natural fibres such as cotton or wool, if possible.

NO

Is the sweating confined to your feet?

YES → Many people have sweaty feet, and this is no cause for concern. Make sure you wash and dry your feet carefully once a day, and avoid wearing socks or shoes made of man-made materials.

NO

Do you notice the sweating only when you are anxious or excited?

YES → Increased sweating is common during times of emotional stress. See ANXIETY, p.300.

NO

Are you in your teens?

YES → It is normal to sweat more at this age. See SPECIAL PROBLEMS OF ADOLESCENTS, p.706.

NO

If you are unable to make a diagnosis from this chart, there is unlikely to be a serious cause for your sweating. However, if you are worried, consult your doctor.

7

GENERAL
over 14 years

Swellings under the skin

Any new lump or swollen area that can be seen or felt under the skin.
For children see chart 96, **Swellings in children**.

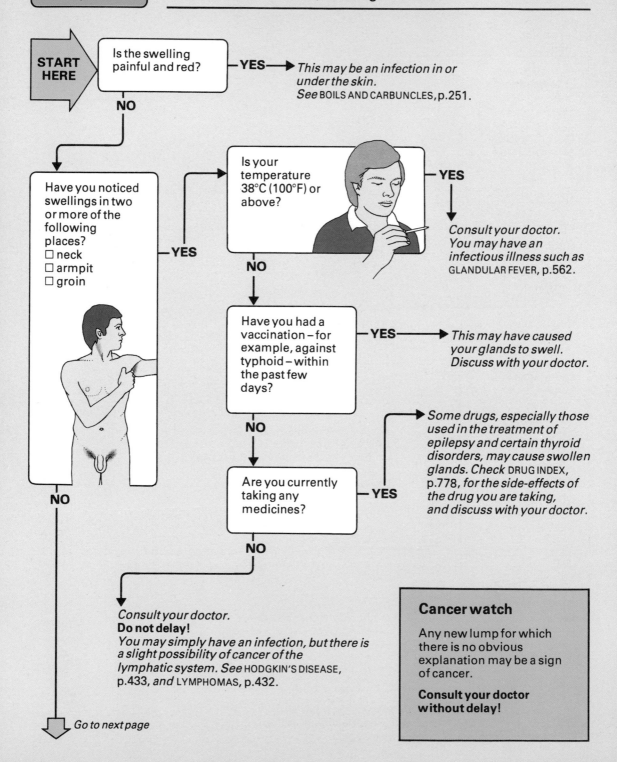

START HERE

Is the swelling painful and red? — **YES** → *This may be an infection in or under the skin.*
See BOILS AND CARBUNCLES, p.251.

NO

Have you noticed swellings in two or more of the following places?
☐ neck
☐ armpit
☐ groin

— **YES** →

Is your temperature 38°C (100°F) or above? — **YES** → *Consult your doctor. You may have an infectious illness such as* GLANDULAR FEVER, p.562.

NO

Have you had a vaccination – for example, against typhoid – within the past few days? — **YES** → *This may have caused your glands to swell. Discuss with your doctor.*

NO

Are you currently taking any medicines? — **YES** → *Some drugs, especially those used in the treatment of epilepsy and certain thyroid disorders, may cause swollen glands. Check* DRUG INDEX, *p.778, for the side-effects of the drug you are taking, and discuss with your doctor.*

NO

NO

Consult your doctor.
Do not delay!
You may simply have an infection, but there is a slight possibility of cancer of the lymphatic system. See HODGKIN'S DISEASE, p.433, *and* LYMPHOMAS, p.432.

Cancer watch

Any new lump for which there is no obvious explanation may be a sign of cancer.

Consult your doctor without delay!

Go to next page

Continued from previous page

Is the swelling on the face between the ear and the angle of the jaw?

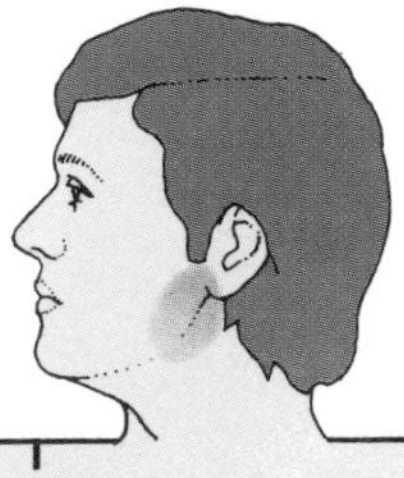

YES → **Is the swelling on both sides?**

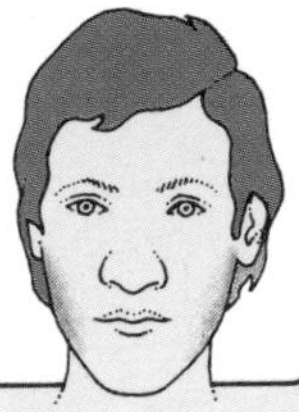

YES → *This may be* MUMPS, p.700.

NO (from "Is the swelling on both sides?")

Consult your doctor.
Do not delay!
One-sided swelling of the face is likely to be due to MUMPS, p.700, *a tooth abscess (see* ABSCESSES IN TEETH, p.439), *or a salivary gland problem such as a* SALIVARY DUCT STONE, p.453. *However, there is a slight chance of a* SALIVARY GLAND TUMOUR, p.454.

NO (from face between ear and jaw)

Is there a swelling on both sides of the back of the neck?

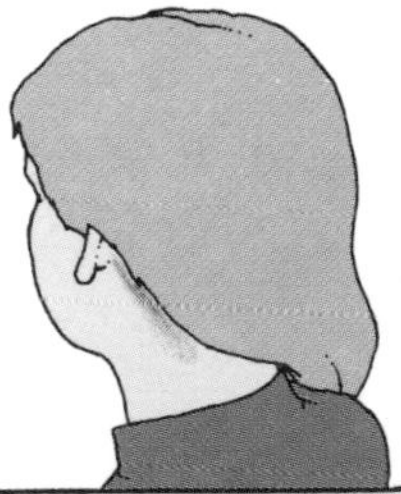

YES → **Do you have a pink rash AND/OR is your temperature 38°C (100°F) or above?**

YES → *You may have* GERMAN MEASLES, p.699.

NO (from pink rash)

NO (from back of neck swelling)

Are there swellings on both sides of the neck?

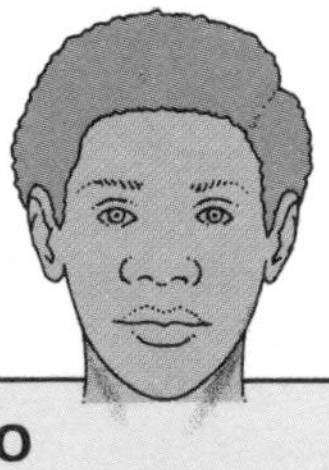

YES → **Is your throat sore?**

YES → *You may have a throat infection (see* PHARYNGITIS, p.350, *and* TONSILLITIS, p.351) *or* GLANDULAR FEVER, p.562.

NO (from throat sore)

Consult your doctor.
Do not delay!
You may simply have an infection, but there is a slight possibility of cancer of the lymphatic system.
See HODGKIN'S DISEASE, p.433, *and* LYMPHOMAS, p.432.

NO (from swellings on both sides of neck)

Go to next page

Swellings under the skin
continued from previous page

Is the swelling at the front of your neck AND does it move when you swallow?

YES → *This may be a* NON-TOXIC GOITRE, p.527, *which occurs as a result of iodine deficiency.*

NO

Is the swelling only in your armpit?

YES → *Consult your doctor. The glands in your armpit may have become swollen as a result of an infection in the arm, possibly from a cut or graze. However, such swelling is occasionally the first sign of* BREAST CANCER, p.589.

NO

Is the swelling in your groin?

YES → **Is it a soft lump that disappears when you press on it AND/OR does it enlarge when you cough?**

YES → *This may be a femoral or inguinal hernia. See* HERNIAS, p.537.

NO → *Consult your doctor. Your glands may have become swollen as a result of infection.*

NO

Do you have a lump in the breast?

YES → *Consult your doctor.* **Do not delay!** *The lump is probably a harmless cyst, (see* LUMPS IN THE BREAST, p.588), *but there is a slight possibility of* BREAST CANCER, p.589.

NO

If you are unable to make a diagnosis from this chart, consult your doctor.

8

GENERAL
over 14 years

Itching without a rash

Irritation of the skin without any change in the appearance of the skin. For children see chart 94, **Itching in children**.

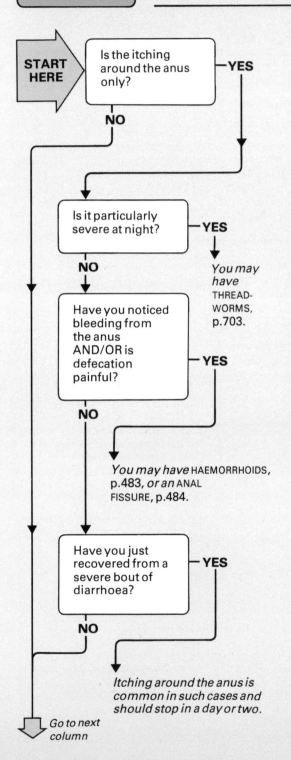

START HERE

Is the itching around the anus only? — **YES**

NO

Is it particularly severe at night? — **YES**

NO

You may have THREAD-WORMS, p.703.

Have you noticed bleeding from the anus AND/OR is defecation painful? — **YES**

NO

You may have HAEMORRHOIDS, p.483, *or an* ANAL FISSURE, p.484.

Have you just recovered from a severe bout of diarrhoea? — **YES**

NO

Itching around the anus is common in such cases and should stop in a day or two.

Go to next column

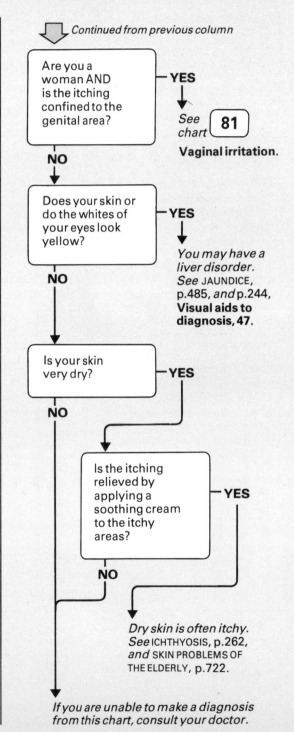

Continued from previous column

Are you a woman AND is the itching confined to the genital area? — **YES**

See chart **81**

Vaginal irritation.

NO

Does your skin or do the whites of your eyes look yellow? — **YES**

You may have a liver disorder. See JAUNDICE, p.485, *and* p.244, **Visual aids to diagnosis, 47**.

NO

Is your skin very dry? — **YES**

NO

Is the itching relieved by applying a soothing cream to the itchy areas? — **YES**

NO

Dry skin is often itchy. See ICHTHYOSIS, p.262, *and* SKIN PROBLEMS OF THE ELDERLY, p.722.

If you are unable to make a diagnosis from this chart, consult your doctor.

9

Feeling faint and fainting

A sudden feeling of weakness and unsteadiness, which may result in brief loss of consciousness.

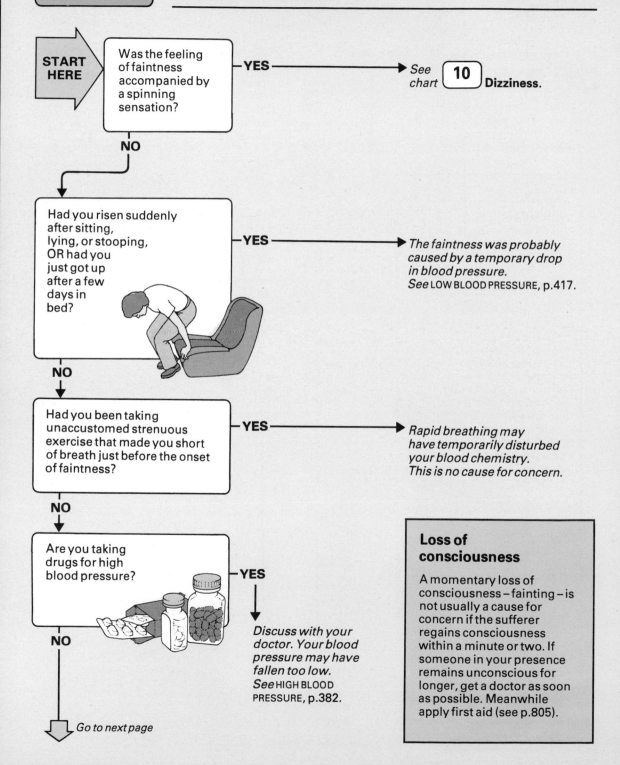

START HERE

Was the feeling of faintness accompanied by a spinning sensation?

— **YES** → *See chart* **10** **Dizziness**.

NO

Had you risen suddenly after sitting, lying, or stooping, OR had you just got up after a few days in bed?

— **YES** → *The faintness was probably caused by a temporary drop in blood pressure. See* LOW BLOOD PRESSURE, p.417.

NO

Had you been taking unaccustomed strenuous exercise that made you short of breath just before the onset of faintness?

— **YES** → *Rapid breathing may have temporarily disturbed your blood chemistry. This is no cause for concern.*

NO

Are you taking drugs for high blood pressure?

— **YES** ↓ *Discuss with your doctor. Your blood pressure may have fallen too low. See* HIGH BLOOD PRESSURE, p.382.

NO

↓ *Go to next page*

Loss of consciousness

A momentary loss of consciousness – fainting – is not usually a cause for concern if the sufferer regains consciousness within a minute or two. If someone in your presence remains unconscious for longer, get a doctor as soon as possible. Meanwhile apply first aid (see p.805).

Continued from previous page

Are you a diabetic OR is it an unusually long time since you last ate something?

YES → *Low blood sugar is probably causing the faintness. A sweet drink or something sugary or starchy to eat will make you feel better. If you are diabetic and have had several such attacks, consult your doctor. (See* HYPOGLYCAEMIA, p.522).

NO

Had you spent several hours in strong sunshine or in very hot or stuffy conditions before you felt faint?

YES → *You may be suffering from heat exhaustion.* For first aid *see* p.810.

NO

Have you noticed one or more of the following symptoms since the attack of faintness?
☐ numbness and/or tingling in any part of the body
☐ blurred vision
☐ confusion
☐ difficulty in speaking
☐ loss of movement in arms or legs

YES → *Consult your doctor.* **Do not delay!** *You may have had a* STROKE, p.268, *or a* TRANSIENT ISCHAEMIC ATTACK, p.270.

NO

Do you have any form of heart disease AND/OR did you notice your heartbeat speed up or slow down before the onset of faintness?

YES → Did you lose consciousness?

NO → *Discuss with your doctor. You may be suffering from a disorder of* HEART RATE OR RHYTHM, p.388.

YES → *Consult your doctor.* **Do not delay!** *You may have had a Stokes-Adams attack, which indicates a disorder of heart rhythm. See* HEART BLOCK, p.390.

NO

Go to next page

Dealing with faintness

If you feel faint lie down with your legs raised

or, if this is not possible, sit with your head between your knees until you feel better.

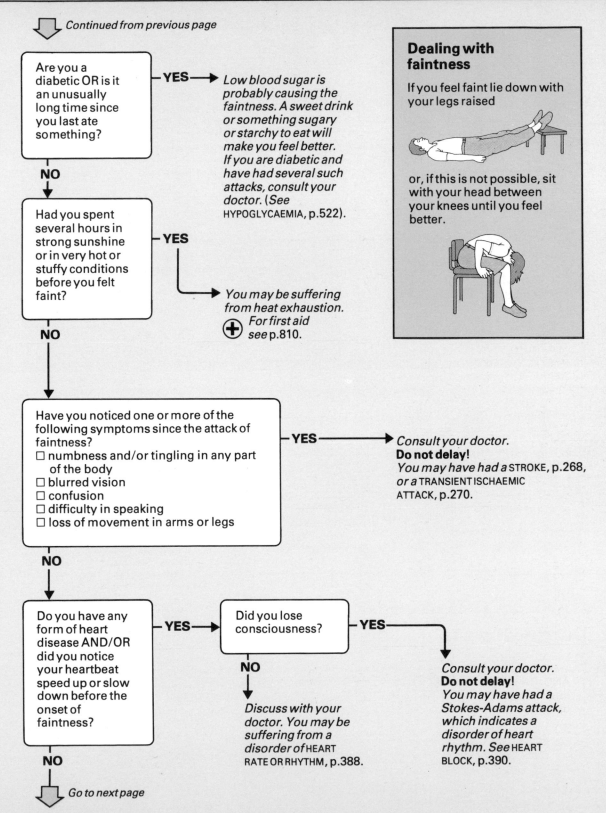

Feeling faint and fainting
Continued from previous page

Were you breathing very deeply or rapidly before you felt faint? — **YES** → *The faintness was probably caused by "overbreathing", possibly as a result of anxiety or stress. See* ANXIETY, *p.300.*

NO

Did you feel faint following an emotional shock? — **YES** → *Emotional upsets can easily affect the nerves that control blood pressure, and this may cause faintness.*

NO

Did you feel faint while you were doing any of the following?
☐ coughing
☐ urinating
☐ stretching
☐ holding your breath
— **YES** → *Any of these activities sometimes affects the supply of oxygen to the brain, causing faintness. This is usually no cause for concern. But if it happens more than once, consult your doctor.*

NO

Are you over 50? — **YES** → **Does turning your head slowly bring on a feeling of faintness?** — **YES** → *These symptoms suggest a disorder affecting the nerves and bones in the neck. See* CERVICAL SPONDYLOSIS, *p.280.*

NO (from Are you over 50?)

NO (from Does turning your head...)

Do you feel inexplicably tired AND/OR are you often short of breath? — **YES** → *You may be suffering from a form of* ANAEMIA, *p.419.*

NO

If you are unable to make a diagnosis from this chart, consult your doctor.

10

GENERAL
all ages

Dizziness

A sense of being dazed and unbalanced accompanied by a sensation of spinning.

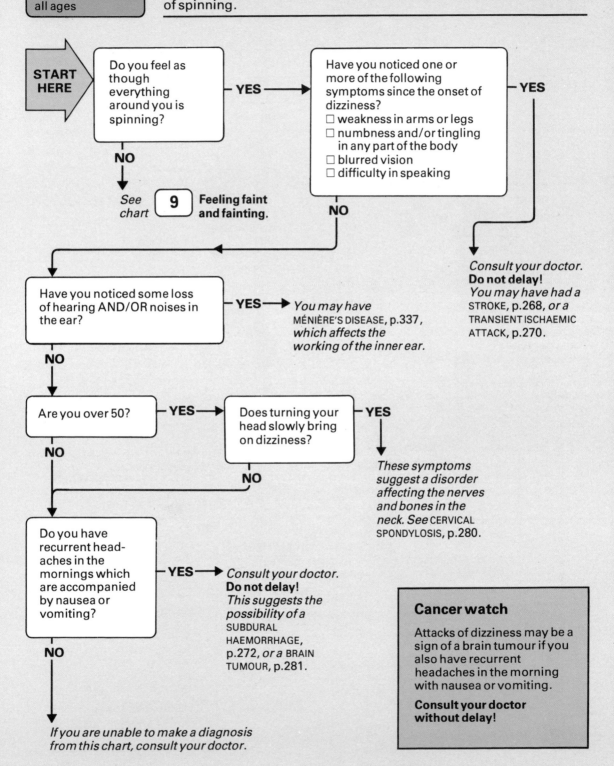

START HERE

Do you feel as though everything around you is spinning?

YES →

Have you noticed one or more of the following symptoms since the onset of dizziness?
☐ weakness in arms or legs
☐ numbness and/or tingling in any part of the body
☐ blurred vision
☐ difficulty in speaking

YES →

Consult your doctor. **Do not delay!** *You may have had a* STROKE, p.268, *or a* TRANSIENT ISCHAEMIC ATTACK, p.270.

NO ↓

See chart **9** **Feeling faint and fainting.**

NO ↓

Have you noticed some loss of hearing AND/OR noises in the ear?

YES → *You may have* MÉNIÈRE'S DISEASE, p.337, *which affects the working of the inner ear.*

NO ↓

Are you over 50?

YES →

Does turning your head slowly bring on dizziness?

YES ↓

These symptoms suggest a disorder affecting the nerves and bones in the neck. See CERVICAL SPONDYLOSIS, p.280.

NO ↓

NO →

Do you have recurrent head-aches in the mornings which are accompanied by nausea or vomiting?

YES → *Consult your doctor.* **Do not delay!** *This suggests the possibility of a* SUBDURAL HAEMORRHAGE, p.272, *or a* BRAIN TUMOUR, p.281.

NO ↓

If you are unable to make a diagnosis from this chart, consult your doctor.

Cancer watch

Attacks of dizziness may be a sign of a brain tumour if you also have recurrent headaches in the morning with nausea or vomiting.

Consult your doctor without delay!

11

GENERAL
all ages

Headache

Pain in the head or forehead may be anything from mild to severe and incapacitating.

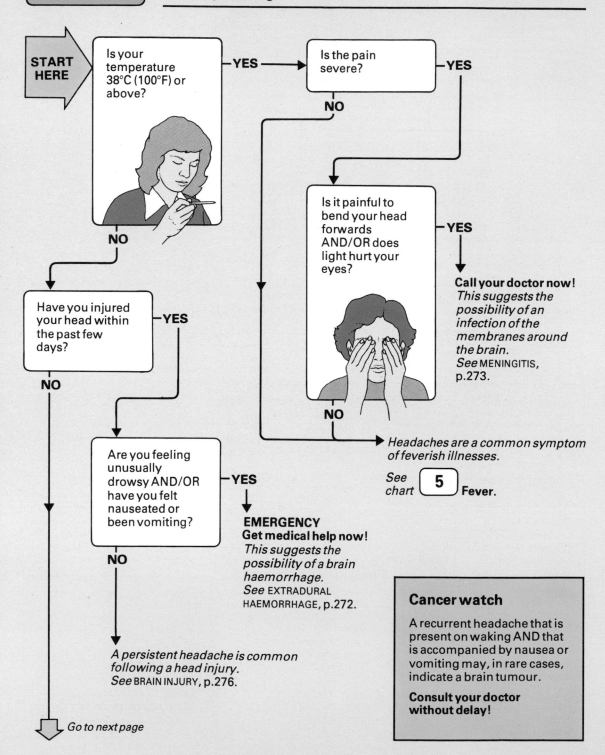

START HERE

Is your temperature 38°C (100°F) or above? — **YES** →

Is the pain severe? — **YES**

NO

NO

Have you injured your head within the past few days? — **YES**

NO

Is it painful to bend your head forwards AND/OR does light hurt your eyes? — **YES**

NO

Call your doctor now! *This suggests the possibility of an infection of the membranes around the brain. See* MENINGITIS, p.273.

Are you feeling unusually drowsy AND/OR have you felt nauseated or been vomiting? — **YES**

NO

EMERGENCY Get medical help now! *This suggests the possibility of a brain haemorrhage. See* EXTRADURAL HAEMORRHAGE, p.272.

Headaches are a common symptom of feverish illnesses.

See chart **5** *Fever.*

A persistent headache is common following a head injury. See BRAIN INJURY, p.276.

Cancer watch

A recurrent headache that is present on waking AND that is accompanied by nausea or vomiting may, in rare cases, indicate a brain tumour.

Consult your doctor without delay!

⇩ *Go to next page*

Continued from previous page

Have you felt nauseated or been vomiting?

— YES → **Do you have severe pain in and around one eye AND is your vision in that eye blurred?**

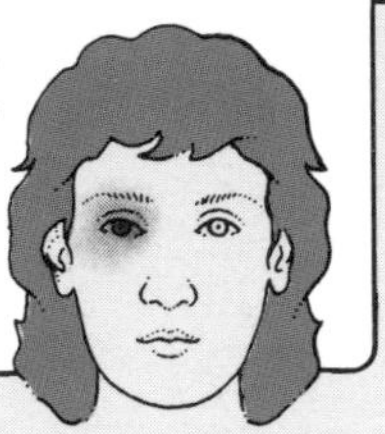

— YES →

Call your doctor now! *This suggests the possibility of raised pressure inside the eye.* See ACUTE GLAUCOMA, p.320.

NO (from nauseated box)

NO (from severe pain box)

Do you have one or more of the following symptoms?
☐ pain when you bend your head forwards
☐ dislike of bright light
☐ drowsiness or confusion

— YES →

EMERGENCY Get medical help now! *These symptoms suggest the possibility of a brain haemorrhage.* See SUBARACHNOID HAEMORRHAGE, p.271.

NO

Did your vision seem disturbed before the onset of pain?

— YES → *You may be suffering from* MIGRAINE, p.285.

NO

Have you had a similar headache on waking on several days over the past week or more?

— YES → **Did the headaches only occur on mornings following evenings during which you drank a lot of alcohol?**

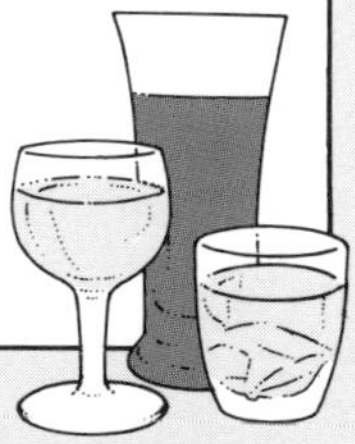

— YES → *You are probably suffering from "hangovers".* See HEADACHE, p.284.

NO (from similar headache box)

NO (from alcohol box)

Are you currently taking any medicines?

— YES → *Some drugs can cause headaches. Check* DRUG INDEX, p.778, *for the side-effects of the drug you are taking, and discuss with your doctor.*

Consult your doctor. **Do not delay!** *Such headaches may be a symptom of tension or* HIGH BLOOD PRESSURE, p.382, *but in very rare cases may indicate a* BRAIN TUMOUR, p.281.

NO

Go to next page

Headache
Continued from previous page

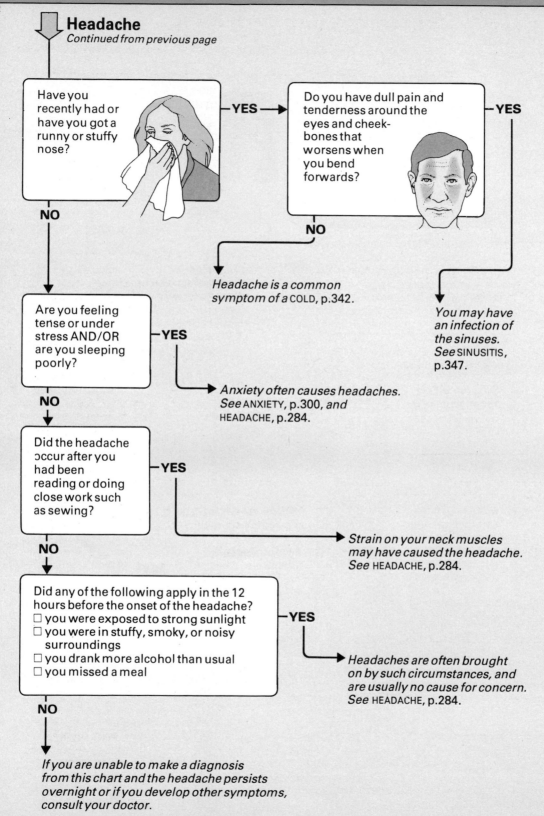

Have you recently had or have you got a runny or stuffy nose?

YES →

Do you have dull pain and tenderness around the eyes and cheek-bones that worsens when you bend forwards?

YES

NO ↓ (from first box)

NO ↓ (from second box)

Headache is a common symptom of a COLD, p.342.

You may have an infection of the sinuses. See SINUSITIS, p.347.

Are you feeling tense or under stress AND/OR are you sleeping poorly?

YES

Anxiety often causes headaches. See ANXIETY, p.300, *and* HEADACHE, p.284.

NO

Did the headache occur after you had been reading or doing close work such as sewing?

YES

Strain on your neck muscles may have caused the headache. See HEADACHE, p.284.

NO

Did any of the following apply in the 12 hours before the onset of the headache?
☐ you were exposed to strong sunlight
☐ you were in stuffy, smoky, or noisy surroundings
☐ you drank more alcohol than usual
☐ you missed a meal

YES

Headaches are often brought on by such circumstances, and are usually no cause for concern. See HEADACHE, p.284.

NO

If you are unable to make a diagnosis from this chart and the headache persists overnight or if you develop other symptoms, consult your doctor.

12
GENERAL
all ages

Numbness and/or tingling

Loss of feeling and/or a prickling sensation ("pins and needles") in any part of the body.

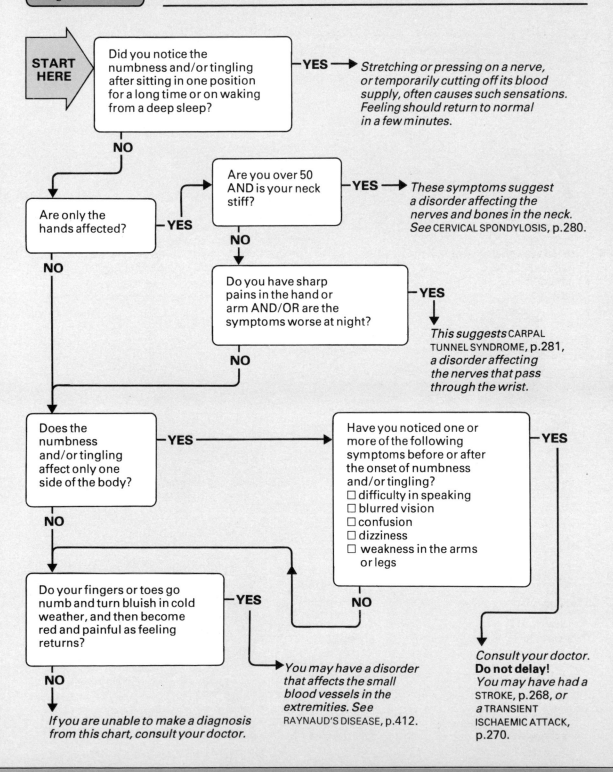

START HERE

Did you notice the numbness and/or tingling after sitting in one position for a long time or on waking from a deep sleep? — **YES** → *Stretching or pressing on a nerve, or temporarily cutting off its blood supply, often causes such sensations. Feeling should return to normal in a few minutes.*

NO

Are only the hands affected? — **YES**

Are you over 50 AND is your neck stiff? — **YES** → *These symptoms suggest a disorder affecting the nerves and bones in the neck. See* CERVICAL SPONDYLOSIS, p.280.

NO

Do you have sharp pains in the hand or arm AND/OR are the symptoms worse at night? — **YES**

This suggests CARPAL TUNNEL SYNDROME, p.281, *a disorder affecting the nerves that pass through the wrist.*

NO

NO

Does the numbness and/or tingling affect only one side of the body? — **YES** →

Have you noticed one or more of the following symptoms before or after the onset of numbness and/or tingling?
☐ difficulty in speaking
☐ blurred vision
☐ confusion
☐ dizziness
☐ weakness in the arms or legs
— **YES**

NO

NO

Do your fingers or toes go numb and turn bluish in cold weather, and then become red and painful as feeling returns? — **YES**

You may have a disorder that affects the small blood vessels in the extremities. See RAYNAUD'S DISEASE, p.412.

NO

If you are unable to make a diagnosis from this chart, consult your doctor.

Consult your doctor. **Do not delay!** *You may have had a* STROKE, p.268, *or a* TRANSIENT ISCHAEMIC ATTACK, p.270.

13
GENERAL
all ages

Twitching and trembling

Any involuntary movements during consciousness, including persistent trembling and shaking or sudden twitching.

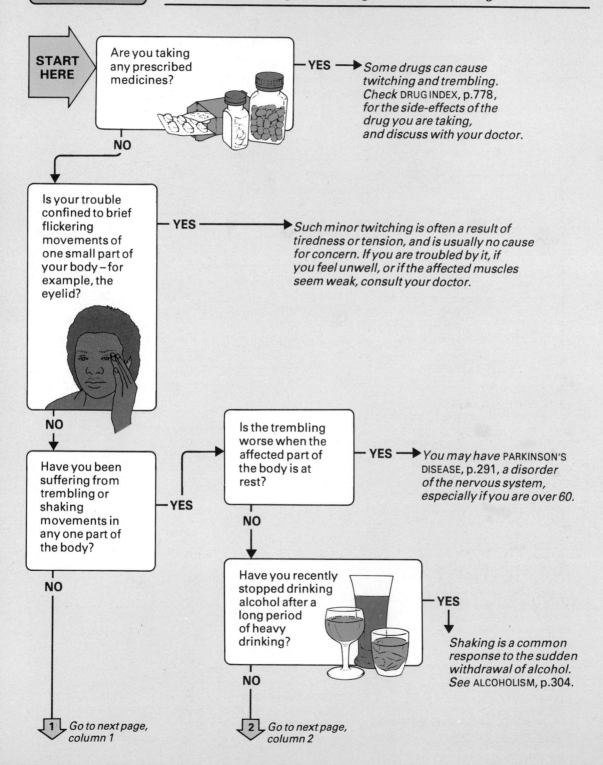

START HERE

Are you taking any prescribed medicines?

YES → *Some drugs can cause twitching and trembling. Check* DRUG INDEX, *p.778, for the side-effects of the drug you are taking, and discuss with your doctor.*

NO

Is your trouble confined to brief flickering movements of one small part of your body – for example, the eyelid?

YES → *Such minor twitching is often a result of tiredness or tension, and is usually no cause for concern. If you are troubled by it, if you feel unwell, or if the affected muscles seem weak, consult your doctor.*

NO

Have you been suffering from trembling or shaking movements in any one part of the body?

YES →

Is the trembling worse when the affected part of the body is at rest?

YES → *You may have* PARKINSON'S DISEASE, *p.291, a disorder of the nervous system, especially if you are over 60.*

NO

Have you recently stopped drinking alcohol after a long period of heavy drinking?

YES → *Shaking is a common response to the sudden withdrawal of alcohol. See* ALCOHOLISM, *p.304.*

NO

NO

1 *Go to next page, column 1*

2 *Go to next page, column 2*

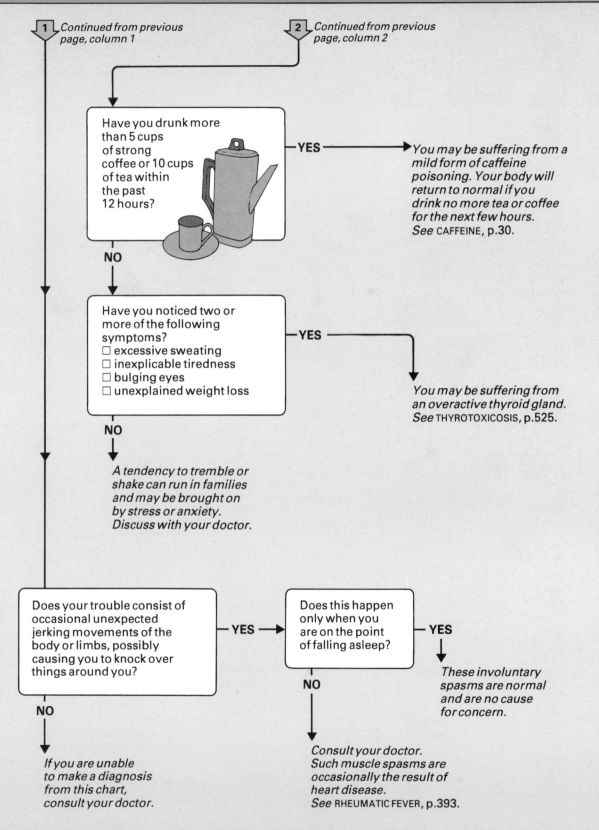

1 Continued from previous page, column 1

2 Continued from previous page, column 2

Have you drunk more than 5 cups of strong coffee or 10 cups of tea within the past 12 hours?

YES → You may be suffering from a mild form of caffeine poisoning. Your body will return to normal if you drink no more tea or coffee for the next few hours. *See* CAFFEINE, p.30.

NO

Have you noticed two or more of the following symptoms?
☐ excessive sweating
☐ inexplicable tiredness
☐ bulging eyes
☐ unexplained weight loss

YES → You may be suffering from an overactive thyroid gland. *See* THYROTOXICOSIS, p.525.

NO

A tendency to tremble or shake can run in families and may be brought on by stress or anxiety. Discuss with your doctor.

Does your trouble consist of occasional unexpected jerking movements of the body or limbs, possibly causing you to knock over things around you?

YES → Does this happen only when you are on the point of falling asleep?

YES → *These involuntary spasms are normal and are no cause for concern.*

NO

Consult your doctor. Such muscle spasms are occasionally the result of heart disease. See RHEUMATIC FEVER, p.393.

NO

If you are unable to make a diagnosis from this chart, consult your doctor.

14

GENERAL
all ages

Pain in the face

Pain in one or both sides of the face or forehead that may be dull and throbbing or intense and stabbing.

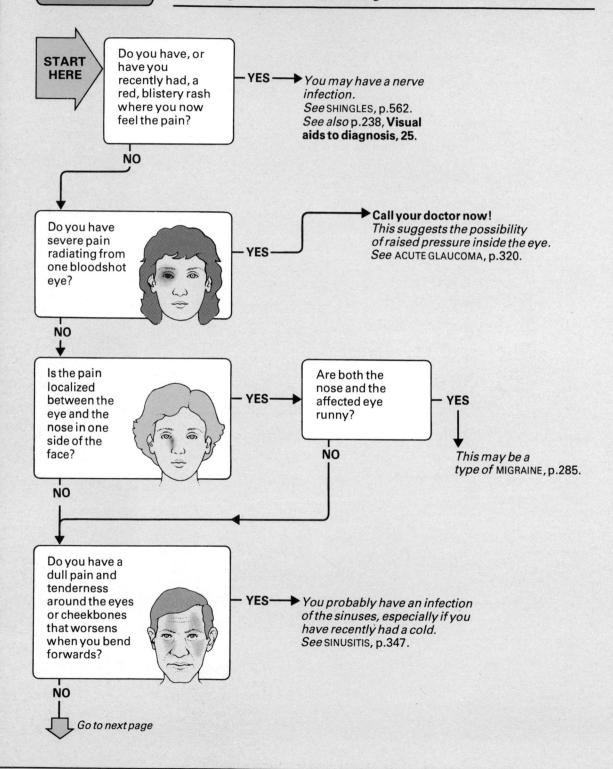

START HERE

Do you have, or have you recently had, a red, blistery rash where you now feel the pain?

YES → *You may have a nerve infection.*
See SHINGLES, p.562.
See also p.238, **Visual aids to diagnosis, 25.**

NO ↓

Do you have severe pain radiating from one bloodshot eye?

YES → **Call your doctor now!**
This suggests the possibility of raised pressure inside the eye.
See ACUTE GLAUCOMA, p.320.

NO ↓

Is the pain localized between the eye and the nose in one side of the face?

YES → **Are both the nose and the affected eye runny?**

YES ↓

This may be a type of MIGRAINE, p.285.

NO (from runny question)

NO ↓

Do you have a dull pain and tenderness around the eyes or cheekbones that worsens when you bend forwards?

YES → *You probably have an infection of the sinuses, especially if you have recently had a cold.*
See SINUSITIS, p.347.

NO ↓

Go to next page

Continued from previous page

Do you have a continuous, throbbing pain on one side of the face?

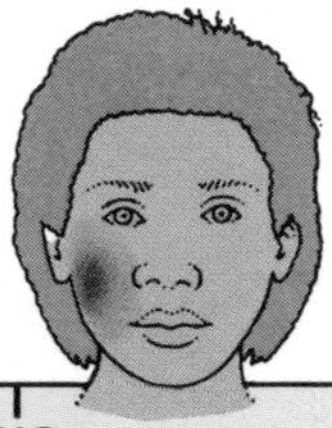

YES → Is the pain worse at night, when you eat, or when you touch a particular tooth?

YES ↓

Consult your doctor or dentist.
Do not delay!
You may have a tooth abscess.
See ABSCESSES IN TEETH, p.439.

NO (from second box)

NO (from first box)

Have you suddenly begun to have a severe throbbing pain in one or both temples?

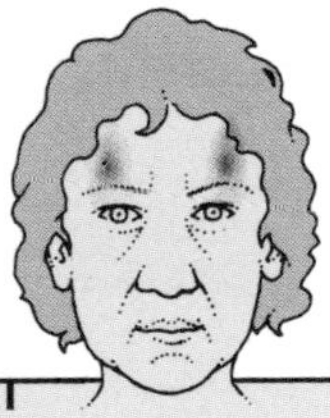

YES → Have you been feeling generally unwell AND/OR is your scalp sensitive to touch?

YES ↓

Consult your doctor.
Do not delay!
You may have inflammation of the arteries in your head.
See TEMPORAL ARTERITIS, p.414.

NO (from second box)

NO (from first box)

Do you have a severe, stabbing pain in one side of the face, brought on by touching the face or by chewing?

YES → *The pain is probably caused by a damaged nerve.*
See TRIGEMINAL NEURALGIA, p.722.

NO ↓

If you are unable to make a diagnosis from this chart, consult your doctor.

15 Confusion

GENERAL
all ages

Confusion may vary from a muddling of times, places, and events, to an alarming loss of contact with reality, known as delirium.

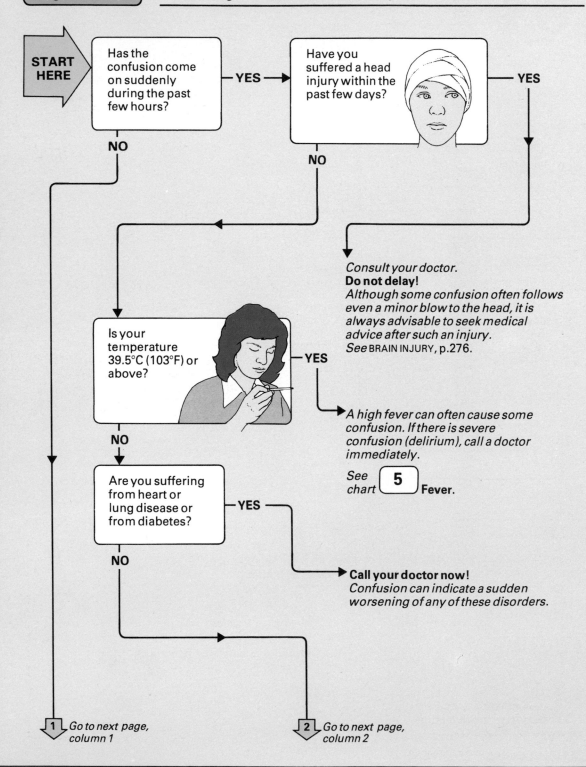

START HERE

Has the confusion come on suddenly during the past few hours? — **YES** → Have you suffered a head injury within the past few days? — **YES** →

NO ↓ (from head injury) **NO** ↓

Consult your doctor.
Do not delay!
Although some confusion often follows even a minor blow to the head, it is always advisable to seek medical advice after such an injury.
See BRAIN INJURY, p.276.

Is your temperature 39.5°C (103°F) or above? — **YES** →

A high fever can often cause some confusion. If there is severe confusion (delirium), call a doctor immediately.

See chart **5** **Fever.**

NO ↓

Are you suffering from heart or lung disease or from diabetes? — **YES** →

Call your doctor now!
Confusion can indicate a sudden worsening of any of these disorders.

NO ↓

1 *Go to next page, column 1*

2 *Go to next page, column 2*

1 Continued from previous page, column 1

2 Continued from previous page, column 2

Have you noticed any of the following symptoms since the onset of confusion?
☐ dizziness
☐ weakness in arms or legs
☐ numbness and/or tingling in any part of the body
☐ blurred vision
☐ difficulty in speaking

YES ⟶ *Consult your doctor.* **Do not delay!** *You may have had a* STROKE, p.268, *or a* TRANSIENT ISCHAEMIC ATTACK, p.270.

NO

Were you drinking alcohol or taking any medicines or drugs before becoming confused?

YES ⟶ *Alcohol and many drugs may cause muddled behaviour. If you think a medicine is causing the problem, discuss with your doctor. See also* THE EFFECTS OF ALCOHOL, p.33, ALCOHOLISM, p.304, *and* DRUG ADDICTION, p.305.

NO

Are you over 65? **YES** ⟶ *See chart* **99** **Confusion in the elderly.**

NO

If you are unable to make a diagnosis from this chart, consult your doctor.

Delirium

If confusion is so marked that the sufferer is unaware of other people, behaving in an over-agitated and disoriented way, or is having hallucinations, he or she is delirious and needs medical attention urgently.

Get a doctor immediately!

16
GENERAL
all ages

Impaired memory

Difficulty in remembering individual events and facts (often called absent-mindedness), or whole periods of time (amnesia).

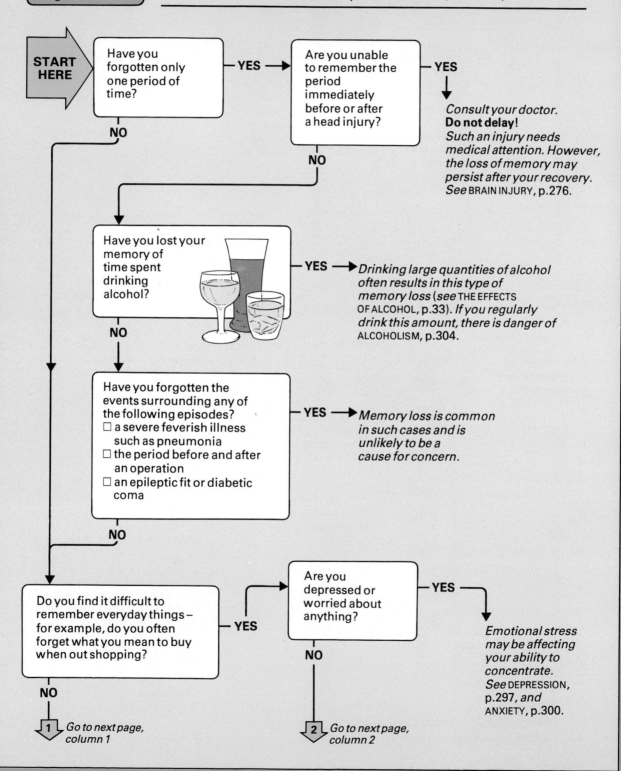

START HERE →

Have you forgotten only one period of time?

— YES → **Are you unable to remember the period immediately before or after a head injury?**

— YES →

Consult your doctor.
Do not delay!
Such an injury needs medical attention. However, the loss of memory may persist after your recovery.
See BRAIN INJURY, p.276.

NO (from head injury box)

NO (from first box)

Have you lost your memory of time spent drinking alcohol?

— YES → *Drinking large quantities of alcohol often results in this type of memory loss (see* THE EFFECTS OF ALCOHOL, p.33). *If you regularly drink this amount, there is danger of* ALCOHOLISM, p.304.

NO

Have you forgotten the events surrounding any of the following episodes?
☐ a severe feverish illness such as pneumonia
☐ the period before and after an operation
☐ an epileptic fit or diabetic coma

— YES → *Memory loss is common in such cases and is unlikely to be a cause for concern.*

NO

Do you find it difficult to remember everyday things – for example, do you often forget what you mean to buy when out shopping?

— YES → **Are you depressed or worried about anything?**

— YES →

Emotional stress may be affecting your ability to concentrate.
See DEPRESSION, p.297, *and* ANXIETY, p.300.

NO

1 *Go to next page, column 1*

NO (under depressed box)

2 *Go to next page, column 2*

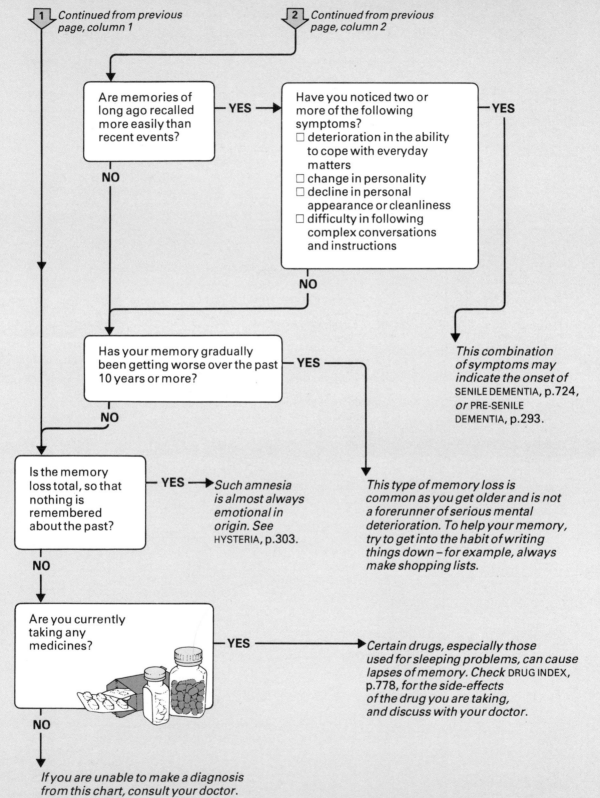

1 *Continued from previous page, column 1*

2 *Continued from previous page, column 2*

Are memories of long ago recalled more easily than recent events?

— **YES** →

Have you noticed two or more of the following symptoms?
- ☐ deterioration in the ability to cope with everyday matters
- ☐ change in personality
- ☐ decline in personal appearance or cleanliness
- ☐ difficulty in following complex conversations and instructions

— **YES**

NO ↓

NO ↓

This combination of symptoms may indicate the onset of SENILE DEMENTIA, p.724, *or* PRE-SENILE DEMENTIA, p.293.

Has your memory gradually been getting worse over the past 10 years or more?

— **YES** —

NO ↓

Is the memory loss total, so that nothing is remembered about the past?

— **YES** →

Such amnesia is almost always emotional in origin. See HYSTERIA, p.303.

This type of memory loss is common as you get older and is not a forerunner of serious mental deterioration. To help your memory, try to get into the habit of writing things down – for example, always make shopping lists.

NO ↓

Are you currently taking any medicines?

— **YES** →

Certain drugs, especially those used for sleeping problems, can cause lapses of memory. Check DRUG INDEX, p.778, *for the side-effects of the drug you are taking, and discuss with your doctor.*

NO ↓

If you are unable to make a diagnosis from this chart, consult your doctor.

17
GENERAL
all ages

Difficulty in speaking
A deterioration in the ability to find, use, or pronounce words.

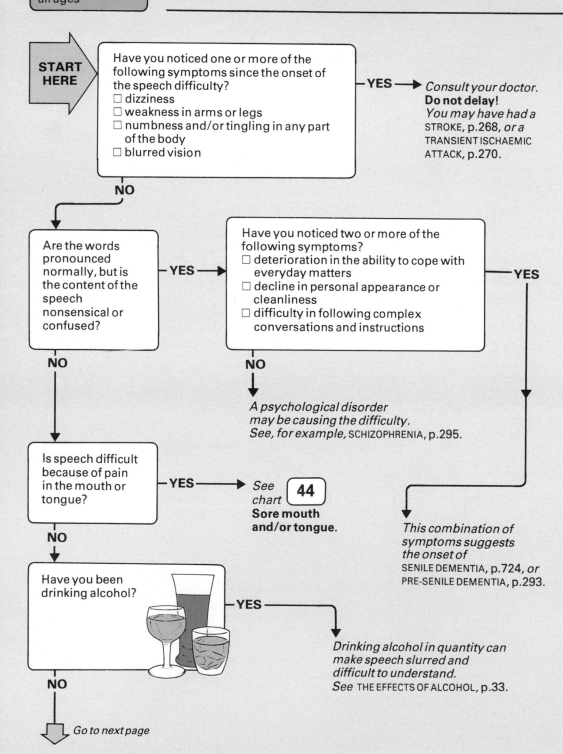

START HERE → Have you noticed one or more of the following symptoms since the onset of the speech difficulty?
☐ dizziness
☐ weakness in arms or legs
☐ numbness and/or tingling in any part of the body
☐ blurred vision

YES → *Consult your doctor.* **Do not delay!** *You may have had a* STROKE, p.268, *or a* TRANSIENT ISCHAEMIC ATTACK, p.270.

NO ↓

Are the words pronounced normally, but is the content of the speech nonsensical or confused?

YES → Have you noticed two or more of the following symptoms?
☐ deterioration in the ability to cope with everyday matters
☐ decline in personal appearance or cleanliness
☐ difficulty in following complex conversations and instructions

YES →

NO ↓

A psychological disorder may be causing the difficulty. See, for example, SCHIZOPHRENIA, p.295.

NO ↓

Is speech difficult because of pain in the mouth or tongue?

YES → *See chart* **44** **Sore mouth and/or tongue.**

This combination of symptoms suggests the onset of SENILE DEMENTIA, p.724, *or* PRE-SENILE DEMENTIA, p.293.

NO ↓

Have you been drinking alcohol?

YES → *Drinking alcohol in quantity can make speech slurred and difficult to understand. See* THE EFFECTS OF ALCOHOL, p.33.

NO ↓

Go to next page

Continued from previous page

Are you currently taking any medicines?

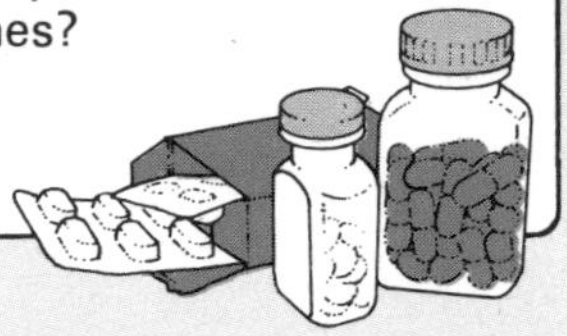

YES → *Some drugs can affect speech. Check* DRUG INDEX, p. 778, *for the side-effects of the drug you are taking, and discuss with your doctor.*

NO

Is speech difficult because you are unable to move the muscles on one side of your face?

YES → *You may have* BELL'S PALSY, p.279, *a disorder of the facial nerves.*

NO

Does your speech lack normal intonation and pauses, so that it sounds expressionless?

YES → **Do your hands tremble?**

YES → *These symptoms suggest* PARKINSON'S DISEASE, p.291, *a degenerative disorder of the nervous system.*

NO

NO

Are you sometimes unable to speak even though you know what you want to say, AND/OR do you sometimes get stuck at the beginning of a word and find yourself repeating the first consonant for several seconds before you can get the whole word out?

YES → *Discuss with your doctor. This stammering or stuttering often develops in early childhood and may recur in an adult under stress.*

NO

If you are unable to make a diagnosis from this chart, consult your doctor.

18

GENERAL
all ages

Disturbing thoughts and feelings

Any thoughts or feelings that may seem (whether to other people or to yourself) to be abnormal or unhealthy.

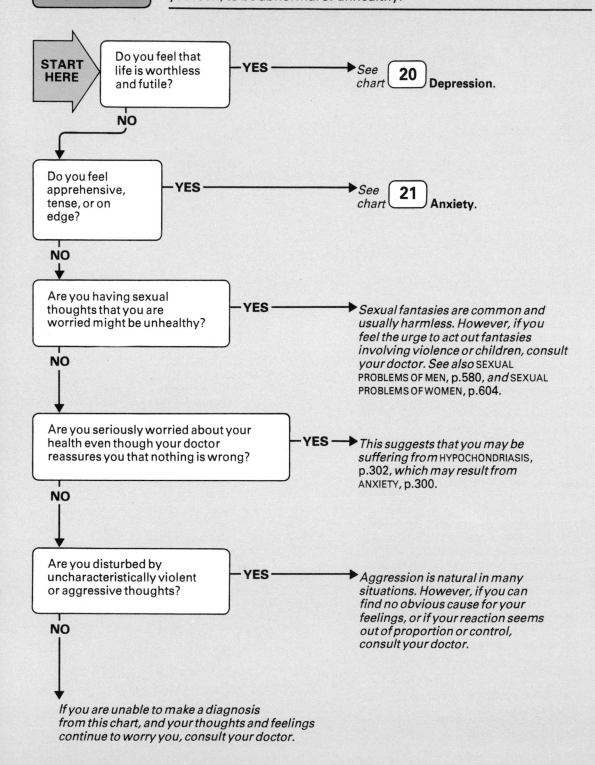

START HERE

Do you feel that life is worthless and futile? — **YES** → *See chart* **20** **Depression**.

NO

Do you feel apprehensive, tense, or on edge? — **YES** → *See chart* **21** **Anxiety**.

NO

Are you having sexual thoughts that you are worried might be unhealthy? — **YES** → *Sexual fantasies are common and usually harmless. However, if you feel the urge to act out fantasies involving violence or children, consult your doctor. See also* SEXUAL PROBLEMS OF MEN, p.580, *and* SEXUAL PROBLEMS OF WOMEN, p.604.

NO

Are you seriously worried about your health even though your doctor reassures you that nothing is wrong? — **YES** → *This suggests that you may be suffering from* HYPOCHONDRIASIS, p.302, *which may result from* ANXIETY, p.300.

NO

Are you disturbed by uncharacteristically violent or aggressive thoughts? — **YES** → *Aggression is natural in many situations. However, if you can find no obvious cause for your feelings, or if your reaction seems out of proportion or control, consult your doctor.*

NO

If you are unable to make a diagnosis from this chart, and your thoughts and feelings continue to worry you, consult your doctor.

19
GENERAL
all ages

Strange behaviour

Any behaviour, whether developing suddenly or gradually, that seems out of keeping with previous behaviour patterns.

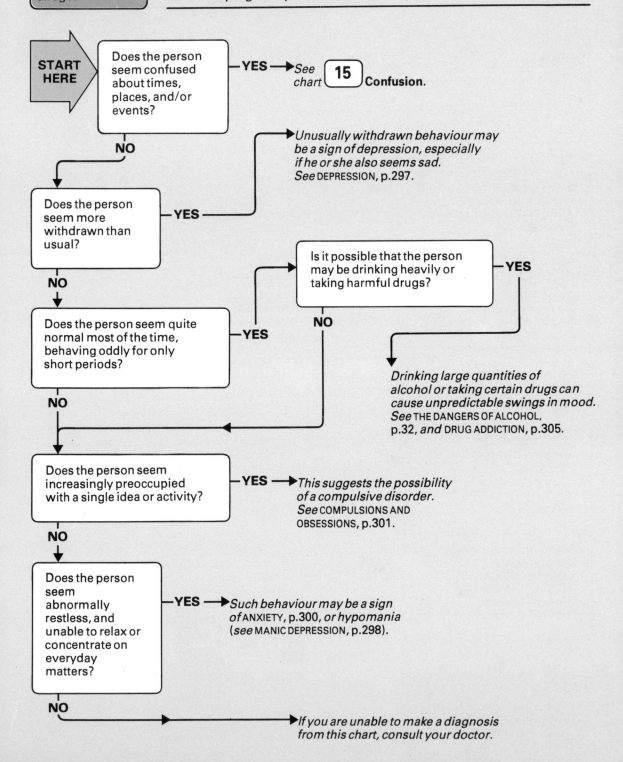

START HERE → Does the person seem confused about times, places, and/or events? — **YES** → *See* chart **15** **Confusion**.

NO ↓

Does the person seem more withdrawn than usual? — **YES** → *Unusually withdrawn behaviour may be a sign of depression, especially if he or she also seems sad. See* DEPRESSION, p.297.

NO ↓

Does the person seem quite normal most of the time, behaving oddly for only short periods? — **YES** → Is it possible that the person may be drinking heavily or taking harmful drugs? — **YES** → *Drinking large quantities of alcohol or taking certain drugs can cause unpredictable swings in mood. See* THE DANGERS OF ALCOHOL, p.32, *and* DRUG ADDICTION, p.305.

NO (from drugs question) ↓

NO ↓

Does the person seem increasingly preoccupied with a single idea or activity? — **YES** → *This suggests the possibility of a compulsive disorder. See* COMPULSIONS AND OBSESSIONS, p.301.

NO ↓

Does the person seem abnormally restless, and unable to relax or concentrate on everyday matters? — **YES** → *Such behaviour may be a sign of* ANXIETY, p.300, *or hypomania (see* MANIC DEPRESSION, p.298).

NO ↓

If you are unable to make a diagnosis from this chart, consult your doctor.

20

GENERAL
all ages

Depression

A feeling of sadness, futility, unworthiness, and/or despair that may make you feel unable to cope with normal life.

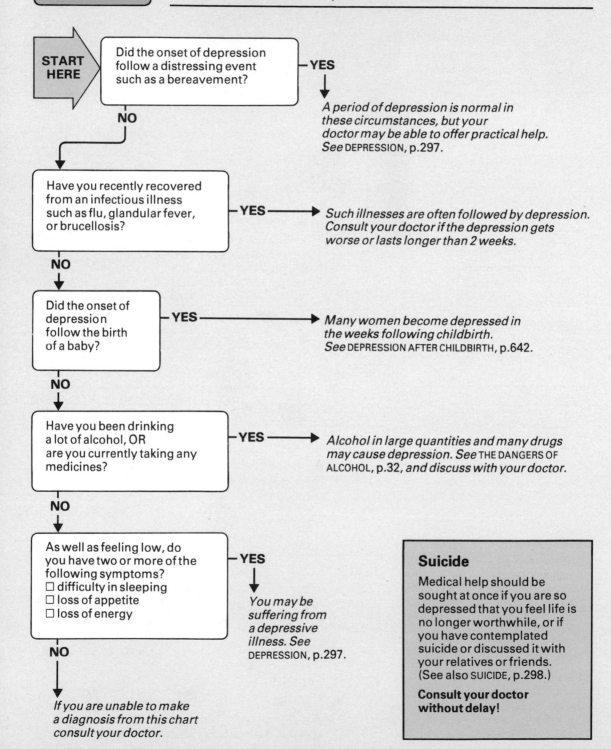

START HERE

Did the onset of depression follow a distressing event such as a bereavement? — **YES**

A period of depression is normal in these circumstances, but your doctor may be able to offer practical help. See DEPRESSION, *p.297.*

NO

Have you recently recovered from an infectious illness such as flu, glandular fever, or brucellosis? — **YES**

Such illnesses are often followed by depression. Consult your doctor if the depression gets worse or lasts longer than 2 weeks.

NO

Did the onset of depression follow the birth of a baby? — **YES**

Many women become depressed in the weeks following childbirth. See DEPRESSION AFTER CHILDBIRTH, *p.642.*

NO

Have you been drinking a lot of alcohol, OR are you currently taking any medicines? — **YES**

Alcohol in large quantities and many drugs may cause depression. See THE DANGERS OF ALCOHOL, *p.32, and discuss with your doctor.*

NO

As well as feeling low, do you have two or more of the following symptoms?
☐ difficulty in sleeping
☐ loss of appetite
☐ loss of energy
— **YES**

You may be suffering from a depressive illness. See DEPRESSION, *p.297.*

NO

If you are unable to make a diagnosis from this chart consult your doctor.

Suicide

Medical help should be sought at once if you are so depressed that you feel life is no longer worthwhile, or if you have contemplated suicide or discussed it with your relatives or friends. (See also SUICIDE, p.298.)

Consult your doctor without delay!

21

GENERAL
all ages

Anxiety

A feeling of tension, apprehension, or edginess, which may be accompanied by physical symptoms such as palpitations or diarrhoea.

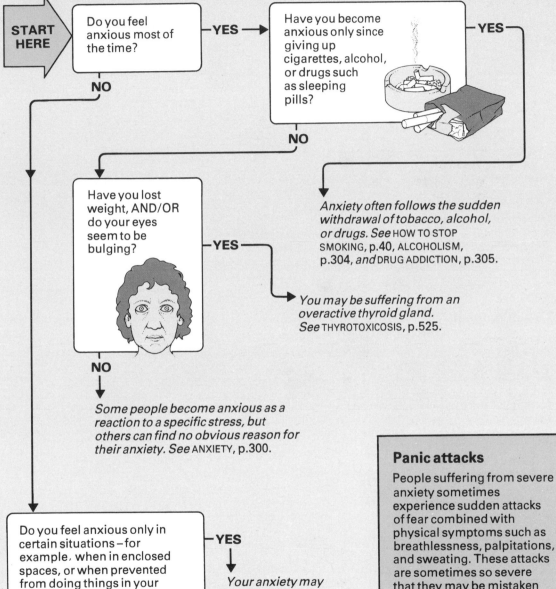

START HERE

Do you feel anxious most of the time?

YES →

Have you become anxious only since giving up cigarettes, alcohol, or drugs such as sleeping pills?

YES

NO

NO

Anxiety often follows the sudden withdrawal of tobacco, alcohol, or drugs. See HOW TO STOP SMOKING, p.40, ALCOHOLISM, p.304, *and* DRUG ADDICTION, p.305.

Have you lost weight, AND/OR do your eyes seem to be bulging?

YES

You may be suffering from an overactive thyroid gland. See THYROTOXICOSIS, p.525.

NO

Some people become anxious as a reaction to a specific stress, but others can find no obvious reason for their anxiety. See ANXIETY, p.300.

Do you feel anxious only in certain situations – for example, when in enclosed spaces, or when prevented from doing things in your usual way?

YES

Your anxiety may be due to a PHOBIA, p.300, *or the result of compulsive behaviour* (*see* COMPULSIONS AND OBSESSIONS, p.301).

NO

If you are unable to make a diagnosis from this chart, consult your doctor.

Panic attacks

People suffering from severe anxiety sometimes experience sudden attacks of fear combined with physical symptoms such as breathlessness, palpitations, and sweating. These attacks are sometimes so severe that they may be mistaken for a heart attack.

If you are in any doubt about the cause of such symptoms, treat the condition as an emergency and follow the first aid measures on p.802.

22

Hallucinations

Mistakenly and repeatedly hearing, feeling, or seeing things that are not heard, felt, or seen by other people.

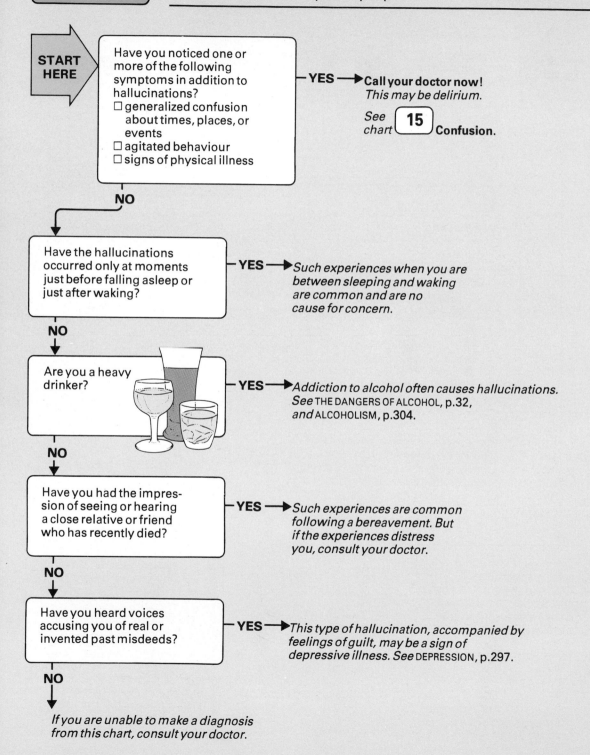

START HERE → Have you noticed one or more of the following symptoms in addition to hallucinations?
- ☐ generalized confusion about times, places, or events
- ☐ agitated behaviour
- ☐ signs of physical illness

YES → **Call your doctor now!** *This may be delirium.*

See chart **15** *Confusion.*

NO

Have the hallucinations occurred only at moments just before falling asleep or just after waking?

YES → *Such experiences when you are between sleeping and waking are common and are no cause for concern.*

NO

Are you a heavy drinker?

YES → *Addiction to alcohol often causes hallucinations. See* THE DANGERS OF ALCOHOL, p.32, *and* ALCOHOLISM, p.304.

NO

Have you had the impression of seeing or hearing a close relative or friend who has recently died?

YES → *Such experiences are common following a bereavement. But if the experiences distress you, consult your doctor.*

NO

Have you heard voices accusing you of real or invented past misdeeds?

YES → *This type of hallucination, accompanied by feelings of guilt, may be a sign of depressive illness. See* DEPRESSION, p.297.

NO

If you are unable to make a diagnosis from this chart, consult your doctor.

23

GENERAL
all ages

Nightmares

Frightening dreams that may be disturbing enough to wake you up.

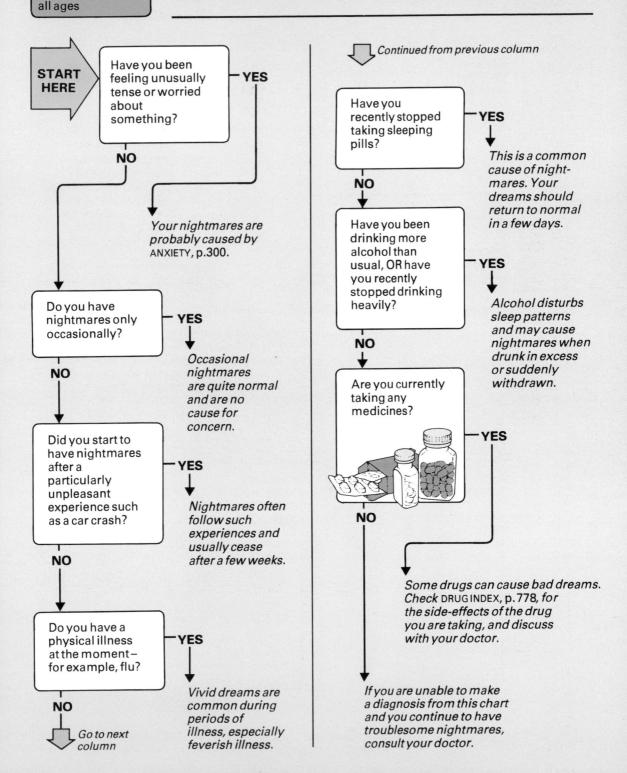

START HERE

Have you been feeling unusually tense or worried about something? — **YES**

NO

Your nightmares are probably caused by ANXIETY, *p.300.*

Do you have nightmares only occasionally? — **YES**

NO

Occasional nightmares are quite normal and are no cause for concern.

Did you start to have nightmares after a particularly unpleasant experience such as a car crash? — **YES**

NO

Nightmares often follow such experiences and usually cease after a few weeks.

Do you have a physical illness at the moment — for example, flu? — **YES**

NO

Go to next column

Vivid dreams are common during periods of illness, especially feverish illness.

Continued from previous column

Have you recently stopped taking sleeping pills? — **YES**

NO

This is a common cause of nightmares. Your dreams should return to normal in a few days.

Have you been drinking more alcohol than usual, OR have you recently stopped drinking heavily? — **YES**

NO

Alcohol disturbs sleep patterns and may cause nightmares when drunk in excess or suddenly withdrawn.

Are you currently taking any medicines? — **YES**

NO

Some drugs can cause bad dreams. Check DRUG INDEX, *p.778, for the side-effects of the drug you are taking, and discuss with your doctor.*

If you are unable to make a diagnosis from this chart and you continue to have troublesome nightmares, consult your doctor.

24

Hair loss

Thinning or loss of hair on all or part of the head.

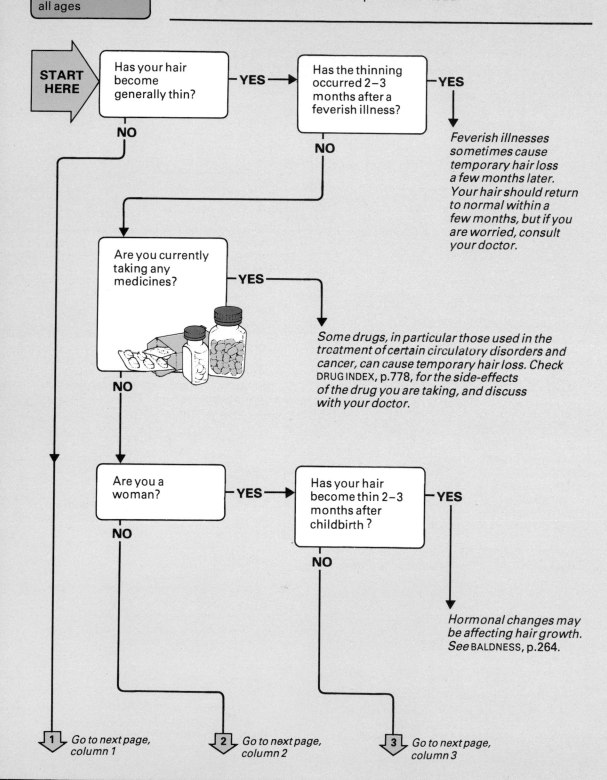

START HERE

Has your hair become generally thin? — **YES** → **Has the thinning occurred 2–3 months after a feverish illness?** — **YES** ↓

Feverish illnesses sometimes cause temporary hair loss a few months later. Your hair should return to normal within a few months, but if you are worried, consult your doctor.

NO (from first box)

NO (from second box)

Are you currently taking any medicines? — **YES** →

Some drugs, in particular those used in the treatment of certain circulatory disorders and cancer, can cause temporary hair loss. Check DRUG INDEX, p.778, for the side-effects of the drug you are taking, and discuss with your doctor.

NO

Are you a woman? — **YES** → **Has your hair become thin 2–3 months after childbirth?** — **YES** ↓

Hormonal changes may be affecting hair growth. See BALDNESS, p.264.

NO (Are you a woman?)

NO (childbirth box)

1 *Go to next page, column 1*

2 *Go to next page, column 2*

3 *Go to next page, column 3*

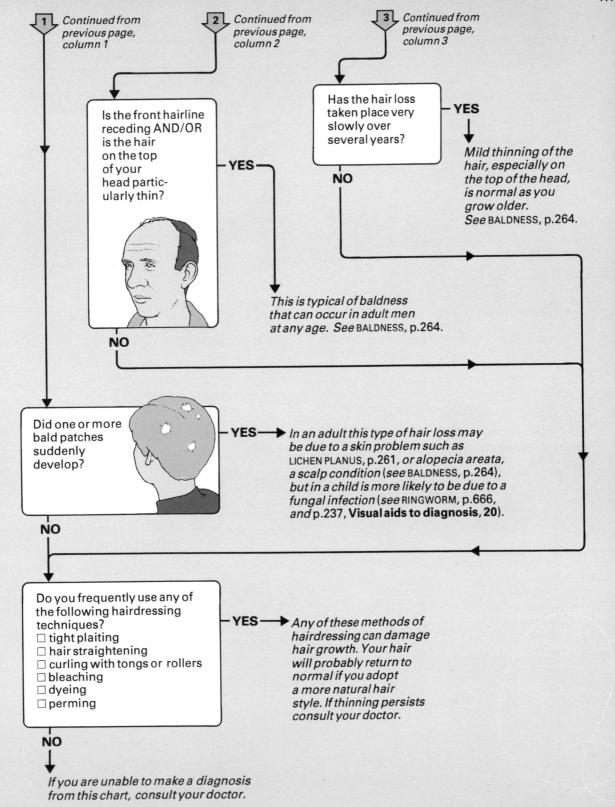

1 Continued from previous page, column 1

2 Continued from previous page, column 2

3 Continued from previous page, column 3

Has the hair loss taken place very slowly over several years?

YES — *Mild thinning of the hair, especially on the top of the head, is normal as you grow older.* See BALDNESS, p.264.

NO

Is the front hairline receding AND/OR is the hair on the top of your head particularly thin?

YES — *This is typical of baldness that can occur in adult men at any age.* See BALDNESS, p.264.

NO

Did one or more bald patches suddenly develop?

YES → *In an adult this type of hair loss may be due to a skin problem such as* LICHEN PLANUS, p.261, *or alopecia areata, a scalp condition (see* BALDNESS, p.264), *but in a child is more likely to be due to a fungal infection (see* RINGWORM, p.666, *and p.237,* **Visual aids to diagnosis, 20**).

NO

Do you frequently use any of the following hairdressing techniques?
☐ tight plaiting
☐ hair straightening
☐ curling with tongs or rollers
☐ bleaching
☐ dyeing
☐ perming

YES → *Any of these methods of hairdressing can damage hair growth. Your hair will probably return to normal if you adopt a more natural hair style. If thinning persists consult your doctor.*

NO

If you are unable to make a diagnosis from this chart, consult your doctor.

25

GENERAL
over 2 years

General skin problems

Any change in the skin, including rashes, spots, etc.
For babies under 2 see chart 89, **Skin problems in infants.**

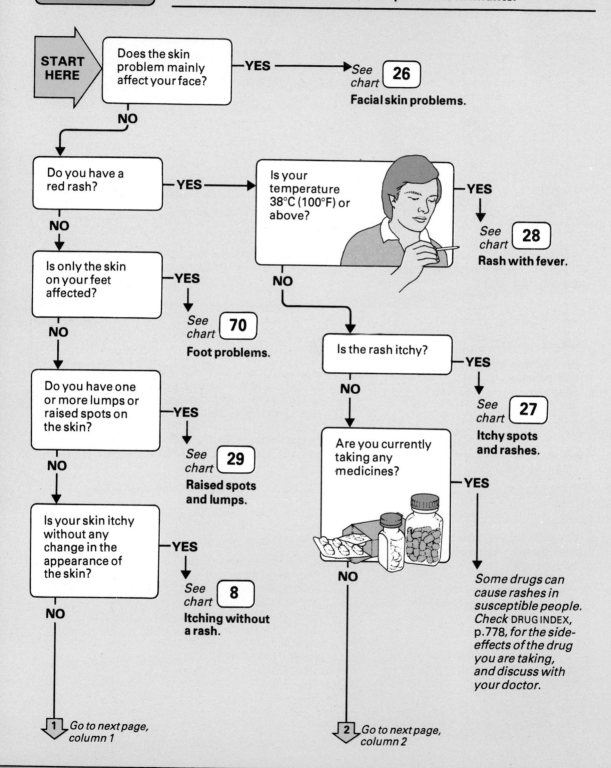

START HERE

Does the skin problem mainly affect your face? — **YES** → *See chart* **26**
Facial skin problems.

NO ↓

Do you have a red rash? — **YES** → **Is your temperature 38°C (100°F) or above?** — **YES** → *See chart* **28**
Rash with fever.

NO ↓ (red rash)

NO ↓ (temperature)

Is only the skin on your feet affected? — **YES** → *See chart* **70**
Foot problems.

NO ↓

Is the rash itchy? — **YES** → *See chart* **27**
Itchy spots and rashes.

NO ↓ (itchy)

Do you have one or more lumps or raised spots on the skin? — **YES** → *See chart* **29**
Raised spots and lumps.

NO ↓

Are you currently taking any medicines? — **YES** → *Some drugs can cause rashes in susceptible people. Check* DRUG INDEX, *p.778, for the side-effects of the drug you are taking, and discuss with your doctor.*

NO ↓ (medicines)

Is your skin itchy without any change in the appearance of the skin? — **YES** → *See chart* **8**
Itching without a rash.

NO ↓

1 ⤓ *Go to next page, column 1*

2 ⤓ *Go to next page, column 2*

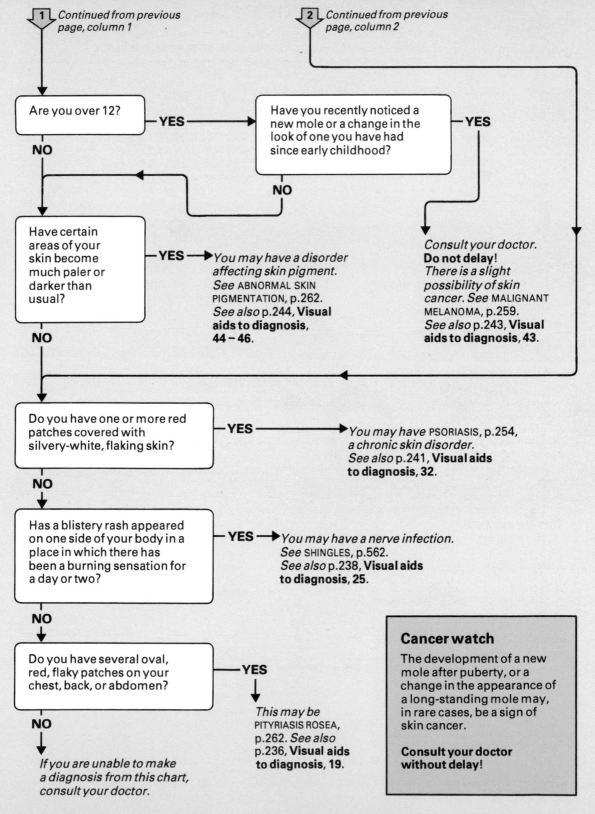

1 *Continued from previous page, column 1*

2 *Continued from previous page, column 2*

Are you over 12? — **YES** → Have you recently noticed a new mole or a change in the look of one you have had since early childhood? — **YES**

NO

NO

Have certain areas of your skin become much paler or darker than usual? — **YES** → *You may have a disorder affecting skin pigment.* See ABNORMAL SKIN PIGMENTATION, p.262. *See also* p.244, **Visual aids to diagnosis, 44 – 46**.

NO

Consult your doctor. **Do not delay**! *There is a slight possibility of skin cancer. See* MALIGNANT MELANOMA, p.259. *See also* p.243, **Visual aids to diagnosis, 43**.

Do you have one or more red patches covered with silvery-white, flaking skin? — **YES** → *You may have* PSORIASIS, p.254, *a chronic skin disorder.* *See also* p.241, **Visual aids to diagnosis, 32**.

NO

Has a blistery rash appeared on one side of your body in a place in which there has been a burning sensation for a day or two? — **YES** → *You may have a nerve infection.* See SHINGLES, p.562. *See also* p.238, **Visual aids to diagnosis, 25**.

NO

Do you have several oval, red, flaky patches on your chest, back, or abdomen? — **YES**

NO

This may be PITYRIASIS ROSEA, p.262. *See also* p.236, **Visual aids to diagnosis, 19**.

If you are unable to make a diagnosis from this chart, consult your doctor.

Cancer watch

The development of a new mole after puberty, or a change in the appearance of a long-standing mole may, in rare cases, be a sign of skin cancer.

Consult your doctor without delay!

26

GENERAL
over 2 years

Facial skin problems

Any rash, spots or change in the skin of the face.
For babies under 2 see chart 89, **Skin problems in infants**.

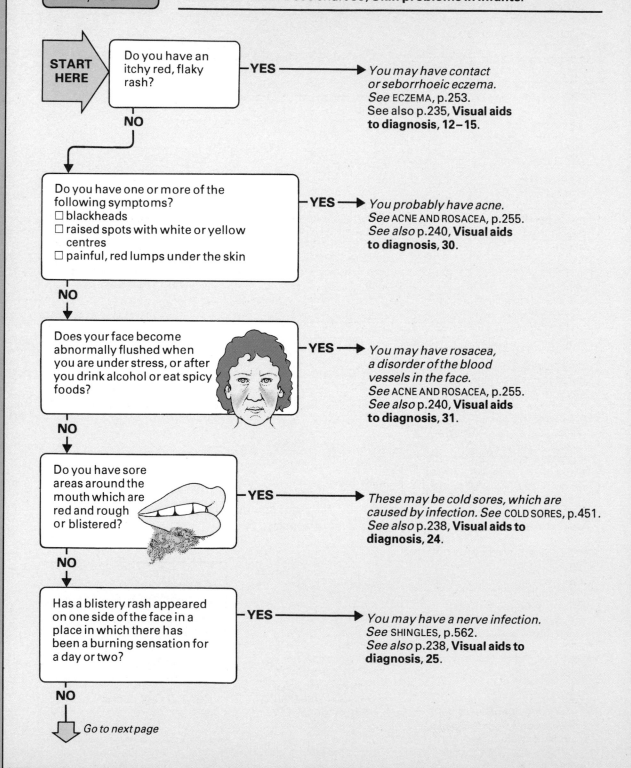

START HERE → Do you have an itchy red, flaky rash? — **YES** → *You may have contact or seborrhoeic eczema.* *See* ECZEMA, p.253. See also p.235, **Visual aids to diagnosis, 12–15**.

NO ↓

Do you have one or more of the following symptoms?
☐ blackheads
☐ raised spots with white or yellow centres
☐ painful, red lumps under the skin

— **YES** → *You probably have acne.* *See* ACNE AND ROSACEA, p.255. *See also* p.240, **Visual aids to diagnosis, 30**.

NO ↓

Does your face become abnormally flushed when you are under stress, or after you drink alcohol or eat spicy foods?

— **YES** → *You may have rosacea, a disorder of the blood vessels in the face.* *See* ACNE AND ROSACEA, p.255. *See also* p.240, **Visual aids to diagnosis, 31**.

NO ↓

Do you have sore areas around the mouth which are red and rough or blistered?

— **YES** → *These may be cold sores, which are caused by infection. See* COLD SORES, p.451. *See also* p.238, **Visual aids to diagnosis, 24**.

NO ↓

Has a blistery rash appeared on one side of the face in a place in which there has been a burning sensation for a day or two?

— **YES** → *You may have a nerve infection.* *See* SHINGLES, p.562. *See also* p.238, **Visual aids to diagnosis, 25**.

NO ↓

Go to next page

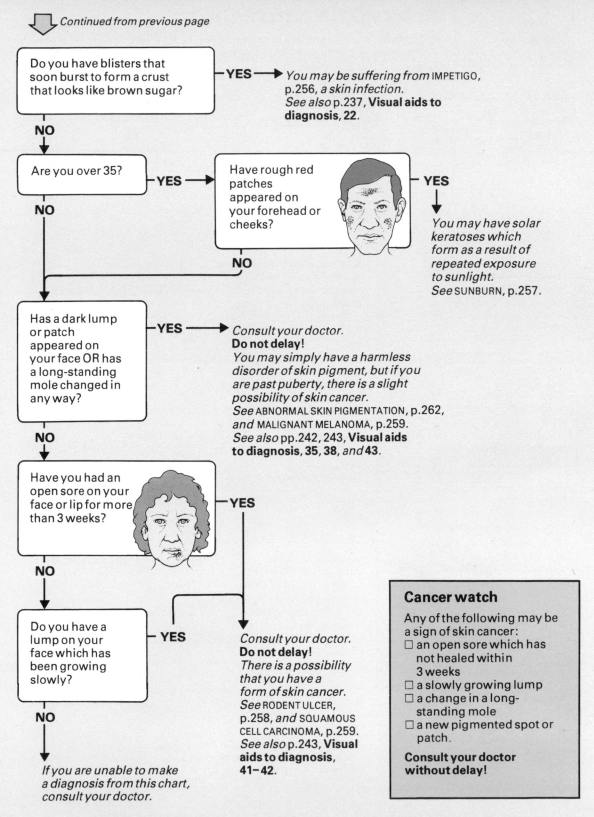

Continued from previous page

Do you have blisters that soon burst to form a crust that looks like brown sugar?

YES → *You may be suffering from* IMPETIGO, *p.256, a skin infection.*
See also p.237, **Visual aids to diagnosis, 22.**

NO

Are you over 35?

YES →

Have rough red patches appeared on your forehead or cheeks?

YES ↓

You may have solar keratoses which form as a result of repeated exposure to sunlight.
See SUNBURN, *p.257.*

NO

Has a dark lump or patch appeared on your face OR has a long-standing mole changed in any way?

YES → *Consult your doctor.*
Do not delay!
You may simply have a harmless disorder of skin pigment, but if you are past puberty, there is a slight possibility of skin cancer.
See ABNORMAL SKIN PIGMENTATION, *p.262, and* MALIGNANT MELANOMA, *p.259.*
See also pp.242, 243, **Visual aids to diagnosis, 35, 38,** *and* **43.**

NO

Have you had an open sore on your face or lip for more than 3 weeks?

YES

NO

Do you have a lump on your face which has been growing slowly?

YES → *Consult your doctor.*
Do not delay!
There is a possibility that you have a form of skin cancer.
See RODENT ULCER, *p.258, and* SQUAMOUS CELL CARCINOMA, *p.259.*
See also p.243, **Visual aids to diagnosis, 41–42.**

NO

If you are unable to make a diagnosis from this chart, consult your doctor.

Cancer watch

Any of the following may be a sign of skin cancer:
- ☐ an open sore which has not healed within 3 weeks
- ☐ a slowly growing lump
- ☐ a change in a long-standing mole
- ☐ a new pigmented spot or patch.

Consult your doctor without delay!

27

GENERAL
over 2 years

Itchy spots and rashes

Discoloured and/or raised areas of itchy skin.
For babies under 2 years see chart 89, **Skin problems in infants**.

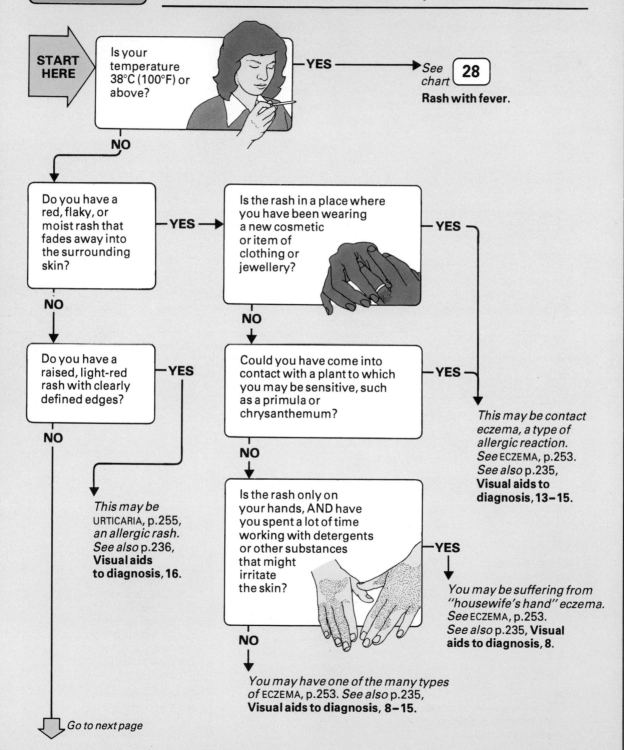

START HERE

Is your temperature 38°C (100°F) or above?

YES → *See chart* **28** **Rash with fever.**

NO

Do you have a red, flaky, or moist rash that fades away into the surrounding skin?

YES → Is the rash in a place where you have been wearing a new cosmetic or item of clothing or jewellery?

YES →

This may be contact eczema, a type of allergic reaction. See ECZEMA, *p.253. See also p.235,* **Visual aids to diagnosis, 13–15.**

NO

Do you have a raised, light-red rash with clearly defined edges?

YES →

This may be URTICARIA, *p.255, an allergic rash. See also p.236,* **Visual aids to diagnosis, 16.**

NO

Could you have come into contact with a plant to which you may be sensitive, such as a primula or chrysanthemum?

YES →

NO

Is the rash only on your hands, AND have you spent a lot of time working with detergents or other substances that might irritate the skin?

YES →

You may be suffering from "housewife's hand" eczema. See ECZEMA, *p.253. See also p.235,* **Visual aids to diagnosis, 8.**

NO

You may have one of the many types of ECZEMA, *p.253. See also p.235,* **Visual aids to diagnosis, 8–15.**

Go to next page

⬇ *Continued from previous page*

Have you started to take any medicines recently?

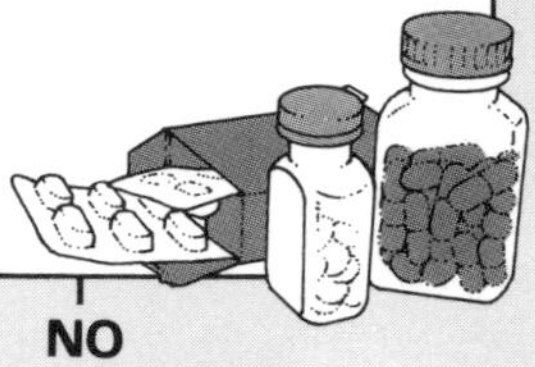

YES ➔ *Some drugs can cause an itchy rash. Check* DRUG INDEX, p.778, *for the side-effects of the drug you are taking, and discuss with your doctor.*

NO

Do you have one or more red, scaly patches spreading out in a ring?

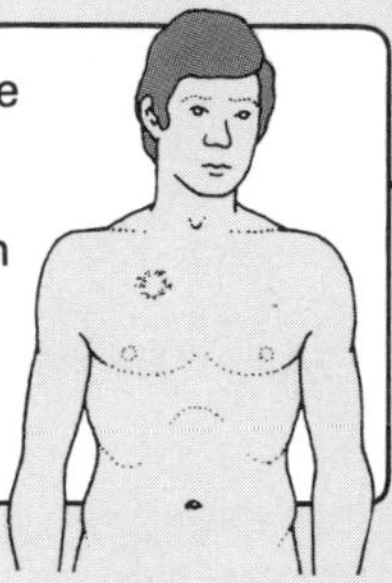

YES ➔ *This may be a fungal infection. See* RINGWORM, p.666. *See also* p.237, **Visual aids to diagnosis, 20.**

NO

Have you a widespread red rash which is particularly itchy at night?

YES ➔ Have you noticed tiny grey lines or red, infected-looking spots between the fingers or on the wrists?

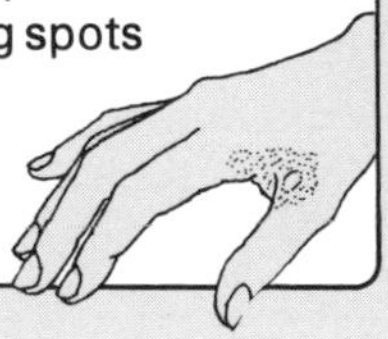

YES
⬇

You may have SCABIES, p.568, *a parasitic infection, especially if someone you are in close physical contact with has the same trouble. See also* p.248, **Visual aids to diagnosis, 67.**

NO ➔

NO

Do you have one or more raised red spots in a small area?

YES ➔ *You may have been bitten by an insect.*
⊕ *For first aid see* p.814.
See also p.248, **Visual aids to diagnosis, 68.**

NO

If you are unable to make a diagnosis from this chart, consult your doctor.

28

Rash with fever

Any spots, discoloured areas, or blisters on the skin combined with a temperature of 38°C (100°F) or above.

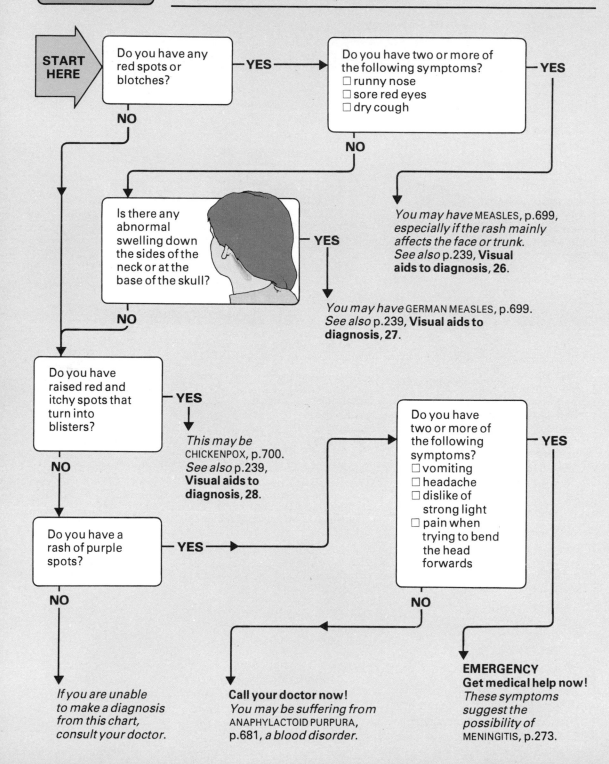

START HERE

Do you have any red spots or blotches? — **YES** → **Do you have two or more of the following symptoms?**
☐ runny nose
☐ sore red eyes
☐ dry cough — **YES**

NO

Is there any abnormal swelling down the sides of the neck or at the base of the skull? — **YES**

NO

You may have MEASLES, *p.699, especially if the rash mainly affects the face or trunk. See also p.239,* **Visual aids to diagnosis, 26.**

You may have GERMAN MEASLES, *p.699. See also p.239,* **Visual aids to diagnosis, 27.**

Do you have raised red and itchy spots that turn into blisters? — **YES**

NO

This may be CHICKENPOX, *p.700. See also p.239,* **Visual aids to diagnosis, 28.**

Do you have two or more of the following symptoms?
☐ vomiting
☐ headache
☐ dislike of strong light
☐ pain when trying to bend the head forwards — **YES**

Do you have a rash of purple spots? — **YES**

NO

NO

If you are unable to make a diagnosis from this chart, consult your doctor.

Call your doctor now! *You may be suffering from* ANAPHYLACTOID PURPURA, *p.681, a blood disorder.*

EMERGENCY Get medical help now! *These symptoms suggest the possibility of* MENINGITIS, *p.273.*

29
GENERAL
all ages

Raised spots and lumps

Any raised spots or lumps on the surface of the skin which may be inflamed, dark, or the same colour as the surrounding skin.

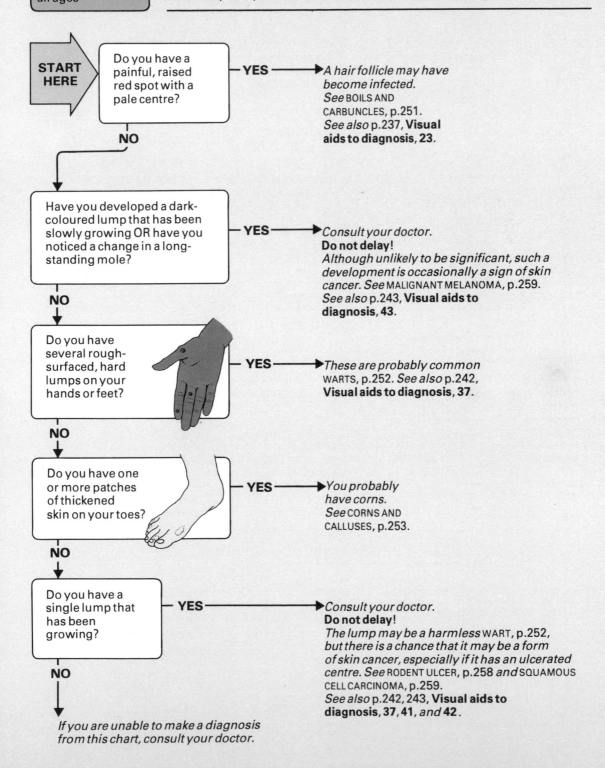

START HERE

Do you have a painful, raised red spot with a pale centre?

— **YES** — ▶ *A hair follicle may have become infected.* See BOILS AND CARBUNCLES, p.251. *See also* p.237, **Visual aids to diagnosis, 23**.

NO

Have you developed a dark-coloured lump that has been slowly growing OR have you noticed a change in a long-standing mole?

— **YES** — ▶ *Consult your doctor.* **Do not delay!** *Although unlikely to be significant, such a development is occasionally a sign of skin cancer.* See MALIGNANT MELANOMA, p.259. *See also* p.243, **Visual aids to diagnosis, 43**.

NO

Do you have several rough-surfaced, hard lumps on your hands or feet?

— **YES** — ▶ *These are probably common* WARTS, p.252. *See also* p.242, **Visual aids to diagnosis, 37**.

NO

Do you have one or more patches of thickened skin on your toes?

— **YES** — ▶ *You probably have corns.* See CORNS AND CALLUSES, p.253.

NO

Do you have a single lump that has been growing?

— **YES** — ▶ *Consult your doctor.* **Do not delay!** *The lump may be a harmless* WART, p.252, *but there is a chance that it may be a form of skin cancer, especially if it has an ulcerated centre.* See RODENT ULCER, p.258 *and* SQUAMOUS CELL CARCINOMA, p.259. *See also* p.242, 243, **Visual aids to diagnosis, 37, 41,** *and* **42**.

NO

If you are unable to make a diagnosis from this chart, consult your doctor.

30

GENERAL
all ages

Painful eye

Pain may be continuous or intermittent and may be felt in or around the eye.

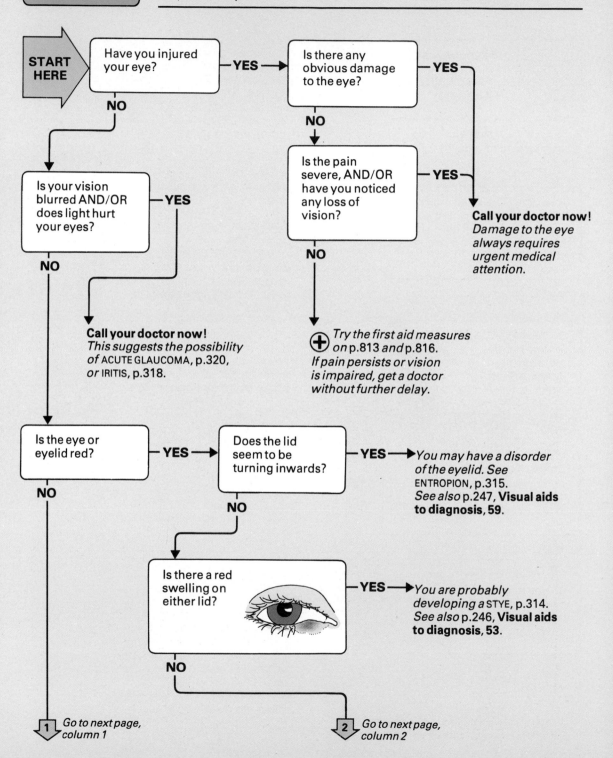

START HERE

Have you injured your eye?

YES →

Is there any obvious damage to the eye?

YES →

NO ↓

NO ↓

Is your vision blurred AND/OR does light hurt your eyes?

YES →

Is the pain severe, AND/OR have you noticed any loss of vision?

YES →

NO ↓

NO ↓

Call your doctor now!
Damage to the eye always requires urgent medical attention.

Call your doctor now!
This suggests the possibility of ACUTE GLAUCOMA, *p.320, or* IRITIS, *p.318.*

✚ *Try the first aid measures on p.813 and p.816. If pain persists or vision is impaired, get a doctor without further delay.*

Is the eye or eyelid red?

YES →

Does the lid seem to be turning inwards?

YES →

You may have a disorder of the eyelid. See ENTROPION, *p.315. See also p.247,* **Visual aids to diagnosis, 59.**

NO ↓

NO ↓

Is there a red swelling on either lid?

YES →

You are probably developing a STYE, *p.314. See also p.246,* **Visual aids to diagnosis, 53.**

NO ↓

1 *Go to next page, column 1*

2 *Go to next page, column 2*

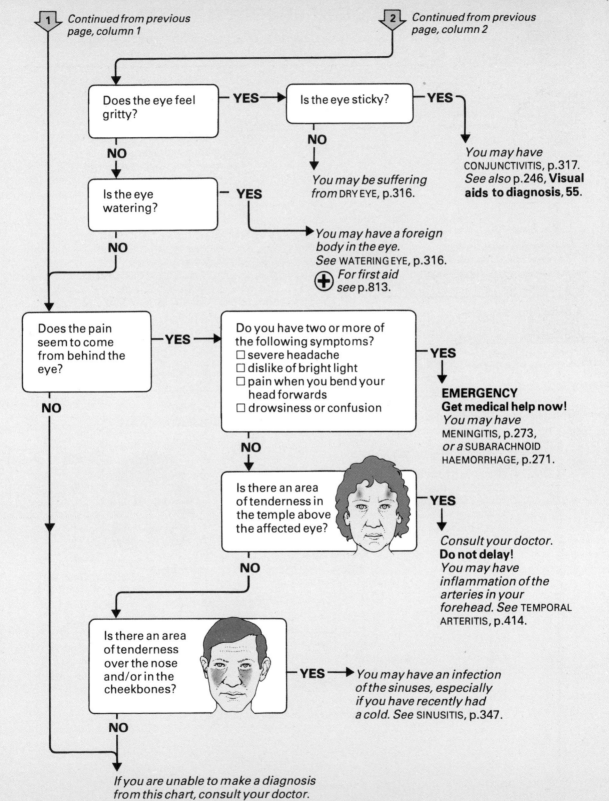

1 *Continued from previous page, column 1*

2 *Continued from previous page, column 2*

Does the eye feel gritty? — **YES** → **Is the eye sticky?** — **YES**

NO ↓ (from "Does the eye feel gritty?")

NO ↓ (from "Is the eye sticky?")

You may be suffering from DRY EYE, *p.316.*

You may have CONJUNCTIVITIS, *p.317. See also p.246,* **Visual aids to diagnosis, 55.**

Is the eye watering? — **YES**

NO ↓

You may have a foreign body in the eye. See WATERING EYE, *p.316.*
✚ *For first aid see p.813.*

Does the pain seem to come from behind the eye? — **YES** → **Do you have two or more of the following symptoms?**
☐ severe headache
☐ dislike of bright light
☐ pain when you bend your head forwards
☐ drowsiness or confusion — **YES**

NO ↓ (from "Does the pain seem to come from behind the eye?")

EMERGENCY
Get medical help now!
You may have MENINGITIS, *p.273, or a* SUBARACHNOID HAEMORRHAGE, *p.271.*

NO ↓ (from symptoms box)

Is there an area of tenderness in the temple above the affected eye? — **YES**

NO ↓

Consult your doctor. **Do not delay!** *You may have inflammation of the arteries in your forehead. See* TEMPORAL ARTERITIS, *p.414.*

Is there an area of tenderness over the nose and/or in the cheekbones? — **YES** → *You may have an infection of the sinuses, especially if you have recently had a cold. See* SINUSITIS, *p.347.*

NO ↓

If you are unable to make a diagnosis from this chart, consult your doctor.

31

GENERAL
all ages

Disturbed or impaired vision

Any reduction in your ability to see, including blurring, double vision, and/or seeing flashing lights or floating spots.

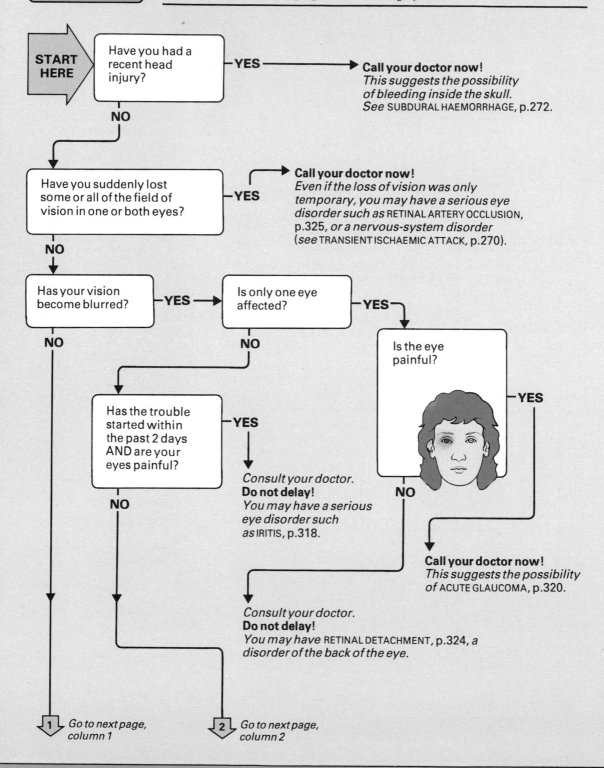

START HERE

Have you had a recent head injury? — YES →

Call your doctor now!
*This suggests the possibility of bleeding inside the skull.
See* SUBDURAL HAEMORRHAGE, p.272.

NO

Have you suddenly lost some or all of the field of vision in one or both eyes? — YES

Call your doctor now!
Even if the loss of vision was only temporary, you may have a serious eye disorder such as RETINAL ARTERY OCCLUSION, p.325, *or a nervous-system disorder* (*see* TRANSIENT ISCHAEMIC ATTACK, p.270).

NO

Has your vision become blurred? — YES → **Is only one eye affected?** — YES

NO

Has the trouble started within the past 2 days AND are your eyes painful? — YES

NO

Is the eye painful? — YES

NO

Consult your doctor.
Do not delay!
You may have a serious eye disorder such as IRITIS, p.318.

Call your doctor now!
This suggests the possibility of ACUTE GLAUCOMA, p.320.

Consult your doctor.
Do not delay!
You may have RETINAL DETACHMENT, p.324, *a disorder of the back of the eye.*

1 ⬇ *Go to next page, column 1*

2 ⬇ *Go to next page, column 2*

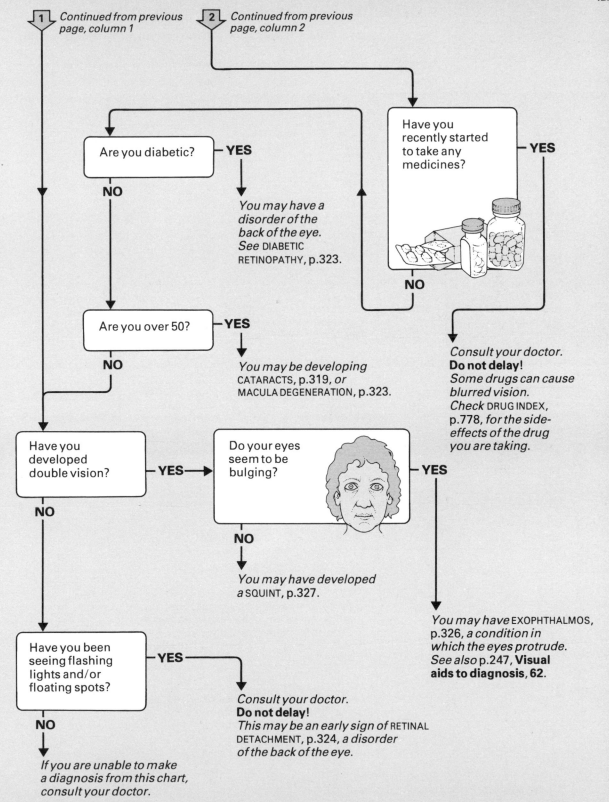

1 *Continued from previous page, column 1*

2 *Continued from previous page, column 2*

Are you diabetic? — **YES**

NO

You may have a disorder of the back of the eye. See DIABETIC RETINOPATHY, p.323.

Have you recently started to take any medicines? — **YES**

NO

Are you over 50? — **YES**

NO

You may be developing CATARACTS, p.319, *or* MACULA DEGENERATION, p.323.

Consult your doctor. **Do not delay!** *Some drugs can cause blurred vision. Check* DRUG INDEX, p.778, *for the side-effects of the drug you are taking.*

Have you developed double vision? — **YES** → **Do your eyes seem to be bulging?** — **YES**

NO

NO

You may have developed a SQUINT, p.327.

You may have EXOPHTHALMOS, p.326, *a condition in which the eyes protrude. See also* p.247, **Visual aids to diagnosis, 62.**

Have you been seeing flashing lights and/or floating spots? — **YES**

NO

Consult your doctor. **Do not delay!** *This may be an early sign of* RETINAL DETACHMENT, p.324, *a disorder of the back of the eye.*

If you are unable to make a diagnosis from this chart, consult your doctor.

32

GENERAL
all ages

Earache

Pain in one or both ears that may be either sharp and stabbing or dull and throbbing.

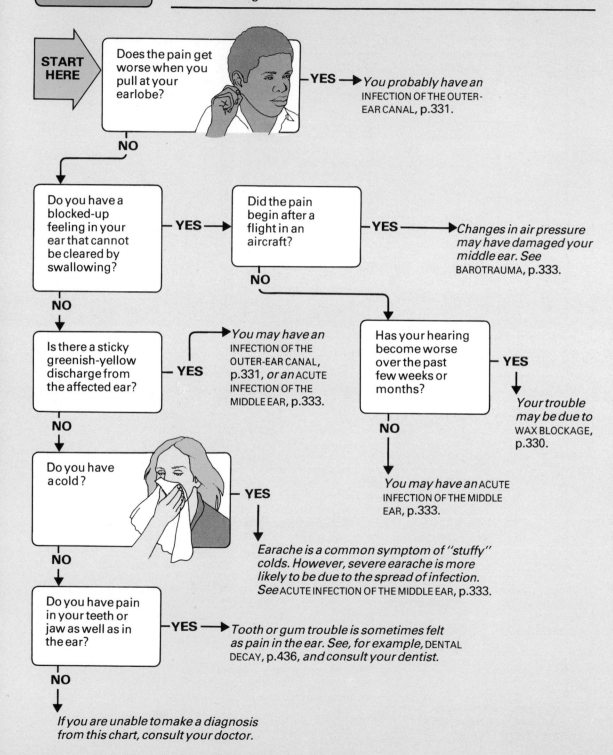

START HERE → Does the pain get worse when you pull at your earlobe? — **YES** → *You probably have an* INFECTION OF THE OUTER-EAR CANAL, p.331.

NO

Do you have a blocked-up feeling in your ear that cannot be cleared by swallowing? — **YES** → Did the pain begin after a flight in an aircraft? — **YES** → *Changes in air pressure may have damaged your middle ear. See* BAROTRAUMA, p.333.

NO

NO

Is there a sticky greenish-yellow discharge from the affected ear? — **YES** → *You may have an* INFECTION OF THE OUTER-EAR CANAL, p.331, *or an* ACUTE INFECTION OF THE MIDDLE EAR, p.333.

Has your hearing become worse over the past few weeks or months? — **YES** → *Your trouble may be due to* WAX BLOCKAGE, p.330.

NO

NO

You may have an ACUTE INFECTION OF THE MIDDLE EAR, p.333.

Do you have a cold? — **YES** → *Earache is a common symptom of "stuffy" colds. However, severe earache is more likely to be due to the spread of infection. See* ACUTE INFECTION OF THE MIDDLE EAR, p.333.

NO

Do you have pain in your teeth or jaw as well as in the ear? — **YES** → *Tooth or gum trouble is sometimes felt as pain in the ear. See, for example,* DENTAL DECAY, p.436, *and consult your dentist.*

NO

If you are unable to make a diagnosis from this chart, consult your doctor.

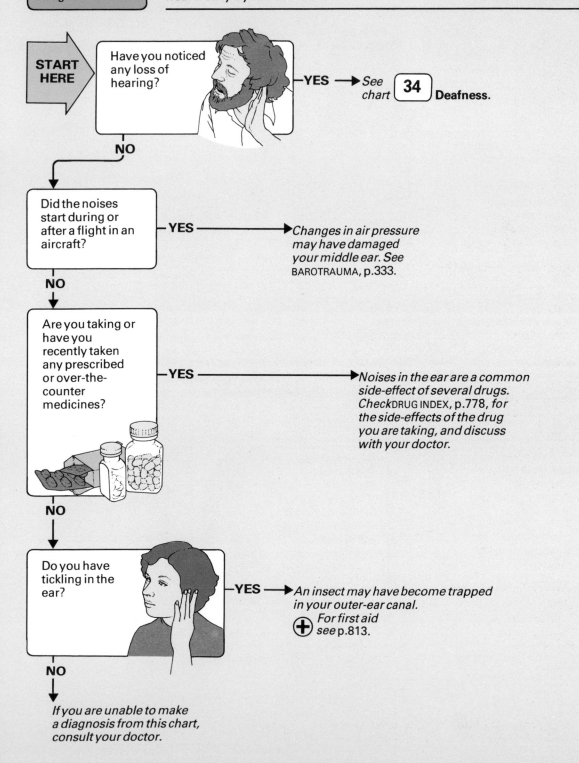

33
GENERAL
all ages

Noises in the ear

Any ringing, buzzing, or hissing (but not speech or music) that can be heard only by the sufferer.

START HERE →

Have you noticed any loss of hearing?

YES → *See chart* **34** Deafness.

NO ↓

Did the noises start during or after a flight in an aircraft?

YES → *Changes in air pressure may have damaged your middle ear. See* BAROTRAUMA, p.333.

NO ↓

Are you taking or have you recently taken any prescribed or over-the-counter medicines?

YES → *Noises in the ear are a common side-effect of several drugs. Check* DRUG INDEX, p.778, *for the side-effects of the drug you are taking, and discuss with your doctor.*

NO ↓

Do you have tickling in the ear?

YES → *An insect may have become trapped in your outer-ear canal.*
⊕ *For first aid see p.813.*

NO ↓

If you are unable to make a diagnosis from this chart, consult your doctor.

34
GENERAL
all ages

Deafness
Deterioration in the ability to hear some or all sounds in one or both ears.

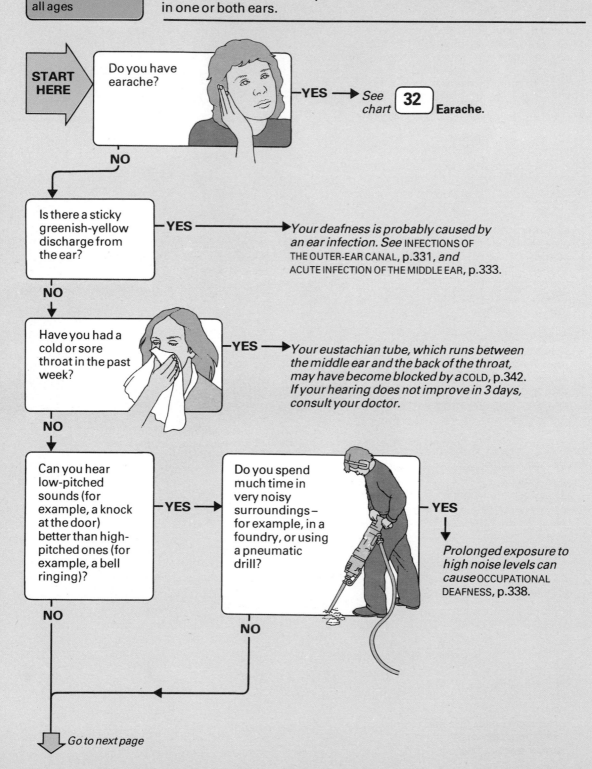

START HERE → Do you have earache? —**YES**→ *See chart* **32** **Earache.**

NO

Is there a sticky greenish-yellow discharge from the ear? —**YES**→ *Your deafness is probably caused by an ear infection. See* INFECTIONS OF THE OUTER-EAR CANAL, p.331, *and* ACUTE INFECTION OF THE MIDDLE EAR, p.333.

NO

Have you had a cold or sore throat in the past week? —**YES**→ *Your eustachian tube, which runs between the middle ear and the back of the throat, may have become blocked by a* COLD, p.342. *If your hearing does not improve in 3 days, consult your doctor.*

NO

Can you hear low-pitched sounds (for example, a knock at the door) better than high-pitched ones (for example, a bell ringing)? —**YES**→ Do you spend much time in very noisy surroundings – for example, in a foundry, or using a pneumatic drill? —**YES**↓ *Prolonged exposure to high noise levels can cause* OCCUPATIONAL DEAFNESS, p.338.

NO ← **NO**

Go to next page

↓ *Continued from previous page*

Have you recently taken any prescribed or over-the-counter medicines? ——**YES**——→ *Hearing loss is a common side-effect of several drugs. Check* DRUG INDEX, p.778, *for the side-effects of the drug you are taking, and discuss with your doctor.*

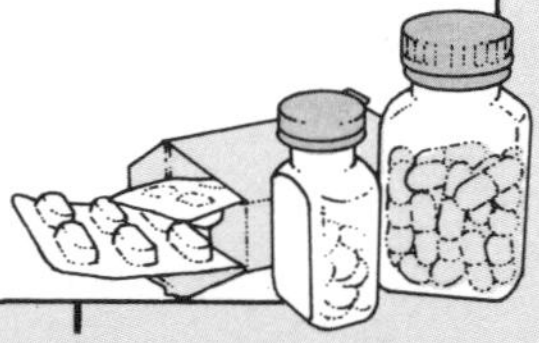

NO
↓

Do you have occasional attacks of dizziness when everything around you seems to spin? ——**YES**——→ *You may have* MÉNIÈRE'S DISEASE, p.337, *which affects the working of the inner ear.*

NO
↓

Are you over 60? ——**YES**——→ *Some degree of deafness is common in later life, but is treatable.* See THE FAILING SENSES, p.721.

NO
↓

Has your hearing been getting worse over a period of several weeks or more? ——**YES**——→ **Have other members of your family suffered from gradual loss of hearing?** ——**YES**——→ *You may have* OTOSCLEROSIS, p.332, *which affects the working of the middle ear.*

NO
↓

Your trouble may be due to WAX BLOCKAGE, p.330.

NO
↓

If you are unable to make a diagnosis from this chart, consult your doctor.

35

GENERAL
all ages

Runny nose

Complete or partial blockage of the nose by a thick or watery discharge.

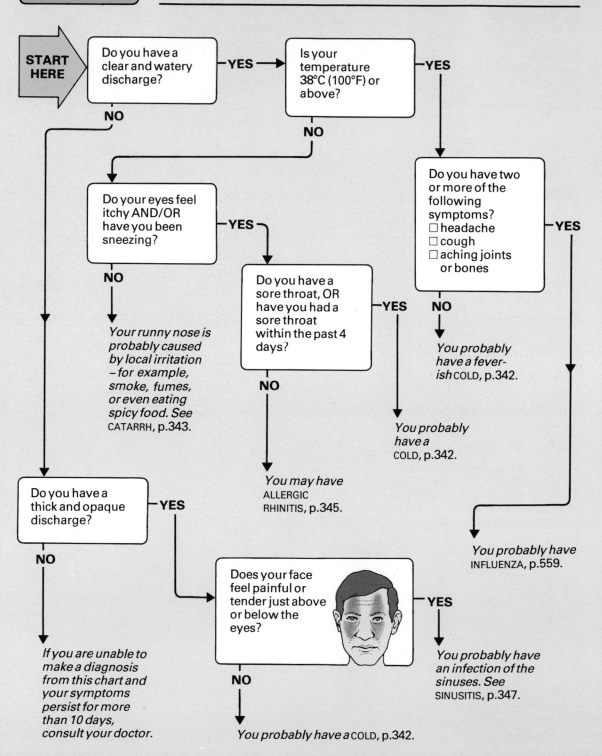

START HERE

Do you have a clear and watery discharge? — **YES** → Is your temperature 38°C (100°F) or above? — **YES**

NO (from clear and watery discharge)

NO (from temperature)

Do your eyes feel itchy AND/OR have you been sneezing? — **YES**

NO

Your runny nose is probably caused by local irritation – for example, smoke, fumes, or even eating spicy food. See CATARRH, p.343.

Do you have a sore throat, OR have you had a sore throat within the past 4 days? — **YES**

NO

You may have ALLERGIC RHINITIS, p.345.

Do you have two or more of the following symptoms?
☐ headache
☐ cough
☐ aching joints or bones
— **YES**

NO

You probably have a feverish COLD, p.342.

You probably have a COLD, p.342.

You probably have INFLUENZA, p.559.

Do you have a thick and opaque discharge? — **YES**

NO

If you are unable to make a diagnosis from this chart and your symptoms persist for more than 10 days, consult your doctor.

Does your face feel painful or tender just above or below the eyes? — **YES**

NO

You probably have an infection of the sinuses. See SINUSITIS, p.347.

You probably have a COLD, p.342.

36
GENERAL
all ages

Sore throat

Any rough or raw feeling in the back of the throat that causes discomfort, especially on swallowing.

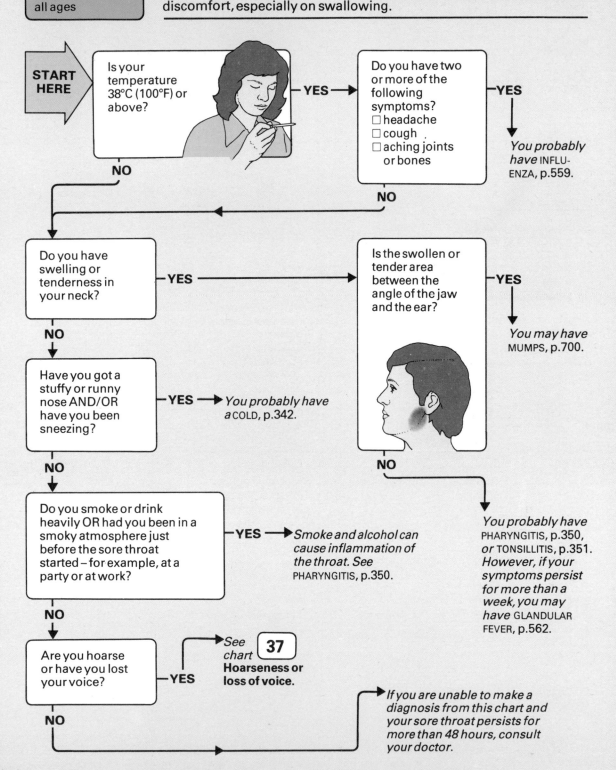

START HERE

Is your temperature 38°C (100°F) or above?

YES → Do you have two or more of the following symptoms?
☐ headache
☐ cough
☐ aching joints or bones

YES → *You probably have* INFLUENZA, p.559.

NO (temperature)

NO (symptoms)

Do you have swelling or tenderness in your neck?

YES → Is the swollen or tender area between the angle of the jaw and the ear?

YES → *You may have* MUMPS, p.700.

NO (swelling)

Have you got a stuffy or runny nose AND/OR have you been sneezing?

YES → *You probably have a* COLD, p.342.

NO (nose)

Do you smoke or drink heavily OR had you been in a smoky atmosphere just before the sore throat started – for example, at a party or at work?

YES → *Smoke and alcohol can cause inflammation of the throat. See* PHARYNGITIS, p.350.

NO (smoke)

NO (jaw/ear) → *You probably have* PHARYNGITIS, p.350, *or* TONSILLITIS, p.351. *However, if your symptoms persist for more than a week, you may have* GLANDULAR FEVER, p.562.

Are you hoarse or have you lost your voice?

YES → *See chart* **37** **Hoarseness or loss of voice.**

NO (hoarse) → *If you are unable to make a diagnosis from this chart and your sore throat persists for more than 48 hours, consult your doctor.*

37

GENERAL
all ages

Hoarseness or loss of voice

Any abnormal huskiness in the voice that may be so severe that little or no sound can be made.

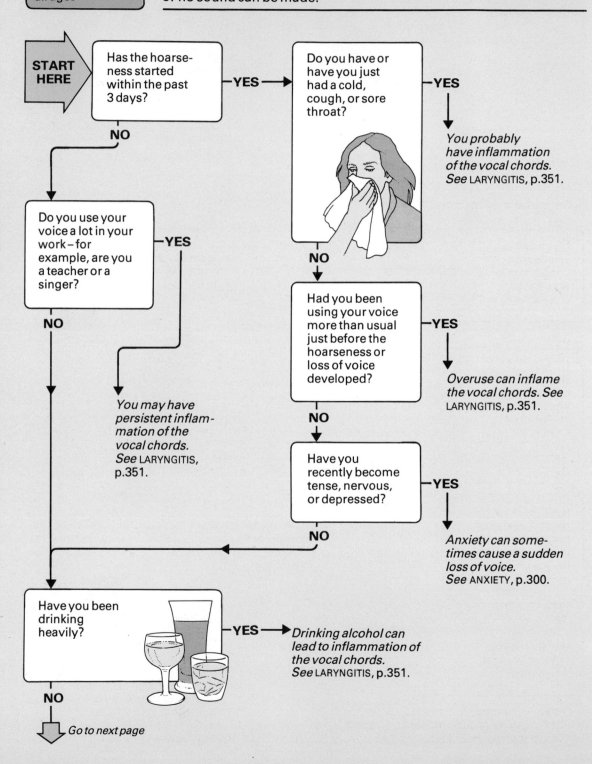

START HERE → Has the hoarseness started within the past 3 days?

— **YES** → Do you have or have you just had a cold, cough, or sore throat?

— **YES** → *You probably have inflammation of the vocal chords. See* LARYNGITIS, *p.351.*

NO (from "Has the hoarseness started...")

Do you use your voice a lot in your work – for example, are you a teacher or a singer?

— **YES** → *You may have persistent inflammation of the vocal chords. See* LARYNGITIS, *p.351.*

NO (from "Do you have or have you just had a cold...")

Had you been using your voice more than usual just before the hoarseness or loss of voice developed?

— **YES** → *Overuse can inflame the vocal chords. See* LARYNGITIS, *p.351.*

NO (from "Had you been using your voice...")

Have you recently become tense, nervous, or depressed?

— **YES** → *Anxiety can sometimes cause a sudden loss of voice. See* ANXIETY, *p.300.*

NO

Have you been drinking heavily?

— **YES** → *Drinking alcohol can lead to inflammation of the vocal chords. See* LARYNGITIS, *p.351.*

NO

⬇ *Go to next page*

⬇ Continued from previous page

Do you smoke?

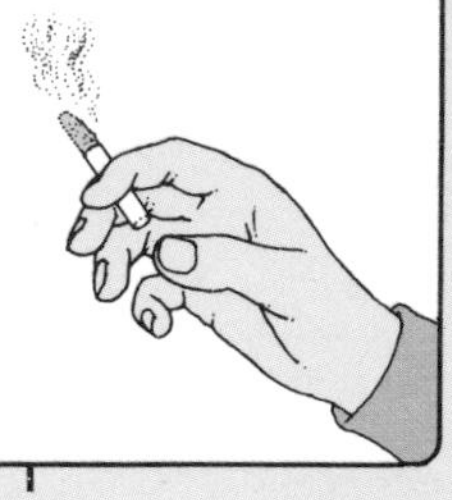

— **YES** ——→ *Smoking can lead to inflammation of the vocal chords.*
See LARYNGITIS, p.351.

NO

Do you have two or more of the following symptoms?
☐ feeling the cold more than you used to
☐ dry skin or hair
☐ weight increase without overeating
☐ inexplicable tiredness

— **YES** ——→ *You may have an under-active thyroid gland.*
See HYPOTHYROIDISM, p.526.

NO

Has your hoarse-ness or loss of voice lasted for more than a week?

— **YES** ——→ *Consult your doctor.*
Do not delay!
Although there is probably a simple explanation for your hoarseness or loss of voice, there is a slight possibility of a growth on the larynx. See TUMOURS OF THE LARYNX, p.352.

NO

Have you had several attacks of hoarseness or loss of voice in the past 6 months?

— **YES**

NO

If you are unable to make a diagnosis from this chart and your hoarseness persists for more than a week, consult your doctor.

Cancer watch

Hoarseness or loss of voice that is recurrent or lasts for more than a week may indicate cancer of the larynx.

Consult your doctor without delay!

38
GENERAL
over 14 years

Coughing

A noisy expulsion of air from the lungs, that may produce phlegm or be "dry". For children see chart 95, **Coughing in children**.

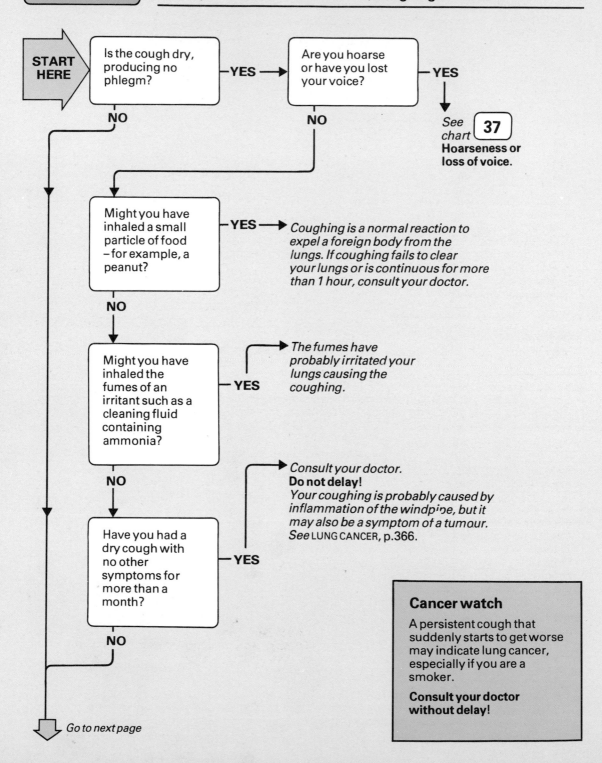

START HERE

Is the cough dry, producing no phlegm? — **YES** → Are you hoarse or have you lost your voice? — **YES** →

See chart **37** **Hoarseness or loss of voice.**

NO (from first box)

NO (from hoarse box)

Might you have inhaled a small particle of food – for example, a peanut? — **YES** → *Coughing is a normal reaction to expel a foreign body from the lungs. If coughing fails to clear your lungs or is continuous for more than 1 hour, consult your doctor.*

NO

Might you have inhaled the fumes of an irritant such as a cleaning fluid containing ammonia? — **YES** → *The fumes have probably irritated your lungs causing the coughing.*

NO

Have you had a dry cough with no other symptoms for more than a month? — **YES** → *Consult your doctor.* **Do not delay!** *Your coughing is probably caused by inflammation of the windpipe, but it may also be a symptom of a tumour. See* LUNG CANCER, p.366.

NO

Go to next page

Cancer watch

A persistent cough that suddenly starts to get worse may indicate lung cancer, especially if you are a smoker.

Consult your doctor without delay!

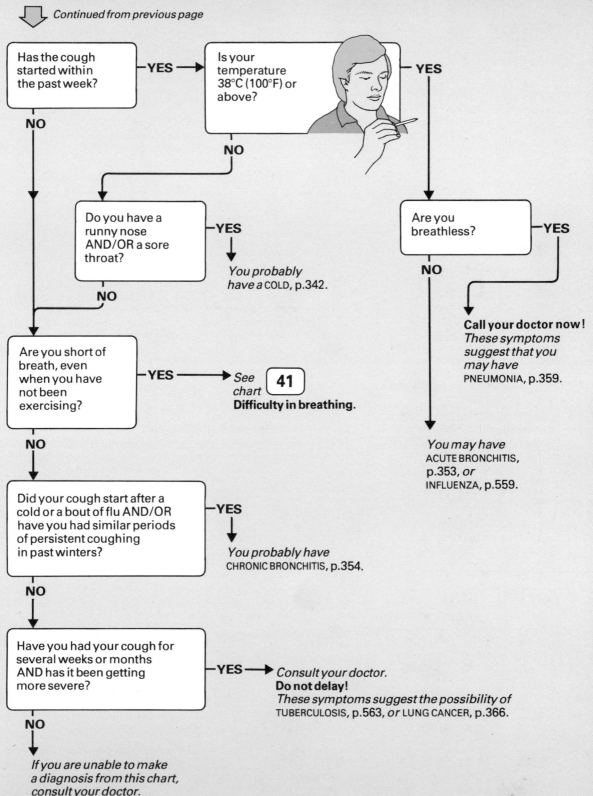

Continued from previous page

Has the cough started within the past week? — **YES** → **Is your temperature 38°C (100°F) or above?** — **YES**

NO ↓

NO ↓

Do you have a runny nose AND/OR a sore throat? — **YES** ↓

You probably have a COLD, p.342.

NO ↓

Are you breathless? — **YES**

NO ↓

Call your doctor now! *These symptoms suggest that you may have* PNEUMONIA, p.359.

You may have ACUTE BRONCHITIS, p.353, *or* INFLUENZA, p.559.

Are you short of breath, even when you have not been exercising? — **YES** → *See chart* **41** **Difficulty in breathing**.

NO ↓

Did your cough start after a cold or a bout of flu AND/OR have you had similar periods of persistent coughing in past winters? — **YES** ↓

You probably have CHRONIC BRONCHITIS, p.354.

NO ↓

Have you had your cough for several weeks or months AND has it been getting more severe? — **YES** → *Consult your doctor.* **Do not delay!** *These symptoms suggest the possibility of* TUBERCULOSIS, p.563, *or* LUNG CANCER, p.366.

NO ↓

If you are unable to make a diagnosis from this chart, consult your doctor.

39

Coughing up blood

Coughing up phlegm that is coloured or streaked bright red or rusty brown, or that is pink and frothy.

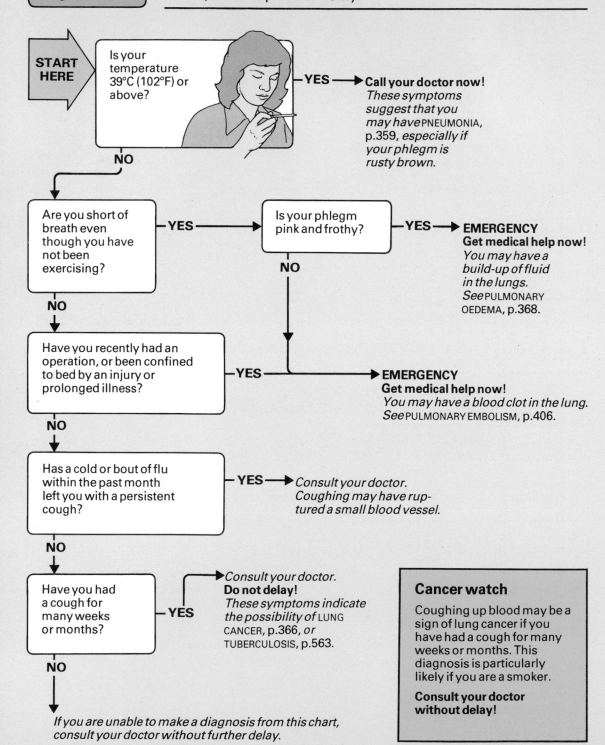

START HERE

Is your temperature 39°C (102°F) or above? — **YES** →

Call your doctor now!
These symptoms suggest that you may have PNEUMONIA, p.359, *especially if your phlegm is rusty brown.*

NO

Are you short of breath even though you have not been exercising? — **YES** → **Is your phlegm pink and frothy?** — **YES** →

EMERGENCY
Get medical help now!
You may have a build-up of fluid in the lungs. See PULMONARY OEDEMA, p.368.

NO (phlegm) / **NO** (short of breath)

Have you recently had an operation, or been confined to bed by an injury or prolonged illness? — **YES** →

EMERGENCY
Get medical help now!
You may have a blood clot in the lung. See PULMONARY EMBOLISM, p.406.

NO

Has a cold or bout of flu within the past month left you with a persistent cough? — **YES** →

*Consult your doctor.
Coughing may have ruptured a small blood vessel.*

NO

Have you had a cough for many weeks or months? — **YES** →

Consult your doctor.
Do not delay!
These symptoms indicate the possibility of LUNG CANCER, p.366, *or* TUBERCULOSIS, p.563.

NO

If you are unable to make a diagnosis from this chart, consult your doctor without further delay.

Cancer watch

Coughing up blood may be a sign of lung cancer if you have had a cough for many weeks or months. This diagnosis is particularly likely if you are a smoker.

Consult your doctor without delay!

40

GENERAL
all ages

Wheezing

Noisy, difficult breathing, particularly when breathing out.

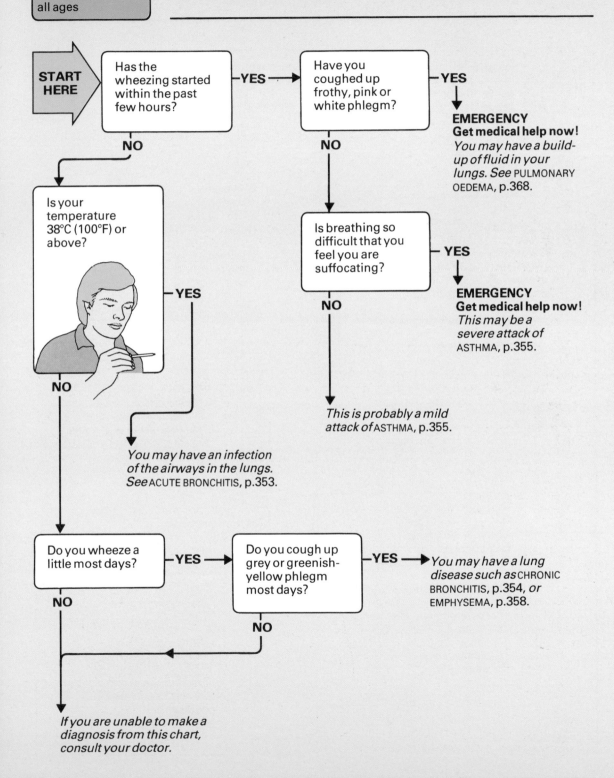

START HERE → Has the wheezing started within the past few hours?

— **YES** → Have you coughed up frothy, pink or white phlegm?

— **YES** →

EMERGENCY
Get medical help now!
You may have a build-up of fluid in your lungs. See PULMONARY OEDEMA, p.368.

NO ↓ (from "frothy phlegm")

Is breathing so difficult that you feel you are suffocating?

— **YES** →

EMERGENCY
Get medical help now!
This may be a severe attack of ASTHMA, p.355.

NO ↓

This is probably a mild attack of ASTHMA, p.355.

NO ↓ (from "started within the past few hours")

Is your temperature 38°C (100°F) or above?

— **YES** →

You may have an infection of the airways in the lungs. See ACUTE BRONCHITIS, p.353.

NO ↓

Do you wheeze a little most days? — **YES** → Do you cough up grey or greenish-yellow phlegm most days? — **YES** → *You may have a lung disease such as* CHRONIC BRONCHITIS, p.354, *or* EMPHYSEMA, p.358.

NO ↓   **NO** ↓

If you are unable to make a diagnosis from this chart, consult your doctor.

41

GENERAL
all ages

Difficulty in breathing

Breathlessness or tightness in the chest which makes you aware of your breathing.

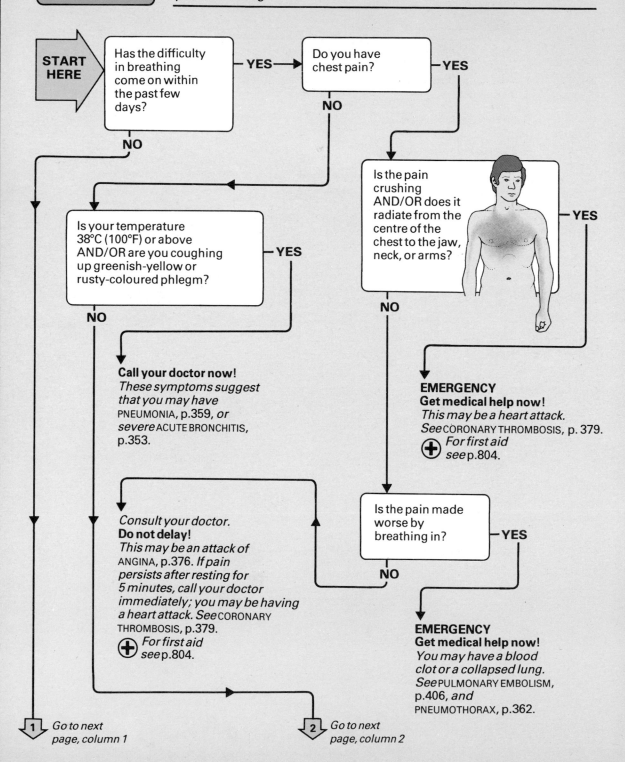

START HERE → Has the difficulty in breathing come on within the past few days?

YES → Do you have chest pain?

— **YES** →

NO (from first box)

NO (from chest pain box)

Is the pain crushing AND/OR does it radiate from the centre of the chest to the jaw, neck, or arms?

— **YES** →

Is your temperature 38°C (100°F) or above AND/OR are you coughing up greenish-yellow or rusty-coloured phlegm? — **YES**

NO

Call your doctor now!
These symptoms suggest that you may have PNEUMONIA, p.359, *or severe* ACUTE BRONCHITIS, p.353.

NO

EMERGENCY
Get medical help now!
This may be a heart attack.
See CORONARY THROMBOSIS, p. 379.
✚ *For first aid see* p.804.

Consult your doctor.
Do not delay!
This may be an attack of ANGINA, p.376. *If pain persists after resting for 5 minutes, call your doctor immediately; you may be having a heart attack. See* CORONARY THROMBOSIS, p.379.
✚ *For first aid see* p.804.

Is the pain made worse by breathing in? — **YES**

NO

EMERGENCY
Get medical help now!
You may have a blood clot or a collapsed lung.
See PULMONARY EMBOLISM, p.406, *and* PNEUMOTHORAX, p.362.

1 *Go to next page, column 1*

2 *Go to next page, column 2*

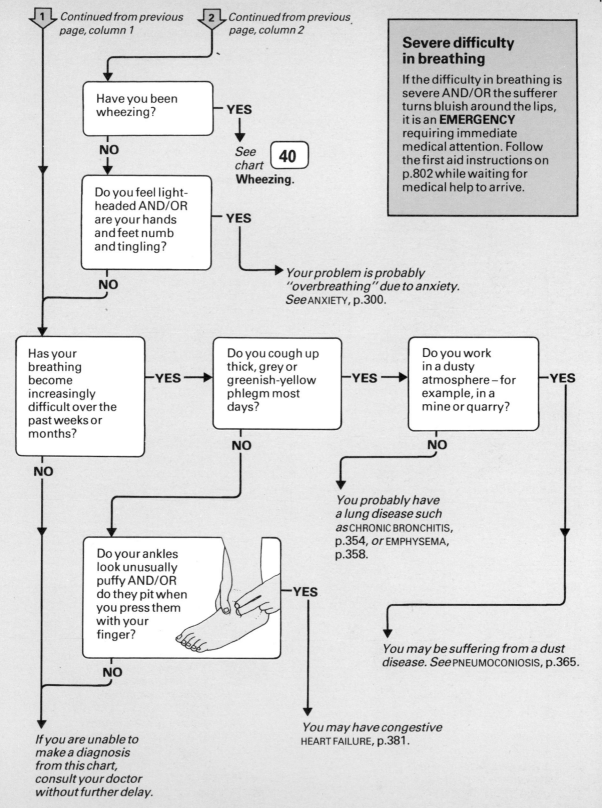

1 Continued from previous page, column 1

2 Continued from previous page, column 2

Have you been wheezing?

YES → See chart **40** Wheezing.

NO

Do you feel light-headed AND/OR are your hands and feet numb and tingling?

YES → Your problem is probably "overbreathing" due to anxiety. See ANXIETY, p.300.

NO

Severe difficulty in breathing

If the difficulty in breathing is severe AND/OR the sufferer turns bluish around the lips, it is an **EMERGENCY** requiring immediate medical attention. Follow the first aid instructions on p.802 while waiting for medical help to arrive.

Has your breathing become increasingly difficult over the past weeks or months?

YES → Do you cough up thick, grey or greenish-yellow phlegm most days?

YES → Do you work in a dusty atmosphere – for example, in a mine or quarry?

YES → You may be suffering from a dust disease. See PNEUMOCONIOSIS, p.365.

NO

NO → You probably have a lung disease such as CHRONIC BRONCHITIS, p.354, or EMPHYSEMA, p.358.

NO

Do your ankles look unusually puffy AND/OR do they pit when you press them with your finger?

YES → You may have congestive HEART FAILURE, p.381.

NO

If you are unable to make a diagnosis from this chart, consult your doctor without further delay.

42

GENERAL
all ages

Toothache

Pain coming from one tooth, or from the teeth and gums generally, felt either as a dull throb or a sharp twinge.

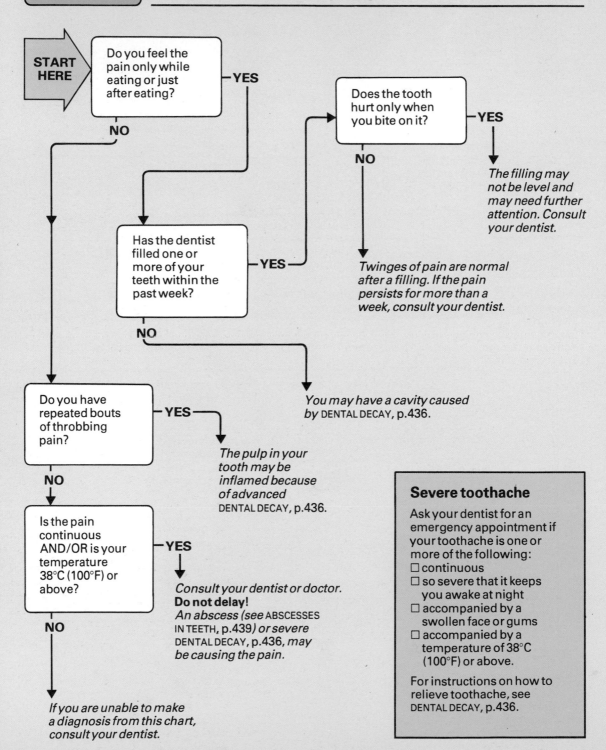

START HERE

Do you feel the pain only while eating or just after eating?
— **YES**
NO

Does the tooth hurt only when you bite on it?
— **YES**
NO

The filling may not be level and may need further attention. Consult your dentist.

Has the dentist filled one or more of your teeth within the past week?
— **YES**
NO

Twinges of pain are normal after a filling. If the pain persists for more than a week, consult your dentist.

You may have a cavity caused by DENTAL DECAY, p.436.

Do you have repeated bouts of throbbing pain?
— **YES**
NO

The pulp in your tooth may be inflamed because of advanced DENTAL DECAY, p.436.

Is the pain continuous AND/OR is your temperature 38°C (100°F) or above?
— **YES**
NO

Consult your dentist or doctor.
Do not delay!
An abscess (see ABSCESSES IN TEETH, p.439*) or severe* DENTAL DECAY, p.436, *may be causing the pain.*

If you are unable to make a diagnosis from this chart, consult your dentist.

Severe toothache

Ask your dentist for an emergency appointment if your toothache is one or more of the following:
☐ continuous
☐ so severe that it keeps you awake at night
☐ accompanied by a swollen face or gums
☐ accompanied by a temperature of 38°C (100°F) or above.

For instructions on how to relieve toothache, see DENTAL DECAY, p.436.

43

GENERAL
all ages

Difficulty in swallowing

Discomfort or pain when swallowing, or difficulty in making food go down at all.

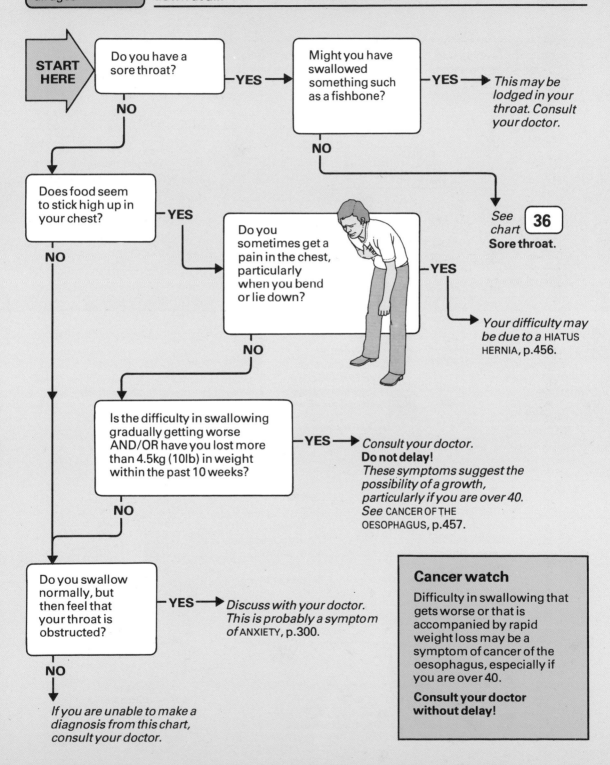

START HERE → Do you have a sore throat?

YES → Might you have swallowed something such as a fishbone? **YES** → *This may be lodged in your throat. Consult your doctor.*

NO

Does food seem to stick high up in your chest?

NO (from sore throat)
See chart **36** **Sore throat.**

YES → Do you sometimes get a pain in the chest, particularly when you bend or lie down? **YES** → *Your difficulty may be due to a* HIATUS HERNIA, *p.456.*

NO ↓

NO ↓

Is the difficulty in swallowing gradually getting worse AND/OR have you lost more than 4.5kg (10lb) in weight within the past 10 weeks?

YES → *Consult your doctor.* **Do not delay!** *These symptoms suggest the possibility of a growth, particularly if you are over 40. See* CANCER OF THE OESOPHAGUS, *p.457.*

NO ↓

Do you swallow normally, but then feel that your throat is obstructed?

YES → *Discuss with your doctor. This is probably a symptom of* ANXIETY, *p.300.*

NO ↓

If you are unable to make a diagnosis from this chart, consult your doctor.

Cancer watch

Difficulty in swallowing that gets worse or that is accompanied by rapid weight loss may be a symptom of cancer of the oesophagus, especially if you are over 40.

Consult your doctor without delay!

44

GENERAL
all ages

Sore mouth and/or tongue

Soreness anywhere inside the mouth and/or on or around the tongue and lips.

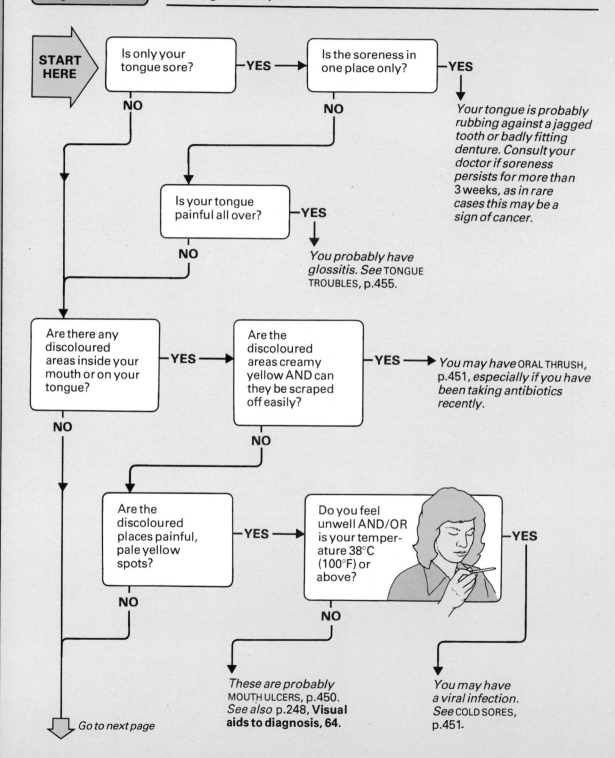

START HERE

Is only your tongue sore?

NO

YES →

Is the soreness in one place only?

NO

YES

Your tongue is probably rubbing against a jagged tooth or badly fitting denture. Consult your doctor if soreness persists for more than 3 weeks, as in rare cases this may be a sign of cancer.

Is your tongue painful all over?

NO

YES

You probably have glossitis. See TONGUE TROUBLES, p.455.

Are there any discoloured areas inside your mouth or on your tongue?

NO

YES →

Are the discoloured areas creamy yellow AND can they be scraped off easily?

NO

YES →

You may have ORAL THRUSH, p.451, *especially if you have been taking antibiotics recently.*

Are the discoloured places painful, pale yellow spots?

NO

YES →

Do you feel unwell AND/OR is your temperature 38°C (100°F) or above?

NO

YES

These are probably MOUTH ULCERS, p.450. *See also* p.248, **Visual aids to diagnosis, 64.**

You may have a viral infection. See COLD SORES, p.451.

⇩ *Go to next page*

Continued from previous page

Are your gums painful, red and swollen?

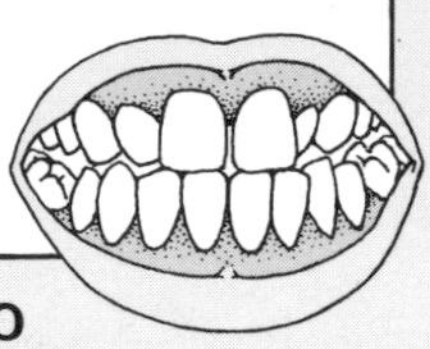

YES → Does your breath smell bad AND/OR do you have a foul, metallic taste in your mouth?

YES → *Consult your dentist. You may have* VINCENT'S DISEASE, p.452, *an infection of the gums.*

NO → *You may have severe* GINGIVITIS, p.445, *or a viral infection (see* COLD SORES, p.451).

NO

Do you have sore places on or around the lips?

YES → Are the sores red, rough, AND/OR blistered?

YES → *You probably have a* COLD SORE, p.451. *See also p.238,* **Visual aids to diagnosis, 24.**

NO

NO → Are there cracks at the corners of your mouth?

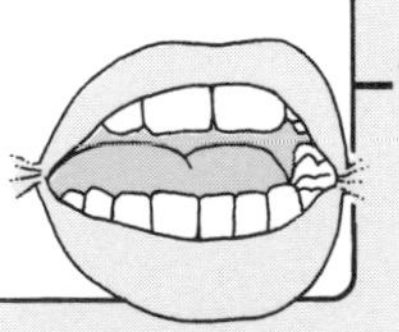

YES → *This soreness may be caused by badly fitting dentures (see* DENTURE PROBLEMS, p.443), *or by vitamin B$_{12}$ deficiency (see* VITAMINS, p.494).

NO

Have you recently started to use any new creams or cosmetics on your lips?

YES → *The soreness may be an allergic reaction to one of the ingredients. See* ECZEMA, p.253.

NO

If you are unable to make a diagnosis from this chart, consult your doctor.

Cancer watch

Any sore area in the mouth or on the tongue may indicate cancer if it fails to heal within 3 weeks.

Consult your doctor without delay!

45

GENERAL
all ages

Bad breath

Offensive-smelling breath of which you may be unaware unless it is mentioned by somebody else.

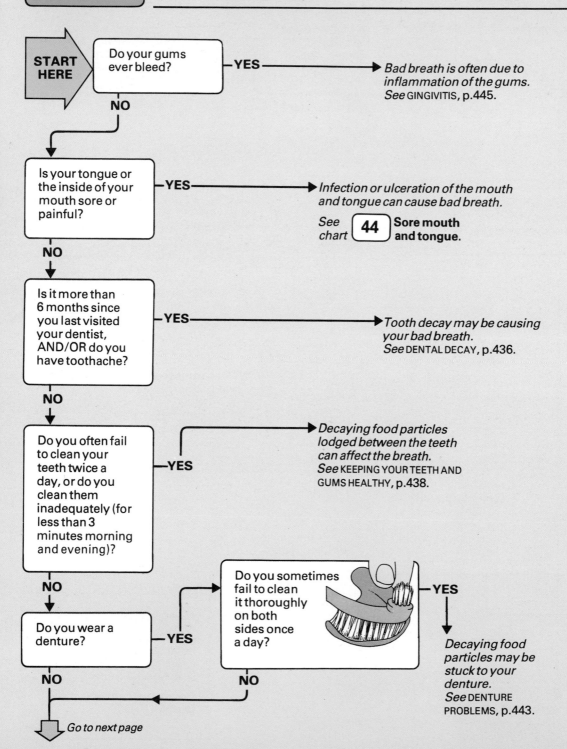

START HERE — Do your gums ever bleed? — **YES** → *Bad breath is often due to inflammation of the gums.* See GINGIVITIS, p.445.

NO ↓

Is your tongue or the inside of your mouth sore or painful? — **YES** → *Infection or ulceration of the mouth and tongue can cause bad breath.*

See chart **44** **Sore mouth and tongue.**

NO ↓

Is it more than 6 months since you last visited your dentist, AND/OR do you have toothache? — **YES** → *Tooth decay may be causing your bad breath.* See DENTAL DECAY, p.436.

NO ↓

Do you often fail to clean your teeth twice a day, or do you clean them inadequately (for less than 3 minutes morning and evening)? — **YES** → *Decaying food particles lodged between the teeth can affect the breath.* See KEEPING YOUR TEETH AND GUMS HEALTHY, p.438.

NO ↓

Do you wear a denture? — **YES** → Do you sometimes fail to clean it thoroughly on both sides once a day? — **YES** → *Decaying food particles may be stuck to your denture.* See DENTURE PROBLEMS, p.443.

NO ↓ **NO** ↓

Go to next page

Continued from previous page

Have you eaten garlic or onions, or drunk alcohol within the past 24 hours?

YES → *These things contain volatile substances which, absorbed into the bloodstream and then released into the lungs, may cause bad breath. Your breath should be back to normal in 24 hours.*

NO

Do you smoke?

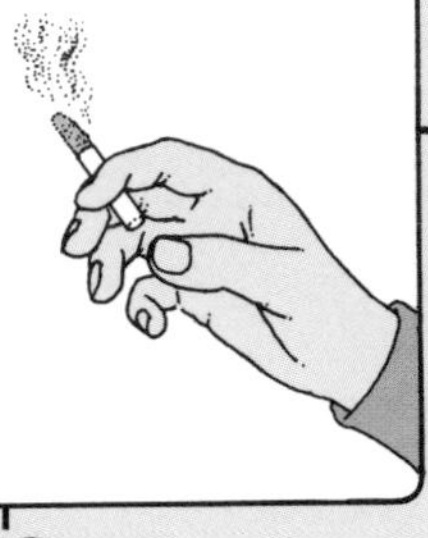

YES → *Smoking almost always causes bad breath.* See THE DANGERS OF SMOKING, p.38.

NO

Is your temperature 38°C (100°F) or above?

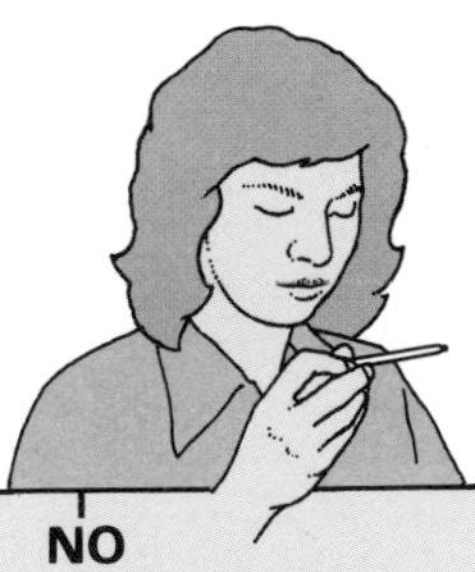

YES → *Bad breath often occurs with feverish illnesses.*

See chart **5** Fever.

For children

see chart **91** Fever in infants

or chart **92** Fever in children.

NO

Do you have a persistent cough that produces foul-smelling phlegm?

YES → *You may have BRONCHIECTASIS, p.363, a chronic lung disease.*

NO

Your bad breath is unlikely to be a symptom of an underlying disease. However, if it persists for more than 3 days, consult your doctor or dentist.

46

GENERAL
over 6 months

Vomiting

Throwing-up of stomach contents that may be preceded by nausea.
For babies under 6 months see chart 87, **Vomiting in infants**.

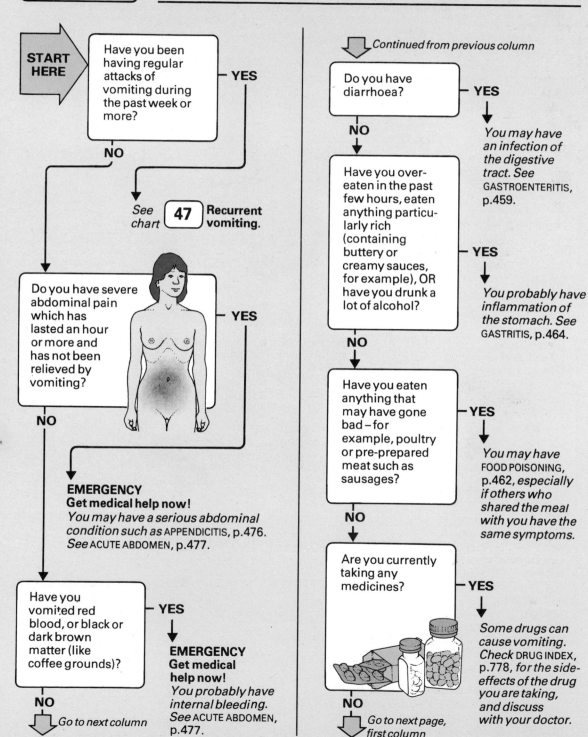

START HERE

Have you been having regular attacks of vomiting during the past week or more? — **YES**

NO

See chart **47** **Recurrent vomiting.**

Do you have severe abdominal pain which has lasted an hour or more and has not been relieved by vomiting? — **YES**

NO

EMERGENCY
Get medical help now!
You may have a serious abdominal condition such as APPENDICITIS, p.476.
See ACUTE ABDOMEN, p.477.

Have you vomited red blood, or black or dark brown matter (like coffee grounds)? — **YES**

NO
Go to next column

EMERGENCY
Get medical help now!
You probably have internal bleeding. See ACUTE ABDOMEN, p.477.

Continued from previous column

Do you have diarrhoea? — **YES**

NO

You may have an infection of the digestive tract. See GASTROENTERITIS, p.459.

Have you over-eaten in the past few hours, eaten anything particularly rich (containing buttery or creamy sauces, for example), OR have you drunk a lot of alcohol? — **YES**

NO

You probably have inflammation of the stomach. See GASTRITIS, p.464.

Have you eaten anything that may have gone bad – for example, poultry or pre-prepared meat such as sausages? — **YES**

NO

You may have FOOD POISONING, p.462, *especially if others who shared the meal with you have the same symptoms.*

Are you currently taking any medicines? — **YES**

NO
Go to next page, first column

Some drugs can cause vomiting. Check DRUG INDEX, p.778, *for the side-effects of the drug you are taking, and discuss with your doctor.*

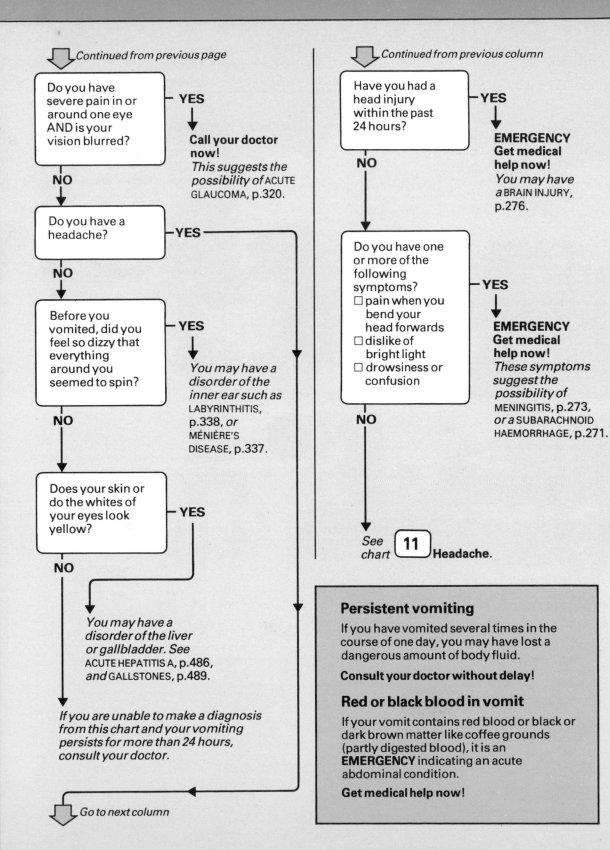

Continued from previous page

Do you have severe pain in or around one eye AND is your vision blurred?

YES →

Call your doctor now!
This suggests the possibility of ACUTE GLAUCOMA, p.320.

NO ↓

Do you have a headache?

YES →

NO ↓

Before you vomited, did you feel so dizzy that everything around you seemed to spin?

YES →

You may have a disorder of the inner ear such as LABYRINTHITIS, p.338, *or* MÉNIÈRE'S DISEASE, p.337.

NO ↓

Does your skin or do the whites of your eyes look yellow?

YES →

NO ↓

You may have a disorder of the liver or gallbladder. See ACUTE HEPATITIS A, p.486, *and* GALLSTONES, p.489.

If you are unable to make a diagnosis from this chart and your vomiting persists for more than 24 hours, consult your doctor.

Go to next column

Continued from previous column

Have you had a head injury within the past 24 hours?

YES →

EMERGENCY Get medical help now!
You may have a BRAIN INJURY, p.276.

NO ↓

Do you have one or more of the following symptoms?
☐ pain when you bend your head forwards
☐ dislike of bright light
☐ drowsiness or confusion

YES →

EMERGENCY Get medical help now!
These symptoms suggest the possibility of MENINGITIS, p.273, *or a* SUBARACHNOID HAEMORRHAGE, p.271.

NO ↓

See chart **11** Headache.

Persistent vomiting

If you have vomited several times in the course of one day, you may have lost a dangerous amount of body fluid.

Consult your doctor without delay!

Red or black blood in vomit

If your vomit contains red blood or black or dark brown matter like coffee grounds (partly digested blood), it is an **EMERGENCY** indicating an acute abdominal condition.

Get medical help now!

47

GENERAL
over 6 months

Recurrent vomiting

Throwing up of stomach contents several times in a week.
For babies under 6 months see chart 87, **Vomiting in infants**.

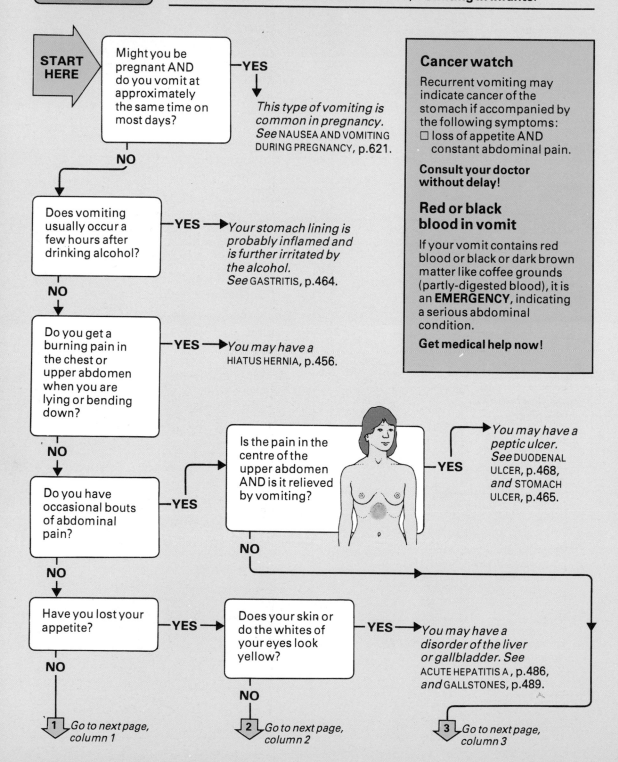

START HERE

Might you be pregnant AND do you vomit at approximately the same time on most days?

YES → *This type of vomiting is common in pregnancy.* See NAUSEA AND VOMITING DURING PREGNANCY, p.621.

NO

Does vomiting usually occur a few hours after drinking alcohol?

YES → *Your stomach lining is probably inflamed and is further irritated by the alcohol.* See GASTRITIS, p.464.

NO

Do you get a burning pain in the chest or upper abdomen when you are lying or bending down?

YES → *You may have a* HIATUS HERNIA, p.456.

NO

Do you have occasional bouts of abdominal pain?

YES → Is the pain in the centre of the upper abdomen AND is it relieved by vomiting?

YES → *You may have a peptic ulcer.* See DUODENAL ULCER, p.468, *and* STOMACH ULCER, p.465.

NO

NO

Have you lost your appetite?

YES → Does your skin or do the whites of your eyes look yellow?

YES → *You may have a disorder of the liver or gallbladder. See* ACUTE HEPATITIS A, p.486, *and* GALLSTONES, p.489.

NO

NO

1 ⬇ *Go to next page, column 1*

2 ⬇ *Go to next page, column 2*

3 ⬇ *Go to next page, column 3*

Cancer watch

Recurrent vomiting may indicate cancer of the stomach if accompanied by the following symptoms:
☐ loss of appetite AND constant abdominal pain.

Consult your doctor without delay!

Red or black blood in vomit

If your vomit contains red blood or black or dark brown matter like coffee grounds (partly-digested blood), it is an **EMERGENCY**, indicating a serious abdominal condition.

Get medical help now!

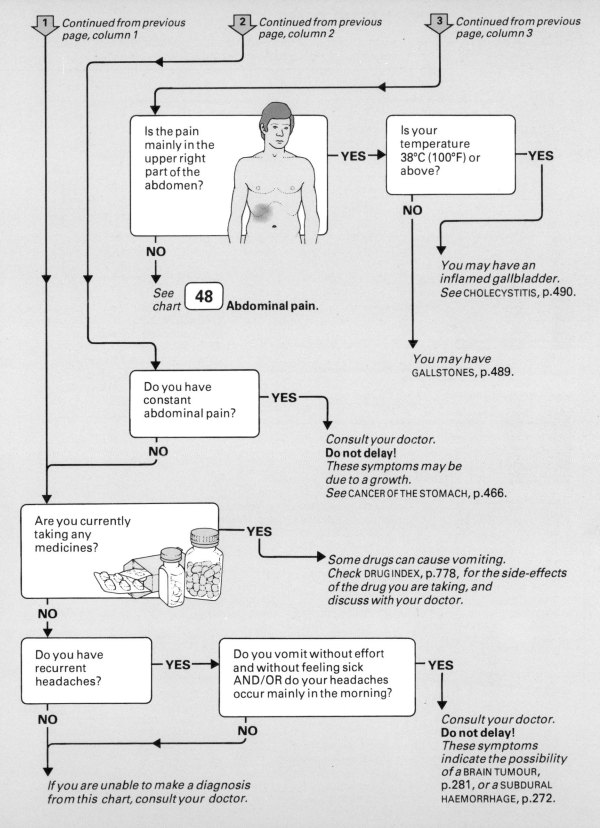

48

Abdominal pain

General or localized pain between the bottom of the ribcage and the groin. For children see chart 93, **Abdominal pain in children**.

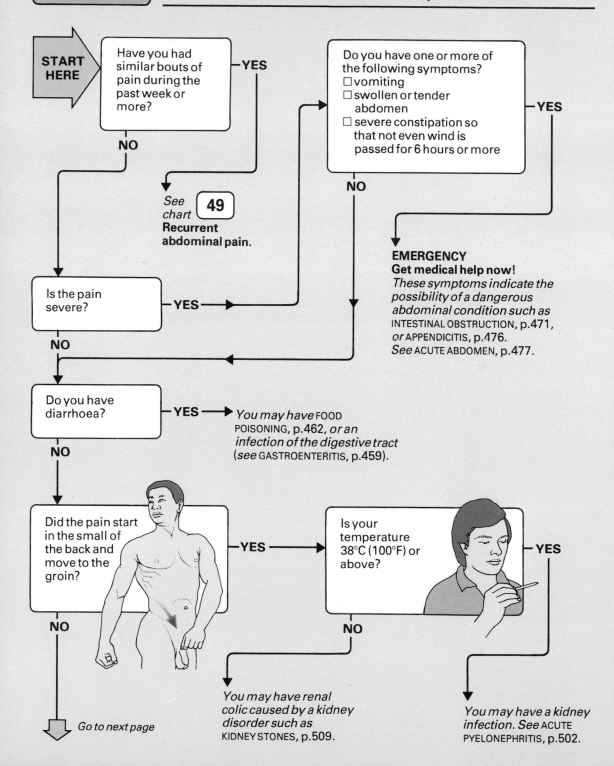

START HERE

Have you had similar bouts of pain during the past week or more?

YES → *See chart* **49** **Recurrent abdominal pain.**

NO ↓

Do you have one or more of the following symptoms?
☐ vomiting
☐ swollen or tender abdomen
☐ severe constipation so that not even wind is passed for 6 hours or more

YES →

NO ↓

Is the pain severe? — **YES** →

NO ↓

**EMERGENCY
Get medical help now!**
These symptoms indicate the possibility of a dangerous abdominal condition such as INTESTINAL OBSTRUCTION, p.471, *or* APPENDICITIS, p.476.
See ACUTE ABDOMEN, p.477.

Do you have diarrhoea? — **YES** →

You may have FOOD POISONING, p.462, *or an infection of the digestive tract* (*see* GASTROENTERITIS, p.459).

NO ↓

Did the pain start in the small of the back and move to the groin? — **YES** →

Is your temperature 38°C (100°F) or above? — **YES** →

NO ↓

You may have renal colic caused by a kidney disorder such as KIDNEY STONES, p.509.

NO ↓

You may have a kidney infection. See ACUTE PYELONEPHRITIS, p.502.

NO ↓
Go to next page

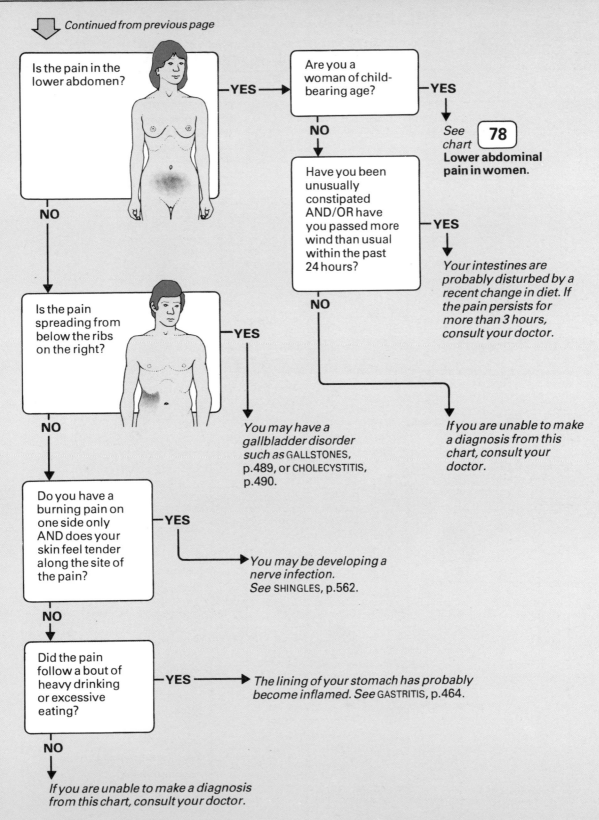

Continued from previous page

Is the pain in the lower abdomen? → **YES** → **Are you a woman of child-bearing age?** → **YES** → See chart **78** **Lower abdominal pain in women.**

NO (below "Are you a woman of child-bearing age?")

↓

Have you been unusually constipated AND/OR have you passed more wind than usual within the past 24 hours? → **YES** → *Your intestines are probably disturbed by a recent change in diet. If the pain persists for more than 3 hours, consult your doctor.*

NO (below the constipation box)

↓

If you are unable to make a diagnosis from this chart, consult your doctor.

NO (below "Is the pain in the lower abdomen?")

↓

Is the pain spreading from below the ribs on the right? → **YES** → *You may have a gallbladder disorder such as* GALLSTONES, *p.489, or* CHOLECYSTITIS, *p.490.*

NO

↓

Do you have a burning pain on one side only AND does your skin feel tender along the site of the pain? → **YES** → *You may be developing a nerve infection.* *See* SHINGLES, *p.562.*

NO

↓

Did the pain follow a bout of heavy drinking or excessive eating? → **YES** → *The lining of your stomach has probably become inflamed. See* GASTRITIS, *p.464.*

NO

↓

If you are unable to make a diagnosis from this chart, consult your doctor.

49

Recurrent abdominal pain

Abdominal pain that has recurred on several days over a week or more. For children see chart 93, **Abdominal pain in children.**

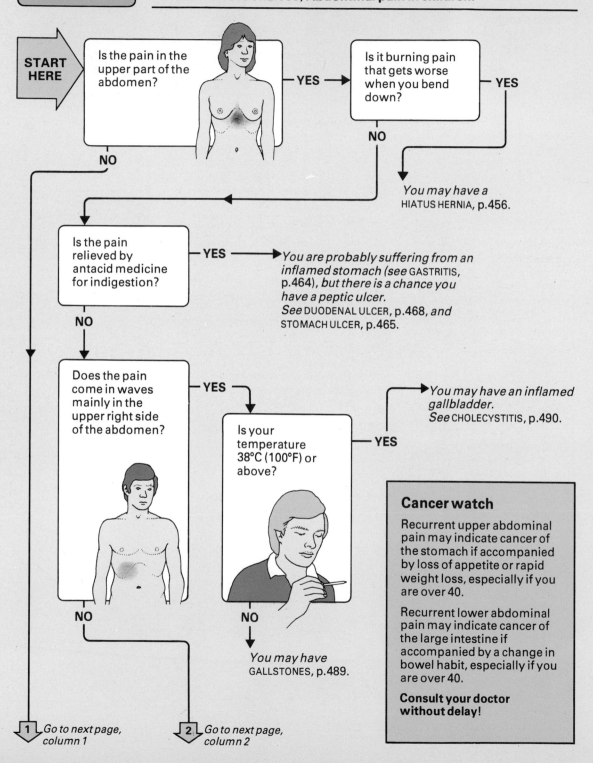

START HERE

Is the pain in the upper part of the abdomen?

YES → Is it burning pain that gets worse when you bend down? → **YES**

NO

NO

You may have a HIATUS HERNIA, p.456.

Is the pain relieved by antacid medicine for indigestion?

YES → *You are probably suffering from an inflamed stomach (see* GASTRITIS, p.464), *but there is a chance you have a peptic ulcer. See* DUODENAL ULCER, p.468, *and* STOMACH ULCER, p.465.

NO

Does the pain come in waves mainly in the upper right side of the abdomen?

YES → Is your temperature 38°C (100°F) or above? → **YES**

You may have an inflamed gallbladder. See CHOLECYSTITIS, p.490.

NO

NO

You may have GALLSTONES, p.489.

Cancer watch

Recurrent upper abdominal pain may indicate cancer of the stomach if accompanied by loss of appetite or rapid weight loss, especially if you are over 40.

Recurrent lower abdominal pain may indicate cancer of the large intestine if accompanied by a change in bowel habit, especially if you are over 40.

Consult your doctor without delay!

1 *Go to next page, column 1*

2 *Go to next page, column 2*

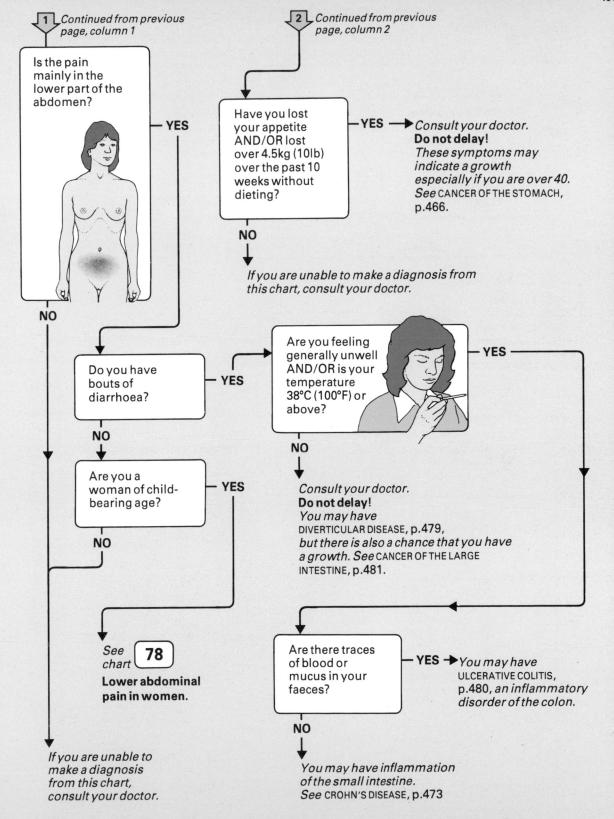

1 Continued from previous page, column 1

2 Continued from previous page, column 2

Is the pain mainly in the lower part of the abdomen?

YES

NO

Have you lost your appetite AND/OR lost over 4.5kg (10lb) over the past 10 weeks without dieting?

YES → *Consult your doctor.* **Do not delay!** *These symptoms may indicate a growth especially if you are over 40. See* CANCER OF THE STOMACH, p.466.

NO

If you are unable to make a diagnosis from this chart, consult your doctor.

Do you have bouts of diarrhoea?

YES

NO

Are you feeling generally unwell AND/OR is your temperature 38°C (100°F) or above?

YES

NO

Consult your doctor. **Do not delay!** *You may have* DIVERTICULAR DISEASE, p.479, *but there is also a chance that you have a growth. See* CANCER OF THE LARGE INTESTINE, p.481.

Are you a woman of child-bearing age?

YES

NO

See chart **78**

Lower abdominal pain in women.

Are there traces of blood or mucus in your faeces?

YES → *You may have* ULCERATIVE COLITIS, p.480, *an inflammatory disorder of the colon.*

NO

If you are unable to make a diagnosis from this chart, consult your doctor.

You may have inflammation of the small intestine. See CROHN'S DISEASE, p.473

50

GENERAL
all ages

Swollen abdomen

Generalized swelling over the whole abdomen between the bottom of the ribcage and the groin.

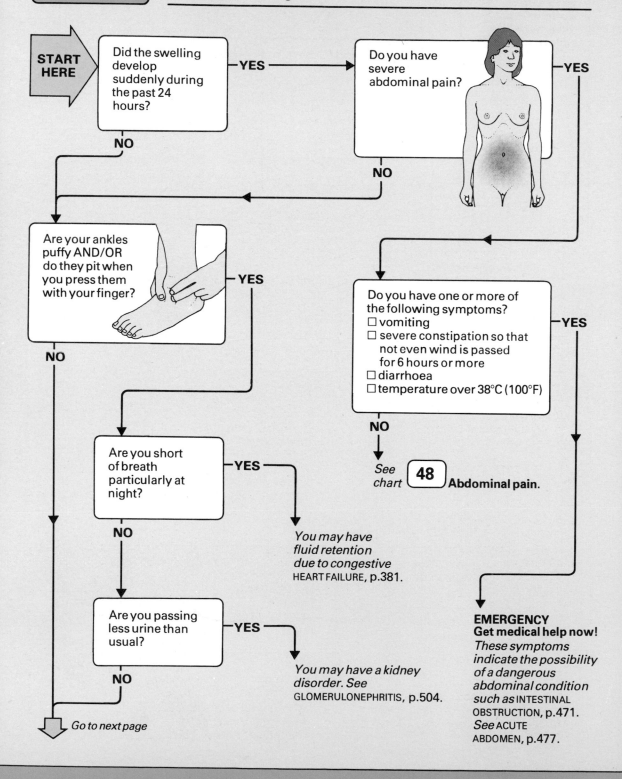

START HERE → Did the swelling develop suddenly during the past 24 hours? — **YES** → Do you have severe abdominal pain? — **YES** →

NO (from "Did the swelling develop suddenly")

NO (from "Do you have severe abdominal pain?")

Are your ankles puffy AND/OR do they pit when you press them with your finger? — **YES** →

NO

Do you have one or more of the following symptoms?
☐ vomiting
☐ severe constipation so that not even wind is passed for 6 hours or more
☐ diarrhoea
☐ temperature over 38°C (100°F)
— **YES** →

NO →

See chart **48** **Abdominal pain**.

Are you short of breath particularly at night? — **YES** →

NO

You may have fluid retention due to congestive HEART FAILURE, p.381.

Are you passing less urine than usual? — **YES** →

NO

You may have a kidney disorder. See GLOMERULONEPHRITIS, p.504.

⬇ *Go to next page*

EMERGENCY
Get medical help now!
These symptoms indicate the possibility of a dangerous abdominal condition such as INTESTINAL OBSTRUCTION, p.471. *See* ACUTE ABDOMEN, p.477.

Continued from previous page

Does your skin or do the whites of your eyes look yellow? —**YES**→ *Consult your doctor.* **Do not delay!** *This suggests a liver disorder such as* CIRRHOSIS OF THE LIVER, p.487.

NO

Are you a woman of child-bearing age? —**YES**→ **Might you be more than 3 months pregnant?** —**YES**→ *Consult your doctor, who will be able to determine whether you are pregnant.* See GENERAL PROBLEMS OF PREGNANCY, p.620.

NO

NO

Did the swelling develop just before or during your period? —**YES**→ *Many women get a swollen abdomen at this time. See* PREMENSTRUAL TENSION, p.585.

NO

Do you suffer from persistent constipation? —**YES**→ *Constipation sometimes causes a swollen abdomen.* See CONSTIPATION AND DIARRHOEA, p.474.

NO

Are you over-weight according to the chart on p.28 AND is your navel deeply sunken? —**YES**→ *Your problem is probably* OBESITY, p.492.

NO

If you are unable to make a diagnosis from this chart and your abdomen remains swollen for more than 2 days, consult your doctor.

Painful swollen abdomen

It is an **EMERGENCY** requiring immediate hospital treatment, if a swollen abdomen is accompanied by severe pain AND one or more of the following symptoms:
☐ vomiting
☐ severe constipation so that not even wind is passed for 6 hours or more
☐ temperature over 38°C (100°F)
☐ diarrhoea.

51

GENERAL
all ages

Wind

The expulsion of air from the digestive tract through the mouth or anus (also called flatulence).

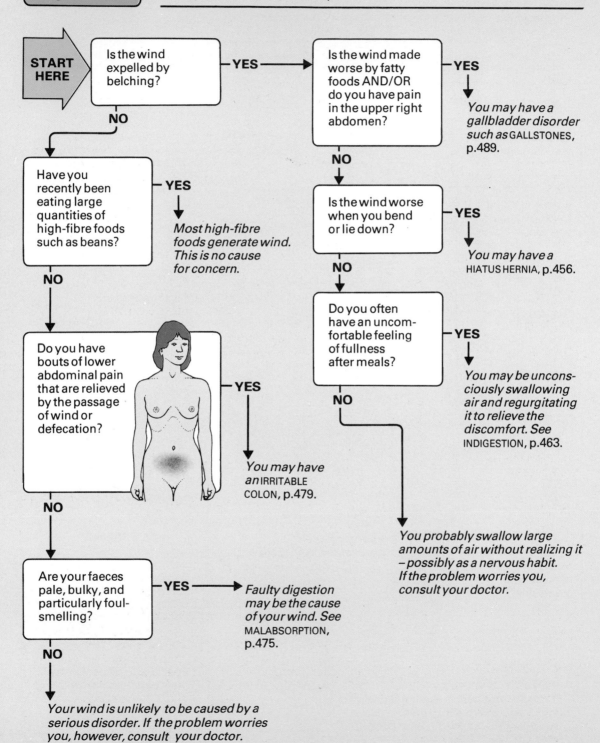

START HERE → Is the wind expelled by belching?

— **YES** → Is the wind made worse by fatty foods AND/OR do you have pain in the upper right abdomen?

— **YES** → *You may have a gallbladder disorder such as* GALLSTONES, p.489.

NO (from belching) ↓

Have you recently been eating large quantities of high-fibre foods such as beans?

— **YES** → *Most high-fibre foods generate wind. This is no cause for concern.*

NO ↓

Do you have bouts of lower abdominal pain that are relieved by the passage of wind or defecation?

— **YES** → *You may have an* IRRITABLE COLON, p.479.

NO ↓

Are your faeces pale, bulky, and particularly foul-smelling?

— **YES** → *Faulty digestion may be the cause of your wind. See* MALABSORPTION, p.475.

NO ↓

Your wind is unlikely to be caused by a serious disorder. If the problem worries you, however, consult your doctor.

Is the wind made worse by fatty foods AND/OR do you have pain in the upper right abdomen?

NO ↓

Is the wind worse when you bend or lie down?

— **YES** → *You may have a* HIATUS HERNIA, p.456.

NO ↓

Do you often have an uncomfortable feeling of fullness after meals?

— **YES** → *You may be unconsciously swallowing air and regurgitating it to relieve the discomfort. See* INDIGESTION, p.463.

NO ↓

You probably swallow large amounts of air without realizing it – possibly as a nervous habit. If the problem worries you, consult your doctor.

52
GENERAL
over 6 months

Diarrhoea
Frequent passing of unusually loose and runny faeces.
For babies under 6 months see chart 88, **Diarrhoea in infants**.

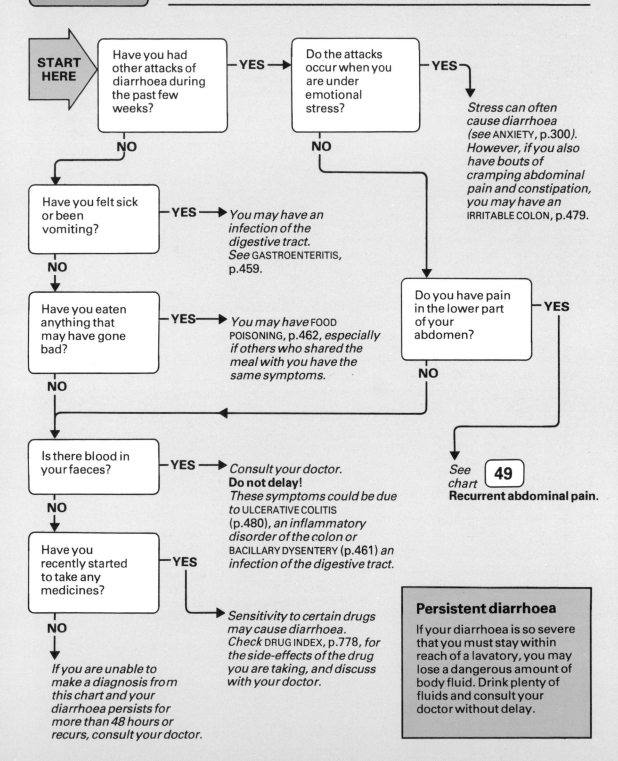

START HERE

Have you had other attacks of diarrhoea during the past few weeks? — **YES** → **Do the attacks occur when you are under emotional stress?** — **YES** →

Stress can often cause diarrhoea (see ANXIETY, p.300). *However, if you also have bouts of cramping abdominal pain and constipation, you may have an* IRRITABLE COLON, p.479.

NO ↓ (first question)

NO ↓ (second question)

Have you felt sick or been vomiting? — **YES** → *You may have an infection of the digestive tract. See* GASTROENTERITIS, p.459.

NO ↓

Have you eaten anything that may have gone bad? — **YES** → *You may have* FOOD POISONING, p.462, *especially if others who shared the meal with you have the same symptoms.*

NO ↓

Do you have pain in the lower part of your abdomen? — **YES** →

NO ↓

Is there blood in your faeces? — **YES** → *Consult your doctor.* **Do not delay!** *These symptoms could be due to* ULCERATIVE COLITIS (p.480), *an inflammatory disorder of the colon or* BACILLARY DYSENTERY (p.461) *an infection of the digestive tract.*

NO ↓

See chart **49**
Recurrent abdominal pain.

Have you recently started to take any medicines? — **YES** → *Sensitivity to certain drugs may cause diarrhoea. Check* DRUG INDEX, p.778, *for the side-effects of the drug you are taking, and discuss with your doctor.*

NO ↓

If you are unable to make a diagnosis from this chart and your diarrhoea persists for more than 48 hours or recurs, consult your doctor.

Persistent diarrhoea
If your diarrhoea is so severe that you must stay within reach of a lavatory, you may lose a dangerous amount of body fluid. Drink plenty of fluids and consult your doctor without delay.

Constipation

Infrequent or difficult passing of hard faeces.

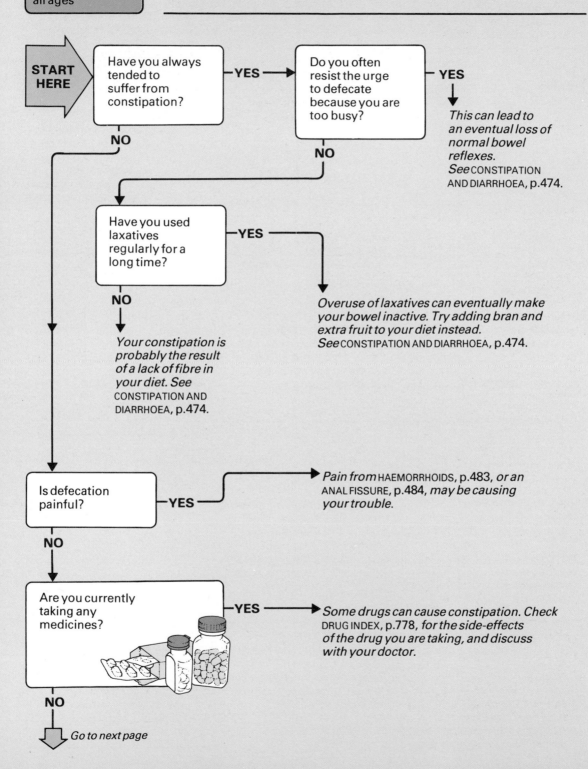

START HERE

Have you always tended to suffer from constipation? — **YES** → **Do you often resist the urge to defecate because you are too busy?** — **YES** ↓

This can lead to an eventual loss of normal bowel reflexes. See CONSTIPATION AND DIARRHOEA, p.474.

NO ↓ (from first box)

NO ↓ (from second box)

Have you used laxatives regularly for a long time? — **YES** →

Overuse of laxatives can eventually make your bowel inactive. Try adding bran and extra fruit to your diet instead. See CONSTIPATION AND DIARRHOEA, p.474.

NO ↓

Your constipation is probably the result of a lack of fibre in your diet. See CONSTIPATION AND DIARRHOEA, p.474.

Is defecation painful? — **YES** →

Pain from HAEMORRHOIDS, p.483, *or an* ANAL FISSURE, p.484, *may be causing your trouble.*

NO ↓

Are you currently taking any medicines? — **YES** →

Some drugs can cause constipation. Check DRUG INDEX, p.778, *for the side-effects of the drug you are taking, and discuss with your doctor.*

NO ↓

Go to next page

Continued from previous page

Are you dieting, or could your diet be short of high-fibre foods such as fruit, vegetables, or wholemeal bread?

YES

There may be insufficient bulk in your diet to stimulate proper bowel action. See EATING AND DRINKING SENSIBLY, p.24.

NO

Are you pregnant?

YES

This trouble is common in pregnancy. See CONSTIPATION DURING PREGNANCY, p.623.

NO

Do you have two or more of the following symptoms?
☐ feeling the cold more than you used to
☐ dry skin or hair
☐ unexplained weight gain
☐ inexplicable tiredness

YES

You may have an underactive thyroid gland. See HYPOTHYROIDISM, p.526.

NO

Do you have lower abdominal pain?

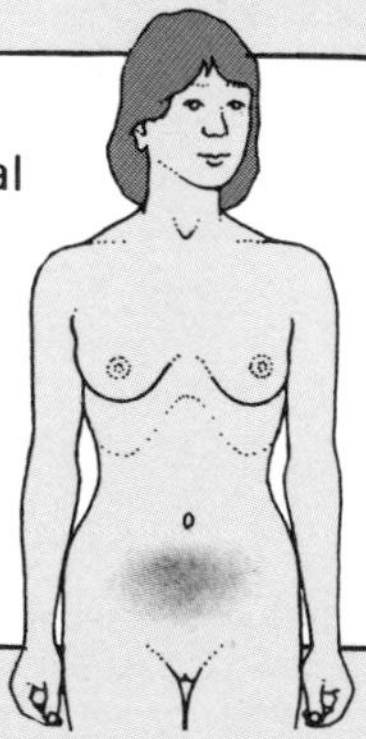

YES

Have you had similar episodes of pain and constipation for many years?

YES → *You probably have an* IRRITABLE COLON, p.479.

NO

Consult your doctor.
Do not delay!
You may have DIVERTICULAR DISEASE, p.479, *but there is a chance that you may have a growth. See* CANCER OF THE LARGE INTESTINE, p.481.

NO

If you are unable to make a diagnosis from this chart and your constipation persists for more than 2 weeks, or if you do not pass any faeces for a week or more, consult your doctor.

Cancer watch

Prolonged attacks of constipation after years of regularity, especially in those over 40, may indicate cancer of the large intestine.

Consult your doctor without delay!

54

Abnormal-looking faeces

Passing faeces that are unusually coloured.

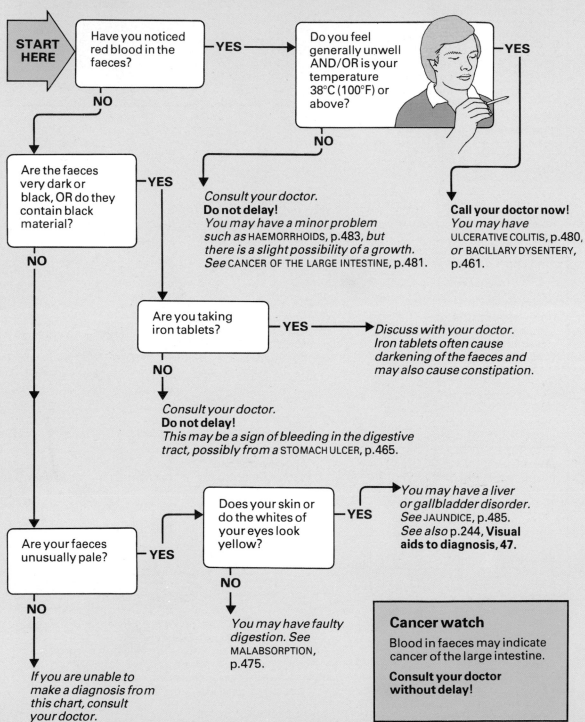

START HERE

Have you noticed red blood in the faeces?

YES →

Do you feel generally unwell AND/OR is your temperature 38°C (100°F) or above?

YES →

Call your doctor now!
You may have ULCERATIVE COLITIS, p.480, *or* BACILLARY DYSENTERY, p.461.

NO ↓ (from "Have you noticed red blood")

NO ↓ (from "Do you feel generally unwell")

Consult your doctor.
Do not delay!
You may have a minor problem such as HAEMORRHOIDS, p.483, *but there is a slight possibility of a growth. See* CANCER OF THE LARGE INTESTINE, p.481.

Are the faeces very dark or black, OR do they contain black material?

YES ↓

Are you taking iron tablets?

YES →

Discuss with your doctor. Iron tablets often cause darkening of the faeces and may also cause constipation.

NO ↓

Consult your doctor.
Do not delay!
This may be a sign of bleeding in the digestive tract, possibly from a STOMACH ULCER, p.465.

NO ↓ (from "Are the faeces very dark")

Are your faeces unusually pale?

YES →

Does your skin or do the whites of your eyes look yellow?

YES →

You may have a liver or gallbladder disorder. See JAUNDICE, p.485. *See also* p.244, **Visual aids to diagnosis, 47.**

NO ↓

You may have faulty digestion. See MALABSORPTION, p.475.

NO ↓ (from "Are your faeces unusually pale")

If you are unable to make a diagnosis from this chart, consult your doctor.

Cancer watch

Blood in faeces may indicate cancer of the large intestine.

Consult your doctor without delay!

55

GENERAL
all ages

Palpitations

A feeling that your heart is beating irregularly, more strongly, or more rapidly than normal.

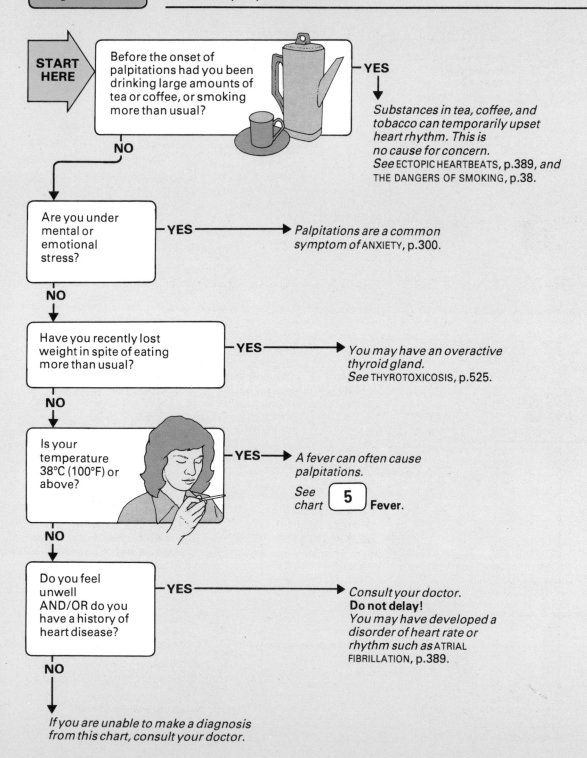

START HERE

Before the onset of palpitations had you been drinking large amounts of tea or coffee, or smoking more than usual?

YES

Substances in tea, coffee, and tobacco can temporarily upset heart rhythm. This is no cause for concern.
See ECTOPIC HEARTBEATS, p.389, *and* THE DANGERS OF SMOKING, p.38.

NO

Are you under mental or emotional stress?

YES

Palpitations are a common symptom of ANXIETY, p.300.

NO

Have you recently lost weight in spite of eating more than usual?

YES

You may have an overactive thyroid gland.
See THYROTOXICOSIS, p.525.

NO

Is your temperature 38°C (100°F) or above?

YES

A fever can often cause palpitations.

See chart **5** Fever.

NO

Do you feel unwell AND/OR do you have a history of heart disease?

YES

Consult your doctor.
Do not delay!
You may have developed a disorder of heart rate or rhythm such as ATRIAL FIBRILLATION, p.389.

NO

If you are unable to make a diagnosis from this chart, consult your doctor.

56

GENERAL
all ages

Chest pain

Pain anywhere between the neck and the bottom of the ribcage which may be dull and persistent, stabbing, burning, or crushing.

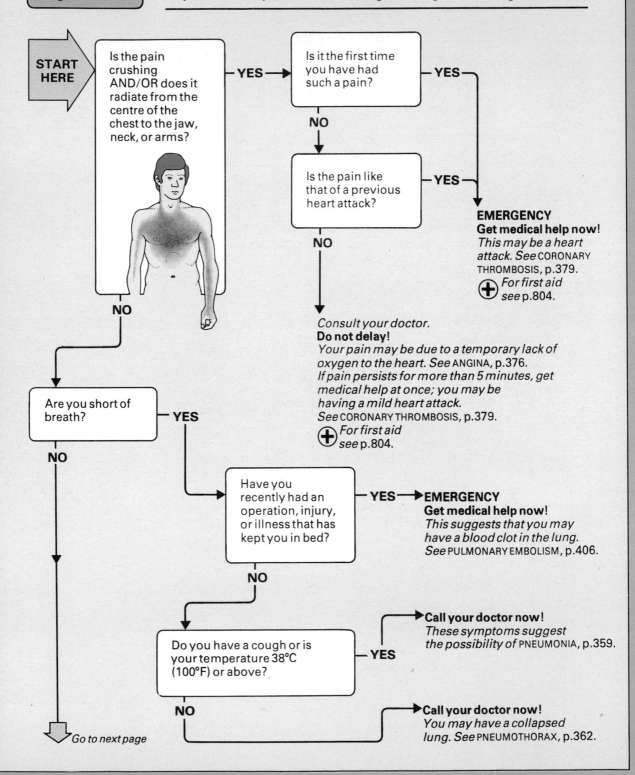

START HERE

Is the pain crushing AND/OR does it radiate from the centre of the chest to the jaw, neck, or arms?

YES → Is it the first time you have had such a pain? — **YES**

NO ↓

Is the pain like that of a previous heart attack? — **YES**

NO ↓

EMERGENCY
Get medical help now!
This may be a heart attack. See CORONARY THROMBOSIS, p.379.
✚ *For first aid see p.804.*

Consult your doctor.
Do not delay!
Your pain may be due to a temporary lack of oxygen to the heart. See ANGINA, p.376.
If pain persists for more than 5 minutes, get medical help at once; you may be having a mild heart attack.
See CORONARY THROMBOSIS, p.379.
✚ *For first aid see p.804.*

NO ↓

Are you short of breath? — **YES**

NO ↓

Have you recently had an operation, injury, or illness that has kept you in bed? — **YES** → **EMERGENCY**
Get medical help now!
This suggests that you may have a blood clot in the lung.
See PULMONARY EMBOLISM, p.406.

NO ↓

Do you have a cough or is your temperature 38°C (100°F) or above? — **YES** → **Call your doctor now!**
These symptoms suggest the possibility of PNEUMONIA, p.359.

NO ↓

→ **Call your doctor now!**
You may have a collapsed lung. See PNEUMOTHORAX, p.362.

Go to next page

⬇ *Continued from previous page*

Have you coughed up greyish-yellow phlegm? —— **YES** ——▶ *You may have an infection of the airways in the lung. See* ACUTE BRONCHITIS, *p.353.*

NO ⬇

Is it a burning pain that worsens when you bend or lie down? —— **YES** ——▶ *You may have a* HIATUS HERNIA, *p.456.*

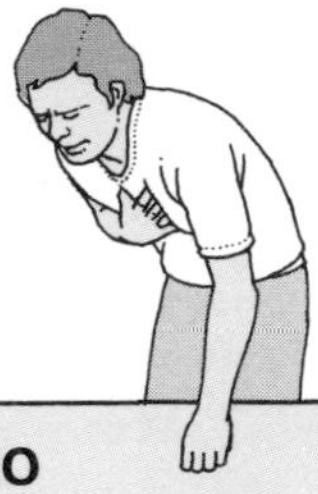

NO ⬇

See chart **43** **Difficulty in swallowing.**

Is the pain worse when you swallow? —— **YES** ——▶

NO ⬇

Is the pain on one side only? —— **YES** ——▶ **Have you recently had a chest injury OR a severe cough?** —— **YES** ——▶ *You may have a* PULLED MUSCLE, *p.532, or a broken rib (see* FRACTURE, *p.534).*

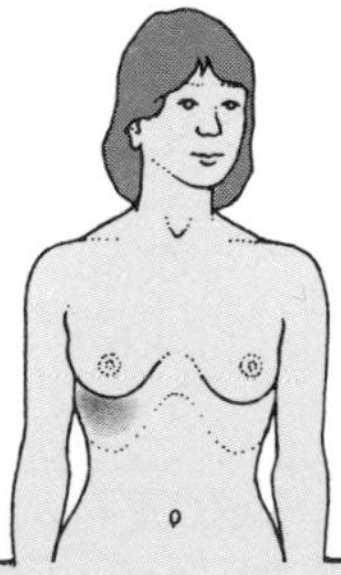

NO ⬇

Does the pain cause a burning feeling in the skin AND is it unaffected by breathing? —— **YES** ——▶ *You may have a nerve infection. See* SHINGLES, *p.562.*

NO ⬇

NO ⬇

If you are unable to make a diagnosis from this chart, consult your doctor without further delay.

57
GENERAL
all ages

Abnormally frequent urination

Feeling the urge to urinate more often than usual, even though little urine may be passed.

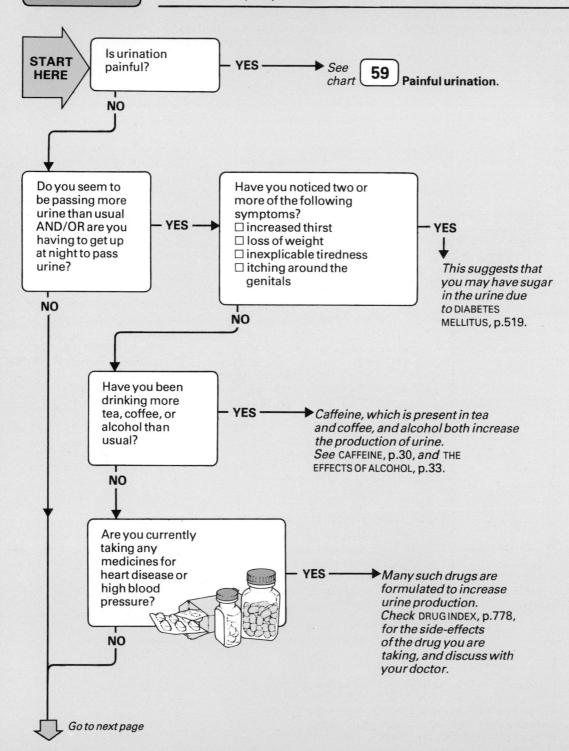

START HERE → Is urination painful? — **YES** → *See chart* **59** **Painful urination**.

NO ↓

Do you seem to be passing more urine than usual AND/OR are you having to get up at night to pass urine? — **YES** → Have you noticed two or more of the following symptoms?
☐ increased thirst
☐ loss of weight
☐ inexplicable tiredness
☐ itching around the genitals — **YES** ↓

This suggests that you may have sugar in the urine due to DIABETES MELLITUS, p.519.

NO (under first box) ↓

NO (under symptoms box) ↓

Have you been drinking more tea, coffee, or alcohol than usual? — **YES** → *Caffeine, which is present in tea and coffee, and alcohol both increase the production of urine. See* CAFFEINE, p.30, *and* THE EFFECTS OF ALCOHOL, p.33.

NO ↓

Are you currently taking any medicines for heart disease or high blood pressure? — **YES** → *Many such drugs are formulated to increase urine production. Check* DRUG INDEX, p.778, *for the side-effects of the drug you are taking, and discuss with your doctor.*

NO ↓

Go to next page

↓ *Continued from previous page*

Is the weather very cold OR are you unusually anxious or excited? — **YES** → *Cold or excitement can cause frequent urination. This is no cause for concern.*

NO ↓

Are you a woman? — **YES** → **Are you pregnant?** — **YES** → *Increased frequency of urination is common in the first three and the last three months of pregnancy. This is unlikely to be a cause for concern.*

NO ↓ (under Are you a woman?)

NO ↓ (under Are you pregnant?)

Are you over 55? — **YES**

NO ↓

Do you have two or more of the following symptoms?
☐ waking to pass urine at night
☐ difficulty in starting to urinate
☐ weak stream
☐ leakage of urine after urination
— **YES** ↓ *You may have a disorder of the prostate gland. See* ENLARGED PROSTATE, p.574.

NO

Do you sometimes have a strong urge to urinate followed swiftly by an uncontrollable leakage of urine? — **YES** ↓ *This is probably "urge incontinence" caused by an* IRRITABLE BLADDER, p.601.

NO

Do you have difficulty in controlling your bladder? — **YES** → *See chart* **60** **Lack of bladder control.**

NO ↓

If you are unable to make a diagnosis from this chart, the increased frequency of passing urine is unlikely to be a cause for concern. Consult your doctor if the increase is such that it wakes you at night or continues for more than a week.

Abnormal-looking urine

Urine that differs from the usual straw colour, or that is cloudy or blood-stained.

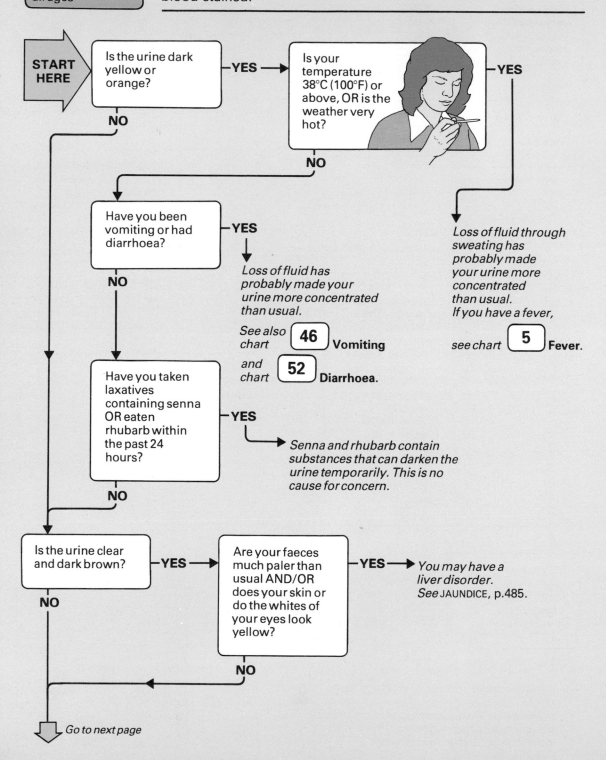

START HERE

Is the urine dark yellow or orange? — **YES** → Is your temperature 38°C (100°F) or above, OR is the weather very hot? — **YES** →

NO

NO

Loss of fluid through sweating has probably made your urine more concentrated than usual.
If you have a fever, see chart **5** Fever.

Have you been vomiting or had diarrhoea? — **YES** →

NO

Loss of fluid has probably made your urine more concentrated than usual.

See also chart **46** *Vomiting*

and chart **52** *Diarrhoea.*

Have you taken laxatives containing senna OR eaten rhubarb within the past 24 hours? — **YES** →

NO

Senna and rhubarb contain substances that can darken the urine temporarily. This is no cause for concern.

Is the urine clear and dark brown? — **YES** → Are your faeces much paler than usual AND/OR does your skin or do the whites of your eyes look yellow? — **YES** → You may have a liver disorder. See JAUNDICE, p.485.

NO

NO

⬇ *Go to next page*

⬇ *Continued from previous page*

Is urination painful? ──**YES**──▶ *See chart* **59** **Painful urination**.

NO

↓

Is the urine pink, red, or smoky-brown? ──**YES**──▶ **Have you started to take any new medicines within the past 24 hours?** ──**YES**

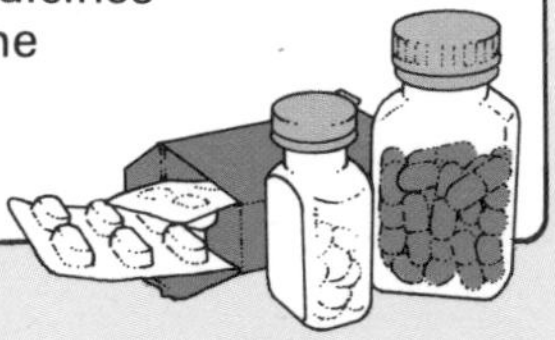

↓

Some drugs can colour the urine. Check DRUG INDEX, *p. 778, for the side-effects of the drug you are taking, and discuss with your doctor.*

NO (under first box)

NO (under medicines box)

↓

Have you eaten beetroot, blackberries, or any foods containing red colouring within the past 24 hours? ──**YES**──▶

Many artificial food dyes and some natural colourings can pass into the urine. This is no cause for concern.

NO

↓

Consult your doctor.
Do not delay!
You may have a urinary-tract disorder such as CYSTITIS (p.505) *or, if you are a man, an* ENLARGED PROSTATE (p.574).
However, there is a slight chance that you have a TUMOUR OF THE KIDNEY (p.508) *or a* TUMOUR OF THE BLADDER (p.508).

Is your urine green or blue? ──**YES**──▶ *The colour is almost certainly due to artificial colouring in food or medicines and is no cause for concern.*

NO

↓

If you are unable to make a diagnosis from this chart, consult your doctor.

Cancer watch

If you pass pink, red, or smoky-brown urine, for no obvious reason, you may have kidney or bladder cancer.

Consult your doctor without delay!

59

GENERAL
all ages

Painful urination

Discomfort when passing urine which may be accompanied by pain in the lower abdomen or urinary passage.

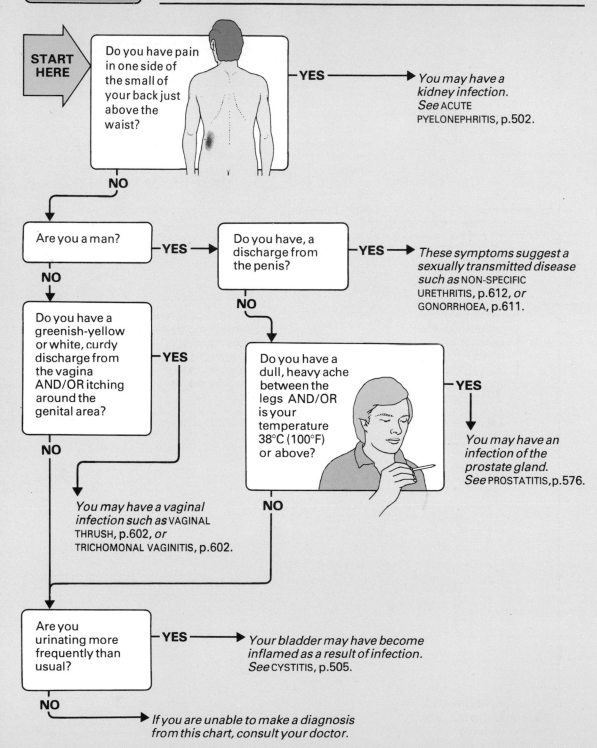

START HERE

Do you have pain in one side of the small of your back just above the waist? — **YES** → *You may have a kidney infection.* See ACUTE PYELONEPHRITIS, p.502.

NO

Are you a man? — **YES** → **Do you have, a discharge from the penis?** — **YES** → *These symptoms suggest a sexually transmitted disease such as* NON-SPECIFIC URETHRITIS, p.612, *or* GONORRHOEA, p.611.

NO

NO

Do you have a greenish-yellow or white, curdy discharge from the vagina AND/OR itching around the genital area? — **YES** → *You may have a vaginal infection such as* VAGINAL THRUSH, p.602, *or* TRICHOMONAL VAGINITIS, p.602.

NO

Do you have a dull, heavy ache between the legs AND/OR is your temperature 38°C (100°F) or above? — **YES** → *You may have an infection of the prostate gland.* See PROSTATITIS, p.576.

NO

Are you urinating more frequently than usual? — **YES** → *Your bladder may have become inflamed as a result of infection.* See CYSTITIS, p.505.

NO

If you are unable to make a diagnosis from this chart, consult your doctor.

60

GENERAL
0–65 years

Lack of bladder control

Involuntary passing of urine.
For those over 65 see chart 98, **Incontinence in the elderly.**

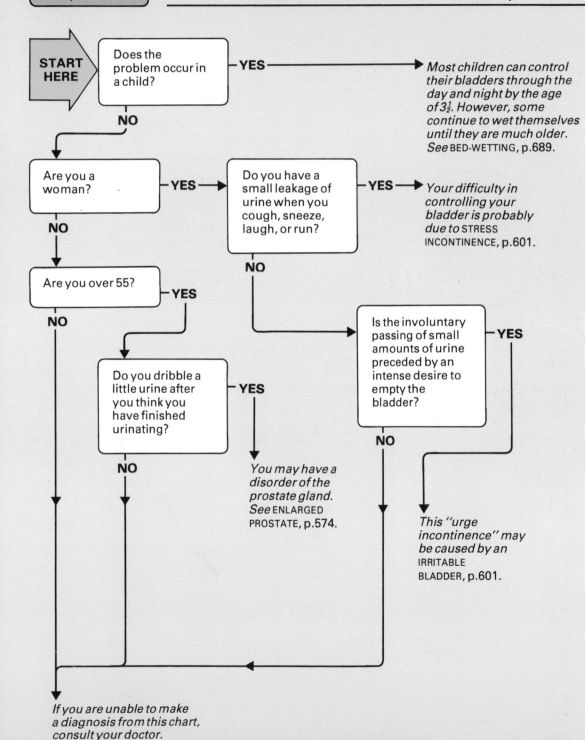

START HERE → Does the problem occur in a child? — **YES** →

Most children can control their bladders through the day and night by the age of 3½. However, some continue to wet themselves until they are much older. See BED-WETTING, p.689.

NO ↓

Are you a woman? — **YES** → Do you have a small leakage of urine when you cough, sneeze, laugh, or run? — **YES** →

Your difficulty in controlling your bladder is probably due to STRESS INCONTINENCE, p.601.

NO ↓ (woman)

Are you over 55? — **YES** →

NO ↓ (over 55)

NO ↓ (small leakage)

Do you dribble a little urine after you think you have finished urinating? — **YES** →

Is the involuntary passing of small amounts of urine preceded by an intense desire to empty the bladder? — **YES** →

NO ↓ (dribble)

You may have a disorder of the prostate gland. See ENLARGED PROSTATE, p.574.

NO ↓ (involuntary passing)

This "urge incontinence" may be caused by an IRRITABLE BLADDER, p.601.

If you are unable to make a diagnosis from this chart, consult your doctor.

61

GENERAL
all ages

Backache

Pain and/or stiffness in the back that may be continuous or intermittent.

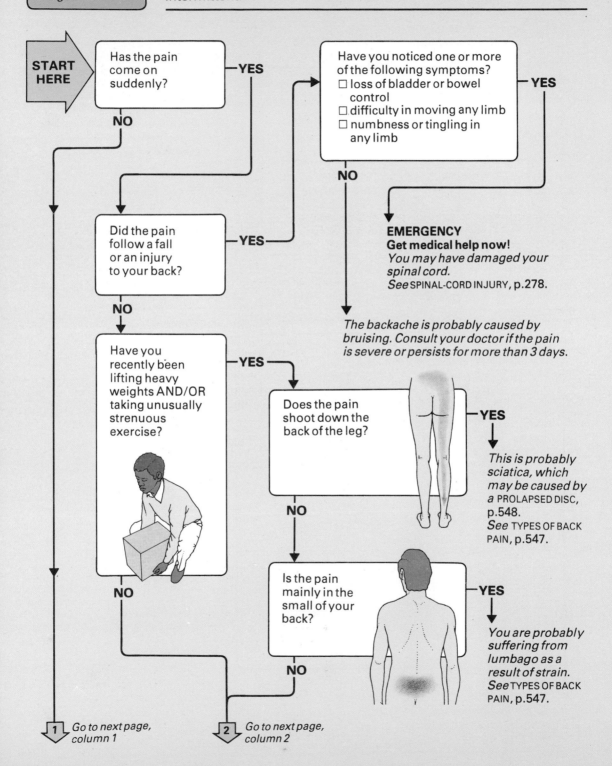

START HERE

Has the pain come on suddenly? — **YES**

NO

Have you noticed one or more of the following symptoms?
☐ loss of bladder or bowel control
☐ difficulty in moving any limb
☐ numbness or tingling in any limb
— **YES**

NO

Did the pain follow a fall or an injury to your back? — **YES**

NO

EMERGENCY
Get medical help now!
You may have damaged your spinal cord.
See SPINAL-CORD INJURY, p.278.

The backache is probably caused by bruising. Consult your doctor if the pain is severe or persists for more than 3 days.

Have you recently been lifting heavy weights AND/OR taking unusually strenuous exercise? — **YES**

NO

Does the pain shoot down the back of the leg? — **YES**

NO

This is probably sciatica, which may be caused by a PROLAPSED DISC, p.548.
See TYPES OF BACK PAIN, p.547.

Is the pain mainly in the small of your back? — **YES**

NO

You are probably suffering from lumbago as a result of strain.
See TYPES OF BACK PAIN, p.547.

1 *Go to next page, column 1*

2 *Go to next page, column 2*

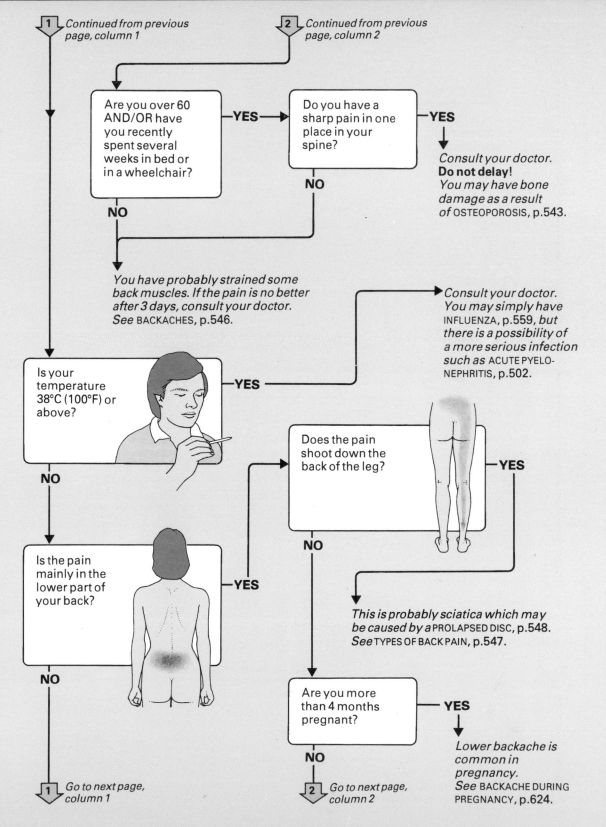

1 *Continued from previous page, column 1*

2 *Continued from previous page, column 2*

Are you over 60 AND/OR have you recently spent several weeks in bed or in a wheelchair? — **YES** → Do you have a sharp pain in one place in your spine? — **YES** →

Consult your doctor. **Do not delay!** *You may have bone damage as a result of* OSTEOPOROSIS, p.543.

NO

NO

You have probably strained some back muscles. If the pain is no better after 3 days, consult your doctor. See BACKACHES, p.546.

Consult your doctor. You may simply have INFLUENZA, p.559, *but there is a possibility of a more serious infection such as* ACUTE PYELO-NEPHRITIS, p.502.

Is your temperature 38°C (100°F) or above? — **YES** →

NO

Does the pain shoot down the back of the leg? — **YES**

NO

Is the pain mainly in the lower part of your back? — **YES**

NO

This is probably sciatica which may be caused by a PROLAPSED DISC, p.548. *See* TYPES OF BACK PAIN, p.547.

Are you more than 4 months pregnant? — **YES**

NO

Lower backache is common in pregnancy. See BACKACHE DURING PREGNANCY, p.624.

1 *Go to next page, column 1*

2 *Go to next page, column 2*

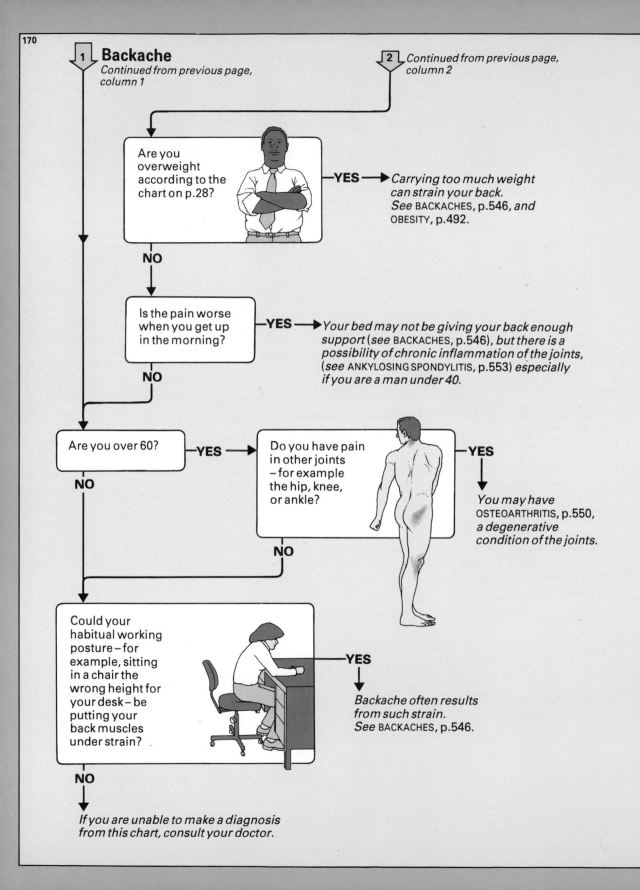

Backache

1 Continued from previous page, column 1

2 Continued from previous page, column 2

Are you overweight according to the chart on p.28?

YES → *Carrying too much weight can strain your back. See* BACKACHES, p.546, *and* OBESITY, p.492.

NO

Is the pain worse when you get up in the morning?

YES → *Your bed may not be giving your back enough support (see* BACKACHES, p.546), *but there is a possibility of chronic inflammation of the joints, (see* ANKYLOSING SPONDYLITIS, p.553) *especially if you are a man under 40.*

NO

Are you over 60?

YES → Do you have pain in other joints – for example the hip, knee, or ankle?

YES ↓

You may have OSTEOARTHRITIS, p.550, *a degenerative condition of the joints.*

NO

Could your habitual working posture – for example, sitting in a chair the wrong height for your desk – be putting your back muscles under strain?

YES ↓

Backache often results from such strain. See BACKACHES, p.546.

NO

If you are unable to make a diagnosis from this chart, consult your doctor.

62

GENERAL
all ages

Cramp

Involuntary, painful tightening of muscles, which usually only lasts a few minutes.

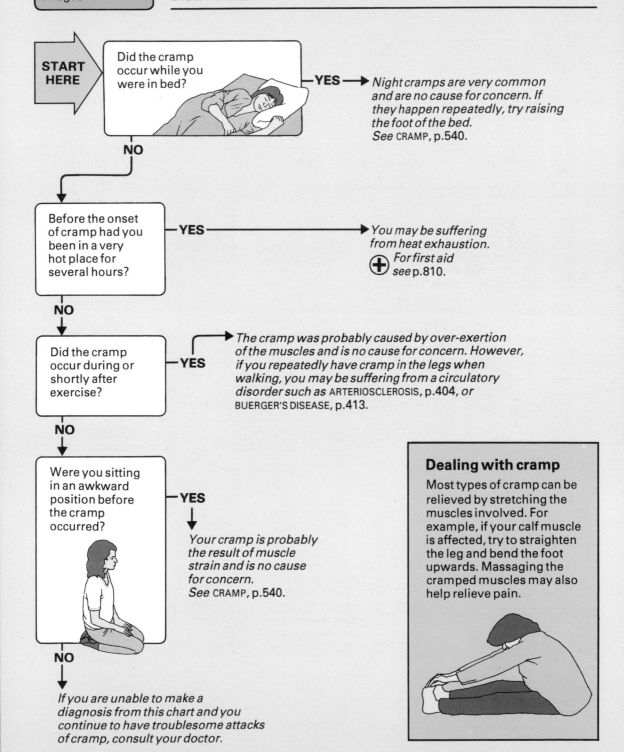

START HERE →

Did the cramp occur while you were in bed?

YES → *Night cramps are very common and are no cause for concern. If they happen repeatedly, try raising the foot of the bed.* See CRAMP, p.540.

NO ↓

Before the onset of cramp had you been in a very hot place for several hours?

YES → *You may be suffering from heat exhaustion.* ⊕ *For first aid see p.810.*

NO ↓

Did the cramp occur during or shortly after exercise?

YES → *The cramp was probably caused by over-exertion of the muscles and is no cause for concern. However, if you repeatedly have cramp in the legs when walking, you may be suffering from a circulatory disorder such as* ARTERIOSCLEROSIS, p.404, *or* BUERGER'S DISEASE, p.413.

NO ↓

Were you sitting in an awkward position before the cramp occurred?

YES ↓

Your cramp is probably the result of muscle strain and is no cause for concern. See CRAMP, p.540.

NO ↓

If you are unable to make a diagnosis from this chart and you continue to have troublesome attacks of cramp, consult your doctor.

Dealing with cramp

Most types of cramp can be relieved by stretching the muscles involved. For example, if your calf muscle is affected, try to straighten the leg and bend the foot upwards. Massaging the cramped muscles may also help relieve pain.

63

Painful and/or stiff neck

Pain (or discomfort) that may or may not be accompanied by a slight headache.

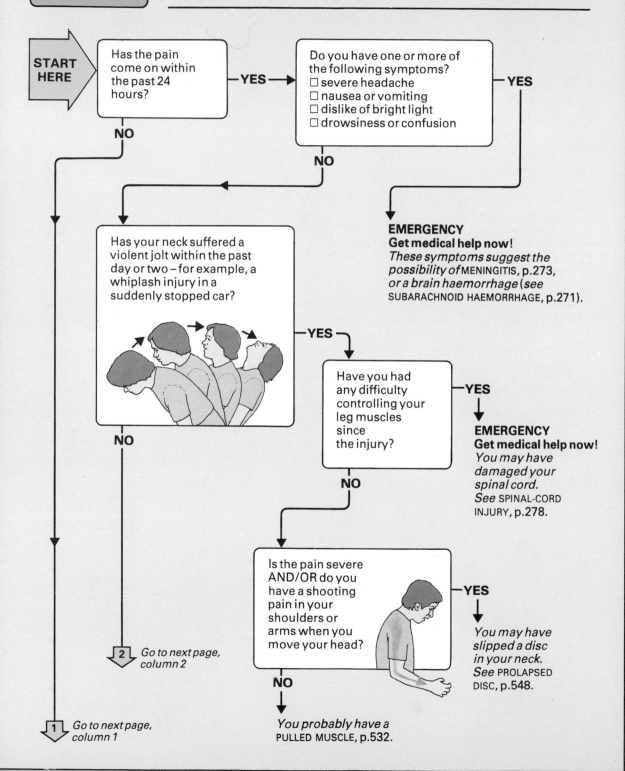

START HERE

Has the pain come on within the past 24 hours?

YES → Do you have one or more of the following symptoms?
☐ severe headache
☐ nausea or vomiting
☐ dislike of bright light
☐ drowsiness or confusion

YES ↓

NO ↓

NO ↓

**EMERGENCY
Get medical help now!**
These symptoms suggest the possibility of MENINGITIS, p.273, *or a brain haemorrhage (see* SUBARACHNOID HAEMORRHAGE, p.271).

Has your neck suffered a violent jolt within the past day or two – for example, a whiplash injury in a suddenly stopped car?

YES →

Have you had any difficulty controlling your leg muscles since the injury?

YES ↓

**EMERGENCY
Get medical help now!**
You may have damaged your spinal cord.
See SPINAL-CORD INJURY, p.278.

NO ↓

NO ↓

Is the pain severe AND/OR do you have a shooting pain in your shoulders or arms when you move your head?

YES ↓

You may have slipped a disc in your neck.
See PROLAPSED DISC, p.548.

NO ↓

2 *Go to next page, column 2*

You probably have a PULLED MUSCLE, p.532.

1 *Go to next page, column 1*

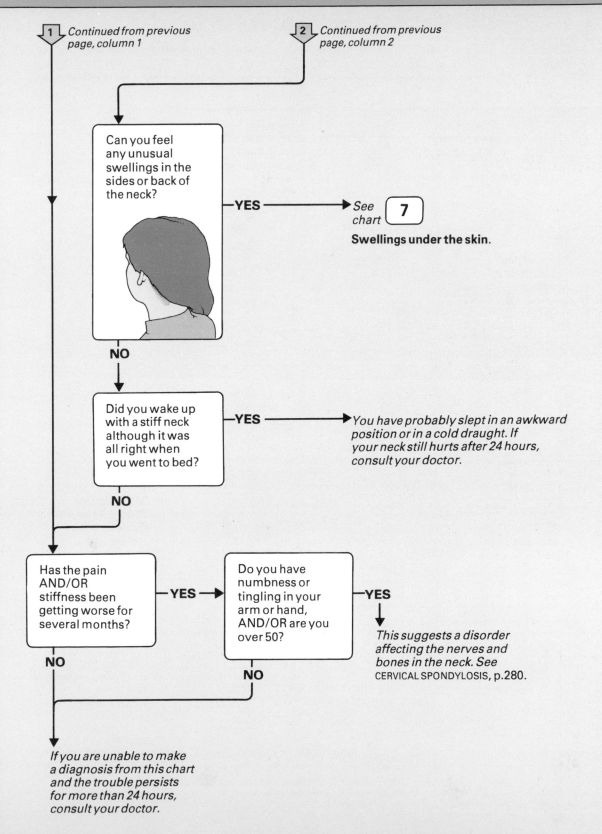

1 _Continued from previous page, column 1_

2 _Continued from previous page, column 2_

Can you feel any unusual swellings in the sides or back of the neck?

YES → _See chart_ **7**

Swellings under the skin.

NO ↓

Did you wake up with a stiff neck although it was all right when you went to bed?

YES → _You have probably slept in an awkward position or in a cold draught. If your neck still hurts after 24 hours, consult your doctor._

NO ↓

Has the pain AND/OR stiffness been getting worse for several months?

YES → **Do you have numbness or tingling in your arm or hand, AND/OR are you over 50?**

YES ↓

This suggests a disorder affecting the nerves and bones in the neck. See CERVICAL SPONDYLOSIS, p.280.

NO

NO ↓

If you are unable to make a diagnosis from this chart and the trouble persists for more than 24 hours, consult your doctor.

64

GENERAL
all ages

Painful arm or hand

Pain in the arm, elbow, wrist, or hand, but not including the shoulder.

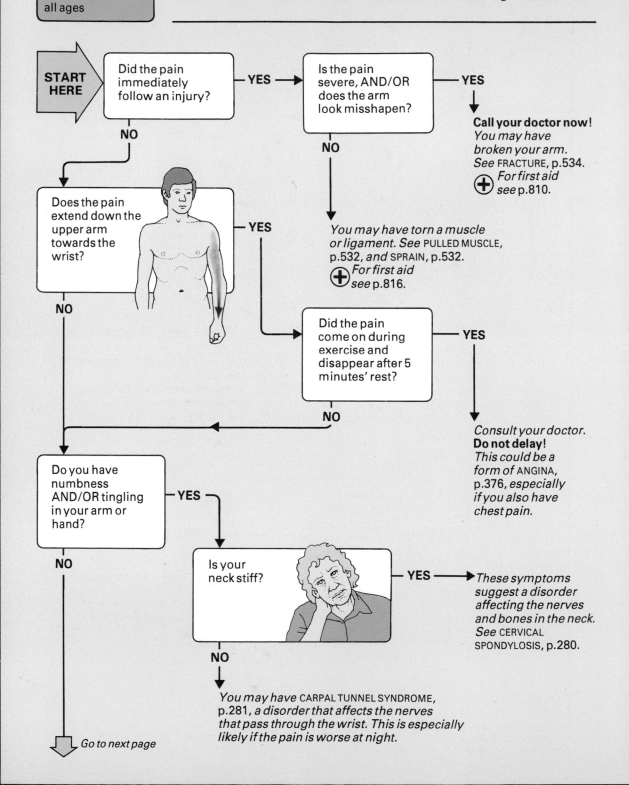

START HERE

Did the pain immediately follow an injury?

YES →

Is the pain severe, AND/OR does the arm look misshapen?

YES →

Call your doctor now! *You may have broken your arm. See* FRACTURE, p.534. *For first aid see* p.810.

NO

NO

Does the pain extend down the upper arm towards the wrist?

YES

You may have torn a muscle or ligament. See PULLED MUSCLE, p.532, *and* SPRAIN, p.532. *For first aid see* p.816.

NO

Did the pain come on during exercise and disappear after 5 minutes' rest?

YES

NO

Consult your doctor. **Do not delay!** *This could be a form of* ANGINA, p.376, *especially if you also have chest pain.*

Do you have numbness AND/OR tingling in your arm or hand?

YES

Is your neck stiff?

YES →

These symptoms suggest a disorder affecting the nerves and bones in the neck. See CERVICAL SPONDYLOSIS, p.280.

NO

NO

You may have CARPAL TUNNEL SYNDROME, p.281, *a disorder that affects the nerves that pass through the wrist. This is especially likely if the pain is worse at night.*

Go to next page

175

Continued from previous page

Is the pain in the elbow, wrist, or finger joints?

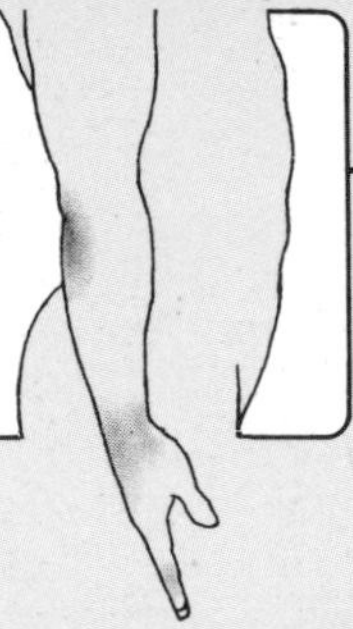

YES → Is the pain accompanied by redness and swelling?

YES → Is only one joint affected?

NO

NO

Is your temperature 38°C (100°F) or above, AND/OR have you recently begun to feel unwell?

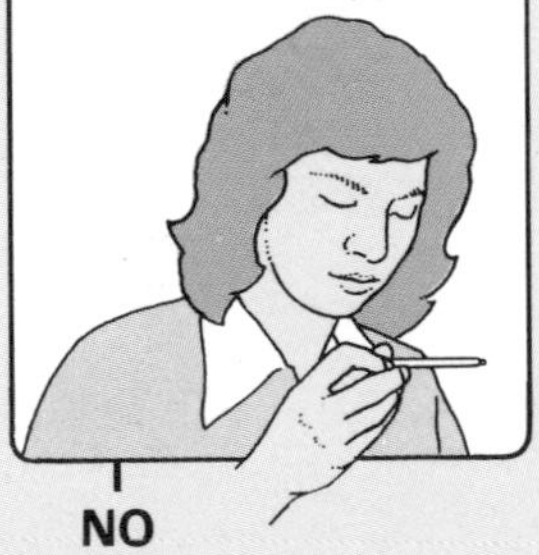

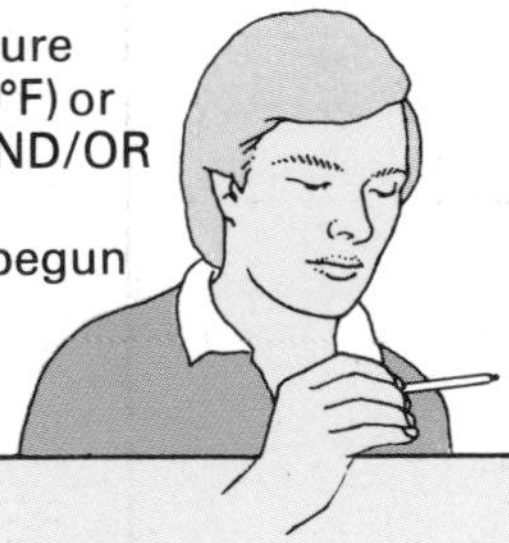

YES → *Consult your doctor.* **Do not delay!** *These symptoms suggest the possibility of* RHEUMATIC FEVER, p.393.

YES

Is your temperature 38°C (100°F) or above, AND/OR have you recently begun to feel unwell?

YES

NO

You may have inflammation of the joints. See RHEUMATOID ARTHRITIS, p.552.

NO

Consult your doctor. **Do not delay!** *You may have a bone infection. See* OSTEOMYELITIS, p.695.

Does the pain occur only when you bend your arm or hand in a certain way?

YES

NO

You may have inflammation of the tendons. See TENDONITIS, p.541.

If you are unable to make a diagnosis from this chart, consult your doctor.

You may have an inflamed joint (see BURSITIS, p.555) *or* GOUT, p.498.

65

Painful leg

Pain in the thigh and/or calf that may be fleeting or continuous.

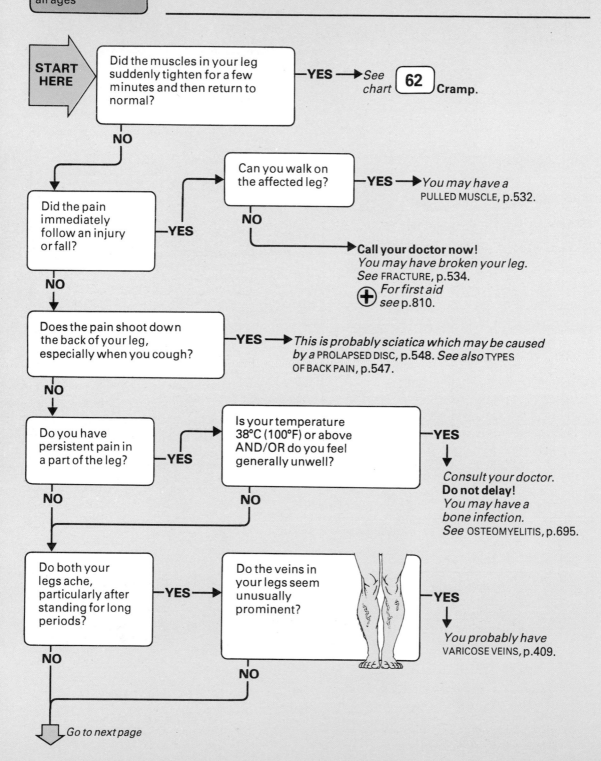

START HERE → Did the muscles in your leg suddenly tighten for a few minutes and then return to normal? — **YES** → *See chart* **62** **Cramp.**

NO ↓

Did the pain immediately follow an injury or fall? — **YES** → Can you walk on the affected leg? — **YES** → *You may have a* PULLED MUSCLE, p.532.

NO ↓ (from "Can you walk on the affected leg?")
Call your doctor now!
You may have broken your leg.
See FRACTURE, p.534.
✚ *For first aid see* p.810.

NO ↓ (from "Did the pain immediately follow an injury or fall?")

Does the pain shoot down the back of your leg, especially when you cough? — **YES** → *This is probably sciatica which may be caused by a* PROLAPSED DISC, p.548. *See also* TYPES OF BACK PAIN, p.547.

NO ↓

Do you have persistent pain in a part of the leg? — **YES** → Is your temperature 38°C (100°F) or above AND/OR do you feel generally unwell? — **YES** ↓

Consult your doctor.
Do not delay!
You may have a bone infection.
See OSTEOMYELITIS, p.695.

NO ↓ (from "persistent pain")   **NO** ↓ (from "temperature")

Do both your legs ache, particularly after standing for long periods? — **YES** → Do the veins in your legs seem unusually prominent? — **YES** ↓

You probably have VARICOSE VEINS, p.409.

NO ↓ (from "Do both your legs ache")   **NO** ↓ (from "veins")

⇩ *Go to next page*

Continued from previous page

Is the hip on the same side as the affected leg painful and/or stiff?

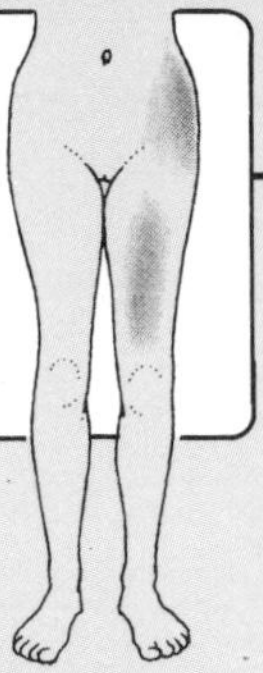

YES → *A disorder of the hip such as* OSTEOARTHRITIS, p.550, *may cause pain in the leg.*

NO

Is the pain mainly in the calf?

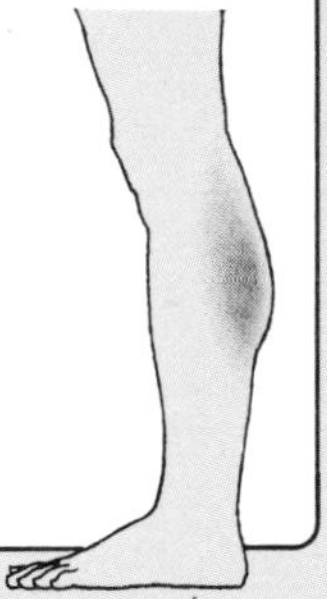

YES → **Is the calf swollen and tender?**

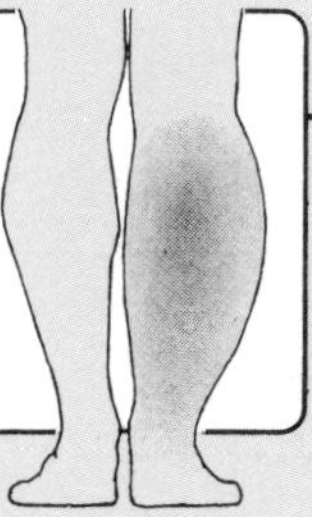

YES ↓

Call your doctor now! *You may have a blood clot in your leg. See* DEEP-VEIN THROMBOSIS, p.405.

NO ↓

Is one of your veins red and inflamed?

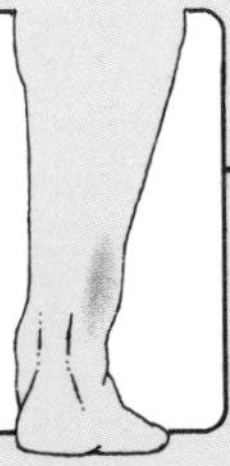

YES ↓

This may be THROMBO-PHLEBITIS, p.407.

NO ↓

NO (from "Is the pain mainly in the calf?")

Did your leg become painful following unusually strenuous exercise?

YES → *You may have a* PULLED MUSCLE, p.532.

NO ↓

Does the leg begin to hurt when you are walking and does the pain disappear with rest?

YES → *Recurrent pain in the calf during exercise may be a sign of a circulatory problem such as* ARTERIO-SCLEROSIS, p.404, *or* BUERGER'S DISEASE, p.413.

NO

If you are unable to make a diagnosis from this chart, and the pain persists for more than 48 hours or gets worse, consult your doctor.

66

GENERAL
all ages

Painful knee

Pain in or around the knee joint that may be accompanied by swelling.

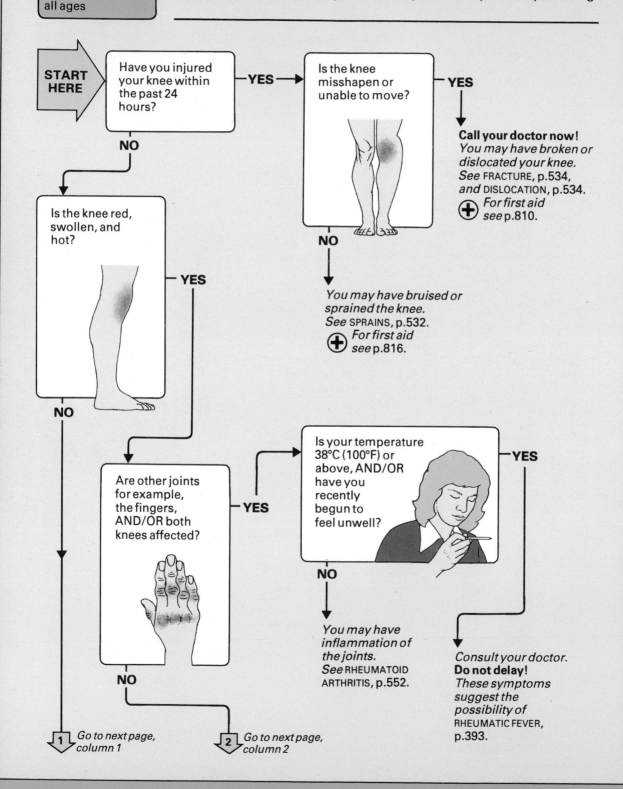

START HERE

Have you injured your knee within the past 24 hours?

YES → Is the knee misshapen or unable to move?

YES →

Call your doctor now!
*You may have broken or dislocated your knee.
See* FRACTURE, p.534, *and* DISLOCATION, p.534.
✚ *For first aid see* p.810.

NO ↓

*You may have bruised or sprained the knee.
See* SPRAINS, p.532.
✚ *For first aid see* p.816.

NO ↓

Is the knee red, swollen, and hot?

YES →

NO ↓

Are other joints for example, the fingers, AND/OR both knees affected?

YES → Is your temperature 38°C (100°F) or above, AND/OR have you recently begun to feel unwell?

YES →

Consult your doctor.
Do not delay!
These symptoms suggest the possibility of RHEUMATIC FEVER, p.393.

NO ↓

*You may have inflammation of the joints.
See* RHEUMATOID ARTHRITIS, p.552.

NO ↓

1 *Go to next page, column 1*

2 *Go to next page, column 2*

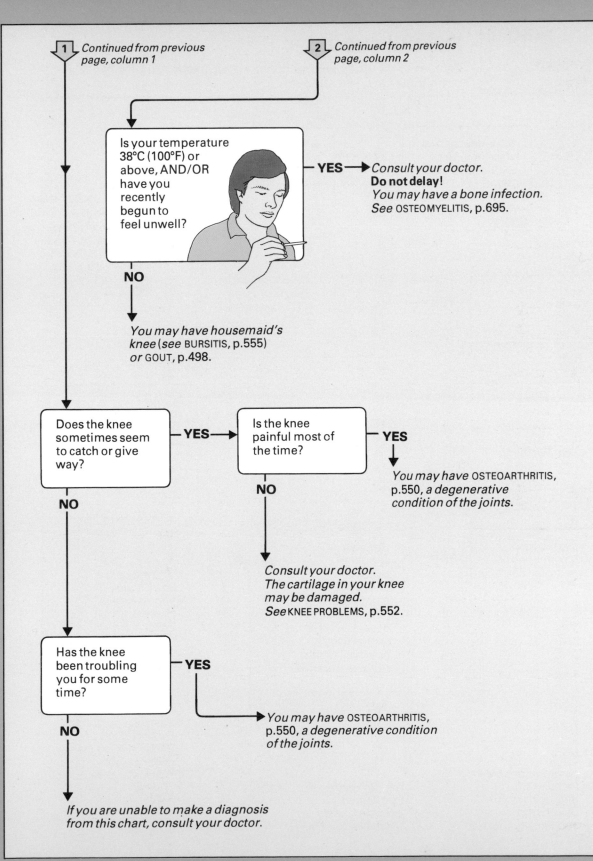

1 Continued from previous page, column 1

2 Continued from previous page, column 2

Is your temperature 38°C (100°F) or above, AND/OR have you recently begun to feel unwell?

YES → *Consult your doctor.* **Do not delay!** *You may have a bone infection.* See OSTEOMYELITIS, p.695.

NO

You may have housemaid's knee (see BURSITIS, p.555) *or* GOUT, p.498.

Does the knee sometimes seem to catch or give way?

YES → Is the knee painful most of the time?

YES

You may have OSTEOARTHRITIS, p.550, *a degenerative condition of the joints.*

NO

Consult your doctor. The cartilage in your knee may be damaged. See KNEE PROBLEMS, p.552.

NO

Has the knee been troubling you for some time?

YES

You may have OSTEOARTHRITIS, p.550, *a degenerative condition of the joints.*

NO

If you are unable to make a diagnosis from this chart, consult your doctor.

Painful shoulder

Pain in the shoulder, which may be accompanied by stiffness that limits upper-arm movements.

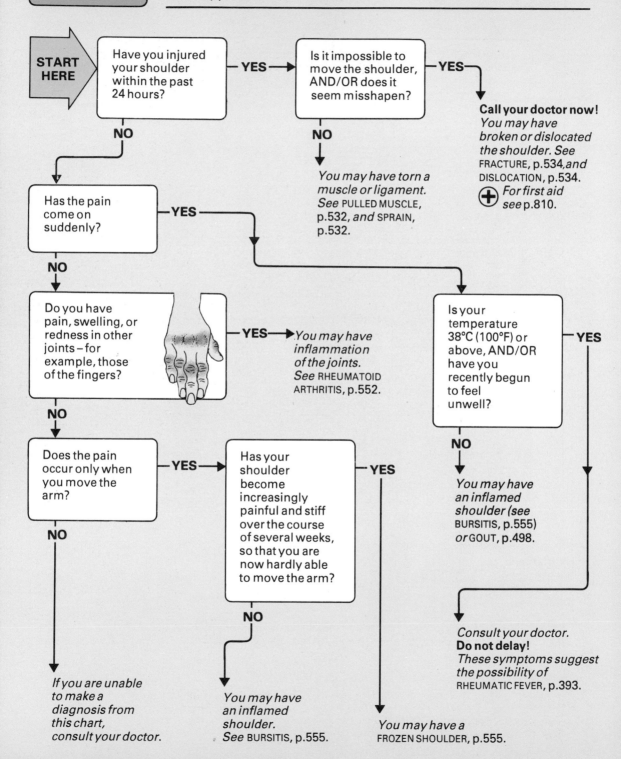

START HERE

Have you injured your shoulder within the past 24 hours?

YES →

Is it impossible to move the shoulder, AND/OR does it seem misshapen?

YES →

Call your doctor now! *You may have broken or dislocated the shoulder. See* FRACTURE, *p.534, and* DISLOCATION, *p.534.* *For first aid see* p.810.

NO ↓

NO ↓

You may have torn a muscle or ligament. See PULLED MUSCLE, *p.532, and* SPRAIN, *p.532.*

Has the pain come on suddenly?

YES →

NO ↓

Do you have pain, swelling, or redness in other joints – for example, those of the fingers?

YES → *You may have inflammation of the joints. See* RHEUMATOID ARTHRITIS, *p.552.*

NO ↓

Is your temperature 38°C (100°F) or above, AND/OR have you recently begun to feel unwell?

YES →

NO ↓

You may have an inflamed shoulder (see BURSITIS, *p.555) or* GOUT, *p.498.*

Does the pain occur only when you move the arm?

YES →

Has your shoulder become increasingly painful and stiff over the course of several weeks, so that you are now hardly able to move the arm?

YES →

NO ↓

NO ↓

If you are unable to make a diagnosis from this chart, consult your doctor.

You may have an inflamed shoulder. See BURSITIS, *p.555.*

You may have a FROZEN SHOULDER, *p.555.*

Consult your doctor. **Do not delay!** *These symptoms suggest the possibility of* RHEUMATIC FEVER, *p.393.*

68

GENERAL
all ages

Painful ankles

Pain, with or without swelling, in or around one or both ankles.

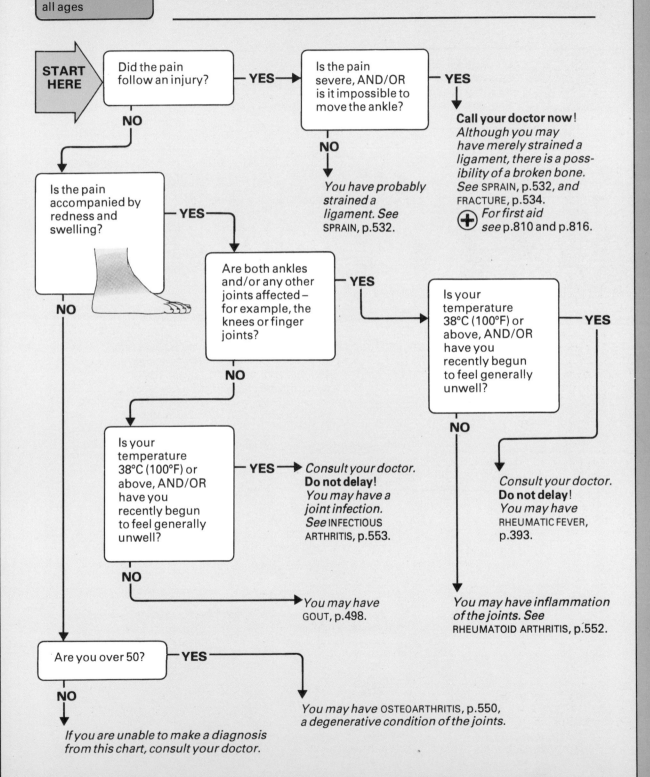

START HERE → Did the pain follow an injury? — **YES** → Is the pain severe, AND/OR is it impossible to move the ankle? — **YES** →

Call your doctor now! *Although you may have merely strained a ligament, there is a possibility of a broken bone. See* SPRAIN, p.532, *and* FRACTURE, p.534. ⊕ *For first aid see* p.810 *and* p.816.

NO ↓ (from "Is the pain severe...")

You have probably strained a ligament. See SPRAIN, p.532.

NO ↓ (from "Did the pain follow an injury?")

Is the pain accompanied by redness and swelling? — **YES** →

Are both ankles and/or any other joints affected – for example, the knees or finger joints? — **YES** →

Is your temperature 38°C (100°F) or above, AND/OR have you recently begun to feel generally unwell? — **YES** →

NO ↓ (from "Is the pain accompanied by redness and swelling?")

NO ↓ (from "Are both ankles...")

Is your temperature 38°C (100°F) or above, AND/OR have you recently begun to feel generally unwell? — **YES** → *Consult your doctor.* **Do not delay!** *You may have a joint infection. See* INFECTIOUS ARTHRITIS, p.553.

NO ↓ (from lower temperature box)

You may have GOUT, p.498.

NO ↓ (from "Is your temperature...unwell?" right box)

Consult your doctor. **Do not delay**! *You may have* RHEUMATIC FEVER, p.393.

You may have inflammation of the joints. See RHEUMATOID ARTHRITIS, p.552.

Are you over 50? — **YES** → *You may have* OSTEOARTHRITIS, p.550, *a degenerative condition of the joints.*

NO ↓

If you are unable to make a diagnosis from this chart, consult your doctor.

69

GENERAL
all ages

Swollen ankles

Swelling may affect one or both ankles.

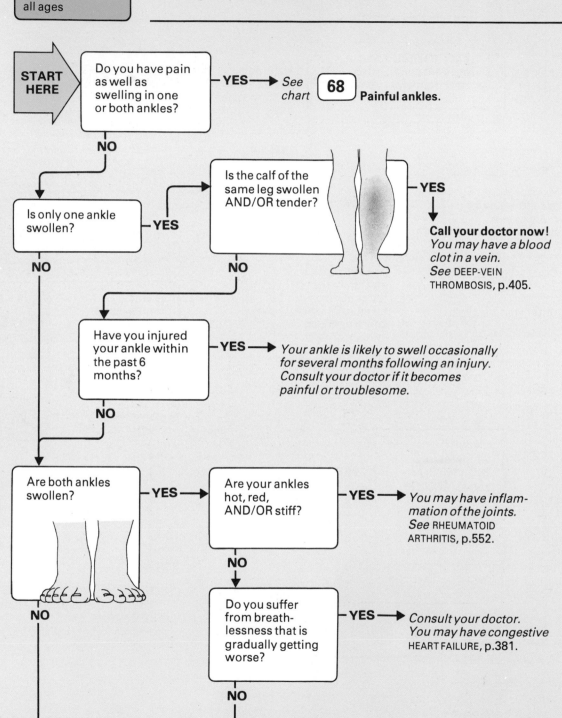

START HERE → Do you have pain as well as swelling in one or both ankles? — **YES** → *See chart* **68** **Painful ankles.**

NO ↓

Is only one ankle swollen? — **YES** → Is the calf of the same leg swollen AND/OR tender? — **YES** ↓

Call your doctor now! *You may have a blood clot in a vein. See* DEEP-VEIN THROMBOSIS, p.405.

NO ↓ (from "Is only one ankle swollen?")

NO ↓ (from "Is the calf...")

Have you injured your ankle within the past 6 months? — **YES** → *Your ankle is likely to swell occasionally for several months following an injury. Consult your doctor if it becomes painful or troublesome.*

NO ↓

Are both ankles swollen? — **YES** → Are your ankles hot, red, AND/OR stiff? — **YES** → *You may have inflammation of the joints. See* RHEUMATOID ARTHRITIS, p.552.

NO ↓

Do you suffer from breath-lessness that is gradually getting worse? — **YES** → *Consult your doctor. You may have congestive* HEART FAILURE, p.381.

NO ↓

1 *Go to next page, column 1*

NO ↓ (from "Are both ankles swollen?")

2 *Go to next page, column 2*

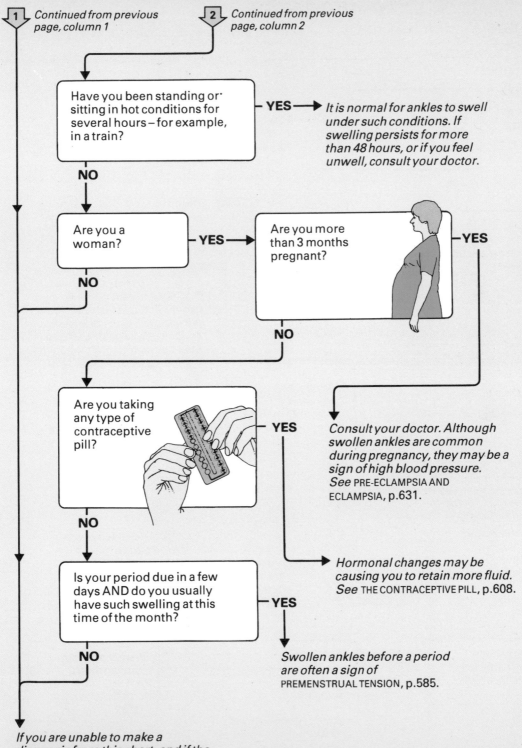

1 Continued from previous page, column 1

2 Continued from previous page, column 2

Have you been standing or sitting in hot conditions for several hours – for example, in a train?

YES → It is normal for ankles to swell under such conditions. If swelling persists for more than 48 hours, or if you feel unwell, consult your doctor.

NO

Are you a woman?

YES → Are you more than 3 months pregnant?

YES →

NO

NO

Are you taking any type of contraceptive pill?

YES →

Consult your doctor. Although swollen ankles are common during pregnancy, they may be a sign of high blood pressure. *See* PRE-ECLAMPSIA AND ECLAMPSIA, p.631.

NO

Is your period due in a few days AND do you usually have such swelling at this time of the month?

YES →

Hormonal changes may be causing you to retain more fluid. *See* THE CONTRACEPTIVE PILL, p.608.

NO

Swollen ankles before a period are often a sign of PREMENSTRUAL TENSION, p.585.

If you are unable to make a diagnosis from this chart, and if the swelling persists for more than 48 hours or if you feel unwell, consult your doctor.

70
GENERAL
all ages

Foot problems
Pain, irritation, or swelling anywhere in one or both feet, but not including the ankles.

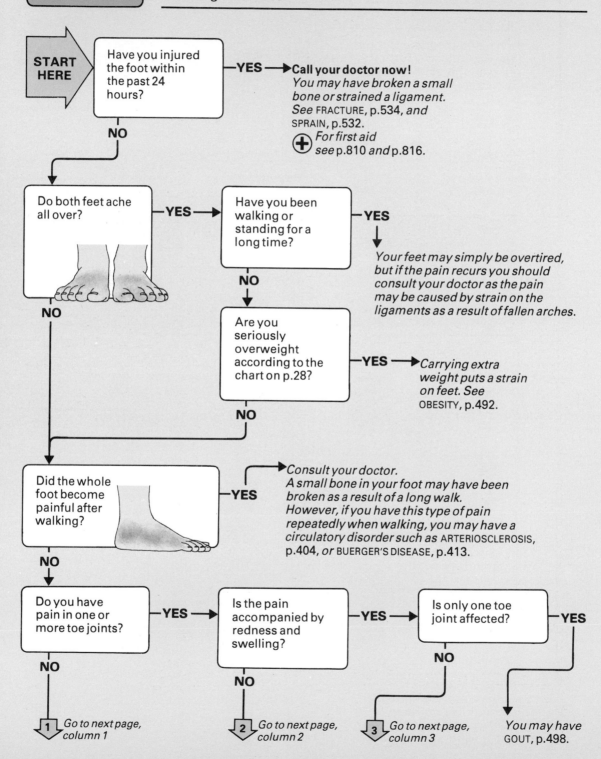

START HERE → Have you injured the foot within the past 24 hours?

— **YES** → **Call your doctor now!** *You may have broken a small bone or strained a ligament. See* FRACTURE, *p.534, and* SPRAIN, *p.532.*
✚ *For first aid see* p.810 *and* p.816.

NO ↓

Do both feet ache all over?

— **YES** → Have you been walking or standing for a long time?

— **YES** ↓

Your feet may simply be overtired, but if the pain recurs you should consult your doctor as the pain may be caused by strain on the ligaments as a result of fallen arches.

NO ↓

Are you seriously overweight according to the chart on p.28?

— **YES** → *Carrying extra weight puts a strain on feet. See* OBESITY, *p.492.*

NO ↓

NO ↓

Did the whole foot become painful after walking?

— **YES** → *Consult your doctor. A small bone in your foot may have been broken as a result of a long walk. However, if you have this type of pain repeatedly when walking, you may have a circulatory disorder such as* ARTERIOSCLEROSIS, *p.404, or* BUERGER'S DISEASE, *p.413.*

NO ↓

Do you have pain in one or more toe joints?

— **YES** → Is the pain accompanied by redness and swelling?

— **YES** → Is only one toe joint affected?

— **YES** ↓

NO ↓

NO ↓

NO ↓

1 *Go to next page, column 1*

2 *Go to next page, column 2*

3 *Go to next page, column 3*

You may have GOUT, *p.498.*

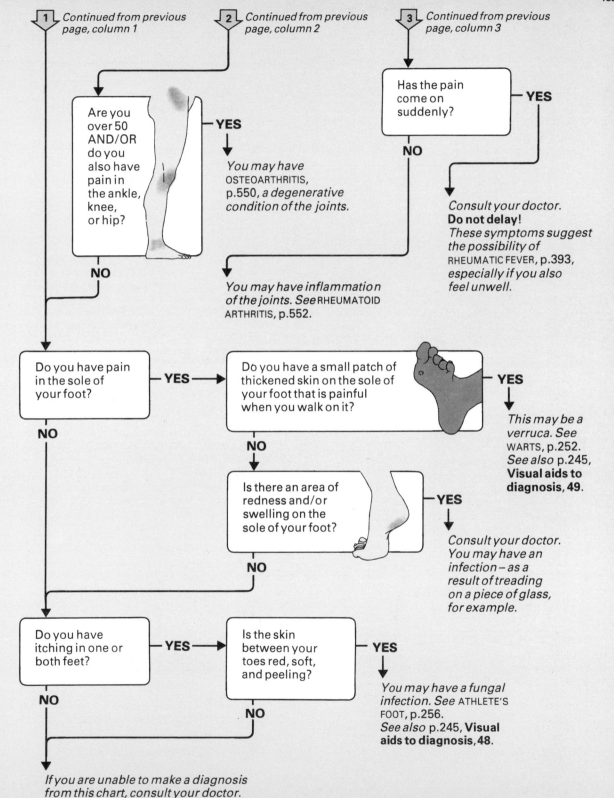

1 Continued from previous page, column 1

2 Continued from previous page, column 2

3 Continued from previous page, column 3

Has the pain come on suddenly? — **YES**

NO

Consult your doctor. **Do not delay!** These symptoms suggest the possibility of RHEUMATIC FEVER, p.393, especially if you also feel unwell.

Are you over 50 AND/OR do you also have pain in the ankle, knee, or hip? — **YES**

NO

You may have OSTEOARTHRITIS, p.550, a degenerative condition of the joints.

You may have inflammation of the joints. See RHEUMATOID ARTHRITIS, p.552.

Do you have pain in the sole of your foot? — **YES** → **Do you have a small patch of thickened skin on the sole of your foot that is painful when you walk on it?** — **YES**

NO

NO

This may be a verruca. See WARTS, p.252. See also p.245, **Visual aids to diagnosis, 49**.

Is there an area of redness and/or swelling on the sole of your foot? — **YES**

NO

Consult your doctor. You may have an infection – as a result of treading on a piece of glass, for example.

Do you have itching in one or both feet? — **YES** → **Is the skin between your toes red, soft, and peeling?** — **YES**

NO

NO

You may have a fungal infection. See ATHLETE'S FOOT, p.256. See also p.245, **Visual aids to diagnosis, 48**.

If you are unable to make a diagnosis from this chart, consult your doctor.

71
MEN

Painful or enlarged testicles

Pain or swelling may affect one or both testicles, or the whole area within the scrotum (the supportive bag).

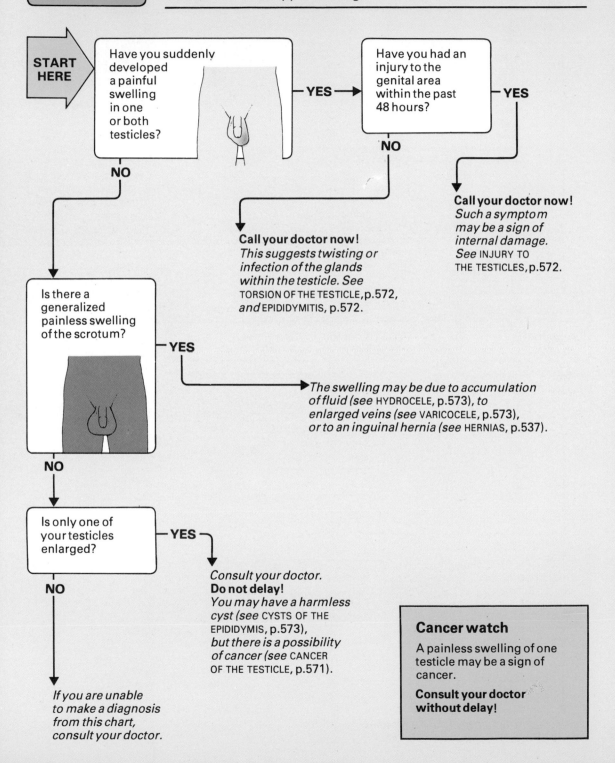

START HERE

Have you suddenly developed a painful swelling in one or both testicles?

YES → **Have you had an injury to the genital area within the past 48 hours?**

YES →

Call your doctor now!
Such a symptom may be a sign of internal damage.
See INJURY TO THE TESTICLES, p.572.

NO ↓ (from injury question)

Call your doctor now!
This suggests twisting or infection of the glands within the testicle. See TORSION OF THE TESTICLE, p.572, *and* EPIDIDYMITIS, p.572.

NO ↓ (from first question)

Is there a generalized painless swelling of the scrotum?

YES →

The swelling may be due to accumulation of fluid (see HYDROCELE, p.573), *to enlarged veins (see* VARICOCELE, p.573), *or to an inguinal hernia (see* HERNIAS, p.537).

NO ↓

Is only one of your testicles enlarged?

YES →

Consult your doctor.
Do not delay!
You may have a harmless cyst (see CYSTS OF THE EPIDIDYMIS, p.573), *but there is a possibility of cancer (see* CANCER OF THE TESTICLE, p.571).

NO ↓

If you are unable to make a diagnosis from this chart, consult your doctor.

Cancer watch

A painless swelling of one testicle may be a sign of cancer.

Consult your doctor without delay!

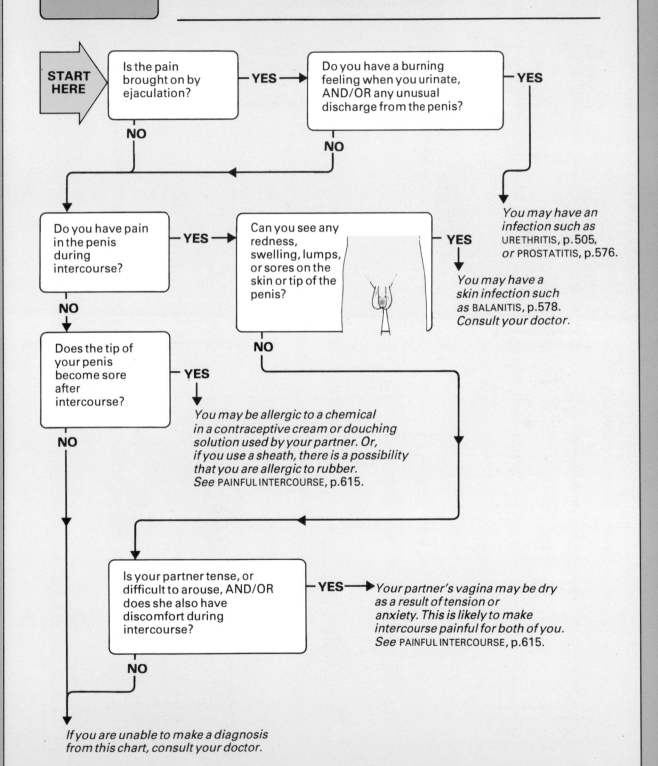

72

MEN

Painful intercourse in men

Pain or discomfort during or just after intercourse.

START HERE

Is the pain brought on by ejaculation?

YES → Do you have a burning feeling when you urinate, AND/OR any unusual discharge from the penis?

YES → *You may have an infection such as* URETHRITIS, p.505, *or* PROSTATITIS, p.576.

NO

NO

Do you have pain in the penis during intercourse?

YES → Can you see any redness, swelling, lumps, or sores on the skin or tip of the penis?

YES → *You may have a skin infection such as* BALANITIS, p.578. *Consult your doctor.*

NO

NO

Does the tip of your penis become sore after intercourse?

YES → *You may be allergic to a chemical in a contraceptive cream or douching solution used by your partner. Or, if you use a sheath, there is a possibility that you are allergic to rubber. See* PAINFUL INTERCOURSE, p.615.

NO

Is your partner tense, or difficult to arouse, AND/OR does she also have discomfort during intercourse?

YES → *Your partner's vagina may be dry as a result of tension or anxiety. This is likely to make intercourse painful for both of you. See* PAINFUL INTERCOURSE, p.615.

NO

If you are unable to make a diagnosis from this chart, consult your doctor.

73
WOMEN

Pain or lumps in the breast

Pain, tenderness, or lumps in one or both breasts, which may be noticed when you examine yourself as described on p.589.

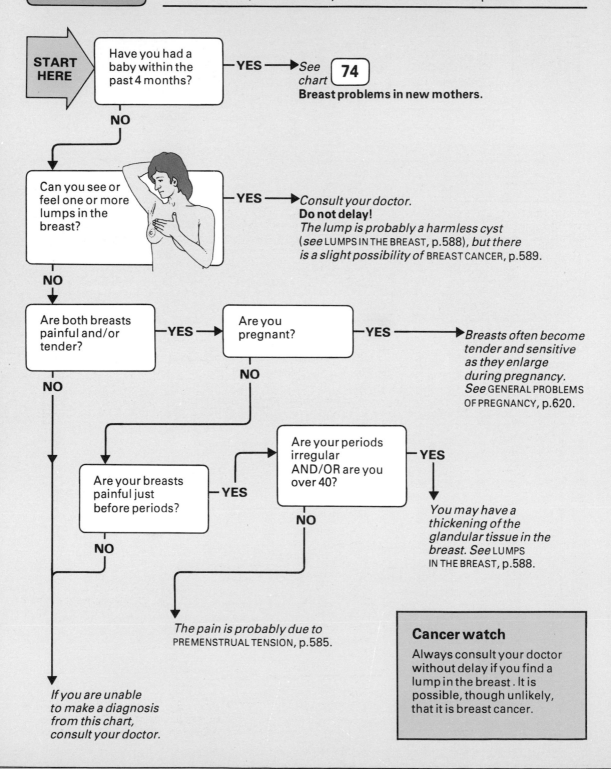

START HERE

Have you had a baby within the past 4 months? — **YES** → *See chart* **74**
Breast problems in new mothers.

NO

Can you see or feel one or more lumps in the breast? — **YES** → *Consult your doctor.* **Do not delay!** *The lump is probably a harmless cyst* (*see* LUMPS IN THE BREAST, p.588), *but there is a slight possibility of* BREAST CANCER, p.589.

NO

Are both breasts painful and/or tender? — **YES** → **Are you pregnant?** — **YES** → *Breasts often become tender and sensitive as they enlarge during pregnancy. See* GENERAL PROBLEMS OF PREGNANCY, p.620.

NO .... **NO**

Are your breasts painful just before periods? — **YES** → **Are your periods irregular AND/OR are you over 40?** — **YES** → *You may have a thickening of the glandular tissue in the breast. See* LUMPS IN THE BREAST, p.588.

NO .... **NO**

The pain is probably due to PREMENSTRUAL TENSION, p.585.

If you are unable to make a diagnosis from this chart, consult your doctor.

Cancer watch

Always consult your doctor without delay if you find a lump in the breast . It is possible, though unlikely, that it is breast cancer.

74
WOMEN

Breast problems in new mothers
Pain, tenderness, or lumps in the breasts of women who have had a baby within the past 4 months.

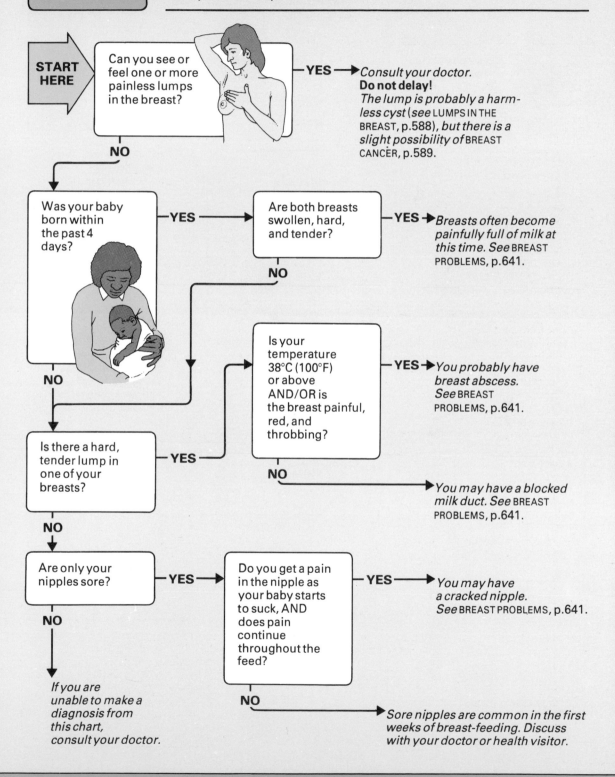

START HERE → Can you see or feel one or more painless lumps in the breast? — **YES** → *Consult your doctor.* **Do not delay!** *The lump is probably a harmless cyst (see* LUMPS IN THE BREAST, p.588), *but there is a slight possibility of* BREAST CANCER, p.589.

NO ↓

Was your baby born within the past 4 days? — **YES** → Are both breasts swollen, hard, and tender? — **YES** → *Breasts often become painfully full of milk at this time. See* BREAST PROBLEMS, p.641.

NO ↓

Is your temperature 38°C (100°F) or above AND/OR is the breast painful, red, and throbbing? — **YES** → *You probably have breast abscess. See* BREAST PROBLEMS, p.641.

NO →

You may have a blocked milk duct. See BREAST PROBLEMS, p.641.

Is there a hard, tender lump in one of your breasts? — **YES** ↑

NO ↓

Are only your nipples sore? — **YES** → Do you get a pain in the nipple as your baby starts to suck, AND does pain continue throughout the feed? — **YES** → *You may have a cracked nipple. See* BREAST PROBLEMS, p.641.

NO ↓

If you are unable to make a diagnosis from this chart, consult your doctor.

NO →

Sore nipples are common in the first weeks of breast-feeding. Discuss with your doctor or health visitor.

75
WOMEN

Absent periods

Absence of periods for at least 2 weeks after a period was due.

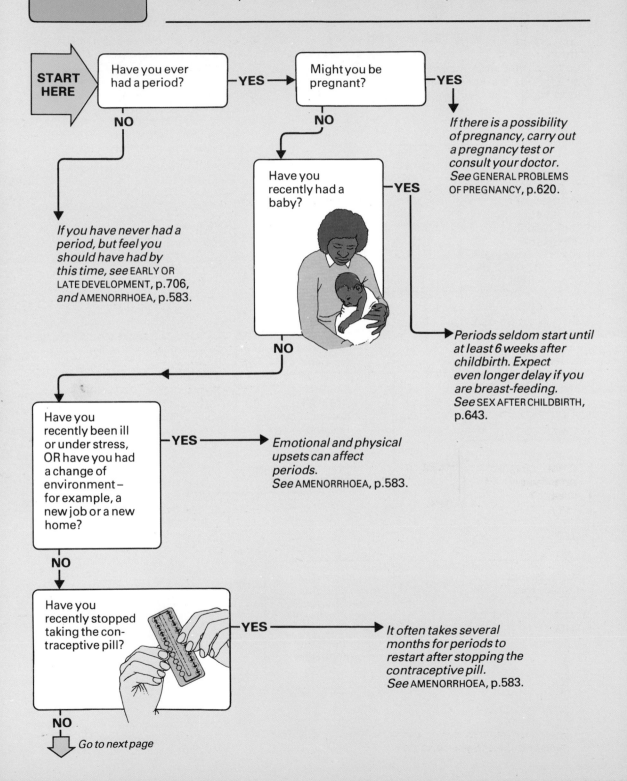

START HERE → **Have you ever had a period?** — **YES** → **Might you be pregnant?** — **YES** ↓

If there is a possibility of pregnancy, carry out a pregnancy test or consult your doctor. See GENERAL PROBLEMS OF PREGNANCY, p.620.

NO ↓

If you have never had a period, but feel you should have had by this time, see EARLY OR LATE DEVELOPMENT, p.706, *and* AMENORRHOEA, p.583.

NO ↓

Have you recently had a baby? — **YES** →

Periods seldom start until at least 6 weeks after childbirth. Expect even longer delay if you are breast-feeding. See SEX AFTER CHILDBIRTH, p.643.

NO ↓

Have you recently been ill or under stress, OR have you had a change of environment – for example, a new job or a new home? — **YES** →

Emotional and physical upsets can affect periods. See AMENORRHOEA, p.583.

NO ↓

Have you recently stopped taking the contraceptive pill? — **YES** →

It often takes several months for periods to restart after stopping the contraceptive pill. See AMENORRHOEA, p.583.

NO ↓

Go to next page

Continued from previous page

Have you lost a lot of weight in a short time through a strict reducing diet or vigorous exercise?

YES → *Sudden loss of weight often results in an absence of periods.* See AMENORRHOEA, p.583.

NO ↓

Are you over 40?

YES → *It is common for women over 40 to begin missing periods.* See MENOPAUSE, p.586.

NO ↓

Do you have two or more of the following symptoms?
☐ increased hairiness
☐ increased spottiness
☐ deepening of the voice
☐ unexplained weight gain

YES → *The delay may be caused by disruption in the production of hormones.* See HYPOTHALAMIC - PITUITARY ABNORMALITIES, p.587.

NO ↓

Are you currently taking any medicines?

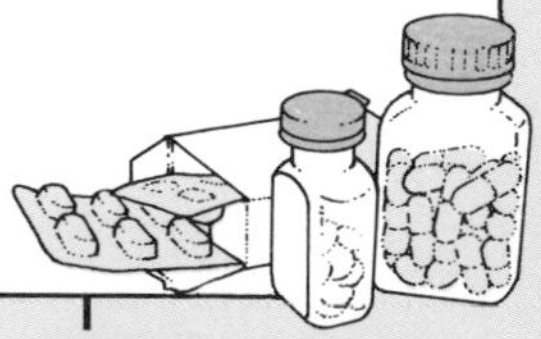

YES → *Some drugs can cause periods to stop.* Check DRUG INDEX, p.778, *for the side-effects of the drug you are taking, and discuss with your doctor.*

NO ↓

If you are unable to make a diagnosis from this chart, consult your doctor.

Heavy periods

Periods that either last more than 7 days or have recently become longer or begun to produce more blood than usual.

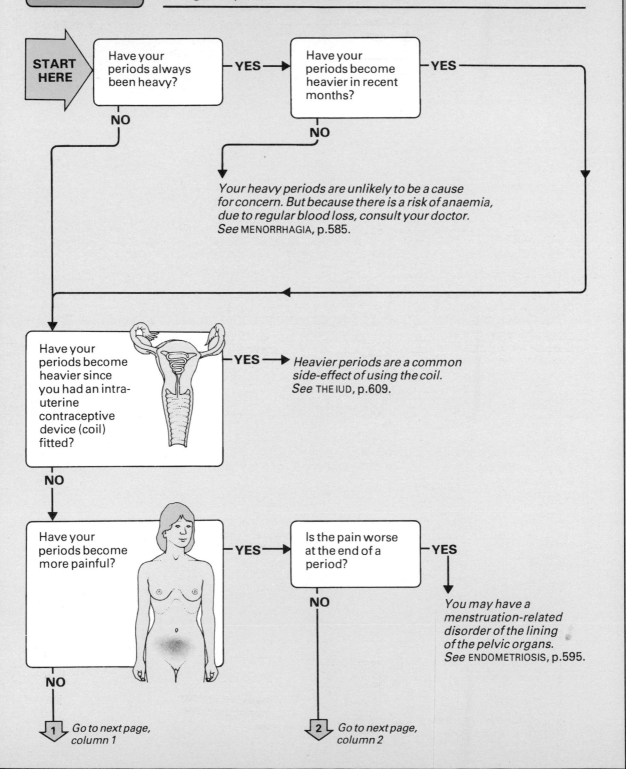

START HERE

Have your periods always been heavy? — **YES** → **Have your periods become heavier in recent months?** — **YES** →

NO

NO

Your heavy periods are unlikely to be a cause for concern. But because there is a risk of anaemia, due to regular blood loss, consult your doctor. *See* MENORRHAGIA, p.585.

Have your periods become heavier since you had an intra-uterine contraceptive device (coil) fitted? — **YES** → *Heavier periods are a common side-effect of using the coil. See* THE IUD, p.609.

NO

Have your periods become more painful? — **YES** → **Is the pain worse at the end of a period?** — **YES** →

NO

NO

You may have a menstruation-related disorder of the lining of the pelvic organs. *See* ENDOMETRIOSIS, p.595.

1 *Go to next page, column 1*

2 *Go to next page, column 2*

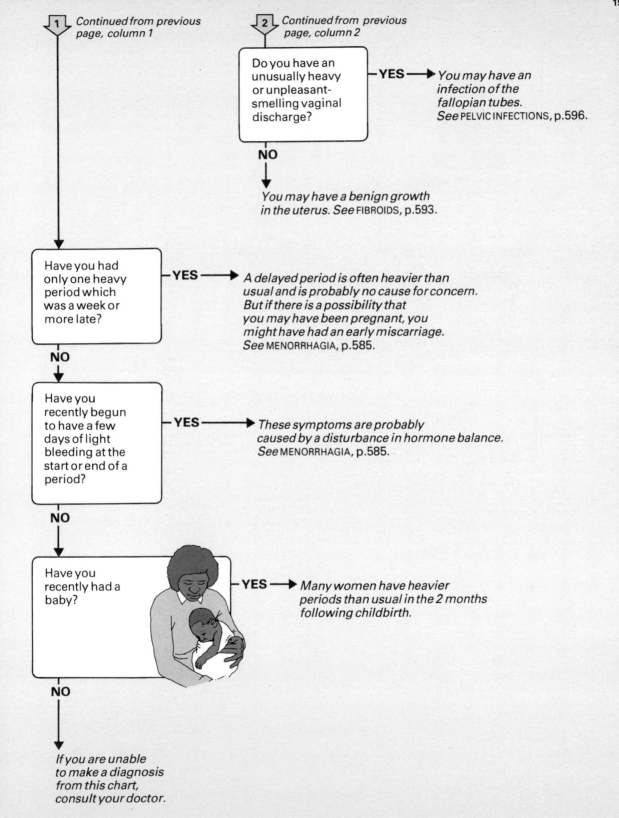

1 Continued from previous page, column 1

2 Continued from previous page, column 2

Do you have an unusually heavy or unpleasant-smelling vaginal discharge?

— YES → *You may have an infection of the fallopian tubes. See* PELVIC INFECTIONS, p.596.

NO

You may have a benign growth in the uterus. See FIBROIDS, p.593.

Have you had only one heavy period which was a week or more late?

— YES → *A delayed period is often heavier than usual and is probably no cause for concern. But if there is a possibility that you may have been pregnant, you might have had an early miscarriage. See* MENORRHAGIA, p.585.

NO

Have you recently begun to have a few days of light bleeding at the start or end of a period?

— YES → *These symptoms are probably caused by a disturbance in hormone balance. See* MENORRHAGIA, p.585.

NO

Have you recently had a baby?

— YES → *Many women have heavier periods than usual in the 2 months following childbirth.*

NO

If you are unable to make a diagnosis from this chart, consult your doctor.

77
WOMEN

Painful periods

Pain associated with menstruation is usually felt as a dull ache or cramping pain in the lower abdomen.

START HERE

Do you have an unusually heavy and smelly vaginal discharge between periods AND/OR is your temperature 38°C (100°F) or above?

YES →

You may have an infection. See PELVIC INFECTIONS, p.596.

NO

Does the pain get worse as the period proceeds?

YES →

You may have a menstruation-related disorder. See ENDOMETRIOSIS, p.595.

NO

Have you started your periods within the past 3 years?

YES →

NO

Have you had painful periods for most of your adult life AND is the pain the same as usual?

YES →

This is primary DYS-MENORRHOEA, p.584. *It is unlikely to be a cause for concern.*

NO

⇩ *Go to next column*

⇩ *Continued from previous column*

Have you recently had an intra-uterine contraceptive device (coil) fitted?

YES →

This sometimes causes an increase in period pain. See THE IUD, p.609.

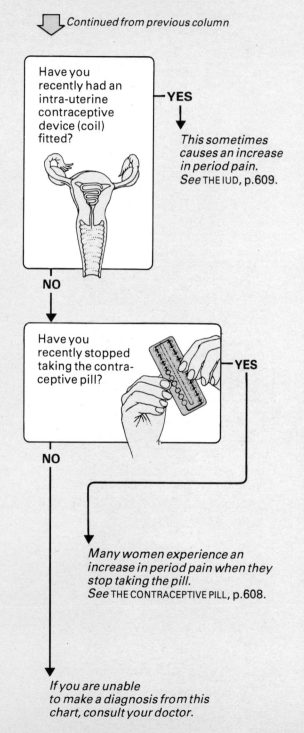

NO

Have you recently stopped taking the contraceptive pill?

YES →

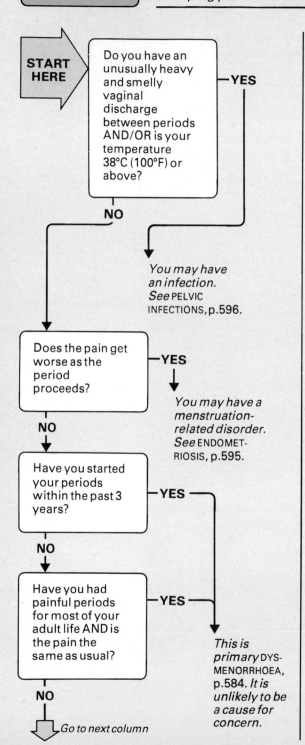

NO

Many women experience an increase in period pain when they stop taking the pill. See THE CONTRACEPTIVE PILL, p.608.

If you are unable to make a diagnosis from this chart, consult your doctor.

78
WOMEN

Lower abdominal pain in women

Pain below the waist in women of childbearing age.
Use this chart only after consulting chart 48, **Abdominal pain**.

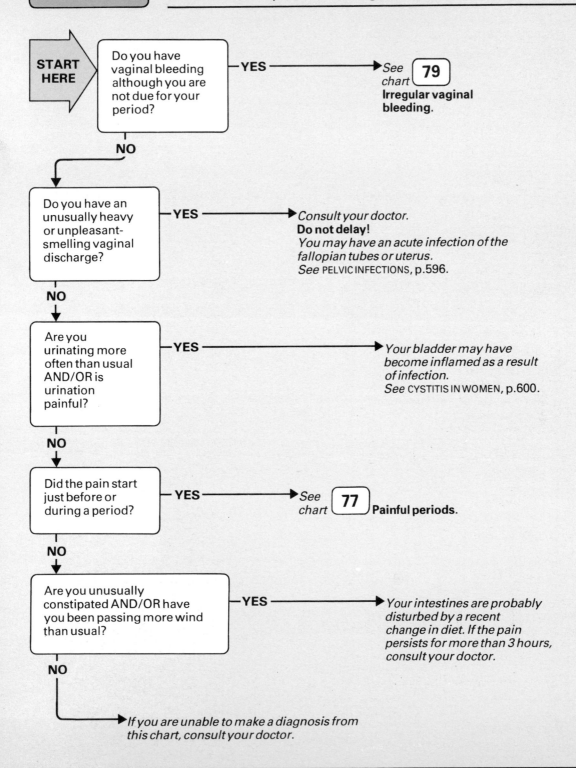

START HERE

Do you have vaginal bleeding although you are not due for your period?

YES → *See chart* **79** **Irregular vaginal bleeding.**

NO

Do you have an unusually heavy or unpleasant-smelling vaginal discharge?

YES → *Consult your doctor.* **Do not delay!** *You may have an acute infection of the fallopian tubes or uterus.* *See* PELVIC INFECTIONS, p.596.

NO

Are you urinating more often than usual AND/OR is urination painful?

YES → *Your bladder may have become inflamed as a result of infection.* *See* CYSTITIS IN WOMEN, p.600.

NO

Did the pain start just before or during a period?

YES → *See chart* **77** **Painful periods.**

NO

Are you unusually constipated AND/OR have you been passing more wind than usual?

YES → *Your intestines are probably disturbed by a recent change in diet. If the pain persists for more than 3 hours, consult your doctor.*

NO

→ *If you are unable to make a diagnosis from this chart, consult your doctor.*

79
WOMEN

Irregular vaginal bleeding

Any bleeding that occurs in between normal menstrual periods, during pregnancy, or after the menopause.

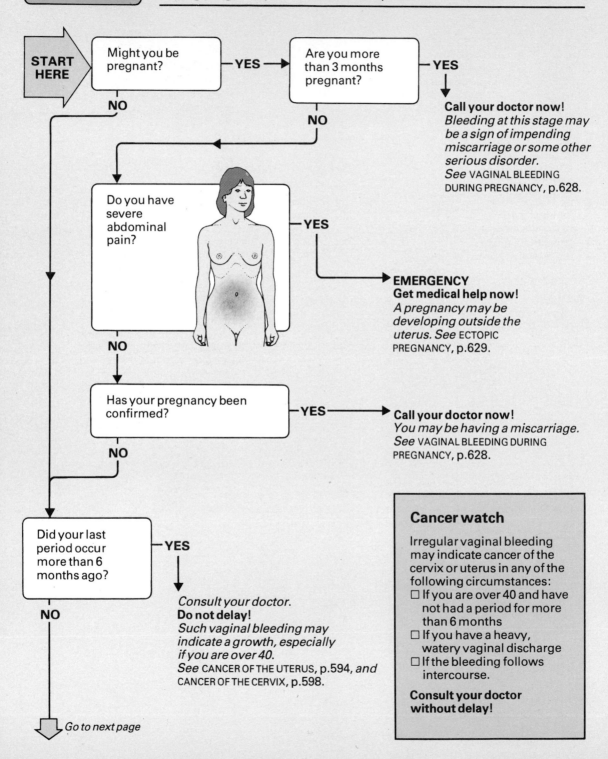

START HERE

Might you be pregnant? — **YES** → **Are you more than 3 months pregnant?** — **YES** →

Call your doctor now!
Bleeding at this stage may be a sign of impending miscarriage or some other serious disorder.
See VAGINAL BLEEDING DURING PREGNANCY, p.628.

NO ↓   **NO** ↓

Do you have severe abdominal pain? — **YES** →

EMERGENCY
Get medical help now!
A pregnancy may be developing outside the uterus. See ECTOPIC PREGNANCY, p.629.

NO ↓

Has your pregnancy been confirmed? — **YES** →

Call your doctor now!
You may be having a miscarriage.
See VAGINAL BLEEDING DURING PREGNANCY, p.628.

NO ↓

Did your last period occur more than 6 months ago? — **YES** →

Consult your doctor.
Do not delay!
Such vaginal bleeding may indicate a growth, especially if you are over 40.
See CANCER OF THE UTERUS, p.594, *and* CANCER OF THE CERVIX, p.598.

NO ↓

Go to next page

Cancer watch

Irregular vaginal bleeding may indicate cancer of the cervix or uterus in any of the following circumstances:

☐ If you are over 40 and have not had a period for more than 6 months

☐ If you have a heavy, watery vaginal discharge

☐ If the bleeding follows intercourse.

Consult your doctor without delay!

Continued from previous page

Do you have a heavy, watery vaginal discharge OR does the bleeding occur immediately after intercourse?

YES → *Consult your doctor.* **Do not delay!** *The bleeding is probably caused by* CERVICAL EROSION, p.598, *but there is a chance that you have* CANCER OF THE CERVIX, p.598, *or* CANCER OF THE UTERUS, p.594.

NO ↓

Have you had an intra-uterine contraceptive device (coil) fitted?

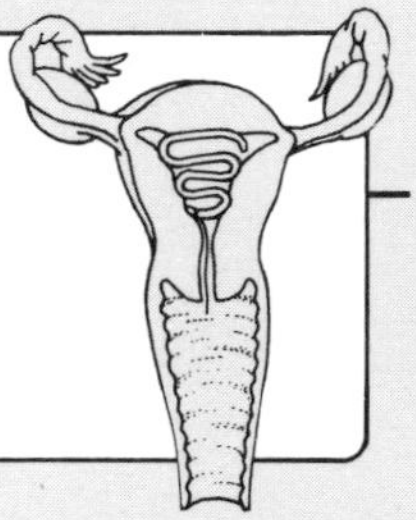

YES → Do you have severe abdominal pain?

YES → **EMERGENCY** **Get medical help now!** *A pregnancy may be developing outside the uterus. See* ECTOPIC PREGNANCY, p.629.

NO ↓ *The coil sometimes causes vaginal bleeding.* *See* THE IUD. p.609.

NO ↓

Are you taking any type of contraceptive pill?

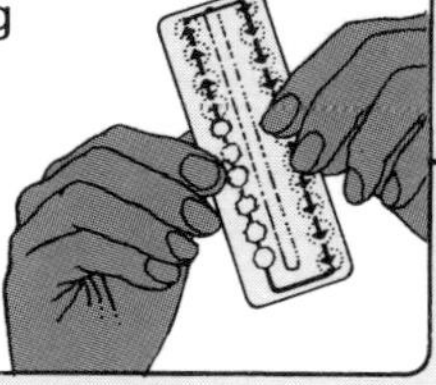

YES → *This is probably "breakthrough bleeding" which is common in women taking the pill.* *See* THE CONTRACEPTIVE PILL, p.608.

NO ↓

Was the bleeding like that of a period?

YES → Have you started your periods within the past 3 years?

YES → *Irregular periods are common during the first 3 years of menstruation. See* MENSTRUATION AND THE MENOPAUSE, p.583.

NO ↓

Are you in your late 30s or in your 40s?

YES → *You can expect irregular periods as you approach the* MENOPAUSE, p.586.

NO ↓

If you are unable to make a diagnosis from this chart, consult your doctor.

80
WOMEN

Abnormal vaginal discharge

Discharge from the vagina that differs in colour, consistency, and/or quantity from what you are used to noticing between periods.

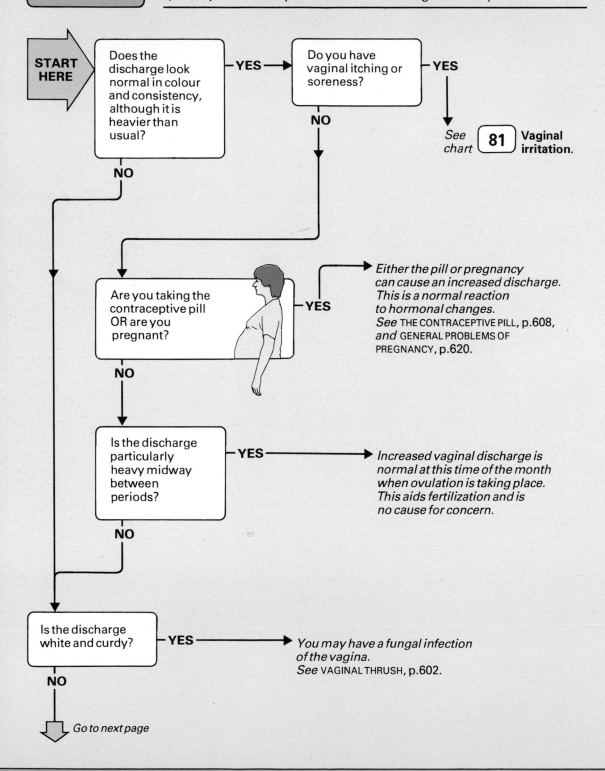

START HERE

Does the discharge look normal in colour and consistency, although it is heavier than usual? — **YES** → Do you have vaginal itching or soreness? — **YES** → *See chart* **81** **Vaginal irritation.**

NO

Do you have vaginal itching or soreness? **NO**

Are you taking the contraceptive pill OR are you pregnant? — **YES** → *Either the pill or pregnancy can cause an increased discharge. This is a normal reaction to hormonal changes. See* THE CONTRACEPTIVE PILL, p.608, *and* GENERAL PROBLEMS OF PREGNANCY, p.620.

NO

Is the discharge particularly heavy midway between periods? — **YES** → *Increased vaginal discharge is normal at this time of the month when ovulation is taking place. This aids fertilization and is no cause for concern.*

NO

Is the discharge white and curdy? — **YES** → *You may have a fungal infection of the vagina. See* VAGINAL THRUSH, p.602.

NO

Go to next page

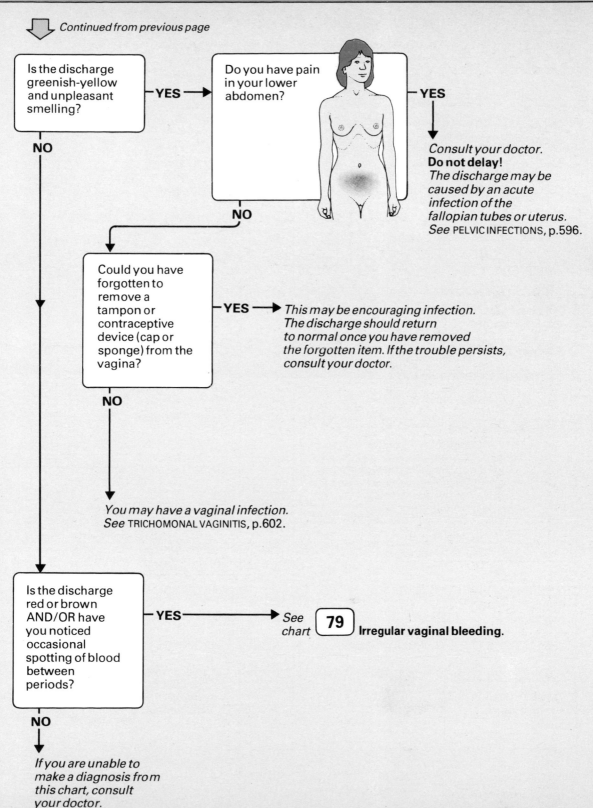

Continued from previous page

Is the discharge greenish-yellow and unpleasant smelling?

YES →

Do you have pain in your lower abdomen?

YES ↓

Consult your doctor. **Do not delay!** *The discharge may be caused by an acute infection of the fallopian tubes or uterus.* See PELVIC INFECTIONS, p.596.

NO ↓

NO →

Could you have forgotten to remove a tampon or contraceptive device (cap or sponge) from the vagina?

YES → *This may be encouraging infection. The discharge should return to normal once you have removed the forgotten item. If the trouble persists, consult your doctor.*

NO ↓

You may have a vaginal infection. See TRICHOMONAL VAGINITIS, p.602.

Is the discharge red or brown AND/OR have you noticed occasional spotting of blood between periods?

YES → *See chart* **79** **Irregular vaginal bleeding.**

NO ↓

If you are unable to make a diagnosis from this chart, consult your doctor.

81 WOMEN

Vaginal irritation

Itching or soreness in the vagina or around the genital area.

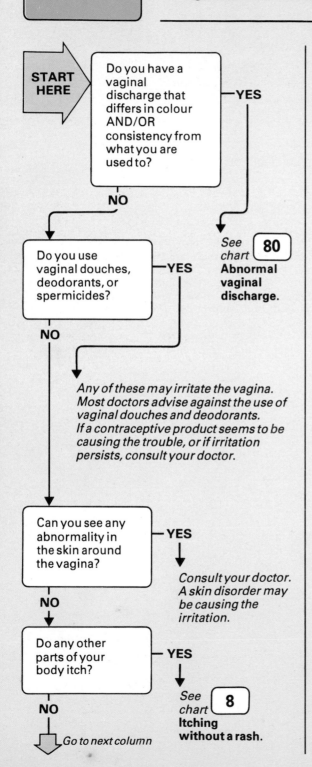

START HERE → Do you have a vaginal discharge that differs in colour AND/OR consistency from what you are used to? — **YES** → See chart **80** Abnormal vaginal discharge.

NO ↓

Do you use vaginal douches, deodorants, or spermicides? — **YES** →

NO ↓

Any of these may irritate the vagina. Most doctors advise against the use of vaginal douches and deodorants. If a contraceptive product seems to be causing the trouble, or if irritation persists, consult your doctor.

Can you see any abnormality in the skin around the vagina? — **YES** → *Consult your doctor. A skin disorder may be causing the irritation.*

NO ↓

Do any other parts of your body itch? — **YES** → See chart **8** Itching without a rash.

NO ↓

Go to next column

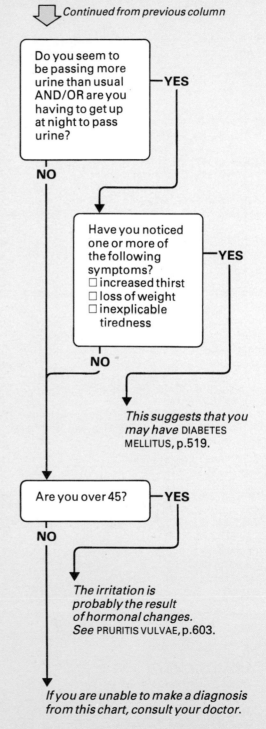

Continued from previous column ↓

Do you seem to be passing more urine than usual AND/OR are you having to get up at night to pass urine? — **YES** →

NO ↓

Have you noticed one or more of the following symptoms?
☐ increased thirst
☐ loss of weight
☐ inexplicable tiredness
— **YES** →

NO ↓

This suggests that you may have DIABETES MELLITUS, p.519.

Are you over 45? — **YES** →

NO ↓

The irritation is probably the result of hormonal changes. See PRURITIS VULVAE, p.603.

If you are unable to make a diagnosis from this chart, consult your doctor.

Abnormal hairiness in women

Any hair growth on the face, limbs, or torso that you consider excessive.

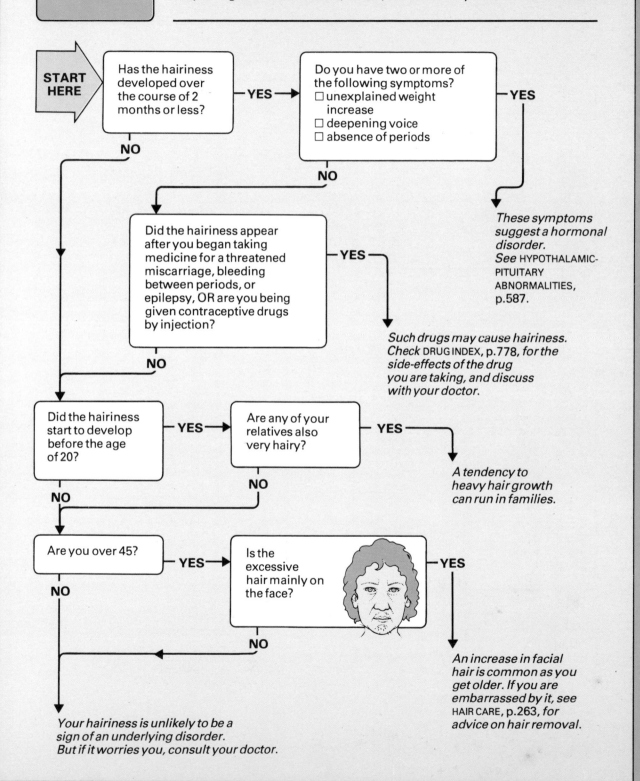

START HERE

Has the hairiness developed over the course of 2 months or less?

YES → Do you have two or more of the following symptoms?
☐ unexplained weight increase
☐ deepening voice
☐ absence of periods

NO

YES →

These symptoms suggest a hormonal disorder.
See HYPOTHALAMIC-PITUITARY ABNORMALITIES, p.587.

NO

Did the hairiness appear after you began taking medicine for a threatened miscarriage, bleeding between periods, or epilepsy, OR are you being given contraceptive drugs by injection?

YES →

Such drugs may cause hairiness.
Check DRUG INDEX, p.778, *for the side-effects of the drug you are taking, and discuss with your doctor.*

NO

Did the hairiness start to develop before the age of 20?

YES → Are any of your relatives also very hairy?

YES →

A tendency to heavy hair growth can run in families.

NO

NO

Are you over 45?

YES → Is the excessive hair mainly on the face?

YES →

An increase in facial hair is common as you get older. If you are embarrassed by it, see HAIR CARE, p.263, *for advice on hair removal.*

NO

NO

Your hairiness is unlikely to be a sign of an underlying disorder. But if it worries you, consult your doctor.

Painful intercourse in women

Pain or discomfort during or just after sexual intercourse.

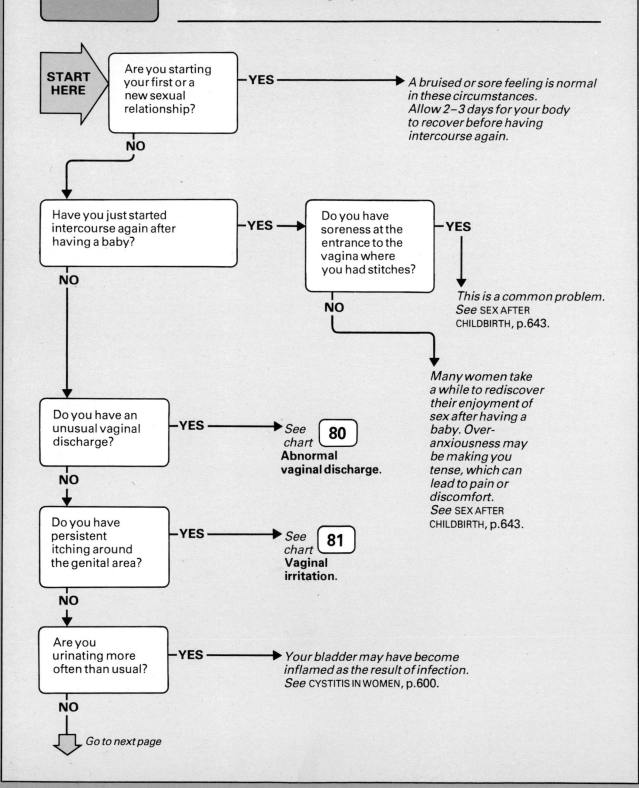

START HERE

Are you starting your first or a new sexual relationship? — **YES** → *A bruised or sore feeling is normal in these circumstances. Allow 2–3 days for your body to recover before having intercourse again.*

NO

Have you just started intercourse again after having a baby? — **YES** → Do you have soreness at the entrance to the vagina where you had stitches? — **YES** ↓

This is a common problem. See SEX AFTER CHILDBIRTH, p.643.

NO

NO

Many women take a while to rediscover their enjoyment of sex after having a baby. Over-anxiousness may be making you tense, which can lead to pain or discomfort. See SEX AFTER CHILDBIRTH, p.643.

Do you have an unusual vaginal discharge? — **YES** → *See chart* **80** **Abnormal vaginal discharge.**

NO

Do you have persistent itching around the genital area? — **YES** → *See chart* **81** **Vaginal irritation.**

NO

Are you urinating more often than usual? — **YES** → *Your bladder may have become inflamed as the result of infection. See* CYSTITIS IN WOMEN, p.600.

NO

⬇ *Go to next page*

Continued from previous page

Is your vagina so dry that penetration is uncomfortable and difficult?

YES → Are you over 45?

YES → *Some dryness is common during and after the* MENOPAUSE, p.586. *See also* PAINFUL INTERCOURSE, p.615.

NO ↓

Anxiety or failure to become aroused may account for your dryness. See PAINFUL INTERCOURSE, p.615.

NO ↓

When your partner penetrates deeply, does it feel as though he is hitting a tender place?

YES → Have your periods become more painful than they used to be?

YES → *You may have a menstruation-related disorder of the lining of the pelvic organs. See* ENDOMETRIOSIS, p.595.

NO ↓

Do you have pain only when you have intercourse in certain positions?

YES → *The pain may be caused by pressure on an ovary during intercourse. See* RETROVERSION OF THE UTERUS, p.597, *and* PAINFUL INTERCOURSE, p.615.

NO ↓

NO ↓

Does your vagina seem too small, so that penetration is difficult?

YES → *Your trouble is probably due to involuntary tightening of the muscles in the vagina. See* PAINFUL INTERCOURSE, p.615.

NO ↓

If you are unable to make a diagnosis from this chart, consult your doctor.

84
COUPLES

Failure to conceive

Failure to conceive after more than 12 months without contraception. In order to make a diagnosis, each partner should read the chart in turn.

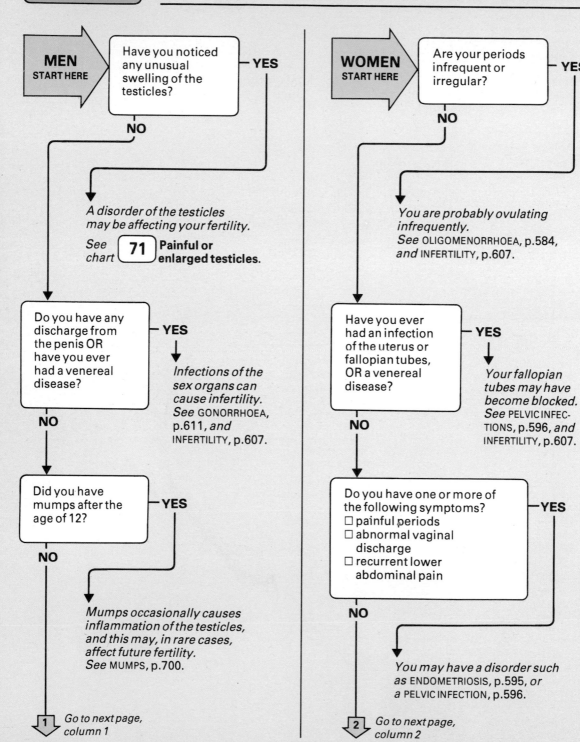

MEN START HERE

Have you noticed any unusual swelling of the testicles? — **YES**

NO

A disorder of the testicles may be affecting your fertility.

See chart **71** **Painful or enlarged testicles.**

Do you have any discharge from the penis OR have you ever had a venereal disease? — **YES**

Infections of the sex organs can cause infertility. See GONORRHOEA, *p.611, and* INFERTILITY, *p.607.*

NO

Did you have mumps after the age of 12? — **YES**

NO

Mumps occasionally causes inflammation of the testicles, and this may, in rare cases, affect future fertility. See MUMPS, *p.700.*

1 *Go to next page, column 1*

WOMEN START HERE

Are your periods infrequent or irregular? — **YES**

NO

You are probably ovulating infrequently. See OLIGOMENORRHOEA, *p.584, and* INFERTILITY, *p.607.*

Have you ever had an infection of the uterus or fallopian tubes, OR a venereal disease? — **YES**

Your fallopian tubes may have become blocked. See PELVIC INFECTIONS, *p.596, and* INFERTILITY, *p.607.*

NO

Do you have one or more of the following symptoms?
☐ painful periods
☐ abnormal vaginal discharge
☐ recurrent lower abdominal pain
— **YES**

NO

You may have a disorder such as ENDOMETRIOSIS, *p.595, or a* PELVIC INFECTION, *p.596.*

2 *Go to next page, column 2*

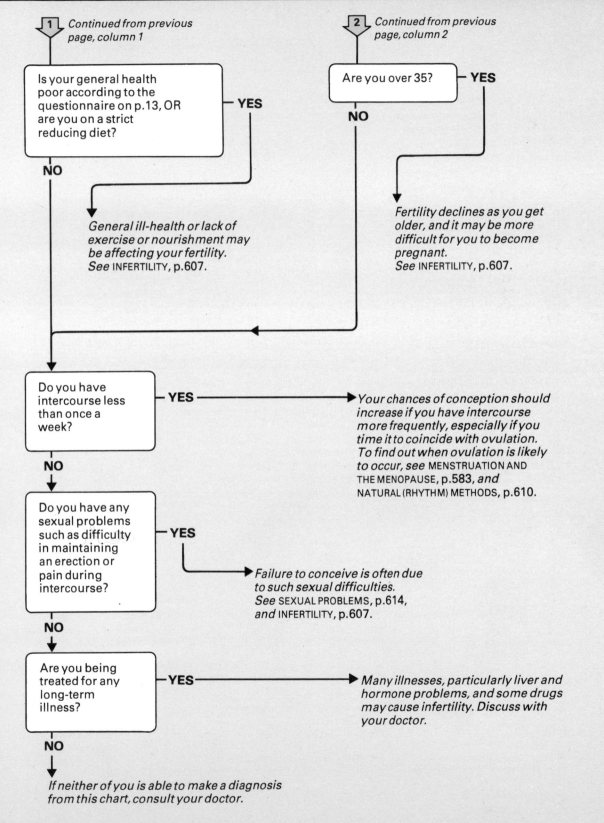

1 Continued from previous page, column 1

Is your general health poor according to the questionnaire on p.13, OR are you on a strict reducing diet?

YES

NO

General ill-health or lack of exercise or nourishment may be affecting your fertility. See INFERTILITY, p.607.

2 Continued from previous page, column 2

Are you over 35? — **YES**

NO

Fertility declines as you get older, and it may be more difficult for you to become pregnant. See INFERTILITY, p.607.

Do you have intercourse less than once a week?

YES

NO

Your chances of conception should increase if you have intercourse more frequently, especially if you time it to coincide with ovulation. To find out when ovulation is likely to occur, see MENSTRUATION AND THE MENOPAUSE, p.583, *and* NATURAL (RHYTHM) METHODS, p.610.

Do you have any sexual problems such as difficulty in maintaining an erection or pain during intercourse?

YES

NO

Failure to conceive is often due to such sexual difficulties. See SEXUAL PROBLEMS, p.614, *and* INFERTILITY, p.607.

Are you being treated for any long-term illness?

YES

NO

Many illnesses, particularly liver and hormone problems, and some drugs may cause infertility. Discuss with your doctor.

If neither of you is able to make a diagnosis from this chart, consult your doctor.

85

CHILDREN
0–5 years

Waking at night

Any waking after the child has gone to sleep for the night that may cause the child to cry or call out.

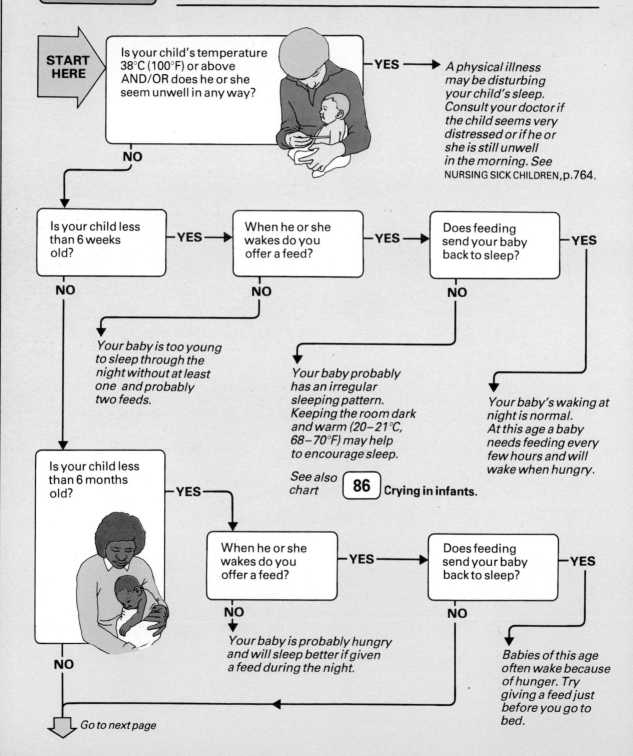

START HERE → Is your child's temperature 38°C (100°F) or above AND/OR does he or she seem unwell in any way?

YES → *A physical illness may be disturbing your child's sleep. Consult your doctor if the child seems very distressed or if he or she is still unwell in the morning. See* NURSING SICK CHILDREN, p.764.

NO

Is your child less than 6 weeks old? — **YES** → When he or she wakes do you offer a feed? — **YES** → Does feeding send your baby back to sleep? — **YES**

NO — **NO** — **NO**

Your baby is too young to sleep through the night without at least one and probably two feeds.

Your baby probably has an irregular sleeping pattern. Keeping the room dark and warm (20–21°C, 68–70°F) may help to encourage sleep.

See also chart **86** **Crying in infants.**

Your baby's waking at night is normal. At this age a baby needs feeding every few hours and will wake when hungry.

Is your child less than 6 months old? — **YES** → When he or she wakes do you offer a feed? — **YES** → Does feeding send your baby back to sleep? — **YES**

NO — **NO** — **NO**

Your baby is probably hungry and will sleep better if given a feed during the night.

Babies of this age often wake because of hunger. Try giving a feed just before you go to bed.

⬇ *Go to next page*

Continued from previous page

Is your child less than a year old?

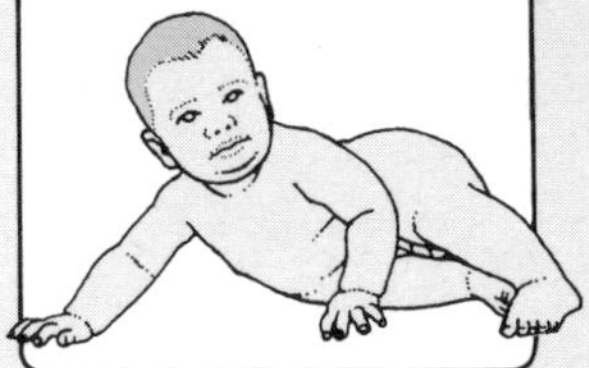

YES →

When you go to your baby in the night, do you find that the bedclothes have been kicked off?

YES → *Your baby is probably woken by the cold. A sleeping bag or a warmer room may solve the problem.*

NO

NO

Does your baby's bottom look red, sore, or spotty?

YES → *Your baby probably has* NAPPY RASH, p.650, *which stings when urine is passed, causing your baby to wake. See also p.234,* **Visual aids to diagnosis, 4.**

NO

Does your baby usually sleep through most of the night, but wake early in the morning?

YES → *Your baby probably does not need any more sleep. Giving a nappy change and a drink, and putting a few toys in the cot may enable you to get some more sleep.*

NO

→ *Your baby probably has an irregular sleeping pattern. See* SLEEPING PROBLEMS IN CHILDREN, p.671.

Does your child seem upset or frightened on waking?

YES → *Nightmares may be waking your child. See* SLEEPING PROBLEMS IN CHILDREN, p.671. *A dim light in the room may help if your child is afraid of the dark.*

NO

Does your child have any cause for worry – for example, the arrival of a new baby, starting a new school, or tension in the home?

YES → *Anxiety may be making your child wakeful. Extra reassurance and affection during the day may help to solve the problem. See* SLEEPING PROBLEMS IN CHILDREN, p.671.

NO

→ *Your child's wakefulness is probably due to an irregular sleeping pattern, and is unlikely to be a sign of any disorder. However, if you are worried by it, consult your doctor.*

86

Crying in infants

Any sobbing, whimpering, or wailing which indicates that your baby is not content.

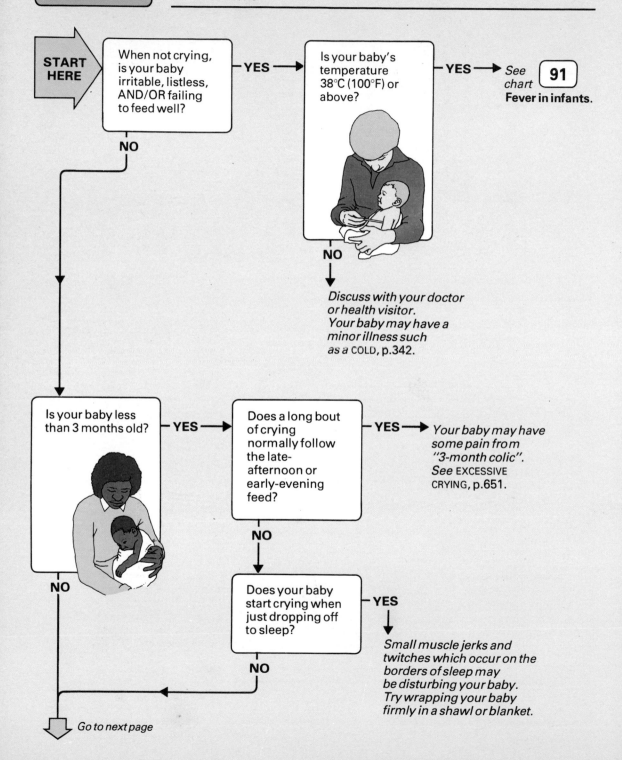

START HERE

When not crying, is your baby irritable, listless, AND/OR failing to feed well? — **YES** →

Is your baby's temperature 38°C (100°F) or above? — **YES** → *See chart* **91** **Fever in infants**.

NO ↓

Discuss with your doctor or health visitor. Your baby may have a minor illness such as a COLD, p.342.

NO ↓

Is your baby less than 3 months old? — **YES** →

Does a long bout of crying normally follow the late-afternoon or early-evening feed? — **YES** → *Your baby may have some pain from "3-month colic". See* EXCESSIVE CRYING, p.651.

NO ↓

Does your baby start crying when just dropping off to sleep? — **YES** ↓

Small muscle jerks and twitches which occur on the borders of sleep may be disturbing your baby. Try wrapping your baby firmly in a shawl or blanket.

NO ↓

NO ↓

⇩ *Go to next page*

Continued from previous page

Is your baby in a cool room, or outside in a pram on a chilly day?

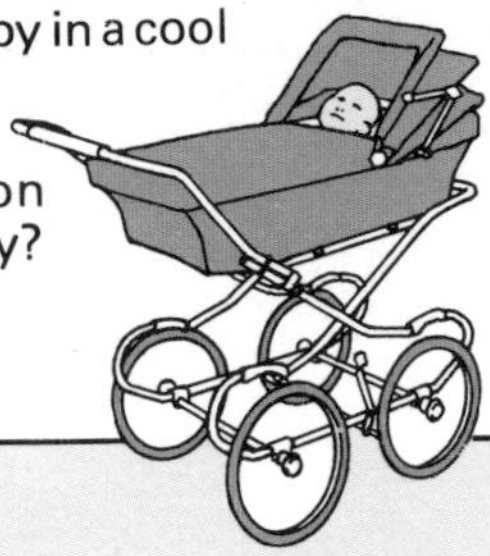

YES → *Your baby may simply be too cold. Moving into a warm room will probably help.*

NO ↓

Does your baby generally stop crying when picked up?

YES → *Your baby is probably bored or lonely. Try giving a little more attention or placing the baby where he or she can see you.*

NO ↓

Does your baby's bottom look red, sore, or spotty?

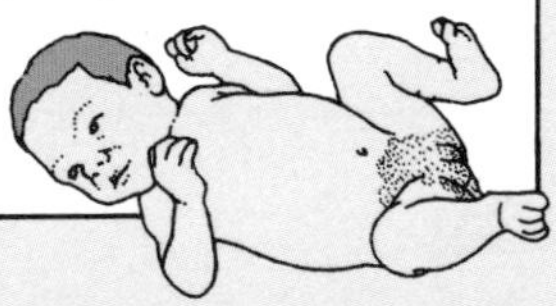

YES → NAPPY RASH, p.650, *may be making your baby uncomfortable. See also* p.234, **Visual aids to diagnosis, 4.**

NO ↓

Does your baby stop crying after being fed?

YES → **Does your baby start crying again less than 2 hours after a feed?**

YES → *You may not be giving enough food. If you are breast-feeding, allow your baby to suck more often and for longer. If bottle-feeding, increase the amount offered. Remember that babies also get thirsty. Giving water between feeds may help to reduce crying. See* FEEDING PROBLEMS, p.649, *and* EXCESSIVE CRYING, p.651.

NO ↓ *Your baby probably cries simply because of hunger. Try offering a feed whenever he or she seems hungry.*

NO ↓ *If you are unable to make a diagnosis from this chart and the crying is worrying you, consult your doctor.*

87

Vomiting in infants

Bringing back or throwing up of stomach contents.

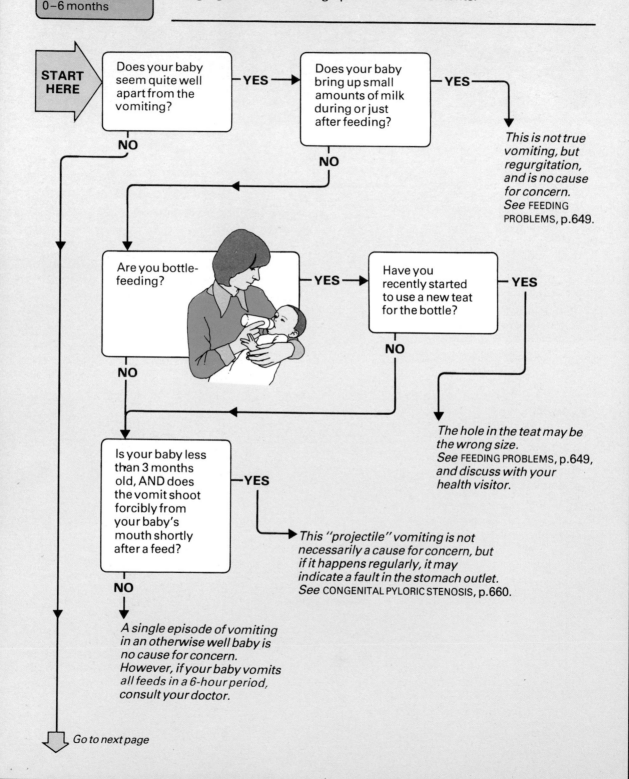

START HERE

Does your baby seem quite well apart from the vomiting? — **YES** →

Does your baby bring up small amounts of milk during or just after feeding? — **YES** →

This is not true vomiting, but regurgitation, and is no cause for concern. See FEEDING PROBLEMS, p.649.

NO ↓ (from first box)

NO ↓ (from second box)

Are you bottle-feeding? — **YES** →

Have you recently started to use a new teat for the bottle? — **YES** →

The hole in the teat may be the wrong size. See FEEDING PROBLEMS, p.649, *and discuss with your health visitor.*

NO ↓

NO ↓

Is your baby less than 3 months old, AND does the vomit shoot forcibly from your baby's mouth shortly after a feed? — **YES** →

This "projectile" vomiting is not necessarily a cause for concern, but if it happens regularly, it may indicate a fault in the stomach outlet. See CONGENITAL PYLORIC STENOSIS, p.660.

NO ↓

A single episode of vomiting in an otherwise well baby is no cause for concern. However, if your baby vomits all feeds in a 6-hour period, consult your doctor.

Go to next page

⬇ *Continued from previous page*

Is your baby passing frequent, watery faeces? — **YES** →

Consult your doctor.
Do not delay!
Your baby may have an infection of the digestive tract.
See GASTROENTERITIS IN INFANTS, p.649.

NO ↓

Is your baby's temperature 38°C (100°F) or above? — **YES** →

See chart **91** **Fever in infants.**

NO ↓

Does your baby have a cough or a runny nose? — **YES** →

A COLD, p.342, *is probably causing the vomiting. This is no cause for concern unless your baby vomits all feeds in a 6-hour period, in which case consult your doctor.*

NO ↓

Is your baby having bouts of loud, uncontrollable crying as if in great pain? — **YES** ↓

EMERGENCY
Get medical help now!
Your baby may have an acute abdominal condition such as INTUSSUSCEPTION, p.683, *or* INTESTINAL OBSTRUCTION, p.471.

NO ↓

If you are unable to make a diagnosis from this chart, consult your doctor.

Persistent vomiting

If your baby's vomiting is persistent (losing all feeds in a 6-hour period) a dangerous amount of body fluid may be lost.
Consult your doctor without delay!

88

Diarrhoea in infants

Passing runny, watery faeces abnormally frequently.

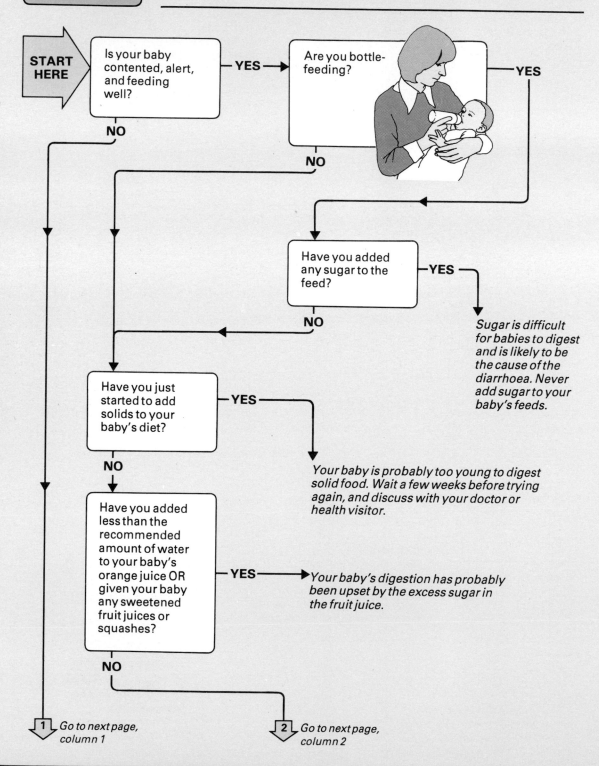

START HERE → Is your baby contented, alert, and feeding well? — **YES** → Are you bottle-feeding? — **YES** →

↓ **NO**

Are you bottle-feeding? ↓ **NO**

Have you added any sugar to the feed? — **YES** →

Sugar is difficult for babies to digest and is likely to be the cause of the diarrhoea. Never add sugar to your baby's feeds.

↓ **NO**

Have you just started to add solids to your baby's diet? — **YES** →

Your baby is probably too young to digest solid food. Wait a few weeks before trying again, and discuss with your doctor or health visitor.

↓ **NO**

Have you added less than the recommended amount of water to your baby's orange juice OR given your baby any sweetened fruit juices or squashes? — **YES** →

Your baby's digestion has probably been upset by the excess sugar in the fruit juice.

↓ **NO**

1 *Go to next page, column 1*

2 *Go to next page, column 2*

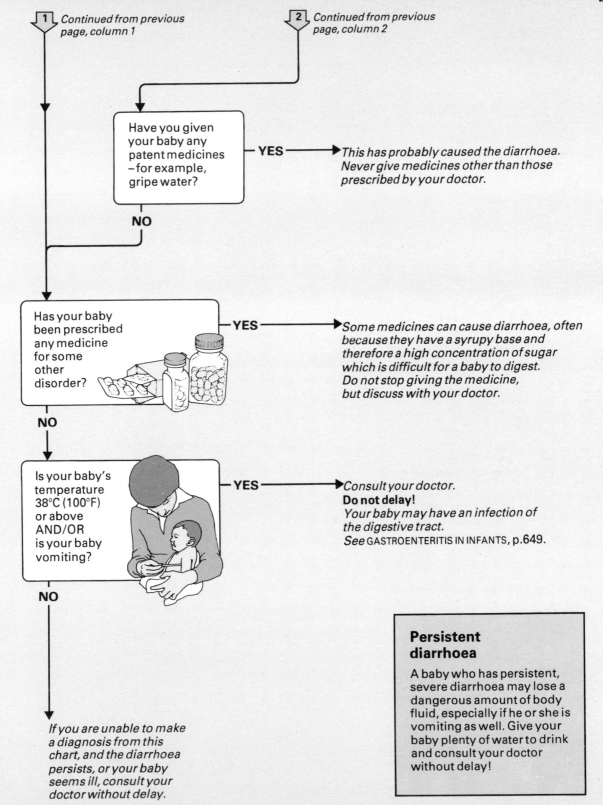

1 Continued from previous page, column 1

2 Continued from previous page, column 2

Have you given your baby any patent medicines – for example, gripe water?

YES → *This has probably caused the diarrhoea. Never give medicines other than those prescribed by your doctor.*

NO

Has your baby been prescribed any medicine for some other disorder?

YES → *Some medicines can cause diarrhoea, often because they have a syrupy base and therefore a high concentration of sugar which is difficult for a baby to digest. Do not stop giving the medicine, but discuss with your doctor.*

NO

Is your baby's temperature 38°C (100°F) or above AND/OR is your baby vomiting?

YES → *Consult your doctor.* **Do not delay!** *Your baby may have an infection of the digestive tract.* See GASTROENTERITIS IN INFANTS, p.649.

NO

If you are unable to make a diagnosis from this chart, and the diarrhoea persists, or your baby seems ill, consult your doctor without delay.

Persistent diarrhoea

A baby who has persistent, severe diarrhoea may lose a dangerous amount of body fluid, especially if he or she is vomiting as well. Give your baby plenty of water to drink and consult your doctor without delay!

Skin problems in infants

Any skin spots, discoloured areas, or blisters that may be sore or itchy.

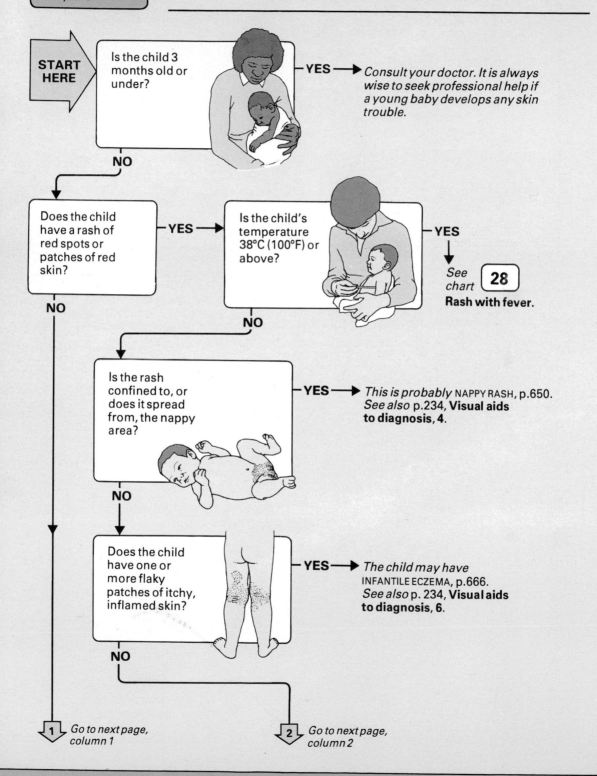

START HERE → Is the child 3 months old or under? — **YES** → *Consult your doctor. It is always wise to seek professional help if a young baby develops any skin trouble.*

NO ↓

Does the child have a rash of red spots or patches of red skin? — **YES** → Is the child's temperature 38°C (100°F) or above? — **YES** ↓ *See chart* **28** **Rash with fever.**

NO ↓ (from red spots box)

NO ↓ (from temperature box)

Is the rash confined to, or does it spread from, the nappy area? — **YES** → *This is probably* NAPPY RASH, p.650. *See also* p.234, **Visual aids to diagnosis, 4.**

NO ↓

Does the child have one or more flaky patches of itchy, inflamed skin? — **YES** → *The child may have* INFANTILE ECZEMA, p.666. *See also* p. 234, **Visual aids to diagnosis, 6.**

NO ↓

1 *Go to next page, column 1*

2 *Go to next page, column 2*

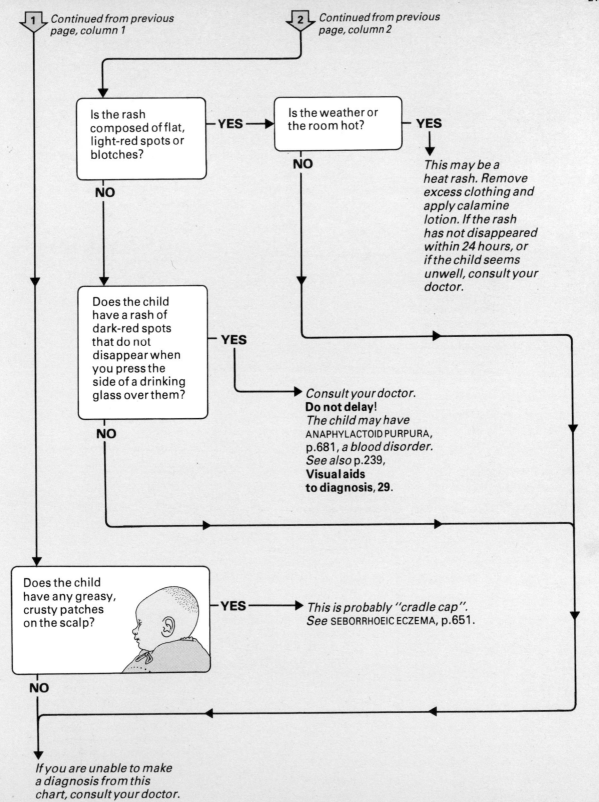

Continued from previous page, column 1

Continued from previous page, column 2

Is the rash composed of flat, light-red spots or blotches? — YES →

Is the weather or the room hot? — YES ↓

NO

This may be a heat rash. Remove excess clothing and apply calamine lotion. If the rash has not disappeared within 24 hours, or if the child seems unwell, consult your doctor.

NO

Does the child have a rash of dark-red spots that do not disappear when you press the side of a drinking glass over them? — YES →

NO

Consult your doctor. **Do not delay!** *The child may have* ANAPHYLACTOID PURPURA, p.681, *a blood disorder.* *See also* p.239, **Visual aids to diagnosis, 29.**

Does the child have any greasy, crusty patches on the scalp? — YES →

This is probably "cradle cap". *See* SEBORRHOEIC ECZEMA, p.651.

NO

If you are unable to make a diagnosis from this chart, consult your doctor.

Slow weight gain

Failure to gain weight or grow at the expected rate (see the box below and the growth charts on p.645).

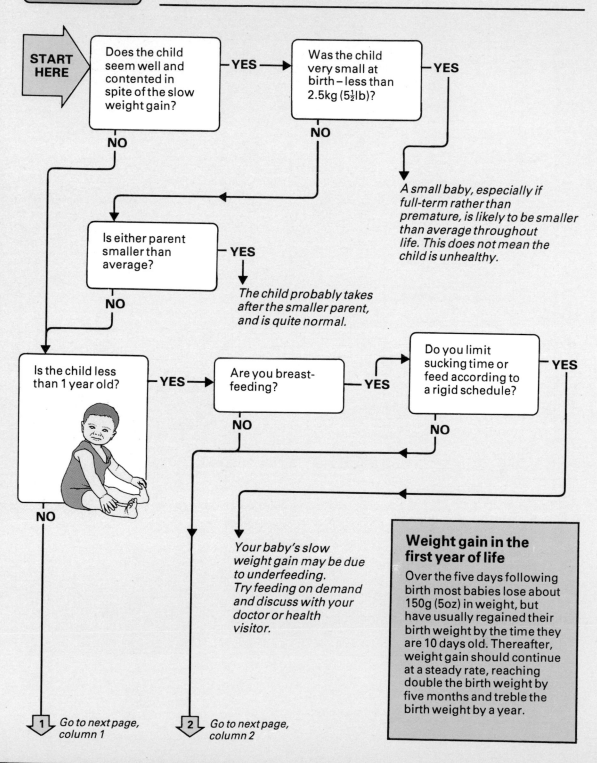

START HERE

Does the child seem well and contented in spite of the slow weight gain?

YES → Was the child very small at birth – less than 2.5kg (5½lb)?

YES → *A small baby, especially if full-term rather than premature, is likely to be smaller than average throughout life. This does not mean the child is unhealthy.*

NO

Is either parent smaller than average?

YES → *The child probably takes after the smaller parent, and is quite normal.*

NO

Is the child less than 1 year old?

YES → Are you breast-feeding?

YES → Do you limit sucking time or feed according to a rigid schedule?

YES

NO

NO

NO

Your baby's slow weight gain may be due to underfeeding. Try feeding on demand and discuss with your doctor or health visitor.

Weight gain in the first year of life

Over the five days following birth most babies lose about 150g (5oz) in weight, but have usually regained their birth weight by the time they are 10 days old. Thereafter, weight gain should continue at a steady rate, reaching double the birth weight by five months and treble the birth weight by a year.

1 *Go to next page, column 1*

2 *Go to next page, column 2*

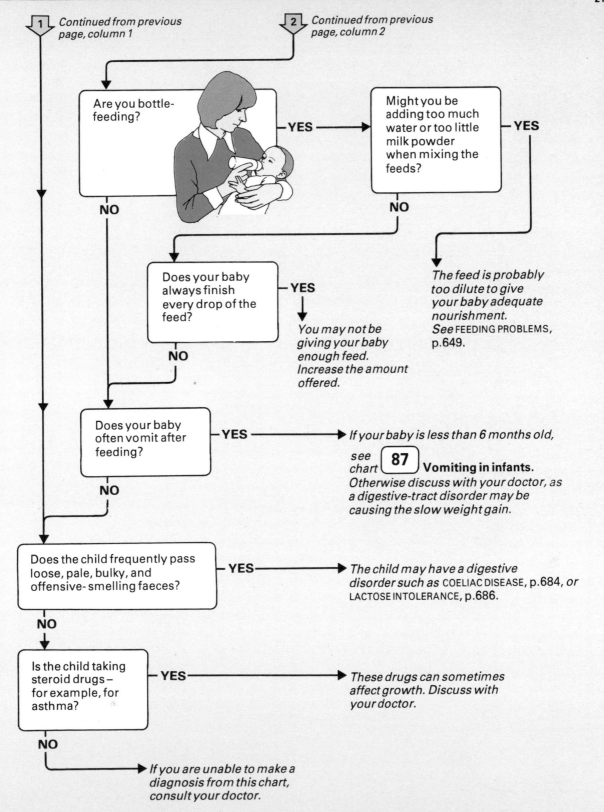

Continued from previous page, column 1

Continued from previous page, column 2

Are you bottle-feeding?

YES → **Might you be adding too much water or too little milk powder when mixing the feeds?**

YES → *The feed is probably too dilute to give your baby adequate nourishment. See* FEEDING PROBLEMS, *p.649.*

NO (Are you bottle-feeding?) →

NO (Might you be adding too much water...) →

Does your baby always finish every drop of the feed?

YES → *You may not be giving your baby enough feed. Increase the amount offered.*

NO →

Does your baby often vomit after feeding?

YES → *If your baby is less than 6 months old, see* chart **87** **Vomiting in infants.** *Otherwise discuss with your doctor, as a digestive-tract disorder may be causing the slow weight gain.*

NO →

Does the child frequently pass loose, pale, bulky, and offensive-smelling faeces?

YES → *The child may have a digestive disorder such as* COELIAC DISEASE, *p.684, or* LACTOSE INTOLERANCE, *p.686.*

NO →

Is the child taking steroid drugs – for example, for asthma?

YES → *These drugs can sometimes affect growth. Discuss with your doctor.*

NO →

If you are unable to make a diagnosis from this chart, consult your doctor.

91

Fever in infants

Temperature of 38°C (100°F) or above, which may make a baby flushed and irritable.

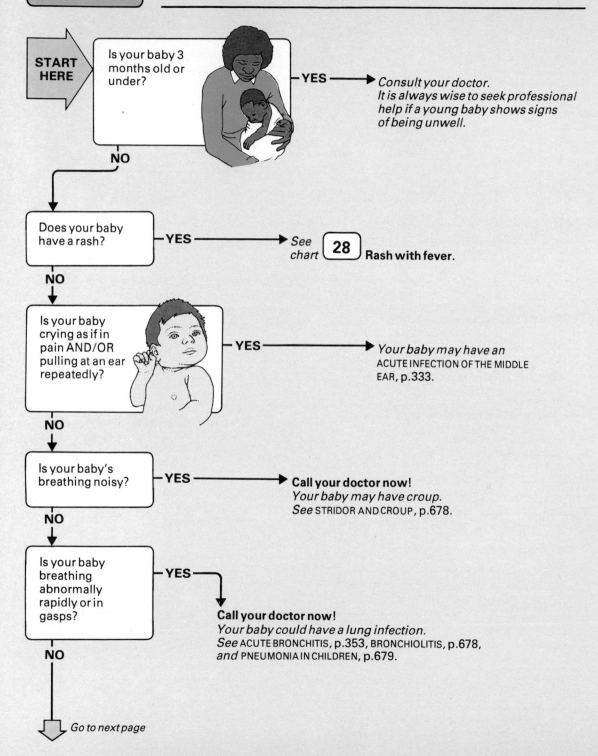

START HERE → **Is your baby 3 months old or under?**

YES → *Consult your doctor.*
It is always wise to seek professional help if a young baby shows signs of being unwell.

NO ↓

Does your baby have a rash?

YES → *See chart* **28** **Rash with fever.**

NO ↓

Is your baby crying as if in pain AND/OR pulling at an ear repeatedly?

YES → *Your baby may have an* ACUTE INFECTION OF THE MIDDLE EAR, p.333.

NO ↓

Is your baby's breathing noisy?

YES → **Call your doctor now!**
Your baby may have croup.
See STRIDOR AND CROUP, p.678.

NO ↓

Is your baby breathing abnormally rapidly or in gasps?

YES → **Call your doctor now!**
Your baby could have a lung infection.
See ACUTE BRONCHITIS, p.353, BRONCHIOLITIS, p.678, *and* PNEUMONIA IN CHILDREN, p.679.

NO ↓

Go to next page

Continued from previous page

Does your baby have diarrhoea? — **YES** →
Consult your doctor.
Do not delay!
This may be an infection of the digestive tract.
See GASTROENTERITIS, p.459.
If your baby is less than 1 year old,
see GASTROENTERITIS IN INFANTS, p.649.

NO

Does your baby have a runny nose? — **YES** → **Has your baby been in contact with measles in the past 2 weeks?** — **YES** →
Your baby may be developing MEASLES, p.699.

NO (runny nose)

NO (measles contact)
Your baby probably has a feverish COLD, p.342.

Is the weather or the room hot AND is your baby warmly dressed? — **YES** →
The fever is probably the result of overheating. Try removing some of your baby's clothing and giving a drink of water.

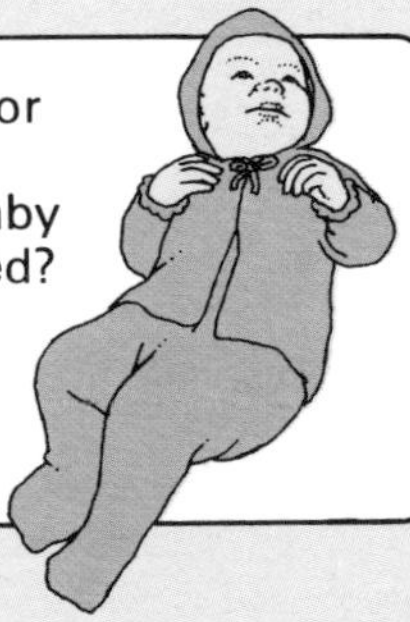

NO

If you are unable to make a diagnosis from this chart, consult your doctor. Do not delay if your baby seems very ill or has a temperature of 39°C (102°F) or above.

Convulsions

Sometimes a high temperature in an infant can cause convulsions. (See CONVULSIONS IN CHILDREN, p.667.) If this happens, or if your baby's temperature reaches 39°C (102°C) or above, call your doctor immediately.

While waiting for the doctor, see p.698 for advice on dealing with a raised temperature.

92

CHILDREN
2–14 years

Fever in children

A temperature of 38°C (100°F) or above, which may make the child flushed, irritable, or sleepy.

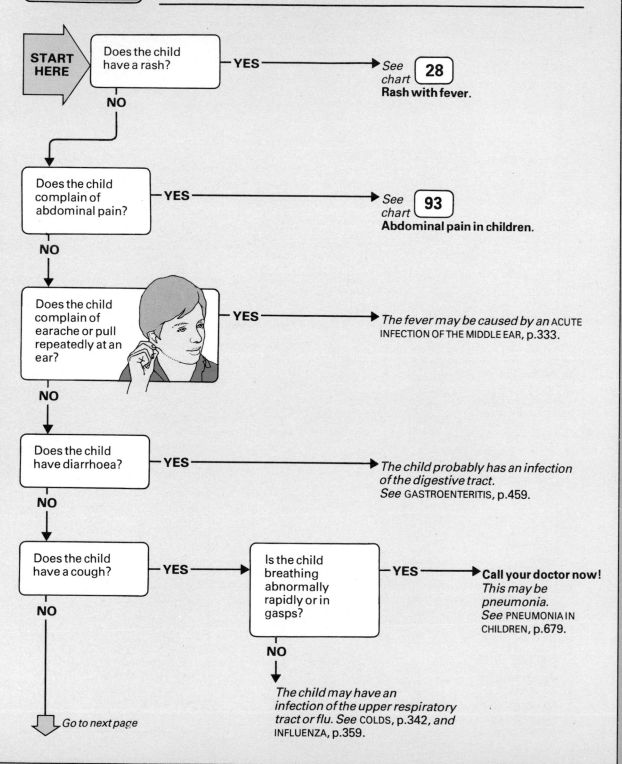

START HERE → Does the child have a rash? — **YES** → See chart **28** **Rash with fever**.

NO ↓

Does the child complain of abdominal pain? — **YES** → See chart **93** **Abdominal pain in children**.

NO ↓

Does the child complain of earache or pull repeatedly at an ear? — **YES** → *The fever may be caused by an* ACUTE INFECTION OF THE MIDDLE EAR, p.333.

NO ↓

Does the child have diarrhoea? — **YES** → *The child probably has an infection of the digestive tract.* See GASTROENTERITIS, p.459.

NO ↓

Does the child have a cough? — **YES** → Is the child breathing abnormally rapidly or in gasps? — **YES** → **Call your doctor now!** *This may be pneumonia.* See PNEUMONIA IN CHILDREN, p.679.

NO ↓ *(from cough branch)*

The child may have an infection of the upper respiratory tract or flu. See COLDS, p.342, *and* INFLUENZA, p.359.

NO ↓ *Go to next page*

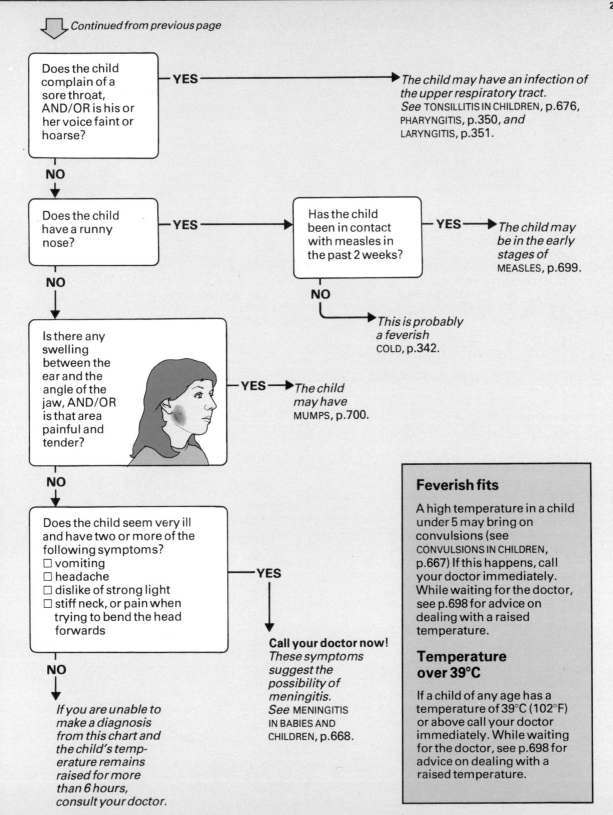

Continued from previous page

Does the child complain of a sore throat, AND/OR is his or her voice faint or hoarse? — YES → *The child may have an infection of the upper respiratory tract.* See TONSILLITIS IN CHILDREN, p.676, PHARYNGITIS, p.350, *and* LARYNGITIS, p.351.

NO

Does the child have a runny nose? — YES → **Has the child been in contact with measles in the past 2 weeks?** — YES → *The child may be in the early stages of* MEASLES, p.699.

NO → *This is probably a feverish* COLD, p.342.

NO

Is there any swelling between the ear and the angle of the jaw, AND/OR is that area painful and tender? — YES → *The child may have* MUMPS, p.700.

NO

Does the child seem very ill and have two or more of the following symptoms?
☐ vomiting
☐ headache
☐ dislike of strong light
☐ stiff neck, or pain when trying to bend the head forwards

— YES → **Call your doctor now!** *These symptoms suggest the possibility of meningitis.* See MENINGITIS IN BABIES AND CHILDREN, p.668.

NO → *If you are unable to make a diagnosis from this chart and the child's temperature remains raised for more than 6 hours, consult your doctor.*

Feverish fits

A high temperature in a child under 5 may bring on convulsions (see CONVULSIONS IN CHILDREN, p.667) If this happens, call your doctor immediately. While waiting for the doctor, see p.698 for advice on dealing with a raised temperature.

Temperature over 39°C

If a child of any age has a temperature of 39°C (102°F) or above call your doctor immediately. While waiting for the doctor, see p.698 for advice on dealing with a raised temperature.

93

Abdominal pain in children

Pain between the bottom of the ribcage and the groin which may vary from a mild "tummy ache" to severe pain.

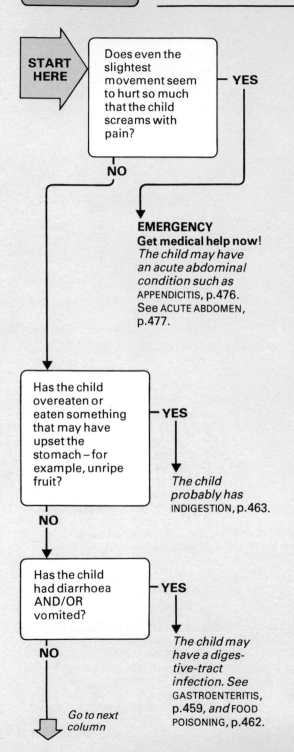

START HERE

Does even the slightest movement seem to hurt so much that the child screams with pain?

YES →

NO

EMERGENCY
Get medical help now!
The child may have an acute abdominal condition such as APPENDICITIS, p.476. See ACUTE ABDOMEN, p.477.

Has the child overeaten or eaten something that may have upset the stomach – for example, unripe fruit?

YES →

The child probably has INDIGESTION, p.463.

NO

Has the child had diarrhoea AND/OR vomited?

YES →

The child may have a digestive-tract infection. See GASTROENTERITIS, p.459, *and* FOOD POISONING, p.462.

NO

Go to next column

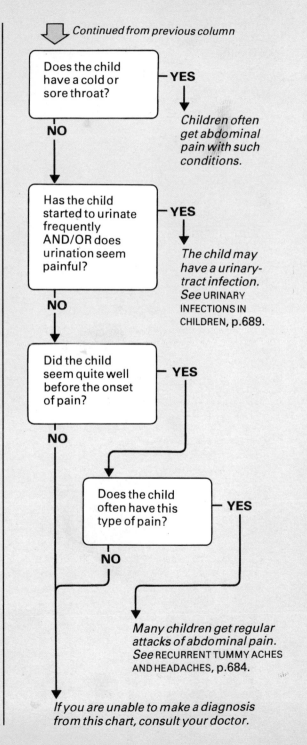

Continued from previous column

Does the child have a cold or sore throat?

YES →

Children often get abdominal pain with such conditions.

NO

Has the child started to urinate frequently AND/OR does urination seem painful?

YES →

The child may have a urinary-tract infection. See URINARY INFECTIONS IN CHILDREN, p.689.

NO

Did the child seem quite well before the onset of pain?

YES →

NO

Does the child often have this type of pain?

YES →

NO

Many children get regular attacks of abdominal pain. See RECURRENT TUMMY ACHES AND HEADACHES, p.684.

If you are unable to make a diagnosis from this chart, consult your doctor.

94
CHILDREN
2–14 years

Itching in children

Generalized or local irritation of the skin, which makes the child want to scratch.

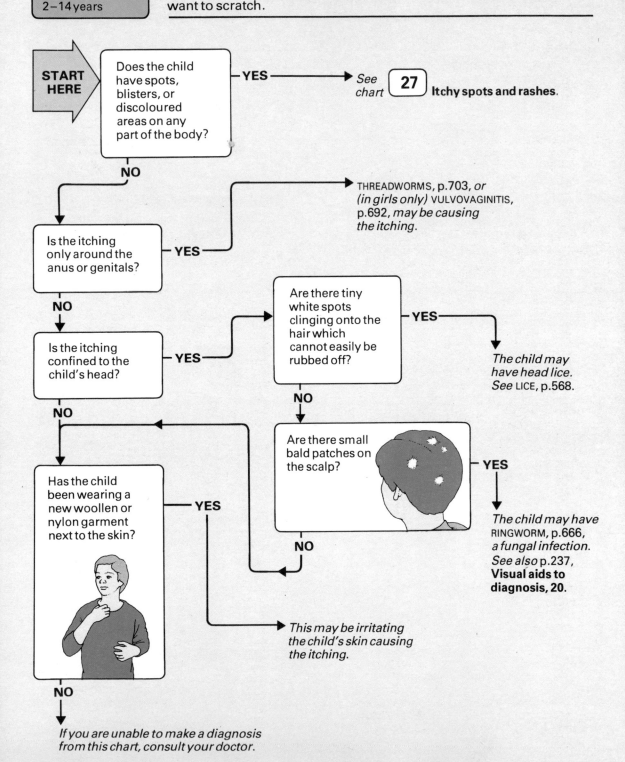

START HERE → Does the child have spots, blisters, or discoloured areas on any part of the body? — **YES** → *See chart* **27** **Itchy spots and rashes**.

NO

Is the itching only around the anus or genitals? — **YES** → THREADWORMS, p.703, *or (in girls only)* VULVOVAGINITIS, p.692, *may be causing the itching.*

NO

Is the itching confined to the child's head? — **YES** → Are there tiny white spots clinging onto the hair which cannot easily be rubbed off? — **YES** → *The child may have head lice. See* LICE, p.568.

NO

Are there small bald patches on the scalp? — **YES** → *The child may have* RINGWORM, p.666, *a fungal infection. See also p.237,* **Visual aids to diagnosis, 20.**

NO

Has the child been wearing a new woollen or nylon garment next to the skin? — **YES** → *This may be irritating the child's skin causing the itching.*

NO

If you are unable to make a diagnosis from this chart, consult your doctor.

95

Coughing in children

Noisy expulsion of air from the lungs.

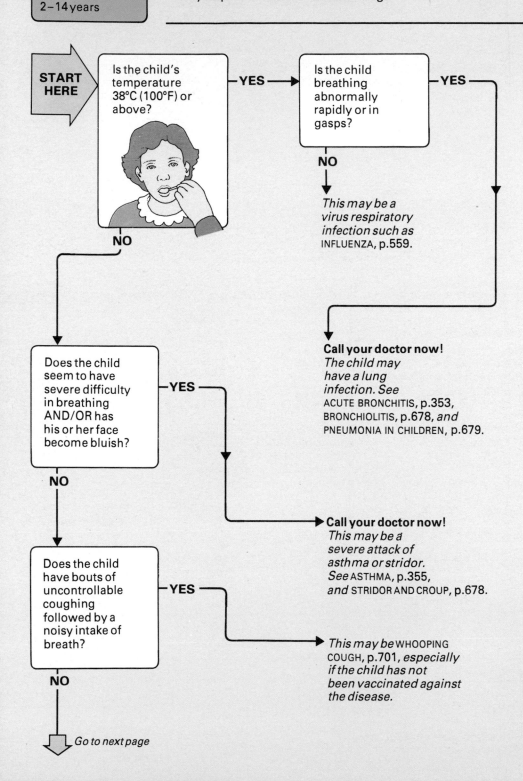

START HERE

Is the child's temperature 38°C (100°F) or above?

YES → Is the child breathing abnormally rapidly or in gasps?

YES →

NO ↓

This may be a virus respiratory infection such as INFLUENZA, p.559.

NO ↓

Does the child seem to have severe difficulty in breathing AND/OR has his or her face become bluish?

YES →

NO ↓

Call your doctor now!
The child may have a lung infection. See
ACUTE BRONCHITIS, p.353,
BRONCHIOLITIS, p.678, *and*
PNEUMONIA IN CHILDREN, p.679.

Call your doctor now!
This may be a severe attack of asthma or stridor. See ASTHMA, p.355, *and* STRIDOR AND CROUP, p.678.

Does the child have bouts of uncontrollable coughing followed by a noisy intake of breath?

YES →

NO ↓

This may be WHOOPING COUGH, p.701, *especially if the child has not been vaccinated against the disease.*

Go to next page

Continued from previous page

Is the child's breathing noisy or wheezy?

— **YES** → **Could the child have choked on or inhaled a small foreign body – for example, a peanut – within the past few days?**

— **YES** → *This may be causing the coughing. See* INHALED FOREIGN BODY, p.678.

NO (from choked question) →

The child may have asthma or croup. See STRIDOR AND CROUP, p.678, *and* ASTHMA, p.355.

NO (from breathing question) ↓

Does the child have a runny or blocked nose?

— **YES** → *Discharge from the back of the nose may be irritating the throat, causing the child to cough. See* RECURRENT COUGHS AND COLDS, p.680 *and* ADENOIDS, p.677.

NO ↓

Has the child had whooping cough within the last 3 months?

— **YES** → *Persistent coughing often follows* WHOOPING COUGH, p.701.

NO ↓

Does anyone in the house smoke heavily OR could the child be smoking?

— **YES** → *Smoking, or even living in a smoky atmosphere, can cause coughing in a child. Giving up smoking will benefit your own and the child's health.*

NO ↓

If you are unable to make a diagnosis from this chart, and the cough persists for more than 2 weeks, consult your doctor.

96

CHILDREN
0–14 years

Swellings in children

Any swellings or lumps in the neck or armpits, which may be tender or painful.

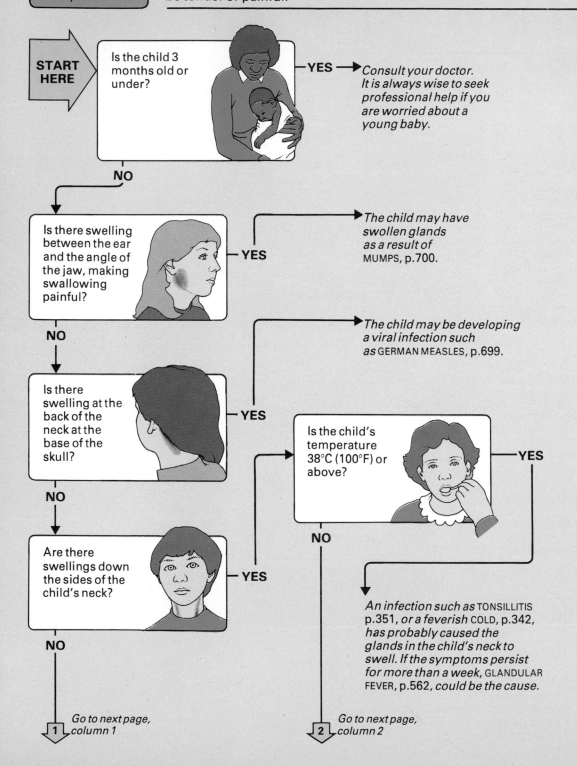

START HERE

Is the child 3 months old or under?

YES → *Consult your doctor. It is always wise to seek professional help if you are worried about a young baby.*

NO

Is there swelling between the ear and the angle of the jaw, making swallowing painful?

YES → *The child may have swollen glands as a result of* MUMPS, p.700.

NO

Is there swelling at the back of the neck at the base of the skull?

YES → *The child may be developing a viral infection such as* GERMAN MEASLES, p.699.

NO

Are there swellings down the sides of the child's neck?

YES →

Is the child's temperature 38°C (100°F) or above?

YES

NO

NO

An infection such as TONSILLITIS p.351, *or a feverish* COLD, p.342, *has probably caused the glands in the child's neck to swell. If the symptoms persist for more than a week,* GLANDULAR FEVER, p.562, *could be the cause.*

1 *Go to next page, column 1*

2 *Go to next page, column 2*

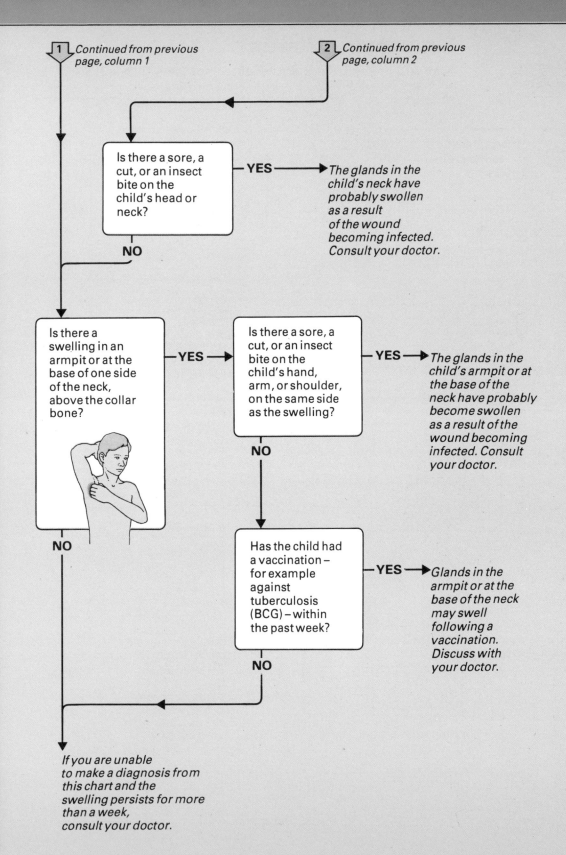

1 Continued from previous page, column 1

2 Continued from previous page, column 2

Is there a sore, a cut, or an insect bite on the child's head or neck?

YES → *The glands in the child's neck have probably swollen as a result of the wound becoming infected. Consult your doctor.*

NO

Is there a swelling in an armpit or at the base of one side of the neck, above the collar bone?

YES → Is there a sore, a cut, or an insect bite on the child's hand, arm, or shoulder, on the same side as the swelling?

YES → *The glands in the child's armpit or at the base of the neck have probably become swollen as a result of the wound becoming infected. Consult your doctor.*

NO

Has the child had a vaccination – for example against tuberculosis (BCG) – within the past week?

YES → *Glands in the armpit or at the base of the neck may swell following a vaccination. Discuss with your doctor.*

NO

NO

If you are unable to make a diagnosis from this chart and the swelling persists for more than a week, consult your doctor.

97

Limping in children

A limp may be accompanied by pain in the affected hip, leg, or foot, and in a young child may result in a reluctance to walk.

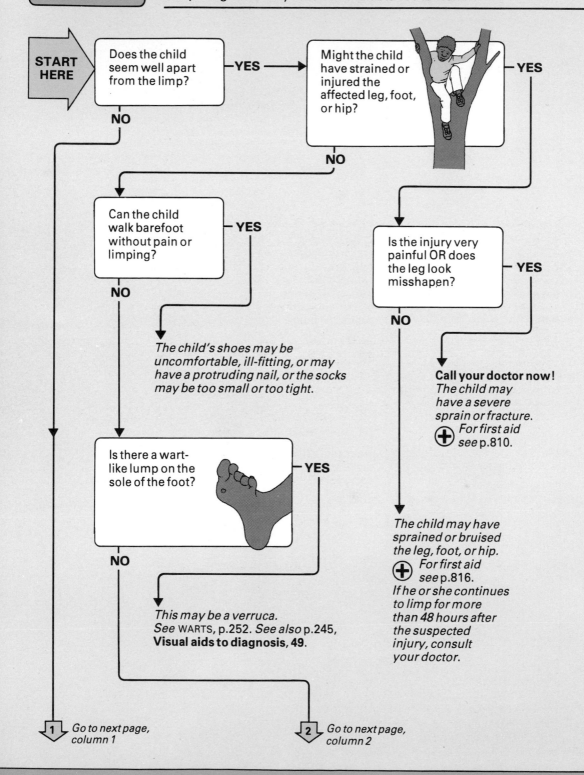

START HERE

Does the child seem well apart from the limp? — **YES** →

Might the child have strained or injured the affected leg, foot, or hip? — **YES**

NO ↓ (from "well apart")

NO ↓ (from "strained or injured")

Can the child walk barefoot without pain or limping? — **YES**

Is the injury very painful OR does the leg look misshapen? — **YES**

NO ↓ (barefoot)

NO ↓ (painful/misshapen)

The child's shoes may be uncomfortable, ill-fitting, or may have a protruding nail, or the socks may be too small or too tight.

Call your doctor now!
The child may have a severe sprain or fracture.
✚ *For first aid see p.810.*

Is there a wart-like lump on the sole of the foot? — **YES**

NO ↓

This may be a verruca. See WARTS, *p.252. See also p.245,* **Visual aids to diagnosis, 49**.

The child may have sprained or bruised the leg, foot, or hip.
✚ *For first aid see p.816.*
If he or she continues to limp for more than 48 hours after the suspected injury, consult your doctor.

1 *Go to next page, column 1*

2 *Go to next page, column 2*

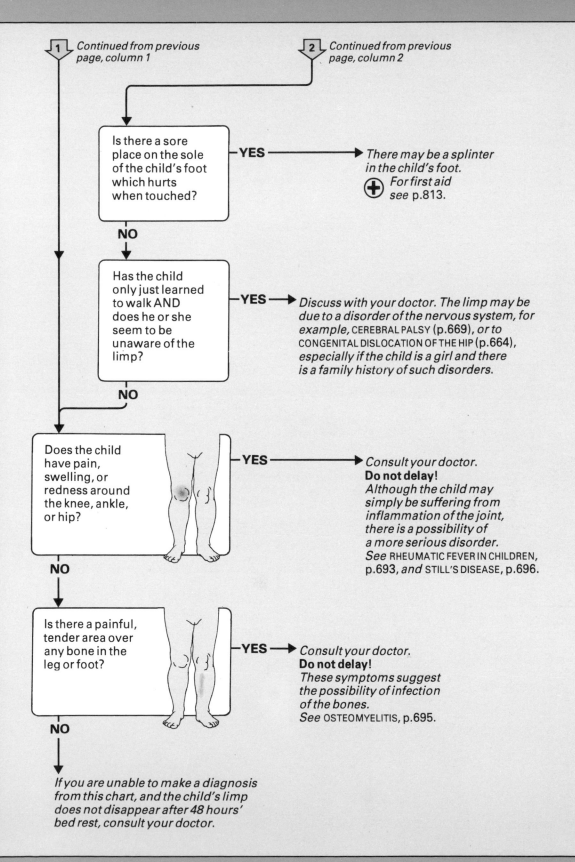

1 Continued from previous page, column 1

2 Continued from previous page, column 2

Is there a sore place on the sole of the child's foot which hurts when touched?

YES → There may be a splinter in the child's foot.
✚ For first aid see p.813.

NO

Has the child only just learned to walk AND does he or she seem to be unaware of the limp?

YES → *Discuss with your doctor. The limp may be due to a disorder of the nervous system, for example,* CEREBRAL PALSY (p.669), *or to* CONGENITAL DISLOCATION OF THE HIP (p.664), *especially if the child is a girl and there is a family history of such disorders.*

NO

Does the child have pain, swelling, or redness around the knee, ankle, or hip?

YES → *Consult your doctor.*
Do not delay!
Although the child may simply be suffering from inflammation of the joint, there is a possibility of a more serious disorder.
See RHEUMATIC FEVER IN CHILDREN, p.693, *and* STILL'S DISEASE, p.696.

NO

Is there a painful, tender area over any bone in the leg or foot?

YES → *Consult your doctor.*
Do not delay!
These symptoms suggest the possibility of infection of the bones.
See OSTEOMYELITIS, p.695.

NO

If you are unable to make a diagnosis from this chart, and the child's limp does not disappear after 48 hours' bed rest, consult your doctor.

98

ELDERLY
over 65 years

Incontinence in the elderly

Involuntary passing of urine that may vary from a small leakage to complete emptying of the bladder.

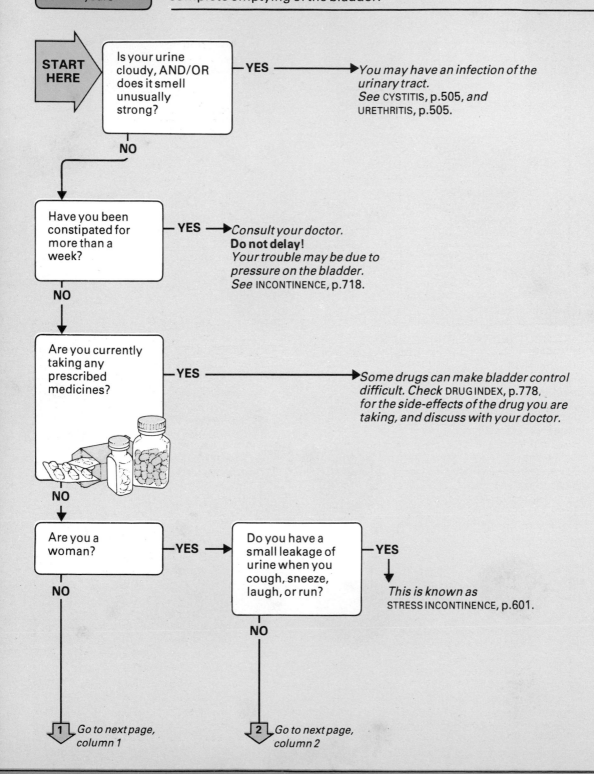

START HERE → Is your urine cloudy, AND/OR does it smell unusually strong? — **YES** → *You may have an infection of the urinary tract.*
See CYSTITIS, p.505, *and* URETHRITIS, p.505.

NO ↓

Have you been constipated for more than a week? — **YES** → *Consult your doctor.*
Do not delay!
Your trouble may be due to pressure on the bladder.
See INCONTINENCE, p.718.

NO ↓

Are you currently taking any prescribed medicines? — **YES** → *Some drugs can make bladder control difficult. Check* DRUG INDEX, p.778, *for the side-effects of the drug you are taking, and discuss with your doctor.*

NO ↓

Are you a woman? — **YES** → Do you have a small leakage of urine when you cough, sneeze, laugh, or run? — **YES** ↓

This is known as STRESS INCONTINENCE, p.601.

NO ↓   **NO** ↓

1 *Go to next page, column 1*   **2** *Go to next page, column 2*

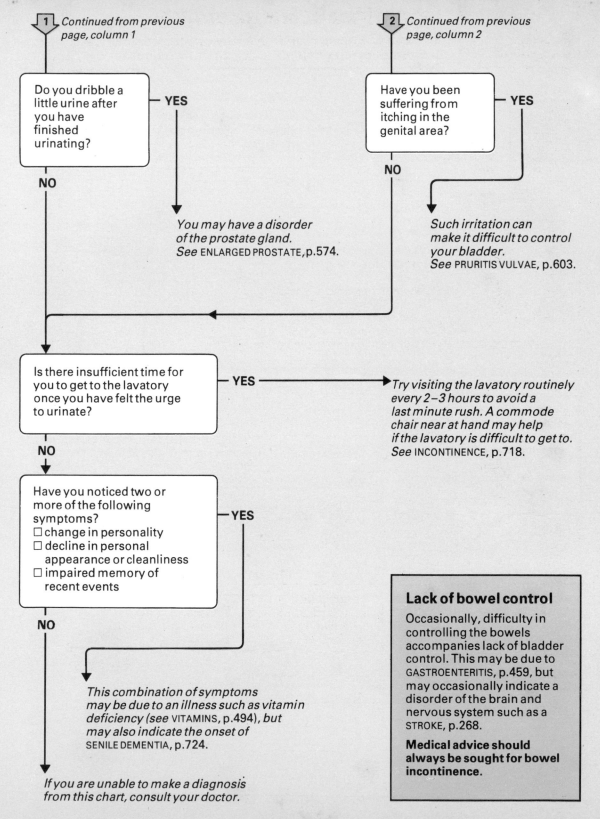

1 *Continued from previous page, column 1*

Do you dribble a little urine after you have finished urinating?

YES — You may have a disorder of the prostate gland. *See* ENLARGED PROSTATE, p.574.

NO

2 *Continued from previous page, column 2*

Have you been suffering from itching in the genital area?

YES — Such irritation can make it difficult to control your bladder. *See* PRURITIS VULVAE, p.603.

NO

Is there insufficient time for you to get to the lavatory once you have felt the urge to urinate?

YES — Try visiting the lavatory routinely every 2–3 hours to avoid a last minute rush. A commode chair near at hand may help if the lavatory is difficult to get to. *See* INCONTINENCE, p.718.

NO

Have you noticed two or more of the following symptoms?
☐ change in personality
☐ decline in personal appearance or cleanliness
☐ impaired memory of recent events

YES — This combination of symptoms may be due to an illness such as vitamin deficiency (*see* VITAMINS, p.494), *but may also indicate the onset of* SENILE DEMENTIA, p.724.

NO

If you are unable to make a diagnosis from this chart, consult your doctor.

Lack of bowel control

Occasionally, difficulty in controlling the bowels accompanies lack of bladder control. This may be due to GASTROENTERITIS, p.459, but may occasionally indicate a disorder of the brain and nervous system such as a STROKE, p.268.

Medical advice should always be sought for bowel incontinence.

Confusion in the elderly

Any muddling of times, places, and events, or loss of contact with reality.
Use this chart only after consulting chart 15, **Confusion**.

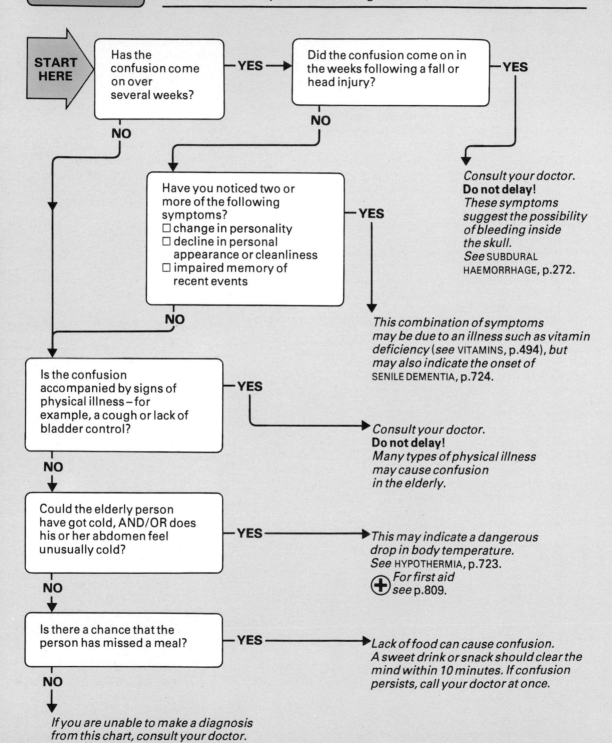

START HERE

Has the confusion come on over several weeks?

— YES → **Did the confusion come on in the weeks following a fall or head injury?** — YES →

Consult your doctor.
Do not delay!
These symptoms suggest the possibility of bleeding inside the skull.
See SUBDURAL HAEMORRHAGE, p.272.

NO ↓   NO ↓

Have you noticed two or more of the following symptoms?
☐ change in personality
☐ decline in personal appearance or cleanliness
☐ impaired memory of recent events

— YES →

This combination of symptoms may be due to an illness such as vitamin deficiency (see VITAMINS, p.494), *but may also indicate the onset of* SENILE DEMENTIA, p.724.

NO

Is the confusion accompanied by signs of physical illness – for example, a cough or lack of bladder control?

— YES →

Consult your doctor.
Do not delay!
Many types of physical illness may cause confusion in the elderly.

NO ↓

Could the elderly person have got cold, AND/OR does his or her abdomen feel unusually cold?

— YES →

This may indicate a dangerous drop in body temperature.
See HYPOTHERMIA, p.723.
⊕ *For first aid see* p.809.

NO ↓

Is there a chance that the person has missed a meal?

— YES →

Lack of food can cause confusion. A sweet drink or snack should clear the mind within 10 minutes. If confusion persists, call your doctor at once.

NO ↓

If you are unable to make a diagnosis from this chart, consult your doctor.

Visual aids to diagnosis

The purpose of this section of the book is to help you identify visible signs of illness. The photographs on the following pages are mainly of disorders with symptoms that show up on the skin, of skin disorders themselves, or of certain nail and eye problems.

The best way to make use of the pictures is to adopt the following procedure: If you are concerned about any symptom, whether visible or not, begin by consulting the appropriate self-diagnosis symptom chart (see p.68). The chart itself may then refer you not only to an article in Part III, but also to a specific illustration in these visual-aid pages. Many kinds of skin trouble look similar, and you might be misled if you examined a picture *before* studying the chart. So do not use a visual-aid illustration as the first or only step in the process of self-diagnosis. And one other word of warning: If the picture you have been referred to does not precisely resemble your own symptom, do not automatically assume your tentative diagnosis is wrong. When in doubt, consult a doctor.

To summarize, remember the following:
- Do *not* use the *Visual aids to diagnosis* as the first step in your diagnosis.
- Consult the appropriate self-diagnosis symptom chart in Part II as the first step in your diagnosis.
- When in doubt, consult your doctor.

Birthmarks

Any area of discoloured skin present from birth or soon afterwards is known as a birthmark. There are two main types: a mass of tiny blood vessels in the skin (a naevus), and a patch of discoloured skin (called a pigmented spot). Birthmarks are not harmful in any way, but they may persist for months or years and some are unsightly. (See *Birthmarks*, p.652.)

1 Strawberry naevus

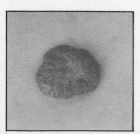

A strawberry naevus (shown above) is a raised, bright-red patch of skin, which grows during the first few months of life. After about 6 months the mark begins to shrink and fade, and, in most cases, has become insignificant by late infancy.

2 Port wine stain

A port wine stain is another type of naevus. It usually consists of a flat or slightly raised patch of purplish-red skin (see the photograph below). Generally this type of birthmark covers quite a large area and occurs singly, most commonly on the face or limbs. Port wine stains usually remain unchanged throughout life, though occasionally they may fade a little. If such a stain is felt to be disfiguring, application of a cosmetic cream to conceal the stain is one remedy or, in some instances, plastic surgery may be advisable.

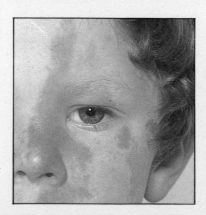

3 Pigmented spot

This type of spot (shown in the photograph below), some kinds of which are called "café au lait" spots, is generally a flat patch of darkened, brownish skin, most often irregularly shaped.

Pigmented spots are usually quite small and occur singly, but rarely they may be large and multiple. They tend to remain unchanged throughout life, so application of a cosmetic skin-coloured cream to conceal the spot may be a solution if the spot is considered disfiguring. In rare cases, plastic surgery may be undertaken.

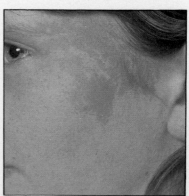

4 Nappy rash

Most babies suffer at some time from this redness around the thighs, buttocks, and genitals. The rash varies in severity from only slight redness to severe, bright-red inflammation. The skin also becomes sore and moist. Ammonia produced by a chemical reaction between faeces and urine is a frequent irritant; another is the detergent present in inadequately rinsed nappies. For mild nappy rash, more frequent changing and sterilization of nappies is often sufficient treatment. Exposing the baby's buttocks to warm air for a few hours each day, and applying a zinc cream, may also help. (See *Nappy rash*, p.650.)

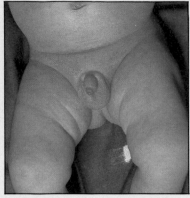

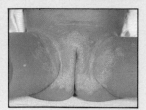

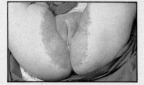

When nappy rash is severe (above) treatment with an antiseptic or barrier cream may be necessary. In a boy, the foreskin may be inflamed, and urination painful.

The two photographs above show how the inflammation is limited to the area of skin covered by the nappy.

Eczema in children

There are many types of eczema (also known as dermatitis). All types are basically skin inflammations which are usually itchy. Babies and children are especially prone to certain types of eczema, perhaps because they have highly sensitive skins. (See the articles on *Eczema*, p.253, *Seborrhoeic eczema*, p.651, and *Infantile eczema*, p.666.)

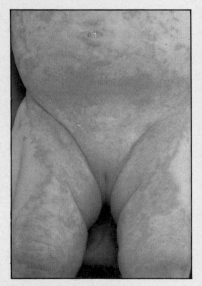

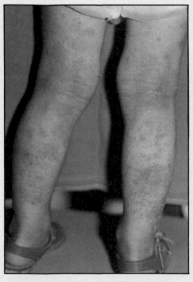

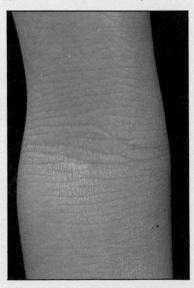

5 Seborrhoeic eczema in infants

This type of eczema usually takes the form of a red, scaly rash on the face and/or body (as shown above). It may also appear as yellowish, greasy-looking scales on the scalp ("cradle cap"). Seborrhoeic eczema usually appears during the first three months of life. Mild cases often clear up on their own, but occasionally the doctor may prescribe a cream to loosen the scales so they can be washed away more easily.

6 Infantile eczema

This red, scaly, itchy skin condition (shown in the photograph above) usually appears as a widespread rash during the first year of life, and improves as the child gets older. Mild forms of the disorder require no specific treatment other than regular applications of a soothing preparation such as petroleum jelly or olive oil. Occasionally, it continues to be a problem in adult life.

7 Skin changes in recurrent eczema

When eczema is a persistent problem, the skin in the affected areas may become dry, leathery, and creased-looking as a result of recurrent inflammation and repeated rubbing. In the photograph above, the changes have occurred on the inside of the elbow (a common site for eczema in children). Such long-term skin changes can occur in adults as well as children, though they only happen in a small proportion of all sufferers.

Eczema in adults

Some types of eczema (also known as dermatitis) are most common in children (see opposite). The types shown below, however, occur chiefly in adults. (See the article on *Eczema*, p.253, for further information.)

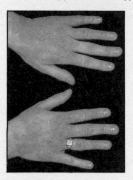

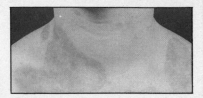

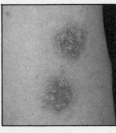

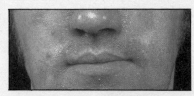

8 Housewife's hand eczema

This type of eczema is common in anyone who constantly handles irritant chemicals in such substances as strong detergents.

9 Eczema in the elderly

Many elderly people suffer from dry skin – particularly on the legs – which may become cracked and itchy. The condition is relieved by application of a moisturizing ointment or cream.

10 Discoid eczema

In this form of eczema round, red, flaky patches form. The photograph above shows the crusting produced when fluid from the patches oozes and then dries. Discoid eczema is a relatively rare type of eczema.

11 Seborrhoeic eczema on the body

In an adult, seborrhoeic eczema often occurs in the form of a red, flaky, itchy rash. It commonly appears on the scalp or the chest (above).

12 Seborrhoeic eczema on the face

When seborrhoeic eczema affects the face (above) it is usually worst by the sides of the nose, on the forehead, and in the eyebrows.

Contact (allergic) eczema

Some types of eczema are caused by certain substances coming into contact with the skin. Touching the substance produces an itchy, flaky rash which is usually limited to the area of contact. Contact eczemas do not affect everyone, however. The reaction occurs only in susceptible individuals who often have other allergic conditions such as asthma or allergic rhinitis. (For further information see *Eczema*, p.253, and *Allergies*, p.705.)

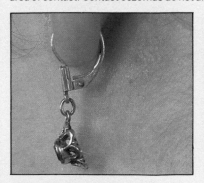

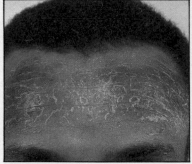

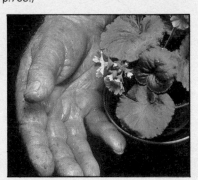

13 Metal contact

Some metals – for example, in earrings, bracelets, watchbands, fasteners, and rings – cause contact eczema. The culprit metals (nickel is a common offender) are often present in small amounts in other metals, such as gold or silver.

14 Hatband contact

Some substances in fabric can occasionally produce contact eczema. The rash shown above was caused by material in the lining of a hat. The lining in gloves has also been known to cause contact eczema.

15 Plant contact

Touching certain plants – primulas and chrysanthemums, for instance – may produce contact eczema that is more severe and widespread than that produced by contact with most other substances.

Allergic reactions

Many people suffer from allergic reactions to external factors. Often the cause is unknown, but food, drugs, infection, contact, heat, and cold are all known offenders. Itchy lumps appear on the skin; they can occur anywhere on the body, and sometimes combine to cover large, patchy areas. Allergic reactions are uncomfortable but not usually harmful. However, in a severe reaction, facial tissues may swell dramatically and endanger breathing.

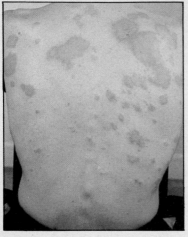

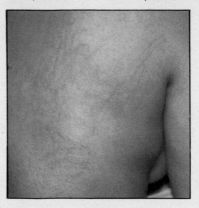

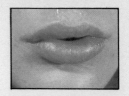

16 Urticaria

Urticaria (p.255) is the most common form of allergic reaction. The rash usually takes the form of one or more raised, light-red patches called weals (above). The weals have clearly defined edges and are itchy. They can occur anywhere on the body and normally disappear within a few hours; sometimes, however, they remain for longer periods. If the weals cause persistent discomfort, a doctor may prescribe antihistamine drugs.

17 Dermographism

Dermographism is a particular form of urticaria usually caused by scratching the skin. It consists of raised weals (as shown above) that exactly follow the lines where scratching or rubbing has occurred. For obvious reasons it is easy to confirm the cause of this type of allergic reaction, even though sometimes the weals do not appear on the skin until several hours after the irritation that caused them.

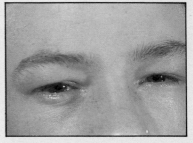

18 Angio-oedema

When urticaria affects the face, considerable swelling may result, especially around the eyes (above) and lips (top). In these circumstances the danger is that the tissues on the inside of the throat may also swell up and cause difficulty with breathing. (For further information see the article on *Urticaria*, p.255.)

19 Pityriasis rosea

The patches which make up the pityriasis rosea rash have a slightly scaly surface. They look red in white skin, and dark brown in black skin. The condition is usually itchy and may persist for up to about three months. It generally disappears of its own accord, though cream may be prescribed to relieve any itching. (See *Pityriasis rosea*, p.262.)

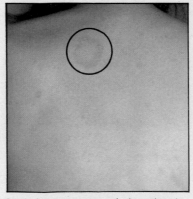

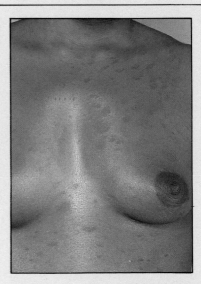

Pityriasis rosea starts as a single, oval patch (known as a herald patch) on the chest or back. (In the picture above the herald patch is circled.) Over the next few days several similar, but usually smaller, patches appear on the trunk (as shown on the right), the upper arms, and the thighs.

Bacterial and fungal infections

The skin may suffer from several types of microbial infection. Two of the most common are shown here: ringworm, which is caused not by a worm but by a fungus; and impetigo, a fast-spreading bacterial infection. *Warts* (p.242) are another type of microbial infection; they are caused by viral infection. Most bacterial and fungal skin infections will not clear up – or will do so only slowly – unless aided by a specific cream, lotion, or paint prescribed by your doctor

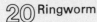 **Ringworm**

This fungal infection often takes the form of a red, itchy rash spreading out in the shape of a ring. It usually appears on warm, moist areas such as the groin or beneath the breasts (below). Within two weeks of the appearance of the first ring other rings appear close to the site of the first one. Ringworm is rarely a serious condition, but it will heal more rapidly with professional help. (See *Ringworm*, p.666.)

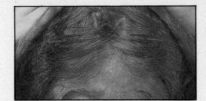

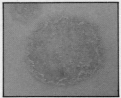

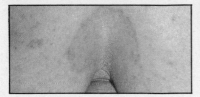

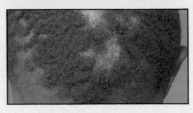

Ringworm on the scalp (above) can lead to temporary bald patches.

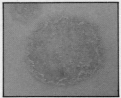 **Animal ringworm**

Some types of ringworm fungus that usually live on pets or farm animals can live on human skin. The ring (above) may appear on any part of the body and is likely to be more red or inflamed than the rings caused by human ringworm. However, it is treated in the same way as human ringworm, and an infected pet should be treated by a vet.

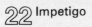 **Impetigo**

This is a bacterial infection, most commonly affecting the area around the nose and mouth. The appearance of groups of small blisters is the first sign of the condition; the blisters then burst to form a yellowy-brown crust. The affected area gradually spreads, and the infection usually has to be treated with an antibiotic.

   Pictured right is a case of impetigo at the early stage of the infection. Far right, the condition is shown at its advanced stage, after the yellowy-brown crust has formed. (See *Impetigo*, p.256.)

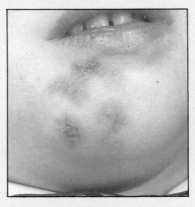

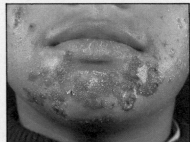

Boils

A boil can result when a hair follicle becomes infected and inflamed. It starts as a red, usually painful lump which gradually becomes swollen with pus. A head forms and the pain generally increases, until eventually the boil bursts. Boils may occur anywhere on the body. (See *Boils and carbuncles*, p.251.)

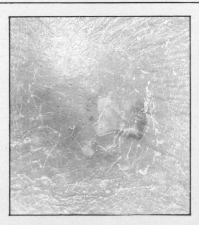

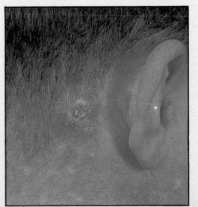

24 Cold sores

Cold sores are small blisters that usually appear on the face, around the lips and nose. The blisters are small areas of infection caused by a virus, herpes simplex. The infection occurs in two stages, as shown in the photographs below. Outbreaks of blisters tend to appear when you are feeling tired and run down, or when you have some other infection such as a cold (hence their name), or when you are exposed to wind or sunshine. (See *Cold sores*, p.451.)

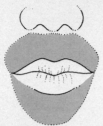

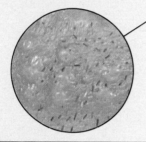

Distribution
Cold sores tend to develop on the skin around the lips or on the lips themselves.

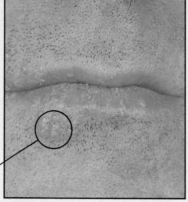

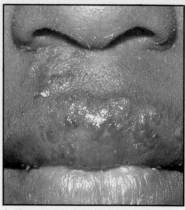

Early stage
In the early stage of cold sores, a group of tiny blisters appears (the inset photograph on the left shows the blisters in more detail). Around the blisters is an area of generally red, inflamed skin. The early stage may produce little or no discomfort in a child; adults tend to suffer itching and irritation.

Late stage
Within a few days of their appearance the blisters (shown above left) enlarge, burst, and dry out. The yellowish crust that forms is similar in appearance to the crust of *impetigo* (p.237). If cold sores persist or recur, see your doctor, who may prescribe a special anti-viral paint to speed healing.

25 Shingles

Like *cold sores* (above), shingles is an infection caused by a herpes virus – in this case, herpes zoster (the same virus that causes *chickenpox* – see opposite). Before the rash appears, there is a burning pain in the affected area of skin. (See *Shingles*, p.562.)

Distribution
Shingles usually develops in a long, thin area on only one side of the body. The trunk and the face are the commonest sites; on the trunk, the rash often affects both the front and back (below).

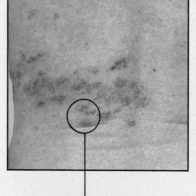

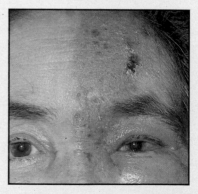

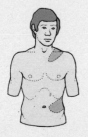

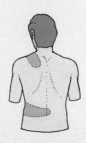

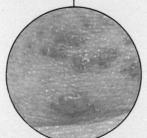

The shingles rash
The rash of shingles (which may be painful) consists of numerous small blisters, shown in detail in the photograph left. Over the course of a few days the blisters become dry, scab over, then slowly fade away over the ensuing weeks. If the rash affects the face near an eye (as shown above), it may affect the eye itself and produce severe pain, redness, and watering. If this happens to you, see your doctor without delay. When the rash affects the body (above left) it tends to occur in a long, narrow strip that follows the line of a rib.

Common childhood infections

Several infectious diseases are usually caught in childhood. Three common examples – measles, German measles, and chickenpox – are shown below. Each of these three infections produces a characteristic rash that helps with identification. Though irritating and uncomfortable, these diseases are not usually serious. (For full information see *Childhood infectious diseases*, p.698, and *Symptom comparison of infectious diseases*, p.702.)

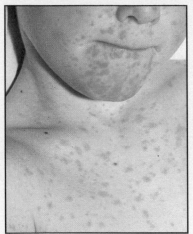

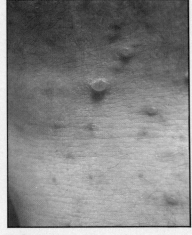

26 Measles

27 German measles

28 Chickenpox

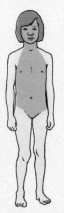

The rash of measles consists of flat, dark-pink spots that often join together to form larger blotches (above). At first the rash affects mainly the face, usually starting on the forehead and behind the ears. Later the rash spreads to cover the trunk (as shown on the left) but it rarely appears on the limbs. (See *Measles*, p.699.)

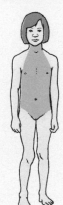

The rash of German measles (shown in the photograph above) tends to be less severe than the measles rash (above left). German measles produces tiny, light-red spots that merge together to form an evenly coloured patch. The diagram on the left shows that the rash spreads over the trunk; it only lasts a few days in most cases. (See *German measles*, p.699.)

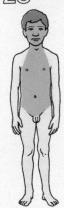

This infection is caused by the same virus that is responsible for *shingles* (opposite). The photograph above shows the crops of small, fluid-filled blisters characteristic of this disease. As shown on the left, the rash covers mainly the face and trunk. The diagrams below show the typical stages in development of the chickenpox rash. (See *Chickenpox*, p.700.)

Development of chickenpox
There are 3 typical stages in the development of the chickenpox rash. In the first, tiny red spots appear. Then the spots enlarge and fill with fluid to form itchy blisters. In the third stage the blisters burst, dry out and crust over; they are still very itchy.

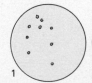

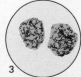

1 Small red spots
2 Fluid-filled blisters
3 Crusted scabs

29 Purpura

A "purpuric" rash may be produced by a number of disorders (listed below) in which blood leaks through the walls of small blood vessels in the skin. The rash consists of many flat, dark-red or purplish spots or blotches. (See *Thrombocytopenia*, p.425, *Anaphylactoid purpura*, p.681, and *Skin problems of the elderly*, p.722.)

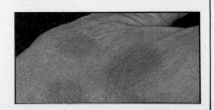

30 Acne

In acne, there is persistent, recurrent development of various types of spot on the skin. The condition is extremely common during adolescence – slightly more so in young men – and in the vast majority of cases it fades away during the late teens or early twenties. (For further information see the article on *Acne*, p.708.)

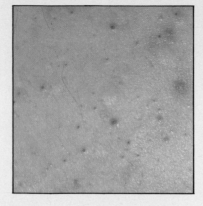

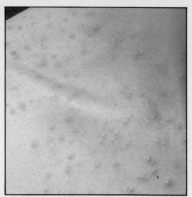

Distribution

The spots of acne commonly appear on the face – chiefly around the mouth – and often on the chest, shoulders, the nape of the neck, and the upper (and occasionally lower) back.

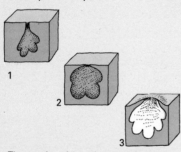

Development of spots

The opening of the sebaceous gland near the surface of the skin becomes blocked (1). There is a build-up of oily sebum within the gland (2); this accumulation leads to localized inflammation (redness and swelling) – the acne spot (3).

Blackheads

One type of spot that appears in acne is the blackhead (shown in the photograph above). Each "black" area is a tiny plug of dark material stuck in a skin pore. Some experts believe that the plug is a mixture of keratin and sebum and the colour is due to melanin (the skin pigment) in it; the "black" of the blackhead is therefore not dirt. Another name for blackheads is comedones.

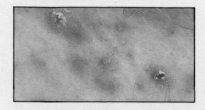

Spots

The typical spots that occur in acne are shown in the above photograph. Some spots develop from blackheads (above left and far left); others develop from whiteheads. If picked or scratched, the spots may become infected and pus-filled. Some spots are just small red lumps, others have white tops. They tend to develop and then fade over the course of about a week.

Severe acne

The most severe form of acne produces painful, fluid-filled lumps called cysts under the skin (see the photograph left). The cysts may be up to 20mm (about ¾in) across, and often persist for many weeks. They may leave pitted, scarred areas of skin when they clear up.

31 Rosacea

In rosacea, sometimes called acne rosacea, the facial skin – principally of the cheeks and nose – becomes abnormally red and flushed. After a time, pus-filled raised spots also appear in the affected skin. Why this condition occurs is not known; the rash tends to spread or become more prominent after eating hot or spicy food, or drinking alcohol. Rosacea is most common in women over 30 years of age. (See *Acne and rosacea*, p.255.)

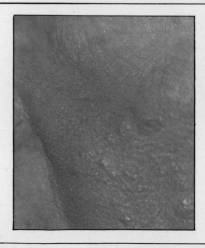

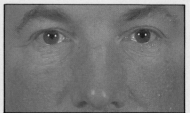

Distribution

Most people who suffer from rosacea have the rash on their cheeks. The sides of the nose may also be affected (see the photograph above).

Abnormal skin formation

A number of skin conditions – some of which are shown below – are characterized by a fault in the normal maintenance of skin tissue. Though not generally harmful to physical health, these conditions can cause sufferers to become embarrassed about their appearance and, in rare cases, may lead to considerable mental stress.

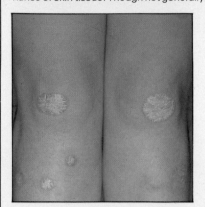

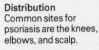

Distribution
Common sites for psoriasis are the knees, elbows, and scalp.

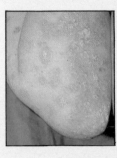

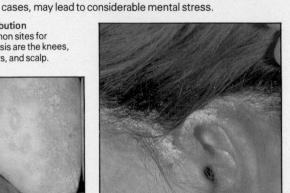

32 Psoriasis

As shown in the photograph above, the rash of psoriasis consists of patches of thickened, silvery-white, scaly skin. The patches often have a red rim. Psoriatic skin generally causes little or no discomfort, but in a few cases it may be sore. (See *Psoriasis*, p.254, for further information.)

Severe psoriasis
In more severe cases of psoriasis (an example is shown in the photograph above) the characteristic smallish patches join together to produce an extensive area of affected skin. The condition may also affect the fingernails and toenails (p.245), causing them to become thickened and roughened.

Psoriasis of the scalp
When psoriasis occurs on the scalp, it leads to the appearance of scaly, sometimes lumpy patches. In the majority of cases the hair of the scalp remains unaffected. It is rare for psoriasis to spread from the scalp and appear on the face.

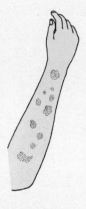

Scar tissue

Whenever the skin is damaged, it is repaired by scar tissue. Scar tissue is formed by special cells called fibroblasts that manufacture collagen and other protein substances; the material they produce is stronger and tougher than ordinary skin, but tends to shrink slightly with age.

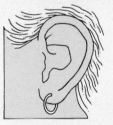

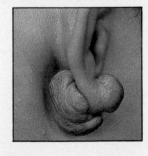

33 Lichen planus

This skin condition is extremely variable in appearance. The photograph above shows one of the more typical guises: a rash of numerous, tiny, purplish-red lumps. The lumps are not scaly but you may be able to see small white marks on the surface of the skin. The cause of the condition is not known. (For further information see *Lichen planus*, p.261.)

Distribution
Lichen planus may occur anywhere on the body, but the usual sites are the arms and wrists and the legs. It can also appear on the lining of the mouth. (See *Oral lichen planus*, p.452.)

34 Keloids

A keloid is formed when scar tissue does not stop growing but continues to increase in size, forming a hardened lump. Keloids can develop after an operation, a vaccination, or accidental injury. In the example shown here, the ear lobe has been pierced for an earring (above left) but a keloid has formed at the site (above right). The growths are more common in people with black skin. (See *Keloids*, p.261.)

Warts and moles

Warts and moles are sometimes thought of as related conditions, and in a few cases they look similar to each other. However, they are in no way related. Warts are small areas of long-standing infection. The infection is caused by a type of virus. Moles are localized areas of skin heavily pigmented with melanin (the substance responsible for general skin colouring). Warts are variable in appearance; four common types are shown below. Both warts and moles are harmless, though very rarely a *malignant melanoma* (opposite) may be mistaken for a mole.

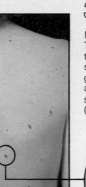
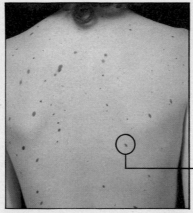

35 Moles

Moles can occur anywhere on the body. They are small, roughly circular areas of skin that are much darker than the surrounding skin. Large moles may have coarse hairs growing out of them (this does not signify anything). Most are present from birth; in some people a few develop in childhood. (See *Abnormal skin pigmentation*, p.262.)

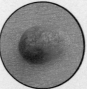

Appearance
The dark patch that constitutes a mole may be flat, or raised above the surrounding skin (as shown in the inset photograph, left).

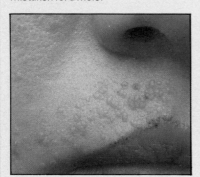

36 Plane warts

Plane warts are slightly raised, brownish spots that usually have a smooth surface. They often appear in groups, and may develop along the line of a scratch. This type of wart is most common in children. The photograph above shows plane warts on the skin near the upper lip – a common site (see *Warts*, p.252).

37 Common warts

This type of wart usually grows on the hands (as shown in the above photograph) or on the feet (where they are known as *verrucas* – see p.245). The typical common wart is a hard lump with a roughened, cauliflower-like surface. Tiny black flecks may be visible in the body of the wart.

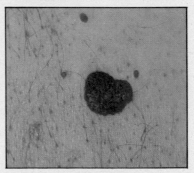

38 Seborrhoeic warts

These warts (above) are dark, sometimes rough-surfaced lumps that often grow in large numbers in later life. Like all warts they are harmless, but because of their similarity to a cancerous *malignant melanoma* (opposite) their appearance should always be reported to a doctor. (See *Abnormal skin pigmentation*, p.262.)

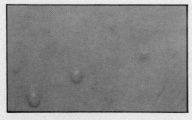

39 Molluscum contagiosum

These tiny, pale lumps are filled with a cheesy fluid. They are not true warts but, like true warts, are caused by a localized area of viral infection. They crop up in groups and tend to affect children (see *Warts*, p.252).

40 Sebaceous cysts

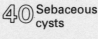

These cysts (right) are sometimes mistaken for warts, though they are not related. A sebaceous cyst typically appears as a soft, smooth, yellowish lump just under the surface of the skin. Sometimes a tiny dark dot can be seen in the skin over the centre of the cyst. The scalp is a common site for these harmless growths. (See *Sebaceous cysts*, p.261, for further information.)

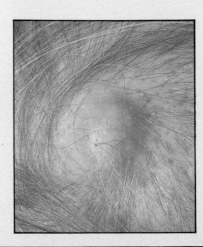

Skin cancers

There are three main types of *malignant* skin growth. These are rodent ulcer, squamous cell carcinoma, and malignant melanoma, as shown below. Skin cancers tend to be rather variable in appearance. As with most other malignant growths, early recognition and surgical removal give a good chance of cure. For this reason, always report any suspicious lump, sore, or ulcer on the skin to your doctor if it persists for more than a week.

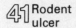Rodent ulcer

This type of skin cancer tends to grow very slowly, and rarely, if ever, spreads to other parts of the body. It is variable in appearance – 3 common versions are shown here. The one on the near right is the ulcerated (open-sore) form. (See *Rodent ulcer*, p.258.)

Common sites
Rodent ulcers almost always appear on the face, often near the eye or the side of the nose.

Encrusted type
The small photograph (right) shows a rodent ulcer that has crusted over to form a scab; when the scab detaches, the ulcer is revealed again.

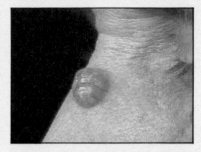

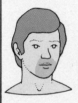

Cystic type
The above photograph shows a cystic type of rodent ulcer growing on the bridge of the nose. It appears as a relatively smooth, skin-coloured lump which gradually enlarges and may have small blood vessels visible inside.

Squamous cell carcinoma

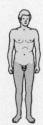

Common sites
Squamous cell growths typically appear on the face – especially on the lips or near the ears – and on the hands. (See *Squamous cell carcinoma*, p.259.)

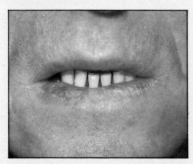

Ulcerated type
The above photograph shows a typical ulcerated type of squamous cell carcinoma – a persistent open sore that slowly enlarges.

Warty type
Squamous cell carcinoma sometimes appears as a small, hard nodule that gradually enlarges into a wart-like lump (as shown in the above photograph). Like the ulcerated type (above left), the warty type of carcinoma does not usually cause pain.

43 Malignant melanoma

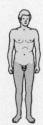

Common sites
This rare but serious type of skin cancer may appear anywhere on the body, but the legs are most often affected. (See the article on *Malignant melanoma*, p.259.)

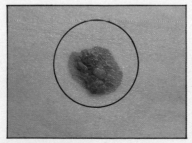

Typical appearance
A malignant melanoma usually takes the form of a dark, slightly raised lump (as shown in the photograph above). Such a malignant growth may also occur in an existing mole, causing it to enlarge and perhaps bleed.

IMPORTANT

Can you tell the difference?
The two photographs above show two harmless skin conditions – a seborrhoeic wart (above left) and a raised mole (above right). The large photograph to the left shows a very similar condition that is life-threatening if not treated in its very early stages – malignant melanoma. Always report a new pigmented spot to your doctor (see *Abnormal skin pigmentation*, p.262).

Abnormal skin coloration

In the conditions shown below, there is an abnormality in the natural colouring of the skin. The conditions are not harmful to general health but may, particularly in the case of vitiligo, cause mental or emotional stress because of the sufferer's appearance. (See *Abnormal skin pigmentation*, p.262, for further information.)

44 Vitiligo

In this skin coloration disorder, irregularly shaped patches of skin lose their normal colour and become much paler than the skin on the rest of the body. The nature of the skin surface and its texture do not alter. In some cases the light areas are symmetrical on the body or limbs (as shown in the small inset photograph, right, of vitiligo on the knees and feet). The exact cause of the condition is not clearly understood, but it is suspected to be an *autoimmune* problem. If appearance of the patches is embarrassing, expert application of special make-up can hide them.

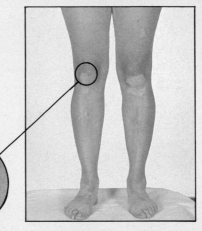

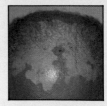

Vitiligo of the scalp
When vitiligo occurs on the scalp (as shown above), it sometimes causes hairs in the affected areas to turn pale or white.

45 Perfume pigmentation

Some perfumes contain chemicals that temporarily increase pigmentation in the areas of skin to which they are applied. The skin returns to normal once the use of the perfume is discontinued. The photograph on the right shows pigmented "perfume spots" on the neck; some people are more susceptible to this condition than others.

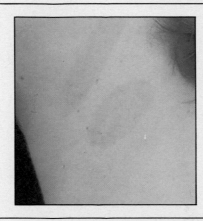

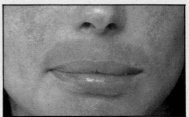

46 Chloasma

This temporary condition is thought to be due to hormonal changes produced by the "pill" or pregnancy. Patches of skin, especially on the face, become darker in colour.

47 Jaundice

Skin colour
Jaundice is not a disease, but a sign of one of several underlying diseases (see *Jaundice*, p.485). It is due to the build-up in the blood of the yellowish-brown substance bilirubin, which is normally extracted from the bloodstream by the liver and excreted in bile. In jaundice, the skin takes on a general yellowish tinge (as shown in the photograph on the right); the whites of the eyes are also affected (far right). The development of jaundice always requires the attention of a doctor.

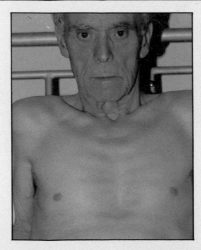

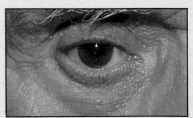

Eye colour
Besides yellowing of the skin (as shown on the left), jaundice also causes the whites of the eyes to take on a yellowish colour. The change in eye coloration, as shown in the above photograph, is usually a more reliable sign of jaundice than yellowing of the skin; the latter is often difficult to discern.

Common foot disorders

The two disorders shown below – athlete's foot and verrucas – are common, harmless, yet irritating conditions. Most other foot problems are also minor, but older people and those with diseases that may affect circulation (for example, diabetes) should beware of neglecting sores and cuts that may become serious without attention.

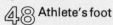 **Athlete's foot**

Athlete's foot is a fungal infection in which the skin of the foot becomes damp, inflamed, and itchy. The infection primarily affects the skin between and underneath the toes. The skin may peel and crack, sometimes producing sore areas. In severe cases (as shown far right) the nails are also infected and take on a thickened, discoloured appearance. (See *Athlete's foot*, p.256.)

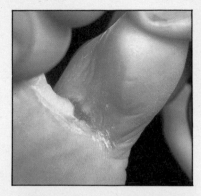

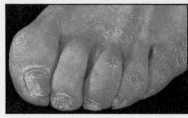

Shown above is an example of severe athlete's foot affecting the toenails.

49 Verrucas

A verruca is simply a common wart on the sole of the foot (see *Warts*. p.252, and *Warts and moles*, p.242). Unlike other warts, the verruca does not usually grow as a raised lump but as a flat area of hard, tough skin. Despite its flat nature, however, walking on a verruca often feels like walking with a stone in your shoe. The photograph on the right shows a verruca growing on the ball of the foot.

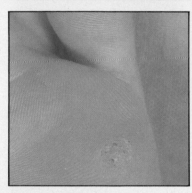

How a verruca develops

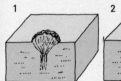

When a verruca first grows, it may be a raised lump like a common wart elsewhere on the body (1). It soon becomes pushed into the surface of the skin (2), though, which makes it more difficult to treat than a common wart elsewhere.

Common nail disorders

Some disorders, such as psoriasis, may affect the nails as well as the skin. In some cases, such as paronychia, it is only the nails, and perhaps the cuticles and nail beds, that are involved. (See *Deformed and discoloured nails*, p.265.)

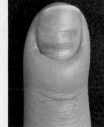

51 Paronychia

In this nail disorder the cuticles and nail fold become swollen and inflamed as a result of infection by bacteria or fungi. If the trouble persists, the nail itself may become darkened and deformed, as shown in the photograph on the left. (See *Paronychia*, p.264, for further information.)

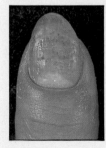

50 Deformed nails

Nails that are deformed in some way (see the photograph on the right) are usually the result of a generalized illness, when healthy nail growth is disrupted, or injury to the nail bed at the base of the nail. Once the cause is removed the nails should grow healthily once again, though it may take some months for the deformed portions to grow out completely (see *Deformed and discoloured nails*, p.265).

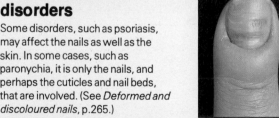

52 Psoriasis of the nails

The photograph above shows how psoriasis may affect the nails, causing them to become pitted and roughened; in other cases, the nails become thickened. Only rarely are the nails alone affected by psoriasis (see *Psoriasis*, p.254, and p.241). Sometimes the nail becomes completely detached from the nail bed.

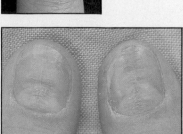

Common eye disorders

The common eye disorders shown below are all treatable. Styes and conjunctivitis are due to infection of the eye; corneal ulcers may be caused by either infection or trauma (physical injury). Several other eye conditions – among them *glaucoma* (p.320) – do not produce obvious change in the appearance of the eye, but do affect vision. Never ignore inexplicable or sudden changes in vision, or sudden pain in the eye.

53 Stye

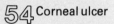

The photograph on the right shows a typical stye – an infected eyelash follicle (see *Stye*, p.314). A stye bears much resemblance to a *boil* (p.251), in that the follicle – the pit in the skin containing dividing cells that make the eyelash – becomes inflamed and pus-filled due to infection by bacteria. Styes are uncomfortable and may be quite painful; they usually clear up within a week.

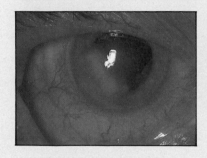

54 Corneal ulcer

An ulcer on the cornea causes pain and discomfort in the eye, and may make the white of the eye turn pink or red. In addition, the ulcer may be visible as a whitish patch (as shown in the photograph on the right) and vision may be misted over or otherwise impaired in the affected eye. In the photograph, the lower eyelid has been pulled down to show the ulcer clearly. (See *Corneal ulcers and infections*, p.316.)

55 Conjunctivitis

In conjunctivitis, the surface of the eye and the inside lining of the eyelids – all of which are covered with a membrane called the conjunctiva – become inflamed and sore. The eye looks red and bloodshot, and there may be a discharge that makes it feel sticky and "gummed up". In the photograph below, the lower eyelid has been pulled down to show the redness of the lower eyelid lining. (See *Conjunctivitis*, p.317.)

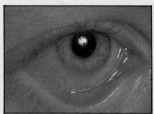

56 Foreign body on the cornea

A speck of grit or other small particle that enters the eye is usually moved by blinking to the edge of the eye, from where you can remove it yourself (see *Accidents and emergencies*, p.813). A corneal foreign body (below) needs expert medical care.

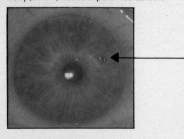

The photograph above shows a foreign body stuck in the cornea, the dome-shaped front of the eye (see diagram right). DO NOT attempt to move a particle embedded in the cornea – get a doctor to do it for you.

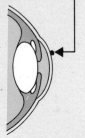

57 Chalazion

A chalazion (also called a meibomian cyst) is a painless swelling on the edge of the eyelid. Chalazions vary in size; some are so small as to be barely noticeable, others grow to be as large as a pea. In this example (right), the chalazion has become inflamed (red and swollen), probably due to infection. Sometimes chalazions disappear of their own accord; in other cases, they are removed surgically. (See *Lumps on the eyelid*, p.315.)

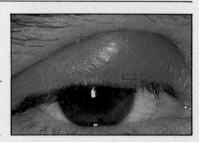

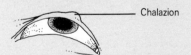

Chalazion

58 Xanthelasma

These are small patches of yellowish-white material that grow on the skin around the eyes, particularly near the nose (see the photograph on the right). In most cases they are unimportant, but rarely they signify an underlying disease, so they should always receive medical attention. The patches are painless. (See *Lumps on the eyelid*, p.315.)

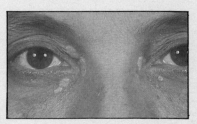

Eye problems in old age

The eye problems illustrated below occur mainly – but not exclusively – in older people. Entropion and ectropion are unlikely to pass unnoticed as they usually cause irritation and discomfort; cataracts are much more insidious in their onset.

59 Entropion

In *entropion* (p.315) the eyelid turns inwards ("in-turned eyelash"), so that the eyelashes rub on the surface of the eyeball. This makes the eye irritated and inflamed, causing much pain and discomfort in some cases. The close-up photograph below clearly shows the redness and swelling.

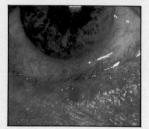

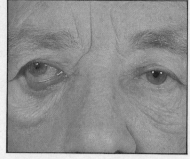

60 Ectropion

In *ectropion* (p.315) the lower eyelid becomes slack and hangs away from the eyeball – this gives the appearance of "out-turned eyelashes" (as shown in the photograph above). The lining of the lid and the eye itself dry out and become sore, and tear fluid cannot drain away properly and runs down the face. Like entropion, ectropion can usually be corrected by minor surgery.

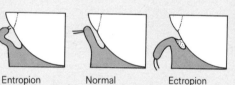

Entropion   Normal   Ectropion

61 Cataract

A cataract is an opaque area in the normally clear tissues of a healthy lens. The photograph below shows a fairly advanced cataract, which is clearly visible as a misty circular area within the normally black-looking pupil. The upper eyelid has been pulled up slightly to give a clearer view of the cataract. (See *Cataract*, p.319.)

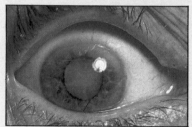

Lens   Cataract in lens

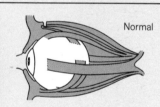

Other eye problems

62 Exophthalmos

Exophthalmos is the technical term for eyeballs that appear bulging, staring, or protruding. Although the eyes appear enlarged, the eyeballs themselves are usually unchanged in size; exophthalmos is due to a build-up of tissue behind the eyeball that pushes it forward within its bony socket set in the skull bone (see diagram, right). An abnormally large amount of the whites of the eyes becomes visible, and it may be difficult to close the eyelids. Exophthalmos is a sign of any one of several underlying disorders. (See *Exophthalmos*, p.326.)

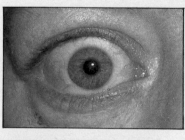

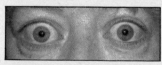

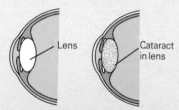

Normal

Exophthalmos

63 Ptosis

In ptosis (right), the upper eyelid of one eye (or both eyes) starts to droop so that the sufferer cannot completely close the affected eye. Occasionally, ptosis affects both eyes. The condition is either present from birth or develops later on, and may signify an underlying disorder. (See *Ptosis*, p.314.)

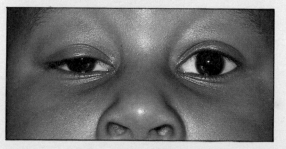

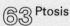

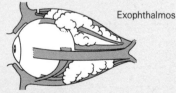

Mouth disorders

Shown below are three disorders that affect the lining of the mouth, the tongue, and lips – mouth ulcers, geographical tongue, and black hairy tongue. None of these disorders is serious; but some ulcer-like growths in the mouth or on the tongue are *malignant*. Early detection of any malignant (cancerous) growth is vital, so it is essential that any lump or raw area that persists for more than three weeks is seen by a doctor. (See *Mouth and tongue*, p.450.)

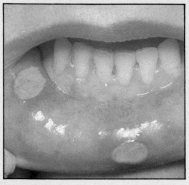

64 Mouth ulcers

These are small, raw, painful areas inside the mouth or on the tongue or lips (see the photograph above, and *Mouth ulcers*, p.450). They may occur as a result of injury (by a toothbrush, for instance) or illness. They usually heal within 7 to 10 days.

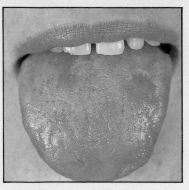

65 Geographical tongue

This is a completely harmless condition (above) in which patches of the tongue's upper surface lose their pinkish, roughened covering. The smooth, dark-red muscular body of the tongue is exposed beneath. Though harmless, geographical tongue may be sore or uncomfortable. (See *Tongue troubles*, p.455.)

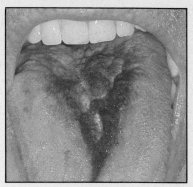

66 Black hairy tongue

The photograph above shows black hairy tongue – a rare, harmless condition in which the hair-like papillae covering the upper surface of the tongue become elongated and stained a dark brown colour. The cause of the condition is not known. (See *Tongue troubles*, p.455.)

Parasites

There are a number of small animals that live on or in human skin and produce characteristic marks there. Shown here are some of the more common ones – though in countries with high standards of hygiene, such as Britain, such problems are relatively rare. (See *Infestations*, p.567.)

Scabies mite
This tiny insect-like creature (right) is responsible for the rash of scabies.

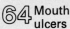

Nits
"Nits" are the eggs of *lice* (p.568); they adhere tenaciously to human hair, as shown right.

Bedbug
This small blood-sucking insect (right) thrives in dirty conditions and feeds mainly at night.

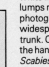

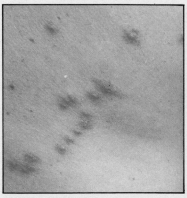

67 Scabies

The photograph above shows a typical infestation of scabies. Sometimes the burrows of the scabies mite can be seen as tiny white lines in the affected skin, and red lumps may also appear in this area (as in the photograph). In most cases there is also a widespread, intensely itchy rash on the trunk. Common sites for this infestation are the hands, wrists, and genitals. (See *Scabies*, p.568.)

68 Insect bites

Many small insects – gnats, fleas, mosquitos, bedbugs, and lice are examples – produce small, inflamed, itchy spots where they bite the skin. People vary in their sensitivity to such bites; some individuals come out in large weals which persist for several days, others may hardly notice a bite from the same insect. Often, several bites appear together, as shown above. (See *Lice*, p.568, and *Fleas*, p.569.)

Part III

Diseases, disorders, and other problems

Skin, hair, and nail disorders
Disorders of the brain and nervous system
Mental and emotional problems
Eye disorders
Ear disorders
Disorders of the respiratory system
Disorders of the heart and circulation
Blood disorders
Disorders of digestion and nutrition
Disorders of the urinary tract
Hormonal disorders
Disorders of the muscles, bones, and joints
General infections and infestations
Special problems of men
Special problems of women
Special problems of couples
Pregnancy and childbirth
Special problems of infants and children
Special problems of adolescents
Special problems of the elderly

Skin, hair, and nail disorders

Introduction

Skin is a supple, elastic tissue that has several important functions. One of these functions is to provide you with information about your surroundings. The information is collected by millions of tiny, specialized nerve endings – receptors – which are buried in the skin and which sense touch, pressure, heat, cold, and pain. Also embedded in skin are minute glands. One type of gland is the sebaceous gland, which produces a waxy substance that keeps your skin surface supple and waterproof and helps to prevent infection. There are also sweat glands, which produce a watery liquid to cool you when you are too hot. To help with this temperature regulation, the small blood vessels in your skin dilate in hot weather to lose heat; this makes you look flushed. The same vessels constrict in cold weather to conserve heat, and you turn pale.

There are thousands of hair follicles in your skin. These are pits of actively dividing cells that continuously make hairs. The largest hairs are found on the scalp, under the arms, and in the pubic region. There is a general body covering of smaller hairs, and in addition there are tiny hairs over most of the body which are too small to be seen by the unaided eye. Fingernails and toenails are also continuously produced by actively dividing cells, situated under the fold of skin at the base of each nail.

Because of the position of skin, hair, and nails – as the outside covering of the body – most people quickly notice any change in their appearance, whether it is due to a skin condition or to another disease which produces symptoms affecting the skin. In fact, most of the skin, hair, and nail problems included here are mainly to do with visual alterations only. There may be, in some cases, additional symptoms such as itching, swelling, or occasionally pain. Generally, however, diseases of the skin, hair, and nails are not life-threatening or harmful to general health. But they can be annoying and, in some instances, cause you to become embarrassed about your appearance.

The disorders dealt with in the following pages can affect virtually anyone, from the very young to the very old. Skin problems that affect only (or chiefly) infants and children – nappy rash, for instance – are covered under *Special problems of infants and children*, p.644.

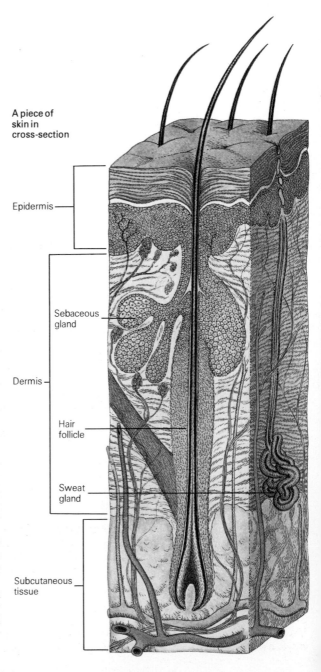

A piece of skin in cross-section

Epidermis

Sebaceous gland

Dermis

Hair follicle

Sweat gland

Subcutaneous tissue

Skin

Skin is composed of two layers. The surface layer that you see is a thin covering called the epidermis. Below the epidermis is a thicker layer, the dermis. The dermis contains many specialized structures such as hair follicles and sweat glands. Below the dermis is a layer of fat, called subcutaneous tissue.

The surface skin layer, the epidermis, is very active. The cells at its base are continuously dividing to produce new cells, which gradually form an accumulation of keratin, a hard substance. As keratin forms, the cells die and move towards the surface of the epidermis, where they replace cells worn away by friction from your clothing or from handling things. In fact, any movement that causes friction means a few skin cells rubbed away.

The continuous production of cells at the base of the epidermis keeps up with the continuous loss of cells from its surface. It takes, on average, about two months for an epidermal cell to complete the journey from base to surface. On parts of the body where pressure and friction are greatest – the palms of the hands and soles of the feet – the epidermis is thicker, and the journey takes longer. A number of skin problems are caused by a fault in the constant turnover of epidermal cells. In psoriasis, for example, there is an abnormally fast rate of cell production in the basal layer of the epidermis.

Skin renewal
The skin consists of 2 layers: the epidermis, a semi-transparent layer of cells; and the underlying dermis, a permanent foundation of fat, supportive tissue, and blood vessels. The cells at the base of the epidermis are constantly dividing to produce new cells, which take about 2 months to reach the surface where they are worn away.

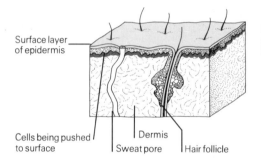

Surface layer of epidermis

Cells being pushed to surface

Sweat pore

Dermis

Hair follicle

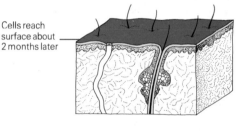

Cells reach surface about 2 months later

Boils and carbuncles

A boil is an infected and inflamed hair follicle (a tiny pit in the skin from which a hair grows). The infection is usually caused by staphylococcus bacteria. White blood cells, which form part of the body's defence system against bacteria, collect at the site to combat the infection. The white cells and bacteria accumulate to form a thick white or yellow pus within the inflamed area.

A carbuncle forms in the same way; it is either an unusually large, severe boil or a group of boils joined together.

Boils and carbuncles are localized infections and are not serious. Recurrent boils, however, can be a sign of the generalized condition *diabetes mellitus* (p.519).

Boils should not be confused with the spots present in *acne* (p.708).

What are the symptoms?
A boil starts as a red, tender lump, which may throb. Over the next day or two, it becomes larger and more painful. As pus collects, it develops a white or yellow centre (head). The pus is under pressure, which increases the pain and tenderness. Eventually, the boil either bursts through the skin or slowly disappears without bursting. In either case, the pain is relieved and the boil heals.

How common is the problem?
Boils are extremely common; they affect almost everyone at some stage. Carbuncles are much less common. Both may recur, because the bacteria that cause the boil or carbuncle may remain on the skin.

There is a risk that if the bacteria find their way from the boil, carbuncle, or skin into warm food, they can multiply; some strains produce *toxins* that cause *food poisoning* (p.462). So if you have a boil, wash your hands thoroughly before preparing food.

What should be done?
Most boils burst or disperse of their own accord within a week. If you have a painful

See p.237,
Visual aids to diagnosis, 23.

boil or recurrent boils, see your doctor. After examining the infection, the doctor may take samples of your blood and urine to rule out the unlikely possibility of diabetes mellitus being responsible for the boils.

What is the treatment?

Self-help: Apply a hot compress (cotton wool soaked in hot salty water) to the boil every few hours; this should reduce tenderness and discomfort.

Professional help: If the boil is about to burst, your doctor may lance it by making a small cut in the centre to allow the pus to drain away. In addition (or perhaps as an alternative), the doctor may prescribe *antibiotics* to kill the bacteria. The usual treatment to prevent recurrent boils is to apply an

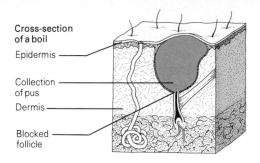

Cross-section of a boil
Epidermis
Collection of pus
Dermis
Blocked follicle

antiseptic or antibiotic to areas of skin where the bacteria live, such as around the mouth or nostrils. You should also add an antiseptic solution to your bath or washing water. This treatment may need to be carried out for several weeks to eradicate the bacteria.

Warts
(including verrucas)

See p.242, **Visual aids to diagnosis 36, 37, and 39,** and p.245, **visual aid 49.**

A wart is a lump on the skin produced by a virus. The virus invades the skin cells and causes them to multiply rapidly. Wart viruses are spread by touch or by contact with the shed skin of a wart.

There are several different types of wart. A common wart (known as a verruca when it develops on the sole of the foot) is a small, hard, horny, whitish or flesh-coloured lump with a cauliflower-like surface. Inside are small clotted blood vessels that resemble black splinters. The common wart can grow anywhere on your body but is most likely to develop on your hands. On the soles of the feet and palms of the hands, it tends to become pushed in so that its surface is level with the rest of the skin. Several warts may appear next to one another on your foot, forming a mosaic-like area that sometimes reaches 25mm (1in) or more across.

Common warts are usually painless. However, a wart on the underside of your foot presses into your foot as you walk and may be quite painful.

Among the other, less common types of wart are plane warts, small brown smooth lumps that occur most often in children; *penile warts* (p.577); and *vulval warts* (p.603). These last two types are probably caused by different strains of wart virus.

Molluscum contagiosum is a wart-like infection that produces tiny white pearly lumps, each with a central depression. These lumps are also most common in children.

How common is the problem?

Warts are common in teenagers and children, but less so in adults. Roughly 1 schoolchild in 20 has one or more warts.

What should be done?

All warts are harmless and disappear naturally in time. But if you consider your warts unsightly, you can, in certain cases, remove them by the self-help measures described below. However, you must consult your doctor if you have penile or vulval warts or if you think you or your child has molluscum contagiosum. You should also see the doctor if you develop any sort of wart and you are over the age of 45, since in older people what looks like a harmless wart may be a more serious skin condition.

What is the treatment?

Self-help: There are many folk remedies for removing warts, but no evidence to show that they work. The best way to treat an unsightly wart is to apply an over-the-counter wart paint, which may destroy the infected tissue. You will usually need to paint the wart daily for several weeks, avoiding the surrounding healthy skin. Between applications, carefully remove the loosened horny skin.

Do *not* treat warts on your face or genitals with wart paint, because the skin on these areas is very sensitive. And never allow the paint to get into your eyes. If you have an unsightly wart that does not respond to wart paint, see your doctor.

Professional help: Your doctor may prescribe a different kind of wart paint. If this fails, or as an alternative, the doctor can remove the wart by freezing it with liquid nitrogen or carbon-dioxide slush. A wart can also be burnt off (*diathermy*) or scraped off (*curettage*) after being numbed by a local anaesthetic. Most warts eventually succumb to treatment, leaving the skin scar-free.

Corns and calluses

Corns and calluses are areas of skin that have thickened because of constant pressure. Corns are small and develop on the toes; calluses are larger and commonly develop on the soles of the feet. Pressure on either causes tenderness in the underlying tissue.

Both corns and calluses tend to develop after you have been wearing a new or ill-fitting pair of shoes. And a callus can also form if you wear high heels, since these cause increased pressure on the ball of the foot. Some people have less cushioning tissue than normal between the bones and skin of their feet and so develop corns and calluses more easily than others.

Calluses may also develop on the fingers and the palms of the hands, especially if you do heavy manual work.

How common is the problem?
Corns and calluses are extremely common. Nearly everyone gets them at some time. But it is unusual for them to become so painful that a doctor has to be consulted. Of those people who do visit their doctor, men outnumber women three to two.

What are the risks?
Usually, corns and calluses are quite harmless. However, if you have *diabetes mellitus* (p.519) and suffer poor sensation in your feet because of this disease, deep ulcers can form under calluses.

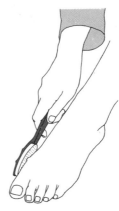

Self-help for corns
If you are prone to corns or calluses, it may be worth investing in a corn file to cut away the upper layers and ease the discomfort.

What is the treatment?
Self-help: Change to shoes that fit more comfortably. After several weeks, the corn or callus should disappear. In the meantime, to ease any discomfort, regularly soften the hard skin with an over-the-counter corn solvent, and then carefully cut away the top layers of the corn or callus with an instrument bought specially for the purpose. To prevent direct pressure on corns, you can buy small spongy rubber rings to put around them. If these self-help measures fail, consult your doctor.
Professional help: The doctor will usually refer you to a *chiropodist*, who will use specialist techniques to slice away the surface of the corn or callus and provide you with more elaborate cushioned dressings.

Eczema
(dermatitis)

The words eczema and dermatitis are virtually interchangeable. For simplicity, the word eczema is used throughout this article.

Eczema is inflammation of the skin that is usually itchy. The itching may be accompanied by redness, flaking, and tiny blisters. There are many types of eczema:
Infantile eczema: This is the commonest type. See p.666 for a description of this type of eczema, which occasionally persists into adult life.
Contact eczema: This eczema is caused by an allergy to certain substances coming into contact with the skin. If the allergy is a strong one – as, for example, in the case of poison ivy or primula – the eczema develops within 48 hours. The skin becomes red and itchy, and tiny blisters develop. These may join to form large blisters, which then break and crust over. If minute traces of chemicals from the plant are transferred from the hands to the face, eczema may develop on the face also.

Some forms of contact eczema are much less pronounced. For example, allergy to nickel (from a metal watch strap, say) produces a red, flaky, itchy patch at the place where the metal touches the skin.
Seborrhoeic eczema: This type of eczema is probably inherited; it is not caused by an allergy. (In infants *seborrhoeic eczema* p.651 is a different, unrelated condition.)

In adults, seborrhoeic eczema causes creases from the sides of the nose to the corners of the mouth to become red, flaky, and itchy. In men, this inflammation may extend to the area of the beard and appear on the hairy parts of the chest and the centre of the back. The condition may also affect other areas such as the groin, armpits, and under the breasts. Seborrhoeic eczema in a mild form on the scalp is the commonest cause of *dandruff* (p.263).
Housewife's hand eczema: Young women (and others) who constantly use washing-up liquids, detergents, household cleaners, and shampoos often suffer damage to the skin on their hands. It becomes red, dry, and rough, particularly over the knuckles. The skin may

See p.234, **Visual aids to diagnosis 7,** and p.235, **visual aids 8-15.**

thicken, crack, flake, and itch. A similar type of eczema occurs among people such as hairdressers and nurses whose jobs necessitate the constant use of irritant chemicals such as those in strong detergents.

Eczema in the elderly: The skin of an elderly person tends to be dry, particularly on the legs. This can lead to mild redness, flaking, cracking, and irritation (see *Skin problems of the elderly*, p.722).

Pompholyx: In this type of eczema, numerous itchy blisters erupt on the palms of the hands and soles of the feet. Some of the blisters may burst and weep, and the area becomes cracked, inflamed, and tender. An attack of pompholyx tends to last for two or three weeks and then clear up of its own accord, though attacks may recur. What causes the disorder is unknown, but it is believed that emotional stress could trigger off attacks in some people.

Discoid eczema: Discs of red, flaking, weeping, itching skin appear, most commonly on the arms and legs. The condition lasts for several months, then usually clears up on its own, permanently. Its cause is not known.

How common is the problem?
Each year 1 person in 30 visits a doctor about some form of eczema. Seborrhoeic eczema and housewife's hand eczema are very common; contact eczema is fairly common; pompholyx is relatively uncommon; and discoid eczema is rare.

What are the risks?
Eczema presents no risk to health, but it can be a great nuisance by causing considerable discomfort. Also, if the skin weeps and is scratched it may become infected by bacteria. The eczema then looks particularly wet or crusted, and unsightly.

What should be done?
If you have housewife's hand eczema, a contact eczema of which you know the cause, or a mild form of any other eczema, try the self-help measures outlined below. If they fail, or if your eczema is severe, see your doctor.

What is the treatment?
Self-help: Any eczema on the hands will improve if you avoid contact with irritants by wearing rubber gloves (unless, of course, you are sensitive to rubber). Dry your hands thoroughly after washing them, and apply a hand cream to protect the broken skin.

If you avoid whatever is causing a contact eczema, the condition should disappear within a few weeks or months.

Professional help: For any of the types of eczema described, your doctor will usually prescribe a *steroid* cream or ointment. Severe itching can be partly relieved by *antihistamine* tablets. These cause drowsiness and impair driving ability, and you may be advised to take them only at night. Any eczema worsened by a bacterial infection will be treated by a course of *antibiotics.*

If your doctor suspects you have a contact eczema, he or she will discuss with you a likely cause. Then *patch tests* (applying suspected substances to the skin) may be carried out to identify the cause; if a patch test is positive, avoiding that substance in the future should improve the eczema.

Steroid-containing skin creams
Many skin conditions are helped by anti-inflammatory *steroid* drugs in special creams or ointments. However, you should always use any such application exactly as prescribed by your doctor. Misuse or overuse of steroid drugs can have harmful effects such as the appearance of a red rash resembling rosacea (p.255), or permanent thinning and reddening of the skin, or other rashes.

Psoriasis

As your skin is worn away, it is replaced by cells produced beneath the surface. In psoriasis, the normal rate of cell production is speeded up, and this does not allow the cells to manufacture the substance keratin that gives skin its hard surface. The result is unsightly flaking of the skin, called psoriasis.

An outbreak of psoriasis is often triggered off by (among other things) a period of mental stress or a throat infection.

See p.241, **Visual aids to diagnosis, 32,** and p.245, **visual aid 52.**

What are the symptoms?
Deep pink, raised patches, covered by white scales, appear on the skin. They usually cause no discomfort but they may be slightly itchy or sore. You may have anything from a single small patch to many large ones. The most common sites are the knees, elbows, and scalp. Less commonly, patches appear in the armpits or under the breasts, on the genitals, and sometimes around the anus.

When psoriasis occurs on the hands and feet, it may be in the form of blisters filled with white (non-infected) pus and thickened, flaky skin. In some cases, the nails are affected and become thickened, pitted, and separated from the skin beneath.

About 7 per cent of psoriasis sufferers develop painful, swollen joints (a condition occasionally termed "psoriatic arthritis" resembling *Rheumatoid arthritis*, p.552).

How common is the problem?
Psoriasis is a common condition. About 1 person in 40 suffers from it to some degree.

It appears most often between the ages of 10 and 30, most cases are mild, and it tends to run in families to a certain extent.

What are the risks?

Psoriasis does not affect general health except occasionally in the very rare, extensive forms of the disease.

What should be done?

If you think you have psoriasis, consult your doctor. Discussion may help pinpoint the factors that trigger off the disease in your case.

What is the treatment?

Self-help: For some sufferers, careful sunbathing or using an ultra-violet lamp helps to clear up psoriasis, but if you have sensitive skin, you must take great care not to become sunburnt because this can easily make the condition much worse.

Professional help: Your doctor will probably prescribe one of several ointments, creams, or pastes to apply to the affected areas. Among them are *steroid* preparations, which are moderately effective. Some applications used to treat psoriasis have to be applied very carefully because they burn unaffected skin, and others may stain bedding and clothing.

In many cases, skin applications improve the condition. If they have little effect, you may receive ultra-violet treatment or a new type of light-ray treatment called *PUVA*, but the possible long-term side-effects of the latter therapy are as yet unknown.

As an alternative you may be advised to enter hospital for about three weeks to receive applications of a skin preparation. Or you may be given a *cytotoxic* drug (one that slows down cell division) if your psoriasis is severe. This last treatment is not used routinely because the cytotoxic drug may affect certain other cells in the body.

For most sufferers, psoriasis is a long-term condition and there is at present no permanent cure. However, modern treatment is largely successful in clearing up each outbreak of the disease.

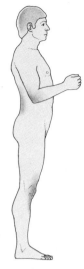

Common sites
of psoriasis

Acne and rosacea

See p.240,
Visual aids to diagnosis, 30–31.

Acne is a condition in which spots of various types appear on the skin. It nearly always develops during puberty, and so it is fully discussed as a special problem of adolescents (see *Acne*, p.708).

Rosacea is an acne-like condition in which the skin of the cheeks and nose flushes easily – after eating hot spicy food, for example, or drinking alcohol or strong tea or coffee. The facial skin of sufferers eventually becomes permanently flushed, and pus-filled spots appear in the affected area. The cause of the condition is not known, though some cases are caused by prolonged application of a *steroid* cream. A few people with rosacea also get sore eyes, caused by a non-infected type of *conjunctivitis* (p.317).

The condition, which is harmless, mainly affects middle-aged people and tends to persist for many years; it may eventually clear up of its own accord.

What should be done?

If you suspect you have acne rosacea, see your doctor, who may prescribe a course of *antibiotic* drugs. This is likely to improve the condition within a few weeks. However, after the drug is discontinued, the condition may well recur and you should return to your doctor for further courses of antibiotics.

Urticaria

(nettle-rash or hives)

See p.236,
Visual aids to diagnosis, 16–18.

In this very common disorder, red itchy lumps, known as weals, develop on the skin. The weals sometimes have pale centres, and they often join together to form large, irregular, raised patches. The weals may occur anywhere on the body.

Urticaria is sometimes triggered off by an allergic reaction to a food – commonly, shellfish, strawberries, nuts, or food additives – or to a drug, such as penicillin. It may also follow an infection or occur at the site of an insect bite. In other people, weals are raised simply when the skin is scratched (this form of urticaria is known as dermographism) or, very rarely, when it is exposed to heat, cold, or sunlight. But in many cases it is impossible to discover what triggers off the condition.

Whatever the cause, tension and stress usually make urticaria worse. Normally, weals clear up in a few hours, but occasionally they recur at intervals for days or months.

Some people suffer from a distressing form of the disorder, called angio-oedema. In this condition the tissues – particularly the lips and skin around the eyes – swell markedly. If the swelling spreads to the throat, suffocation becomes a possibility. In the majority of cases, however, urticaria is an irritating but harmless condition.

What should be done?

If your urticaria is due to a food allergy, you will probably be able to identify the food responsible, because weals will appear within a few minutes of eating it. But it may well be that you cannot identify the triggering factor and so prevent outbreaks of urticaria. In that case, consult your doctor. You can relieve any itching yourself by applying calamine lotion to the weals. Avoid taking aspirin as this can make urticaria worse and can sometimes start an attack. Consult your doctor if the rash has not disappeared within four hours. If your lips and the skin around your eyes start to swell and this swelling spreads to the throat, contact the doctor immediately.

To control troublesome urticaria, the doctor will prescribe *antihistamine* tablets. If you have severe angio-oedema, the doctor may give you an injection of a *steroid* or the hormone *adrenalin* to bring down the swelling and so remove any risk of suffocation.

Athlete's foot

See p.245,
Visual aids to diagnosis, 48.

In this harmless condition, a fungus (tinea) grows in the skin between and under the toes – especially the fourth and fifth toes. The skin becomes red, flaky, and itchy. Sweat or water makes the top layer of skin white and soggy. The fungus may also affect other parts of the foot and the nails. The latter become thickened and yellow in colour. Some sufferers find it difficult to eradicate the condition.

The same type of fungus may infect the skin of the groin and around the anus; the tinea fungus also affects the scalp, where it causes *ringworm* (p.666).

Athlete's foot is very common, but each year only 1 person in 400 finds it troublesome enough to visit a doctor. Men are affected more than women.

What should be done?
If you have the symptoms described above, try the following self-help measures; if they fail, consult your doctor.
Self-help: Apply an over-the-counter antifungal cream, spray, or powder; if the skin is soggy, use an antifungal powder. Some doctors consider that measures to keep the feet dry – for example, by wearing absorbent socks, made of natural not artificial fibres, and open sandals or shoes with porous soles and uppers – help clear up athlete's foot, but the value of these precautions is not universally accepted.
Professional help: The doctor will probably prescribe a more effective *antifungal* preparation than the one you have been using. If this produces no improvement, a prescribed four- to six-week course of antifungal tablets is usually effective in clearing up the problem.

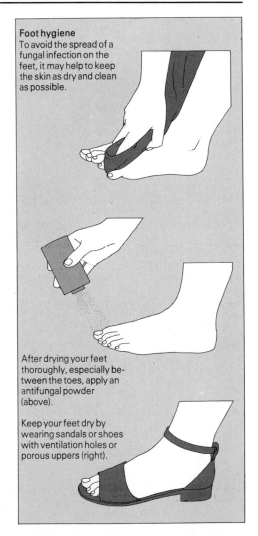

Foot hygiene
To avoid the spread of a fungal infection on the feet, it may help to keep the skin as dry and clean as possible.

After drying your feet thoroughly, especially between the toes, apply an antifungal powder (above).

Keep your feet dry by wearing sandals or shoes with ventilation holes or porous uppers (right).

Impetigo

See p.247,
Visual aids to diagnosis, 22.

Impetigo is a bacterial skin infection. It can occur almost anywhere, but usually affects the area around the nose and mouth.

What are the symptoms?
A small patch of tiny blisters appears. The blisters soon break, exposing a patch of red, moist, weeping skin beneath. Gradually, the area becomes covered by a golden crust that looks like demerara sugar. The infection then spreads at the edges, and new infected areas may appear elsewhere.

Impetigo is a *contagious* (catching) disease, especially among children.

How common is the problem?

Impetigo is a common condition, and is more prevalent among children than adults. Each year about 1 person in 100 sees a doctor concerning the problem.

What are the risks?

Impetigo is not a serious disease except in newborn babies, when it can produce large blisters and make extensive areas of the skin become red and start to peel. The baby will probably be generally ill. Certain types of impetigo lead to *glomerulonephritis* (p.504).

What should be done?

If you have impetigo, keep your own towel and other wash things, to avoid spreading the infection to others. You should always consult your doctor if you have the symptoms described above, because, left untreated, the condition spreads and may persist.

What is the treatment?

Self-help: Gently wash away the crusts of impetigo with soap and water and gently pat the area dry with a clean towel.

Children should stay away from school until their impetigo has healed. People with the condition should always wash their hands before preparing food.

Professional help: Your doctor will probably prescribe an *antibiotic*, either as a course of tablets or as an ointment. This should clear up the impetigo within a few days.

Cellulitis

(erysipelas)

Cellulitis is a skin infection caused by streptococcal bacteria which probably enter the skin tissue through a small cut or sore. They produce special chemicals (*enzymes*) that allow the infection to spread through the skin tissues. Any part of the body can be affected but it is usually the face or lower leg that is affected by this condition.

What are the symptoms?

A red, tender, swollen area appears and spreads gradually over a day or two. Red lines may appear on your skin, running from the infected area along lymph vessels to nearby lymph glands such as those in your groin. Your temperature rises and you become feverish and feel generally unwell.

What are the risks?

If the infection is not treated, the bacteria may get into the bloodstream and cause *blood poisoning* (p.421). So consult your doctor as soon as you become aware of the possibility that cellulitis might develop.

What is the treatment?

The doctor will put you on a course of *antibiotics*, which should clear up the infection. If your leg is affected, rest it and keep it raised to reduce the swelling.

Sunburn

Sunburn is inflammation of the skin caused by over-exposure to ultra-violet rays from the sun. The affected area becomes red, hot, and tender, and in bad cases blisters may form. You are much more likely to become sunburnt if you have light-coloured skin.

You need not sit under a blazing sun to get sunburnt. Prolonged sunbathing in hazy conditions will also produce sunburn, even when you feel deceptively comfortable.

How common is the problem?

Mild sunburn is common. Most fair-skinned people suffer it on their first exposure to strong sun in the summer. People from temperate climates who take a short summer holiday in a hot country and attempt to get a quick suntan are especially at risk.

What are the risks?

Repeated sunburn, or regular exposure to strong sun over many years, breaks down the elastic tissues in the skin and makes it look prematurely old and wrinkled. In addition, it can cause solar *keratoses* (roughened, red patches of skin) to appear on exposed places, especially in fair-skinned people. Long-term exposure to strong sun increases the risk of skin cancer (see, for example, *Squamous cell carcinoma*, p.259).

What should be done?

Prevent sunburn by sunbathing sensibly. If you have fair skin and the sun is strong, have only 15 minutes exposure on the first day. Increase this by about 30 minutes each day until you are beginning to tan noticeably – which usually takes four or five days. People with darker skin can usually sunbathe for slightly longer. During this early period, it is important to use an over-the-counter sunscreen (rather than suntan) lotion. Once your tan is under way, use plenty of suntan oil or lotion to prevent your skin from becoming dry. If you get sunburn, adopt the following self-help measures. Protect sunburnt skin – even while swimming – by wearing clothing. Apply calamine lotion or a similar soothing cream, and take paracetamol to relieve discomfort. Do not sunbathe until the redness and tenderness have disappeared (for further information and first-aid measures see *Accidents and emergencies*, p.815).

If the sunburn is very painful, consult a doctor. An anti-inflammatory *steroid* cream should help the condition heal faster.

Effects of ultra-violet rays on the skin
Ultra-violet rays from the sun can penetrate the semi-transparent epidermis to reach the underlying dermis.

The capillaries under the epidermis dilate, allowing more blood to flow near the surface and causing the skin to look red in colour.

The ultra-violet rays eventually stimulate certain cells to produce more melanin, a skin pigment that shades the underlying tissues. Melanin in the epidermis causes the skin to look darker.

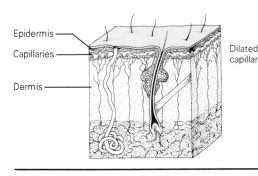

Epidermis
Capillaries
Dermis

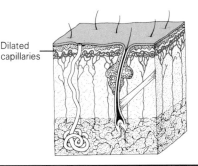

Dilated capillaries

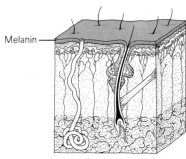

Melanin

Rodent ulcer
(basal cell carcinoma)

See p.243,
Visual aids to diagnosis, 41.

A rodent ulcer is the most common of the three types of skin cancer (the other two are *squamous cell carcinoma* and *malignant melanoma*, opposite). Changes in the dividing cells in skin cause a *malignant* tumour to develop, which then becomes ulcerated. The cell changes usually seem to be brought about by long-term exposure to strong sunlight, but it may be many years before this produces a rodent ulcer. The ulcer grows very slowly over several years, destroying the tissue as it spreads. Unlike many other malignant growths, it does not spread (*metastasize*) to other parts of the body.

What are the symptoms?
A small, flesh-coloured, sometimes pearly-looking lump appears on the skin. The commonest site is the face, especially next to the eye or nose. The lump grows slowly and may develop into an ulcer with a raised border and a raw, moist centre, which may bleed. Scabs repeatedly form on and fall from the ulcer, but it does not heal.

In a few cases the ulcer appears without any obvious lump, and sometimes the rodent ulcer does not even look like an ulcer but a red, flaky patch of skin which slowly enlarges.

How common is the problem?
Rodent ulcers affect those with light skin, most commonly middle-aged and elderly people who have spent many years in strong sunlight. The ulcers are rare in people with dark skin because the extra melanin (skin-colouring pigment) in their surface skin cells shields underlying skin cells from sunlight.

What are the risks?
Because they grow so slowly and do not metastasize, rodent ulcers cause problems only if they are neglected for many years. A large untreated ulcer will grow relentlessly and can destroy part of a nearby structure such as an eye or ear. Death resulting from a rodent ulcer is extremely rare. It occurs only when a large, neglected ulcer erodes some vital underlying structure, such as an artery.

What should be done?
If you suspect you have a rodent ulcer, see your doctor, who will probably make the diagnosis after a visual examination. There are several ways to remove a rodent ulcer. It may be cut out, frozen by *cryosurgery*, destroyed by *radiotherapy*, scooped out with a sharp spoon-like instrument (*curetted*), or treated by special cream. All these methods have a high success rate, and leave only a slight mark on the skin where the ulcer was.

After treatment, your doctor may advise regular check-ups, because a few ulcers recur, usually within about two years. If this happens, the ulcer is simply treated again.

Squamous cell carcinoma

See p.243,
Visual aids to diagnosis, 42.

This is one of three types of skin cancer. (The other two are *rodent ulcer*, opposite, and *malignant melanoma*, below.) In squamous cell carcinoma, skin cells develop into a *malignant* tumour (lump). As with the other types of skin cancer, years of exposure to strong sunlight seems to be one of the main causes of damage. A less common cause is long-term exposure to industrial tar. Very rarely, a squamous cell carcinoma arises from a solar *keratosis* (see *Sunburn*, p.257).

What are the symptoms?
A firm, fleshy, hard-surfaced lump develops, and grows steadily. In some cases it looks like a wart; in others it forms an *ulcer*. A squamous cell carcinoma usually appears on a place exposed to sunlight. The lower lip, ear, and hand are common sites.

How common is the problem?
Together with rodent ulcers (which are more common), the carcinomas occur at the rate of 1 new case per 1,500 people each year. You are most at risk if you have lived in a sunny country for many years, have light skin, and are middle-aged or elderly. The disorder is rare in people with darker skin.

What are the risks?
If the cancer is allowed to reach an advanced stage, it may spread to other parts of the body (*metastasize*). If this happens, the outlook is poor. Normally, the problem is detected early, and treatment is simple and effective.

What should be done?
Go to your doctor without delay if you develop any lump for no apparent reason. After examining you, the doctor may then want to remove a small sample of the suspected carcinoma for laboratory analysis (*biopsy*).

What is the treatment?
Most squamous cell carcinomas are easily removed by cutting them away. This is usually a minor operation. When the carcinoma is large, a skin graft (see *Plastic surgery*, p.260) will be needed to cover the scar.

Alternative treatments for squamous cell carcinoma are freezing the area (*cryosurgery*) and *radiotherapy*.

Over 90 per cent of patients with this condition are completely cured, and regular check-ups are given over the next few years so that any recurrence of the cancer can be detected and further treatment given.

Malignant melanoma

See p.243,
Visual aids to diagnosis, 43.

Malignant melanoma is the most serious of the three types of skin cancer (the other two are *rodent ulcer*, opposite, and *squamous cell carcinoma*, above). This is because, unlike the others, malignant melanoma often spreads throughout the body (*metastasizes*).

The tumour sometimes develops from pigment cells in a mole, sometimes from pigment cells in ordinary skin. As with rodent ulcer and squamous cell carcinoma, many years of exposure to strong sunlight seems to play a part in the development of the disease, but this is a less definite factor than in the other two types of skin cancer.

What are the symptoms?
The most common symptom is that a mole which has been present since childhood changes in one of several ways. It may begin to grow; to become patchy, or lighter, or darker; to develop a black margin that spreads into the surrounding skin; to bleed spontaneously; or to itch. Another common symptom is the development of a new mole at any time after puberty. Sometimes a flesh-coloured or red lump may appear on the skin. A malignant melanoma may also develop in the dark, irregular freckles which sometimes occur on the skin of elderly people. Most malignant melanomas tend to arise in areas of skin that have been exposed to the sun. But they sometimes occur on other sites, such as the soles of the feet.

How common is the problem?
This form of skin cancer is not as common as the other two. In Britain there is about 1 new case per 6,000 people each year. It is extremely rare before the onset of adolescence – so it is highly unlikely that a child who develops a new mole is suffering from the disease. The tumours are more prevalent among middle-aged or elderly people with light skin who have spent much of their lives in strong sunlight – for example, Australians are especially susceptible.

What are the risks?
Because the cancer can spread (hence the name *malignant* melanoma), early recognition, diagnosis, and treatment are essential, otherwise the outlook is poor.

What should be done?
It may well be that the change in a person's mole is not a malignant one but due simply to some minor injury. In the same way, a change in pigmentation of an area may be the result

of some harmless skin condition. However, a person who develops any of the symptoms described should take no chances and should see a doctor immediately. Even if the doctor thinks the mole or lump is harmless, he or she may still decide to have it removed and examined under a microscope (*biopsy*) for signs of cancerous cells. If the diagnosis is then confirmed, treatment of the melanoma in hospital will start right away. The melanoma is cut out along with a wide margin of adjacent skin. A skin graft (see *Plastic surgery*, below) to cover the area is often carried out at the same time. In some cases, sessions of *radiotherapy* or some other specialized treatment may also be given.

Plastic surgery

Plastic surgery is done to repair or reconstruct a part of the body that has suffered an injury (a severe burn, for example) or that is malformed due to faulty development (for instance, to mend a cleft palate). It usually involves the technique of skin grafting and sometimes surgery on underlying tissues such as muscle and bone. Plastic surgery may also be done with the sole purpose of improving a person's appearance; in such situations it is called cosmetic surgery.

Skin grafts

A wound resulting from an accident, severe burn, or an extensive operation may need a skin graft. Skin for grafting is taken from suitable areas elsewhere on the patient's body. This means that skin that survives the transplantation will not then be attacked by the body's immune system (see *Transplants*, p.402).

The most common method of skin grafting – split-thickness grafts – is to shave a thin layer of skin off a healthy, large area, such as the thigh or back, and bandage it in place over the wound for a week to 10 days until it attaches itself to the underlying tissues. The area from which the skin has been taken usually heals in 1 to 3 weeks.

In a situation where such a graft is not likely to "take", a pedicle flap graft may be done. One type of pedicle flap graft involves loosening a strip of skin from a donor site near the area to be covered and pressing it over the damaged area, while leaving it attached to the donor site by one of its edges so that it is still supplied with blood. Depending on its size, the area from which the skin has been taken may be stitched together or may need a split-skin graft.

With recent advances in skin-culture techniques, it is now possible to take a small area of skin from a donor site and culture it under artificial conditions until it is large enough, when replaced, to cover a damaged site of virtually any size.

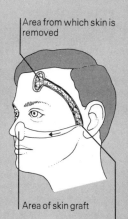

Area from which skin is removed

Area of skin graft

Point of attachment

Pedicle flap graft
The pedicle (the stalk-like attachment) keeps the grafted skin supplied with blood until it "takes" on the new area.

Cosmetic surgery

Cosmetic surgery is available under the National Health Service only if the defect is causing psychological problems; it is usually expensive if done privately. Before having cosmetic surgery consult your GP and ask to be referred as a private patient to an NHS consultant who does private work. Do not risk having cosmetic surgery at a clinic that advertises its services but is not recommended by your doctor.

The most common operations are nose reconstruction (rhinoplasty), facelift, and breast enlargement (augmentation mammoplasty). Most involve only a few days' stay in hospital and, with the exception of facelifts – which last anything from 2 to 10 years – are permanent and leave few noticeable scars.

Varicose (venous) ulcers

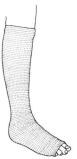

An elastic bandage can help speed up sluggish blood flow.

If you have poor circulation – which becomes more likely as you grow older – the blood flow through the lower parts of your body, especially your calves and ankles, becomes sluggish. You may already have *varicose veins* (p.409). In addition, any small injury or crack that appears in the skin is unlikely to heal quickly because the tissues are filled with stagnant fluid and are poorly served by fresh blood. The injury or crack may enlarge and gradually become a varicose ulcer.

What are the symptoms?
The ulcer is a flat area where the skin surface breaks down to leave a pale, weeping centre. The commonest site for a varicose ulcer is the skin on the inside of the leg, just above the ankle. Sometimes both legs are affected. The skin next to the ulcer usually becomes red, flaky, and itchy, and the surrounding area turns brown and looks mottled. In a young person ulcers usually heal in a few weeks, but in an older person they may persist for months or even years.

How common is the problem?
Each year about 1 person in 700 sees a doctor about the problem. Twice as many women as men are affected. Though a varicose ulcer is not serious, it can persist and be troublesome for several years. So if you think you have a varicose ulcer, make an appointment to see your doctor, and meanwhile adopt the self-help measures described below.

What is the treatment?
Self-help: Whenever you sit or lie down, raise the affected ankle as high as possible. Avoid prolonged standing, and take some moderate walking exercise.
Professional help: Your doctor may provide a knee-high elastic bandage or thick elastic

stocking to wear during the day. If the ulcer is severe, your doctor or nurse will treat it by cleaning it daily with a mild antiseptic and covering it with a dressing. In some instances this still fails to clear up the problem, in which case you may be advised to go into hospital for a few weeks. There you can rest in bed in the proper position, and you and your ulcer will be under constant supervision and treatment. To hasten healing, surgery on the veins or a skin graft (see *Plastic surgery*, opposite) may be advisable.

Sebaceous cysts

See p.242, **Visual aids to diagnosis, 40**.

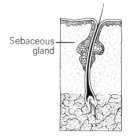

Sebaceous gland

A sebaceous *cyst* is a small, fluid-filled sac that develops in the skin. Why sebaceous cysts appear is not known. The cyst is filled with a thick white fluid that slowly accumulates and causes the cyst to grow slowly over many years. It can be seen as a pale lump beneath the skin; the scalp is a common site. In some cysts, a narrow pore connecting the cyst and the skin surface is marked by a tiny dark central dot.

Sebaceous cysts occur singly or in groups. They are usually painless and harmless, quite common, and first noticed in adult life.

What are the risks?
If a sebaceous cyst is infected by bacteria, it becomes enlarged, red, inflamed and tender. It may eventually burst and release a foul-smelling pus. After this, the inflammation recedes but the cyst still remains and may become re-infected later.

What should be done?
Most people with small cysts simply accept them. If a cyst becomes infected, or if you want one removed because it is unsightly, see your doctor. A course of *antibiotics* is usually given for an infected cyst. An obtrusive cyst can be removed by surgery during a simple out-patient operation, for which you will be given a local anaesthetic. If, however, even a small part of the cyst is left behind after surgery – as is sometimes unavoidably the case – it can recur.

Keloid

See p.241, **Visual aids to diagnosis, 34**.

A keloid is an excessive growth of the fibrous tissue that forms a scar. It can occur in any kind of scar – for example, after an injury, an operation, a burn, a vaccination, or the piercing of an ear lobe. At first, the scar seems to heal normally, but after several weeks it grows and becomes noticeably larger and thicker. Occasionally, a keloid develops on a scar that has remained dormant for many years, or even appears on an area of skin with no previous scar.

All keloids are harmless but some are unsightly. They tend to be quite common in people with dark or black skin, and less common in those with light skin.

What should be done?
If you want a keloid treated for cosmetic reasons, consult your doctor, who will probably give a course of injections into the keloid; this sometimes makes it smaller. Alternative treatments are *cryosurgery* (freezing with a probe), *radiotherapy*, or *plastic surgery* (opposite). A keloid cannot simply be cut out as this would leave a scar which might very well eventually turn into another keloid.

Lichen planus

See p.441, **Visual aids to diagnosis, 33**.

Lichen planus is an itchy skin rash, the cause of which is unknown. It consists of small, shiny, violet spots that appear suddenly, but fade gradually over weeks or months and leave a flat brown mark. When lichen planus occurs on the inside of the mouth (termed oral lichen planus) a white lacy pattern appears on the lining. Lichen planus can also affect fingernails and toenails (see *Deformed and discoloured nails*, p.265). If it occurs on the scalp, it can cause hair loss.

How common is the problem?
Lichen planus is rare; it occurs most often in middle-aged people. Although it is harmless, if you suspect you have it, you should always consult your doctor.

What is the treatment?
Most doctors diagnose lichen planus on sight. To treat the condition, the doctor will probably prescribe a *steroid* ointment to relieve the irritation and reduce the rash.

Severe lichen planus tends to be unaffected by steroid ointment and so is treated by a two- or three-week course of steroid tablets, but the condition has a tendency to recur when the course is finished.

For further information on *oral lichen planus* see the article on p.452.

Pityriasis rosea

See p.236,
Visual aids to diagnosis, 19

The cause of this skin rash is unknown, though some doctors suspect that a virus is responsible. It starts as one or more small red spots, generally on the trunk. Over the next few days more spots appear and spread to cover the trunk and upper arms (a "T-shirt" distribution) and the upper legs. The spots become oval patches of red or copper-coloured skin with scaly margins. The patches may be itchy. The condition affects mainly children and young adults.

There are no risks attached to pityriasis rosea, but you should visit your doctor to ensure that you do not have some other similar skin disorder. Your doctor may advise you to wait for the rash to disappear naturally – which often happens over several weeks or months. Any minor itching you can relieve yourself by applying calamine lotion. If the rash is very bad, the doctor may prescribe a *steroid* cream, and severe itching can be lessened by *antihistamine* tablets.

Ichthyosis

Ichthyosis is a rare, inherited skin condition. In infancy or early childhood the skin becomes extremely dry all over, and is broken up into diamond-shaped plates resembling fish scales. Often the skin is darker than normal. The condition usually improves during adolescence, though a few adults find it troublesome. It presents no risk to health.

What should be done?
Take your child to the doctor if you suspect he or she has the condition. There is no cure, but there are various creams and special soaps your doctor can recommend to make the skin less dry. Cold weather makes the condition worse, so make sure your child wears warm clothing.

Abnormal skin pigmentation

See p.242,
Visual aids to diagnosis 35 and 38, and p.244,
visual aids 44–46.

Normal skin contains an evenly distributed population of special cells, called melanocytes, which produce the brown skin-colouring pigment melanin. The amount of melanin produced increases with exposure to sunlight. In certain skin conditions the melanocytes are either abnormally formed or abnormally distributed in the skin, or make less or more melanin than normal, and the result is very pale or very dark skin.

Albinism: This is a rare, inherited condition. The melanocytes are unable to make melanin, so albino people are very pale-skinned and have white hair and pink or pale-blue eyes. They are advised to wear dark glasses and to avoid bright sunlight because sun hurts their eyes and burns their skin.

General darkening of the skin: Certain diseases (*Addison's disease*, p.524, for example) can provoke a widespread darkening ("suntan") without exposure to sun. If your skin begins to darken for no obvious reason, see your doctor for diagnosis and treatment of the underlying problem.

Vitiligo: Vitiligo is thought to be an *autoimmune* condition. Pale, irregular patches of skin appear on the body. It is rare, and sometimes occurs along with another autoimmune disease such as *hypothyroidism* (p.526).

Pityriasis (tinea) versicolor: This common fungal infection causes patches of pale or dark, often flaking skin to develop over various parts of the trunk.

Chloasma: Hormonal changes during pregnancy or while taking the contraceptive pill cause some women to develop patches of darker skin on the face, particularly on the cheeks. The condition sometimes improves after childbirth or when the pill is stopped.

Moles: These are small dark areas of skin composed of dense collections of melanocytes. They usually develop during childhood and may be flat or raised; some moles are hairy. Very occasionally a mole may become *malignant*. For further details see *Malignant melanoma*, p.259.

Seborrhoeic warts: These are not true *warts* (p.252), but small, round or oval patches of dark skin. They are common and often develop after middle age. They usually have a crusty, greasy appearance.

What should be done?
Most of the above-mentioned conditions are harmless, but if you are distressed or suspicious (especially about a mole or seborrhoeic wart) consult your doctor.

Self-help: Make-up and cosmetics are often the most satisfactory way of dealing with patches of light or dark skin.

Professional help: There are specific treatments available for some of the above conditions. Pityriasis versicolor can be cured by an *antifungal* ointment; disfiguring moles may be cut out or their hairs removed by *electrolysis*; and special cosmetics are available to cover various skin blemishes. Your own doctor may treat you; otherwise, ask him or her to refer you to an appropriate specialist for further information.

Hair and nails

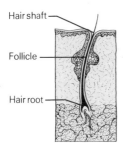

Hair shaft

Follicle

Hair root

Hair and nails are specialized hardened structures that are basically very similar in composition to the surface layer of skin. Hairs grow from follicles (pits of actively dividing cells in the skin), nails grow from the fold of skin at the base of the nail. The substance that gives both hair and nails their hardness is a protein called *keratin* (which is found in smaller amounts in the skin itself).

Because hair has little real function, diseases that affect it generally cause cosmetic rather than medical problems. Similarly, fingernails and toenails are not essential to life; nail disorders can be unsightly and irritating but are not harmful to health.

The articles in the following pages deal with several of the more common conditions that affect hair, nails, and associated tissues.

Dandruff

Dandruff is the abnormal production of small flakes of dead skin on the scalp. The two main causes of this are a mild form of seborrhoeic *eczema* (p.253), or, less commonly, *psoriasis* (p.254) of the scalp. The hairs on the scalp are usually unaffected.

Dandruff is common, and carries no health risk whatsoever; it is simply unsightly and may lead to cosmetic embarrassment.

What is the treatment?
Self-help: Use an anti-dandruff shampoo, following the instructions on the bottle. Frequent shampooing (once every two or three days) is usually necessary, at least to start with, and use of the anti-dandruff shampoo often needs to be continued to prevent the dandruff returning.

Professional help: If the above treatment does not work, your doctor will probably prescribe a special lotion containing a *steroid*, which acts to suppress the underlying cause of the dandruff.

If the scaling is thick and sticks to your scalp, the doctor may prescribe a lotion containing a mild acidic substance, which loosens the abnormal skin. This allows the anti-dandruff shampoo to work effectively.

Hair care

Normal shampooing and brushing of the hair will not damage it. However, various hairdressing procedures – particularly frequent perming and dyeing, and excessive heat used in drying or setting the hair – tend to make the hair look dull, become fragile so that it breaks easily, and develop split ends. So-called "hair conditioners" do little to repair this type of damage.

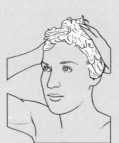

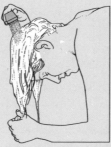

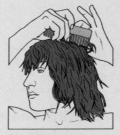

Washing your hair
Unless your hair is very dirty, one application of shampoo will suffice. You can water down the shampoo by half. Wet your hair completely, apply the shampoo, and massage the lather gently but thoroughly into your scalp. Rinse with clean water. If you wish, use a special rinse or conditioner at this stage, but remember that over-use will make your hair lank and greasy. Wrap your dripping hair in a towel, and then comb it out gently to keep damage to a minimum.

Drying your hair
Hand-held or hood dryers are unlikely to burn or otherwise damage hair, but heated rollers or curling tongs should not be used too hot or too frequently. The best way to dry your hair is to leave it, and let it dry on its own.

Removing unwanted hair
Many women (and most men) regularly remove hair from certain areas. Hair is usually removed if it is considered unsightly, especially if it is dark. Whether hair is unsightly is really a matter of personal and social preference – removal of unwanted hair is unlikely to improve hygiene or general health.

Most methods of removing unwanted hair are simple and painless, but have only a temporary effect. The most commonly used methods are:
Shaving: suitable for most parts of the body. Contrary to popular belief the hair does not grow thicker as a result.
Depilatory creams and sprays: suitable for all parts of the body, but may irritate areas of sensitive skin.
Abrasives: suitable for most parts of the body but may cause soreness if used on the face.
Plucking: normally used for small areas, often individual hairs (eyebrows); gives long-lasting results.
Waxing: suitable for most areas; gives long-lasting results. Often carried out at beauty salons.
Electrolysis: usually permanent. Should only be done by an expert, generally on small areas (especially the face).

Baldness
(including alopecia areata)

In the vast majority of cases, baldness is a natural process. In men, it tends to run in the family. The normal pattern is for the front hairline to recede while hair thins over the crown. In some men these areas eventually meet, and the thinning may carry on to affect the whole scalp.

In many women, there is a gradual but slight and diffuse thinning of the hair that begins in young adult life. Again, this is a natural process and should not be regarded as abnormal. Occasionally the hair thins about three months after having a baby; this is a fairly common occurrence and the hair grows back over the following months.

Rarely, baldness is due to some underlying disorder. It can occur after a severe, sudden illness. Many hairs stop growing during the illness and then fall out about three months later. Again, they will regrow. In certain severe or prolonged illnesses, such as thyroid diseases (see *Thyroid and parathyroid glands*, p.525) and *iron-deficiency anaemia* (p.419), diffuse hair loss also occurs. In most of these cases, effective treatment of the underlying disease will restore hair to normal. Certain diseases that affect the scalp, such as *lichen planus* (p.261), may destroy the hair follicles and, unless treated early, produce patches of permanent baldness. Some forms of treatment – in particular *cytotoxic* drugs used to slow down cell growth, especially against cancer – can cause loss of hair. The hair usually grows back when the treatment ceases. There are certain fungal scalp infections that produce bald patches with flaky skin and a few broken-off hairs.

Finally, there is a specific disease that can cause hair loss; most people affected have only patchy loss, but in a few cases the loss is complete. The disease is called alopecia areata. Round, bald patches appear suddenly; the exposed scalp looks normal and may contain a few fine, white hairs and/or "exclamation mark" hairs which are narrower at the base than at the tip. The cause is unknown.

How common is the problem?
Natural hair loss happens to everyone, but to some more than others. Each year 1 person in 400 sees a doctor about unusual or severe baldness; the numbers are equally divided between men and women.

What should be done?
Most people accept natural balding as part of the ageing process. Some people undergo hair transplantation, which is not available under the National Health Service and is not always successful. For balding that has been caused by disease or medical treatment, you can obtain a toupee or wig free under the National Health Service.

Baldness caused by a fungal infection can be treated with *antifungal* tablets. Bald areas due to alopecia areata usually regrow hairs within a few months. Your doctor may advise you to wait for this natural recovery or may attempt to hasten it by a course of *steroid* injections into the scalp.

Male-pattern baldness
Baldness that occurs naturally in men generally runs in the family. The front hairline may recede first and often meets a growing bald patch at the crown.

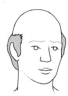

Paronychia
(including whitlow)

A paronychia is an infection of the skin adjacent to a nail. It occurs particularly in people who spend a lot of time with their hands in water. The infecting microbes may be bacteria or yeast (a type of fungus). The bacteria usually cause acute (sudden and severe) infections. Fungi – particularly candida, which causes thrush (see *Oral thrush*, p.451) – are usually responsible for chronic infections, which are slow to develop and less painful but often very persistent and occasionally difficult to cure even with prolonged treatment.

What are the symptoms?
In acute infections, your nail fold becomes swollen, red, and painful. The cuticle may lift away from the base of the nail, and if you press on it you may expel pus from beneath.

A blister of pus (often called a whitlow) may develop alongside the nail. Chronic infections produce similar, but less marked, symptoms. Often the skin around several nails is affected. The nail-forming area, no longer protected by the cuticles, is damaged, and this causes *deformed or discoloured nails* (opposite). Occasionally, the nails themselves are attacked by the fungi and become thick, ridged, and discoloured, perhaps with a soft, powdery surface.

What should be done?
You can help to prevent paronychia by protecting your hands when they are immersed in water. Wear rubber gloves with cotton gloves inside them, or use a dusting of talcum powder inside the outer gloves.

See p.245,
Visual aids to diagnosis, 51.

What is the treatment?

If you go to the doctor with an acute infection in the early stages, a course of *antibiotics* may clear up the problem. If pus has collected, the doctor may pierce the blister, allowing pus to drain away and relieving the pain. If the infection is chronic, your doctor will probably prescribe an *antifungal* cream or paint to apply to the affected nail(s) just after you wash your hands.

After several months of treatment, the swelling usually subsides completely and any raised cuticles and unsightly nails should have returned to their normal condition.

Deformed and discoloured nails

(including ingrowing toenail)

See p.245,
Visual aids to diagnosis, 50.

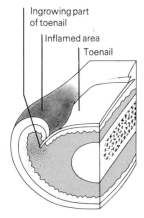

Ingrowing part of toenail

Inflamed area

Toenail

Ingrowing toenail
An ingrowing toenail curves into the sides of the toe.

Nails may become deformed or discoloured because of injury or illness. Injury to the nail-forming area beneath the cuticle – which is sometimes caused by continuous pressure from too-tight shoes – can lead to thickening of the whole nail. Many disorders can produce nail deformities. *Psoriasis* (p.254), and fungal infections such as *paronychia* (opposite) can cause separation of the trimmed end of the nail from the underlying skin. Bacteria entering this space may make the nail turn blackish-green. *Iron-deficiency anaemia* (p.419) can make nails spoon-shaped, and some disorders, notably *lung cancer* (p.366) and *congenital heart disorders* (p.656) can cause *clubbing* – the nails growing round the enlarged ends of the fingers and sometimes toes. After any illness, temporarily poor nail growth may cause a crosswise groove to appear in nails; this gradually grows out.

Discoloration is caused by one of various illnesses. The nail bed appears pale in *anaemia* (p.419), and white in some forms of liver disease. Small, black, splinter-like areas appear under the nails in infections of the *heart valves* (p.392). And in certain fungal nail infections the nail becomes thickened, discoloured, and has a white, crumbly surface; the free end of the nail may become separated from the nail bed.

A knock to the nail can cause one or more small white patches to appear in the nail and move with the nail as it grows. Finally, the nail of the big toe sometimes curves under at the sides. This is an ingrowing toenail. It is believed that the condition is caused by wearing tight shoes or cutting the toenails in a curve and down at the sides, rather than straight across at the end.

What should be done?

Deformities and discoloration caused by an underlying illness often grow out after the illness is treated. Nails badly damaged by injury usually grow again naturally in about nine months but may be deformed. A nail which persistently grows in a deformed manner should be seen by your doctor, who may refer you to a *chiropodist* for advice on how to trim it so that it causes fewest problems. Fungal nail infections sometimes respond to *antifungal* tablets from your doctor.

If you have an ingrowing toenail, try the following self-help measures. Wear well-fitting shoes; keep the affected area clean and dry; cut the nail straight across the top, and be careful not to leave splinters at the edges.

Occasionally, your doctor or chiropodist may recommend a minor operation to remove the ingrowing edge of the nail and the nail fold which produces it. After the operation, you should follow the self-help treatment described above, so that the condition does not recur.

Nail Care

For healthy nails, observe the following advice.

Protect hands from prolonged immersion in water, especially soapy water; wear rubber gloves with a dusting of talcum powder on the inside, and dry your hands afterwards.

Keep nails short to prevent them from splitting and getting dirty.

Trim your nails regularly with scissors or special nail clippers – a good time is after a bath, when they are fairly soft.

Either leave cuticles alone or else push them down with a cuticle stick or the thumbnail of the opposite hand – again after a bath, while they are relatively soft.

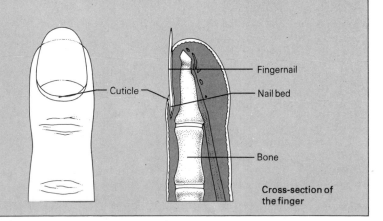

Cuticle

Fingernail

Nail bed

Bone

Cross-section of the finger

Disorders of the brain and nervous system

Introduction

Imagine the most complex and sophisticated electronic computer yet built. Your brain is far more complex and sophisticated than this, and your entire nervous system is even more so. It consists of two parts – a central system and a peripheral system. The central system includes the brain together with the spinal cord, a column of nerve tracts running down the protective bony canal of the spine. The peripheral system comprises the vast network of nerves that run through the rest of the body. The peripheral nerves that run throughout the body are of two types. The *sensory* nerves convey nerve impulses from sensory organs to the brain. Besides the fairly obvious examples of sensory organs – the eye, ear, nose, and taste buds – there are numerous sense receptors in the skin that detect touch, pressure, pain, and temperature. There are also specialized sense receptors, called stretch receptors, in your muscles. These tell you how stretched or contracted each of your muscles is, and consequently let you know in what position your limbs and body are at any time virtually without your having to think about it. The other type of nerve is the *motor* nerve. Motor nerves carry messages from the brain to the various muscles of the body, "ordering" them to contract or relax to a greater or lesser degree. The peripheral nerves connect with the spinal cord at different levels, and it is by way of the spinal cord that information to and from the peripheral nerves is fed to and from the brain. This system controls all your conscious activities and profoundly affects even unconscious processes such as heartbeat rate, breathing rate, and bowel functions.

Like the rest of the body, the nervous system is vulnerable to various problems. Defects in its blood supply (vascular disorders) can injure it; and it can be damaged by infections, degeneration, structural defects, and tumours. Because of the nervous system's complexity, the symptoms of brain or nerve damage can be varied. Among these symptoms, which may come and go, are headache, dizziness, loss of balance or coordination, weakness, numbness, tingling, memory loss, difficulty finding or understanding words, fits, tremors, loss of consciousness, and loss of bowel or bladder control.

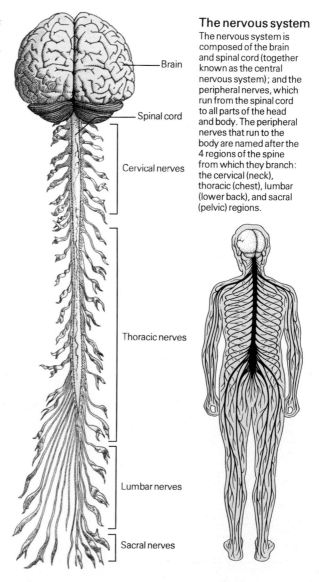

Brain

Spinal cord

Cervical nerves

Thoracic nerves

Lumbar nerves

Sacral nerves

The nervous system

The nervous system is composed of the brain and spinal cord (together known as the central nervous system); and the peripheral nerves, which run from the spinal cord to all parts of the head and body. The peripheral nerves that run to the body are named after the 4 regions of the spine from which they branch: the cervical (neck), thoracic (chest), lumbar (lower back), and sacral (pelvic) regions.

The brain

The brain lies well protected within the rigid, bony case of the skull. It is divided into 3 main parts – the cerebral hemispheres, the cerebellum, and the brain stem. The cerebral hemispheres are responsible for controlling "higher functions" such as speech, memory, and intelligence. Some functions are controlled by specific areas, such as the speech centre. If the speech centre is damaged by a stroke, the ability to translate your thoughts into words vanishes. Other functions, such as memory, cannot be localized and seem to be controlled by the cerebral hemispheres generally. Under the cerebral hemispheres is the cerebellum, which controls certain subconscious activities, especially co-ordinating movement and keeping your balance. The brain stem merges into the top of the spinal cord and maintains the "vital functions" of the body, such as breathing and circulation. Nerve signals travel up and down the spinal cord, which links the brain to the rest of the body.

The diagram on the right shows some of the better-defined areas of the brain and their functions.

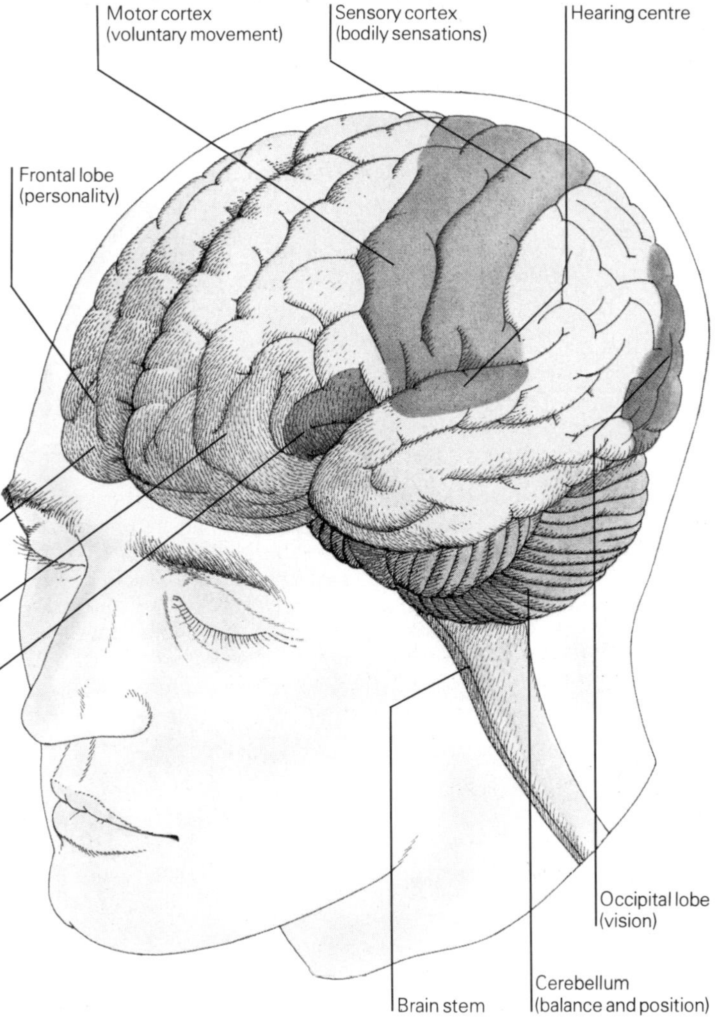

Motor cortex (voluntary movement)

Sensory cortex (bodily sensations)

Hearing centre

Frontal lobe (personality)

Right cerebral hemisphere

Left cerebral hemisphere

Speech centre

Occipital lobe (vision)

Cerebellum (balance and position)

Brain stem

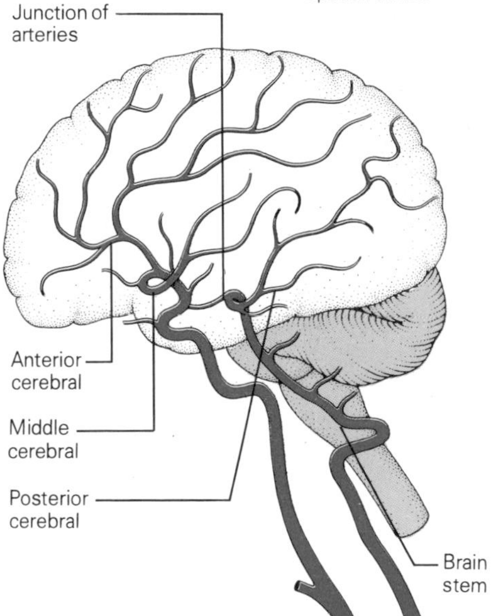

Junction of arteries

Anterior cerebral

Middle cerebral

Posterior cerebral

Brain stem

Vertebral

Carotid

The main arteries of the brain (above)

The 2 vertebral arteries and the 2 carotid arteries run up the neck to supply the brain with blood. At the bottom of the brain, they form a circular junction from which other arteries – the anterior cerebral, the middle cerebral, and the posterior cerebral – run to other parts of the brain.

Inside the brain (right)

In this sectional view of the brain, the corpus callosum – the part that links the cerebral hemispheres together – is shown as a band of tissue near the centre. The cerebral hemispheres lie in folds on either side. Each hemisphere consists of a core of white matter surrounded by a layer of grey matter. The hypothalamus at the base of the brain is concerned with sleep, appetite, and sexual desire.

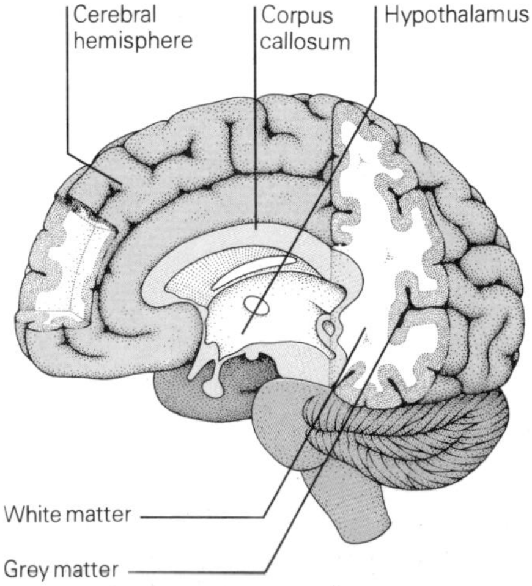

Cerebral hemisphere

Corpus callosum

Hypothalamus

White matter

Grey matter

Vascular disorders

Four major blood vessels supply your brain with blood carrying oxygen and essential nutrients. There are two arteries in your neck (the carotids) and two running up protective bony canals in the neck section of your spine (the vertebrals). These major arteries join to form a roughly circular arrangement at the base of your brain, and branches from the circular arrangement run to all its parts. Areas that depend on only a single branch are especially vulnerable to a disturbance in the flow of blood, such as that caused by a *thrombosis*. The following articles deal with the main ways in which the brain can be affected by defects in this vascular (blood-supply) system. Strokes and other disorders caused by inadequate blood supply or by bleeding in the brain tissues from diseased arteries are among the most common disorders in patients admitted to hospital in Western countries and they account, in one way or another, for one-third of all deaths.

Stroke

A stroke occurs when part of the brain is damaged because its blood supply is disturbed, with resultant deterioration of the physical or mental functions controlled by the injured area. The disturbance may be due to one of three types of vascular disorder: *thrombosis*, *embolism*, or *haemorrhage*.

The first of these, cerebral thrombosis, can happen if an artery supplying blood to the brain is narrowed, usually because of *atherosclerosis* (p.372). Blood flow through the narrowed and roughened portion of the artery becomes so disrupted that the blood coagulates, forming a clot (*thrombus*) that partially or completely blocks the artery.

A cerebral embolism is also a blockage, but it occurs when disease elsewhere releases into the bloodstream a small blood clot (*embolus*) which is swept along until it becomes wedged in an artery supplying the brain.

In a cerebral haemorrhage the artery is not blocked but bursts. Blood seeps from the rupture into surrounding brain tissue and continues to do so until prevented by a build-up of pressure and the process of clotting. The initial effects of haemorrhage may be more severe than those of thrombosis or embolism, but long-term effects of all types of stroke are similar. The results of a stroke, whatever the cause, depend on which part of the brain is mainly affected.

What are the symptoms?

If you suffer a stroke, you may wake up to find you have lost the power of speech or movement of part of the body; or you may, while conscious, feel an arm or leg become heavy and useless. Sometimes a stroke begins with sudden loss of consciousness. Among the many other possible symptoms are numbness, blurred or double vision, confusion, and dizziness. Often it is the functions of only one side of the body that fail. This is because damage is usually limited to one side of the brain; and the right side of the brain controls the left side of the body, and the left the right.

On the surface of each hemisphere of the brain there are specific areas that control definite parts of the body, or functions such as vision, movements, and speech. Thus there is a characteristic pattern of symptoms that indicate which cerebral artery is malfunctioning. For example, you may have weakness or numbness only in your arm or hand, or on one side of your face. If a crucial control centre such as the brain stem (which connects

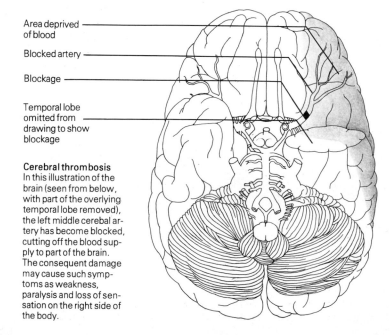

Area deprived of blood

Blocked artery

Blockage

Temporal lobe omitted from drawing to show blockage

Cerebral thrombosis
In this illustration of the brain (seen from below, with part of the overlying temporal lobe removed), the left middle cerebal artery has become blocked, cutting off the blood supply to part of the brain. The consequent damage may cause such symptoms as weakness, paralysis and loss of sensation on the right side of the body.

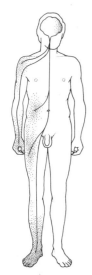

Brain and body
Each side of the body is controlled by the opposite side of the brain. This means that damage to the left side of the brain results in paralysis or loss of sensation in the right side of the body.

the brain and spinal cord) is involved, there may be a complex combination of symptoms or loss of consciousness. In any event, the symptoms (unlike those of a *transient ischaemic attack*, p.270) persist for at least 24 hours – and normally much longer.

How common is the problem?
Strokes cause more deaths in Western society than any group of disorders other than heart disease (see, for example, *coronary artery disease*, p.374). Both problems are often the result of atherosclerosis.

In an average year, 1 person in 500 in Britain will have a stroke. Most sufferers are people over 65 (more often male than female) whose blood vessels have been narrowed by atherosclerosis and who tend to have *high blood pressure* (p.382). An abnormally high blood pressure at any age can bring on a stroke by weakening arterial walls and by encouraging the formation of blood clots; indeed, high blood pressure is the major cause of cerebral haemorrhage.

Whether or not your blood pressure is dangerously high, you are more likely than others to suffer a stroke if you smoke heavily. Strokes are also more prevalent among diabetics and people with a high level of *cholesterol* (p.27) in the blood.

What are the risks?
About one in three strokes is fatal; one in three causes permanent damage or disability; and one in three has no lasting ill-effects. A person who survives a stroke may be partially paralysed for months before improvement becomes apparent. Even a mild stroke is a danger signal; it may be the first of a succession of increasingly severe attacks.

What should be done?
If you develop symptoms suggestive of a stroke, get medical help immediately. Except in very mild cases, when weakness, numbness, or dizziness may last for only a day or two, people who have had a stroke usually need to be admitted to hospital. To assess the situation fully, your doctor will probably require an *electrocardiogram* (*ECG*) and skull and chest *X-rays*. Although treatment of all three forms of stroke is essentially the same, different types of investigation may be needed in order to determine the cause and location of the disturbance. If there is reason to believe that the stroke has been caused by cerebral embolism, the doctor may want special X-rays of the neck arteries (carotid *arteriograms*). This is because surgery to prevent further strokes is sometimes possible if

the possible source of the embolus can be tracked down to a carotid artery (see "What is the treatment?" below).

If someone loses consciousness in your presence, it may be because of a stroke. Whatever the cause, carry out first-aid measures (see *Accidents and emergencies*, p.805) while waiting for assistance. Remember that in cases of stroke an apparently unconscious person often senses what is going on nearby. So do not panic, but try to remain calm, and comfort and reassure the sufferer.

What is the treatment?
Self-help: You can do nothing once you have had a stroke, but you can do much to guard against strokes or prevent recurrence. Have your blood pressure checked routinely. If it is high, be sure to take the drugs your doctor prescribes. Do not smoke or eat too much fatty food, and take some moderate regular exercise (see *Eating and drinking sensibly*, p.24, and *Keeping physically fit*, p.14).
Professional help: The doctor's first priority is to assess the severity of the attack and to carry out necessary life-saving procedures to maintain breathing and circulation. But most people admitted to hospital following a stroke are not unconscious, and their main requirement is *physiotherapy*, which aims to restore function to affected areas of the body. It often takes extreme patience and support, both physical and moral, to help the sufferer gradually relearn old skills.

The nerves of a severely damaged portion of the brain cannot be regenerated. An undamaged area, however, can often be "taught" to take over the control of an affected function, and such "teaching" is the aim of most rehabilitation programmes. If a stroke weakens your legs, for example, you may be given exercises that slowly progress from using parallel bars to walking with a frame or stick to walking freely without help. Your relatives and friends may eventually be involved in the process, which is likely to continue long after you leave hospital. Similarly, if your speech is impaired, the *speech therapist* will try to retrain you in skills of vocalization and pronunciation that you once assumed were as natural as breathing.

Prevention of further strokes is obviously of prime importance. You will be warned not to smoke and will probably need to have regular doses of drugs such as a *beta-blocker* to keep your blood pressure down. If the cause of your stroke is determined to have been an embolism, tests may show that the source of the embolus is the roughened surface of part of a carotid artery that has been narrowed by the accumulation of *plaque* formed as a result of atherosclerosis. It is often possible to locate, clean out, and open up that section of the artery. This operation, which is done under a general anaesthetic, is usually successful; and further strokes from the same source are unlikely to occur. If surgery is not feasible, your doctor may prescribe a lifetime course of *anticoagulants* to guard against the formation of clots. Recovery from a stroke is more likely in people who are determined to get well. Many people who have had strokes gain valuable advice, support, and motivation from the *Disabled Living Foundation* (p.768) and from various local self-help organizations ("Stroke clubs") – your doctor will provide you with names and addresses.

Transient ischaemic attack

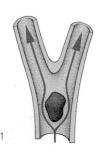

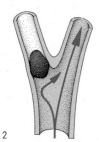

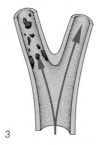

How the attack occurs
A transient ischaemic attack is caused by a collection of blood cells (1) blocking off a small artery in the brain (2). The attack is only temporary because the blood cells are soon broken up and swept away (3), and blood flow is restored.

Ischaemia is a condition in which body tissues receive an inadequate supply of oxygen because the flow of blood through vessels that service those tissues is impeded. An ischaemic attack in the brain resembles a stroke due to cerebral *embolism* (see *Stroke*, p.268), but a "transient" attack differs in that stroke-like symptoms last for only a short time. A sudden onset of weakness and numbness down one side of the body, for example, may last a few minutes or hours and then disappear, whereas the symptoms of stroke last for more than 24 hours. It is important to understand this difference; if transient ischaemic attacks are recognized and treated, more serious damage (in other words, a stroke) can sometimes be averted.

The narrowing or obstruction of arteries to the brain may result from any of several causes. Most often, though, an ischaemic attack occurs because a small clot or a piece of *plaque* (see *Atherosclerosis*, p.372) breaks away from the wall of an artery or heart valve and is carried into the cerebral circulation. As the clot or piece of plaque (called an *embolus*) passes through blood vessels in the brain, it temporarily impedes the flow to an area of brain tissue, with consequent ill-effects. Circulation is soon restored, however, and the temporarily deprived tissues recover. The embolism is therefore transient. But transient embolisms are likely to recur.

What are the symptoms?
Symptoms are like those of a stroke but do not last. If the embolus lodges in an artery supplying an eye, there may be a loss of vision due to *retinal artery occlusion*, p.325.

How common is the problem?
Because many transient ischaemic attacks go unrecognized, no dependable estimate of incidence is possible. Certainly they are quite common, particularly among people over 60.

What are the risks?
Recurring transient ischaemic attacks increase the likelihood of a stroke. Nearly half of all sufferers from transient ischaemic attacks have a stroke within a period of five years after the first attack.

What should be done?
If you have had stroke-like symptoms or sudden loss of vision in one eye, do not delay in consulting your doctor, who may, after examining you, refer you to a *neurologist*. The first diagnostic step will be to identify the source of a possible embolus. A likely source of emboli is one of the two carotid arteries in your neck. To search for signs of narrowing of the carotid arteries, your doctor may listen with a *stethoscope* to various places in your neck. The stethoscope may also be placed at your chest to pick up any sounds of an abnormal heart valve or irregularity in heartbeat rhythm. You may then need to undergo an *electrocardiogram* (*ECG*), a chest *X-ray*, and possibly other scanning tests, and the doctor may want to take special X-rays (called *arteriograms*) of blood vessels that may be the source of the trouble.

What is the treatment?
Self-help: The purpose of the treatment is to try to prevent a stroke. Preventive measures depend largely on age and general state of health, but there are several simple steps anyone can take. If you smoke, give it up. Try to avoid eating fatty foods, and take regular exercise. Make sure you have your blood pressure checked regularly so that any increase can be treated promptly (see *High blood pressure*, p.382).
Professional help: Medical treatment may consist simply of two aspirin tablets once a day for the rest of your life; aspirin is a good weapon against recurrence of attacks since it prevents blood particles from sticking together. Powerful *anticoagulant* drugs are also available on prescription, and in some cases surgery is advisable. If the precise location of the narrowing of an artery has been identified, that part of the artery can sometimes be surgically "re-bored" so as to improve the flow of blood.

Subarachnoid haemorrhage

As with cerebral haemorrhages (one form of *stroke* – see p.268), the cause of a subarachnoid haemorrhage is a ruptured blood vessel. The disorder differs from a cerebral haemorrhage in that blood escapes to spread over the surface of the brain instead of seeping into the brain tissue itself.

The surface of the brain has three thin, membranous layers (the meninges) covering it. The outside membrane (called the dura) adheres to the skull; the innermost one (pia) adheres to the brain; the middle one (arachnoid) is much closer to the dura than to the pia. Thus there is a space between the arachnoid and the pia, and this "subarachnoid" space is filled with fluid.

A subarachnoid haemorrhage occurs when blood leaks into the subarachnoid space. This is usually caused by a burst *aneurysm* (p.407) in a cerebral-artery wall. The blood either remains in the fluid or gradually seeps through the pia into the brain tissue.

What are the symptoms?
The main symptom is a sudden headache, which is likely to be far more painful than an ordinary *headache* (p.284) or even *migraine* (p.285). A stiff neck and inability to endure bright light (*photophobia*) often follow, and there may also be fainting, dizziness, confusion, drowsiness, nausea, and vomiting. A major attack can cause the sufferer to lose consciousness suddenly.

How common is the problem?
Subarachnoid haemorrhage accounts for 1 in 12 cases of vascular brain trouble. It is most common in people aged 40 to 60 and is slightly more common in women than it is in men. Anyone who has *high blood pressure* (p.382) is especially susceptible.

What are the risks?
Up to 45 per cent of major attacks (those causing unconsciousness) are fatal, and one in three sufferers who survive a first attack has further attacks. There is a risk of permanent brain damage due to the pressure of blood on the brain tissues. In about half of all cases, blood spreads into the brain itself, causing stroke-like symptoms.

What should be done?
If you get a sudden severe headache, especially if accompanied by a stiff neck and sensitivity to light, call a doctor without delay. If someone in your presence complains of a sudden headache and then lapses into unconsciousness, two possible causes are stroke or subarachnoid haemorrhage. In either case follow the first-aid advice given in *Accidents and emergencies* (p.805), while waiting for a doctor.

With an unconscious person, the doctor's first step is to initiate life-saving procedures – ensuring that breathing is not obstructed. Once the sufferer is out of danger, the next need is an accurate diagnosis. If a physical examination suggests the probability of subarachnoid haemorrhage, the best way to confirm the diagnosis is to do a *lumbar puncture*, which involves taking a specimen of cerebrospinal fluid. This watery fluid circulates in the subarachnoid space of both the brain and spinal cord, and the easiest place to take a specimen in order to see whether it contains blood is in the lumbar region (the area at the base of the spine).

What is the treatment?
If blood is found in cerebro-spinal fluid, the doctor's chief concern will be to prevent further bleeding. No drug treatment can heal a burst artery; but if you survive the few days following a subarachnoid haemorrhage, the rupture that caused the trouble has probably been sealed (at least temporarily) by natural clotting of blood, and healing is under way. The basic treatment now is several weeks of bed rest, usually in hospital. During this period the doctor may prescribe a painkiller such as paracetamol to relieve headaches. If blood pressure is high, you will also have to take one of the *beta-blocker* group of drugs.

Within three days of the attack, the major arteries that supply your brain will probably be subjected to special *X-rays* called *arteriograms* in order to locate the site of the aneurysm and any other defective spots in arterial walls. If arteriograms indicate a danger of further attacks, surgery to prevent more leakages may be advisable. Such surgery usually involves sealing off an aneurysm by means of a tiny metallic or plastic clip.

What are the long-term prospects?
If you regain consciousness after a major attack and survive for six months without further trouble, you are probably out of danger. Chances of full recovery from surgery are also good. Residual symptoms after an attack vary according to the areas of the brain affected. Partial paralysis, weakness, or numbness may linger or even be permanent, as may difficulties with sight and speech (for further information on these types of problem see the article on stroke). After an initial attack, blood pressure should be checked regularly; high blood pressure can strain an already weak vessel wall.

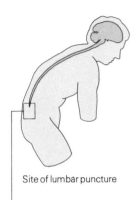

Site of lumbar puncture

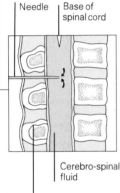

Needle | Base of spinal cord

Cerebro-spinal fluid

Backbone

Diagnosing subarachnoid haemorrhage
A sample of cerebrospinal fluid is taken from the base of the spine by a lumbar puncture. Blood in the fluid indicates that a subarachnoid haemorrhage has occurred.

Subdural haemorrhage

Subdural haemorrhage is leakage of blood from vessels in the dura – the outermost of the three layers (meninges) covering the brain. It differs from *extradural haemorrhage* (below) in that the ruptured blood vessels are (as the name of the disorder implies) on the underside, rather than the outside, of the dura. Because these inner vessels are smaller than the outer ones, there is likely to be less profuse leakage of blood; it tends to seep quite slowly into the space between the dura and the arachnoid (the middle layer of the three meninges). Often, therefore, quite a long time – up to several weeks – will elapse before gradually mounting pressure on underlying brain tissues causes noticeable symptoms. Among eventual symptoms of subdural haemorrhage are drowsiness, confusion, visual disturbance, weakness or numbness down one side of the body, and persistent or recurrent headaches and nausea. During a period of days or weeks such symptoms may come and go, but if they are caused by a subdural haemorrhage, they will gradually become worse.

Subdural haemorrhage is a very rare complication of a head injury (see *Brain injury*, p.276, and *Accidental falls*, p.719). It most often occurs in elderly people who have fallen, and who may well have forgotten the accident by the time symptoms develop.

What should be done?

Consult your doctor without delay if you develop the symptoms described above. Because they are similar to those of a minor *stroke* (p.268), be sure to tell the doctor if you have recently had a head injury (even a slight one). You will probably be admitted to hospital for diagnostic tests such as *X-rays*, *arteriography*, *radio-isotope scan*, and possibly a brain scan (known as a *CAT scan*) to determine the cause of your symptoms. If the trouble is diagnosed as subdural haemorrhage, treatment is similar to the treatment for extradural haemorrhage.

Subdural haematoma
A subdural haemorrhage – bleeding between the dura and arachnoid, 2 of the 3 layers covering the brain – results in a subdural haematoma, which may cause symptoms similar to those of stroke or dementia.

Haematoma
Dura
Arachnoid
Skull
Brain tissue compressed

Extradural haemorrhage

Extradural haemorrhage occurs when blood vessels in the dura – the outermost of the three layers (meninges) covering the brain – rupture and blood flows outwards over the surface of the brain. The trouble usually results from a head injury that causes some of the blood vessels in the outer surface of the dura to burst (see *Brain injury*, p.276). Because these vessels are large, a substantial amount of blood flows away, and the symptoms of an extradural haemorrhage are likely to appear within 24 hours of the blow that caused it. (For *subdural haemorrhage*, in which blood leaks inwards instead of outwards, see above.) Even if the original injury seemed trivial when it happened, the symptoms are severe. They include a sudden bad headache; nausea, which often culminates in vomiting; and increasing drowsiness, which may lead to unconsciousness.

How common is the problem?

About one million head injuries are treated in the accident and emergency departments of British hospitals every year, but only 10 per cent of these require hospital admission, and only 1 or 2 per cent develop extradural haemorrhage as a complication. It is a serious complication, however, because potentially damaging pressure on the brain mounts as more and more blood floods into the narrow space between brain and skull.

What should be done?

If you or anyone in your presence shows symptoms of extradural haemorrhage, get medical help fast, especially if there has been a blow to the head within the past day or so. Unless the sufferer is treated promptly, there is danger of permanent brain damage or even death. You will be admitted to hospital immediately for diagnostic tests, such as an *X-ray* of the skull and a *CAT scan*, and general treatment for the injury. If tests indicate the presence of extradural haemorrhage, you will need to undergo surgery to stop the bleeding. The operation involves removal of a portion of skull bone in order to release leaked blood and permit the surgeon to repair ruptured blood vessels. When the operation is done promptly, it is likely to result in complete recovery.

Infections

Infections of the nervous system are less frequent than infections of, say, the respiratory system because the brain and spinal cord are well sealed from the outside world. Infections gain entry through the bloodstream, or via the air spaces in the ears, or through head injuries. Most nervous-system infections cause obvious, serious illness; early diagnosis is important since prompt treatment can save life and prevent long-term damage to the brain, spinal cord, or nerves. You should familiarize yourself with the symptoms of nervous-tissue infection so that you can act quickly if anyone in your family is affected.

Meningitis

Meningitis is inflammation of the coverings of the brain and spinal cord (the meninges) as a result of bacterial or viral infection. Many of the potentially causative bacteria are constantly present in the noses and throats of most people who do not, however, develop the disease. It seems that a person's natural resistance has to be lowered before the infection can become established. There are a number of ways in which infection can reach the meninges. For example, microbes may spread via the bloodstream from some other infected part of the body, such as the lungs. They can also spread to the brain through the cavities in bone from an infected ear or infected sinuses. Or if you have a head injury in which you suffer a fractured skull, this provides an easy entry for infection.

There are many forms and degrees of meningitis. Much depends on the type of bacterium or virus that causes the disease.

Infection of the meninges
The brain and spinal cord are surrounded by cerebro-spinal fluid, contained between the arachnoid and the pia, 2 of the 3 sheets of fibrous tissue called the meninges.

Meningitis occurs when, for some reason, microbes spread to infect the cerebro-spinal fluid, causing inflammation of the meninges themselves.

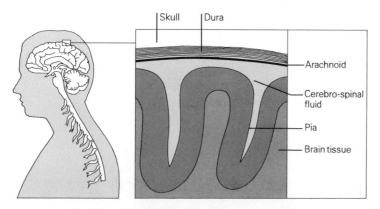

Skull | Dura

Arachnoid

Cerebro-spinal fluid

Pia

Brain tissue

What are the symptoms
Fever, headache, nausea and vomiting, a stiff neck, and *photophobia* (inability to bear bright light) usually develop over the course of a few hours. An occasional additional symptom is a deep-red or purplish rash over most or all of the body. If the infection continues unchecked, the sufferer becomes confused and then drowsy and may eventually lose consciousness.

Symptoms may be less obvious in infants and young children. For a full discussion of *meningitis in babies and children* see p.668.

How common is the problem?
Meningitis is a very rare illness in Britain. The most common form, a viral infection, spreads from person to person through the air. It therefore tends to occur in epidemics, often in winter, as do many viral illnesses. It may affect anybody, at any age, male or female. Such epidemics rarely last for more than a few weeks; in those weeks there may be several cases of meningitis in a hospital that has none at all during the rest of the year. There may also be epidemics of bacterial meningitis, but individual cases are equally common. Meningitis is more common in tropical countries, particularly where *tuberculosis* (p.563) is still prevalent, as tuberculosis itself can cause meningitis.

What are the risks?
The sooner treatment of bacterial meningitis is started, the better the results. Untreated bacterial meningitis may well be fatal. Most people recover completely, but a few are left with permanent damage including deafness, blindness, or mental deterioration. In very rare cases an *epidural abscess* (p.275) may develop even when meningitis is diagnosed and treated promptly. Babies and elderly people are most in danger of either failing to recover or being left with residual damage. The reasons for this may be the increased

likelihood of delay in diagnosis at these ages and impaired powers of resistance.

Viral meningitis, fortunately, tends to be a less severe illness than the bacterial type. Full recovery, with no after-effects, can be confidently expected in most cases.

What should be done?

If you or anyone in your family develops symptoms of meningitis – particularly a combination of severe headache, stiff neck, and photophobia – consult your doctor without delay. A tentative diagnosis of meningitis can be confirmed by an examination, in hospital, of a sample of the cerebro-spinal fluid that bathes your central nervous system. If the sample, which is obtained by means of a *lumbar puncture*, looks cloudy and contains pus cells, this indicates infection of the meninges. Further tests of the sample should identify the offending organism.

What is the treatment?

In most cases sufferers should remain in hospital until the meningeal infection has been dealt with. If your infection is bacterial, you will be given large doses of *antibiotics*, which may be fed directly into a vein by means of an *intravenous drip*. This process may continue for as much as two weeks. Because any one of a number of bacteria may have caused bacterial meningitis, the exact treatment may well vary from case to case. For the same reason, the possible complications of the disorder, and the speed and eventual degree of recovery, can also vary.

Since most viruses are not affected by antibiotics, most cases of viral meningitis must be left to run their course. You can expect to be fully recovered in two or three weeks (depending on the severity of your attack). Tubercular meningitis is treated by a long-term course of special antibiotics.

While in hospital, you will be made as comfortable as possible. Bed rest in a darkened room, plenty of fluids – given through a drip if you are very ill – and drugs to lower your temperature and ease the pain of headaches will help your defence mechanisms to overcome the viruses.

Encephalitis

Encephalitis is inflammation of brain cells. The usual cause is a viral infection. In some cases, the virus spreads to the nervous system from an infection such as mumps, measles, or glandular fever. In most cases, however, encephalitis is the only result of the infection. There are a few other kinds of brain infection which are not caused by viruses – for example, African sleeping sickness, which is caused by a single-celled animal transmitted by the tsetse fly – but such diseases are virtually unknown in Britain.

What are the symptoms?

Encephalitis varies enormously in its severity. In mild cases the symptoms are those of any viral infection – fever, headache, and loss of energy and appetite. In more severe cases brain function is more obviously affected, with irritability, restlessness, drowsiness, and perhaps *photophobia*. In the most severe cases there may be loss of muscular power in the arms or legs, double vision, impairment of speech and hearing, and eventually coma.

How common is the problem?

Mild encephalitis is quite common. However, the symptoms can mistakenly be thought to indicate a mild bout of flu or may be indistinguishable from the symptoms of the underlying illness, and so many people are unaware that they have had it. About 1 in 1,000 cases of measles causes mild encephalitis. Severe attacks are extremely rare.

What are the risks?

Much depends on the age of the sufferer and on the kind of microbe that causes the disease. Encephalitis in babies and the elderly may be fatal, but people in other age groups often recover completely, even after serious and prolonged illness. Although there is a risk of permanent brain damage, only a small number of cases have serious consequences.

What should be done?

If you develop symptoms indicative of encephalitis, and especially if you have recently had a virus infection such as measles, consult your doctor, who will probably order diagnostic tests, including blood tests, a skull X-ray, and an *electroencephalogram* (*EEG*). An essential test for infection of the nervous system is examination of cerebro-spinal fluid taken by means of a *lumbar puncture*.

What is the treatment?

Since viruses do not usually respond to *antibiotic* drugs, the basic treatment consists of measures to ease symptoms and allow the body's natural defence system to overcome the infection. For the most part, you are simply kept comfortable and well nourished. Sometimes *steroid* drugs can help suppress inflammation. In severe cases feeding is done by a *nasogastric* tube, and breathing may have to be assisted by a *respirator*.

Recovery from a severe attack may be slow, and you may need the help of a *physiotherapist* to relearn fundamental skills such as clear speech or the ability to use a knife and fork. In such cases – which are rare – you may well be dependent on medical and family aid for up to a year.

Polio
(poliomyelitis)

This viral infection, which attacks *motor* (muscle-controlling) nerves, used to be universally dreaded since a small proportion of its victims were left permanently paralysed. But with modern preventive techniques the disease has been virtually stamped out in the Western world; most years, there are no cases in Britain, where children are routinely given doses of anti-polio vaccine from early infancy onwards (see *Immunization*, p.701).

If you are planning to travel abroad to a polio-risk area, ask your doctor about the availability of further preventive doses of the vaccine. Where polio exists, it is spread by personal contact or by eating or drinking food or liquids that have been contaminated by sewage. Its early symptoms are headache, sore throat, and fever, followed by pain in the neck and back muscles. In severe cases, muscular weakness may lead to paralysis.

Anyone who has recently been abroad, especially in the Tropics, and who subsequently develops the above symptoms should see a doctor without delay.

Epidural abscess

An epidural *abscess* is a collection of pus in the space between the skull or the spinal bones and the dura, which is the outermost of the three membranes (meninges) that cover the brain and spinal cord. The pus is usually due to bacterial infection, which may have spread from an infected ear or sinuses or may have travelled to the brain from some other area via the bloodstream. As pus collects it exerts pressure on nerve tissue, and it may

Where the abscess forms
An epidural abscess is a localized collection of pus between the skull or spinal bones and the dura. The abscess is prevented from spreading over a large area, and causing consequent damage to more nervous tissue, because of the dura's close attachment to these bones.

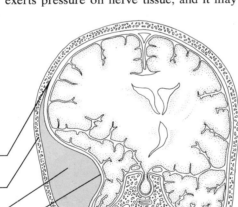

Dura attached to skull

Skull

Epidural abscess

Dura

damage the dura by the action of harmful chemicals (*toxins*) produced by the bacteria.

What are the symptoms?
An abscess on the spinal cord can cause loss of muscular power in the legs and numbness of the entire lower part of the body. An abscess in the brain may mimic a *stroke* (p.268), causing weakness down one side of the body or difficulty with speech. The onset of stroke-like symptoms is seldom rapid; they usually come on over the course of several hours. In addition you may have general symptoms caused by the infection – raised temperature, confusion, and perhaps delirium or convulsions.

How common is the problem?
Epidural abscesses are extremely rare nowadays. This is because it has become increasingly easy to combat the infections that used to cause them by the use of *antibiotics*. Such infections include *acute infection of the middle ear* (p.333) and *sinusitis* (p.347).

What should be done?
If you suspect an abscess, consult your doctor, who, after considering your history of previous infection, will probably order diagnostic tests. Among them may be blood tests to identify the invading bacteria, skull *X-ray*, and perhaps an *electroencephalogram* (*EEG*). In addition, *arteriography*, a *CAT* brain scan, and an examination of the spinal cord (*myelography*) may also be advisable.

What is the treatment?
To combat infection, your doctor will prescribe an *antibiotic*. In some cases, however, this will not effect a cure and surgery will be necessary. This involves making an opening in the skull or vertebral bone through which pus can be removed. Following such an operation, antibiotic treatment is continued. If the original cause of infection is also dealt with, you have a good chance of full recovery.

Structural disorders

A structural disorder of the nervous system is one in which part of the system is in some way physically distorted or damaged – by injury, for example, or by a tumour. While the skull provides protection from external damage, the brain may also be damaged because of the skull's very inflexibility. A small tumour on the brain cannot expand outwards because of the rigidity of the skull, and so the brain itself becomes compressed.

Occasionally, the peripheral nerves that emerge from spaces between the vertebrae are pinched where the spaces have become narrowed for some reason, or where the nerves themselves have become inflamed. The pinching causes pain and tingling. These sensations are felt in areas of the body serviced by affected nerves. For example, if peripheral nerves emerging from the lumbar spine are affected, pain is felt in the legs.

Brain injury

A blow on the head or a powerful crushing force can sometimes damage the brain, jolting and bruising it even though the protective skull is not fractured. In such cases the area of the brain that is damaged may be much larger than the area of the skull which sustained the blow. This is because sometimes, when a blow is forceful enough to shake the brain about within the skull, the area of the brain immediately beneath the blow is damaged, as is the area on the opposite side, where it has been jolted up against the skull. The resultant swelling of brain tissues may produce symptoms because outward expansion is obstructed by the rigid confines of the skull. If the skull *is* fractured, brain damage is much more likely. The extent of the damage and the question of whether it will be temporary or permanent depend chiefly on the type and force of the injury.

What are the symptoms?
Symptoms depend on where and how strongly the blow falls. Generally, however, a minor injury is followed almost immediately by a headache. A simple headache that clears up within a day or two signals rapid repair of brain tissues and – in all but rare cases – complete recovery. A more severe injury usually causes immediate unconsciousness, which may last only a few seconds (so-called "concussion") or persist for weeks (when the sufferer is said to be "in a coma").

A person who has been temporarily knocked out is always dazed and confused upon regaining consciousness. There may also be loss of memory (*amnesia*), further headaches, mental lapses, and muscular weakness or paralysis (including difficulty with speech). Such symptoms tend to disappear gradually as healing progresses, but in extreme cases there may be residual damage that leads to lasting physical or psychological problems such as paralysis, abnormal irritability, depression, or decreased mental alertness.

How common is the problem?
In an average year about 100,000 people (that is, 1 person in 500) are admitted to British hospitals because of head injuries that involve possible brain damage. In about 1 per cent of cases, the damage is severe enough to result in permanent mental or physical disability. The injuries are most often caused by traffic accidents (especially of young motorcyclists), industrial accidents, falls, fights, and explosions or gunshot wounds.

What are the risks?
A severe head injury may rupture one or more blood vessels, causing a *subdural, extradural,* or – rarely – *subarachnoid haemorrhage* (see p.271, and p.272 for symptoms and other information). The symptoms of haemorrhage resulting from an injury may not appear until hours, days, or even weeks after the injury occurs. If the skull is fractured, there is an additional danger. Microbes may enter through the fracture and infect brain tissues, causing *meningitis* (p.273). Finally, there is a possibility that lasting brain damage from a serious injury may bring on recurrent fits or convulsions (see the article on *Epilepsy*, p.287).

What should be done?
If you are present when someone loses consciousness because of an injury, follow the first-aid instructions given in *Accidents and emergencies* (p.805) and summon medical help at once. An injured person who does not lose consciousness but has other symptoms of brain damage should see a doctor as soon as possible. If you are the victim and you do not

The CAT scan

The CAT (computerized axial tomography) scanner enables special X-rays to be taken of soft tissues in the body, such as the brain, which do not form clear images on conventional X-rays. The special X-ray pictures are taken from many angles and then combined by a computer to show a two-dimensional "slice" of the tissues under examination. CAT scans can detect soft-tissue abnormalities such as an injury or a tumour. The procedure is completely painless.

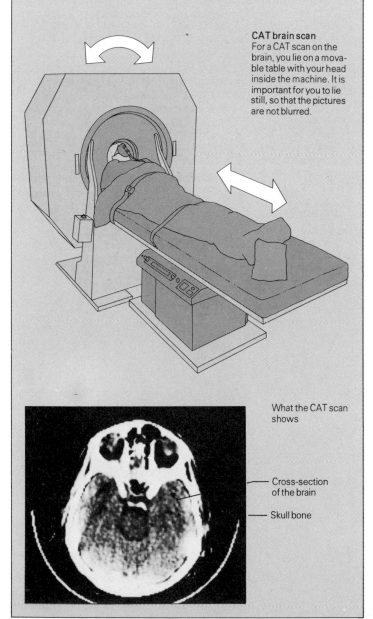

CAT brain scan
For a CAT scan on the brain, you lie on a movable table with your head inside the machine. It is important for you to lie still, so that the pictures are not blurred.

What the CAT scan shows

— Cross-section of the brain

— Skull bone

remember precisely what happened, it will help if someone who saw the incident can go with you in order to describe it to the doctor. The extent of any amnesia that has occurred will indicate the severity of the head injury – the longer the gap in the subject's memory, the more severe the injury.

If you develop a headache for no apparent reason and at the same time you begin to feel weak or mentally confused, think back over the past few days. Have you recently banged your head or had a slight accident? In any case, you should consult your doctor. Depending on the severity of symptoms and the results of your doctor's own observations, you may need some hospital diagnostic tests to discover the extent of the damage. The first of these will certainly be one or more skull *X-rays* to detect a possible fracture. Then – especially if symptoms persist – you may be required to undergo a computerized brain scan (known as a *CAT scan*) and perhaps *arteriography* to look for evidence of a ruptured blood vessel.

What is the treatment?

Self-help: There are various drugs that can counteract mild symptoms of brain injury – for example, *analgesics* for pain and sedatives for confusion. But they should never be taken by someone who was knocked unconscious unless a doctor has been consulted. If you have had a fairly hard knock, your doctor may want you to spend a night or two in hospital for observation, just in case of complications. Most minor damage is self-healing, though, and two or three days of rest after a slight accident should be sufficient treatment in the majority of cases.

Professional help: An unconscious person should be in hospital, where professional intensive care is of paramount importance. A *steroid* drug may be administered through an *intravenous drip* to reduce the inflammation of brain tissues. In cases of skull fracture, urgent surgery to relocate and stabilize bone fragments may be necessary.

What are the long-term prospects?

Recovery from severe brain injury usually takes many weeks, but chances for complete cure are fair. A few sufferers are left with some reminder of their injury in the form of slurred speech or muscular weakness in an arm or leg. Encouragement and support from family and friends are an important part of the recovery process for these people, most of whom will also need *physiotherapy* to overcome paralysis, muscle weakness, or disrupted coordination.

Spinal-cord injury

The bony vertebrae (backbones) that protect your spinal cord are separated from one another by discs of flexible cartilage. The discs permit a certain amount of bending and twisting of your back. Injuries that primarily affect the bones or cartilage (such as the condition known as a *prolapsed disc*, p.548) are discussed in another section of this book. In this article our concern is with damage to the spinal cord itself.

The bundles of nerves (the nerve tracts) that make up the spinal cord transmit nerve impulses between your brain and body. This allows you to control your movements and detect sensations such as touch or heat. If the spinal cord is damaged by an accident, part or parts of the body below the point of injury may be affected. The damage may be only temporary, but it occasionally leads to permanent disability.

What are the symptoms?

The bodily area affected depends on the location of spinal-cord damage. There may be numbness, weakness, or paralysis of all muscles below the level of the injury, including those that control bowel and bladder activity.

Less often, muscles on only one side of the body are affected. Pain is not an inevitable symptom of injury to the spinal cord, but accompanying injury to nearby nerves sometimes causes extreme pain – as, for example, in sciatica (see *Types of back pain*, p.547).

Unlike the symptoms of certain types of *brain injury* (p.276), which may become apparent only after a long delay, symptoms of spinal-cord damage almost always appear immediately following the injury.

How common is the problem?

Spinal-cord injuries are much less common than brain injury. Even so, they account for about 10,000 hospital cases in Britain every year. Most spinal-cord injuries are due to falls or traffic accidents; a major cause of disability is the whiplash type of injury that occurs when a car is stopped abruptly at high speed and the spinal cord in the neck is damaged by a sudden wrenching of the head.

What are the risks?

Injury to the spinal cord in the neck can be fatal if it damages nerves that control breathing; or it can result in total paralysis of both

The spine and its nerves

Nerve signals pass from the brain up and down the spinal cord to the peripheral nerves. These emerge from the spinal cord as 2 roots (the posterior and the anterior roots) in the gap between each vertebra, then join together to relay the nerve signals to and from specific parts of the body. The peripheral nerves that emerge in the cervical region of the spine supply both the neck and the arms; those that emerge in the thoracic region supply the ribcage and abdominal wall; and those from the lumbar region the legs. The nerves that emerge from the sacral region control the bowels and bladder.

Posterior root
Anterior root
Spinal cord

Peripheral nerve
Vertebra (backbone)
Intervertebral disc

Cervical nerves
Thoracic nerves
Lumbar nerves
Sacral nerves

arms and legs, as well as general numbness from the neck down. Injuries to other parts of the cord are not normally fatal but may be permanent and cause severe disability. Bladder paralysis often leads to recurrent urinary-tract infections (see *Infections, inflammation, and injury,* p.502); numb parts of the body are especially susceptible to various kinds of injury; and pressure sores (see *Preventing bedsores,* p.760) can be a problem for immobilized sufferers. Spinal-cord injury can also affect sexual activity – for example, by making ejaculation difficult for a man.

What should be done?

Serious injury to the spinal cord obviously requires urgent admission to hospital. If a person who has had an accident is unable to move the legs or complains of numbness, get professional help immediately. Do not try to move the victim; the wrong kind of movement can further injure nerves. Ambulances are equipped with special stretchers for carrying badly injured people. Your best role is to stand by the sufferer, giving reassurance that help is on the way. (See *Accidents and emergencies,* p.811, for further information.)

As soon as possible, the spine will be *X-rayed* in order to discover the site and extent of damage. Doctors will probably test lower parts of the body for numbness, usually by simply touching them with a pin. In some cases a *myelogram* will be carried out. The objective is to determine whether the spinal cord is merely bruised and has a good chance of recovering without specific treatment, or whether there is more serious damage.

What is the treatment?

Self-help: Spinal-cord injury with lasting effects inevitably makes a drastic change in life style. If you suffer such an injury, your stay in hospital may be as long as several months. With the aid of various medical workers you will be learning new ways to move about and to cope with the problems of daily life. Some modifications may be necessary in your house – you may not be able to negotiate stairs, for instance – but you should do everything possible to carry on with your former working routine. If this is not possible, ask your doctor or a social worker for information about training courses and helpful associations for disabled people – for example, the *Disabled Living Foundation* (p.768).

Professional help: The treatment of suspected spinal damage starts right from the time of the injury. If there is severe damage to vertebrae, surgery is sometimes advisable, but bed rest alone is often enough to allow healing. Severely damaged nerve tracts, however, do not heal of their own accord and cannot be medically or surgically treated. At first you will be kept fairly immobile and under constant observation to see if your symptoms improve. If the neck has been injured, the head will be supported at either side to prevent unnecessary movement. While under observation, you will need intensive nursing care so as to be fed, turned regularly to prevent pressure sores, and have your bladder and bowels attended to.

This stage may last several weeks, after which, if you remain disabled, a team of doctors, nurses, *physiotherapists,* and *occupational therapists* will start the process of rehabilitation. Their aim will be to help you make good use of the power left in your muscles. Various mechanical and electrical aids are available to help develop a disabled person's physical skills and improve his or her independence. If the lower back has been injured, and the arms are therefore not affected, a reasonable amount of independence can be hoped for, although it is likely that the sufferer will have to use a wheelchair for getting about. The aims and manner of any treatment obviously depend on the degree of injury, but you should not be ashamed to seek counselling and guidance on coping with, for example, sexual problems.

What are the long-term prospects?

It is important for the sufferer and his or her family not to lose patience. It may be three or four months before the degree of disability and future recovery can be assessed. Courage, determination, and good will during this long and difficult period can play a large part in your recovery.

Bell's palsy

This is a condition – usually only temporary – in which the muscles on one side of the face become paralysed because of a fault in the nerve that controls them. On each side of the skull the facial nerve runs out from the brain through a small hole in the skull near the ear. Bell's palsy occurs when one of the nerves becomes swollen and is pinched at the point of exit from the skull. We do not yet know what causes the condition.

What are the symptoms?

The characteristic symptom is weakness of one side of the face. The corner of the mouth droops, it may become impossible to close one eye, and any facial gesture such as a smile or frown is misshapen since there is virtually no movement of muscles from forehead to mouth on the paralysed side. The attack usually happens suddenly, often overnight, and it is sometimes accompanied by pain in the ear or on the affected side of the face.

How common is the problem?
In an average year about 1 person in 3,000 in Britain suffers an attack of Bell's palsy. It can occur in people of any age but seems to be most common among young adult males. A middle-ear infection (such as *Acute infection of the middle ear*, p.333) sometimes appears to bring on the problem.

What are the risks?
Though disfiguring, this is not a dangerous condition. The main risk is irritation of or injury to the eye; because it cannot close properly, it is exposed to dust. It can also develop ulcers if left unprotected for any length of time and allowed to dry out (see *Corneal ulcers and infections*, p.316).

What should be done?
If you have symptoms of Bell's palsy, consult your doctor, who can recognize this disorder by simply looking at you. Do not delay.

What is the treatment?
If Bell's palsy is diagnosed within a day or two of its onset, a short course of *steroid* tablets increases the chances of a swift cure. Otherwise recovery may take up to several weeks. Until fully recovered, the sufferer may need to wear a protective eye patch and to apply moisturizing drops to the eye.

What are the long-term prospects?
Most sufferers from Bell's palsy make a complete recovery even without early treatment. When, as infrequently happens, facial disfigurement persists, an operation may help to relieve the physical disability and improve facial appearance.

Cervical spondylosis

Cervical spondylosis is a disorder that affects some of the seven vertebrae of the neck (the cervical vertebrae) and the flexible discs of cartilage sandwiched between them. Bony growths develop on the vertebrae, frequently accompanied by a misalignment or hardening of the washer-like discs. As a result, the neck becomes stiff and the nerves in the upper part of the spinal cord – especially those running between the cord and the arms and hands – are subjected to an abnormal amount of pressure (see *Neuralgia*, p.290). We do not know the cause of this disorder, which is particularly prevalent among middle-aged and elderly people. We do know, however, that bones in many parts of the body become roughened and distorted with age.

What are the symptoms?
The main symptom of cervical spondylosis is a stiff, painful neck. Resultant pressure on the nerves to your hands and arms may cause such symptoms as tingling, pins and needles, numbness, and – occasionally – pain (usually somewhere in the hands). These symptoms are likely to occur on only one side of the body at any one time.

Pressure within the neck may in time affect further portions of the spinal cord. Thus, if cervical spondylosis becomes increasingly severe, there may be a gradual weakening of the legs, and perhaps urinary disorders. Sometimes, too, blood vessels that run through the neck vertebrae to the brain can become constricted because of this disorder, causing symptoms such as headache, dizziness, unsteadiness, or double vision, especially if you try to bend your neck.

How common is the problem?
Cervical spondylosis is a common condition, especially in the elderly. Each year in Britain about 1 person in 150 is diagnosed as having the disorder. There are many others who have it in a mild form and do not seek help from their doctor. Men and women are equally susceptible.

What are the risks?
Minor symptoms of cervical spondylosis cause discomfort but present no serious problems. In most cases the symptoms do not worsen. If they do, and if lower parts of the spinal cord become affected, there is a risk of serious and irreversible damage, perhaps leading to paralysis of the lower half of the body in severe cases.

What should be done?
If minor symptoms persist and seem to be worsening, consult your doctor who, after examining you, may arrange for an *X-ray* of your neck. If your legs appear to be weakening, you will probably also need to undergo *myelography* in order to determine the extent of damage to the cord.

What is the treatment?

The treatment for troublesome symptoms of cervical spondylosis is regular daytime use of a supportive plastic collar; a more comfortable soft collar is substituted at night. The collar prevents extreme movements of the head and supports it in a position that minimizes pressure on the cervical nerves and blood vessels. The collar is usually worn for about three months, and in most cases there are no further problems. During the periods while you are wearing the collar, you may be advised to take *analgesics* such as aspirin or paracetamol, and your doctor may also prescribe a tranquillizer to relax you and keep your neck muscles from tightening up.

If, as rarely happens, symptoms persist or new ones develop, you may have to enter hospital for *traction* or for an operation. Surgery involves an enlargement of nerve pathways in the spinal cord and/or a fusing together of some of the cervical vertebrae. Either or both of these procedures will usually give considerable relief from symptoms, but you may be left with a reduced ability to twist or bend your neck.

Carpal tunnel syndrome

At certain points in the body, nerves run through confined spaces where they are apt to become severely pinched if surrounding tissues become swollen. A major nerve particularly subject to this kind of damage is the one that carries signals between the hand and brain. As it travels through the wrist this nerve passes through a tunnel formed by the wrist bones (known as the carpals) and a tough membrane on the underside of the wrist which binds the bones together. This passageway – the carpal tunnel – is rigid; if tissues within it swell for some reason, they press on and pinch the nerve. This nerve compression leads to the painful condition called carpal tunnel syndrome.

may lead to an accumulation of fluid – and consequent swelling – in the wrists at the time of the menopause. It can also occur during pregnancy if fluid retention is a problem.

What are the symptoms?

Symptoms of carpal tunnel syndrome consist of tingling and intermittent numbness of part of the hand, often accompanied by pains shooting up the arm from the wrist. The pains are generally worse at night and may be severe enough to wake you from a deep sleep; some relief may be gained if you hang your hand over the side of the bed and rub or shake it. If the condition is severe it can result in permanent numbness and weakness of the thumb and one or more fingers. One or both hands may be affected.

What is the treatment?

In some cases the condition clears up of its own accord. In others a splint worn on the affected wrist at night seems to help. To reduce the amount of fluid in the swollen tissues, your doctor may prescribe a *diuretic*; and an injection of a *steroid* drug at the wrist can help combat inflammation. But if you are in great pain and it persists, the best possible treatment is an operation. The surgeon frees the pinched nerve by cutting through the tough membrane, creating more space for the nerve. This is usually a highly successful procedure, which gives immediate relief, requires a hospital stay of only one or two days, and leaves a barely noticeable scar on the inside of the wrist.

Symptoms of carpal tunnel syndrome
Pressure of swollen tissue on the median nerve where it passes through the carpal tunnel can result in loss of sensation in the hand, chiefly in the thumb and first 3 fingers.

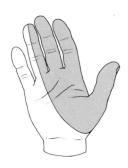

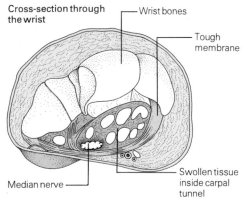

Cross-section through the wrist — Wrist bones — Tough membrane — Swollen tissue inside carpal tunnel — Median nerve

Carpal tunnel syndrome is a fairly common disorder, especially among women approaching middle age. There is some evidence that a change in the balance of female sex hormones

Brain tumour

An excessive or abnormal growth of tissue in the brain is a serious matter whether the growth is *benign* or *malignant*. This is because the protective bones of the skull make it impossible for any type of tumour to expand outwards, and so the soft brain tissue becomes dangerously compressed as the growth develops. The distinction between benign and malignant tumours that develop in the brain is therefore somewhat less clear-cut than it is for growths that appear in other parts of the body.

What are the symptoms?
As a tumour enlarges, it causes increased pressure within the skull. The result is frequent headaches, which are often most painful when the sufferer is lying down. The headaches are generally accompanied by nausea and vomiting. Sometimes, however, the vomiting that is symptomatic of a brain tumour seems to occur suddenly, without even the warning of a spell of nausea. Because the build-up of pressure can affect the nerves at the back of the eye, there may also be blurred or double vision. Other possible symptoms depend on the location of the growth in the brain. They include weakness down one side of the body, general unsteadiness, loss of the sense of smell, loss of memory, or even a drastic personality change. These last symptoms may be very mild at first, then become gradually more severe over a period of days or even weeks. In some cases the presence of a brain tumour may also cause epileptic fits (see *Epilepsy*, p.287). In the rare cases when a child develops a brain tumour, the tumour is most commonly situated at the back of the brain, causing the development of headaches followed after a while by unsteadiness.

How common is the problem?
Brain tumours are much less common than tumours of the breast, lung, or intestinal tract. However, spread of cancers from these parts of the body to the brain is relatively common. Secondary tumours (those that have *metastasized* from elsewhere in the body) are more common in later life, when cancers in general are most likely to occur. They enlarge and produce symptoms in the same way as primary tumours.

What are the risks?
Tumours of the brain will, if untreated, lead to permanent damage of brain tissues, and most will eventually prove fatal. If a benign growth is discovered and treated early enough, however, there is often an excellent chance for a full recovery.

What should be done?
If you have any of the characteristic symptoms (especially a headache that worsens when you lie down and is accompanied by vomiting), consult your doctor, who may refer you to a *neurologist* for diagnostic tests. In addition to *X-rays* (including X-rays of the chest, since secondary brain tumours frequently arise from malignant tumours of the lung), you may be given a computerized brain scan (known as a *CAT scan*), along with *angiography* and perhaps also a *radio-isotope scan* of the brain tissues.

What is the treatment?
Surgery to remove a benign tumour is often possible, and may well be completely successful. Even when the tumour involves a crucial part of the brain, it is sometimes feasible to remove a portion of the growth in order to reduce pressure and relieve symptoms. Surgery, whether for full or partial removal, is sometimes followed by *radiotherapy* to kill any remaining tumour cells and prevent recurrence of the symptoms.

Surgical treatment is usually less successful in the case of malignant brain tumours. But even in such cases there are ways of relieving symptoms and making sufferers more comfortable. *Steroid* drugs may help diminish the swelling of brain tissue – and thus the pressure – around the growth. *Anticonvulsant* drugs can be prescribed for epileptic fits. And there are various *analgesics* that reduce the pain of severe headaches.

Spinal-cord tumour

Tumours of the spinal cord are similar to *brain tumours* (p.281), but they produce different symptoms. Persistent back pain is one possible symptom. More often, though, you may develop sensations of numbness or coldness as well as muscle weakness in one or more of your limbs, or you may have difficulty in urinating or defecating. Precise symptoms depend on exactly which nerves are damaged by the tumour.

What should be done?
Spinal-cord tumours are even rarer than brain tumours. If you have symptoms that suggest the possibility of a growth on the spinal cord, your doctor will probably refer you to a *neurologist* for a physical examination, *myelogram* (a special *X-ray* of the spine), and perhaps other diagnostic tests. If a tumour is found, an operation to chip away the surrounding vertebrae may be carried out. By relieving the pressure on spinal nerves, such operations generally result in immediate relief of pain and may also restore the use of affected muscles and limbs. As with brain tumours, further treatment and prospects depend on various factors such as the type, size, and site of the growth.

Peripheral neuropathy

Damage to the peripheral nerves (nerves in the body other than those in the brain and spinal cord) is technically known as peripheral neuropathy. The damage sometimes occurs as a complication of a long-term disorder such as diabetes mellitus, alcoholism, certain vitamin deficiencies, or tumours in certain parts of the body. There are many other possible causes of peripheral nerve damage – for example, overdoses of certain drugs and over-exposure to certain chemicals (especially arsenic, mercury, lead, and the so-called "organo-phosphorus" chemicals found in weed-killers). Certain infections can also directly attack the peripheral nerves – perhaps the most common being *leprosy* (p.565), although diphtheria, polio, and tetanus can have the same effect. In very rare cases severe peripheral neuropathy may develop following a mild virus infection. This is usually followed by complete recovery.

What are the symptoms?

In most forms of peripheral neuropathy, symptoms come on gradually over the course of many months (for a dramatic exception see *Guillain-Barré syndrome*, below). One common pattern is for a tingling sensation that begins in the hands and feet to spread slowly along all four limbs to the trunk. Then, following the same course, numbness may develop. In some cases the muscles waste away and there is a gradual weakening of muscle power throughout the body.

How common is the problem?

In Britain each year, about 1 person in 400 is diagnosed as having some degree of peripheral neuropathy. The disease is relatively common among alcoholics and diabetics. Cases caused by a build-up of *toxic* chemicals are rare in the general population but occur with some frequency among workers in certain industries and on farms. There is evidence that some types of peripheral

neuropathy which develop for no obvious reason may be inherited abnormalities.

What are the risks?

If a numbed part of your body is injured, you may remain unaware of the injury until infection or ulceration occurs. When the disorder has been caused by leprosy, fingers and toes may be damaged beyond repair. And a gradual wasting away of the muscles may result in weakness or paralysis.

What should be done?

Because slow damage to nerves is normally irreversible, early diagnosis is important. If your hands and feet are tingling (especially if any of the factors that can cause this condition are applicable in your case), see your doctor, who will probably refer you to a *neurologist* for tests. The neurologist will want your medical and personal history and will examine your body for signs of numbness or muscle weakness. Special tests depend on the suspected cause of your trouble.

What is the treatment?

No direct medical or surgical treatment is possible. But if the cause of nerve damage is found to be some other disorder, stricter treatment of the underlying problem should slow or halt the progress of peripheral neuropathy. If toxic chemicals are at fault, you will be advised to stop – or at least reduce – your exposure to the offending substance. This may well involve a change of occupation.

In severe cases, where muscles have been badly weakened, such aids to mobility and independence as *physiotherapy*, walking sticks or frames, and bath rails may be prescribed. You will also be warned to remain aware of the possibility of unnoticed wounds on your numb limbs and to consult your doctor whenever you have a bruise or an open sore. Engage a chiropodist to take care of your feet and wear well-fitting shoes.

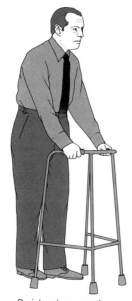

Peripheral-neuropathy sufferers may find a walking frame useful.

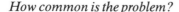

Guillain-Barré syndrome

This is an extremely rare and sudden form of *peripheral neuropathy* (above), which can follow some viral infections or even a vaccination. Several hundred cases occurred in the United States as a complication of vaccination against "swine" influenza in 1976. Why it occurs is not clear, but some doctors think it may be caused by an unpredictable allergic reaction to the viral illness. The symptoms come on a few days after the causative illness has cleared up, and they are often severe. Within hours, a sensation of tingling, then

numbness, then weakness or paralysis may spread from the hands and feet to the rest of the body. Often the paralysis is so extensive that it affects breathing, and intensive care in hospital becomes necessary.

Unlike other, longer-term forms of peripheral neuropathy, the nerve damage of the Guillain-Barré syndrome is usually only temporary. With appropriate hospital care, full recovery from severe attacks is probable, but the sufferer may require *physiotherapy* for many months.

Functional disorders

The following group of disorders have one feature in common: they are generally caused not by a detectable fault in the structure of the central nervous system, but by something wrong in the way it functions. Typical symptoms are mainly localized in the head – a sense of dizziness, for example, or the pain of certain kinds of headache. Pain usually serves the protective function of warning the sufferer that something is wrong, but in the case of migraine and many types of headache, it causes distress for no explicable reason. But malfunctioning of the brain can often cause a disturbing reaction of the whole body, such as a blackout or a fit.

The physical reasons for functional disorders such as migraine, epilepsy, and even the common headache, remain largely unknown in spite of intensive research. This is why the conditions themselves are usually identified by their characteristic symptoms rather than by the somewhat mystifying processes that produce them. One achievement of modern medical research, however, has been the discovery of effective ways to relieve the symptoms of many of these disorders – generally by the use of drugs – even though actual cure is not yet possible. As a result, many sufferers from conditions such as epilepsy can now lead nearly normal lives.

Headache

Headaches are occasionally a symptom of an underlying disorder. In fact, up to a quarter of the hundreds of disorders discussed in this book number headache among possible symptoms. However, if you get headaches, the strong probability is that they occur "on their own", developing gradually (often without apparent cause) and clearing up in a few hours, leaving no after-effects. In other words, most headaches indicate nothing seriously wrong within the head or elsewhere.

Your headaches, however painful, are likely to be insignificant and temporary, brought on by some sort of tension that puts a strain on muscular tissues or blood vessels in the head or neck. Brain tissues, incidentally, never ache; they are insensitive to pain since the brain itself does not contain *sensory* nerves. Sensitivity in this area exists only in the meninges that overlie the surface of the brain, the skin and muscles that cover the skull, and the many nerves that run out of the skull into the head and face.

There are some types of headache that are neither symptoms of underlying disorders nor insignificant and fleeting, but which can be considered as a specific disease (for a familiar example see *Migraine*, opposite). But the headaches discussed in the following paragraphs are not of that kind. They are simple, ordinary headaches, so common as to be almost universal.

Depending on your physical and mental make-up, your headaches may be due to any of several factors. These include stress, too little or too much sleep, overeating or drinking, a noisy or stuffy environment, heavy work indoors or outdoors, and so on. You may or may not be able to put your finger on what has caused a given attack. From a physiological standpoint, however, there are two important – and related – causes of the pain of these headaches. The first is tension deriving from strain on facial, neck, and scalp muscles; the second is swelling of local blood vessels that results in strain within their walls. These are called tension headaches and vascular headaches, respectively. If you have been under emotional stress, for example, you may think that worry or grief has given you a headache. In fact, the strain may have in some way affected your posture, creating a physical tension that results in pain. Similarly, if you have spent hours of concentration on desk-work, the resultant headache probably comes from your crouching position, not the mental effort.

The typical "morning-after" headache that follows an episode of over-indulgence in alcohol may be due to a widening of the blood vessels in the brain. Alcohol in itself is a *vasodilator* drug, acting to dilate (widen) blood vessels in the body. A tension headache may also develop because vascular pain leads to a straining of head muscles.

What should be done?

If you have had headaches from time to time for several years, you probably know already whether they are migraines. If they have begun recently, however, your first priority is to decide what they might signify. As a starting point, consult the "Headache" Self-diagnosis symptom chart in this book. This is especially important if you have become aware of other symptoms beside head pains.

A headache that relents overnight is likely to be no cause for concern. But if you have headaches that last for more than 24 hours or that recur as often as two or three times a week, you should consult your doctor. The doctor will ask you for a detailed description of your headaches, so that he or she can assess their significance. You will be asked how long each headache lasted, which particular area of your head was affected, how often the headache occurred, whether it was related to a particular time of day, and whether it was accompanied by other symptoms, such as nausea or visual disturbance. The doctor may also want to know whether your headaches are aggravated by a change in position or a bout of coughing. After examining you, the doctor may refer you to a *neurologist* for diagnostic tests to make sure there is no underlying disorder of the central nervous system or elsewhere.

Relieving a headache
Relaxation is the best cure for a tension headache. Have a leisurely, warm bath or lie down in a darkened room and let all your muscles relax.

What is the treatment?
Self-help: One or more of the following measures should ease a simple tension or vascular headache. First, try to relax. Stretch and massage the muscles of your shoulders, neck, jaws, and scalp. Have a hot bath, lie down, placing a warm, dry cloth – or, if it feels better, a cold, wet one – over the aching area. Drink plenty of fruit juices or other non-alcoholic liquids, and take a mild painkiller such as aspirin or paracetamol. The oldest, time-honoured remedy is often the best: a good night's sleep.

Professional help: If your headaches are diagnosed as indicating no serious underlying disease, your doctor can do little but recommend the above self-help measures. One possibility, though, is the prescription of another, more powerful type of painkiller.

Migraine

If you suffer from this disorder you have periodic headaches, generally along with other symptoms such as nausea and disturbed vision, that virtually put you out of action for as long as they last. In spite of intensive medical research, we do not know why only some people are subject to such attacks or what triggers them off. Certain factors do appear to be involved, at least in many cases. For instance, susceptibility to migraine headaches tends to run in families. Sometimes certain foods – perhaps cheese, or chocolate, or red wine – have been found to provoke attacks. Often there is a relationship between the recurrent headaches and menstruation, stress, or even the anticipation of relaxation after stress. But your own case may well seem to be unaffected by any of these, or indeed any other obvious factors.

The effects of an attack are probably the result of the way the arteries leading to the brain react to the triggering factors, whatever they are. For some reason the arteries become first narrowed, then swollen, causing a disturbance in blood flow to the brain (compare this to the description of vascular headaches – see *Headache*, opposite).

What are the symptoms?
Migraine is basically a condition in which severe headaches are both preceded and accompanied by other symptoms. The nature of each recurrent attack varies from person to person, but there is usually a "warning" period during which you feel abnormally tired and out of sorts. This is followed by nausea, vomiting, and sometimes diarrhoea. You may find bright lights unbearable (a condition called *photophobia*). You may also have some sort of visual disturbance (usually worse on one side) such as misting over, or zig-zag distortion, or shimmering lights. Early symptoms can last for several hours or up to a few days.

When the headache comes, the warning symptoms tend to fade away. You are likely to have intense, gripping pain which starts at one side of the forehead but gradually spreads, though the pain usually remains confined to one side of the head. While the migraine persists, your eyes may be bloodshot and you will look pale and clearly unwell. In some cases the pain is centred between the nose and eye, and both the nose and eye tend to run.

The length of each attack and the length of migraine-free periods between attacks are variable. Most sufferers tend to have groups of attacks. For a while they occur every few days or weeks; then, at last, there comes a rest period of months or even years. The times are unpredictable, but you can generally predict the nature and duration of each of your own attacks. Among less common symptoms experienced by some sufferers are numbness or tingling in the arm or down one side of the body, dizziness, a ringing in the ears, and temporary mental confusion.

How common is the problem?

Migraine is a common complaint. Estimates suggest that in Britain 1 person in 10 suffers from it. Migraine headaches rarely start before adolescence, but the unexplained recurrent abdominal pains of some children (see *Recurrent tummy aches and headaches*, p.684) are sometimes an indication that they will have migraine attacks in later life. Only rarely does a first attack occur after the age of about 40. In fact, some sufferers stop having attacks after reaching middle age.

You are most likely to have migraine if it runs in your family and you are female; three out of four sufferers are women.

What are the risks?

Although migraine causes considerable suffering, it is not a dangerous disease. In a few people some accompanying numbness, weakness, or visual disturbance has been known to become permanent. This is an exceptionally rare occurence, however.

What should be done?

If you have recurrent headaches that you cannot control by means of painkilling drugs such as aspirin or paracetamol, you should consult your doctor. There are no satisfactory diagnostic tests for determining whether headaches are in fact migraines; the doctor will probably be able to base a diagnosis on the description of your symptoms.

What is the treatment?

Self-help: Try to make an objective study of your condition; in particular, give some thought after each attack to what you were doing, thinking, feeling, eating, and drinking prior to the onset of symptoms. You may discover that you indulged your special fondness for cheese or chocolate or some other food before falling ill. Then, if you are lucky, you can prevent further attacks by striking the offending substance off all future menus. Or you may find that you tend to have attacks just after emerging from periods of extra-hard work or stress. In that case try taking things easy; avoid a crowded appointments schedule, and leave time for relaxation.

For some women the contraceptive pill appears to be a trigger factor. If you began to have migraine headaches at about the same time as you went on the pill, discuss the matter with your doctor. A change of pill or of contraceptive method may be the answer.

As you come to recognize the early warning signs of an attack, you may be able to fend it off. The moment you suspect that migraine might be coming on, splash your face with cold water, take two *analgesic* (aspirin or paracetamol) tablets, lie down in a darkened room, and stay there for two or three hours. Do not worry about the migraine during those hours. Simply relax, listen to a favourite record (do not read), or meditate.

A good way to help fellow-sufferers as well as yourself is to join a self-help organization such as the *Migraine Trust* or the *British Migraine Association* (for details see p.768).

Professional help: Although migraine cannot be cured, it can be relieved by modern drugs. There are two basic types of treatment. After a discussion of the illness as it affects you, your doctor will decide on the kind of treatment that is likely to be most helpful. If your migraines are only fairly heavy and not unbearably frequent, the first method is probably best for you. This consists of drugs that ease an attack after it has begun. The doctor may prescribe pills, suppositories, or injections of one or more drugs. The drugs include *vasoconstrictors* which act to narrow blood vessels, perhaps combined with *antihistamines*. You may also be advised to take an *anti-emetic* in order to control vomiting. It is important to take drugs only when necessary, and precisely as prescribed. Overdose can have several unpleasant side-effects –

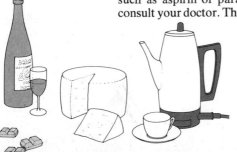

Some causes of migraine
Many foods, notably cheese, chocolate, red wine, and coffee, may precipitate migraine attacks. Even so, someone who has attacks after eating chocolate may be able to eat cheese without any ill-effects.

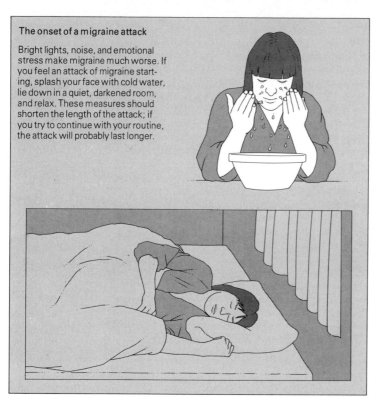

The onset of a migraine attack

Bright lights, noise, and emotional stress make migraine much worse. If you feel an attack of migraine starting, splash your face with cold water, lie down in a quiet, darkened room, and relax. These measures should shorten the length of the attack; if you try to continue with your routine, the attack will probably last longer.

among them, headaches that are as bad as, or worse than, the migraine itself.

The second type of treatment is preventive. It is designed for people whose migraines are so severe and frequent as to considerably disrupt their everyday lives. It consists of continuous medication that helps you avoid attacks. Regular small doses of some *anti-hypertensive* may be combined with a *diuretic*, a mild tranquillizer, or an *antidepressant*, to prevent attacks from occurring. There are many alternative preparations, and your doctor may need a trial-and-error period in order to find the most effective drugs for you.

A natural method for relieving or even preventing migraine is being researched today in some hospitals. The method is based on the fact that during an attack of migraine most people's body temperature drops. Groups of volunteers, using *biofeedback* methods for recording their body temperatures, are taught to maintain temperature control by relaxation. Only certain sufferers are considered suitable for the course, but so far results have been promising. Migraines may still occur, but the sufferer is able to dispel them after about 30 minutes using relaxation techniques. In some people who practise daily, migraines do not recur.

Epilepsy

There are many forms of epilepsy, each with characteristic symptoms. Whatever its form, the disease results from a functional problem in the brain's communication system. Normally, the brain's nerve cells communicate by sending tiny electrical signals back and forth. In someone with epilepsy, the signals from one group of nerve cells occasionally become too strong – so strong that they overwhelm neighbouring parts of the brain. This excessive electrical discharge may occur suddenly throughout the brain or may start locally and either spread or remain confined to the area where it began. It is this sudden, excessive electrical discharge that brings on the behaviour we know as an epileptic fit. The fit may take different forms, depending on the position and extent of the area of the brain tissues affected.

It is not yet known what causes the brain's communication system to misfire in the above fashion, or why it happens recurrently in some people. Exhaustive research projects, including the testing of great numbers of sufferers, have shown that roughly two out of three epileptics have no detectable or identifiable structural fault in the brain. As for the remaining one-third, their condition can generally be traced back to an underlying problem such as brain damage at birth, severe head injury, or brain-tissue infection.

Occasionally (especially when epilepsy develops in adulthood) the condition may be caused by a *brain tumour* (p.281).

What are the symptoms?

The basic symptom of epilepsy is a brief, abnormal phase of behaviour commonly known as a fit or convulsion. It is important to realize that a single such episode does not indicate that you are suffering from epilepsy. By definition, epileptic fits recur. Of the many forms of the disease, two major types are worth singling out: these are known as petit mal and grand mal.

Petit mal epilepsy is a disease of childhood that does not normally linger on past late adolescence. Your child is probably suffering from this form of epilepsy if, from time to time, he or she suddenly stares blankly around for a few seconds (sometimes up to half a minute), interrupting whatever activity might have been under way. During the blank interval the child is unaware of what is happening, and will not respond if questioned. There may be a slight jerking movement of the head or arm, but youngsters with petit mal do not generally fall to the ground during this type of convulsion. When it ends, they carry on as if nothing has happened, often without realizing that they have had a brief blank spell. (For further information see *Convulsions in children*, p.667.)

The most characteristic symptom of grand mal epilepsy is a fit in which the unconscious sufferer falls to the ground, the entire body first stiffening, then twitching or jerking about uncontrollably. This may last for a few minutes and is usually followed by a period of deep sleep or mental confusion. During the fit some sufferers actually lose bladder control and pass urine.

In many cases the sufferer gets a warning of an impending seizure by having certain strange sensations before losing consciousness. Any such warning that occurs just before a fit is called an aura; abnormal sensations in the hours before a fit are termed a prodrome. The sensations may consist of nothing but a feeling of tension or some other ill-defined experience; but some sufferers have quite specific sensations – for example the impression of smelling unpleasant odours, hearing peculiar sounds, distorted vision, or an odd bodily feeling, particularly in the stomach. Some epileptics learn to recognize their particular warning signs, and this may give them time to avoid accidents (see "What are the risks?" below).

Other types of epilepsy are less common than petit mal and grand mal. One of these is "focal" epilepsy. Someone with focal epilepsy does not necessarily lose consciousness when the fit starts; depending on the part of the brain affected, he or she has an uncontrollable twitching of one part of the body or an abnormal sensation such as seeing flashes of light. Twitching may spread, so that if the thumb of one hand starts to jerk, this may be followed by the jerking of the entire arm and then of the rest of that side of the body.

Another type of epilepsy is "temporal-lobe" epilepsy, named after the part of the brain in which the abnormal electrical activity takes place. A sufferer from temporal-lobe epilepsy is likely to have an aura lasting only a few seconds. Then, without being aware of it, he or she does something entirely out of character, interrupting normal activity with some sort of bizarre behaviour. Strange chewing movements of the mouth often occur throughout any such episode.

How common is the problem?
In Britain, surveys show that roughly 1 person in 200 is epileptic. Both sexes are equally

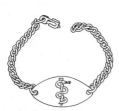

Identification aid
If you suffer from epilepsy, it is a good idea to wear a bracelet engraved with information about your case. If you have a fit, anyone coming to your assistance will be able to read the bracelet for advice on what action to take.

susceptible, and the disease seems to run in families. Petit mal epilepsy occurs only in children, and epilepsy generally is more common in children than in adults. This is partly because some children grow out of the condition during their teens.

It should be emphasized that isolated, non-recurrent (and therefore non-epileptic) *febrile* fits, which are quite common in children, may be caused by an infection which brings on a high temperature.

Focal epilepsy is an exception to the rule that epilepsy is more common among children, since it occurs more commonly among the middle-aged and elderly.

What are the risks?
Fortunately, modern drug treatment keeps most forms of epilepsy under control, and epileptic people can generally lead virtually normal lives. If occasional seizures do occur, however – usually because the disorder is not receiving adequate treatment – there is an obvious danger that they may happen in the wrong place at the wrong time. If your condition is not successfully controlled, you risk your life – and perhaps the lives of others – if you climb ladders, handle dangerous machinery, or drive a car. For this reason you must declare your epilepsy to the car-licensing authorities. To qualify for a driving licence, a person with epilepsy must show himself or herself to be free of fits during the day for at least three years while undergoing treatment. Those people who are no longer subject to fits during the day but occasionally have a fit at night may still qualify for a licence.

Even in a safe place on the ground, accidents can happen to a person having a fit. The sufferer may accidentally bite his or her tongue while clenching the jaw uncontrollably, for instance; and as the sufferer jerks about unconsciously he or she may come into harmful contact with sharp objects.

Recurrent, uncontrolled epilepsy has been known to lead to more generalized brain damage, but with modern preventive treatment this is rare.

What should be done?
If you think someone in your family may have epilepsy, consult your doctor, who will want a full description of the convulsions and details about frequency from both the observer and the sufferer. If there has been no recent illness or injury that might cause fits, the doctor can probably diagnose the condition as epilepsy on the strength of the given facts. In some cases, an *electroencephalogram* (*EEG*) will be carried out to confirm the diagnosis.

And if there seems a possibility that some identifiable brain damage or infection is causing the apparent epilepsy, there may also be a skull *X-ray*, blood tests, and a computerized brain scan (*CAT scan*). Most of the testing will be done in hospital under the direction of a *neurologist*.

What is the treatment?

Self-help: If anyone in your family has epilepsy and is taking medicine for it, be sure that the drugs are taken exactly when and how the doctor prescribes.

Once the diagnosis of epilepsy is confirmed, try to join the *British Epilepsy Association* (p.768). The association provides advice and assistance for epileptics and their families. Ask the association or your doctor about how to obtain a card or tag that will tell strangers you are epileptic if you ever suffer an unexpected attack. Some cards or tags carry a telephone number or advice on what action an observer should take. Carry it at all times. Do not be ashamed to tell your schoolmates or fellow-workers about your condition. Onlookers may panic at their first sight of a fit if not forewarned; they are much less likely to be frightened and more likely to be of help if they know about your condition and what action they should take.

Professional help: Except in the relatively rare cases of epilepsy caused by treatable brain damage, tumours, or infection, epilepsy cannot be cured. Regular, sensible use of *anticonvulsant* drugs, however, effectively prevents most sufferers from having fits, and as about one-third of patients with epilepsy cease having convulsions as they grow older, drug treatment is regularly reviewed and can be discontinued in these cases.

There are many anticonvulsant drugs to choose from, and your doctor will prescribe the drug (sometimes more than one) most appropriate for your case. You will need to take medication for epilepsy at regular intervals for as long as your fits persist; this may mean for life.

Anticonvulsants occasionally have unpleasant side-effects, especially if taken in excessive amounts. So your doctor will need to see you from time to time and will perhaps want occasional blood tests in order to check on whether you are having the correct dose of the prescribed drug. If it is not proving wholly effective, the doctor may increase the dose or may decide to try a different type of anticonvulsant for a trial period. If your condition is clearly due to an underlying nervous-system disorder, that disorder will also require treatment, of course.

How to help someone who has a fit

As explained in this article, some epileptic fits are merely momentary blackouts in which the posture of the body remains virtually unaffected. If someone (probably a child suffering from petit mal epilepsy) has such an attack in your presence, it is generally wise to ignore it. Just guide the sufferer gently towards safety if a petit mal convulsion occurs in a potentially dangerous situation – while crossing the street, for example. This advice applies equally in cases of temporal-lobe epilepsy where, instead of falling to the ground, the

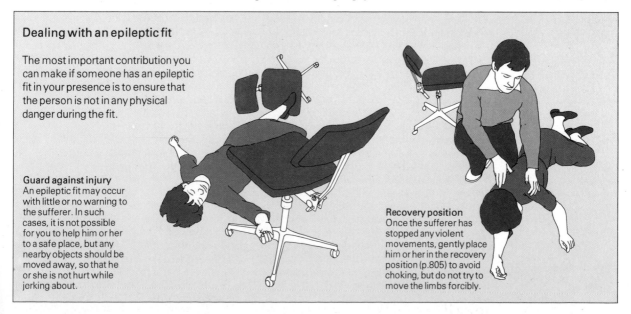

Dealing with an epileptic fit

The most important contribution you can make if someone has an epileptic fit in your presence is to ensure that the person is not in any physical danger during the fit.

Guard against injury
An epileptic fit may occur with little or no warning to the sufferer. In such cases, it is not possible for you to help him or her to a safe place, but any nearby objects should be moved away, so that he or she is not hurt while jerking about.

Recovery position
Once the sufferer has stopped any violent movements, gently place him or her in the recovery position (p.805) to avoid choking, but do not try to move the limbs forcibly.

person may act strangely in any of a variety of ways; just remember that, no matter how active he or she may seem to be, the sufferer is in reality unaware of what is happening, and should be gently guided away from danger, not scolded or reasoned with.

Someone who has a grand mal epileptic fit will start to twitch or jerk, and may well fall to the ground. If this happens, you can help by taking the following steps:

1. Gently guide or move the person to a safe place *only* if he or she seems to be in immediate danger – near a fire, for example. Otherwise, do *not* interfere.

2. Move nearby objects or place padding (coats, blankets) over immovable ones so that they cannot cause injury. Do *not* attempt to hold down or restrain the person.

3. Most fits last only a minute or two. If a fit continues for more than about three minutes, or if another fit starts a few minutes after the first, summon medical help immediately. The person may be carrying a card or tag giving emergency information.

4. Many epileptics fall deeply asleep shortly after having had a fit. If this happens, allow the person to wake naturally. If possible, move him or her to somewhere quiet to allow undisturbed sleep, and check from time to time that everything is all right.

There is a common belief that the main thing you should do for someone having a fit is to force something between their teeth so as to keep them from biting or choking on the tongue. Do *not* attempt this manoeuvre – it may damage the sufferer's mouth.

Vertigo

Vertigo is not a disease. It is a symptom of a disturbance in the brain and/or the organs of balance in your inner ears (see *Ear disorders*, p.328, for more about the organs of balance). The disturbance may be caused by any of several underlying disorders.

What are the symptoms?
If you have vertigo, you get a sensation of either spinning about or being stationary while everything around you spins. This may be no worse than a mild spell of dizziness; but you may be so severely affected that you feel nauseated, vomit, lose your balance and fall down, or even faint. (Vertigo is often incorrectly used to mean fear of heights. The correct term for fear of heights is "acrophobia".)

Vertigo is sometimes caused by a specific disease such as *labyrinthitis* (p.338) or *Ménière's disease* (p.337). It is more usual, however, for the disorder that causes it to be minor and only temporary, and so the vertigo itself is only minor and temporary. In such cases, though, it may be impossible to discover the cause of the difficulty, especially in older sufferers.

What should be done?
If you have a severe attack or repeated attacks of vertigo, consult your doctor, who may want special diagnostic tests to determine whether anything is seriously wrong.

What is the treatment?
The best way to deal with vertigo is to lie down until the dizziness (and nausea, if any) passes away. If there is no identifiable underlying cause of persistent attacks, the doctor may prescribe a drug that helps to stabilize the balancing mechanism in your inner ears.

Neuralgia

Neuralgia is pain from a damaged nerve. Several possible kinds of damage can lead to this disorder. The trouble may be temporary and mild, as in the pain sometimes brought on by minor inflammation of a nerve (see *Peripheral neuropathy*, p.283). Or it may be recurrent and severe, as in sciatica (see *Types of back pain*, p.547) and *trigeminal neuralgia* (p.722), a facial pain that mainly afflicts the elderly. The pain of neuralgia tends to be sharp and hard to bear. You feel it shooting along the course of the damaged nerve; it usually lasts only a few seconds, but several attacks may occur in quick succession.

What is the treatment?
Treatment of neuralgia depends on the location of the damaged nerve or nerves and on the cause of the damage. If you have occasional attacks that are only mildly painful, you can probably relieve the pain with *analgesics* such as aspirin or paracetamol. But if the pain becomes intolerable, consult your doctor, who may prescribe a stronger painkilling drug. The doctor may also decide to refer you to a *neurologist* for diagnostic tests and further treatment. In some very rare cases surgery may be recommended to control persistent pain.

Degenerations

Grouped under this heading are diseases in which nerve cells degenerate and die – usually slowly, over months or years. Such degeneration may be caused by either temporary inflammation that leaves nerves permanently damaged or the slow loss of nerves that die for no apparent reason. The symptoms of the various diseases differ widely, depending on the area of the brain or spinal cord in which the degeneration occurs. The results are always distressing and often tragic, but it is encouraging that our understanding of these disorders is being gradually broadened by research into causes and treatments.

Parkinson's disease
(Paralysis agitans, shaking palsy)

Parkinson's disease is due to gradual deterioration in nerve centres within the brain that control movement, particularly semi-automatic movements such as swinging the arms while walking. Deterioration of these nerve centres upsets the delicate balance between two chemicals, dopamine and acetylcholine (known as neurotransmitters), essential for controlling the transmission of nerve impulses within this part of the nervous system. The resultant lack of control produces the symptoms of Parkinson's disease.

We do not know what generally causes the more common forms of the illness. An extremely rare form of *encephalitis* (p.274) can lead to a particular type of Parkinson's disease. In rare cases the nerve degeneration results from such factors as carbon-monoxide poisoning or high levels of certain metals in body tissues. High doses of some drugs used in treating psychiatric conditions such as *schizophrenia* (p.295) sometimes produce Parkinson's disease, but symptoms disappear when doses of the drug are reduced.

What are the symptoms?
One characteristic symptom is a type of tremor (sometimes incorrectly spoken of as "palsy" – a word that actually means "paralysis") and this is usually one of the first signs of the disorder. There is an involuntary, rhythmic shaking of the hands and/or head, often accompanied by a continuous rubbing together of thumb and forefinger. Such tremors are worst when the affected part of the body is not consciously in use; once it is put into motion to do a specific act, the tremor disappears or diminishes.

If the disorder worsens, there is a gradual loss of almost automatic physical movements such as the swinging of arms that makes for smooth walking, or the ability to write legibly or speak clearly. It becomes increasingly difficult to initiate new movements, or to change from one position to another. Over the years the sufferer develops a characteristic shuffling walk. There is no pain, numbness, or tingling – simply an increasing poverty of movement. Falls may be frequent because sufferers cannot retain their balance while walking. Easy activities such as rising from a chair can become hard to manage. Further symptoms include excessive salivation, abdominal cramps, and – in later stages of the disease – deterioration of memory and thought processes.

How common is the problem?
Every year about 1 person in 1,000 develops Parkinson's disease. Most sufferers are elderly or in late middle age. Men are slightly more susceptible than women, and there is evidence that this disease runs in families.

What are the risks?
Because the disease does not affect nerves that supply the heart or other vital organs, it is not immediately life-threatening. But it can lead to extreme mental depression.

What should be done?
There is no immediate cause for concern if, after the age of 50, you develop a mild tremor; many people do so as they grow older. Consult your doctor, though, if you have further symptoms of Parkinson's disease or if the tremor worsens. Your doctor should be able to make a diagnosis on the strength of a general physical examination; special tests are rarely necessary unless symptoms occur in someone well under 50.

What is the treatment?
Self-help: Much can be done in the way of family support, encouragement, and practical changes in the house. Mobility is assisted, for example, by bath-rail supports, special banisters along habitual routes, and chairs with high arms. If you have Parkinson's disease, try to take some regular exercise, and keep up

your morale by remaining as actively engaged as possible in your everyday routine.

Professional help: Modern drug treatment can do much to relieve symptoms, particularly stiffness and immobility. In mild cases drugs are not generally prescribed, for they may have troublesome side-effects. But your doctor will probably want to see you every six months or so in order to observe the progress of your condition. If drug treatment becomes necessary, the widely used preparations are those that re-establish the balance of dopamine and acetylcholine within the affected area of the brain. Among possible side-effects, such as nausea, some of these drugs tend to make the mouth unpleasantly dry – but that may seem almost like a benefit if excessive salivation is a symptom. New drugs are constantly being developed, but none has yet proved effective against the characteristic tremor.

What are the long-term prospects?

As yet no treatment seems to slow down the progress of Parkinson's disease, but the relief from symptoms that various treatments give has kept millions of sufferers in reasonable health. If you develop Parkinson's disease after the age of 60 you will probably live out your normal life expectancy.

Multiple sclerosis

Many nerves in the brain and spinal cord are enclosed in a protective covering called myelin sheath. The sheath feeds nutrients to the delicate nerve fibres within and also speeds up the passage of electrical impulses. If the myelin sheath becomes inflamed and swollen, it damages the internal nerve fibres; and if this affects a number of nerves in your central nervous system, you have the disease known as multiple sclerosis. Any part of the brain or spinal cord containing myelin-covered nerves can be affected. There is some evidence that the damage may be due to a virus, and another possibility is that the cause may be a deficiency or abnormality of the fatty substance that makes up myelin.

What are the symptoms?

Myelin is so widespread in the nervous system that multiple sclerosis can manifest itself in many different ways. Most commonly, it begins with a vague, transient symptom which clears up completely within a day or two. For example, you may get a feeling of tingling and numbness or weakness which may be patchy or affect only one limb or one side of the body. Temporary weakness of a limb may cause you to fumble or drop things or to drag a foot when you walk. This type of symptom may be especially apparent after a hot bath or exercise. As any numbness fades, it may be followed by a sensation of increased sensitivity in the area that was numb.

Other possible indications of multiple sclerosis include *ataxia* (general physical unsteadiness), temporary blurring of vision (see *Optic neuritis*, p.326), slurred speech, difficulty in passing urine, or incontinence. All symptoms may disappear after the first episode. In some cases there is no further trouble. But for other sufferers there are repeated attacks; recovery is less complete after each episode, and permanent disability such as weakness of limbs or general paralysis gradually develops.

How common is the problem?

About 1 person in 2,000 in Britain has multiple sclerosis. Contrary to popular belief, there is no reliable evidence to suggest that the disease runs in families. In two-thirds of all cases, attacks start to occur in the age group 20 to 40. They virtually never begin in children or in people over 60. Women sufferers slightly outnumber men.

What are the risks?

Repeated attacks of multiple sclerosis can cause severe disability or even death, but this is not an inevitable outcome. If one of your symptoms is loss of bladder control (urinary incontinence), there is a risk of infection of the urinary tract.

What should be done?

If you have symptoms of multiple sclerosis, your doctor will probably refer you to a *neurologist*. There is no specific diagnostic test for this elusive disease, but certain tests – for instance, *ophthalmoscopy*, *lumbar puncture*, and skull and chest *X-rays* – will help rule out other possible disorders.

What is the treatment?

Self-help: The best thing anyone with severe multiple sclerosis can do is to try to come to terms with the disease. Those who approach this problem most optimistically and constructively succeed best at making necessary changes. You should join the nearest branch of the *Multiple Sclerosis Society* (p.768).

Professional help: Some doctors believe that in some cases the severity of symptoms is lessened by *steroid* injections or tablets.

There are certain other treatments available – for example, a diet rich in sunflower oil (which supplies extra amounts of a chemical necessary for the growth and repair of myelin). Treatments of this type may reduce the frequency and severity of attacks.

Muscle-relaxant drugs sometimes relieve muscular stiffness or pain, and surgery for relief of spasms is occasionally advisable. With particularly troublesome urinary incontinence it is best to have a *catheter* introduced into the bladder. Urine drains into a bag, which is emptied and cleaned daily. Finally, your doctor may advise *physiotherapy* to strengthen your muscles and *occupational therapy* to help you remain active and alert.

Only a limited number of sufferers are crippled by multiple sclerosis. Many people have transient symptoms, which pass without leaving ill-effects; many others are left with minor disabilities but lead essentially normal lives. Indeed, about 70 per cent of sufferers will still be actively engaged in their normal pursuits five years after diagnosis.

Motor neurone disease

This exceedingly rare condition results from the dying off of certain nerve cells (*motor neurones*) that run from the brain stem to the muscles and control their movements. Unstimulated and unused, the affected muscles gradually waste away, and the affected part of the body becomes increasingly weak and uncoordinated. The disease can cause difficulty in swallowing, breathing, walking, or any other muscle-powered activity (in other words, virtually any physical function).

Motor neurone disease most often occurs in people over 50. Little is known about its cause, and it cannot be cured. Treatment is directed at easing symptoms and helping sufferers to remain relatively mobile and independent. In most cases death occurs within 5 to 10 years of the onset of the disease.

Huntington's chorea

Huntington's chorea is a very rare degenerative nerve disease that starts in middle age. Uncontrollable body movements gradually develop and are followed by mental deterioration such as loss of memory and a change of personality. No treatment to halt the progress of the disease or control its symptoms has yet been discovered. The word "chorea" means "dance" and is a rough description of the swift, jerky movements that occur in this disease. (A similar disorder, Sydenham's chorea, has the familiar common name St Vitus's dance.)

Huntington's chorea is inherited (see *Genetics*, p.704). Unfortunately, it does not produce symptoms before middle age, and so someone with Huntington's chorea may well be unaware of the fact when becoming a parent. If you know of anyone in your family who has had the disease, consult your doctor or a *genetic counsellor* (p.619) about possible risks for yourself and your children.

Friedreich's ataxia

This is an exceedingly rare inherited disease in which certain groups of nerve fibres gradually deteriorate. The main symptom is *ataxia* (loss of coordination of movement and balance), especially when walking. Gradually it also becomes difficult for the sufferers to stand still, speak, or use their arms – which may begin to shake just when the afflicted individual intends to move them (an *intention tremor*). Symptoms usually become apparent between the ages of 5 and 15. Only a dozen or so people succumb to the disease in Britain in an average year. As yet there is no treatment.

Friedreich's ataxia runs in families; if it affects any of your relatives, you should seek advice from your doctor, *genetic counsellor* (p.619), or the *Friedreich's Ataxia Group* (p.768) before starting a family.

Pre-senile dementia

Whereas *senile dementia* (p.724) is primarily a disease of the elderly, pre-senile dementia is a similar disease – leading to intellectual and emotional disintegration – which occurs in someone well under 60. It may well be due to an underlying disorder such as *hypothyroidism* (p.526) or a *brain tumour* (p.281), which, if discovered in time, can sometimes be successfully treated. If this is not the case, reasoning powers, memory, and various physical processes tend to deteriorate much more swiftly than in senile dementia. The disease in a comparatively young person generally proves fatal in about five years.

Mental and emotional problems

Introduction

In general, if you are able to keep your mental balance during periods of emotional stress, you can call yourself mentally healthy. If you lose your balance, you are, at least to some extent, ill. The articles in this section are designed to help you recognize some of the warning signs of common forms of mental trouble, not only in yourself but in others. The arrangement of articles is based on two groupings. First, there are illnesses that arise primarily from internal influences – for example, schizophrenia, depression, and compulsions. The actual causes are not known, but among them may be hereditary factors, personality factors, slight variations in the amount and type of chemicals in the brain, and – occasionally – physical disorders. Secondly, there are addictions – mental problems triggered off by external influences such as alcohol or other drugs. Certain personality types appear to be especially susceptible to the various addictive illnesses.

Some people are overwhelmed by trivial crises such as a minor marital squabble; others manage to retain their balance in daunting circumstances such as the break-up of a once happy home. Your mental breaking point and the way you respond to stress depend in part on your heredity and upbringing. Much also depends on whether you are flexible, whether you accept reality (seeing things as they are, rather than as you would like them to be), and whether you sometimes give your attention to other people's problems instead of dwelling on your own. You can identify and encourage healthy attitudes in yourself and thus stand a better chance of coping with the problems of living (see *Keeping mentally fit*, p.18).

Some helpful definitions

There is a quite special vocabulary relating to psychological problems and their treatment. Many general terms used in these pages have clearly defined meanings for medical people, but laymen sometimes find it difficult to distinguish among them. Here are some definitions:

Psychiatrist: A psychiatrist is a medically qualified doctor and, as such, may diagnose and prescribe drugs for any type of illness; but, as a psychiatrist, he or she specializes in mental problems.
Psychologist: A psychologist has not been trained as a medical doctor, but, as a student of normal human psychology, may be able to help by counselling people through critical periods of their lives. Psychologists are not licensed to prescribe drugs.
Psychoanalyst: Psychoanalysts are so called because they treat mental disorders by probing into and analysing the unconscious, as well as the conscious, contents of the minds of their patients. A psychoanalyst may or may not be a medically qualified doctor (see *Psychoanalysis*, p.299).

Psychotherapy: Psychotherapy is a general term applied to the treatment of mental disorders by primarily mental means – such as suggestion, analysis, and persuasion. Any such treatment may be applied by general practitioners as well as those who specialize in psychological problems (see *Psychotherapy*, p.299).
Neurotic: Neurotic people are notably susceptible to mental or emotional stress; they may sometimes become depressed, for example, or have an irrational fear of flying or of meeting strangers. But their illness does not become so severe that they lose contact with the realities of daily life.
Psychotic: A person is or has become psychotic if he or she has lost contact with reality and is (whether occasionally or always) incapable of rational behaviour.
Psychosomatic: A *psychosomatic illness* (p.301) is a real physical illness caused by a mental or emotional problem.
Psychopathic: Psychopathic people may seem on the surface to be normal, but they are mentally or emotionally irresponsible, and their behaviour is chronically – often dangerously – antisocial (see *Psychopathy*, p.303).

Mental illnesses

The chemistry of the brain probably plays an important part in causing mental illness. That is why drugs are generally used along with *psychotherapy* in treating the disorders discussed below. But most cases of illness such as anxiety or hypochondriasis are largely the result of personality factors. Many people, for example, are by nature *neurasthenic*; they tire easily, are over-sensitive, and lack energy. When under stress, such people sometimes succumb to depression or anxiety. Many others are *cyclothymic*; they have swings in mood from elation and energy to lethargy and withdrawal. When under stress, such people may become manic-depressive. Most of us, however, overcome the drawbacks of negative personality traits and manage to face up to emotional problems without a doctor's help. If you have a neurasthenic or cyclothymic personality, you are by no means on the verge of a mental illness. Also, do not assume that mental illness can be treated only in mental hospitals. "Madness", in the commonly accepted sense of the word, is rare. Nearly 15 per cent of the average general practitioner's patients have consulted the doctor mainly because of a mental or emotional problem. And the physical disorders of many others are in some way related to underlying psychological stress. In fact, about 40 per cent of the average GP's patients are either *neurotic* and temporarily in need of help or are suffering from *psychosomatic* symptoms such as palpitations, headache, or indigestion (for definitions of terms see *Some helpful definitions*, opposite).

It is only when people lose touch with reality and behave in bizarre and perhaps life-threatening ways that they can be considered *psychotic* rather than merely neurotic. It is usually best to treat such sufferers in hospital. But relatively few people are likely to have a severe mental illness during the course of their lives.

Schizophrenia

Schizophrenia (literally "split mind") is often thought of as a split or dual personality. However, this disease is more correctly defined as a disorganization of normal thought and feeling. It is probably caused by malfunctioning of certain cells within the brain. Symptoms usually appear in late adolescence or early adulthood, sometimes triggered off by extreme mental stress. The illness is lifelong, but acute attacks tend to come and go, usually occurring at times of emotional upheaval or personal loss.

What are the symptoms?

An attack begins with a gradual – or occasionally sudden – withdrawal from day-to-day activities. The schizophrenic's speech may become increasingly vague, and he or she may seem unable to follow a simple conversation. An acute attack happens unexpectedly, but more often the onset is so gradual that it is difficult to know when *psychotic* symptoms appear. Among such symptoms are disturbances in thoughts and feelings and sometimes disorders of movement (see below). The thought processes of schizophrenics may be disturbed so that they do not follow each other logically, and the associations between them seem strange and unconnected. They may experience "thought blocking", in which there is a sudden cessation of all thoughts and the mind seems suddenly to stop and remain empty; or "thought insertion", in which thoughts may arise spontaneously as if they have been placed in the mind by someone else.

Schizophrenics often believe that others hear and "steal" their thoughts. Sometimes they fear they have lost control of bodily movement as well as thought, as if they were puppets. They frequently hear voices, often hostile ones. Less commonly, they have hallucinations of odd physical sensations or of being given poisoned food. In time many build up an entire set of beliefs in a fantasy world in order to make sense to themselves of all these strange experiences and sensations. They may express exaggerated feelings of happiness, puzzlement, or despair. They may laugh at a sad moment or cry without cause. Or they may seem devoid of feeling, so that it becomes impossible to make emotional contact with them. Disorders of movement sometimes occur, when the muscles become fixed and stiff, or the sufferer may take up bizarre postures, such as standing on one leg for several hours.

There are several types of schizophrenia, according to the symptoms that predominate, but the only practical distinction that most doctors now make is between the *paranoid* and other types. The main symptom of paranoid schizophrenia is constant suspicion and resentment, with a fear that people are plotting to destroy the sufferer.

How common is the problem?

Most young and middle-aged patients in mental hospitals are there because they are schizophrenic. About 1 person in 100 has some degree of the disorder. Men and women are equally prone. In middle-aged and elderly sufferers, paranoid schizophrenia is the most common type.

The abnormality of brain chemistry that underlies schizophrenia can be inherited; but if it runs in your family, you will not necessarily have schizophrenic attacks. You may, however, have a "schizoid personality" (a tendency towards shyness and withdrawal) or a "paranoid personality" (a tendency towards over-sensitivity and distrustfulness). People with a paranoid personality who then go on to develop schizophrenia usually have paranoid schizophrenia. If you have a schizophrenic parent, you stand a 30 per cent chance of having a schizoid or paranoid personality, but only a 15 per cent chance of developing schizophrenia. Even if both parents are schizophrenic, you have a 50 per cent chance of escaping the illness.

What are the risks?

During severe attacks of schizophrenia sufferers can do physical harm to themselves or others, or may try to commit suicide.

What should be done?

If you suspect that someone in your family is schizophrenic, persuade him or her to see a doctor. It may not be easy. People who are becoming mentally ill often refuse to admit the fact. Even those who realize that something is wrong have a fear of being "put away". But medical care is vital. Never leave sufferers who seem extremely disturbed alone. The presence of a relative or friend to reassure them – or even keep them from hurting themselves – is essential until help arrives. People with symptoms of schizophrenia are usually admitted to hospital for a preliminary period of observation. During this time tests are carried out to make sure the symptoms are not due to a physical illness such as a *brain tumour* (p.281).

What is the treatment?

Severe cases must be treated in hospital. Treatment usually involves drugs, some form of *psychotherapy*, and rehabilitation.

The most effective drugs are regular doses of special tranquillizers to modify abnormal brain chemistry. As symptoms gradually disappear, doses are reduced, and all medication is sometimes discontinued when an acute attack ends. Some people, however, need long-term medication. They may either take pills regularly or be given an injection every two to four weeks. Some sufferers also need *anti-depressant* drugs; and, rarely, *electroconvulsive therapy (ECT)* may be necessary.

The final stage of treatment is rehabilitation, which helps people recovering from attacks to regain normal skills and behaviour patterns. In the early stages of hospital treatment schizophrenics are generally given *occupational therapy*. As their condition improves, they are given increasingly complex tasks and pressures to cope with, and these eventually approximate to the tasks and pressures of the outside world. Once the acute phase of the illness is over, the schizophrenic prepares for a return to the outside world by having periodic visits from hospital to home or to a hostel associated with the hospital. Some are even able to resume their normal jobs while still in hospital. In this way they can come to terms with normal pressures gradually.

What are the long-term prospects?

Many people recover from an attack of schizophrenia well enough to return to relatively normal life. But they are apt to have further attacks if subjected to undue stress. In some people the condition becomes chronic. Such sufferers will always be withdrawn and emotionally unresponsive, but they can usually avoid the recurrence of bad attacks with the aid of constant medication.

What is a "nervous breakdown"?

People who say that someone has had a nervous breakdown are using a phrase that doctors avoid. To speak of a nervous breakdown is to express a precise, often rather harsh fact in an imprecise, gentle way. The fact is that anyone with a "nervous breakdown" has become unable to cope with day-to-day events because of a specific mental problem such as schizophrenia, depression, or anxiety. If someone you know is under treatment for any such disorder, you may prefer to avoid naming the problem and to say that he or she has had a nervous breakdown. But remember that there is no more reason to feel shame about a mental than about a physical illness.

Depression

Most people feel depressed once in a while. There is no question of their being mentally ill, though, if they carry on with their daily routine and gradually brighten up. The difference between "feeling depressed" and having the mental illness known as depression is that people who are actually ill cannot lift themselves out of their misery; their depression persists, deepens, and eventually interferes with their ability to lead normal lives. If you or others in your family have occasional periods of down-heartedness that ease up after a few days or weeks, you have no cause for concern. The symptoms of true depressive illness are described below. (See also *Manic depression*, p.298.)

There are two main types of depressive illness. The first type, "reactive" depression, is caused by extreme reaction to a specific emotional blow such as the death of a loved one, the end of a love affair, or financial loss. *Neurotic* people sometimes over-react to such misfortunes, and the result may be mental breakdown. The second type of depression is called "endogenous" (a word that means "growing from within"). Endogenous depression usually occurs without apparent cause, but it has sometimes been known to follow a viral infection such as *glandular fever* (p.562). It may also result from the hormonal changes after childbirth (see *Depression after childbirth*, p.642) or may be associated with *schizophrenia* (p.295).

There are certain periods of particular susceptibility to depressive illness in almost everyone's lifetime. Late adolescence, middle age, and the post-retirement years are such periods. Youngsters often find the transition from adolescence to adulthood difficult, especially when under intense educational or work pressures. A menopausal woman may equate her loss of fertility with loss of femininity. A man in late middle age may brood over the realization that he can advance no further in his career and has lost much of his virility. And depressive illness among elderly people is extremely common.

Every severe depression, especially of the endogenous type, is probably accompanied by a chemical change that affects the way the brain functions.

What are the symptoms?

Symptoms of depressive illness include not only overriding melancholy but physical changes such as loss of energy and appetite for food and sex, insomnia, and sometimes indigestion, constipation, and headaches. In addition, people suffering from endogenous depression are liable to have severe psychological symptoms. They may lose touch with reality, may feel guilty and worthless without cause, may believe that they are being justifiably persecuted or that their bodies are rotting away, and may have hallucinations. Sometimes acute *anxiety* (p.300) accompanies the depression, and resultant restlessness and agitation may mask the more obvious symptoms of depression.

Intensity of symptoms often varies with the time of day. Typically, a sufferer from endogenous depression wakes early in a sad mood that brightens as the day progresses. But reactive depressions are often worst at night. As the illness progresses, depression may deepen until it never lifts. The sufferer then becomes totally withdrawn, spending much of the day huddled in bed.

How common is the problem?

About 1 person in 25 is likely to experience at least one period of depression severe enough to require medical help, though the symptoms may not be specifically identified as those of depressive illness. A tendency to endogenous depression runs in families.

What are the risks?

The gravest risk is suicide, the last resort of someone who finds life unbearable (see *Suicide*, p.298). Depression causes two-thirds of the 4,000 suicides in Britain each year. In rare cases the illness can unbalance sufferers' minds to such a degree that they feel forced to kill others as well as themselves, to spare them the agony of being alive.

What should be done?

If you recognize the symptoms of increasing depressive illness (not just passing sadness) in yourself, see a doctor now; do not be ashamed to tell him or her about your fears. If you recognize the symptoms in other people, try to persuade them to accept medical help. Too many sufferers reach the point of no return because their relations and friends fail to interpret warning signs correctly or ignore repeated threats of suicide. *Always* take suicide threats seriously.

What is the treatment?

Self-help: If you think a mild form of depression is lasting too long or beginning to deepen, a change of scene or a treat such as an evening out may provide the necessary lift. It is not possible to do this, however, in cases of true depressive illness. If a member of your family seems severely affected, try gentle but firm persuasion to get him or her to a doctor. The threat of suicide should be considered an emergency even if the person has made such threats before and you suspect that he or she is probably just seeking attention.

Professional help: Much depends on the type and severity of symptoms. Your family doctor may or may not refer you to a specialist for treatment, which is likely to consist of a combination of drugs and *psychotherapy. Antidepressants*, the most commonly used drugs, usually begin to relieve a mild depression in two or three weeks. In severe cases, especially when there is a risk of suicide, the doctor may advise admission to hospital, where the severity of symptoms can be monitored and drug treatment and psychotherapy can be closely supervised. In rare cases of persistent illness *electroconvulsive therapy* (*ECT*) may become necessary.

In all cases treated in a mental hospital, the aim is not only to cure your depression but to prepare you for a return to normal life. Along with psychotherapy you will probably be given *occupational therapy*.

What are the long-term prospects?
People with depressive illness nearly always respond well to treatment. Unfortunately, this does not assure freedom from further attacks. Endogenous depressions are often recurrent. Emotional stress may lead to reactive depressions if you are susceptible. Yet many people who have repeated bouts of depressive illness manage to function satisfactorily by seeking treatment early in each attack. The frequency of attacks may be reduced by long-term drug treatment.

Manic depression
(including mania)

A normal person has moods – shifting from moderate liveliness to moderate lethargy – depending largely on circumstances. A sufferer from manic depression has extreme moods unrelated to external events. Manic-depressive illness tends to be cyclical, with periods of elated overactivity (mania) irregularly alternating with deep *depression* (p.297). Periods of normality, sandwiched between the extremes, may last for a short time or for years. There is some evidence that this illness may be caused partly by a flaw in brain chemistry.

Extreme stress may trigger off a sudden attack of mania or depression, particularly in people who seldom have acute attacks.

Often, however, there is no direct cause, and phases of the illness begin gradually. Very rarely it is caused by severe infection, a stroke, or brain injury.

What are the symptoms?
Close associates are more likely than sufferers themselves to recognize the beginning of the manic phase, which starts gradually with hypomania (a moderate degree of mania). People in this phase begin to wake earlier and earlier, until they find themselves leaping vigorously out of bed at 4 am. But their output of work falls because they are easily distracted and increasingly restless. They may be abnormally promiscuous sexually, go on spending sprees, and enthusiastically start (but rarely finish) new projects. They are often irritable, given to sudden rages.

Hypomania seldom reaches a fully manic stage. If it does, one result may be wild speech, full of rhyming, punning, and illogical word associations. Some sufferers sing and dance or laugh uproariously for no reason. At times an underlying sadness may break through in fleeting moments of withdrawal. Because manic people lack concentration, they often forget to eat; so they tend to lose weight and become exhausted. Eventually, there may be delusions of grandeur or intense anger at inability to carry out wild schemes.

The depressive phase is like depression, but symptoms are often more severe in the manic depressive. The onset is gradual. Sufferers become increasingly withdrawn. Sleep is frequently disturbed; but although there may be early-morning wakefulness, late rising becomes habitual. Sex drive decreases, speech and movement slow down, and any

Suicide
Each year about 200,000 people in this country try to kill themselves, but only about 4,000 succeed. Those who fail often want to fail; a botched attempt at suicide may well be a lonely or frustrated person's way to attract attention. You can never be certain, though, that someone who tries to commit suicide and fails will not succeed some day. So if anyone you know seems emotionally disturbed and threatens to attempt suicide, try to get him or her to see a doctor. If quick action seems necessary, telephone the local branch of the Samaritans, an organization experienced in dealing with this problem; they are on call 24 hours a day. While waiting for help, encourage the suicidal person to talk, and listen patiently without passing judgement. Never leave such people alone before professional help arrives.

If you find someone lying unconscious or semi-conscious, whatever the cause, dial 999 and ask for an ambulance. Disturbed individuals often seek death by taking an overdose of sleeping pills. If you find tablets or tablet containers anywhere near the person, be sure to give them to the ambulance crew when they arrive. Meanwhile apply first aid (see *Accidents and emergencies*, p.801).

imagined problems multiply. After a time some sufferers, feeling unable to face the world, simply stay shut in their rooms.

How common is the problem?
Manic-depressive illness is rarer than depression, affecting only about 1 person in 250. It tends to run in families, affects three times as many women as men, and is especially apt to develop in some women after childbirth or during the menopause.

What are the risks?
Although sufferers may threaten suicide during depressions, they usually lack energy or conviction to do it. The danger increases with emergence from deep depression, when renewed energy accompanies a continuing death-wish. In the manic phase, outrageous behaviour may ruin social and professional relationships, and lack of judgement can lead to financial disaster.

What should be done?
If you suspect that someone is manic-depressive, persuade him or her to see a doctor. If necessary, ask your own doctor for advice. If you think that you yourself may be becoming manic-depressive, see the doctor without delay; the illness. is most easily treated in its early stages.

What is the treatment?
In mild cases drugs may be prescribed to be taken at home; tranquillizers are given for the manic phase and *antidepressants* for the depressive phase. Your doctor may also refer you to a specialist for *psychotherapy*. In severe cases – especially when there is a risk of suicide, or irrational behaviour gets out of hand – treatment in hospital is usually necessary. Lithium, a chemical that alters brain chemistry, is now generally used for preventing manic-depressive attacks. Because of possible side-effects, however, sufferers must undergo blood, kidney, and thyroid-gland tests before being started on treatment with this chemical. *Electroconvulsive therapy (ECT)* may also be advisable.

As treatment in hospital begins to show results, sufferers are also given *occupational therapy* to prepare them for a return to normal routine. If somebody in your family has been in hospital, you will be told how to recognize signs of an impending attack and how to reduce strains upon the sufferer so as to lessen the risk of further attacks. After release from full hospital care, many manic depressives must continue taking lithium; they are given monthly check-ups to make sure there are no harmful side-effects.

What are the long-term prospects?
Not long ago about 80 per cent of people who had one episode of manic-depressive illness could expect to have further attacks, which might become increasingly severe. However, this gloomy outlook can now often be brightened by the long-term use of lithium to prevent further attacks.

Psychoanalysis

Psychoanalysis is not only one kind of *psychotherapy* (right); it is the technique from which all others have stemmed. Developed by a Viennese neurologist, Sigmund Freud, in the late nineteenth century, it is based on Freud's theory that adult behaviour is largely determined by early-childhood conflicts. There are numerous variants of Freud's basic theory and technique, but all have the same goal: to help mentally insecure or disturbed patients recall old memories buried deep in the subconscious mind. Once the root causes of a problem are recollected and understood, the problem may lose its force.

Treatment of this sort requires many meetings with the analyst, during which such matters as present and past dreams, recollections, thoughts, and feelings are unremittingly discussed, analysed, and interpreted. Because full treatment involves several hour-long sessions per week for at least two or three years, psychoanalysis is not generally feasible except for people with time and money to spare. Moreover, it has proved to be less effective than its early practitioners hoped. Many doctors now believe that the main value of Freud's work is that it provided a framework for modern psychiatry in emphasizing the vital influence of early experience upon patterns of adult behaviour. An understanding of this relationship is essential for all forms of psychotherapy.

Psychotherapy

Psychotherapy is treatment by verbal means. The original verbal technique for treating mentally ill people was *psychoanalysis* (left); modern techniques stem from the need to develop less time-consuming methods. These vary widely but usually involve a number of counselling sessions, during which the therapist discusses the special problems of the sufferer and offers help and advice without making a detailed investigation of childhood experiences. Sometimes people are treated in groups. The advantage of group psychotherapy is that members of the group learn from one another, and pressure to adopt a healthier attitude towards daily stresses can be brought to bear on individuals by the group as a whole. This type of therapy is particularly helpful for people who are not mentally ill but who do have personality problems.

Anxiety

For most people, anxiety is a temporary reaction to stress. It becomes an illness only when it persists, preventing you from leading a normal life. Some anxiety states are caused by severe stress. But in anxiety-prone people only slight stresses, or none at all, may be involved. Sufferers from the disorder known as "free-floating" anxiety live in a constant state of apparently causeless uneasiness.

What are the symptoms?

If you have an attack of anxiety, you will probably feel apprehensive and tense, unable to concentrate, to think clearly, or to sleep well. You may have frightening dreams and occasional symptoms of fear such as a thudding heart, sweating palms, trembling, loss of voice, difficulty in swallowing, and even diarrhoea. Some people in a state of anxiety find it hard to breathe, as if their lungs are under constant pressure. And they may also become hypochondriacs (see *Hypochondriasis*, p.302), convinced that they have heart or stomach trouble. Sexual activity can also be affected; males may have trouble maintaining an erection or may suffer from *premature ejaculation* (p.614). In so-called "panic attacks", which can occur apparently without cause at any time, the physical symptoms of fear intensify frighteningly.

How common is the problem?

Anxiety is a very common form of psychological disorder. It is slightly more common in women than men, and adolescents and the elderly are especially susceptible.

What are the risks?

If severe anxiety is untreated, sufferers may gradually sink into *depression* (p.297) or may, over the long term, succumb to stress-related physical illness.

What should be done?

If your anxiety is caused by a specific stress, try to remove it. For example, consider changing jobs if your current work makes you tense. If there is no way to deal with the stress, or if severe anxiety persists, consult your doctor, who will examine you to determine whether your symptoms may be due to a physical condition such as an overactive thyroid gland (see *Thyrotoxicosis*, p.525). If your trouble is clearly mental, you may be referred to a specialist.

The first time you have a panic attack, you may think you are having a heart attack. To be on the safe side, call your doctor; if he or she is unavailable, ask for an ambulance.

What is the treatment?

Self-help: Various methods of relaxation can lessen the severity of symptoms. Whenever you feel tense and troubled, try the relaxation exercises recommended in *How to relieve tension*, p.19, or sit and read or listen to music.

Professional help: Your doctor may suggest a course of exercises to relax tense muscles. In addition, or alternatively, you may be given an anti-anxiety drug. To ease physical symptoms the doctor may also prescribe a *beta-blocker* drug. Severe cases need some form of *psychotherapy*.

What are the long-term prospects?

If your disorder is due to a stress that can be dealt with, you have a good chance of permanent cure. But if you are anxiety-prone or have free-floating anxiety, recurrent attacks are likely. You may be able to avoid them – or at least minimize symptoms – by continuing relaxation exercises even when not actively anxious. Ask your doctor for help as soon as you feel the onset of an attack.

Phobias

A phobia is an irrational fear of a specific object or situation. For instance, you may dread the sight or touch of a spider, or you may have a morbid fear of heights (acrophobia). Such fears do not usually prevent you from leading a normal life; you simply avoid spiders or high places. Fear of confined spaces (claustrophobia) is more troublesome since it may make you unable to face such psychological hazards as cars, trains, and lifts, but most claustrophobic people manage to overcome their fears. Some phobias, however, may make normal life impossible. A common example is agoraphobia, which is generally defined as fear of public places.

For an agoraphobic person a public space may be not just an avoidable park or shopping centre but anywhere outside the home. The phobia may also involve abnormal shyness – a fear of society – which is closely associated with the withdrawal symptoms of *depression* (p.297). Severe agoraphobia is an illness. If you suffer from this or any other phobia, the need to face whatever you fear can bring on the symptoms of *anxiety* (above), including "panic attacks".

What is the treatment?

Self-help: To combat a relatively mild phobia, try forcing yourself to come to grips with it gradually – a process termed *desensitization*. If you abhor spiders, for example, start by looking at pictures of them; next, make yourself stay in a room with one; next, look at one closely; then let one run over your hand. Or, if agoraphobia makes you dread shopping, begin by going to small neighbourhood shops and gradually widen your horizons until the large city stores no longer terrify you.

Professional help: If your symptoms are those of a general anxiety state, treatment is much as for anxiety. For agoraphobia associated with depression many doctors prescribe *antidepressants*. Another common type of treatment is *behaviour therapy*, given either in or out of hospital. There are two kinds of behaviour therapy. The first, desensitization, has been described above. If you are unable to desensitize yourself, professional guidance may help. The second technique, "flooding", is too drastic to be used as a self-help measure.

Whereas desensitization is like entering a cold sea gingerly, flooding is like the shock of a quick plunge. You are suddenly confronted with the feared object or placed in the feared situation, with no chance of escape, although you are reassured by the therapist's presence. Thus, having experienced your phobia at its fullest intensity, you come to realize that the dreaded thing is not truly dangerous. As you can imagine, flooding is risky; only a competent therapist should attempt it.

Psycho-somatic illness

Almost every physical disorder has some connection with emotional factors. Even accidental injuries such as broken bones seem to happen more often to children with disturbed home backgrounds than to others. A psychosomatic disease is one in which emotional factors are not just present but dominant; for example, in many skin disorders, migraine, some types of asthma, and some gastrointestinal disorders. Psychosomatic illnesses are not imaginary; they are real physical conditions. (For apparently physical disorders entirely stemming from mental illness see *Hysteria*, p.303.)

You know from experience that your state of mind affects your body. For instance, your heart beats faster when you are emotionally aroused, a stomach ache often follows an emotional upset, fright can make you sweat, and so on. These are very simple examples, but there are far more complex links – between chronic anxiety and duodenal ulcers, for instance – that certainly exist, though nobody quite understands the mechanism of the linkage. Certain psychosomatic disorders may be due to genetic factors, and it is significant that a tendency to disorders such as asthma, eczema, irritable colon, or migraine seems to run in families.

What is the treatment?

If you develop a disorder known to have a psychosomatic element, your doctor may ask questions about your life style, and if straightforward medical treatment does not relieve your symptoms, he or she may well begin to concentrate on helping you to handle the stresses of your day-to-day life. The very knowledge that you can probably ease some symptoms by avoiding certain emotional strains should be of help to you. Relaxation exercises (see *How to relieve tension*, p.19), together with changes in daily routine, can be particularly helpful in treating *vascular* disorders, such as high blood pressure, that are made worse by stress. Many migraine sufferers, too, are able to stave off threatened attacks by making a conscious effort to relax.

Compulsions and obsessions

A compulsion is an irresistible need to behave in a certain way even though you know it is absurd; an obsession is an idea or thought that seizes your mind and will not let go. Obsessional mental activity often leads to compulsive behaviour, and that is why compulsions and obsessions are discussed together in the following paragraphs.

At one time or another most people have minor obsessions and compulsions. On a certain day, for example, you cannot get a popular tune out of your head. Or you perhaps irrationally feel that you "must" always walk to work on the same side of the street. Such things are unimportant. Obsessions and compulsive actions become disorders only when they are so intense and persistent that they interfere with normal life.

What are the symptoms?

Obsessions take hold gradually. You become interested in something – a single aspect of politics, perhaps, or religion, or hygiene. Next you find yourself brooding about it. Eventually you can think of little else. Usually, then, the obsession begins to affect your behaviour. If, for instance, you have become obsessed with the notion that housebreaking is rampant, you may feel a compulsion to test your front door again after locking it securely. This is a comparatively harmless compulsion. Some people, however, might carry it beyond the bounds of normality by getting out of bed repeatedly during the night to test the door lock over and over again.

Compulsive disorders often centre on irrational fears. Some people, for example, obsessed with fear of "germs", wash their hands endlessly. Sufferers realize they are behaving irrationally, but their attempts to resist an overwhelming compulsion cause them intense anxiety.

How common is the problem?

Severe compulsive disorders are rare. Only about 1 person in 2,000 requires treatment for the condition. It is most likely to develop in people who are under 30, and it affects twice as many women as men.

What should be done?

If you feel that any of your ideas or actions are slipping out of control – so that, for example, you cannot bring yourself to go to work because your customary route has been closed – consult your doctor, who will probably refer you to a specialist for *psychotherapy*. Treatment for mild cases may be based on an effort to reassure sufferers while trying gradually to discover what lies behind the compulsive behaviour. Compulsions can sometimes be cured by *desensitization* therapy (see *Phobias*, p.300).

Medical opinion is divided on the effectiveness of drugs to treat serious obsessional or compulsive disorders. *Antidepressants* and tranquillizers, however, help to reduce accompanying symptoms of depression and anxiety. For an extremely severe obsession or compulsive behaviour involving violence, the only hope may be surgery to cut certain nerve pathways in the brain. But this is rarely done since the results are uncertain.

Hypo-chondriasis

Most healthy people are scarcely conscious of the internal workings of their bodies. If you suffer from hypochondriasis (commonly called hypochondria), you are morbidly aware of them, concentrating on them so much that they have come to seem constantly troublesome. Mild cases of hypochondria are extremely common and do not generally require treatment. An exaggerated concern about health becomes a form of mental illness, however, if it causes a person to lose interest in virtually everything but his or her imagined ailments. The disorder usually occurs as a complication of an underlying mental condition such as *anxiety* (p.300).

The hypochondriac usually buys and uses great quantities of patent medicines, repeatedly visits doctors, and, if dissatisfied with conventional medical help, is apt to try various types of fringe medicine. If hypochondriasis is due to an underlying anxiety state, the sufferer tends to interpret the symptoms of anxiety – for example, rapid heartbeat, trembling, breathlessness, and disturbed sleep – as signs of severe physical illness. People whose hypochondriasis is associated with depressive illness (see *Depression*, p.297) are often convinced that their bodies are degenerating – that, for instance, they have cancer or blocked bowels.

If you are constantly worried that you have a serious illness, and you are not convinced by your doctor's repeated reassurances, try to accept that you may have a psychological problem. If you can at least admit the possibility and discuss it with your doctor, you are halfway to resolving the problem. If your hypochondriasis is due to an underlying mental illness such as depression, successful treatment of the basic disorder will usually cure the hypochondriasis. When hypochondriasis is the only problem, it is almost impossible to treat. Mild tranquillizers are sometimes prescribed, and in some cases *psychotherapy* helps. In the main, though, hypochondriasis is part of an individual's personality.

Organic psychosis

Psychosis is mental illness so severe that the sufferer loses contact with reality. It is usually due to malfunctioning brain cells or is brought on by extreme stress. Sometimes, however, psychoses may be caused by physical factors – for instance, a brain illness, pneumonia, or a reaction to certain drugs. In such cases the psychosis is said to be *organic*.

Organic psychoses cause obvious signs of illness such as a dazed expression and confused speech. Visual hallucinations (seeing imaginary events) are common. The only satisfactory treatment is to deal with the underlying physical problem. If this is impossible, tranquillizers may give temporary relief from the more severe symptoms.

Hysteria

Hysteria is a type of over-reaction to an experience or situation. You are not hysterical in the medical sense of the word if you normally react to moments of stress by weeping uncontrollably or shrieking. Many people tend to over-dramatize their feelings, and they are not mentally ill because of this tendency. The illness known as hysteria occurs when someone (who may or may not be normally highly strung) reacts to severe stress by developing physical symptoms not due to physical factors.

Such sufferers do not realize that their symptoms are hysterical. They – and usually their families and friends – simply assume they have been afflicted with a genuine physical illness. The affliction is often of a kind that helps the sufferer to escape from the stressful situation. For example, people who see a frightful accident at their place of work sometimes develop a weakness of the legs that prevents them from leaving home. Or a total loss of memory (*amnesia*) follows an incident that the sufferer yearns to forget.

Do not confuse hysteria with *psychosomatic illnesses* (p.301), which, though affected by stress, are actual physical disorders.

What are the symptoms?
The hysterical reaction may be fairly mild (for instance, vague pains, weakness, or dizziness) or extremely severe (paralysis of the limbs, say, or sudden blindness). Less commonly, there may be loss of memory.

How common is the problem?
In an average year only about 1 person in 600 is diagnosed as suffering from hysteria. The problem is four times more common in women than men and is most prevalent among young adults.

What should be done?
If you suspect that the disability of someone in your family is due to hysterical reaction to some experience or situation, consult your doctor. Whether or not your suspicion is correct, never accuse anyone of faking symptoms. Hysterical people are ill and often super-sensitive. Because hysteria is extremely difficult to diagnose, your doctor will probably want in-hospital tests to rule out the possibility of a physical cause of the symptoms. If the condition is established as being probably hysterical, your relative will then be referred to a specialist.

What is the treatment?
The aim is to discover the underlying problem and help the sufferer solve it. No medical treatment can cure symptoms of hysteria, and so everything depends on sympathetic and patient *psychotherapy*. The only drug that may be prescribed for most sufferers is a tranquillizer to help them relax while the underlying trouble is being uncovered and symptoms coaxed away. In rare cases a treatment known as "abreaction", which docs involve drugs, may be advisable. It works best for people whose hysteria is due to a single, sharp emotional shock.

Sufferers undergoing abreaction must lie in a quiet, darkened room. To overcome their resistance to discussing a painful subject, they are put into a hypnotic state by either being given ether to breathe or being injected with a special drug. Then, when fully relaxed, they are asked to recall in detail the incident that triggered off their hysterical reaction. Just re-living in this way a suppressed experience sometimes removes symptoms of hysteria. Nobody quite knows why this should happen, but it does.

Psychopathy
(antisocial personality)

A psychopathic person is by nature incapable of accepting the restraints of the outside world. Psychopaths tend to be irresponsible, unable to hold down jobs, and incapable of having satisfactory relationships. Psychopathy might be called a long-term mental illness, which may or may not become a problem for the sufferer and society. Some psychopaths achieve material or creative success in spite of their personality disorder. Most, however, are inadequate people who merely drift along unhappily. And a fair number become violent when frustrated, or habitually break the rules that create social order. Such psychopaths spend much of their time in prison or under state care.

As yet, no way of altering the psychopath's personality has been discovered. It is possible to treat the disorders to which psychopaths are susceptible (such as extreme depression, alcoholism, and drug addiction) but not the basic personality. Some people who are extremely antisocial when young, however, become more emotionally mature in middle age. If you think the behaviour of someone in your family reflects a psychopathic personality, do not hesitate to consult your doctor, who can help you seek further guidance. Psychopathy usually starts in adolescence; so if an adult suddenly shows abnormal antisocial behaviour, the cause is more likely to be an organic brain disorder.

Addictions

Addictions are, or can become, mental illnesses in that an addict's craving for some sort of drug or pleasurable activity is uncontrollable. The necessity to have whatever it is that addicts crave prevents them from living normal lives. And addiction often leads to lack of mental balance even when it does no physical damage. Of the many possible types of addiction, three are singled out for discussion in the following pages: drugs, alcohol, and the psychological stimulant of gambling. Alcohol is itself a drug, of course, but it is discussed separately because, although addiction to alcohol has features in common with addiction to other drugs, alcoholism is a special and common disorder in its own right. Alcohol is more easily available than most other drugs, and so alcoholism is a more widespread problem than drug addiction.

Smoking, the most widespread of all addictions, is not included in this group of articles because it is fully – and frequently – discussed elsewhere. For a general discussion of smoking, along with advice on how to give it up, see *The dangers of smoking*, p.38. For further information see the sections on *Disorders of the respiratory system* (p.340) and *Disorders of the heart and circulation* (p.370).

Alcoholism

People who become addicted to alcohol usually begin to drink heavily in order to find relief from personal, business, or social stress. Since they generally find what they are looking for, even though only temporarily and at the cost of occasional hangovers, they gradually take to drinking whenever they feel slightly tense. The more they drink, the less tension they can tolerate without alcohol; and so an occasional need to relax at stressful moments becomes a motiveless addiction. You can consider yourself an alcoholic – or in danger of becoming one – if you have reached a point where you need to drink not to relieve tension but simply to make yourself feel "normal". And your illness is severe and requires immediate treatment if drinking has begun to affect health and interfere with personal and business affairs (see *Are you drinking too much alcohol?* on p.32) .

Some people can drink more, and more often, than others before reaching this stage. Much depends on one's physical tolerance for alcohol (see *The dangers of alcohol*, p.32). The shift from social drinking to alcoholism can happen almost imperceptibly over the course of many years, or it can occur with dramatic rapidity. Drinking habits, too, vary widely. Some alcoholics are "binge" drinkers, who go on two- or three-day sprees separated by a "dry" week or so. Others drink constantly and are never quite sober. Some drink only wine, or gin, or beer, while others will gulp down anything alcoholic.

For all such reasons it is virtually impossible to generalize about what "causes" this addiction or how it "develops". It is often true, though, that people in the early stages of alcoholism can tolerate greater amounts of alcohol without showing symptoms of the disorder than they can in the later stages.

What are the symptoms?

Even relatives and close friends of people who are becoming alcoholics seldom notice the early symptoms. The alcoholic seems merely to drink rather too heavily, chiefly on social occasions. Sometimes, though, such drinkers will admit to having blackouts, waking in the morning with no memory of what happened the night before. If this happens to someone in your family, you should recognize it as a sign of approaching trouble. Before long the drinking will start earlier in the day and last longer. The alcoholic then begins to mix larger and stronger drinks while drinking the same number.

In later stages the drinking may become secretive. Glasses of fruit juice may be surreptitiously spiked with gin. Bottles may be hidden around the house. Alcoholics, feeling guilty about their addiction, often have periods of uncharacteristic behaviour when they become irritable and aggressive, and may combine repeated assertions that they are giving up drink with denials that they have a drinking problem. They may have hallucinations, or become depressed, jealous, resentful, or even *paranoid*. Eventually there is likely to be loss of memory and concentration, along with inability to meet the demands of a steady job. Physically, an increasing dependence on alcohol is apt to lead to a flushed, veiny face; bruises on body and limbs; a husky voice; trembling hands; and chronic *gastritis* (p.464).

How common is the problem?

In Britain about 1 person in 100 is an alcoholic. The disorder is five times more common in men than in women; and people with alcoholic parents seem to be particularly susceptible, probably because of both environmental and genetic factors. Some sufferers have symptoms of alcoholism in adolescence or even earlier, but most alcoholics are between 35 and 55.

What are the risks?

Heavy drinking damages the body, and alcoholism may affect every one of the body's systems. About 1 in 5 heavy drinkers develops *cirrhosis of the liver* (p.487). Heavy drinking also makes the liver particularly liable to infection and may cause serious diseases of the stomach, heart, and brain. Because alcoholics seldom eat adequately, they are likely to suffer vitamin deficiencies, particularly of vitamin B (see *Vitamins*, p.494). And a pregnant woman who drinks more than three double measures of spirits, or six large glasses of wine, a day has a nearly 1 in 3 chance of having a mentally retarded or physically deformed baby.

What should be done?

If you detect signs of an early stage of alcoholism in yourself, cut down on the amount and frequency of social drinking. If you find this impossible, seek help without delay. Get in touch with your family doctor or the nearest branch of *Alcoholics Anonymous* (p.768), a helpful worldwide organization for people with drinking problems. If someone close to you shows symptoms of alcoholism but denies that he or she is drinking too much (as alcoholics often do), consult a doctor about the matter. You cannot force an unwilling person to seek help, but persuasion by a doctor or social worker may be effective.

What is the treatment?

For treatment to be successful, the sufferer must recognize the existence of the problem and be determined to grapple with it. The most satisfactory solution, of course, is simply to control one's drinking. Unfortunately, though, total abstinence from alcohol is the only possible answer for many addicts. Some people are able to give up on their own, but it is seldom an easy thing to do; withdrawal only too often leads to symptoms of *anxiety* (p.300). Self-help is rarely possible; in the early stages most alcoholics refuse to admit there is a problem. For people in a later stage of alcoholism, a "drying-out" process in hospital is usually necessary. Such sufferers are completely deprived of alcohol, as a result of which they may have minor withdrawal symptoms such as trembling of the limbs or feelings of anxiety. Tranquillizers will suppress the major withdrawal symptoms – including hallucinations, fits, and *delirium tremens* (popularly known as DTs) – which occur when alcohol is suddenly withdrawn without medical supervision. Alcoholics who are being weaned off the drug may also be given vitamins, to replace those in which they have become deficient.

Psychotherapy is the most successful way of continuing treatment after the initial drying-out period. And alcoholics are usually referred to a branch of Alcoholics Anonymous when they leave the hospital. In a few cases a special drug is also prescribed. The sufferer takes one tablet each morning; this discourages drinking because the combination of alcohol with the drug produces nausea, vomiting, and sweating. No such treatment will work, however, unless the alcoholic desperately wants it to and never "forgets" to take a tablet, which is effective for only 24 hours.

What are the long-term prospects?

The general outlook for alcoholics depends to a large extent on themselves. If you drink too much, it may be because of nearly irresistible social and business pressures. But if you are determined to give up alcohol, you will probably succeed, even if you can do so only by changing your job and your friends.

Drug addiction

People usually start to take drugs for one of two reasons. They may be prescribed by a doctor to relieve physical or mental distress; or they may simply be taken to provide a pleasurable mental effect – perhaps the warm, carefree drowsiness induced by heroin, or even the mild alertness produced by caffeine in coffee or tea. Whether or not a given drug is addictive varies considerably, not only from drug to drug but from person to person. Mildly addictive drugs such as codeine (together with apparently non-addictive drugs such as cannabis) are commonly known as *soft* drugs. *Hard* drugs are drugs that can lead to severe addiction, and it is with these that this article deals. Anyone who habitually takes a hard drug must do so in gradually increasing doses in order not only to maintain the pleasurable effects of the drug but to keep from breaking down both

Drugs and their effects

A drug is, literally, any non-nutritional chemical substance that can be absorbed into the system. As commonly used, the word "drug" may mean either a medicine or something taken (usually voluntarily) to produce a temporary (usually pleasurable) mental effect. Sometimes the two categories overlap. Morphine may be prescribed as a medical treatment for relief of pain; self-administered by an otherwise healthy person, it gives an impermanent sense of well-being. Some drugs – morphine is one – are strongly addictive and harmful. Even such "innocent" substances as tea and coffee may be not only addictive, but capable of doing harm to some people. The following list of commonly used drugs does not include caffeine, alcohol, nicotine, or minor tranquillizers (such as Valium), all of which are discussed elsewhere.

Type of drug	What it does	Outward signs of use	Some long-term effects
Amphetamines, including methedrine and dexamphetamine (often called pep pills or speed).	Speeds up physical and mental processes, producing extreme energy and unusual excitement.	Weight loss, dilated pupils, insomnia, diarrhoea, trembling.	Paranoia and violent behaviour; possible death from an overdose.
Barbiturates (often called downers).	Produces extreme lethargy and drowsiness.	Slurred and confused speech, lack of physical coordination and balance.	Disruption of normal sleeping pattern; double vision; possible death from an overdose, especially in conjunction with alcohol; often ulcers at injection site.
Cannabis, including marijuana and hashish (often called dope, hash, or grass).	Relaxes the mind and body, heightens perception, and brings on mood swings.	Red eyes, dilated pupils, lack of physical coordination, lethargy, sometimes obvious nausea.	Long-term physical effects uncertain; possible psychological damage through dependence.
Cocaine (often called snow).	Stimulates nervous system, producing heightened sensations and sometimes hallucinations.	Dilated pupils, trembling, apparent intoxication, hallucinations, and insomnia.	Ulceration of nasal passages if drug is "sniffed"; generalized itching, producing open sores.
Opiates, including opium, morphine, heroin, methadone, pethidine.	Relieves physical and mental pain, producing temporary euphoria.	Weight loss, lethargy, mood swings, sweating, slurred speech, sore eyes, and pallor.	Loss of appetite leading to malnutrition; extreme susceptibility to infection; amenorrhoea in women; usually death from an overdose of the highly addictive drug.
Psychedelic drugs, including lysergic acid (LSD) and mescaline (often called acid).	Unpredictable. Usually produces hallucinations, which may be pleasant or frightening.	Dilated pupils, sweating, trembling, altered behaviour, sometimes fever and chills.	Possible irresponsible behaviour; although apparently not addictive, a single dose may cause long-term psychological upset.
Volatile substances (inhaled fumes of, for example, glue and cleaning fluids).	Produces hallucinations, dizziness, temporary euphoria, and sometimes unconsciousness.	Obvious confusion, dilated pupils, flushed face.	Risk of brain, liver, or kidney damage; possible suffocation from inhalation.

physically and emotionally. The large amounts *tolerated* by a long-term addict would kill someone taking them for the first time. If the addict's need for the drug is unsatisfied, intense *anxiety* (p.300), along with other physical and psychological effects, known as withdrawal symptoms, will result.

What are the symptoms?

Every type of drug produces its own kind of mental and physical symptoms (see the table *Drugs and their effects*, opposite). In general, though, any addiction is likely to cause a gradual deterioration of the addict's standards of work and personal relationships. The behaviour of addicts is often erratic and their moods changeable, with periods of restlessness and irritability perhaps alternating with extreme drowsiness. There is often loss of appetite, and the sufferer may seem unreasonably tired and surly. If someone close to you has some of the above symptoms, they do not necessarily indicate drug addiction. But if, in addition, he or she spends increasing amounts of time away from home and seems to be always out of funds without an obvious reason, you may well have good cause for suspicion.

How common is the problem?

There are no reliable statistics on the number of drug addicts in this country. We know, however, that more than 50 per cent of all people charged with offences involving drugs are in the 17 to 24 age group, and that twice as many men as women are involved.

What are the risks?

Hard drugs taken habitually will violently upset the body's chemical system. In extreme cases the end result is serious physical or mental illness, or even death.

What should be done?

Anyone addicted to a drug is in need of help, but addicts are unlikely to seek help unless they have become desperate. If you have cause for concern about yourself or anyone else, consult your doctor or get in touch with an organization such as *Release* or the *Samaritans* (p.768).

What is the treatment?

Self-help: None is possible for severe addiction. If you seem to be becoming dependent on regular doses of some prescribed drug such as a tranquillizer, do not hesitate to speak to your doctor about the matter. The doctor will either allay your fear of possible addiction or will recommend appropriate measures to break the habit.

Professional help: Hospital treatment, if possible in a special drug unit, is essential for addicts. The addictive drug is withheld from the sufferer either immediately or gradually, according to the severity of withdrawal symptoms. Once the addict is free of withdrawal effects, the second stage of treatment consists of an attempt to prevent renewed addiction by means of *psychotherapy* and *occupational therapy*. But it is not easy to "kick" a drug habit permanently. Before discharge from hospital, "cured" addicts are usually offered temporary accommodation in a reliable new environment and advised to break with drug-taking friends and form new relationships. On discharge from hospital, addicts determined to remain healthy often join *SCODA* (the *Standing Conference on Drug Abuse*), an organization of former addicts (p.768).

Addictive gambling

There are many kinds of relatively harmless mental addiction – watching old films on TV, for example, or collecting autographs or old china – but some can be extremely harmful. Perhaps the most common such addiction is obsessive gambling. Obsessive gambling is an addiction, not a *compulsion* (p.301), in that gambling gives pleasure to the gambler, whereas a need for pleasure is not an important element in most compulsive activities. Obsessive gamblers are people who cannot resist the pleasurable excitement of, for example, a card game, the roulette table, or betting on sports events. Unlike most of us who enjoy an occasional fling, they no longer play primarily in order to win. Their gambling is an addiction because they cannot resist the constant repetition of periods of exciting tension that gambling provides. As a result, many obsessive gamblers gamble so recklessly that they bring financial ruin upon themselves and their families.

This addiction is more common than is generally recognized. It affects many more men than women (the ratio is about 20 to 1).

What should be done?

If you have an obsessive gambler in your family, try to get him or her to seek help from *Gamblers Anonymous* (p.768). If your addicted relative refuses to do so, you yourself should consult an organization called *Gam-Anon* (p.768), which has been set up to advise the families of addicts.

Eye disorders

Introduction

By far the most important of the five main senses is sight. Your eyes tell you much more about the world around you than your other senses do; and the part of the brain that deals with sight is far larger than the parts of the brain dealing with the other senses.

The eye is a complex, intricate, and fairly delicate structure (see the diagram opposite). Each eyeball is a sphere about 25mm (1in) in diameter. The outer part of the eyeball consists of three concentric layers of tissue. The tough outermost layer, the sclera, is visible as the white of the eye. Its exposed surface at the front of the eye has a transparent covering, the conjunctiva, which also lines the inner surface of the eyelids. At the front of the eye the sclera and conjunctiva give way to the cornea, a dome-shaped, transparent structure sometimes called the "window" of the eye.

Beneath the sclera is the choroid, a layer rich in blood vessels that supply the outer half of the retina (see below) with oxygen and nutrients. Towards the front of the eye the choroid thickens to form the ciliary body. From the front of the ciliary body extends a circular area of muscular fibres, the iris, whose colour varies from person to person. In the centre of the iris is a hole, the pupil, which is seen as a black disc. Through this, light enters the eye. The amount of light is controlled by the contraction or dilation (enlargement) of the pupil – a process regulated by the muscles of the iris. Immediately behind the iris and pupil is a transparent, elastic lens, which is attached to the ciliary body. Muscles in the ciliary body thicken or narrow the lens, to focus the eye on objects at varying distances. The space between the cornea and lens is filled with a watery transparent substance called aqueous humour. Behind the lens, and constituting the bulk of the eyeball, is a transparent jelly-like substance, vitreous humour.

The third, innermost layer, the retina, lines the rear three-quarters of the eyeball. The retina includes a layer of light-sensitive nerve cells, the rods and cones (so-called because of their shape). Light passes through the pupil and lens to the retina, forming an upside-down image of whatever you are looking at. The rods are very sensitive to light intensity and enable you to see in dim light; the cones detect colour and fine detail. Between them, the rods and cones (of which there are around 125 million and 7 million respectively in each eye) transform the sensations of colour, form, and light intensity that they receive into nerve impulses. These impulses are then transmitted along retinal nerve fibres to the optic nerve, a stalk-like collection of nerves connecting the rear of the eyeball to the brain. (The area where the optic nerve leaves the retina is known as the optic disc.) The brain then interprets the impulses received from the eyes.

The eye disorders covered in this section are dealt with in four groups. The first consists of errors of refraction – problems such as short sight and long sight. The second group is concerned with disorders of those parts of the eye you can see – chiefly the eyelids, eyelashes, sclera, iris, and lens. The third group deals with two forms of the disease glaucoma, which arise from a fault in the drainage of aqueous humour. The final group is concerned with disorders affecting the structures towards the rear of the eye – primarily the retina and its blood supply, but also the muscles and other tissues that surround the eyeball in its bony socket, known as the orbit.

Drugs and the eye

Drugs used to treat existing eye conditions can have side-effects that also affect the eye. Although most such side-effects are inconvenient rather than dangerous, some can be serious and may, in some cases, cause *cataract* (p.319), *glaucoma* (p.320), or even, rarely, blindness. For this reason, drugs used to treat eye conditions should only be administered by an expert.

The eyes can also be affected by some drugs used to treat general disorders. For example, *steroids* can cause cataract, while tranquillizers taken by old people may precipitate acute glaucoma. Such side-effects do not occur in all cases, but should be suspected if you are taking drugs for some other disorder and find that you are beginning to suffer from eye problems.

The eye

The diagram (below) shows the main parts of the eye in horizontal cross-section. The bony socket is not shown.

Ciliary body and muscle

Sclera

Choroid

Retina

Conjunctiva

Iris

Cornea

Pupil

Aqueous humour

Lens

Optic nerve

Vitreous humour

Image reception

When the eye focuses on an object, the image projected through the pupil on to the retina is upside down and back to front. The brain then interprets the image in terms of the real world.

Object

Cornea

Lens

Image focused on retina

Stereoscopic vision (below)

Each eye sees a slightly different view of the same object, and it is the brain that coordinates the 2 views that it receives, to form a 3-dimensional, "solid" image of the object in view.

Image received by left eye

Image received by right eye

Brain

Combined 3D image

Colour blindness

All the colours we see are made up of combinations of the 3 colours red, green, and blue in the light rays that enter our eyes. Cells in the retina called *cones* each contain a light-sensitive substance that responds to one of these colours. But in people with defects of colour vision there is either a partial or complete lack of one or more of the light-sensitive substances in the cones.

Colour blindness is the popular but incorrect term for the very common condition of being unable to distinguish between certain colours. Literal colour blindness – seeing everything in shades of grey – is extremely rare.

The most common defect is an inability to distinguish in dim light between reds and greens. In clear light the colours are seen normally; many colour-blind people believe that everyone sees these colours in the same

way they do in dim light, and so are unaware that they have a defect unless tested for colour vision. The second most common defect is to have the same inability even in clear light. Anyone who has this condition will almost certainly be aware of it and will have learned how to deal with the problem as it affects daily life. For example, red and green on traffic lights are distinguished by their position.

Defects of colour vision affect 8 per cent of the male population, only 0.5 per cent of females. The defects are almost always hereditary and therefore present from birth (rarely they can result from an eye disease later in life), and are passed on only by women. There is no cure for colour blindness; but it is a condition that does not seriously interfere with daily life.

Errors of refraction

Refraction
The eye focuses on an object with both its cornea and its lens. Each of these acts as a convex lens and bends ("refracts") the light rays received in order to direct them on to the retina. If the eyeball is small, hypermetropia (long sight) may result; if it is too large, myopia (short sight) is a problem.

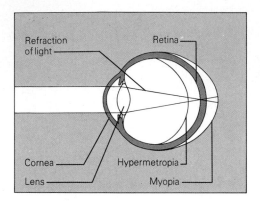

The way that light from objects is focused through the eye into an image on the retina is called refraction. In a normal eye, light reflected from what you are looking at is brought to a focus exactly on the retina by a process called accommodation, and a clear image is seen. In some eyes, however, light is focused either behind or in front of the retina, so that the image is blurred.

The four most common disorders of refraction are short sight (myopia), long sight (hypermetropia), astigmatism, and presbyopia. Unlike the first three, presbyopia always affects both eyes equally.

Short sight
(*myopia*)

Correcting short sight
In short sight, the light rays refracted from a distant object through the cornea and lens are focused short of the retina, producing a blurred image. A concave lens held in front of the eye corrects the error.

Medical myth

Too much reading causes short sight.

Wrong. There is no medical evidence for this.

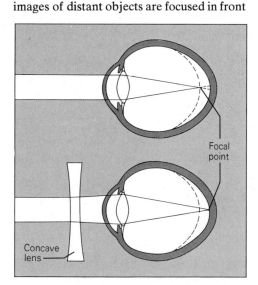

In short sight the eye is too long from front to back or, less usually, the focusing power of the cornea and lens is too great. As a result, images of distant objects are focused in front of the retina and are blurred. Near objects, however, are seen clearly. In short sight, the eye cannot counteract blurring as it sometimes can in *long sight* (below).

Short sight is very common; about 1 person in 6 is affected by the problem. It usually develops during late childhood and may worsen until about the age of 20. The condition tends to run in families.

What should be done?
If you think you are short-sighted, consult an optician (see *Going to the optician*, p.312). If, after tests, your suspicion is confirmed, the optician will prescribe spectacles (or contact lenses) with concave (inwardly curved) lenses. These will move images of distant objects back on to the retina and bring them into clear focus.

Once you have reached the age of 20 or thereabouts, short sight is unlikely to get much worse; but you should visit your optician every two years or so to enable any subsequent changes to be detected.

Long sight
(*hypermetropia*)

In long sight the eye is too short from front to back. Or, less commonly, there is a weakness in focusing by the cornea and lens. In either case, images of objects at any distance are focused behind the retina and so the images that are received by the brain appear blurred. Images of near objects are even more blurred, and so close vision (such as reading) is often severely affected.

Long sight is generally present from birth and is usually diagnosed after a child has

complained of eye fatigue; like *short sight* (above) it tends to run in families.

What are the symptoms?
Many people with mild long sight have no symptoms. Others suffer from eyestrain (aching or discomfort in the eye), because they constantly have to use the ciliary muscles to focus and see clearly. People with moderate to severe long sight have continuous blurred vision and may also have eyestrain. Neither

Correcting long sight
In long sight, the focal point of the image received is beyond the retina. A convex lens held in front of the eye reinforces the eye's own convex lens and focuses the image on the retina.

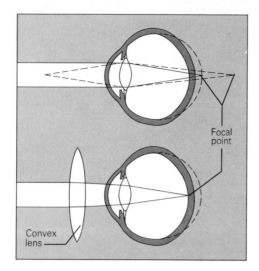

Focal point

Convex lens

symptom can permanently damage vision although it is advisable to obtain treatment early, before a child's education suffers.

What should be done?
If you suffer from blurred vision or eyestrain, visit an optician (see *Going to the optician*, p.312). If the optician establishes that you have long sight, he or she will prescribe for you spectacles (or contact lenses) with convex (outwardly curved) lenses. These reinforce the focusing power of the cornea and lens of your eye and enable you to see clearly, so removing any eyestrain.

What are the long-term prospects?
With increasing age, the ciliary muscles may weaken, and as a result you may need stronger lenses every few years.

Presbyopia

At rest, a normal eye is focused for distance vision. To enable the eye to focus on closer objects, the ciliary muscles contract and so thicken the lens, a process known as accommodation. With age, the lens of the eye hardens, and consequently its ability to change shape to focus on near objects is gradually reduced. This deterioration in the elasticity of the lens is called presbyopia.

What are the symptoms?
The condition is usually first noticed in the mid-40s and becomes increasingly pronounced. If it is uncorrected, you can read printed matter only by holding it further and further from your eyes, until eventually it cannot be made out even at arm's length. People with *short sight* (opposite) may notice that they need to take their spectacles off to read print at normal distance.

What should be done?
If you find that nearby objects appear slightly blurred unless you hold them at arm's length, you should consult an optician (see *Going to the optician*, p.312).

What is the treatment?
If you have presbyopia, the optician will prescribe spectacles with convex (outwardly curved) lenses to reinforce the power of the natural lenses of your eyes and enable you to see near objects clearly.

What are the long-term prospects?
Every few years, you will need slightly stronger spectacles, to compensate for the decreasing power of your natural lenses.

If you also have *long sight* (opposite), short sight, or *astigmatism* (p.313), and as a result are already wearing spectacles for distance vision, you can, to avoid the need for two pairs of spectacles, have a pair of bifocals. One part of each lens is for distance viewing, the other part for close-to vision.

Treatment for presbyopia
The treatment for people whose eyesight was normal until they developed presbyopia is the same as for those who are longsighted – convex lenses to reinforce the eyes' own lenses.

Focal point

Convex lens

Bifocal lenses
A bifocal lens is a combination of 2 lenses – the lower lens enables you to see near objects clearly and the upper lens, distant objects.

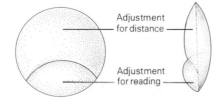

Adjustment for distance

Adjustment for reading

Going to the optician

Why should you go?

It is not only people with defective vision who should visit an optician; even if there is nothing apparently wrong with your eyes, you should have regular sight tests – ideally, once every 2 years. This is because some serious eye diseases, such as certain types of glaucoma (which can cause blindness), are symptomless in the early stages and can be detected at their onset only by an eye examination; with early detection they can then be treated and cured.

Any sudden, serious changes in eyesight should be reported immediately to your doctor, not an optician.

Where do you go?

You go either to a doctor called an ophthalmic medical practitioner, at an NOTB (National Ophthalmic Treatment Board) medical eye centre, normally located at a dispensing optician's; or to an ophthalmic optician. You can go straight to either; you do not need to be referred to them by your doctor.

Lists of NOTB medical eye centres and ophthalmic opticians can be obtained from the telephone directory (NOTB centres under "Medical", opticians in the yellow pages), or from main post offices, libraries, or the offices of your local Family Practitioner Committee (see *General practice*, p.729).

What does the optician do?

The doctor or optician tests your sight in various ways. He or she will test the sharpness (*acuity*) of your vision by asking you to read the 8 rows of letters on a Snellen chart. The result is given as 2 figures. The first refers to the distance in metres – usually 6m (about 20 feet) at which you are asked to read the letters. The second figure refers to the lowermost row of letters that you were able to read correctly, and indicates the optimum distance in metres at which a person with normal vision could read that row. So the result 6/12 means that the lowest row of letters you were able to read at a distance of 6m was one that a person with normal vision could read at 12m. (This result of 6/12 is the equivalent of the minimum acuity of vision required for driving a private car.)

The doctor or optician also looks at each eye through an instrument called an *ophthalmoscope*. With this, the backs of the eyes can be examined to see if you have any internal eye disorder, such as *glaucoma* (p.320) or *retinal detachment* (p.324), or whether there are signs of any general disorder, such as high

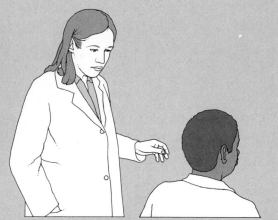

blood pressure or diabetes. In addition, the examiner may also test the balance of the muscles that control the movements of the eyes, to detect any *squint* (p.327).

If the examiner discovers a disorder of refraction, spectacles or contact lenses may be prescribed. If a more serious eye disorder or a general disorder has been detected, you will be given a note to take to your GP.

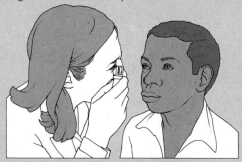

How do you obtain your spectacles?

If your test reveals that you need spectacles, you are given a prescription to hand to the dispensing or ophthalmic optician on the premises or to take to an optician elsewhere. The optician takes the necessary measurements of your eyes and head, and you choose the type of lenses (glass or plastic) and frame you want. (Plastic lenses are lighter than glass, and are safer for those engaged in a lot of physical activity; but they scratch more easily.)

Spectacles take about 2 to 3 weeks to be made up. When you return to the optician to collect them, any necessary adjustments to the frame can usually be made on the premises. You wear them for a trial period, and if you find the lenses are not satisfactory, you will be tested again. For information on contact lenses see opposite.

Snellen chart
The letters on a Snellen chart (named after its inventor) are a standard size and meant to be read from a distance of 6m (approximately 20ft).

Examining the eye
The optician examines the back of your eye by shining the light from an ophthalmoscope through the pupil. A series of lenses in the ophthalmoscope allows the optician to estimate roughly the strength of the lenses needed to correct any refractive errors.

Astigmatism

Astigmatism is distorted vision caused by uneven curvature of the cornea. Vertical but not horizontal lines are in focus, or vice versa, depending on which rays of light are bent by the irregular curvature. Diagonal lines may also be out of focus. Astigmatism usually occurs in conjunction with *short sight* or *long sight* (p.310). It is usually present from birth and does not grow worse with age.

Medical myth

Watching too much television or working for a long time in poor light can harm the eyes.

Wrong. Extensive use of healthy eyes can never damage them, just as extensive walking cannot damage the legs.

What should be done?

If you suspect your vision is not normal, visit an optician (see *Going to the optician,* opposite). If tests establish you have astigmatism, the optician will prescribe spectacle lenses shaped to the curvature required to correct the unevenness of the cornea. Such lenses are called cylindrical lenses because of their shape. These will enable you to see normally.

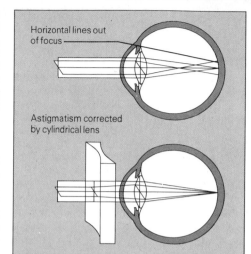

Horizontal lines out of focus

Astigmatism corrected by cylindrical lens

Contact lenses

Contact lenses are an alternative to spectacles. They have become very popular in recent years, especially among sportspeople and those who do not want to wear spectacles for reasons of appearance.

Each contact lense is a circular plastic lens that fits snugly over the front of the eye, to correct any errors of refraction. There are two types of contact lens: the hard lens, which is made of a plastic that is tough and hard-wearing but which some people do not find comfortable to wear; and the soft lens, which is often more comfortable but which becomes scratched and worn more easily.

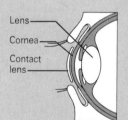

Contact lens

Lens

Cornea

Contact lens

Contact lenses, placed directly on the cornea, perform the same function as spectacle lenses.

How do you obtain contact lenses?

Contact lenses cannot be obtained on the National Health Service unless a hospital specialist prescribes them. You must pay for them privately. It is always wise to insure them against loss or damage.

To set about trying to obtain contact lenses, you should, in the first instance, have a private sight test at a medical eye centre or ophthalmic optician's. At the test it will be decided, first, whether your eyes are suitable for contact lenses (if you have hay fever, for example, they may not be), and then, if they are suitable, whether you should wear hard lenses or soft ones. Once you are wearing contact lenses permanently, you will be advised to see the lens specialist once a year for a check-up.

Inserting contact lenses

With clean hands, rinse your contact lenses thoroughly when you take them out of their storage solution.

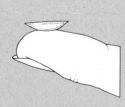

Place a lens, lubricated with wetting agent, cup side up on the tip of your forefinger.

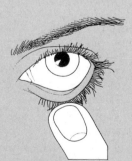

Hold your lower lid down or both lids well apart with the fingers of the other hand.

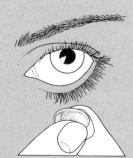

Look straight ahead or directly at the contact lens as you bring it up towards your eye.

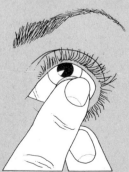

Place the lens gently over the cornea. Look downwards and then release your lids.

Eyelids and the front of the eye

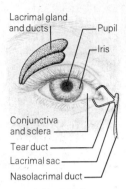

Lacrimal gland
and ducts
Pupil
Iris
Conjunctiva
and sclera
Tear duct
Lacrimal sac
Nasolacrimal duct

The visible eye represents only about one-tenth of the surface area of the entire eyeball. The eyelids act as protective covers for this segment of the eye. Muscles in the lids open and close them, and act with fibrous tissue in the lids to keep them taut against the eyeball. The lid margins and the eyelashes are lubricated by a row of small glands, called the meibomian glands, on each lid margin.

The exposed surface of the eye (except for the cornea) and the inner surface of each lid are lined by a sensitive transparent membrane called the conjunctiva. They are also covered by a thin film of watery fluid called tears, produced by the lacrimal glands above each eyeball. Apart from being a physical sign of emotion, tears have two main functions: to lubricate the eye so that the lids can move over it smoothly, and to wash away foreign bodies. Tears drain away from each eye along two tear ducts. A tiny hole at the inner end of both lid margins marks the opening of these ducts. The ducts lead to the lacrimal sac at the side of the nose, and from the sac the tears pass down the much larger nasolacrimal duct into the nose.

Ptosis

See p.247,
**Visual aids to
diagnosis, 63.**

Drooping eyelid
Consult your doctor if a previously normal upper eyelid starts to droop and partially cover the eye. This may be a symptom of an underlying muscular disorder such as myaesthenia gravis.

Drooping of the upper eyelid so that it partially or completely covers the eye is known as ptosis. It is due to weakness of the muscle that raises the lid. Ptosis may be present from birth, but can develop at any age if damage occurs to the nerve controlling the lid muscle or to the muscle itself. The nerve can be affected by injury or by one of several diseases, including *diabetes mellitus* (p.519) and *aneurysms* (p.407) within the skull. Muscle damage can be caused by muscular diseases such as *myaesthenia gravis* (p.540). In all these cases, ptosis may affect one or both eyes and may vary in severity during the course of the day. Finally, ptosis may occur as old age weakens the muscles of one or both of the upper eyelids. Ptosis can often be accompanied by double vision.

Ptosis can be unsightly, and if severe it will block the vision of the affected eye. In children this may lead to the development of a "lazy" eye (see *Squint in children*, p.674).

Always consult a doctor about ptosis. Successful treatment of any underlying disease may cure the disorder. In other cases, either an operation to strengthen the muscle may be carried out or, if an operation is inadvisable, the lid can be kept raised by a support incorporated into spectacles or a contact lens.

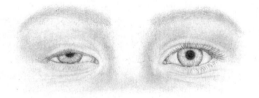

Stye

See p.246,
**Visual aids to
diagnosis, 53.**

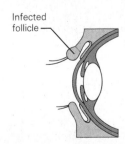

Infected
follicle

Like all hairs, eyelashes grow from follicles – pits in the skin. It is quite common for one of these to become infected. Such an infection is usually caused by a staphylococcus bacterium. When this happens, a red, painful swelling like a *boil* (p.251) develops on the lid margin, around the base of the eyelash. A white head of pus appears on the swelling, which is known as a stye (sometimes also called a hordeolum); within a few days it bursts, relieving the pain and causing the loss of the eyelash.

The stye subsides about seven days after it first appeared and the eyelid returns to normal. However, styes often recur within a short period, and sometimes several styes may develop on the lids at the same time. In both cases, this is probably because the bacteria that caused the initial stye have spread and infected other eyelash follicles.

What should be done?
You can hasten the relief of pain by making the stye burst early. As soon as the inflammation appears, apply hot compresses to it three times a day. Do this by wrapping a clean pad around a wooden spoon, dipping it in hot water, and pressing the back of the spoon gently on the stye. When these applications draw the pus to a head, pull out the eyelash and the pus will be released. Wash the eye carefully to ensure that all the pus is removed.

If styes keep recurring, see your doctor, who may decide you need an *antibiotic*.

Lumps on the eyelid

See p.246,
Visual aids to diagnosis, 57–58.

The most common kinds of lump that can develop on the eyelid are *styes* (opposite), chalazions, papillomas, and xanthelasma.

A chalazion (sometimes called a meibomian *cyst*) is a painless swelling on the lid margin. It is caused by the blockage of one of the meibomian glands, which lubricate the lid margin. Small chalazions usually disappear naturally within a month or two. You can speed up the process yourself by gently massaging the lid towards the margin and so emptying the gland of its blocked-up material. Larger chalazions, which may grow to the size of a small pea, often do not disappear spontaneously and are then treated surgically. An incision is made in the eyelid from the inside and the contents of the chalazion are removed. This is done in a hospital outpatient department and requires only a local anaesthetic. A chalazion can become infected, in which case it will become more swollen, red, and painful. In many cases it will disappear of its own accord. If not, an incision will need to be made in the eyelid to enable the pus to drain away.

A papilloma is a harmless outgrowth of skin, ranging in colour from pink to black, anywhere on the eyelid or lid margin. It may increase in size very slowly. If it is unsightly it can be removed surgically after you have been given a local anaesthetic.

Xanthelasma consists of yellow patches of fatty material that accumulate beneath the outer skin of the lids, especially near the nose. Rarely they may be a feature of an inherited abnormality of body *metabolism* (see *Hyperlipidaemia*, p.499) but in most cases the condition is harmless. If the patches are unsightly they can be removed, but even then they may recur some time later.

Other less common lumps which may occur on the lid include a form of *birthmark* (p.652) called an angioma, and a skin growth known as a *rodent ulcer* (p.258).

Entropion

(in-turned eyelashes)

See p.247,
Visual aids to diagnosis, 59.

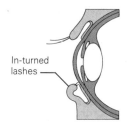

In-turned lashes

This is a condition in which the lid margin of the lower eyelid turns inwards so that the lashes rub on the surface of the eyeball – the conjunctiva and cornea. This causes irritation and may result in *conjunctivitis* (p.317) or *corneal ulcers* (p.316). Persistent entropion can permanently damage the cornea and affect vision. Entropion of the upper lids does occur but it is unusual for it to be found in temperate climates.

How common is the problem?
The condition affects chiefly old people. The fibrous tissue in the lower lids becomes lax, allowing the muscle in the lid margin to contract excessively and pull the margin in on the eye. Occasionally, entropion occurs at any age, when it is not caused by muscle laxity but by a pre-existing problem causing constant irritation of the eye (as in conjunctivitis) that causes the lids to be screwed up.

What should be done?
If there has been any pre-existing irritation of the eye, see your doctor to have it treated. Otherwise, turn the lid outwards and keep it in this position by attaching one end of a piece of adhesive plaster to the skin beneath the lower lashes and the other end to the cheek. After a few days remove the plaster and see if the condition clears up of its own accord. If the disorder does not clear up using this method, consult your doctor, who may arrange for you to have a minor operation of the eyelid (usually under a local anaesthetic) to treat the problem.

Ectropion

(out-turned eyelashes)

See p.247,
Visual aids to diagnosis, 60.

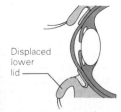

Displaced lower lid

In ectropion the lower lid hangs away from the eyeball, so that the lower half of the exposed surface of the eyeball and the lining of the lower lid become dry and sore. In addition, the tears lubricating the lining of the upper lid and the front of the eye may be prevented from entering the tear duct in the lower lid – and they then run down the cheek.

How common is the problem?
Ectropion is usually a complaint of old age. The muscle in the lower lid that keeps the lid taut against the eyeball becomes weak. The condition can also be caused at any age by a scar on the lower lid or cheek that has contracted and pulled down the lid.

What are the risks?
If ectropion is untreated, *corneal ulcers* (p.316) may develop on the exposed cornea and damage it permanently.

What should be done?
The condition rarely disappears of its own accord, and you should see your doctor, who may arrange for you to have an operation on the tissues beneath the eye. This is a minor procedure requiring a local anaesthetic.

Blepharitis

Blepharitis is an inflammation of the lid margins that causes a persistent and unsightly redness and scaliness of the skin on and around the margins. The disorder is often associated with seborrhoeic eczema (p.253) of the scalp and eyebrows, and the flakes of skin resemble the flakes from dandruff. In some cases, bacteria infect the area and make the condition worse.

In bad cases, small ulcers may develop on the lid margins, and eyelashes may fall out. Often flakes of skin from the lid margin enter the eye and cause *conjunctivitis* (opposite).

What should be done?

Try treating the condition yourself by washing away the scales, morning and night, with a cotton-tipped applicator soaked in warm salt water or a warm solution of sodium bicarbonate. Washing the scalp with an anti-dandruff shampoo can also help. If this does not improve the condition within two weeks, consult your doctor, who may prescribe a combined *antibiotic* and *steroid* ointment for you to rub into the lid margins after washing. Blepharitis is a disorder that often recurs and needs repeated treatment.

Dry eye

This condition is due to a deficiency of tear production by the lacrimal glands. The white of the eye becomes red, and the eye feels gritty. Usually both eyes are affected. Dry eye may occur in people with *rheumatoid arthritis* (p.552), but in many instances it occurs for no known reason.

The condition is most common in middle age and affects women more than men. There is usually no threat to sight, but the condition can be extremely irritating.

What is the treatment?

To relieve the discomfort, your doctor will prescribe artificial tear drops for you to apply to your eye whenever they seem necessary. In a few cases this treatment may need to be continued for life.

Watering eye

Continuous watering of the eye is usually caused by a blockage in the ducts that drain tears from the eye into the nose. Sometimes blockage follows injury to the bone at the side of the nose, sometimes it is caused by repeated swelling of the lining of the ducts and lacrimal sac, as in long-standing *sinusitis* (p.347), but often the cause is unknown. One or both eyes can be affected.

Blockage of the tear duct can lead to infection of the lacrimal sac. This causes a red and painful swelling in the skin beside the nose. In some babies, the tear duct has failed to open up and watering and discharge may start to occur soon after birth.

Watering eye due to blockage is uncommon. It usually occurs in middle age or later.

What should be done?

If your eye keeps watering, see your doctor. The doctor will probably refer you to an eye specialist, who will carry out tests to discover the cause of the trouble. If the tear ducts are found to be blocked and the condition is in an early stage, the ducts can sometimes be cleared by syringeing.

If blockage of the tear duct is at too advanced a stage for syringeing to clear it and the symptoms are very troublesome, you will need an operation to create an artificial duct that bypasses the blockage. If the lacrimal sac is infected, you may have to take a course of *antibiotics* to settle the infection before treatment is attempted. (A probe is used to open up a closed duct in an infant.)

Corneal ulcers and infections

See p.246,
Visual aids to diagnosis, 54.

The cornea, a transparent section of the eye's outer covering at the very front of the eye, is, because of its position, the part of the eyeball most susceptible to injury and infection.

When an ulcer (an open sore) occurs on the cornea, infection often follows, and vice versa. When an ulcer forms first, it is usually the result of a foreign body striking or scratching the cornea; the ulcer then becomes infected by bacteria. When an infection occurs first, it is very often a virus that is responsible – usually herpes simplex, the virus that also produces *cold sores* (p.451) around the mouth. (For this reason, if you have a cold sore never put your fingers to your eyes after touching your mouth.)

In nearly all cases, only one eye is affected.

What are the symptoms?

You experience discomfort or pain in the eye (because the cornea is well supplied with *sensory* nerves), the white of the eye becomes pink or red, and your sharpness of vision is impaired to a degree dependent on the size of

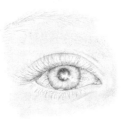

A corneal ulcer caused by bacteria may sometimes be visible as a white patch on the cornea.

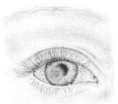

A dendritic ulcer of the cornea (usually caused by the herpes simplex virus) is invisible unless stained.

the ulcer. In cases of bacterial infection you can sometimes see the ulcer, if you look at the eye closely in a mirror, as a whitish patch. Herpes simplex infection produces what is called a dendritic ulcer, which has a branching pattern and is extremely difficult to see with the naked eye.

Symptoms are much more pronounced in bacterial than in viral infections.

How common is the problem?
Each year about 1 person in 1,000 suffers from a corneal ulcer infection. Many of those affected are people engaged in work such as metal grinding, which exposes their eyes to a spray of flying particles.

What are the risks?
If an ulcer is not treated promptly, a scar can form on the cornea and perhaps reduce vision if the centre of the cornea is affected. A neglected ulcer may *perforate* the cornea, cause pain and loss of vision, and allow infection to enter the eyeball with the consequent risk of loss of the eye.

What should be done?
Always wear protective goggles or a mask when engaged in grinding, hammering, or similar work, to protect your eyes from flying particles. Because of the serious risks involved, see your doctor as soon as possible if you suspect a corneal ulcer or infection. If the doctor suspects herpes simplex infection, he or she will apply drops that stain and reveal any dendritic ulcer present.

What is the treatment?
Ulcers caused by injury to the cornea and the bacterial infections that often follow them are treated with *antibiotics*, given as drops, ointment, tablets, or injections near the eye. For viral infections and the ulcers they produce, antiviral drops and ointments are prescribed. Dendritic ulcers tend to recur.

If scars from ulceration drastically reduce vision, you may need a corneal transplant – an operation to graft a new cornea on to the eye (see *Transplants*, p.402). If an ulcer has perforated the cornea, immediate surgery will be required to seal off the hole.

Conjunctivitis

See p.246, **Visual aids to diagnosis, 55.**

Conjunctivitis is inflammation of the conjunctiva, a transparent membrane that lines the eyelids and the outer eye up to the edge of the cornea. The disorder can be caused by an infection or an allergy.

An infection is usually caught from contaminated fingers, towels, or face cloths. However, in babies up to about three days old it may have been caught from the mother's birth canal; this condition, known as ophthalamia neonatorum, is serious.

What are the symptoms?
In all cases of infective conjunctivitis, the white of the eye turns red and feels sore. There is then a discharge of yellow pus from the eye. Overnight this glues the eyelashes together and forms a crust. Bacterial infection usually affects both eyes and produces a marked discharge, whereas viral infection is usually limited to just one eye and causes only a slight discharge.

Allergic conjunctivitis is caused by an allergy to pollen, cosmetics, or other substances. There is usually a long-standing redness and itchiness of the white of the eye, without, however, any discharge of pus; the form that occurs in children and young adults all year round, but more severely in the pollen season, is known as spring catarrh (see *Allergic rhinitis*, p.345). Less commonly, there is a sudden puffiness of the conjunctiva – usually during the pollen season – which disappears after a few hours.

Conjunctivitis is very common. Each year about 1 person in 50 visits a doctor because of it. It is a troublesome disorder but, except in the case of ophthalamia neonatorum, not usually serious.

What should be done?
If you suspect conjunctivitis, see your doctor without delay. If the symptoms are those of infective conjunctivitis, avoid spreading the disease: wash your hands after you have touched your eyes, and have your own separate face cloth and towel.

What is the treatment?
In cases of infective conjunctivitis caused by bacteria, your doctor will prescribe *antibiotic* drops or ointment to be applied to your eyes after you have bathed away any discharge from the lids with warm water. One or two weeks of this treatment should clear up the condition. Viral infections usually disappear spontaneously, though in some cases they last for several weeks. A child with ophthalamia neonatorum will be treated in hospital with antibiotic drops.

If you can identify the cause of allergic conjunctivitis, it may be possible to treat it using *antihistamine* eye drops, which you can obtain without a prescription.

Episcleritis

Surrounding the eyeball is a transparent tissue called the episclera. At the front of the eye it lies between the sclera (the white of the eye) and the conjunctiva (the transparent membrane overlying the sclera). In some young adults the tiny blood vessels in the episclera become inflamed.

What are the symptoms?
The symptoms of episcleritis are a diffused or patchy redness over the white of the eye and a feeling of slight discomfort in the eye. One or both eyes may be affected. The condition is not serious and usually disappears of its own accord after a week or two – though it may recur from time to time.

What is the treatment?
Natural healing of the inflammation can be hastened by anti-inflammatory drugs which will be prescribed by your doctor, either as eye drops or ointment.

Scleritis

Scleritis is inflammation of the sclera, the tough outer coat of the eyeball that you can see as the white of the eye. The inflammation often accompanies *rheumatoid arthritis* (p.552) or one of certain disorders of the digestive system, including *Crohn's disease* (p.473). It can affect one or both eyes.

What are the symptoms?
The symptoms are one or more areas of intense redness on the white of the eye – except when the inflammation is at the back of the eye – and a dull pain in the eye. If the back of the eye is inflamed, there may be some loss of vision caused by inflammation of neighbouring structures within the eyeball.

How common is the problem?
Scleritis is an uncommon disorder that occurs mainly in people between about 30 and 60. More women than men are affected and, as well as affecting people who have or have had rheumatoid arthritis, it may occur in those with *ulcerative colitis* (p.480).

What are the risks?
If the condition is not treated, there is a risk that where the sclera is inflamed the tissue will become thinned and possibly *perforated*. It is therefore essential that if you suspect you have scleritis, you see your doctor right away.

What is the treatment?
The inflammation can usually be cleared up in mild or moderate cases with anti-inflammatory drugs, either in tablet form or applied to the eye as drops. In severe cases, *immunosuppressive* drugs will be prescribed. If the sclera has become perforated, surgery will be needed to repair the damage.

Iritis
(anterior uveitis, iridocyclitis)

Iritis is inflammation of the iris. The disorder causes microscopic white cells from the inflamed area, together with an increase in protein leaked from the small blood vessels of the iris, to float in the aqueous humour between the iris and the cornea. If there are a lot of floating cells, they may attach themselves to the back of the cornea or settle to the bottom of the aqueous humour.

The cause of iritis is not known, but the disorder can sometimes occurs in conjunction with one of a range of other diseases, including, for example, *rheumatoid arthritis* (p.552) and *ankylosing spondylitis* (p.553). One or both eyes may be affected.

What are the symptoms?
There is a feeling of discomfort in the eye, which becomes reddened. This is accompanied by a slight reduction in vision. If there is a rise of pressure in the eye, the condition may become painful, although most commonly any symptoms are mild.

How common is the problem?
Iritis is an uncommon disorder. Each year only about 1 person in 2,000 visits a doctor because of the complaint. It affects people of all ages, but is most common in young adults.

What are the risks?
If treated early, iritis is not usually a serious problem. However, if you fail to consult a doctor, then complications are likely to develop. So many white cells may accumulate in the aqueous humour that they block the opening through which the liquid drains out of the eye, causing a type of *glaucoma* (p.320). This complication may also develop if the back of the inflamed iris sticks to the front of the lens and as a result aqueous humour is trapped behind the iris. Long-standing iritis can cause *cataract* (opposite).

What should be done?
At any sign of redness, discomfort, and loss of vision in an eye, however slight, see your

doctor. If you are found to have iritis, the earlier treatment is started the easier it is to clear up an attack and the less likely it is that complications will occur.

What is the treatment?
Steroid eye drops or ointment are given to reduce the inflammation; in more severe cases, a steroid drug may be injected between the conjunctiva and sclera after the use of a local anaesthetic. You will also be given eye drops to enlarge the pupil and so prevent the back of the inflamed iris from sticking to the front of the lens. Any rise in pressure in the eye is controlled by tablets.

Even when treated early, iritis may often recur, though in most cases the disorder eventually disappears completely.

Cataract

A cataract is the gradual clouding up of the jelly-like substance that forms the lens of the eye. The cataract blocks or distorts light entering the eye and so progressively reduces vision; but in some cases the loss of vision never becomes severe enough to warrant treatment. Both eyes are usually affected – in most cases, one is more advanced than the other.

The most common cause of a cataract is deterioration of the lens in old age. Other causes include *iritis* (opposite), injury to the eyeball (when only the injured eye will be affected), *diabetes mellitus* (p.519), and *steroid* drugs taken orally for some other, unrelated, complaint or used in eyedrops over a long period of time. (For further information see *Drugs and the eye*, p.308.) The disorder tends to run in families and in some cases is present from birth or shortly after.

What are the symptoms?
The main symptom in all cases is a lessening or distortion of vision in the affected eye; in some cases this is worse in bright sunlight. Other than in some advanced cases, cataracts cannot easily be seen by an observer; in advanced cases, the lens may become white and opaque and visible through the pupil. Rarely, a very advanced cataract produces painful inflammation and pressure within the eye.

How common is the problem?
Cataracts are fairly common, and you are more likely to have them as you get older and your lenses deteriorate. Each year about 1 person in 500 develops the problem.

See p.247,
Visual aids to diagnosis, 61.

Advanced cataract
A cataract is not a growth but a change in the quality of the lens itself. In severe cases, the whole lens may eventually be affected, making the pupil in front of it look white.

What are the risks?
The disorder may lead to severe deterioration of vision, but this can be rectified at any time by surgery.

What should be done?
If you experience any lessening or distortion and blurring of vision, see an optician. The optician may diagnose a cataract or may not suspect it until glasses fail to improve your vision. In either case, the optician will then refer you to your doctor.

What is the treatment?
The only treatment possible for a cataract is the removal of the diseased lens (this is the most common of all operations on the eye). So if your vision is not too badly affected, your doctor will do nothing but ensure that your optician is providing you with glasses that give you the maximum benefit. Usually a specialist will consider recommending an operation for an adult if both eyes are affected and vision worsens to the extent that performing everyday activities becomes difficult; or if only one eye is affected but you need good vision in both eyes for your job. A fully developed cataract in a baby or young child will be treated as soon as possible to prevent the development of a permanently "lazy" eye (see *Squint in children*, p.674).

Either a general or a local anaesthetic is given for the operation. Usually the entire lens is taken out, but in some cases only the substance within the lens is removed, through a small needle, and the transparent capsule of the lens is left behind. This last procedure is more suitable for children.

Removal of the lens from an eye makes the eye very long-sighted (see *Long sight*, p.310). This is corrected by spectacles, a contact lens, or a plastic lens placed in the eye at the time of the operation. If vision is then not as good as was anticipated, this is usually due to a fault in the retina at the back of the eye, which was obscured before the operation by the opacity of the lens. The most common retinal fault is *macula degeneration* (p.323).

Glaucoma

Glaucoma is one of the most common and severe eye disorders in people over 60. Early treatment is vital, or the condition may eventually lead to blindness.

The ciliary body in the eye is constantly producing a fluid called aqueous humour, which circulates from behind the iris, through the pupil, and into the chamber between the iris and the cornea. In a healthy eye the fluid drains out of the eye through a network of tissue in the drainage angle (the junction of the iris and the cornea) and then into a channel (Schlemm's canal) which leads to small veins on the outside of the eye. But in some eyes the drainage is defective. As a result of the defect, the aqueous humour flows away more slowly than it is produced – or fails to flow away at all – and its pressure builds up within the eyeball.

The pressure causes the collapse, at the back of the eye, of tiny blood vessels whose function is to nourish the nerve fibres of the optic disc. It is these nerve fibres that carry impulses from the eye to the brain. Robbed of blood, the nerve fibres begin to die, and, as they do so, vision begins to fade. The damage to the nerve fibres is irreversible and results in loss of vision from the affected part. For this reason it is important that glaucoma is diagnosed and treated as early as possible, so that loss of vision is kept to a minimum.

The cause, extent, and type of glaucoma vary considerably. (Certain drugs can hasten the onset of the condition; see *Drugs and the eye*, p.308.) The two most common types of the disease, and those described here, are acute glaucoma (also known as angle-closure glaucoma) and chronic simple glaucoma (also known as open-angle glaucoma).

The development of glaucoma

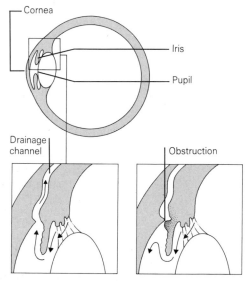

Normally, fluid circulates constantly through the pupil, between the iris and cornea, to be drained into veins via a drainage channel. In glaucoma, the drainage of the fluid becomes obstructed, resulting in a build-up of fluid.

Acute glaucoma

(angle-closure glaucoma)

This is a glaucoma in which the drainage angle between the cornea and the iris becomes blocked suddenly (see *Glaucoma*, above, for a general explanation of how glaucoma occurs). It affects mainly long-sighted elderly people. In long sight the distance between the cornea and iris is shorter than normal, and so the drainage angle is narrower. With age, the lens of the eye gradually enlarges and pushes the iris forward, and this narrows the angle further. In cases of extremely narrowed drainage angle, blockage can then occur at any time. What blocks the angle is the iris when it retracts to enlarge the pupil – either in dim light or during an emotional reaction. Aqueous humour, which is produced in the chamber behind the iris, cannot then drain away, and pressure builds up in the eyeball. The iris may recede from the drainage angle spontaneously, to make the pupil smaller. If it fails to recede and is caught fast in the angle, the pressure in the eyeball continues to mount, causing the symptoms of acute glaucoma.

Usually, only one eye is affected, but the other eye is highly susceptible to an attack at some later date.

What are the symptoms?

In some cases there are short preliminary attacks months or weeks before a fully developed attack of acute glaucoma occurs. The attacks usually happen in the evening, when the light is dim, and last for as long as the iris blocks the drainage channel – usually for an hour or two. Your vision becomes blurred, you may see haloes round lights, the cornea begins to look hazy (as pressure in the eyeball forces aqueous humour into it), and often there is some pain and redness in the eye; but no permanent damage to the vision occurs at this stage.

A fully developed attack is signified by the same symptoms occurring but persisting and becoming increasingly worse. Severe pain, resulting from the build-up of pressure in the eyeball, may be felt in the head as well as the eye, and is often accompanied by vomiting and even prostration. The cornea appears increasingly hazy as fluid is forced into it by the high pressure, and it sometimes looks grey and granular. The eyeball may feel very tender and hard to the touch.

How common is the problem?
Acute glaucoma is a common condition, especially in the elderly. In Britain, in the 40 to 65 age group 1 person in 100 is affected by some form of glaucoma, and in the over-65s the figure rises to 1 person in 20. Men and women are equally prone. About half of those sufferers who seek medical attention do so because of the warning symptoms that occur before a fully developed attack.

Acute glaucoma is about as common as *chronic simple glaucoma* (p.322) and is one of the commonest disorders of the eye requiring emergency treatment.

What are the risks?
If a fully developed attack of acute glaucoma is treated early, vision in the eye will return almost to normal. But once an attack is well under way, the fibres of the optic disc at the back of the eye are often damaged, causing some permanent loss of vision; and, if an attack is neglected altogether, the eye may well become totally blind.

What should be done?
Because of the risks to sight involved, early treatment is essential; most people seek this anyway, because of the extreme discomfort of the symptoms.

At the first signs of an attack see your doctor at once. If the attack occurs out of surgery hours, contact the doctor on emergency duty or go to the casualty department of the nearest hospital. The doctor will arrange for you to be admitted to hospital under the care of an eye specialist.

What is the treatment?
In hospital you will be given eye drops, to encourage the iris to withdraw from the drainage angle. To reduce the production of aqueous humour, you will receive an injection of a drug and possibly also be given a *dehydrating* agent, in the form of tablets or, in urgent cases, *intravenous drip*.

Usually, the above treatment brings down the pressure in the eye within hours. A day or two after this has been achieved, a simple operation called an iridectomy, for which you are given a local or general anaesthetic, is performed to prevent any further attack (see the box on this page). A tiny artificial channel for the drainage of aqueous humour is made through the iris and directly into the drainage angle. The channel is pierced through the outer edge of the iris, usually beneath the upper eyelid, so that it does not show. Since your other eye may well be affected by glaucoma later, you will be strongly advised to have an iridectomy performed on that eye while you are still in hospital for the operation on the affected eye. The success rate of

---

OPERATION: **Iridectomy**

An iridectomy is commonly performed to treat glaucoma. Because glaucoma usually affects both eyes eventually, the operation will probably be done on both eyes, though symptoms may have occurred in only one.

During the operation You are given either a local or general anaesthetic. The surgeon then makes an incision at the border of the conjunctiva and the cornea. A piece of iris is gently pulled through the incision and snipped off. This provides an artificial channel and allows the aqueous humour to drain away, so relieving the symptom-producing pressure in the eye. The incision is then closed up. The operation takes about 30 minutes for each eye.

After the operation You will be given eye drops to suppress inflammation and will wear a patch over the eye for a few days. You should be able to leave hospital after about 7 days.

Convalescence You should soon be able to resume normal activities but will be advised not to bend down or lift any heavy weights for a month afterwards.

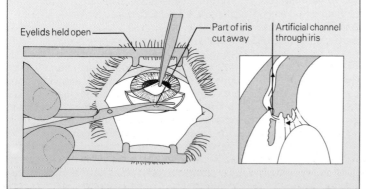

Eyelids held open — Part of iris cut away | Artificial channel through iris

iridectomy in preventing any further attacks of glaucoma is extremely high.

If you have delayed in obtaining treatment, it may no longer be possible to move the iris from the drainage angle, which will then be permanently obstructed. You will then need more complex surgery – a glaucoma drainage operation – in which aqueous humour is allowed to drain directly to the outside of the eye, beneath the conjunctiva. Either a local or a general anaesthetic is used. Again, this operation has a high rate of success.

What are the long-term prospects?
In the majority of cases when a glaucoma drainage operation is only partially successful, either a second, similar operation is performed or lifelong drug treatment, together with the partial drainage achieved by the operation, should control the pressure.

Chronic simple glaucoma
(open-angle glaucoma)

In this insidious eye disease the network of tissue in the drainage angle between the iris and the cornea gradually becomes blocked, by an obstruction of unknown nature, over a period of years. It becomes increasingly difficult for aqueous humour, produced in the chamber between the iris and the lens, to drain out of the eye through the network of tissue, and so there is a slow and steady build-up of pressure by the aqueous humour on the rest of the eyeball (for a general explanation of *glaucoma* see p.320). In most cases, both eyes are affected simultaneously. In chronic simple glaucoma it is the drainage channels themselves that become blocked, rather than the access to them (the drainage angle) as in *acute glaucoma* (p.320). So a doctor examining the eyes for signs of glaucoma will see a normal drainage angle.

What are the symptoms?
The development of the disorder is so gradual that the only symptom that occurs in the early stages is too slight to be noticeable. This is the loss of small areas of the outer field of vision in each eye, caused by pressure in the eyeball damaging the fibres of the optic nerve. Gradually, other areas of the outer field are lost, the areas lost increase in size, and they join together. At some point in this process, you may become aware that your field of vision is no longer so wide as it was.

If the disease is allowed to continue unchecked, the entire outer field of vision of both eyes is lost; then the ability of each eye to see straight ahead is diminished until both eyes become totally blind.

How common is the problem?
Chronic simple glaucoma tends to run in families, partly because its predisposing factors, such as long sight, also run in families. It increases in incidence from middle age onwards. If you are over 40 and have blood relatives who have (or have had) the disease, you should be especially alert to the possible onset of the condition.

What are the risks?
Since any vision that is lost through the disease can never be regained, the sooner you receive treatment the better. Do not wait until your vision has deteriorated considerably before seeking medical help.

What should be done?
As there is no way for anyone suffering from the early stages of this glaucoma to know that he or she has it, it is advisable for every adult to have a regular eye examination at least once every two years (see *Going to the optician*, p.312). If you have a close relative who has had chronic simple glaucoma, you should have an inspection once every year. And you should ask your doctor whether there is in your area one of the hospitals that run special clinics to look for early signs of the disorder.

If the doctor at the eye centre or the clinic suspects glaucoma, you will be referred via your own doctor to an eye specialist for further diagnosis. The specialist will examine the optic disc at the back of the retina which, in chronic simple glaucoma, becomes hollowed out like a saucer.

What is the treatment?
The treatment is to try to reduce the pressure in the eyeball. You will be given eye drops to open up the network of tissue in the drainage angle or to reduce the production of aqueous humour. Tablets or capsules for the same purpose are sometimes also given.

What are the long-term prospects?
All drops generally have to be taken for life, and you will also need lifelong check-ups by your doctor. Taking the drugs soon becomes part of your daily routine, and provided you do not lapse in this respect you should not suffer any further loss of vision.

If drugs fail to reduce the pressure in the eye sufficiently, the specialist may recommend that you have a glaucoma drainage operation, already described as part of the treatment for acute glaucoma.

Back of the eye and eye orbit

The function of the back of the eye is to receive the light that is focused by the front of the eye and to transform it into nerve impulses. These impulses are then passed along the optic nerve, which leads from the back of the retina to the brain. The structure that receives the light is the retina, a layer of light-sensitive nerve cells that lines the rear three-quarters of the eyeball. There are two types of nerve cell, known as the rods and the cones because of their shapes.

Cones detect fine detail and colour. They are most highly concentrated in the centre of the retina (an area known as the macula), at the very back of the eye – which is why, to see an object clearly, you have to look straight at it. Rods, most of which are on the rest of the retina, detect much less detail and no colour but are more sensitive to the degree of light entering the eye; you can often see an object more clearly in dim light by looking not directly at it but slightly to one side.

The bony socket of each eyeball is called the orbit. The eyeball swivels in the orbit by means of muscles attached to the outside of the eyeball and the inside of the orbit. An imbalance between these muscles causes the disorder known as squint. A squint that develops in adult life tends to have a different cause from the squint that appears in a child; the former is covered here, the latter is dealt with as a special problem of infants and children (see *Squint in children*, p.674).

Disorders of the back of the eye and eye orbit are particularly difficult to diagnose with any speed because these structures are invisible from outside the eye except with the help of special equipment.

Macula degeneration

The macula, near the optic nerve at the rear of the eye, is tightly packed with cones and is the part of the retina that distinguishes fine detail at the centre of the field of vision. In some elderly people, the small blood vessels of the choroid, which lies beneath the retina, become constricted and reduce the blood supply to the macula. This causes degeneration of the macula, which results in blurring of the central vision. In many cases both eyes are affected, either simultaneously or one after the other.

Macula degeneration usually develops gradually and is always painless. When both eyes have become affected, reading and other activities requiring sharp vision are impossible. Eventually, central vision disappears altogether, but the outer field of vision in each eye always remains.

What should be done?
Most cases of the disease are untreatable, but anyone who notices symptoms should still see a doctor right away. Vision can sometimes be improved by spectacles with powerful magnifying lenses, and occasionally treatment by a *laser beam* can halt the degeneration if it is caught early enough.

Diabetic retinopathy

In a small proportion of people who suffer from *diabetes mellitus* (p.519), many of the capillaries (tiny blood vessels) of the retina disintegrate, usually from both eyes. The remaining vessels may leak blood and tissue fluid into the retina, causing a permanent reduction in sharpness of vision. In other sufferers, fragile new blood vessels may grow on the retina and in many cases bleed into the vitreous humour (the jelly-like bulk of the eyeball), dimming or obliterating the vision for a variable length of time. The blood is usually reabsorbed from the vitreous humour through the retina, but scar tissue forms around the damaged blood vessels and this distorts or obliterates parts of the retina, leading to permanent loss of vision. The disorder occurs more often in diabetics who fail to control their level of blood glucose properly; but all diabetics are susceptible and should have regular eye checks.

What is the treatment?
Modern treatment is quite effective in controlling diabetic retinopathy. The development of the fragile vessels that leak blood can often be prevented by the use of a *laser beam*.

Bleeding into the vitreous humour that has not cleared within a year can be treated by draining the eye of vitreous humour with special instruments and replacing the humour with an artificial substitute.

Retinal detachment

The retina is the delicate layer of light-sensitive cells lining the rear three-quarters of the eyeball. Underlying the retina, and providing it with nutrients and oxygen, is a layer of blood vessels called the choroid.

Retinal detachment is the lifting away of the retina from the underlying choroid. What causes the detachment in most cases is the formation of a hole in the retina, due either to degeneration of the retina or to the vitreous humour (the jelly-like bulk of the eyeball) shrinking away from the retina and tearing it. The hole usually forms near the front edge of the retina. Fluid from the vitreous humour seeps through the hole and starts to detach the retina from the choroid. Left untreated, this process continues, more and more retina being lifted away. Eventually it is attached only at the front of the eye to the ciliary body (an extension of the choroid), and at the rear of the eye to the edge of the optic disc (the end of the optic nerve).

Both eyes may be affected, though hardly ever at the same time.

What are the symptoms?
The only symptoms are abnormalities of vision in the affected eye. But because the other eye is almost always normal, early symptoms are not always noticed. The first signs of the disorder may be flashes of light, which often occur shortly before a hole in the retina develops. Floating, black, often cobweb-like shapes may be seen when the hole is actually formed. Once detachment starts, you may notice the loss of part of the outer field of vision in the affected eye. This often appears as a black curtain being drawn over the eye. If detachment continues unchecked, the entire field of vision is lost.

Treating a detached retina
Fluid can seep through one or more holes in the retina, causing it to become detached from the underlying choroid (right). To treat a detached retina, the surgeon pushes the choroid against the retina at the point of each tear (below right) and seals the layers with a freezing probe (cryosurgery). The rest of the retina reattaches itself as the fluid drains away.

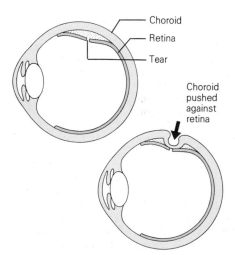

Choroid
Retina
Tear

Choroid pushed against retina

How common is the problem?
Retinal detachment is rare. Each year in Britain, about 1 person in 10,000 develops the condition. It occurs mainly from middle age onwards, and men and women are equally affected. You are particularly at risk if you are short-sighted (because your retina is likely to be stretched due to the shape of your eyeball – see *Short sight*, p.310); if you suffer an eye injury; or if you have the lens of your eye removed because of a *cataract* (p.319).

What are the risks?
If the disorder is neglected, there is a risk of permanent blindness in the affected eye. Also, detachment in one eye is sometimes followed by detachment in the other; measures can be taken during treatment to prevent this (see "What is the treatment?" below).

What should be done?
If you experience any of the symptoms described, see your doctor without delay. The doctor will be able to detect retinal detachment by looking into your eye through an instrument called an *ophthalmoscope*.

What is the treatment?
If a hole in the retina is discovered before detachment has started, the hole is sealed permanently by freezing or a *laser beam* after local anaesthetic has been given. If retinal detachment has begun, you will require surgery under a general anaesthetic. The outer layers of the eyeball in the region of the retinal hole are pushed in towards it and the hole is permanently sealed by freezing. The fluid between the retina and choroid may then be absorbed by them – or, if not, it is drained off – and the retina sinks back to its normal position.

If surgery is carried out before detachment has involved the macula (the central part of the retina), vision usually returns to normal after the operation. If detachment is more extensive and central vision has been impaired, then, although the full field of vision will usually be restored, vision will be permanently blurred to some extent. In 10 per cent of cases of complete detachment, the retina fails to sink back against the choroid after the operation, and the eye remains blind. After surgery, retinal detachment recurs in only a small minority of cases.

Following detachment in one eye, there is a considerable risk of the condition developing in the other, and you will need to have this eye examined; any weak areas in the retina can be detected and treated, often at the same time as the eye with the detached retina.

Retinal artery occlusion

The blood required by the nerve fibres of the retina is supplied by the central retinal artery, a tiny vessel that enters the rear of the eye with the optic nerve. Sometimes – usually in middle-aged or elderly people – the artery or one of its branches becomes blocked, either by a blood clot resulting from *thrombosis* or by an *embolus* that has travelled from a diseased blood vessel elsewhere in the body (see *Arterial embolism*, p.415).

What are the symptoms?
If the main artery is blocked, there is immediate blindness in the affected eye; if a branch of the artery is blocked, only part of the vision, usually either the upper or lower half, is blacked out.

What should be done?
If you suddenly lose all or part of the vision of one eye, you must see your doctor or go to hospital *immediately*, since if treatment can be given within a few hours, it is occasionally possible to restore some of the sight in the eye. This is done either by emergency surgery or by drugs that allow the clot or embolus to be pushed further along the blood vessel to a position where less of the retina is affected by the blockage.

Whatever happens to the eye, your doctor will set out to discover the cause of the blockage so that it can be treated to prevent the possibility of the other eye being affected. To this end, you may be given an *electrocardiogram* (*ECG*), an *arteriogram*, and other tests.

Retinal vein occlusion

The central retinal vein carries used blood away from the retina. In rare cases, mainly from middle age onwards, the vein or one of its branches can become blocked by a blood clot. When this happens, blood and tissue fluid begin to leak out of the blocked vessel and cause vision to become blurred over the course of a few hours.

The disorder is often associated with the early stages of *chronic simple glaucoma* (p.322) or with *high blood pressure* (p.382). Rarely, it is caused by a blood disease in which the blood tends to clot more readily than normal – for example, it can be caused by *polycythaemia* (p.429).

The younger you are, the more likely it is that the leaked blood will be reabsorbed naturally, through the wall of the retina, and that as a result vision will improve over several months. If reabsorption does not occur, the blurring will be permanent, since there is no treatment presently available for the disorder. Sometimes new blood vessels form and create complications. Any that grow on the retina itself are fragile and tend to rupture and bleed, causing further blurred vision which, again, may improve spontaneously, especially in younger people. If vessels grow on the surface of the iris, they can cause a form of *glaucoma* (p.320) that may lead to complete loss of vision in the affected eye.

A retinal vein occlusion that has not been noticed by the sufferer – because only a small branch of the vein has been blocked – is sometimes detected by an examination of the eye with an *ophthalmoscope* during a routine eyesight test. This is one good reason for having such a test regularly (see *Going to the optician*, p.312). More effective control of any underlying cause – high blood pressure, for instance – may then prevent the eye from being further affected.

Choroiditis

Choroiditis is inflammation of the choroid, a layer of blood vessels beneath the retina. When the inflammation subsides after treatment, the choroid and retina are left scarred.

Often the exact cause of the disorder cannot be discovered. Some cases are the result of infection by a microbe acquired before birth. In a small proportion of children who are affected, the disorder is due to infection by a worm-like microbe that enters the system after the child has touched dirt fouled by a dog or, less commonly, a cat, and then carried the infection into his or her mouth. The inflammation causes blurring of the central vision. The condition is painless. If you experience any blurring of vision, see your doctor without delay. The doctor will arrange for blood tests and *X-rays* to be carried out, in a search for an underlying cause.

What is the treatment?
Steroids are given to clear up the inflammation and blurred vision. In a severe case not caused by infection, *immunosuppressive* drugs may also be prescribed.

If scarring of the choroid and retina occurs away from the macula, near the front of the eye, there will be some loss of the outer field of vision, which may well not even be noticed. But if the central choroid and retina, at the rear of the eye, is affected, there will be a varying degree of loss of central vision.

Tumours of the eye

Tumours are abnormal growths of tissue. They may be *malignant* – in which case they usually spread – or *benign*, when they remain localized. Tumours of the eye are rare, generally malignant, and usually painless.

Malignant melanoma of the eye

This is a tumour similar to a form of skin cancer (see *Malignant melanoma*, p.259). It occurs mainly in the choroid (a layer of blood vessels beneath the retina) or the ciliary body (a forward extension of the choroid). Occasionally it grows in the iris. Only one eye is affected. More than half of all cases are discovered during a routine examination by an optician. The rest are reported by the sufferer because of a gradual loss of part of the vision in the affected eye. The doctor treating the case will arrange for *diagnostic angiography* to be carried out. This shows up the nature of the tumour. The usual treatment for young adults is to remove the affected eye to prevent the spread of the tumour to other parts of the body. In elderly people in whom the tumour is growing very slowly and is not causing any loss of vision, it is usually considered best to leave the eye alone; if signs of definite growth are observed, it is advisable to remove the eye.

Secondary tumours of the eye

In some cancers, secondary tumours spread (*metastasize*), via the bloodstream or lymphatic system, from a primary growth in, for example, the breast or lung, and affect other parts of the body. Secondary tumours in the eye develop during the late stages of such a cancer. If they grow behind the eyeball, they may cause bulging of the eye (see *Exophthalmos*, below). Their effect on vision will vary according to their position in the eye and their rate of growth.

A secondary tumour in the eye can sometimes be destroyed by *radiotherapy*, but in some cases this is not feasible.

Retinoblastoma

This is a malignant tumour of the retina that occurs in one or both eyes, usually in children under five. The child will not complain of any symptoms. If the central vision of only one eye is affected, the child may squint – which is why all cases of squint must be examined by a doctor (see *Squint in children*, p.674). If the tumour is not discovered during its early growth, it may become visible through the pupil as a white area in the interior of the eye. The disease is often inherited. If you know that it runs in your family, it is sensible, before having children, to seek the advice of your doctor, and essential, if you already have a child, to tell the doctor about the family history of retinoblastoma so that the baby can have regular eye examinations. If the tumour is detected in the early stages, treatment by *radiotherapy* is very effective. But if the tumour is advanced, the eye will have to be removed to prevent secondary tumours spreading to other parts of the body and endangering the child's life.

Optic neuritis

In some young adults between about 20 and 40 the optic nerve in one eye becomes inflamed, for unknown reasons. The inflammation causes a gradual or sudden blurring of vision in the affected eye (in severe cases, the blurring progresses within a few days to temporary blindness). Often the eye is painful when you move it.

What should be done?

Consult your doctor without delay if your vision becomes blurred. If your doctor then suspects you have optic neuritis, he or she will send you to hospital to have an examination to confirm the diagnosis. The treatment of the disorder is usually injections of *steroids*. These hasten the spontaneous recovery that usually takes place and, with it, a return to normal vision. The problem sometimes recurs, however – in either eye. After several recurrences the vision may not recover completely. A small proportion of people affected with optic neuritis develop *multiple sclerosis* (p.292) later on.

Exophthalmos

See p.247,
Visual aids to diagnosis, 62.

Exophthalmos is bulging of one or both eyeballs. It is brought about by a swelling of the soft tissue that lines the bony orbit in which the eyeball lies. The eyeball is pressed forward, exposing an abnormally large amount of the front of it, which tends to become dry and feel gritty. Eye movement is restricted as the swelling tissue affects the external eye muscles, resulting in double vision. And in severe cases, the eye is pressed forward so much that its blood supply is restricted and vision becomes seriously blurred; the lids may be unable to close; and *corneal ulcers* (p.316) may develop. The most common cause of the swelling is an abnormality in the production of thyroid hormones (see *Thyrotoxicosis*, p.525). Other cases of exophthalmos may be caused by a tumour that is growing behind the eyeball (see *Tumours of the eye*, opposite) or inflammation of the tissue there (see *Orbital cellulitis*, below).

Blood tests, *X-rays*, and an examination of the eye are carried out to discover which factor is responsible for the disorder.

What is the treatment?
If the thyroid gland is found to be the source of the condition, treatment will be for that disorder. Such treatment may, however, fail to control the exophthalmos, in which case *steroid* drugs may be given, or part of the lids may be stitched together as a protection against future corneal ulcers. In severe cases, an operation may be carried out to relieve the pressure behind the eyeball.

Orbital cellulitis

The bony orbit in which the eyeball lies is lined with soft tissue. In rare cases, bacteria enter the tissue – usually from infected sinuses in the nose (see *Sinusitis*, p.347) or from a boil near the eye – and cause it to become inflamed. Usually only one eye is affected.

The pressure of the swollen tissue pushes the eyeball forward (see *Exophthalmos*, opposite). Other symptoms are severe pain and redness in the eye, swollen eyelids that you may be unable to close, and usually fever; in some cases the eye exudes pus. The condition may resemble very severe *conjunctivitis* (p.317). Vision is affected by the swelling and discharge but generally returns to normal after treatment. There is a very slight risk of the infection spreading backwards to the brain and causing *meningitis* (p.273).

Treatment – which is usually successful – consists of high doses of *antibiotics*, given as tablets or by injection. If infected sinuses are the source of the trouble, you may later need an operation to have them drained, to prevent recurrence of the cellulitis.

Squint

Normal eyes move in conjunction, so that each looks at the same object. This is achieved by the brain sending instructions via nerves to muscles attached to the outside of each eyeball. A squint occurs when this co-ordination is absent: one eye looks at what you want to observe, the other elsewhere.

Most squints develop in infancy or early childhood (see *Squint in children*, p.674). They are not associated with any other disease; but squints that develop after childhood – those discussed here – almost always occur because of a disorder elsewhere in the body. Among such disorders are diabetes mellitus, high blood pressure, temporal arteritis, brain injury, and myaesthenia gravis.

What are the symptoms?
The disorder affects the nerves connecting the brain to the eye muscles or, less commonly, the muscles themselves, and in almost all cases double vision occurs. You may also have other symptoms, such as headache, from the underlying disorder.

What should be done?
If you start seeing double and have never suffered from squint, see your doctor. As a temporary measure to prevent double vision, cover one eye with a patch, which you can buy over the counter. To discover the underlying cause of the squint, the doctor will probably take your blood pressure, ask you to provide urine and blood samples for testing, and arrange for you to have various *X-rays*.

What are the long-term prospects?
In the majority of cases, good response to treatment of the underlying disorder causes the squint gradually to disappear within a few months. If some degree of squint then remains, this can be corrected by spectacles containing prisms if the squint is slight, or, if it is marked, by surgery on the eye muscles.

Movements of the eye
Each eye is controlled by 6 muscles arranged in 3 pairs. Each pair moves the eye in different directions (right). An underlying illness affecting the nervous control of these muscles can cause a squint to develop.

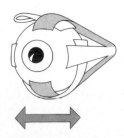
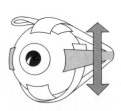
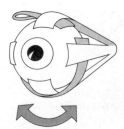

Ear disorders

Introduction

As well as enabling you to hear, your ears are important as organs of balance. Each ear consists of three parts: the outer ear, middle ear, and inner ear.

The outer ear is made up of the ear that we see – the folds of skin and cartilage known as the pinna – and of the outer-ear canal, a passage about 20mm ($\frac{3}{4}$in) long which leads from the pinna to the eardrum. The part of the outer-ear canal nearest the surface is made of cartilage covered with skin cells that produce wax and hairs; the deeper part of the canal has a thin lining surrounded by bone. The eardrum, which separates the outer ear from the middle ear, is a membrane stretched across the end of the canal.

The middle ear is a small cavity between the eardrum and the inner ear, bridged by three small, connected bones: the hammer (malleus), anvil (incus), and stirrup (stapes), so-named because of their shape. The hammer is attached to the inner lining of the eardrum, and the stirrup to a membrane covering an opening known as the oval window, which leads to the inner ear. There are various connecting passages leading from the middle ear: those to the air spaces in the mastoid process, a bone behind the pinna; those into the inner ear; and one, known as the eustachian (or auditory) tube, which leads to the cavity at the back of the nose. The main function of this tube is to channel air from the nose to the middle-ear chamber, so that air pressure on the inside of the eardrum equals that on the outside. Sometimes the tube becomes blocked – when you have a cold, for example – and you can detect when the tube becomes clear because the sudden equalization of pressure makes the ear "pop".

The inner ear consists of a series of membrane-lined chambers filled with fluid. It can be broadly divided into the labyrinth and the cochlea. The labyrinth is made up of three semicircular tubes, called canals. They are set at right angles to one another so that each canal is on a different horizontal or vertical plane. The cochlea starts on the inner side of the oval window and curls round like a snail's shell. It is the inner ear that controls balance, although like the other parts, it is vital to the ear's main function, hearing.

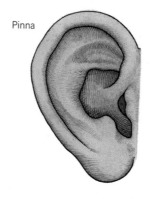

Pinna

The structure of the ear
The ear consists of 3 parts: the outer ear, which collects and funnels sound waves along the outer-ear canal; the middle ear, which receives these waves and passes them on to the inner ear; and the inner ear, which converts the sound waves into nerve impulses and transmits them to the brain. The inner ear also contains the mechanism by which the body keeps its balance.

Outer ear	Middle ear	Inner ear
Pinna	Eardrum	Cochlea
Outer-ear canal	Hammer	Labyrinth
	Anvil	
	Stirrup	
	Eustachian tube	

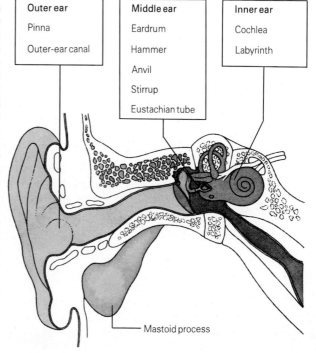

Mastoid process

How the ear works

How you hear

Objects in motion disturb the air, producing sound waves (see *Sound and noise levels*, p.339). The visible ear gathers these waves, which then travel down the outer-ear canal and strike the eardrum, making it vibrate. The vibrations pass through the hammer, anvil, stirrup, and oval window into the fluid in the cochlea. Tiny hairs lining the cochlea transform the vibrations in the fluid into nerve impulses, which are transmitted to the brain along the auditory nerve. This, the main form of hearing, is supplemented by the conduction of vibrations through the bones of the skull to the inner ear. This secondary hearing plays a large part in the way you hear your own voice.

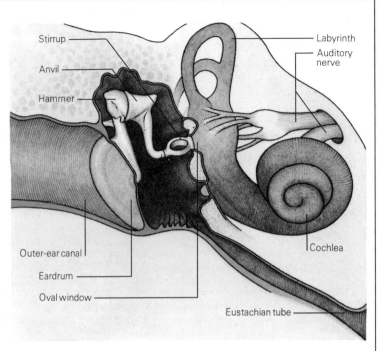

Stirrup — Labyrinth
Anvil — Auditory nerve
Hammer —
Outer-ear canal —
Eardrum —
Oval window —
Eustachian tube —
Cochlea

How you keep your balance

Your brain is continually monitoring the positions and movements of your head and body so that you are able to keep your balance. In each inner ear is a structure called the labyrinth, which detects the positions and movements of the head by means of three semicircular canals. Each canal is at right angles to the other two, so whichever way you move your head – whether you nod it (A), shake it (B) or tilt it (C) – one or more semicircular canals detects the movement, and relays the information to the brain. The brain coordinates this information with information from your eyes, and from the muscles in your body and limbs, to assess your exact position and the movements you need to make to keep your balance.

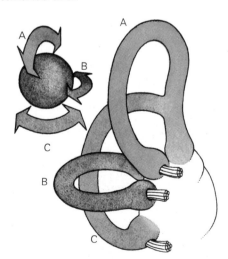

Each semicircular canal in the labyrinth, above right, detects movement in one of the three directions shown above left.

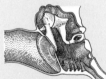

Conductive deafness
This occurs because of a mechanical defect in the middle ear (above) which prevents sound from being conducted to the inner ear.

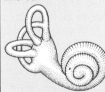

Perceptive deafness
Damage to the cochlea in the inner ear (above) can cause perceptive deafness. Sounds received are not passed on to the brain.

Deafness and vertigo

Contrary to general belief, deafness and vertigo are not disorders in themselves but symptoms of disorders.

There are two kinds of deafness, conductive and perceptive. In conductive deafness sounds do not reach the inner ear, as a result of, for example, *wax blockage* (p.330) in the outer ear, or the immobilization of the stirrup bone in the middle ear (see *Otosclerosis*, p.332). In perceptive deafness sounds reach the inner ear but are not transmitted to the brain, usually because of damage to the cochlea or the auditory nerve, as happens in some forms of *occupational deafness*, p.338 .

Vertigo is a false sense that either you or your surroundings are spinning round. Vertigo often causes loss of balance. It is a common symptom of an inner-ear disorder, which is where the organs of balance are situated. (For details see *Vertigo*, p.290.)

Outer ear

The lining of the outer-ear canal is simply an extension of the skin of the visible ear, therefore most disorders of the outer ear, apart from the problem of wax blockage, are skin disorders. For this reason, they are generally not as serious as middle- and inner-ear diseases, which affect the delicate mechanisms that control hearing and balance.

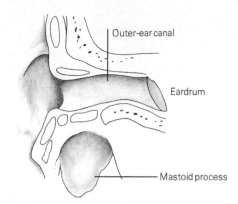

Outer-ear canal

Eardrum

Mastoid process

Wax blockage

Wax is produced by glands in the outer-ear canal to clean and moisten the canal. The amount produced varies considerably from person to person. Some people produce so little that it never accumulates in the outer canal. In others, wax blocks the entire canal every few months.

Symptoms of wax blockage include a feeling of fullness in the ear, partial deafness or ringing in the ear, and, less commonly, earache and some vertigo (dizziness).

What is the treatment?

Self-help: You can often remove wax by gently manipulating a cotton-wool bud in the ear. If the wax is hard, first soften it with olive oil (or a proprietary product made for the purpose) warmed to hand temperature. Apply drops of olive oil for several nights until the wax is soft enough to wash out.

If you work in very dusty conditions and are prone to wax blockage, consider wearing ear plugs at work.

Professional help: If you cannot remove the wax, your doctor will flush (syringe) the ear with warm water, which washes out the wax. The wax is often softened first with ear drops. When wax is very difficult to remove, the doctor may dislodge it with a probe or electric suction apparatus.

Syringeing the ear
A blockage of wax in the outer-ear canal can be removed by syringeing. The doctor directs a syringe containing warm water into and towards the top of the canal. The water flows along the top of the canal to bounce off the eardrum and flow back along the bottom of the canal, flushing the wax out with it.

Protruding ears

Normally, the ears lie almost flat against the side of the head; but in some people they protrude, and, in extreme cases, may be at right angles to the head. In Britain, 1 person in 200 has ears that protrude to some extent. Most people are untroubled by or even unaware of the condition. However, it may cause real embarrassment and distress, especially if the protrusion is severe. Such distress should not be underestimated. Unfortunately, strapping the ears back at night has no effect on protruding ears.

If you have protruding ears and this distresses you, discuss the problem with your doctor who may well be able to reassure you. You can conceal the "disfigurement" simply by growing your hair longer. In extreme cases, the doctor may recommend surgery. Two incisions a few millimetres apart are made in the crease of the skin behind the ear,

Correcting protruding ears
The ears can be pulled flat against the head by removing a strip of skin from behind the ear, and sewing together the 2 raw edges. It is simple surgery, but is an unwise operation before the age of 5, because the ears are not fully developed until that time.

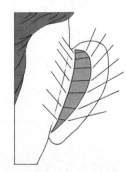

and the strip of skin between them cut away. The ear is pulled towards the head, and the two cut edges are sewn together. The result of the operation is invariably excellent, and because of their position behind the ears, no scars are visible. It is a simple procedure and you will need to stay in hospital for only one or two days.

Infections of the outer-ear canal

(otitis externa)

An infection of the outer-ear canal may be localized – a boil or *abscess*, for example – or generalized, affecting the whole lining of the canal. Ear infections often occur after swimming as damp skin is particularly susceptible to any infection that may be present in the water. Another cause of both localized and generalized infections is scratching the inside of the ear to relieve itching or while attempting to remove wax.

The first symptom is irritation in the ear, usually followed by pain. There may be a discharge from the ear. If pus blocks the outer-ear canal, there is some loss of hearing. And any movement of the pinna (the ear flap itself) causes pain.

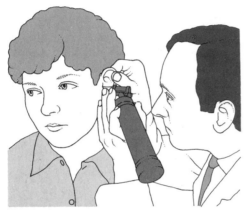

Inspecting the outer-ear canal
To check whether there is anything wrong with the outer-ear canal or eardrum, the doctor examines the ear through an otoscope (auriscope) while pulling the top of the ear upwards and backwards. This gives a view of the whole canal.

Infections of the outer ear are very common, especially in young adults. Each year, 1 person in 100 consults a doctor with the problem. If the infection is untreated, it can occasionally spread and affect underlying cartilage and bone.

What is the treatment?

Self-help: Take a painkiller such as aspirin and place a warm, dry cotton-wool pad over the ear to help to relieve the pain until you can see the doctor.

Professional help: The doctor will look into the ear with an *otoscope*, and may take a swab of pus, which is sent to a laboratory for analysis. The ear is first cleaned with a cotton-wool-coated probe; you will find that this procedure considerably relieves irritation and pain. The doctor may then prescribe tablets or ear drops made up of *antibiotics* and *steroids*. Together with gentle daily cleaning of the ear with a cotton-wool bud, the drops or tablets should clear the condition. If the pain is severe, the doctor may prescribe a painkiller to be taken until the infection clears up.

In all cases, you must keep the infected ear dry. This means no swimming, and wearing ear plugs or a bathing hat when taking a bath or shower.

Occasionally the infection recurs and needs further treatment. This often happens if the microbes causing the infection are fungi, or if you have developed an allergy to the microbes (see *Allergies*, p.705). If this happens a steroid cream or ear drops will probably be prescribed, and should eventually clear the trouble.

Tumours of the outer ear

Ear tumours
Occasionally lumps that appear on the ear are malignant, such as this rodent ulcer.

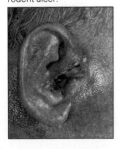

Like all tumours, those of the outer ear may be *benign* or *malignant*. Malignant tumours are the same as those found in *squamous cell carcinoma* (p.259) or *rodent ulcer* (p.258).

A benign tumour occurs on the visible ear as a painless wart or, in the canal itself, as a hard growth of underlying bone tissue (*osteoma*). With an osteoma, there may be either no symptoms at all, simply an accumulation of wax, or the symptoms of an *infection of the outer-ear canal* (see above).

Malignant tumours on the visible ear start, like benign tumours, as warty growths. They usually bleed easily if knocked and eventually become painful. Malignant osteomas in the canal cause intense earache and a blood-stained discharge.

Tumours of the outer ear are very rare; but the dangers of a malignant tumour are those of any malignant growth, so if you notice any of the symptoms described above, see your doctor without delay.

What is the treatment?

Benign tumours can be removed in hospital, usually under local anaesthetic. In the case of malignant tumours, *radiotherapy* may get rid of a growth at an early stage. If this fails, the tumour – and, with it, part or all of the visible ear – may be removed in hospital; the operation is sometimes followed by further *X-ray* treatment. Tumours in the canal require both an operation and X-ray treatment. These operations require a hospital stay of one to two weeks. If the tumour is treated at an early stage, the prospects for recovery are good. *Plastic surgery* (p.260) is available to reconstruct the visible ear.

Middle ear

The most common disorders of the middle ear are infections and damage to the eardrum. Infections are caused by bacteria or viruses, which enter the middle ear either through a perforated eardrum or along the eustachian tube. The delicate bones that conduct sound vibrations to the inner ear are vulnerable to damage, so some deafness (see *Deafness and vertigo*, p.329) is a symptom in many middle-ear disorders.

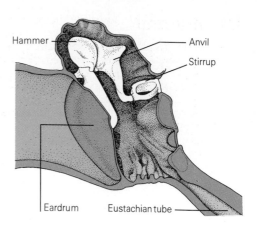

Hammer · Anvil · Stirrup · Eardrum · Eustachian tube

Otosclerosis

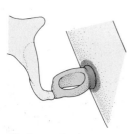

The bones of the middle ear vibrate to transmit sound from the eardrum to the inner ear. In otosclerosis, the base of the stirrup is prevented from moving by an abnormal growth. This results in a form of conductive deafness.

In otosclerosis, abnormal growth of honey-combed bone occurs at the entrance to the inner ear, and immobilizes the base of the stirrup, a tiny bone which vibrates after sound waves have struck the eardrum. The result is that few or none of the sound waves that enter the ear are passed on to the inner ear, causing conductive deafness. In about 80 per cent of people with the disease, both ears are affected, either simultaneously or one after the other.

What are the symptoms?
If the disease is untreated, there is usually a slow progression towards total deafness in both ears over a period of 10 to 15 years. But in a few cases (usually children) the progression is rapid. Sometimes, however, it stops well short of total deafness – for example, loud speech can still be heard. For some reason, hearing is often better when there is background noise.

As the disease progresses, some perceptive deafness (see *Deafness and vertigo*, p.329) may occur. A symptom of this is *tinnitus* (noises in the ear) and the sufferer may speak more loudly to compensate. Otosclerosis may become worse during pregnancy.

How common is the problem?
About 1 person in 250 suffers from otosclerosis; it affects twice as many women as men. Fifty per cent of cases have a family history of the disorder, which usually appears between the ages of 20 and 40.

What are the risks?
The risks are those of total deafness and of the social isolation that the sufferer sometimes has to endure. Because the disease does not usually develop until adulthood, there is no risk of defective speech.

What should be done?
If you experience any deafness or ringing in the ears, see your doctor, who will examine your ears and carry out some simple hearing tests. If otosclerosis is suspected – particularly if you have a blood relative who has the disease – special hearing tests (see *Hearing loss and hearing aids*, p.335) will be arranged for you to attend.

What is the treatment?
When some degree of deafness is present in only one ear, a hearing aid is usually prescribed. But this is simply an aid – not a cure. The usual treatment to halt or cure otosclerosis is an operation called *stapedectomy*. This improves conduction by replacing the fixed stirrup. Stapedectomy improves hearing significantly in 90 per cent of cases. But in about 2 to 5 per cent of operations the result is total deafness in the ear operated on. Sometimes hearing does not improve until any blood clot left in the middle ear after the operation has been absorbed. Your doctor will take into account the risk of deafness when assessing the likelihood that your hearing will be improved by the operation. For example, in those with rapidly progressive otosclerosis in both ears, the operation is advised as an emergency to prevent rapid onset of total deafness. Usually only one ear is operated on so that should the operation fail, some hearing is preserved.

In stapedectomy, the eardrum is perforated, and the diseased stirrup is removed and replaced by a tiny metal or plastic substitute. The eardrum heals naturally in one to two weeks. The patient, who usually feels dizzy after the operation, leaves hospital after a week or two, and can usually return to a normal daily routine after another two to three weeks.

Barotrauma

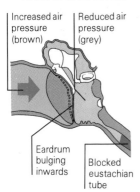

Increased air pressure (brown)

Reduced air pressure (grey)

Eardrum bulging inwards

Blocked eustachian tube

Normally, because of air passing along the eustachian tube, air pressure within the middle ear is balanced with that in the outer ear. But if a severe imbalance occurs, the eardrum can be damaged by the force of the unequal pressures (barotrauma).

Barotrauma often takes place when someone who has an infection of the nose or throat, such as a bad cold, is on board an aircraft. During flight the air pressure in the cabin (and, therefore, in the outer-ear canal), is lowered to that which exists at 2,000m (about 6,000ft). Usually air from the middle ear travels down the eustachian tube and out through the nose or mouth to equalize the pressure. Even when the tube is blocked by catarrh or pus, the pressure of the outgoing air enables it to force its way through the fluid. Barotrauma occurs as the aircraft is repressurized before touchdown. Air may be unable to travel back along the blocked auditory tube to the middle ear, and consequently the eardrum is pushed inwards.

Symptoms of barotrauma are pain in the ear (sometimes severe), a feeling of blockage, and some loss of hearing. There may also be noises in the ear and mild vertigo. The symptoms normally clear up within a few hours.

What should be done?

If you have a nose or throat infection and the flight is unavoidable, take with you a decongestant nasal spray. Use this and suck sweets to encourage swallowing as often as possible. This will usually keep the eustachian tube open and prevent any problems.

If you think you have developed barotrauma, and your symptoms do not clear within 24 hours, consult your doctor, who may perforate the eardrum to allow any fluid to drain from the middle ear. The eardrum heals naturally in a week or so.

Ruptured eardrum

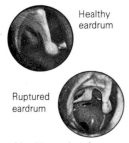

Healthy eardrum

Ruptured eardrum

A healthy eardrum is almost transparent; when ruptured, the middle-ear bones are clearly visible.

The most common causes of rupture of the eardrum are a sharp object poked into the ear to relieve irritation, a blast from an explosion, and a blow to the ear. Although a great deal of pressure is needed to break an eardrum, that pressure can be produced simply by a hard slap on the ear. Other causes of eardrum rupture are a fractured skull and, more commonly, a middle-ear infection. And in some forms of ear surgery the eardrum must be perforated to gain access to the middle ear.

Symptoms of a ruptured eardrum are pain (usually slight) in the ear, sometimes partial loss of hearing and noises in the ear, and, occasionally, slight bleeding from the ear. The symptoms usually last only a few hours. There is also a risk that infection may enter the middle ear through the rupture. If you suspect that you have a ruptured eardrum, see your doctor as soon as possible.

What is the treatment?

Self-help: To relieve pain, cover the affected area with a clean, dry pad and take a painkiller such as paracetamol.

Professional help: The doctor will prescribe tablets or capsules of an *antibiotic* either to prevent or act against any infection. The ear will be kept under observation until it heals naturally – usually in one or two weeks. If it has not healed after three months, a minor operation is carried out to graft a tiny piece of your own body tissue on to the eardrum. This usually cures the trouble. A ruptured eardrum, when healed, causes no problems and does not affect hearing.

Acute infection of the middle ear

(acute otitis media)

An infection, either viral or bacterial, enters and inflames the middle-ear cavity. The inflammation causes the eustachian tube – which connects the middle-ear cavity with the back of the nose – to become swollen and blocked. In a bacterial infection, pus will form in the middle-ear cavity.

The disorder often develops after an infection of the nose and throat region, such as a cold, when microbes travel along the eustachian tube to the middle ear. In a few cases, the infection is caused by microbes gaining access through a *ruptured eardrum* (see above). Repeated attacks – usually in children – can cause *glue ear* (p.675).

What are the symptoms?

There is usually a feeling of fullness in the ear, accompanied by a severe stabbing pain that may prevent sleep. Other symptoms include raised temperature and some loss of hearing in the affected ear. If the infection is caused by bacteria and remains untreated, the pressure of pus within the middle ear may eventually burst the eardrum, producing sudden relief from pain accompanied by a discharge of pus from the ear.

How common is the problem?

In Britain about 1 person in 30 suffers from the disorder each year. The problem is very

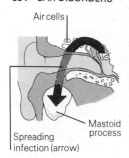

Air cells

Mastoid process

Spreading infection (arrow)

The spread of infection from the middle ear Infections of the middle ear can spread to the air cells in the mastoid process. If antibiotic treatment is unsuccessful, the only way of curing this problem is by mastoid drainage.

common in children: at least half have an infected middle ear at some time. This is because their narrow eustachian tubes and large *adenoids* (p.677) are more susceptible to infection, and also because their eustachian tubes are shorter than in adults, which makes it easier for infections from the nose and throat (for example, the common cold virus) to reach the middle ear.

What are the risks?
If the infection is viral, the risks are minimal. But if the infection is bacterial and treatment is delayed too long, there is a danger that it may become chronic (see *Chronic infection of the middle ear*, below) or may spread to the air cells in the mastoid process, in which case an operation known as *mastoid drainage* (p.336) may be necessary.

What should be done?
The infection does not require emergency treatment, but see your doctor as soon as possible. The doctor will examine your ears closely with an *otoscope*, and will usually be able to diagnose the condition straight away, without any further tests.

If you have a cold, it is possible to reduce the chances of getting an infection in the middle ear by taking the following measures. Suck mentholated pastilles to keep your nasal passages free – this reduces the chance of the eustachian tubes swelling and becoming susceptible to the spread of infection – and avoid getting water in your ear.

What is the treatment?
Self-help: To provide some relief from pain, take aspirin and, to avoid the possibility of further infection, place a clean, dry pad over the affected ear.

Professional help: A *vasoconstrictor* drug may be prescribed, as nose drops or spray, to help unblock the eustachian tube and thus allow pus, produced by the infection, to trickle down into the nose and throat. The doctor may also prescribe a course of an *antibiotic*, which usually clears up a bacterial infection completely. If the infection is viral, an antibiotic will prevent any secondary bacterial infection from taking a hold.

If the eardrum is bulging, the doctor may make a small cut in it, to relieve the pressure of the pus, and with it the pain. In the case of a child, this will be done in hospital, with the child under a general anaesthetic. The eardrum heals naturally in one to two weeks and hearing will return to normal.

Chronic infection of the middle ear
(chronic otitis media)

A chronic infection is one that persists over a long period. Unlike an acute infection, which flares up suddenly and often painfully but usually causes little damage, a chronic infection is slow, relentless, and can cause serious damage. Chronic infection of the middle ear is often the result of an untreated ear infection in childhood (see *Glue ear*, p.675); the infection either never completely clears up, so that some microbes (usually bacteria) always remain, or it eventually clears up but leaves a site susceptible to any further microbes entering the system. Continual production of pus from the chronic infection eventually eats away a hole in the eardrum, and often damages or destroys the small bones of the middle ear; the eventual result can be loss of hearing.

Cholesteatoma (p.336) is another form of the disorder, which is potentially more dangerous because the infection can spread through the skull bones to the brain.

What are the symptoms?
There are periodic discharges of greyish or yellowish pus from the ear. There may be some deafness, depending on how long the infection has been present. Such chronic infections are far less common than they used to be. Only 1 person in 400 is treated for this disorder each year.

What are the risks?
If the infection reaches an advanced stage, it may spread to the air cells in the mastoid process and require an operation called a *mastoid drainage* (p.336). The bones of the middle ear may be damaged, resulting in a degree of permanent deafness.

What should be done?
See your doctor, who will examine your ears with an *otoscope* and probably arrange for *X-rays* of your head to discover if the infection has spread to the mastoid area.

What is the treatment?
Self-help: Keep the ear dry and clean. Wipe away any discharge with a cotton-wool bud.

Professional help: The doctor will clean the ear with a cotton-wool-covered probe, and will probably prescribe tablets containing an *antibiotic* and ear drops containing a *steroid* as well as an antibiotic. This treatment is aimed at drying up the ear and preventing any discharge for three months, after which time an

Hearing loss and hearing aids

Are you becoming hard of hearing?
Deafness or hearing loss is not in itself a disease, but a symptom of an underlying disorder. Some hearing loss is quite normal as you get older (see *The failing senses*, p.721), but if you are under 50 and you are becoming hard of hearing, you should see your doctor without delay. The doctor will examine your ears with an *otoscope*, and may carry out some simple hearing tests in the surgery; you usually listen to a watch, a tuning fork, or even a whisper. If the tests indicate that your hearing is impaired to a serious degree, you will need to attend hospital for more specialized hearing tests – *audiometry* and *impedance testing*.

Audiometry
There are two parts to this test. The first part measures your ability to hear sounds conducted through the air. You listen through earphones, one ear at a time, to sounds of various frequencies (from low notes to high notes). For each frequency, the sound starts at an inaudible level, then increases to a "threshold" volume at which you can just hear it. The results show which frequencies you can hear, and the threshold volume at which you can hear each frequency.

The second part of the test measures your ability to hear sounds conducted through the bones of the head. The procedure is the same as in the first part, but this time you wear special earphones which vibrate against your skull – usually against the mastoid process just behind the outer ear. Your thresholds in both tests are recorded on a graph called an *audiogram*.

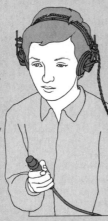

Impedance testing
Impedance testing measures the ability of the eardrum to reflect sound waves. In a healthy ear, the pressure on one side of the eardrum equals that on the other. This allows the eardrum to vibrate freely when sound waves hit it. The vibrations are passed on through the middle ear and are also reflected back into the air. Unequal pressures on the eardrum, as happens in some middle-ear disorders, cause the eardrum to become too stiff to conduct – and reflect – sounds properly. A probe, covered with a soundproof material such as cork, is inserted into the outer-ear canal and seals up the entrance to the ear. Pressure in the canal sweeps from high to low, by the regulation of air pumped through the probe, and while this happens, sounds are aimed at the eardrum by means of a transmitter in the probe. The reflections of these sounds are measured by a receiver in the probe. From the degree of reflection at various pressure readings, it is possible to detect any damage to the ear and to deduce what ear disorder has caused the damage.

Hearing aids
Modern hearing aids use electric power from a small battery to increase the volume of sound. A tiny microphone collects the sound and transforms it into electrical signals; an amplifier increases the strength of the signals; and an earphone turns the signals back into sound, now amplified, and transmits it to the ear (see diagram right).

Hearing aids are supplied free by the National Health Service at the ear, nose, and throat department of hospitals and at audiology clinics. You can also buy an aid privately at a commercial hearing aid centre which will offer a wider range of styles. It is important to choose both the right kind of aid and one that fits snugly into your ear; the advice of your doctor or ear specialist is invaluable in this respect. Also your doctor or specialist should be told immediately of any change in your hearing that occurs between regular check-ups.

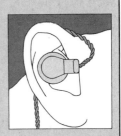

Behind-the-ear aid
The microphone, amplifier, and tiny battery are contained in a small, light plastic case worn behind the ear. The earphone fits into your outer-ear canal and seals it up so that no amplified sound is lost. It is connected to the rest of the apparatus by a short plastic tube.

Bone-conduction aid
In cases of marked conductive deafness (see *Deafness and vertigo*, p.329) – when, for example, the middle-ear bones are damaged (see *Otosclerosis*, p.332) – sound is transmitted from the apparatus not through an earphone but through a vibrating pad touching the mastoid process behind the ear. The vibrations pass through the bone to the inner ear.

Body-worn aids
In some more powerful hearing aids, the amplifier and battery are housed in a larger plastic case worn on the body. They are connected to the earphone by a thin plastic-covered wire.

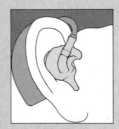

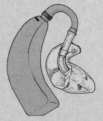

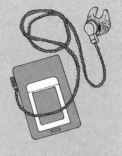

operation is performed to improve hearing. If, however, the discharge persists, a preliminary operation has to be carried out to clean the middle ear and remove any infected areas nearby, such as the tonsils or the adenoids.

The main operation, requiring a hospital stay of up to two weeks, can be performed once the infection has been eradicated. This operation involves mending the tiny bones in the middle ear, or replacing them with metal or plastic substitutes if they are past saving. Then the eroded eardrum is repaired by a tiny tissue graft from, for example, a vein; it cannot heal naturally because of the build-up of scar tissue resulting from repeated damage. In 70 per cent of cases, damage to the middle ear can be made good and at least some hearing restored.

Cholesteatoma

This disorder is a more serious form of *chronic infection of the middle ear* (p.334). Following repeated, untreated infections, a matted ball of tissue called a cholesteatoma grows in the middle ear. As the cholesteatoma grows, it can become infected, damaging the eardrum, producing pus, and damaging the delicate bones in the middle ear.

The symptoms of cholesteatoma are slight deafness, earache, and pus discharged from the ear. Headache, weakness of facial muscles and dizziness can also occur.

Cholesteatoma is not very common. It affects only those who do not seek treatment for long-standing ear trouble. The main risk is that, if unchecked, it can eat away the roof of the cavity of the middle ear, sometimes causing an *epidural abscess* (p.275) or *meningitis* (p.273).

OPERATION: Mastoid drainage
mastoidectomy

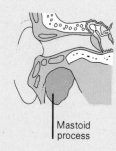

Mastoid process

This is a short operation to remove infected tissue from the mastoid process – a honeycombed area of bone behind the ear. It is usually done when an infection of the middle ear has spread to the mastoid process and cannot be cured by *antibiotic* drugs.

During the operation The hair behind your ear is shaved off, then you are taken to the operating theatre and given a general anaesthetic. The specialist ear surgeon makes an incision behind the flap of the ear, and delicately pares away the infected bone. The incision is then closed with stitches or clips. The usual operating time is 1 to 2 hours.

After the operation For a few days a drainage tube draws excess fluid from the site of the operation. You will probably stay in hospital for about 7 days.

Convalescence You should take 2 or 3 weeks away from work and must not get water in your ear for at least 2 months. Your hair gradually grows over the scar.

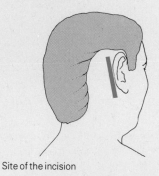

Site of the incision

What should be done?

If you have any of the symptoms described, especially if you have a childhood history of ear trouble, see your doctor. If a cholesteatoma is suspected, you will need to see a specialist for an ear examination and an audiometry test to assess your hearing (see *Hearing loss and hearing aids*, p.335). *X-rays* of the mastoid process will be needed to discover whether the infection has spread. Your doctor will choose a course of treatment depending on how easily the cholesteatoma can be removed. If the cholesteatoma is small, it may be possible to remove it and clean out the middle-ear cavity by means of a minor operation under a local anaesthetic.

If damage to the middle ear is extensive, the cavity is opened and cleaned out. Then a hole is drilled behind the visible ear, into the middle-ear cavity, to provide an outlet for the pus. In a further operation the tiny bones in the middle ear are restored or replaced with metal or plastic substitutes, and the eardrum is repaired. The operation, which normally necessitates about two weeks' stay in hospital, usually improves hearing significantly in most sufferers.

In about 20 per cent of people, there are recurrences of infection. These are not dangerous if treated right away; your doctor will probably examine your ears at least once a year to check for signs of infection. If your hearing is permanently damaged by the disease, a hearing aid may help.

Inner ear

Disorders of the inner ear affect two sensitive structures – the cochlea, which transforms sound vibrations into electrical signals that are then sent to the brain by way of the auditory nerve; and the labyrinth, which controls balance. If the cochlea and labyrinth are damaged, it is impossible to repair them because they are extremely delicate, and surgery is not yet possible. The result is that perceptive deafness, caused by damage to the delicate structures in the inner ear, is rarely curable (unlike conductive deafness – see *Deafness and vertigo*, p.329).

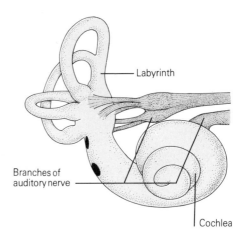

Labyrinth

Branches of auditory nerve

Cochlea

Ménière's disease

In Ménière's disease there is an increase in the amount of fluid in the labyrinth. The labyrinth, a fluid-filled chamber in the inner ear, constantly monitors the position and movements of the head, and relays the information to the brain so that you can maintain your balance. The increased pressure caused by the excess fluid distorts or even ruptures the nerve cells in the labyrinth wall, disturbing the sense of balance. The adjacent cochlea may also be damaged and, as a result, the hearing impaired.

The disease attacks one ear, then, in about half of sufferers, the other.

What are the symptoms?
Symptoms may be absent or mild for most of the time but attacks occur periodically. These vary in frequency from every few weeks to every few years, and in length from hours to several days. The main symptom of an attack is vertigo (dizziness), which can last for any period from a few minutes to a few hours and is often accompanied by noises in the ear and by muffled or distorted hearing (especially of low notes). At the same time, there may be severe nausea and vomiting. Sometimes you feel pressure in the affected ear before or during an attack. In persistent cases the attacks become less severe as time goes by, although some deafness and noises in the ear may remain between attacks, often becoming serious.

How common is the problem?
Ménière's disease is not common; there is only 1 case per 2,000 people each year. For some reason, it affects mainly fair-skinned, blue-eyed people.

What are the risks?
In most people, the disorder is mild and clears up spontaneously, but in a few cases complete deafness can occur in one or both ears. In these severe cases, anxiety and migraine may also occur. There are also risks associated with the dizziness which can easily cause the sufferer to be involved in accidents.

What should be done?
If you have the symptoms described, see your doctor without delay. The doctor will probably send you to hospital for tests, which may take two or three days.

The first test will probably be audiometry (see *Hearing loss and hearing aids*, p.335). If the results suggest but do not confirm a diagnosis of Ménière's disease, the test may be repeated after you have been *dehydrated* by not being allowed to drink or by being given a *diuretic* drug. Either method reduces the amount of fluid (and therefore pressure) in the labyrinth. If the second test shows your hearing has improved by a certain amount, this is strong evidence that you have Ménière's disease.

If there is still doubt about the diagnosis, you may be given further tests. In one, called a vestibular function test, the ear is flooded with water at different temperatures. After each flooding, you experience a whirling sensation that makes the eyes flicker. The length of the flickerings indicates whether the labyrinth is diseased.

In rare cases, a third test called cochleography may be necessary; this requires a general anaesthetic. A needle-like probe is inserted through the eardrum and registers the electrical activity of the cochlea.

What is the treatment?

Self-help: Lying still during an attack can ease symptoms. Cutting down generally on fluids (and salt) can reduce the frequency and severity of attacks by reducing the volume of fluid in the labyrinth.

Professional help: In most cases, the doctor will prescribe a *vasodilator* drug to reduce the excess fluid in the labyrinth; and, for acute attacks, you may also receive a tranquillizer to reduce any anxiety which may be exacerbating the attack.

If, despite treatment, there is so much fluid in the labyrinth that it is being progressively damaged, although your hearing has not yet been badly affected, then an operation is performed. A hole is drilled through the bone of the middle ear into the labyrinth, releasing fluid. In about 70 per cent of cases the vertigo is cured, and the operation not only prevents further loss of hearing in the affected ear but in some cases improves it.

If the disease is so severe that the vertigo it causes is disabling, the labyrinth can be destroyed by surgery or *ultrasound*. This cures the vertigo but brings on total deafness in the affected ear; however, deafness would be inevitable even without treatment.

Before deciding on such drastic operations, doctors take into account many factors, including the condition of the patient's other ear and also his or her age.

In some cases of Ménière's disease, the condition may clear up without treatment.

Labyrinthitis

The labyrinth, a group of fluid-filled chambers that control balance, can become infected in a number of ways – most commonly by a virus spreading from the nose or throat along the eustachian tube into the middle ear and then to the inner ear. Such an infection inflames the labyrinth and totally disrupts its functioning.

What are the symptoms?

The main symptom is vertigo: you feel extremely dizzy, and everything seems to be spinning round rapidly. Your eyes move slowly sideways, then flick back to their original position. Any movement of the head makes the vertigo worse. In some cases, there is extreme nausea and vomiting.

How common is the problem?

Labyrinthitis is uncommon. Each year only 1 person in 1,000 goes to the doctor for advice about this complaint.

What should be done?

If you have severe vertigo, see your doctor at the first opportunity. If you cannot travel, ask your doctor to visit you. The doctor will examine your ears with an *otoscope* and will question you about any recent respiratory infections, in order to determine whether the vertigo is caused by labyrinthitis (see also *Vertigo*, p.290).

What is the treatment?

You will need to lie quietly in bed for a week or more and take tranquillizers. Your doctor may prescribe *anti-emetic* drugs. The symptoms can be frightening, but your doctor will reassure you that they will soon disappear. Most cases clear up within three weeks.

Occupational deafness

Prolonged periods of loud noise at or above 90 dB (see *Sound and noise levels*, opposite), especially if high-pitched, can damage the sensitive hair cells lining the cochlea, the innermost part of the ear. This results in some degree of hearing loss. Among occupations particularly hazardous to unprotected ears are boiler-making, driving a tractor, using a pneumatic drill, and playing in, or even listening to, a loud rock group.

What should be done?

Perceptive deafness (see *Deafness and vertigo*, p.329), caused by damage to the cochlea, is irreversible. Therefore, prevention is all-important. If you are exposed to dangerous levels of noise, you must wear suitable ear protectors. Ear muffs are the most effective. They resemble headphones and almost totally insulate the ears from noise. If the wearer needs to communicate with colleagues – as on the flight deck of an aircraft – a small microphone and earphones can be added to the muffs. The next most effective protectors are ear plugs, of foam, plastic, wax, or rubber.

If you work in very noisy conditions, see a doctor at regular intervals, to have hearing tests. Loss of hearing can be detected at an early stage and steps taken to prevent further exposure to the noise responsible. If you think that the noise level where you work is too high and is endangering your health, contact the Health and Safety Executive and ask for the noise to be measured.

Sound and noise levels

What is sound?

Sound is a series of air-pressure waves – alternate peaks of high pressure and troughs of low pressure travelling through the atmosphere. Noise is a vague term that people usually use to mean loud, unpleasant sound.

How is loudness measured?

Loudness (volume) of sound is measured in units called decibels (dB) by a decibel meter. The microphone of the meter measures the peaks of high air pressure. Sound loud enough to cause immediate damage to the ears is usually above 130 dB. At the other end of the scale, sounds quieter than 10 dB cannot be heard by humans (but can be heard by some animals). See the diagram below for more details.

How loud is "painfully loud"?

Generally speaking, sound at 90 dB or above can cause pain in the ears. This pain warns you that your ears are in imminent danger of suffering damage – probably permanent – unless the sound source is removed. There are recommended sound limits and times of exposure (see table below) for various noisy occupations where the decibel measurement is over 80. If you are habitually exposed to sound levels of 90 dB or above, read the article on *Occupational deafness* on the facing page.

Note: Measurements on the decibel scale do not equate with our own perception of loudness; a rock concert registering 100 dB is much more than twice as loud as a stream registering 50 dB.

Legal limits of exposure to loud noise		
Noise level (decibels)	UK limit (hours)	US limit (hours)
90	8	8
92	5	6
94	3	—
95	—	4
96	2	—
99	1	—
100	0.5	2
110	—	0.5
115	—	0.25

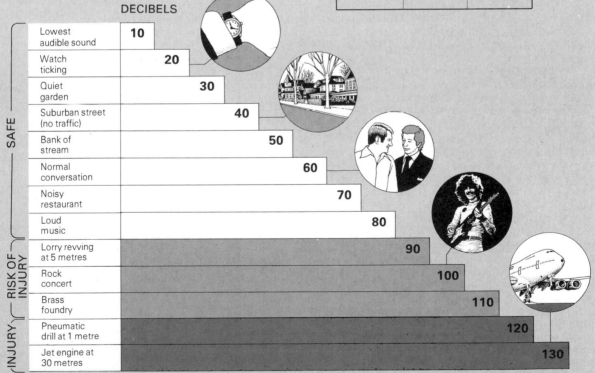

DECIBELS

Lowest audible sound	**10**
Watch ticking	**20**
Quiet garden	**30**
Suburban street (no traffic)	**40**
Bank of stream	**50**
Normal conversation	**60**
Noisy restaurant	**70**
Loud music	**80**
Lorry revving at 5 metres	**90**
Rock concert	**100**
Brass foundry	**110**
Pneumatic drill at 1 metre	**120**
Jet engine at 30 metres	**130**

SAFE

RISK OF INJURY

INJURY

Disorders of the respiratory system

Introduction

You breathe in order to supply your body with the oxygen essential for energy production, and to get rid of carbon dioxide, which is a waste product of energy production. At the centre of the respiratory system are the lungs, where breathed-in oxygen is exchanged for carbon dioxide from the blood. The channel along which air is breathed into and out of the lungs (the respiratory tract) consists primarily of the nose, throat, and trachea (windpipe). Deep in the chest the trachea divides into two main bronchi, one for each lung, and each bronchus divides within the lung, into increasingly smaller bronchioles. At the tip of all bronchioles are balloon-like cavities called alveoli – about 300 million of them in each lung. The vital exchange of oxygen for carbon dioxide occurs through minute blood vessels in the thin alveoli walls.

Air is sucked into the lungs by muscular action. The main muscle concerned is the diaphragm (a dome-shaped muscular sheet attached to the lower ribs), which divides the chest cavity from the abdomen. When the diaphragm contracts, along with other muscles between the ribs, air is sucked in; when the muscles relax, air is forced up the respiratory tract and out of the body (usually through the nostrils) by the elastic recoil of the lungs. If this mechanism works well, breathing is an almost unnoticeable activity. But a number of things can go wrong with the lungs, with essential parts of the respiratory tract, or with the muscular "bellows" action.

The articles in this section are arranged in three groups, each concentrating on disorders affecting one area of the respiratory system. The first group deals with problems affecting the nose and air spaces behind it (the nasal passage and sinuses). The second group consists of disorders of the throat, including the larynx (the voice-box at the top of the trachea) and the pharynx (the tube that leads from the nasal cavity down to the place where the oesophagus separates from the trachea); the larynx and pharynx are so closely related that, in practical terms, pharyngeal and laryngeal disorders are virtually indistinguishable. The third group comprises all the most common diseases of the lungs and chest, including the trachea, bronchi and bronchioles, and alveoli.

The main parts of the respiratory system

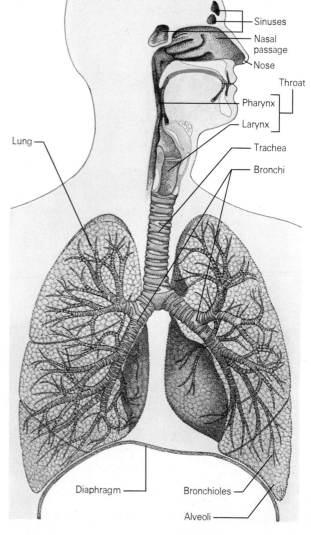

Sinuses
Nasal passage
Nose
Throat
Pharynx
Larynx
Lung
Trachea
Bronchi
Diaphragm
Bronchioles
Alveoli

How the respiratory system works

How you breathe

Air breathed in through the nose is warmed and moistened by small blood vessels very close to the surface of the nasal cavity before it passes into the lungs. Also the tiny hairs that line the nose provide a filtering system to stop foreign bodies such as dust particles from entering the lungs. When you breathe in, your diaphragm, which is dome-shaped when relaxed, is pulled flat (right). At the same time, muscles between your ribs contract and pull your ribcage upwards and outwards. These movements increase the volume of your chest, causing your lungs to expand and air to be sucked into them. The stronger the muscle action, the more air enters your lungs. Your rate of breathing in and out is determined mainly by the amount of carbon dioxide needing to be expelled from your bloodstream. When you breathe out, your chest muscles and diaphragm relax (far right). This causes your ribcage to sink and your lungs – which are very elastic – to contract, squeezing out air. The air that you breathe out still contains some oxygen. If this were not so, mouth-to-mouth artificial respiration would be unsuccessful.

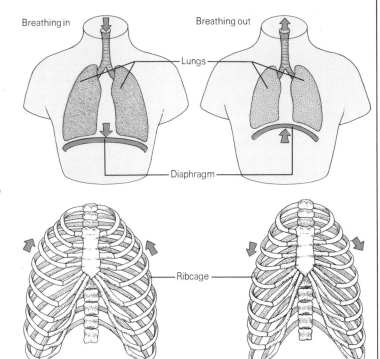

Breathing in

Breathing out

Lungs

Diaphragm

Ribcage

Breathing and swallowing (below)

As you breathe, the top of your oesophagus is kept closed by a ring of muscles which prevents air entering your digestive tract. When you swallow, the top of your oesophagus opens and the top of the trachea closes off to prevent food being inhaled into the lungs.

The pleurae (below)

Each lung is surrounded by a thin membranous coating called the pleura. This is folded back on itself to form a double layer all around the lung. There is a tiny space between the 2 layers which contains a small amount of fluid and forms a vacuum. The inner layer is attached to the lung and the outer layer is attached to the ribcage. The main function of the pleura is to act as a lubricating mechanism, allowing smooth, uniform expansion and contraction of the lung. When you breathe in and your ribcage lifts up and out, your lungs are also pulled up and out.

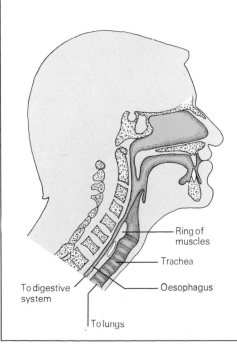

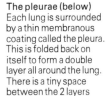

Ring of muscles

Trachea

Oesophagus

To digestive system

To lungs

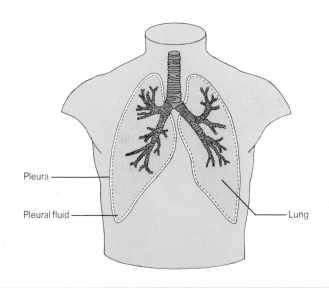

Pleura

Pleural fluid

Lung

Nose

The nose is the main entrance to the respiratory system, and is lined with a hairy mucous membrane that contains many tiny blood vessels close to the surface. This ensures that the air you breathe is filtered, moistened, and warmed as it goes through the nasal passage towards your throat and lungs. The nasal passage runs along the top of the palate (the shelf separating the nose from the mouth) and turns downwards to join the passage from the mouth to the throat. But the nasal passage is not a simple tube. Pairs of air-filled cavities (the sinuses) branch from it into the bones of the skull at various points, and the lining of the nose extends into these cavities. Thus nasal infections sometimes spread into the sinuses as well as into the rest of the respiratory system.

The nose is also, of course, the organ of smell, and you are apt to suffer a temporary loss of the ability to detect odours whenever a disorder of the respiratory system gives you a stuffy nose. However, permanent loss of sense of smell (*anosmia*) is rare and far less of a disability than loss of sight or hearing.

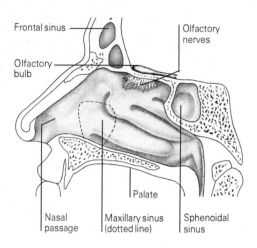

The nasal passage and sinuses
The nasal passage is linked to three pairs of sinuses – air-filled cavities inside the skull bones. Projecting into the top of the nasal passage are the sensitive hair-like endings of the olfactory nerves, which detect odours in the air in the nose and pass the information to the olfactory bulb at the base of the brain.

Colds

The disease we call the common cold is, in fact, a group of minor illnesses caused by any of nearly 200 different viruses. Normally, a common (or "head") cold is confined to the nose and throat, but these viruses can also infect the larynx (causing *laryngitis*, p.351) and the lungs (causing *acute bronchitis*, p.353). The viral infections sometimes pave the way to more serious bacterial infections of the throat, ears, or lungs (see "What are the risks?" below). All of us get colds, and we are likely to have our first cold during our first year of life. For the next year or two most children are extremely susceptible to nasal viral infection; then they gradually become immune to many of the viruses common in their surroundings. Frequency of attack increases again during the early school years because the new environment contains new types of virus. As people get older, they acquire more immunity and catch fewer and less severe colds. (See also *Recurrent coughs and colds*, p.680.)

What are the symptoms?
To some extent the symptoms depend on the virus responsible for the cold. The major

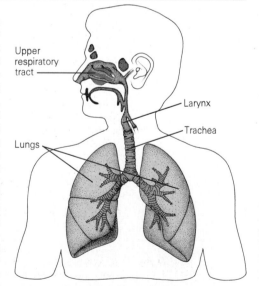

Effects of the common cold
A cold can affect almost any part of the respiratory system. Sneezing and a runny nose mean that the upper respiratory tract is affected. The infection may also irritate the trachea, causing a cough, or the larynx, making the sufferer's voice hoarse. Occasionally the lungs become infected, leading to bronchitis.

symptoms include one or more of the following: sneezing, watering eyes, sore throat, hoarseness, coughing, and – above all – a runny nose. The nasal discharge begins by being rather watery, then becomes thick and greenish in colour. You may also have a headache and become slightly feverish; this rise in temperature may cause shivering and a feeling of being chilled. A very high temperature and general body pains are more likely to be symptoms of *influenza* (p.559).

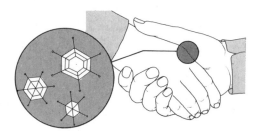

Spreading colds
Although it is not known exactly how cold viruses are spread, hand-to-hand contact is a possibility. If you have a cold, you may hold your hand in front of your mouth when you cough or sneeze and may then pass on the virus by touching hands.

How common is the problem?
Everybody will get an occasional cold – perhaps one or two a year – throughout life. Nobody is quite sure how colds are caught. One important way seems to be through hand-to-hand contact, but the viruses are also sprayed by coughs and sneezes into the air we breathe. Colds occur far less frequently in isolated communities, where everyone soon becomes immune to the viruses in circulation; an outbreak is apt to follow the arrival of strangers.

Besides the fact that there are so many different cold-causing viruses, the viruses themselves are constantly changing (*mutating*) as they multiply, so new kinds of virus to which we have not built up any resistance are constantly appearing.

What are the risks?
An ordinary cold often clears up in three to four days; even with bacterial infection a head cold should not last longer than a week. But because the respiratory tract is a series of spaces connected by passages, the infection can spread to the middle ear, sinuses, larynx (voice-box), trachea (windpipe), and lungs (see, for example, *Acute infection of the middle ear*, p.333).

What should be done?
Anyone with a cold should stay at home and, if convenient, in isolation. This is chiefly for the sake of other people. Consult your doctor only if the cold lasts over 10 days, or if it seems that infection has spread beyond the nose and throat, or if you are prone to bronchitis or ear infections.

What is the treatment?
Self-help: There is no way to cure a common cold, but there are measures you can take to ease the symptoms. Stay at home, in a warm (but not overheated) room, and moisten the atmosphere by means of some type of humidifier; steam from a basin of hot water will do. Drink plenty of fluids, preferably in the form of fruit juices, and take an aspirin or two at night to help you sleep. Commercial "cold cures" and nasal sprays may also give temporary relief. But use patent medicines only in moderation, and do not expect them to cure your cold.

Professional help: There is no point in asking a doctor to treat a normally healthy person who has a cold. Your doctor will not generally prescribe *antibiotics* since viruses are not affected by them; antibiotics might actually make matters worse by producing side-effects such as diarrhoea or swollen lips and throat. Anyone prone to recurrent attacks of bronchitis or ear infection, however, should see a doctor at the first sign of a head cold. For such persons an antibiotic will give some protection against complications due to the secondary bacterial infection that can often follow a viral illness.

Catarrh

"Catarrh" is a vague, non-scientific term meaning different things to different people, but virtually all sufferers experience a blocked nose that occasionally discharges fluid. The fluid may be thin and clear but is more usually thick and opaque. There is discomfort and breathing is difficult. At night the nostril on the side the sufferer lies on gets blocked and disturbs sleep, or the discharge drops back into the throat, bringing on a fit of coughing. Depending on its cause, the condition may persist for weeks, or come and go in the space of a few days.

The most common causes of catarrh are viral infections, such as a common *cold* (opposite). Children in their first years at school, when they are first exposed to many viruses, are particularly prone to attacks of

Self-help for a blocked or runny nose

Although viral infections such as the common cold cannot be cured, the nasal discomfort they cause can be eased by using the simple self-help advice given here. In addition, always remember that the lining of the nasal passageways is fragile and has many tiny blood vessels just under its surface; be careful not to blow your nose too hard, thereby adding a nosebleed to your problems.

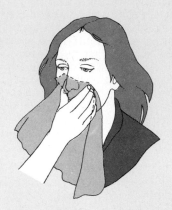

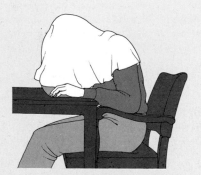

Blowing your nose

Blow into a clean handkerchief or disposable paper tissue. First clear one nostril, keeping the other nostril closed by pressing on that side of the nose (above left). Then repeat for the other nostril (above right). A common fault is to press both nostrils almost closed as you blow. This forces air that cannot escape through the nose along the eustachian tube to the middle ear, where it may rupture the eardrum. Mucus may also be pushed along the eustachian tube to the middle ear, spreading the infection to the ear.

Steam inhalation

There are several over-the-counter inhalation preparations available; they usually contain menthol or a similar substance. When dissolved in hot water and breathed through the nose they loosen mucus which can then be cleared by blowing your nose thoroughly.

Nasal decongestants

These over-the-counter preparations are intended to shrink and dry out the swollen, mucus-producing tissue inside the nose and sinuses, and liquefy and free remaining mucus. They are available as tablets, spray or drops. Never exceed the maximum dose advised on the packet because over-use can lead to a "rebound" reaction when the tissues respond to the drug in the decongestant by producing even more mucus than before. And prolonged use can eventually damage and scar the nasal tissues, causing further problems.

Substances that trigger off allergic rhinitis

Pollen

The pollen from any plant, particularly grass and trees, may trigger off an allergy. Symptoms appear when the plant or plants to which you are allergic produce pollen, usually between March and September.

Animal fur

If you are said to be allergic to animal fur you are not, in fact, affected by the fur itself but by the tiny skin flakes also shed by the animal.

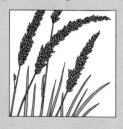

Mites in house dust

House-dust mites are found in almost every house. If anyone in your family is allergic to these mites, you should keep your house as dust-free as possible.

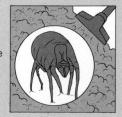

Feathers

An allergy to feathers is probably one of the easiest to deal with. Simply avoid anything that is stuffed with feathers, such as some pillows and sleeping quilts.

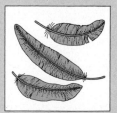

catarrh. By the age of eight most children are more resistant to such infections.

Other conditions which may cause catarrh include *allergic rhinitis* (below), *nasal polyps* (p.348), and any distortion of the nasal passages (see *Deviated septum*, p.348). When the underlying condition is dealt with, the catarrh will usually clear up as well. Catarrh may be brought on by local irritation from dust, an over-dry atmosphere, gas or oil fires, or airborne chemicals. Certain drugs may also stimulate the nose to produce a discharge. For hints on how to relieve a blocked or runny nose, see opposite.

Allergic rhinitis
(hay fever)

Allergic rhinitis is similar to *asthma* (p.355) except in one respect. Whereas in asthma an airborne substance causes an allergic or hypersensitive reaction in the lungs and chest, the reaction in allergic rhinitis occurs in the eyes, nose, and throat. Exposure to the airborne irritant (known as the *allergen*) triggers off the release of *histamine* (a body chemical), and this causes inflammation and fluid production in the cells of the fragile linings of the cavities in and behind the nose and in the eyelids and surface layer of the eyes (see *Conjunctivitis*, p.317).

Nobody knows why certain people are hypersensitive to an otherwise harmless pollen grain or other airborne particles. The response depends on the function of the body's natural immune system (see *Allergies*, p.705). And since allergy-based diseases such as asthma, *eczema* (p.253), and allergic rhinitis often run in families, the cause is probably partly genetic.

If you have allergic rhinitis, you react to specific allergens (even though you may not yet know what they are). For example, if you suffer from hay fever, the most familiar variety of the disease, you may be sensitive to grass pollen, which is produced most abundantly in early summer; or you may be particularly sensitive to tree pollen, which abounds in spring; or you may literally suffer from exposure to autumnal hay. Almost any airborne substance derived from a living organism can cause allergic rhinitis: hair, skin, or feathers from a domestic pet, for example. You may be allergic to house dust – or, rather, to the mites that infest the dust. You may even react to a certain smell (which is carried through the air by molecules of the substance that causes it).

Allergic rhinitis may be either seasonal (for example, hay fever, which occurs for only a few weeks when the offending pollen abound) or perennial (occurring all year round and caused by exposure to airborne allergens more or less constantly present).

What are the symptoms?
You sneeze frequently, your nose runs, and your eyes are red, itchy, and watery. Rubbing the eyes makes them worse. Itching skin, dry throat, and wheezing can also occur. If you have hay fever, the symptoms are most severe when the amount of pollen in the air (the "pollen count") is highest. Symptoms tend to be especially severe for a 15- to 30-minute period – a so-called "attack" of allergic rhinitis – and then to subside for a while.

Because airborne allergens are generally too small to be visible, it is difficult to predict when, or even why, you may suffer an attack. For example, if you are allergic to cats, you may start to sneeze on entering an empty room which has been frequented by a cat. The reason is that tiny, unseen pieces of cat skin are still floating about in the room.

How common is the problem?
Allergic rhinitis is very common. In Britain about 1 person in 90 suffers badly enough (usually from hay fever) to consult a doctor, and many other people have the disorder in a milder form. Although there is a widespread belief that young people tend to grow out of allergic rhinitis in their late teens or early twenties, this is not necessarily so. Anyone can have the disorder or can grow into it or out of it at any age. You are particularly susceptible, though, if you are under 40 and have another allergic condition such as asthma or eczema, or if any such condition runs in your family. Many people suffer from more than one variety of allergic rhinitis, both seasonal and perennial.

What are the risks?
Although it can be a lifelong scourge, allergic rhinitis does not normally endanger the sufferer's general health.

What should be done?
If you find that allergic rhinitis interferes with your daily routine, see your doctor. You will be asked questions to ascertain how badly you are affected and, depending on your answers, you may be advised against any professional treatment. This is because possible side-effects and the inconvenience of some kinds of treatment may be more troublesome than the condition itself. If you

do not know what causes your rhinitis, the doctor may arrange for a skin test that will help to identify the allergens so that you can try to avoid them. The test involves putting drops of liquid, each containing a common allergen, on your forearm and pricking the skin under each drop. If the skin under a given drop turns red and itchy, then you are allergic to that substance. Treatment is more likely to be successful if you are allergic to only one or two substances.

What is the treatment?

Self-help: If you get hay fever regularly, stay indoors as much as possible during the hay-fever season. When you go outdoors, it may help to wear sunglasses; but avoid contact lenses, which can irritate your eyes, and resist all temptation to rub them. Keep track of the pollen count as given on television and radio and in many newspapers. If your allergic rhinitis is not seasonal, try to discover what you are allergic to, and take steps to avoid or minimize exposure. Self-help recommendations for asthmatics also apply for people with perennial allergic rhinitis.

Regardless of whether your condition is seasonal or perennial, there are many preparations for easing symptoms that can be bought without a doctor's prescription. The most commonly used drugs are *antihistamine* tablets, which are generally effective for both preventing and stopping attacks. To be fully effective, antihistamines must be taken regularly at four- to six-hour intervals, often for several days at a time, and the side-effects of drowsiness and dryness of nose and throat may be more troublesome than the rhinitis itself. In any event, because such tablets make you sleepy, you should never take one if you intend to drive a vehicle or operate machinery within the next few hours.

For swift relief from a runny or blocked nose, you may want to use decongestant nose drops or a nasal spray, which can ease symptoms within minutes. Do not use such preparations often or regularly, however; they eventually aggravate the very symptoms they are supposed to suppress.

Professional help: There is a wide range of symptom-suppressing drugs that can be procured only with a prescription. If you get relief from none of the self-help measures suggested above, your doctor may prescribe a kind of antihistamine that is more suitable for you than any you have yet tried. There are various types of drug, some of them *steroids*, which will not stop an attack after symptoms have started. Taken several times a day, they act as a preventive measure when exposure to a known allergen is imminent. Steroids are normally given as nasal sprays, because when applied only to the site of irritation (the lining of the nose), they do not have the unpleasant side-effects often associated with steroid tablets, which affect the entire body.

All drug treatments merely suppress symptoms and do not alter the basic allergic reaction. The only possible cure for allergic rhinitis is a course of "desensitizing" injections. If a skin test has succeeded in identifying the offending substance or substances, your doctor can give you a series of allergen-concentrate injections in an attempt to get your body to stop reacting to the allergens. This treatment sometimes works well, but sometimes does not.

Treatment for allergic rhinitis

Sometimes an allergy may be cured by a course of desensitizing injections. Most treatments prescribed by your doctor are designed simply to relieve symptoms of the allergy rather than the underlying cause. Irritation of the eyes and nose can be soothed by various antihistamine drops and sprays. There are also some preparations available that prevent the allergy from being triggered off, but these are only effective if taken regularly before and during exposure to a known allergen.

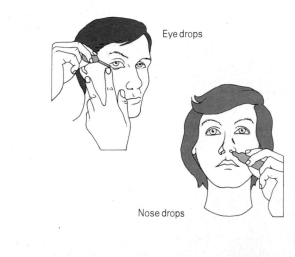

Eye drops

Nose drops

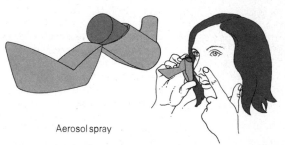

Aerosol spray

Sinusitis

Sinusitis is inflammation of the mucous membranes of the sinuses resulting from bacterial or viral infection. Of the several linked sinuses (air spaces around the nose), those most likely to be affected are the frontal sinuses (in the forehead just above the eyes) and maxillary sinuses (in the cheek-bones). The mucous membranes of the main nasal cavity are continuous with those that line the sinuses, and the organisms that cause sinusitis spread to the sinuses from the nose. This generally happens when a common cold, which is a viral infection, becomes complicated by a secondary infection of bacteria (see *Colds*, p.342).

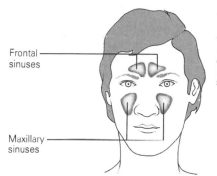

Frontal sinuses

Maxillary sinuses

Headache over one or both eyes indicates that your frontal sinuses are inflamed. Less commonly, your cheeks hurt if your maxillary sinuses are affected.

Examining the sinuses by X-ray

If you suffer from persistent sinus trouble, your doctor may arrange for you to have your sinuses examined more thoroughly by X-rays before attempting to drain them. Several X-rays taken from different angles show the exact position of the sinuses. Healthy air-filled sinuses show up as dark patches surrounded by grey areas of bone. Any fluid in these sinuses can be seen on the X-rays as white areas below the black, air-filled spaces.

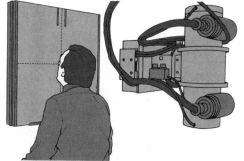

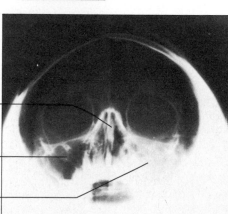

Nasal passage

Healthy, air-filled sinus

Fluid-filled sinus

X-ray picture

What are the symptoms?

After a few days of a cold, when you would expect it to get better, the blockage in your nose worsens and the greenish discharge increases. Later, because the passageways between the nose and sinuses also become blocked, the discharge may cease, and your nose is more stuffed up than ever. You have to breathe through your mouth, your speech becomes nasal, and you feel generally ill. If frontal sinuses are affected, a major symptom is headache over one or both eyes; it is most painful when you wake in the morning. The under-surface of your forehead just above the eyes feels tender, and you may get a stab of pain when you bend your head forwards.

If maxillary sinuses are affected, one or both cheeks will hurt. You may feel as if you have a toothache in the upper jaw. Occasionally, sinusitis follows dental treatment because infection spreads from the roots of a tooth through the bone into the sinus (see *Abscesses in teeth*, p.439).

How common is the problem?

Sinusitis is common, but susceptibility varies enormously. Some people never get it; others succumb whenever they have a bad cold; others can get it simply by jumping into water without holding their nose. Damage to nasal bones, or even a foreign body caught in a nostril, may bring on an attack. A deformity of the nose such as a *deviated septum* (p.348) may increase susceptibility by obstructing the nasal passageways.

What are the risks?

Risks are minimal if sinusitis is treated with *antibiotics*. Before these were discovered, infection sometimes spread through the mucous membrane of the sinuses into the bones and even into the brain. Such complications are now almost non-existent.

What should be done?

Try the self-help measures recommended below. If, after three or four days, symptoms persist, consult your doctor, who will probably confirm the diagnosis of sinusitis by examining your mouth and nose and gently pressing the floor of the sinuses above the eyes or behind the cheeks.

What is the treatment?

Self-help: Stay indoors, in a room with an even temperature and high humidity; dry, overheated rooms aggravate the symptoms. Blow your nose gently with tissues, destroying them after use. To relieve pain, take aspirin or paracetamol, and inhale steam from a basin of hot water (see *Self-help for a blocked or runny nose*, p.344).

Professional help: In addition to prescribing a "broad-spectrum" *antibiotic*, your doctor may suggest the use of a decongestant, either in tablet form or as nasal drops or spray. Decongestants shrink the swollen mucous membrane, thus widening the airways, but they should be used only as directed on the package or as advised by your doctor; if used incorrectly, they can do more harm than good. Further treatment is unnecessary

unless sinusitis persists, when a minor operation under local anaesthetic may be advisable. The procedure involves piercing a bone between the nose and the sinuses so as to open an extra passageway, then washing the sinuses out with sterile water. This relieves the obstruction, and the washings are usually analysed in order to identify the invading organisms and determine the best way to combat them. Further minor surgery to improve drainage may be needed if infection recurs, but this rarely happens.

Nasal polyps

If part of the mucous membrane that lines the nose becomes distended and protrudes into the nasal cavity, the growth that it forms is known as a polyp. Polyps are caused by over-production of fluid in the cells of the membrane resulting from a condition such as *allergic rhinitis* (p.345). The polyps are harmless, but a big one or several little ones can obstruct the nasal airway and make breathing difficult, and impair your sense of smell. If the opening between the nasal cavity and one of the sinuses is blocked, you may have headaches or facial pains similar to those occurring in *sinusitis* (p.347).

What should be done?
If your nose is gradually becoming blocked, you may have polyps. Examine the lining of your nose in a mirror while shining a light up your nostrils – the polyps look like pearly grey lumps. But polyps are often at the back of the nose, where they can be seen only with a special instrument. If you suspect that you

may have nasal polyps, you should visit your doctor who, if the diagnosis is confirmed, may refer you to a specialist for surgery; the only way to treat them is to remove them. This minor operation is usually done under local anaesthetic, with virtually no risk of complications, and is generally successful; though in a few cases the polyps may recur and require further minor surgery.

Examining the nose
To examine the inside of your nose, the doctor separates your nostrils with a special instrument – a nasal speculum – that looks like a pair of sugar tongs.

Deviated septum

If the nasal septum (the wall between the nostrils) is very crooked, the air passage on one side is narrowed, and this can make breathing slightly difficult, with the flow of air through the narrow passage sometimes becoming blocked. Substantial deviation of the septum is not a common complaint; it usually happens as the result of an injury, and the nose often looks quite straight. There are no significant symptoms other than the mild breathing problem and, rarely, an increased tendency to *sinusitis* (p.347).

What is the treatment?
The septum can be easily straightened by surgery if the deviation is producing troublesome symptoms. Most people, however, simply learn to live with the condition and any minor symptoms it causes.

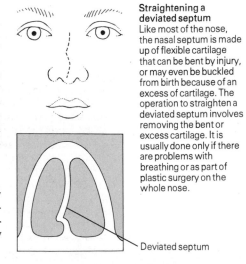

Straightening a deviated septum
Like most of the nose, the nasal septum is made up of flexible cartilage that can be bent by injury, or may even be buckled from birth because of an excess of cartilage. The operation to straighten a deviated septum involves removing the bent or excess cartilage. It is usually done only if there are problems with breathing or as part of plastic surgery on the whole nose.

Deviated septum

Anosmia

"Anosmia" is the technical term for loss of the sense of smell (and, incidentally, of taste) that persists even when there is no obvious cause, such as a head cold. Most commonly, anosmia results from a chronic condition like *allergic rhinitis* (p.345) or from *nasal polyps* (opposite). Very rarely it may be a symptom of a *brain tumour* (p.281) or may occur as the result of a head injury that ruptures the olfactory nerves (the nerves that run from the top of the nasal passage and carry smell sensations from the nose to the brain).

What should be done?

If you have lost your sense of smell or taste, consult your doctor, who will probably find that you have a nasal condition that can be treated, thereby curing the anosmia. If there is no sign of abnormality in your nose, the doctor may refer you to a neurologist, who will perform various diagnostic tests. It is unlikely that your olfactory nerves have been damaged; if they have, it is unlikely that the damage can be repaired.

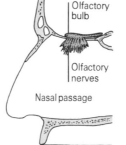

The position of the olfactory nerves
The olfactory nerves, well protected at the top of the nose just below the base of the brain, convert smells into nerve impulses. These travel via the nerves to the olfactory bulb in the brain.

Olfactory bulb
Olfactory nerves
Nasal passage

Nosebleed

The nose begins to bleed, usually quite suddenly and from only one nostril. This may occur quite often. The nasal lining is easily damaged by infections (such as colds) and the crusting that often accompanies them. In most cases, though, unless the nose has been injured, bleeding simply seems to "happen". There is seldom cause for concern, since a nosebleed is unlikely to be a symptom of any other disorder. A generalized bleeding disorder such as *thrombocytopenia* (p.425) may, rarely, cause nosebleeds, but in such cases there is usually a good deal of bleeding elsewhere – for instance, from the gums or mouth, or under the skin.

What is the treatment?

Self-help: Sit down, lean forward, and breathe through your mouth. Close the lower part of the nose on the bleeding side by pressing it with the ball of the thumb. Keep pressing for 5 to 10 minutes. This stops most nosebleeds. Do not blow your nose for about 12 hours; thereafter blow gently so as not to dislodge the clot that has formed and stopped the bleeding.

Professional help: If bleeding continues, consult your doctor or go to the casualty department of a hospital. The doctor will probably pack a strip of gauze into the nostril and tell you to leave it in for several hours. If bleeding persists or keeps recurring, the bleeding area may have to be *cauterized*, and the doctor may take a specimen of your blood to make sure you do not suffer from *anaemia* (p.419). This is unlikely; generally, despite appearances, relatively little blood is lost through nosebleeds. If your nosebleed was caused by a fairly substantial injury, it is possible that you may have sustained a *deviated septum* (opposite), which may cause breathing difficulties. Ask your doctor for a nasal examination if you are worried about this possibility.

Medical myth

Nosebleeds are often due to high blood pressure and are nature's way of lowering it.

Wrong. If a doctor whom you consult about nosebleeds takes your blood pressure, it is partly to reassure you and partly because it is always wise to test blood pressure.

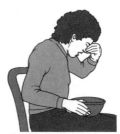

Sit with your head forward

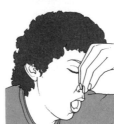

Pinch the fleshy part of your nose

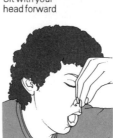

Doctor packs the nostril with gauze

Treatment for a nosebleed
If you have a nosebleed, sit down with a bowl held under your nose. Pinch the fleshy part of your nose firmly between your index finger and thumb for about 5 minutes, while breathing through your mouth. This pressure allows a blood clot to form and seal the damaged blood vessels. Do not blow your nose for several hours after the bleeding has stopped, as this may dislodge the blood clot and bleeding may start again. If the bleeding has not stopped after 20 minutes, go to your doctor. The doctor will use a special instrument to pack strips of gauze into the affected nostril, and so apply constant pressure to the ruptured blood vessels.

Throat

The throat is a multi-purpose tube leading from the back of the nose and mouth down to the trachea (windpipe) and oesophagus (gullet). When you breathe, air passes through your throat into the trachea on its way to the lungs. When you swallow, chewed food lubricated with saliva slips down the throat into the oesophagus on its way to the stomach. And when you speak, you use your larynx (voice-box), which is located in the throat at the top of the trachea. Air passing over the vocal cords (stretched flaps of tissue in the larynx) causes them to vibrate, producing the sounds that your mouth shapes into speech.

Like the rest of the respiratory system, the throat is chiefly at risk from infection, which often spreads upwards or downwards throughout the system. The symptom "sore throat" accounts for up to 12 per cent of all visits to general practitioners. It is not always a disorder in its own right, though; a sore throat sometimes indicates an infectious or inflammatory condition such as *acute bronchitis* (p.353) elsewhere in the system.

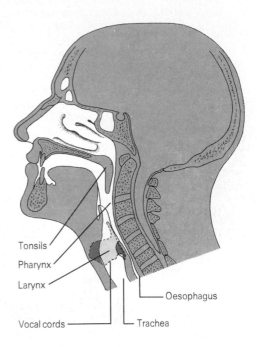

Tonsils
Pharynx
Larynx
Vocal cords
Oesophagus
Trachea

Pharyngitis

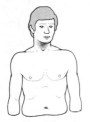

Site of the pain

A sore throat
Although a sore throat is rarely a serious disorder, it can make breathing, swallowing, and speaking painful and difficult.

Your pharynx is the part of your throat between your tonsils and your vocal cords (larynx). Acute (sudden) inflammation of the pharynx, like acute inflammation of the tonsils, is caused by infection with bacteria and viruses. The only difference is that pharyngitis tends to be less severe than *tonsillitis* (opposite), and some medical authorities simply speak of both conditions as "acute sore throat". Persistent infection (chronic pharyngitis) occurs when a chronic infection of surrounding organs – usually a respiratory, sinus, or mouth disorder – spreads to the pharynx and remains there. But pharyngitis can also be caused simply by irritation and inflammation of the pharynx without infection – for example, by cigarette smoke, alcohol, or excessive use of the voice.

What are the symptoms?

If you have acute pharyngitis, your throat is sore, you have trouble swallowing, and you probably feel feverish. As in tonsillitis, your throat is red and angry-looking. If you have chronic pharyngitis, the symptoms are usually less severe. In either form your voice may sound hoarse if the inflammation has affected your larynx.

How common is the problem?

Pharyngitis is a very common complaint. Statistics show that, on average, each person in Britain consults a doctor once a year because of an acute sore throat (pharyngitis and/or tonsillitis).

What should be done?

Try the self-help advice detailed below if you suspect you have pharyngitis. If, despite these measures, your sore throat persists for more than a few days, you should then consult your doctor.

What is the treatment?

Self-help: Whether your pharyngitis is acute or chronic, do not smoke. Give your throat a rest by having a mostly fluid diet. Commercial lozenges, mouthwashes, and gargles should relieve the symptoms of acute pharyngitis, and aspirin or paracetamol may ease generalized aches and pains.

Professional help: For an acute and particularly troublesome attack, *antibiotics* in tablet form are usually prescribed. For chronic pharyngitis your doctor will try to find and treat the primary source of infection. Your pharyngitis should then disappear.

Tonsillitis

Tonsillitis (acute infection of the tonsils) is primarily a children's disease (see *Tonsillitis in children*, p.676). It occurs occasionally in adults, however, with symptoms so similar to those of influenza that sufferers may assume they have a "touch of flu". If you are generally unwell, have a sore throat and a headache, and feel alternately hot and shivery, examine your throat. If your tonsils are red and inflamed and seem larger than usual, you probably have tonsillitis.

What should be done?

Stay in bed for a day or two, take one or two aspirins every four hours, and drink plenty of fluids. Consult your doctor if sore throat and fever last for more than 48 hours. Your doctor may, in certain cases, prescribe a course of *antibiotics* to relieve the problem.

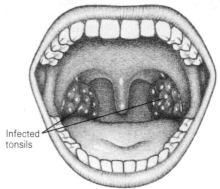

Infected tonsils

The tonsils
The tonsils are glandular swellings at either side of the throat which help to trap and destroy micro-organisms. If they become swollen and inflamed in the process, you have a "sore throat".

Laryngitis

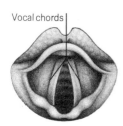

Vocal chords

Laryngitis is usually caused by bacterial or viral infection of the larynx (voice-box), which is situated at the top of the trachea (windpipe). The infection tends to follow a cold or sore throat, and it causes generalized inflammation and swelling of the mucous membrane of the larynx, including the vocal cords. Because the opening of the larynx in young children is very narrow, the swollen membrane sometimes interferes with breathing (see *Stridor and croup*, p.678) but this is not a problem of adult laryngitis. Occasionally laryngitis is caused simply by irritation and inflammation of the larynx without infection – for example, by cigarette smoke, alcohol, or excessive use of the voice.

What are the symptoms?

The main symptom is hoarseness, which may lead, over the course of two or three days, to loss of voice; speaking may even be painful. There may be fever or other flu-like symptoms. Most people recover in a few days, but laryngitis sometimes becomes persistent, especially for sufferers from *sinusitis* (p.347) or *chronic bronchitis* (p.354).

What are the risks?

The main risk of apparent laryngitis is that it may be a symptom of a tumour (see *Tumours of the larynx*, p.352). In rare cases when painful swallowing and earache are associated with hoarseness, the source of the trouble may be *tuberculosis* (p.563).

What should be done?

If you obviously have laryngitis and are otherwise healthy, stay at home, resting your

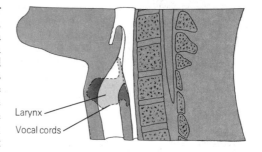

Larynx

Vocal cords

The effects of laryngitis
An infection of the upper-respiratory tract may affect the vocal cords, causing them to become inflamed. When air passes over these swollen cords during speech, the sounds you make are distorted – producing the hoarseness common to laryngitis. Over-use of the voice can also cause the cords to swell.

voice and not smoking or drinking alcohol until the inflammation clears up and you can talk normally. This should take no more than four or five days. If hoarseness persists for over a week, consult your doctor, who will question you about your general health and will examine your throat for signs of inflammation. If there are no such signs, your trouble is probably not laryngitis and further diagnostic procedures will be required, perhaps meaning a visit to hospital.

If it becomes evident that you are suffering from chronic bronchitis, sinusitis, or tuberculosis, treatment of the underlying condition should cure the laryngitis. The doctor will also advise you, if appropriate, to give up smoking, moderate your drinking habits, and even perhaps change your job.

Tumours of the larynx

A growth on the larynx may be either *benign* or *malignant*. There is a fine distinction between two types of benign growth – papillomas, of which there are usually several, and polyps, of which there is generally only one. Both types can be removed without permanent ill-effects; they appear to be caused by misuse (perhaps over-use) of the vocal cords. Malignant tumours (cancers) occur chiefly in heavy smokers and are found only rarely in non-smokers.

What are the symptoms?

Hoarseness is usually the only symptom. There are no flu-like symptoms as in *laryngitis* (p.351). If the tumour is malignant, the spreading cancer may eventually make swallowing difficult; and there may be an increasingly obvious lump in the neck. In a child,

Examining the larynx
To examine your vocal cords, the doctor uses a system of mirrors. Light is reflected from a special eyepiece, which is basically a mirror with a hole in it for the doctor to look through. Another small mirror attached to a long handle is held at the back of your throat to reflect the light on to your vocal cords.

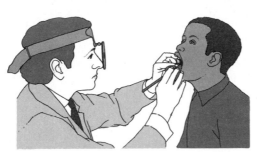

because the airway through the larynx is narrow, tumours on the larynx often give the voice a high-pitched, crowing sound (see *Stridor and croup*, p.678).

Hoarseness due to benign growth tends to be intermittent, but hoarseness due to cancer is continuous and gradually worsens. Since it is not painful and comes on slowly, the sufferer may scarcely notice it at first.

How common is the problem?

There are about 2,000 new cases of cancer of the larynx every year in Britain. Benign tumours are slightly less common; they occur chiefly in people, such as singers, who misuse or over-use the vocal cords.

What are the risks?

The main risk is that you may ignore slowly increasing hoarseness until it is too late to deal successfully with cancer of the larynx, which can nearly always be cured if diagnosed early. If not discovered in time, it can either spread locally or get into the bloodstream and produce secondary cancers (*metastases*) elsewhere in the body.

What should be done?

Do not ignore inexplicable vocal changes. If you remain hoarse for over a week, or if hoarseness keeps returning after periods of normality, consult your doctor. If your throat shows no signs of the inflammation that accompanies laryngitis, the doctor will probably refer you to a specialist, who will examine your larynx by means of light reflected from a mirror held at the back of the throat. If swelling or any other abnormality is apparent, the specialist will probably do an *endoscopic* examination, along with a *biopsy* to determine whether or not your tumour is in any way malignant.

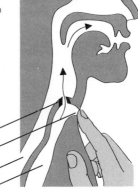

Voice production following larynx removal
You may be given surgery to create a breathing hole in your throat and a valve made of oesophageal tissue. When you want to speak, you place a finger over the hole, causing air from your lungs to pass through the new valve, making it vibrate.

Path of air during speech
Valve
Breathing hole
Oesophagus
Trachea

What is the treatment?

Benign growths, whether papillomas or polyps, can usually be snipped out in a minor operation done under local anaesthetic. Malignant tumours discovered early are generally treated – and in most cases cured – by *radiotherapy*. If the cancer is more advanced, the larynx may need to be surgically removed. Even then there is a 50 per cent chance of cure. To regain your voice, however, you will have to work, perhaps for several months, with a speech therapist, who will teach you how to use the oesophagus as a substitute larynx. An alternative, recently devised technique involves surgery to create a flap-like valve between the oesophagus and trachea. The valve permits air to be breathed out of the lungs, through the valve, and up the oesophagus, where speech sounds are produced. The process of taking air into the stomach and "breathing out" from the stomach in order to speak is thus avoided (see the diagram above).

Lungs and chest

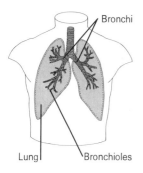

Bronchi

Lung

Bronchioles

The body needs a constant supply of oxygen in order to stay alive. In the lungs oxygen is absorbed from the air, to be transported to all parts of the body by the blood. The main airway, or bronchus, leading into each lung divides into smaller and smaller airways called bronchioles; eventually each bronchiole ends in a cluster of tiny air sacs called alveoli. Deoxygenated blood is pumped to the lungs through the pulmonary arteries, which branch in a similar way. Each alveolus contains several small capillaries, whose thin walls allow oxygen and carbon dioxide to diffuse between the air and the blood.

Because of this intricate structure, the lungs are especially at risk from particles floating in the air we breathe. Microbes such as bacteria (causing, say, pneumonia), irritants such as tobacco smoke (which can cause lung cancer), and *allergens* (causing asthma) can all interfere with the essential process of obtaining oxygen.

Acute bronchitis

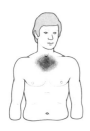

Site of the pain

Pollution in the atmosphere
Bronchitis occurs more often in areas with atmospheric pollution.

Inflammation of the mucous lining of the main air passages of the lungs is called bronchitis. Anyone with a respiratory infection may develop acute bronchitis, since infection with the same viruses that cause *colds* (p.342) and *pharyngitis* (p.350) can spread down into the airways of the lungs (the bronchi and bronchioles). The resultant inflammation usually clears up in a few days; this is the basic difference between acute and *chronic bronchitis* (p.354), in which prolonged, recurrent attacks of the infection cause gradual deterioration of the lungs.

What are the symptoms?
The main symptom is a cough that brings up greyish or yellowish sputum (phlegm). Other symptoms are breathlessness, wheezing, and a raised temperature. There is often pain in the upper chest, made worse by coughing.

How common is the problem?
Virtually everyone gets an occasional attack of acute bronchitis. If you do not smoke cigarettes and have no chronic lung or heart trouble, you are unlikely to have an attack more than once every few years. Smokers, people with chest disorders such as *asthma* (p.355), and residents of places with high atmospheric pollution are susceptible to more frequent attacks, as are people whose lungs are congested (waterlogged) because of *heart failure* (p.381).

What are the risks?
There is little risk if a healthy non-smoker has a single attack of acute bronchitis. But anyone whose susceptibility to bronchitis is increased by smoking, asthma, or a lung disease such as *bronchiectasis* (p.363) is likely to have repeated attacks. In time the attacks will damage the lining of the bronchi, impairing the normal process of clearing mucus from the air passages. This further increases susceptibility and may lead to chronic bronchitis.

What should be done?
Do not ignore repeated attacks of acute bronchitis. Consult your doctor, who may be able to find an explanation. If this is your first attack, or your first for several years, follow the self-help procedures suggested below.

What is the treatment?
Self-help: If you have a raised temperature, take a couple of aspirins three or four times a day to bring it down. Almost any over-the-counter cough medicine, taken according to the instructions on the label, should help soothe your cough, and a hot-water bottle placed on the chest may also help. Stay at home, not necessarily in bed but in a warm –

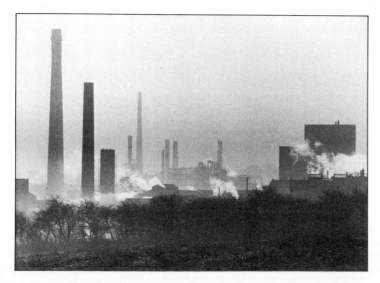

not hot or stuffy – room. It may help to clear your nasal and bronchial passages if you add humidity to the atmosphere by means of a humidifier or steam from hot water. This simple treatment is usually all that is needed; but call your doctor if you become breathless, if you cough up blood, if your temperature rises above 38.5°C (101°F), or if you do not improve 48 hours after the onset of symptoms. If you have had several bouts of bronchitis, remember that cold, damp living or working conditions are bad for anyone susceptible to this disease; so consider changing your place of residence or your job.

Professional help: Because acute bronchitis is usually a viral infection, no specific treatment is possible or advisable. If, however, your breathing is wheezy, the doctor may prescribe a *bronchodilator* drug to be inhaled in aerosol form. You may be prescribed a cough-suppressant medicine if your chest is sore from repeated attacks of coughing or if the cough is dry. And if your sputum becomes greenish yellow, indicating the probability of secondary bacterial infection, the doctor will give you an *antibiotic*. In fact, some doctors prescribe such antibiotics as a precaution against secondary bacterial infection.

Chronic bronchitis

Chronic bronchitis differs from *acute bronchitis* (p.353) in that bronchial inflammation persists and worsens. This dangerous disease starts so insidiously that many people in the early stages do not know they have it. Repeated infections of the bronchi and bronchioles thicken and distort the lining of these tubes, which are also narrowed and obstructed by over-secretion of mucus and excessive contraction of muscles in their walls.

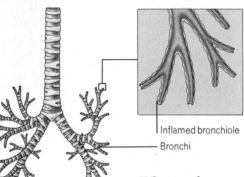

Some risks of chronic bronchitis
Repeated infections of the bronchi and bronchioles damage the linings of these tubes, leaving the lungs susceptible to further infection. Infection can also spread from the tubes to the alveoli, leading in some cases to pneumonia.

Inflamed bronchiole
Bronchi

What are the symptoms?
The first symptom is a morning cough that brings up sputum (phlegm). Smokers often regard the cough as a "normal" smoker's cough. Over the years the amount of sputum gradually increases, and coughing begins to occur throughout the day. Breathlessness and wheeziness gradually become increasingly troublesome.

In the early stages, only bad colds or attacks of influenza cause flare-ups. Eventually, though, every minor head cold brings on a severe attack. Many sufferers have several flare-ups every winter. Indeed, an accepted medical definition of chronic bronchitis is that it is a recurrent cough with sputum production that occurs on most days during at least three months a year (usually in winter) for at least two consecutive years. In the late stages, coughing, breathlessness, and wheezing are severe and nearly continuous.

How common is the problem?
In Britain about 30,000 people (that is, about 1 person in 2,000) die of chronic bronchitis every year. Around a million others have the disease, many without realizing it. Smoking is the main cause. Even the children of heavy smokers may be affected; as infants they seem notably prone to attacks of acute bronchitis and *pneumonia* (p.359), and such attacks increase the risk of chronic bronchitis. The disease is much more common in men than in women; deaths of men from it outrun deaths of women by 3 to 1. An important factor is air pollution; the disease is more common in industrialized countries and in urban areas. Britain has the highest rate in the world – which explains why chronic bronchitis has been termed the "English" disease.

What are the risks?
Once the condition is established, a vicious circle of bronchial infection causing more extensive lung damage leading to increased liability to further infection becomes almost inevitable. Among major diseases to which chronic bronchitis can lead are *pulmonary hypertension* (p.416), *emphysema* (p.358), and right-sided *heart failure* (p.381). If infection spreads into the alveoli, the result is likely to be pneumonia.

Some chronic-bronchitis sufferers gradually become blue about the lips and face because of the lack of oxygen, and eventually develop respiratory failure – their lungs can no longer supply their bodies with enough oxygen. Others succumb to *lung cancer* (p.366), not because chronic bronchitis causes cancer but because smoking is so often the cause of both diseases. A decline in the condition of a person with chronic bronchitis

– for instance, an increase in the degree of breathlessness and a change in the nature of the cough – may be the first signs of developing cancer of the lung.

What should be done?

If you have a morning cough with sputum and if you smoke, stop smoking. If bronchitis persists, consult your doctor, who will examine you and, after considering such factors as your smoking habits and place of residence, may decide that further investigation is advisable. Tests are likely to include a chest *X-ray* and various lung function tests (see *Asthma* below).

What is the treatment?

Self-help: In addition to giving up cigarettes, avoid smoke-filled rooms. Stay away from people with colds. What is a mere cold to a person with healthy lungs may spark a troublesome flare-up of bronchitis in someone with this problem. If you work in a polluted atmosphere, it would be wise to change your job and even, if possible, to move to a place with a warm, dry climate. Chronic bronchitics are at greater risk if they spend their winters in cold, damp places.

Professional help: Treatment depends largely on how far the disorder has progressed before you consult your doctor. If you are already suffering from breathlessness, the doctor will probably prescribe an aerosol inhaler, which will help you, if you use it three or four times a day, by relaxing the wall muscles of your bronchi, thus widening the airways. If you are having a bad attack of infection and coughing up phlegm, you will probably be given an *antibiotic*, normally in the form of tablets or capsules to be taken three or four times daily. In serious flare-ups, injection is the quickest way of getting antibiotics to the source of the infection.

Your doctor may prescribe small doses of an antibiotic throughout a period of weeks or months as a preventive measure. Or you may be advised to take a full dose only at the first sign of a flare-up. There is no consensus among doctors about the best way to treat chronic bronchitis. Although antibiotics are not effective against viral infection, they are often prescribed even when a virus rather than a bacterium is responsible for an attack. The reason for this is that viral infections increase the susceptibility of the lungs to bacterial invasion.

Asthma

Asthma is a long-term condition marked by occasional, often frequent and sustained, attacks of breathlessness. The cause is a partial obstruction of the bronchi and bronchioles, which is due to contraction of their wall muscles. In contrast to bronchitis, in which there is constant wheeziness, attacks of asthma come and go, with wide variations in the degree of obstruction at different times. Although the condition cannot be cured, each attack can be relieved by treatment or, if untreated, usually ends naturally.

Asthma generally starts in childhood or adolescence, but in rare cases the first attack may be delayed until middle age or later. Some attacks occur for no apparent reason. Others are triggered off by allergic reactions to such things as pollen, cat or dog fur, and house dust (see *Allergies*, p.705); by infections (especially of the respiratory tract); certain drugs; inhaled irritants; exercise; and emotional or psychological upsets.

What are the symptoms?

The main symptom is breathlessness accompanied by a feeling of painless tightness in the chest, along with wheezing, the amount of which varies greatly. Sometimes only a doctor's *stethoscope* can catch the sound of wheezing – or it may be loud enough to carry across a crowded room. In severe cases the effort of breathing out (which is when the wheezing is most pronounced) may cause sweating, an increase in pulse rate, and severe anxiety. Often the sufferer finds that it helps to sit up straight, with the arms held stiff to support the chest. With increased breathlessness, breathing becomes increasingly shallow and fast, and wheezing sounds grow louder. In very severe attacks the face and lips may turn bluish (*cyanosis*), because of the diminishing supply of oxygen in the circulation, or the skin may become very pale and clammy.

Some attacks of asthma are accompanied by a thick cough, due to the accumulation of sputum (phlegm) in the lungs.

How common is the problem?

Asthma is quite common among British schoolchildren, about 10 per cent of whom have at least an occasional mild attack. Most children outgrow the condition by puberty, but a small proportion develop it again in adult life. About 2 to 3 per cent of the adult population are asthmatic.

Your chances of having asthma are greatest if there is a history of asthma, hay fever (see *Allergic rhinitis*, p.345), or *eczema*

Self-help during an asthma attack
During an asthma attack, it may help to sit with your elbows resting on the back of a chair. This lifts and stabilizes the top of your ribcage, allowing your chest muscles to force air out more efficiently.

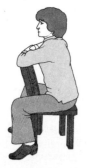

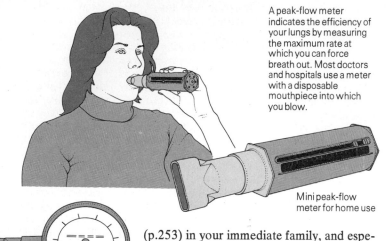

A peak-flow meter indicates the efficiency of your lungs by measuring the maximum rate at which you can force breath out. Most doctors and hospitals use a meter with a disposable mouthpiece into which you blow.

Mini peak-flow meter for home use

Peak-flow meter for hospital use

(p.253) in your immediate family, and especially if you yourself have an allergic condition such as hay fever or eczema.

What are the risks?

A succession of severe asthmatic attacks can be very disabling; about 2,000 people die in Britain every year during the course of an attack (though they are mostly elderly and already ill from other causes). With recent medical advances (see "What is the treatment?" below), there is little risk of lasting disability or death for people who take the problem seriously and regularly consult a doctor about their asthma.

Repeated severe attacks in children may stunt their growth and also cause a protrusion of the chest (popularly known as "pigeon chest") that can predispose them to *emphysema* (p.358) in later life.

What should be done?

Do not accept asthmatic attacks stoically, as a cross you must bear. Study your own disease, take the self-help measures recommended below, and see your doctor whenever you have a severe and persistent period of breathlessness. Asthma is an illness that the doctor can easily control, but only with your co-operation. Because you can never be sure that the symptoms you have at home will be apparent half an hour later when the doctor puts a stethoscope to your chest, you must be able to give a clear description of what seems to cause your breathlessness and of the sort of breathlessness you get. If, for instance, you already have *chronic bronchitis* (p.354), your breathlessness may be ascribed to bronchitis – the sounds heard with a stethoscope are similar – unless you tell the doctor that your breathlessness comes and goes, unlike the continuous breathlessness that is a symptom of chronic bronchitis.

What is the treatment?

Self-help: Because asthma is most often due to some form of allergy, your first step is to try to identify the *allergen* (the substance or substances responsible) in your case. Your doctor may be able to help by arranging skin tests with suspected allergens, but you can do much detective work yourself. Does your asthma vary with the season of the year, and do you also have hay fever? If so, the allergens are probably pollen grains. Do your attacks occur more often on certain days of the week than on others? This might suggest a link with dusts at work (flour in a bakery, for example) or with a hobby (for instance, flowers in a greenhouse). Is the asthma worse in one room of your house than another? Many asthmatics are allergic to fur or feathers from a domestic pet, or to mites in house dust (the mites live on skin that has been shed).

Other possibilities worth considering are allergies to food or drink. Shellfish, eggs, and chocolate, for example, have all been proved to bring on attacks in susceptible people.

Whatever you suspect, you can test your theory by keeping a record of the frequency and severity of your attacks and seeing how often they coincide with your exposure to the

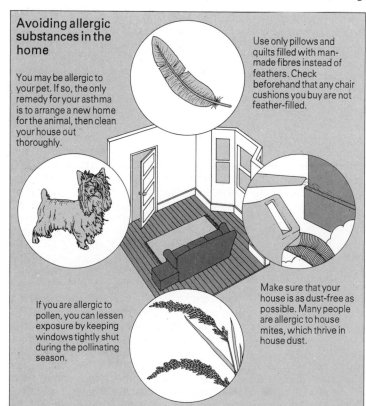

Avoiding allergic substances in the home

You may be allergic to your pet. If so, the only remedy for your asthma is to arrange a new home for the animal, then clean your house out thoroughly.

Use only pillows and quilts filled with man-made fibres instead of feathers. Check beforehand that any chair cushions you buy are not feather-filled.

If you are allergic to pollen, you can lessen exposure by keeping windows tightly shut during the pollinating season.

Make sure that your house is as dust-free as possible. Many people are allergic to house mites, which thrive in house dust.

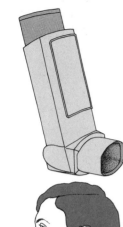

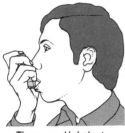

The aerosol inhalant
Some aerosol inhalants (top) are prescribed to prevent asthma attacks; others relieve symptoms. You breathe out, and make an airtight seal with your mouth around the mouthpiece (above). Then, as you breathe in, you press the top down, so that a fine spray of the prescribed drug is released and inhaled into your lungs.

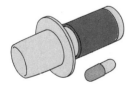

How to use a spinhaler
With the mouthpiece pointing downwards, unscrew the body of the spinhaler and insert the drug capsule into the centre of the propeller (1). Screw the body back onto the mouthpiece and slide the outer part of the body down until it pierces the capsule (2). Breathe out. Make an airtight seal around the mouthpiece with your lips, then tilt your head back and breathe in to activate the propeller and release the drug (3).

Spinhaler and drug capsule

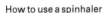

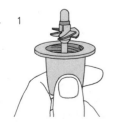
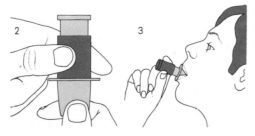

1   2   3

suspect allergen or allergens. The best way to measure the severity of an attack is by means of a small *peak-flow meter* (your doctor may be able to lend you a mini-meter if you cannot buy one). By measuring the maximum flow of air when breathing out, such meters help asthma sufferers to keep precise records of the amount of narrowing of the air passages in their lungs.

Once you have identified an allergen, the ideal solution is to avoid further exposure to it. This is no problem if the allergen is a single foodstuff or a domestic animal, but can be very difficult if it is pollen; on days when the pollen count (the amount of pollen in the atmosphere) is high, there is no way of avoiding it, short of staying indoors all day. Most of your symptoms will have to be controlled in cooperation with your doctor.

Even if you cannot identify the allergen, you may have fewer attacks if you reduce the amount of dust in your house. Have feather pillows replaced and airtight plastic covers put on mattresses, in which house-dust mites thrive. Make sure that dust is removed from crevices with a vacuum cleaner, and have rugs or carpets that can be kept dust-free. Be aware, too, of other factors that can bring on attacks, such as some forms of exercise or psychological stresses.

Professional help: Once the diagnosis is made (and the accuracy of your account of symptoms and probable allergens may help your doctor make it without requiring allergy tests), much can be done for you. In the past few years the treatment of asthma has been improved enormously with the introduction of new drugs, which can be taken as pills, liquid medicine, or inhalants. Some (known as the *prophylactics*) are taken regularly

to prevent asthma attacks from occurring. *Steroid* prophylactics are inhaled three or four times a day. Because it is inhaled, the drug acts directly on the lungs, and only on the lungs; the more generalized side-effects of a tablet or injection are thus avoided. Other drugs (the *bronchodilators*) are best for people who get only occasional attacks, and are taken once the attack has started. The doctor will decide which type to prescribe on the strength of your description of how and when breathlessness occurs.

The best way to use prophylactics or bronchodilators is by inhaling them, since an inhalant gets right to the site of the obstruction; but they can be taken orally by those people who find inhalants difficult to use. Sometimes, if no pill, liquid, or inhalant succeeds in relieving a severe case of asthma, the drug is injected into the bloodstream, and this method almost always works.

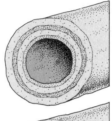

Cross-section of bronchiole treated with bronchodilator drug to unblock airway.

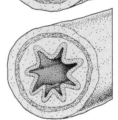

Cross-section of untreated bronchiole with blocked airway

If your asthmatic attacks are clearly due to some allergen such as grass pollen, it is possible to desensitize the lungs against that allergen by means of a long course of injections. But the drugs already discussed are proving so effective that doctors seldom recommend desensitization as a treatment for asthma, chiefly because its success rate is fairly low and somewhat unpredictable.

Despite the success of modern treatment with drugs, however, an attack of asthma is sometimes severe enough to warrant admission to hospital, where various types of treatment can be given more easily than at home. Some drug treatments are most effective when given in the form of a fine mist through a breathing apparatus that requires professional maintenance. If necessary, a hospital patient can be given muscle-relaxant drugs and connected to a mechanical *respirator*. This form of treatment abolishes spasms in the air passages inside the lungs and rests

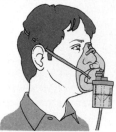
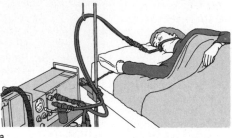

Hospital treatment for asthma

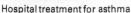

If your asthma attack is so severe that your normal dosage of drugs is ineffective, you may have to wear a specially designed oxygen mask (above left) which allows you to breathe in a fine mist of the drug combined with oxygen. If your condition still does not improve, you will be connected to an artificial respirator (above right) which forcibly pumps air in and out of your lungs. This treatment is usually given in combination with muscle-relaxant drugs and is rarely necessary for longer than 24 hours.

chest muscles, since the work of breathing is done by the machine. The presence of nursing and medical staff 24 hours a day may also relieve the anxiety that aggravates the attack.

What to do for a severe attack of asthma

A sudden, severe attack of asthma can be frightening for the sufferer and his or her family. In most cases the doctor will have prescribed an inhalant of a bronchodilator drug, or of a steroid. If one inhalation does not relieve the wheezing quickly, the dose should be repeated. If the second dose is ineffective, the inhalant should not be used again (over-dosage may be dangerous). Instead, a member of the family should act *immediately* as follows:

1. If the sufferer has turned blue, or pale and clammy, dial 999. Emergency admission to hospital is essential.

2. If there is no blueness, unnatural pallor, or clamminess, telephone your doctor or the emergency asthma unit of your local hospital. Then get the drugs and inhaling apparatus together, and note the time the sufferer takes the first dose of his or her drug.

In all cases, while you are waiting, help 'the asthmatic to find the most comfortable position. Sufferers are usually best off when they sit up, leaning slightly forward, resting on their arms, and are given plenty of fresh air. And don't allow other people to stand around in a worried group; this increases the asthmatic's anxiety. Delegate the job of staying with the sufferer to one, sensible person.

Emphysema

Emphysema is a disorder in which the lungs become less and less efficient because of damage to some of the millions of bubble-shaped alveoli in which the exchange of oxygen and carbon dioxide takes place. Healthy lungs have an elastic, spongy texture that permits them to contract and expand fully, but their springy nature is gradually destroyed if the alveoli become stretched, lose their elasticity, or burst and blister. This type of damage occurs when the alveoli are constantly subjected to pressure that is higher than normal, as in the case of people with long-standing lung disease. *Chronic bronchitis* (p.354) or *asthma* (p.355), for example, causes narrowing of the airways into the lungs, which can be overcome only by forceful breathing that strains and weakens the elastic strands in alveoli walls.

What are the symptoms?

The main symptom is shortness of breath, which is likely to worsen through the years. If you have emphysema, your chest is probably distended into a barrel shape. If you also wheeze, cough, and bring up sputum, these are symptoms of other kinds of lung trouble, not of emphysema.

How common is the problem?

About 1 in 100 people in Britain suffers from some degree of emphysema. It seldom occurs, however, in people who are not also bronchitic or asthmatic. It is 10 times as common in men as in women, and your chances of having it increase if you smoke or live in a polluted atmosphere. An inherited defect in the chemical make-up of your lungs can predispose you to the disease. People whose jobs require exceptionally forceful use of lung power – glass blowers and trumpet players, for instance – are also susceptible.

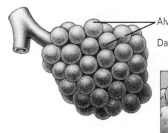

Alveoli

Damaged alveoli

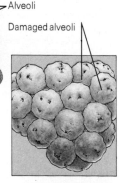

Breathlessness in emphysema
Damaged alveoli (air sacs in the lungs) may burst and merge to make fewer, larger alveoli with a consequent reduction in surface area. With each breath, less oxygen is able to travel through the walls of the alveoli into the bloodstream, and the lungs have to work harder to maintain the correct oxygen level in the blood.

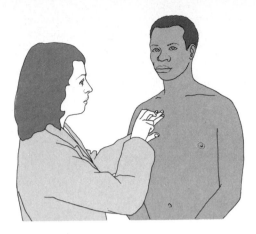

Percussing the chest
Because sufferers from emphysema have enlarged air sacs in the lungs, the doctor can detect the condition by percussing the chest. This involves placing 2 fingers on the chest and tapping them with the fingers of the other hand. The enlarged air sacs produce a hollower sound than usual.

What are the risks?

Increasing shortness of breath entails a risk of eventual non-functioning of the lungs (*respiratory failure*). People who have already developed emphysema are also more prone to chest infections. There is, too, a serious risk of a *pneumothorax* (p.362). And since blood cannot flow freely through damaged alveoli, the right side of the heart (the side responsible for pumping blood into the lungs) is strained, leading to *heart failure* (p.381).

What should be done?

If troubled by breathlessness, consult your doctor, who will *percuss* your chest and listen to it with a *stethoscope*. You may also be asked to blow hard into a machine (a *peak-flow meter*) to assess your breathing capacity, and the doctor may want to see a chest *X-ray* before making a firm diagnosis.

What is the treatment?

Self-help: If you smoke, stop; avoid places with polluted air; keep away from people with coughs or colds. Take moderate exercise in fresh, clean air.

Professional help: Doctors can relieve the symptoms and delay the progress of emphysema but cannot cure it. If you have bronchitis along with emphysema, you may be told to inhale a *bronchodilator*, which widens the airways and helps prevent further inflation of alveoli. This will make your breathing less difficult. Since bronchitis and lung infection of any kind aggravate emphysema, the best way to control the disease is to take what measures your doctor advises to prevent respiratory infection. Thus your doctor may prescribe *antibiotics* as a preventive measure even at times when no infection is apparent.

Pneumonia

Pneumonia is not a specific disease; it is a general term that *pathologists* use for several kinds of inflammation of the lungs. The tissue becomes swollen, red, hot, and painful, just like any other inflamed body tissue. Pneumonia is usually the result of microbial infection – by some sort of bacterium or virus, for example – but it can also be caused by chemical damage from inhaled liquid or poisonous gas such as chlorine. And the lung inflammation can be anything from a mild complication of an upper-respiratory-tract infection to a life-threatening illness.

The course of an attack of pneumonia, its impact, and its outcome depend partly on the cause, partly on the general health of the

DIFFERENT KINDS OF PNEUMONIA

Microbe responsible	Onset of symptoms	Temperature	Breath-lessness	Other symptoms	Mortality rate in young adults
Influenza virus	within hours of the flu starting	40°C (104°F) or above	marked	bad cough; blood-stained sputum; *cyanosis*	has been 50% in epidemics
Other viruses	4 to 5 days after infection	about 38.5°C (101°F)	some	dry cough	less than 5%
Mycoplasma (bacterium-like)	3 to 4 days after infection	about 38.5°C (101°F)	none	dry, troublesome cough; headache	less than 1%
Pneumococcus bacterium	within a few hours of infection	40°C (104°F) or above	marked	chills; chest pain; possible *cyanosis* followed by cough with blood-stained sputum	less than 5%

person concerned, and partly on other factors; viral pneumonia, for instance, does not respond to treatment with *antibiotics*. For a comparison of the causes and likely results of four of the most common types of pneumonia, see the table on p.359.

The variability of the "disease" has led to all manner of popular and medical descriptive terms. If you are told you have "double" pneumonia, it means that both your lungs are affected. If your attack is due to a bacterium-like microbe belonging to the genus Mycoplasma, you may be said to have "atypical" pneumonia. "Bronchopneumonia" is patchy inflammation of one or both lungs, whereas "lobar" pneumonia affects the entire area of one or more lobes (segments) of the lung.

What are the symptoms?

No single symptom is characteristic. You should consider the possibility of pneumonia, however, if someone in your family who already has a respiratory illness – with, for instance, a cough and fever – becomes short of breath while at rest, with no physical activity to account for the breathlessness. Additional symptoms to watch for (apart from coughing and raised temperature) are chills, sweats, chest pains, a bluish tinge to the skin (*cyanosis*), blood in the phlegm, and even mental confusion or delirium. Obviously, the larger the lung area affected, the more severe the symptoms.

The swiftness of onset of symptoms and their relative prominence vary according to the cause of the infection. An especially virulent strain of the influenza virus, for example, can kill an old, feeble person within 24 hours. In a healthy young adult, pneumonia resulting from a mild respiratory microbe might cause symptoms no worse than those of an ordinary common cold.

How common is the problem?

In Britain each year, 1 person in 300 catches pneumonia and about one-third of such cases are fatal. One reason for the comparatively high proportion of deaths is that pneumonia is often the final complication of some other debilitating disorder. Anyone whose resistance is already low is an easy prey; thus, where heart failure, cancer, stroke, or chronic bronchitis may be the terminal illness, often the actual cause of death is pneumonia. Infection of the lungs is virtually inevitable in anyone who is semi-conscious or paralysed. This is because the normal coughing reflex that keeps the lungs clear of mucus and stagnant fluid is much reduced, or even absent, under such conditions.

You are more likely to get pneumonia – and, having got it, to be seriously ill – if you belong in any of the following categories: you are very young (under two) or very old (over 75); you suffer from a chronic chest disease such as asthma or you have a chronic illness, such as rheumatoid arthritis or kidney failure, which reduces your body's resistance to infections; or you are a heavy smoker or drinker. Also highly susceptible are people under long-term treatment with *immunosuppressive* or anti-inflammatory drugs, especially *steroids*. These drugs suppress the body's normal defences against microbes.

What are the risks?

Because pneumonia varies so much, no generalizations can be made about its risks. In old, or weak, or debilitated people, the main risk is death. Any type of pneumonia may lead to *pleurisy* (opposite), or *empyema* (p.364). The most dangerous type of pneumonia is that caused by viruses such as the influenza virus, which do not respond to antibiotics. (Compare its mortality rate in the table on p.359 with that of a similarly virulent form of pneumonia caused by the pneumococcus bacterium, which can be treated with antibiotic drugs.) Clearly, with increasing age or chronic illness, your chances of surviving even a mild attack are correspondingly lessened.

What should be done?

Consult your doctor without delay if you suspect you may have pneumonia – you become short of breath even when lying down, if your chest hurts when you breathe, or if you cough up blood-stained sputum. The doctor will listen to your chest through a *stethoscope*, will *percuss* the chest, and will ask you questions about the onset of symptoms as well as your smoking and drinking habits. It may be possible to make a firm diagnosis of pneumonia – and even of the type of pneumonia – on the basis of such an examination. More probably, further tests such as a chest *X-ray* and laboratory examination of blood and sputum samples will be necessary.

What is the treatment?

Because pneumonia can become severe in a matter of hours, admission to hospital is often advisable. The best treatment may be no more dramatic than a combination of warmth, soothing cough medicines, and antibiotics; but close professional supervision and observation are highly desirable during the early stages of the attack, especially if there is some doubt about the precise nature and extent of the inflammation and the general health of the sufferer is poor.

Antibiotic drugs may be taken as tablets or capsules, or – in severe cases – they may be given by injection. There is a wide variety of antibiotics to choose from, and the choice for your case will depend largely on the doctor's findings about the probable microbial cause of your illness. Laboratory tests of your blood and sputum should provide the required information as to which organism (or organisms) is causing your infection. And the doctor will need to find out whether you may be allergic to certain antibiotics or peculiarly responsive to others.

Analgesics such as aspirin help to relieve chest pain. If breathlessness and cyanosis become conspicuous, you are probably in need of oxygen, which is generally supplied by means of a face mask or a tube held in the mouth. If your lungs remain troublesome in spite of all such measures, your doctor will doubtless arrange for further tests. In particular, he or she may require *bronchoscopy* to exclude the possibility of the presence of *lung cancer* (p.366).

A healthy young person should recover completely from pneumonia within two to

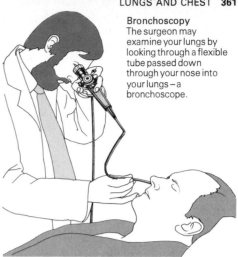

Bronchoscopy
The surgeon may examine your lungs by looking through a flexible tube passed down through your nose into your lungs – a bronchoscope.

three weeks. Even in cases of viral pneumonia, chances of serious complications are minimal since, although antibiotics do not combat the primary infection, they effectively ward off the menace of secondary bacterial infection. On the other hand, recovery may take several months, or the disease may be fatal, in heavy cigarette smokers or people who are in some other way vulnerable.

Pleurisy
(and pleural effusion)

In normal breathing the lungs expand and contract easily and rhythmically within the ribcage. To facilitate this movement and lubricate the moving parts, each lung is enveloped in a moist, smooth, two-layered membrane (the pleura). The outer layer of this membrane lines the ribcage; and

The pleurae
Each pleura is a double-layered membrane wrapped around one lung. The left pleura (and lung) is slightly smaller than the right one, because the heart takes up some of the space in the left side of the ribcage.

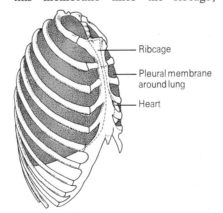

Ribcage

Pleural membrane around lung

Heart

between the layers is a virtually imperceptible space (the pleural space) that permits the layers to glide gently across each other. If either of your pleurae becomes inflamed and roughened the gliding process is impeded, and you are suffering from pleurisy.

Pleurisy is actually a symptom of an underlying disease rather than a disease in itself. The pleurae may become inflamed as a complication of a lung or chest infection such as *pneumonia* (p.359) or *tuberculosis* (p.563); or the inflammation may be due to a slight *pneumothorax* (p.362) or chest injury. The pleural inflammation sometimes creates a further complication by causing fluid to seep into the pleural space, resulting in a condition known as pleural *effusion*. But pleurisy is not the only condition that can lead to pleural effusion; it may also be produced by diseases such as *rheumatoid arthritis* (p.552), liver or kidney trouble, or *heart failure* (p.381). Even cancer spreading from the lung, breast, or ovary can cause pleural effusion.

What are the symptoms?
If you have pleurisy, it hurts to breathe deeply or cough, and chest pain (one-sided, not centralized) is likely to be severe. Accompanying the pain are any other symptoms associated with the underlying disorder. The pain will disappear if a pleural effusion occurs as a consequence of pleurisy, because fluid stops the layers of the pleura from rubbing against each other; but you may become breathless as the fluid accumulates.

How common is the problem?
Thanks to *antibiotics*, pleurisy and pleural effusion due to infection have become rare disorders. In an average year, 1 person in 1,000 visits a doctor because of one or both of these disorders, and fatalities are now extremely rare. Pleurisy is four times as common as pleural effusion.

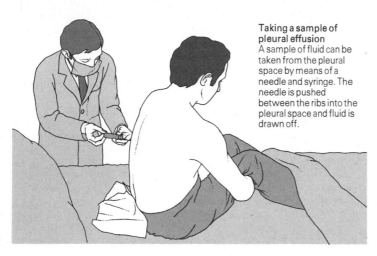

Taking a sample of pleural effusion
A sample of fluid can be taken from the pleural space by means of a needle and syringe. The needle is pushed between the ribs into the pleural space and fluid is drawn off.

What are the risks?
In most cases the risks are those of the underlying cause. A big pleural effusion can compress the lungs and cause breathlessness. Any effusion may lead to *empyema* (p.364).

What should be done?
Consult your doctor if breathing becomes painful, you have a fever (no matter how slight), and seem unusually short of breath. After questioning you about symptoms and previous illness, the doctor will listen to your chest through a *stethoscope* and will *percuss* the chest, alert for characteristic sounds of irritated pleurae and pleural effusion. A chest *X-ray* may be required. And if you have a pleural effusion, one way to diagnose the cause is to study the composition of the fluid; so a sample of fluid for microscopic examination may be taken from the pleural space with a needle and syringe.

What is the treatment?
Because pleurisy and pleural effusion are symptoms of basic disorders, the only way to ensure a cure is to treat the underlying disease. Meanwhile, to ease chest pains, the doctor may recommend use of an *analgesic*.

Pneumo-thorax

As a healthy lung expands and contracts, each of the two layers of the pleura slips smoothly over the lubricated surface of the other. Pneumothorax occurs when air gets into the pleural space between the layers and

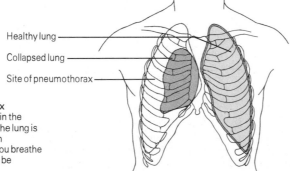

Healthy lung
Collapsed lung
Site of pneumothorax

Pneumothorax
If air is present in the pleural space, the lung is prevented from expanding as you breathe in and is said to be collapsed.

forces them apart. As a result, the lung – or, more commonly, part of the lung – collapses (that is, loses its elasticity and is therefore deprived of air). The cause of the trouble may be a chest injury or, more often, air may escape into the pleura from the lung itself. A small pneumothorax will often disappear of its own accord; but sometimes more air enters the pleural space, with consequent collapse of a larger and larger part of the lung.

What are the symptoms?
The major symptoms are breathlessness and chest pain, generally on the affected side but sometimes at the bottom of the neck. The pain is usually sudden and sharp, though it sometimes is hardly more than a sensation of general discomfort in the chest.

There may also be a feeling of tightness across the chest. Severity of symptoms depends on the size of the damaged area and your general health. If you are young and in good condition, you may have little pain and little difficulty in breathing even if you have a large pneumothorax and a wide expanse of collapsed lung. If you are middle-aged and a chronic bronchitic, a small pneumothorax can be extremely painful and cause acute difficulty in breathing.

How common is the problem?
Pneumothorax is relatively rare. In an average year, about 1 in 5,000 consults a doctor because of the problem. It occurs chiefly in otherwise healthy young men (nobody knows why) and in middle-aged people, both male and female, whose lungs are already damaged by asthma, chronic bronchitis, emphysema, or some other serious lung condition.

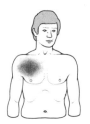

Site of the pain

What are the risks?

Much depends on how air is finding its way into the pleura. Often a small pneumothorax is inconsequential and self-healing. But if there is a hole that permits the pneumothorax to increase in size, there will be increasing breathlessness and pain as more and more of the lung collapses. If the disorder remains untreated, *respiratory failure* is likely.

What should be done?

If you suspect you have this condition, consult your doctor. Examination of your chest with a *stethoscope* will quickly detect a large pneumothorax, but the doctor may need a chest *X-ray* to find a small one. In any case, even if there is only a suspicion of trouble, you will probably be admitted to hospital for specialist observation.

What is the treatment?

Treatment depends on the size of the pneumothorax and the state of your lungs. Since the disorder is often self-healing, you may need no more than a few days of X-ray observation and bed rest to make sure that the pleural air has gone and that the collapsed portion of the lung is no longer deprived of air. Treatment, if required, consists primarily of an effort to suck out the pleural air by means of a tube (a *catheter*) inserted between the ribs into the pleural space. If catheterization fails to improve the condition, your doctor will need to get a clearer idea of the source of the trouble. This may involve the use of a *thoracoscope* to inspect the inner side of each layer of the pleura. When a thoracoscope is inserted between the ribs into the pleural space, the specialist may be able to find the hole through which air is seeping and seal it up by chemical means.

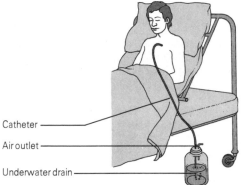

Treatment for pneumothorax
To remove pleural air, a catheter is inserted into the pleural space. As you breathe out, the air between your lungs and your deflated ribcage is squeezed out along the catheter. An underwater drain ensures that the air travels only one way.

Catheter
Air outlet
Underwater drain

Bronchi-ectasis

Bronchiectasis is a widening or distortion of one or more bronchi, usually occurring in adulthood as a result of frequent infections in childhood. In this disorder, the drainage of the fluid secreted by bronchial cells is impaired, and fluid accumulates and stagnates in the bronchi, leading to further infection.

Bronchiectasis can also develop at any time if one of the bronchi is blocked by a foreign body for a long period or if part of it has been much narrower than normal since birth.

What are the symptoms?

The main symptom is a frequent cough that brings up large quantities of green or yellow sputum (phlegm), sometimes spotted with blood. The quantity of sputum may increase when you change position, especially when you lie down. You are more likely to get repeated lung infections whenever you catch a cold. And you may have bad breath.

How common is the problem?

Bronchiectasis is now rare because many childhood infections that were once its main cause, such as sinusitis and the chest infections that often followed measles or whooping cough, are prevented by immunization or effectively treated by *antibiotics*. Similarly, tuberculosis, which also used to damage the lungs, has become extremely rare. Even people who have bronchiectasis can usually lead normal lives because of antibiotics given at the first sign of further infection.

What should be done?

If you repeatedly cough large amounts of green or yellow phlegm, consult your doctor, who will examine your chest with a *stethoscope* and may also want a chest *X-ray* and *bronchoscopy* in order to make a diagnosis.

What is the treatment?

Self-help: There is nothing you can do until the condition has been diagnosed. If you find that you are bronchiectatic, make a special effort to avoid colds and sore throats. Do not smoke or subject your lungs to the atmosphere of smoke-filled rooms. If the lower part of your lung is infected – as it usually is in people with this disorder – your doctor will explain the self-help technique of postural drainage, which is a method of getting rid of bronchial secretions by placing oneself in a position in which the bronchus leading to the affected lobe is upside down, so that fluid drains out under the force of gravity and can then be coughed up. Lying on a bed with your head and chest hanging over the edge for five to 10 minutes twice a day can keep your lungs fairly clear.

Professional help: At the first sign of infection your doctor will probably put you on antibiotics and will emphasize the need to complete the prescribed course even if the infection seems to clear up more quickly than expected. If your condition is very localized, or if a lot of blood is mixed with the sputum, surgical removal of the affected part of the lung may be advisable.

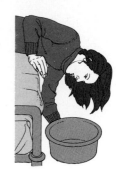

Draining phlegm from affected lungs
Because it is difficult to cough up bronchitic phlegm, a doctor or physiotherapist will teach you how to lie in the best position to drain the affected area of your lungs. The phlegm drains into your trachea, and you then cough it up. This procedure is called postural drainage.

Lung abscess

An *abscess* in the lung is usually due to one of two conditions. It may be a complication of some type of *pneumonia* (p.359), or it may result from inhaling foreign material, such as a fragment of tooth or food, while unconscious. This sometimes happens when a person is under a medical anaesthetic or has passed out after drinking excessive amounts of alcohol. *Antibiotic* treatment has made abscesses associated with pneumonia very rare; lung abscesses occur today most often among chronic alcoholics and people suffering from malnutrition.

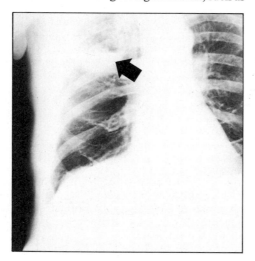

X-ray diagnosis of a lung abscess
An abscess in the lung is at least partially filled with fluid. The fluid-filled area shows up on an X-ray as a pale patch (arrow) surrounded by a dark area, the air-filled lung.

What are the symptoms?
The main symptoms are alternating chills and fever, but there may also be chest pain and a cough that brings up thick, pus-like sputum, often blood-stained.

What should be done?
Admission to hospital is essential for diagnostic tests. A chest *X-ray* will locate the site of the abscess, and further tests will identify the microbes that have caused it. Treatment with appropriate antibiotics should give complete recovery.

Empyema

Empyema is, technically, an accumulation of pus in any body cavity; but the term as used by doctors generally refers to a pleural effusion (see *Pleurisy*, p.361) that has become infected, so that the watery fluid in the space between the layers of the pleura has thickened into pus. This can happen as a complication of an infectious disease of the lungs such as *pneumonia* (p.359) or of an abdominal infection that spreads into the chest. There are no special symptoms, and the diagnosis depends on an examination of a sample of fluid taken from the pleural space by means of a needle and syringe.

What should be done?
Empyema has become extremely rare since the advent of *antibiotics*, and most people who develop it do so as a complication of an underlying lung disorder. Treatment and prospects for full recovery depend on what that disorder is.

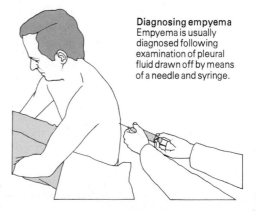

Diagnosing empyema
Empyema is usually diagnosed following examination of pleural fluid drawn off by means of a needle and syringe.

Pneumo-coniosis

(and other dust diseases)

"Pneumoconiosis" means "dust in the lungs", and the disease is actually a number of occupational diseases, all of which are caused by inhaling various kinds of dust particles. If you have been continually inhaling such particles over the course of many years, little patches of irritation may have formed in one or both of your lungs; you are suffering from some type of pneumoconiosis if the resultant scar tissue has made the lungs less flexible and porous, with consequent shortness of breath. The most common form of the disorder in this country is appropriately named coal-miner's pneumoconiosis. Slightly less widespread is silicosis, which affects workers in quarries, stone masons, metal grinders, and miners engaged in rock drilling. Among others exposed to some degree of pneumoconiosis are people who work with products such as aluminium, asbestos, beryllium, iron, talc, and certain synthetic fibres. It should be emphasized that these diseases are caused only by prolonged and constant exposure. It normally takes at least 10 years' continual daily exposure to produce a dust disease (though some men working under poor conditions succumb to asbestosis in only five years). Coal-miner's pneumoconiosis sometimes takes up to 25 years to develop.

What are the symptoms?
Breathlessness on exertion is the dominant symptom. In sufferers from silicosis it usually becomes progressively more severe, and there are likely to be associated symptoms of *tuberculosis* (p.563). In all cases of dust disease there is usually a cough with sputum. The sputum of coal miners is often black.

How common is the problem?
There is likely to be *X-ray* evidence of a small degree of pneumoconiosis in nearly everyone who is subjected for many years to any dust that irritates the lungs. Recent figures, however, indicate that only about 20,000 people in Britain are suffering severely enough to require medical attention. There are 40 male victims for every female.

What are the risks?
Silicosis can severely damage the lungs and is liable to lead to tuberculosis. Rarer, but still possible, are dangerous respiratory-system complications such as *lung cancer* (p.366) from asbestosis. But industrial regulations and preventive medicine have made severe illness from pneumoconiosis and its complications much less likely than it used to be.

What should be done?
Give up smoking. If you work at a place where you are exposed to dust, make a point of finding out what the dust is and whether it carries some risk of pneumoconiosis. If it does, make sure you have a routine chest X-ray once a year, and consult your doctor if at any time you find yourself increasingly short of breath. The doctor will probably want an immediate chest X-ray, which will indicate whether or not you are becoming severely affected. If the answer is yes, it may be advisable to change your job. Even in a new and different job, continue having periodic chest X-rays for the rest of your life so that in the unlikely event of later complications of your dust disease they will be discovered while still in an early stage.

Farmer's lung

The disease known as farmer's lung, which is caused by frequent exposure to a fungus that grows in mouldy hay or grain, attacks only people who are allergic to the fungus. Because, like *pneumoconiosis* (above), the allergy causes lung inflammation that narrows the air passages and thickens the alveoli walls, farmer's lung is sometimes called *organic* pneumoconiosis. A similar allergic reaction to certain kinds of fungus occurs among workers who deal with malt, mushrooms, and other substances, as well as among people who handle animals in laboratories, pigeon breeders, and others closely associated with birds (fungi often flourish in the droppings).

What are the symptoms?
The main symptom is breathlessness, which becomes troublesome several hours after exposure to the *allergen* and usually passes away after another few hours. The breathlessness is usually accompanied by a dry cough. Since there may also be symptoms such as fever, chills, and headache, farmer's lung is often mistakenly thought to be persistent or recurring flu.

How common is the problem?
Farmer's lung and similar allergic reactions are rare since they are suffered only by a small proportion of those who are in constant contact with the mouldy substances that cause the symptoms.

What are the risks?
If, as often happens, the sufferer fails to discover the true cause of the constantly recurring symptoms and continues to remain

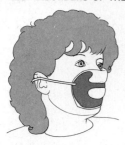

Avoiding farmer's lung
If you are often exposed to the types of fungus that cause farmer's lung, you should wear a protective face mask at work to filter out the tiny particles that may cause the damage.

exposed to the allergen, the condition may well worsen. When untreated over a long period, inflammation of the lungs will destroy the elastic lung tissue, which is replaced by stiff scar tissue. The result is permanent, progressive breathlessness, which can lead to a serious condition such as *respiratory failure* or *heart failure* (p.381).

What should be done?

Consult your doctor if you get repeated attacks of breathlessness, and if you are frequently exposed to any substance that can cause farmer's lung, be sure to point this out. Diagnostic tests will include a chest *X-ray* and skin tests, and you may be asked to blow into a *peak-flow meter* in order to see how well your lungs are functioning.

What is the treatment?

Self-help: Avoid further exposure to the allergen. Change your job if possible; if not, at least wear a protective mask over your nose and mouth whenever you are likely to be exposed to the substance. In most cases no other treatment is necessary. Without further exposure your breathlessness will probably disappear and your lungs return to normal over the course of a few weeks.

Professional help: If you have had the condition for some time, it may be much more difficult to cure than at an earlier stage. The most effective treatment is likely to be *steroid* tablets given for several months. Your doctor will gradually decrease an initially high dose by prescribing fewer tablets or tablets of lower dosage.

Lung cancer

(bronchial carcinoma)

There are several kinds of lung cancer, but only one – known as bronchial carcinoma – is common. It accounts for 99 in 100 cases and is nearly always caused by smoking. Only about 3 in 1,000 cases of bronchial carcinoma occur in lifelong non-smokers.

Smoking damages the cells that line the bronchi, and many scientists believe that the damaged cells represent an early stage of cancer. Some of these cells may gradually form a wartlike tumour, which is the starting point of bronchial carcinoma. As the tumour grows, it spreads into the lungs, and the cancer cells often get into the bloodstream and are carried to other parts of the body such as the brain, liver, bone, and skin.

What are the symptoms?

The first symptom is usually a cough, nearly always an increase in the usual smoker's cough. The disease is closely associated with *chronic bronchitis* (p.354), and more than half the people who get lung cancer have had bronchitis for years before cancer develops. Along with the cough there is generally some sputum, which may be blood-stained. There may be a little breathlessness. Often you will have chest pains, either sharp (and becoming sharper when you take a deep breath) or dull and persistent. And you may sometimes wheeze when you breathe out.

When lung-cancer cells have spread to other organs, the first symptoms may be due to the secondary cancers (called *metastases*). This happens in about 1 in 8 cases, and it is the secondary cancer that alerts the doctor to the primary cancer of the lung. The symptoms of secondary cancer depend on where the cancer cells have settled. If they are in the

brain, the sufferer may get headaches, feel mentally confused, or have an epileptic fit or a stroke. In the bone the symptoms are pain, swelling, or even fracture; in the skin *cyst*-like swellings appear; in the liver the symptoms are likely to be indigestion, dyspepsia, and – later – jaundice.

How common is the problem?

Bronchial carcinoma is the most common form of cancer in the Western world, with the highest death rate in Britain, where it causes 1 in every 18 deaths. At present it affects more men than women, probably because lung cancer takes a long time to develop and men smoked much more heavily than women 20 to 30 years ago. There has recently been a drop in the incidence of the disease among males and a rise in the incidence among females. The probable reason is that men have been smoking less than they used to, whereas large numbers of women only began to smoke heavily after the last war. In fact, statistics indicate that lung cancer now seems likely to surpass breast cancer as the main killer cancer among women.

Your chances of having the disease vary according to the number of cigarettes you smoke. Light smokers are 10 times as susceptible as non-smokers; heavy smokers are 25 times as susceptible. If cancer has not already started to develop, then as soon as you stop smoking, the danger begins to decrease. After 5 years of non-smoking you can feel nearly as secure as if you had never started. If, however, you spend most of your time in an atmosphere heavily contaminated with tobacco smoke, your risks are increased by this so-called "passive" smoking.

Medical myth

There is no point in giving up smoking if you have smoked for years; if you are going to get lung cancer, it can no longer be avoided.

Wrong. There is firm evidence that people who have smoked heavily for many years improve their chances by stopping.

Deaths caused by lung cancer

Lung cancer was a rare disease before cigarette smoking became such a popular habit. Since records of deaths from lung cancer have been kept the numbers continued to rise steadily and steeply for men until only a few years ago. The numbers of women who died of lung cancer rose only slightly between 1900 and 1940 but in the last 40 years there has been a steady increase. This is because it has gradually become more socially acceptable for women to smoke since the Second World War. This increase is reflected in the relatively rapid rise in the number of women who have since died of lung cancer. Despite this rise, however, there are still approximately 4 times as many male as female fatalities from lung cancer in Western society. Tobacco smoking has been linked with many illnesses besides lung cancer. For further information on how cigarettes (and other forms of tobacco) can damage health see *The dangers of smoking*, p.38.

OPERATION:

Lung removal
(pneumonectomy or lobectomy)

Pneumonectomy is an operation to remove a lung. If only part of the lung is removed, it is called a lobectomy. Either operation is done to treat cancer of the lung when the disease is diagnosed at an early stage, and occasionally for tuberculosis or bronchiectasis.

During the operation You are given a general anaesthetic. The specialist chest surgeon makes an incision from front to back on the affected side along the line of a lower rib. One rib is usually removed and the affected lung or part of the lung is removed through the gap. The operation usually takes between 1 and 3 hours.

After the operation You will spend a few days in the intensive-care unit. While there, you will have a drip in your arm and at least 2 drainage tubes leading from the incision. You may have to breathe through an oxygen mask. You can help yourself best by coughing frequently to bring up any secretions. The usual hospital stay is about 2 to 3 weeks.

Convalescence You will need to convalesce for several months after you leave hospital and will be advised to give up smoking for life.

See also information on operations, p.738.

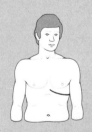

Site of the incision

What are the risks?

If lung cancer is discovered early – as soon as the symptoms develop, or by a routine chest *X-ray* – the affected portion of the lung can sometimes be removed surgically. Only about 5 per cent of the people who get lung cancer are cured by surgery, however. By the time most sufferers seek help, the cancer has spread and surgery no longer suffices for a cure. Smokers should understand that they are also courting needlessly early death from other diseases associated with smoking (coronary artery disease, stroke, or chronic bronchitis, for example).

What should be done?

Stop smoking now, even if you do not have a smoker's cough. The tumour takes years to develop, and removing the cause may slow or even halt the process. If you are experiencing symptoms such as worsening of smoker's cough, chest pains, and blood in the sputum, see your doctor, who will listen to your chest with a *stethoscope* and will probably arrange for a chest X-ray. You may then be referred to a chest specialist, who will probably use a *bronchoscope* to search for cancerous growths in your bronchi.

What is the treatment?

Self-help: Give up smoking now.

Professional help: Surgical removal of the cancer offers the best possible results, but about two-thirds of bronchial-carcinoma cases are too advanced for total removal when the chest is opened. Treatment by *radiotherapy* slows down the progress of the cancer and can relieve the symptoms for months or sometimes years.

Another possibility is treatment by *cytotoxic* drugs, which act against cancer cells. This form of treatment is similar to methods that have proved effective in cancers such as *Hodgkin's disease* (p.433) and *leukaemia* (p.426). Treatment extends over several months, and cytotoxic drugs have unpleasant side-effects, but the results so far are promising. Since this treatment is comparatively new, long-term results of research trials are not yet available, but this type of therapy offers the best prospect for cure in cases where surgery is not feasible.

The choice of which treatment is most suitable for an individual depends on several factors: the extent of the disease, laboratory examination of a specimen of tumour (*biopsy*), and the person's general health. Discuss the possibilities with your doctor. Although a diagnosis of lung cancer is serious, you should not view it as an inescapable death sentence.

Interstitial fibrosis

Fibrous tissue in the alveoli walls
Healthy alveoli (below left) have thin walls that allow oxygen to pass into the bloodstream. In interstitial fibrosis the alveoli walls become thickened by a fibrous material (below right) that reduces the amount of oxygen which can pass through into the bloodstream.

In interstitial fibrosis (also known as diffuse interstitial fibrosis or pulmonary alveolar fibrosis) the efficiency of the lungs as gas-exchange organs is greatly impaired by an accumulation of fibrous matter that obstructs bronchioles and thickens alveoli walls. The fibrous material stiffens the lungs so that they expand and contract less easily.

What are the symptoms?

Interstitial fibrosis may be either acute or chronic. In the acute form, the major symptom is increasingly severe shortness of breath. At first this occurs only on exertion, but as the disease advances it is present even during periods of rest. There is also a cough that may or may not bring up blood-stained sputum, and there may also be chest pains. The progress of the disease is so rapid that most sufferers die within a year.

The chronic, more usual form starts in middle age, and symptoms – the most important of which is breathlessness – develop much more slowly. An additional symptom of chronic interstitial fibrosis is a deformity of the fingertips – clubbing – which also occurs in other chronic lung diseases. The appearance of this symptom does not mean that the disease is at an advanced stage, since clubbing can occur surprisingly early in the illness.

How common is the problem?

The precise cause of this rare, serious disorder is unknown, but it accounts for no more than 1 in 100,000 deaths in Britain.

What is the treatment?

Both acute and chronic forms of this condition end in *respiratory failure*. But treatment with *steroid* drugs relieves symptoms and slows the progress of the disorder.

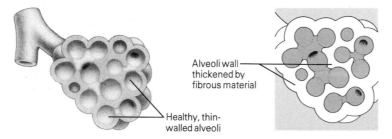

Alveoli wall thickened by fibrous material

Healthy, thin-walled alveoli

Clubbed fingers
A symptom of chronic lung disease is deformed fingers. Your cuticles seem to disappear and your fingernails curve round the ends of your fingers. The tips of your fingers may also flatten out to become spatula-shaped. In particularly bad cases the ends of your toes may be similarly affected. The reason why chronic lung disease sometimes produces this strange deformity is not known.

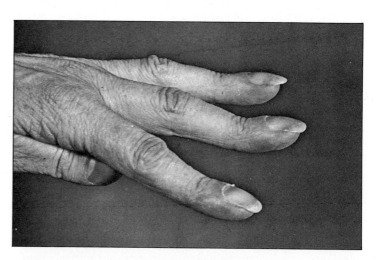

Pulmonary oedema

Pulmonary oedema is not a disease; it is an acute, dramatic, and sometimes life-threatening symptom of *heart failure* (p.381). The oedema (swollen tissue) results from inefficient pumping action of the left ventricle, which causes back pressure of blood in the pulmonary veins (those that bring oxygenated blood to the heart from the lungs). As the pressure rises in the veins and their tributaries in the lungs, fluid diffuses from the blood vessels into the alveoli, and an accumulation of fluid leads to swollen lungs. When there is a sudden flare-up of acute breathlessness, the sufferer is said to have an attack of pulmonary oedema. This sometimes happens suddenly and without warning to a person who is not even aware that he or she is suffering from heart failure.

What are the symptoms?

An attack of pulmonary oedema manifests itself in breathlessness that becomes progressively worse over the course of a few hours. This often occurs in the middle of the night, when the sufferer may have a frightening sense of the need to fight for breath and may rush outside or to an open window. There is generally a cough, which is dry and tickling in the early stages, but which may eventually bring up blood-stained, frothy sputum. In a severe attack there is also likely to be *cyanosis* (indicated by the lips beginning to turn blue) because of insufficient amounts of oxygen in the blood.

How common is the problem?
Statistics indicate that about 1 person out of every 1,000 in Britain has an attack of pulmonary oedema in an average year. Attacks are not always severe, however.

What should be done?
If you have an attack of pulmonary oedema, you may already be under treatment for heart failure. At the first sign of sudden severe breathlessness, send for your doctor; this is an emergency that will respond to treatment, but delay may be fatal. While waiting for the doctor, do not throw away your sputum, since an examination of it will assist the diagnosis. Upon arrival, the doctor will take your blood pressure, make a rapid examination of your chest with a *stethoscope*, and ask whether you have chest pain; pain in addition to breathlessness indicates that there may be an underlying *coronary thrombosis* (p.379) rather than pulmonary oedema.

What is the treatment?
Self-help: Try to keep calm. Sitting up in a chair rather than lying down will make breathing easier for you.

Professional help: If coronary thrombosis is not suspected, the main objective is to relieve the breathlessness as quickly as possible. This is usually done best in hospital, where you can be given oxygen to prevent cyanosis. The doctor has several choices of drugs, any of which can be injected directly into a vein so as to act swiftly. An injection of morphine for slowing and deepening breathing is a possibility. Or the doctor may prefer to give you a *diuretic* (which will help to drain fluid from your lungs and thus make breathing easier) or a *bronchodilator* (which opens up blocked air spaces in the lungs). If you are not already receiving treatment for heart failure, your doctor may consider giving you drugs to strengthen the action of your heart. In some cases, if the attack of pulmonary oedema has been triggered off by a chest infection, *antibiotics* must be taken in addition to the other medicines.

If pulmonary oedema is treated rapidly and efficiently, and if your attack has not been brought on by coronary thrombosis, your stay in the hospital should be no longer than a week or so. Once you have left hospital, it will be necessary for your doctor to continue to treat you for heart failure so that the chances of pulmonary oedema recurring are lessened.

Sarcoidosis

This is a rare disease in which sarcoids (fleshy patches of inflammation) suddenly appear in one or several parts of the body – frequently in the lungs. The word "sarcoid" should not be confused with *sarcoma*. The inflamed tissues of sarcoidosis are not due to infection, nor are they a kind of tumour. And doctors do not know why the disease occurs or why it clears up, as it usually does, of its own accord. Symptoms vary according to the tissues or organs affected; often the disease is symptomless. If the lungs are affected, there may be some shortness of breath, and scar tissue from the sarcoids may lead to bacterial infection or *bronchiectasis* (p.363).

Sarcoidosis tends to affect men and women equally, and about two-thirds of sufferers are under 40 years of age.

What should be done?
Because sarcoidosis is often symptomless, the condition is usually detected at a routine check-up. If your doctor suspects you may have sarcoidosis, diagnosis can be made following a chest *X-ray*. Untreated sarcoidosis will generally disappear in two or three years. Your doctor may think it advisable, however, to treat you with an anti-inflammatory *steroid* drug to relieve any troublesome symptoms.

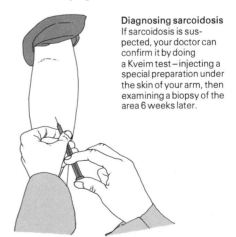

Diagnosing sarcoidosis
If sarcoidosis is suspected, your doctor can confirm it by doing a Kveim test – injecting a special preparation under the skin of your arm, then examining a biopsy of the area 6 weeks later.

Disorders of the heart and circulation

Introduction

The blood is the body's transport system. Its main function is to carry both fuel and the oxygen for burning the fuel to every living tissue. It also carries waste matter away from the tissues and helps maintain body temperature. To do all this it must circulate continuously.

At the centre of the circulatory system is the heart, whose steady beating propels at least 5 litres of blood through a full circuit of the body every minute. Basically, the heart consists of two pumps side by side. Blood is pumped from the right side to the lungs, where waste gases are removed and oxygen added. Freshly oxygenated blood returns to the left side, from which it is pumped to all organs and tissues. Blood flows away from the heart, either to the lungs or the rest of the body, through arteries, which branch again and again, getting smaller. These branching, smaller arteries are called arterioles. The arterioles go on branching and getting narrower and narrower until they become tiny capillaries. As the blood continues its journey, it passes through capillaries that join together, getting larger until they become veins, which carry "used" blood back to the heart.

Disorders of the heart and circulation are many and varied; only the most common are covered in this chapter. One that has become especially common in our century is coronary artery disease, the underlying cause of which is atherosclerosis, a thickening of the internal lining of the blood vessels. The exact cause of this condition is still uncertain, but doctors have a fairly clear picture of various factors linked with it: heavy cigarette smoking, obesity, lack of exercise, and a fatty diet. Coronary artery disease, which can lead to what is commonly called a heart attack, accounts for almost 1 out of every 3 deaths in the Western world today.

In a healthy person the two sides of the heart beat steadily, but some disorders cause the beats to become uncoordinated, or abnormally fast or slow. These disorders of rhythm can usually be cured by drugs or by attaching a pacemaker to the heart to regulate the heartbeat. The heartbeat may also be disturbed by disorders of the heart muscle, which provides the force required for pumping the blood.

To ensure that the blood flows in one direction only, the heart contains one-way valves. If these do not function properly, the result is a form of valvular heart disease. Malfunction of a heart valve causes fluid retention in body tissues, and can lead to heart failure. Fortunately, surgeons can repair or even replace damaged valves.

Finally, even if the heart itself is sound, damaged blood vessels can cause any of a number of disorders.

Treatment of heart and circulation disorders has improved enormously in the past 20 years, largely as a result of advances in surgical techniques. In too many cases, however, the first symptom of serious trouble is permanent disability or even death. Since several kinds of circulatory-system disease are preventable, doctors are increasingly emphasizing the importance of a healthy life style *before* rather than *after* trouble begins.

For congenital heart disease see the series of articles on *Congenital heart disorders*, p.656.

How blood circulates
The heart acts as a pump to propel blood through the body. Deoxygenated – "used" – blood (grey) has made a full circuit of the body and is pumped from the right ventricle into the lungs. There it exchanges carbon dioxide for oxygen. The newly oxygenated blood (brown) returns to the left side of the heart. It is then pumped out of the left ventricle to all of the body tissues.

Body tissues

Lungs

Right ventricle

Left ventricle

The structure of the heart and blood vessels

The heart

The heart is basically a muscular bag consisting of 2 pumps. Each pump is divided into 2 compartments linked by valves. The principal compartment is the left ventricle, which pumps blood, freshly oxygenated by the lungs, through the aorta to all parts of the body. "Used" blood returns to the heart through the veins, which drain into 2 large channels (the superior and inferior venae cavae). Both of these drain into the right atrium. From there the blood passes through the tricuspid valve into the right ventricle. It is then pumped through the pulmonary artery into the lungs, where it receives oxygen. This oxygenated blood flows back to the left atrium of the heart via the pulmonary veins. From the left atrium it passes through the mitral valve into the left ventricle.

Blood vessels

Blood vessels, leading to and from the heart, carry blood to all parts of the body. For a detailed illustration of how the blood circulates around the body, see p.403.

Arteries

Arteries carry blood away from the heart. The walls of the arteries need to be strong, because blood is forced along them under high pressure from the heart. Arteries are made up of 4 layers: the fibrous outer coating, strong muscle, a tough layer of springy elastic tissue, and a smooth, membranous inner lining.

Capillaries

Capillaries – tiny, very thin-walled projections of the smallest arteries – carry blood to every cell of the body. Oxygen and other nutrients in the blood permeate the capillary walls to reach body tissues, while waste matter from the tissues is taken up and carried through the veins back to the heart.

Veins

Veins carry blood to the heart. Since this blood is under much less pressure than the blood in the arteries, veins have thinner, less elastic, and less muscular walls. Compression of the walls by muscle action squeezes the blood on its way. Valves in the veins (bottom left) stop blood from flowing in the wrong direction. Veins are composed of 3 layers: the fibrous outer coating, a thin layer of muscle and elastic tissue, and a membranous lining.

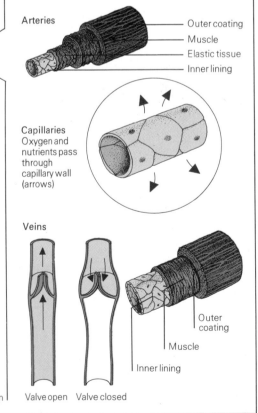

Superior vena cava

Aorta

Pulmonary artery

Pulmonary veins

Inferior vena cava

Tricuspid valve

Right atrium

Pulmonary valve

Right ventricle

Left ventricle

Aortic valve

Mitral valve

Left atrium

Arteries
Outer coating
Muscle
Elastic tissue
Inner lining

Capillaries
Oxygen and nutrients pass through capillary wall (arrows)

Veins
Outer coating
Muscle
Inner lining

Valve open   Valve closed

Major disorders

Deaths from heart disease account for one-third of the total mortality in Western countries, and most of these deaths are due to coronary artery disease and *hypertension*. Coronary artery disease is caused by atherosclerosis – narrowing and hardening of arteries by *atheroma*. These disorders and their complications – shock, heart failure, angina, and coronary thrombosis – are discussed in the opening pages of this chapter because of their close inter-relationships and their importance as causes of severe illness.

Athero-sclerosis

Your arteries are muscular-walled vessels that carry blood from the heart to the rest of the body. If they are healthy, their walls are smooth on the inside and are elastic enough to accommodate extreme variations in blood pressure, so that blood passes through freely. Sometimes, though, fatty streaks appear on the inner wall, possibly starting at stress points where an artery branches or where the wall is slightly damaged. As a fatty streak grows, it further damages the arterial wall, and in time the streak can become a hard mass of fatty tissue, which erodes the wall, diminishes the elasticity of the artery, narrows the passageway, and interferes with the flow of blood. The fatty tissue is known as *atheroma*; a large mass of atheroma is called a *plaque*; and the name of the disorder, atherosclerosis, means, literally, "hardening from atheroma". Atherosclerosis is an important contributory factor in the development of *arteriosclerosis* (p.404).

What are the symptoms?

There are rarely any symptoms until damage becomes extensive. When you do develop symptoms – generally after a number of years – it is because a particular part of your body is being deprived of blood, and the symptoms depend on which part is affected. You may merely have cramps in your legs after exercise, or you may have a stroke, kidney failure, angina, or a heart attack. See "What are the risks?" below.

How common is the problem?

Atherosclerosis is common in Western societies. So much of it is symptomless that accurate figures are unavailable, but postmortem examinations on people killed in road accidents indicate that some degree of the disorder is almost universal, especially in men. Even children are affected. A major reason for this is that atherosclerosis is associated with a high level of fats and *cholesterol* in the bloodstream. Most people in the Western world eat a great deal of fatty or cholesterol-rich foods such as meat, butter, and eggs, and this diet is probably the main cause of the frequency of atherosclerosis.

Your chances of having the disease are higher if, in addition to eating a lot of fatty food, you are a man of any age or a woman over 35; if you smoke; or if you have a condition such as diabetes, kidney trouble, or high blood pressure. Naturally, the severity of atherosclerosis increases with age.

What are the risks?

Severe atherosclerosis can exist without apparent ill-effects. Many parts of the body are supplied with blood not only by a particular

Atheroma in the arteries

Atherosclerosis is the build-up of patches of fatty tissue (atheroma) in and on the inner walls of arteries. Atheroma tends to form at the point at which an artery branches and the smooth flow of blood is naturally disturbed. As increasing amounts of atheroma build up, the artery is substantially narrowed, and this further disturbs blood flow, causing even more fatty deposits to form. Atheroma that has accumulated into a mass (plaque) roughens the arterial wall. This also speeds up the process of atherosclerosis.

Roughened artery wall
Atheroma
Blood flow

artery and its branches, but also by minor branches of neighbouring arteries; and these may be unaffected even though the major supply channel is badly damaged. As the supply of blood from the major artery dries up, other arteries can sometimes compensate by enlarging, thus allowing total blood supply to remain almost unaffected. Even for some body tissues that rely on the supply from a single artery, the channel can often be narrowed considerably without ill-effects because the normal supply of blood usually exceeds actual need.

Thus atherosclerosis may do you little or no harm for many years. It is more than likely, though, that as an artery becomes narrowed by the development of plaque, the part of your body dependent on that artery or one of its branches will eventually suffer from lack of blood. If this happens in the coronary arteries, which supply the heart, you are in danger of having *angina* (p.376) or a heart attack (see *Coronary thrombosis*, p.379). If the cerebral arteries (those supplying the brain) are affected, you may have a *stroke* (p.268). Or you can suffer either kidney damage, leading to *kidney failure* (p.511), or *dry gangrene* (p.415) in an arm or leg.

What should be done?

Do not wait for symptoms to develop before doing something about atherosclerosis. The only symptoms that will appear are those of the consequences, and by the time the disease produces troublesome consequences it will have been gaining ground for years. Assume *now* that you and your children are at risk, and that the risk may be greater if any of your near relations has had a heart disorder or a stroke. Now is the time to begin taking the self-help measures recommended below. They will help you to prevent or slow down the development of atherosclerosis.

Research studies suggest that a fatty streak on the lining of an artery can be made to disappear, but that nothing can be done about an established plaque. After a certain point in the development of atherosclerosis vigorous treatment can still reduce the likelihood of strokes, but there is a stage after which nothing seems to make a heart attack less likely. This is not to suggest that you should ask your doctor for immediate tests of whether you already have atherosclerosis. Such tests are complicated and expensive, and self-help measures should be enough for almost everyone.

Consult your doctor, however, if there is a family history of heart or circulatory disorders, if you know that some of your near relations have high levels of fat in the blood, or if you are diabetic. In any such case you might reasonably ask whether you ought to have diagnostic tests as a possible preliminary to undergoing drug treatment. Your doctors may consider it advisable for you to have a blood-cholesterol test (as preparation for which you will need to fast for a few hours). Other possible tests – apart from the obvious check of your blood pressure – include a chest *X-ray* to estimate heart size and to look for deposits of calcium in suspected areas of atherosclerosis; an *electrocardiogram* (*ECG*); and *arteriograms*.

What is the treatment?

Self-help: Because the risk of developing severe atherosclerosis is related to the level of cholesterol in your blood, reduce your intake of animal fats and other *saturated* (dairy) fats. Eat poultry and fish instead of pork, beef, and lamb. Remove fat from the animal flesh that you do eat, and grill rather than fry it. Since one egg gives you almost a day's quota of cholesterol, restrict yourself to three eggs a week. Avoid cream and sweets; use margarine high in *polyunsaturated* fats instead of butter; eat more fruit and vegetables; and use cooking oils labelled "high in polyunsaturates" – for example, corn oil and sunflower oil – not oil labelled "vegetable oil" without further explanation.

No clear-cut link between obesity or smoking and atherosclerosis has been established. But people who are overweight as well as being heavy smokers are known to be peculiarly susceptible to most of the disorders that can be caused by atherosclerosis. So be prudent. Give up cigarettes, even if you are not overweight, since you are also risking *lung cancer* (p.366). If you are also overweight, follow a reducing diet to help you lose that dangerous excess fat.

Finally, take regular exercise. A programme of moderate physical activity can impede the development of atherosclerosis and lessen your chance of succumbing to one of the serious consequences. Do not overdo it, however. Get advice from your doctor if you suspect that exercise may harm you (see *Keeping physically fit*, p.14).

Professional help: Your doctor can help by keeping a watch on your blood pressure and treating you for *hypertension* if necessary. If you have an abnormally high blood-cholesterol level, the doctor may prescribe a drug that will lower it if taken regularly (though some such drugs have side-effects, such as slight increase in the risk of gallbladder disease).

Coronary artery disease

(also called coronary atherosclerosis, ischaemic heart disease, or coronary heart disease)

The heart muscle requires a constant flow of oxygen- and nutrient-rich blood, just as other body organs do. This blood reaches the heart through two coronary arteries, which nourish the heart muscle by means of a network of branches over its surface. If fatty deposits (*atheroma*) are formed in the arteries, these passageways become narrowed and fail to provide the heart with the right amount of oxygen and food. Moreover, the narrowing of the coronary arteries can lead to clotting of the blood flowing through them; and a clot (or *thrombus*) can block an artery. When, in response to physical or nervous stress, the heart beats faster and thus requires increased oxygen and food, severely narrowed or blocked arteries cannot cope, and the result is *angina* (p.376). If the flow of blood to part of the heart muscle is reduced by a clot in one of the coronary arteries, the result is a heart attack (see *Coronary thrombosis*, p.379).

What are the symptoms?

Often there are no symptoms of coronary artery disease, especially in the early stages. For symptoms that do occur, see the articles on angina and coronary thrombosis.

How common is the problem?

Coronary artery disease is common in the Western world, where it accounts for 30 per cent of all deaths. More men than women are affected. In Britain about 1 in every 170 men aged 45 to 64 dies as a result of the disease each year; the comparable figure for women is 1 in 500. The incidence is much lower in less affluent countries. Some additional facts:

1. More men than women suffer from coronary artery disease; but the risk to women increases after the menopause, and women over 60 are nearly as susceptible as men.

2. Cigarette smokers are at least twice as susceptible as non-smokers. In fact, deaths from the disorder among people aged 34 to 45 are *five* times more common in smokers.

3. There is increased risk for people with high blood pressure and diabetics. Male diabetics are twice as susceptible as other men, and female diabetics are five times as susceptible as other women.

4. The disease runs in families. You are more at risk if members of your family have had it.

5. Also more at risk are people who overeat – particularly if they eat large quantities of fatty foods.

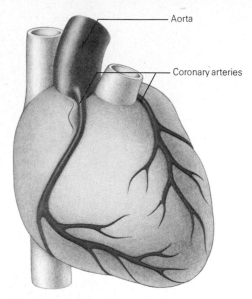

Aorta

Coronary arteries

The coronary arteries
The heart has its own blood supply to keep it contracting regularly and strongly. Some of the freshly oxygenated blood that is pumped out of the aorta flows into the 2 coronary arteries. These form a branching network over the surface of the heart and supply its tissues with blood.

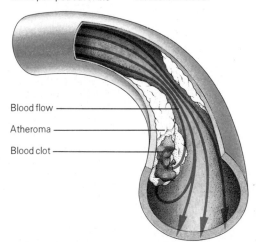

Blood flow

Atheroma

Blood clot

How blood clots form in the arteries
Although plaque can form anywhere along the length of an artery, it builds up most commonly wherever the smooth flow of blood is naturally interrupted. As the atheroma forms, it roughens the arterial wall and causes increasing turbulence in the flow of blood. This turbulence may trigger off the blood's clotting mechanism. Any blood clot (thrombus) so formed may partly or completely block the artery, or a fragment of the clot (embolus) may be swept into the bloodstream to block the artery at a narrower point. In a coronary artery, such a blockage can lead to a heart attack.

6. People with sedentary jobs appear to be more susceptible than people who do hard physical work.

7. Women over 35 who are taking the contraceptive pill are much more at risk than women using other forms of contraception.

8. People who live in soft-water areas seem to be more susceptible than those in hard-water areas.

What are the risks?

If coronary artery disease remains untreated and the arteries are increasingly blocked, blood supply to the heart may be so reduced that there is a risk of heart attack – possibly a fatal one. But even after a major attack the heart can often be restored to health. Furthermore, many people live for years with coronary artery disease and have no trouble; and even though others are forced to restrict their activities because of recurrent attacks of angina, these people can also lead relatively active lives as long as they keep the disease under control.

Sometimes, however, the heart muscle is damaged so much that pumping action is weakened, causing *heart failure* (p.381).

What should be done?

For advice on what to do if you experience either of the main symptoms of coronary artery disease, see the articles on angina and coronary thrombosis. If you are simply worried that you may be susceptible, start taking preventive measures. Too often, sudden death is the first symptom of the disease. The following recommendations for self-help (see "What is the treatment?" below) are useful not only if you already have heart trouble but also if you want to improve your chances of avoiding it.

If you want to check the state of your heart, see your doctor, who, after examining you, may order some of the tests mentioned in the article on angina. If you are over 40, you should also have your blood pressure checked (see *High blood pressure*, p.382).

What is the treatment?

Self-help: There is, as yet, no way to dissolve atheroma that has formed in the coronary arteries, but you can take steps to prevent or slow down further accumulations. If you smoke, give it up, or at least change your cigarettes to cigars or a pipe. If you are overweight, choose a moderate reducing diet and follow it consistently. There are definite links between the kinds of food eaten in a country

and its incidence of coronary artery disease. As a result, heart specialists have drawn up certain dietary guidelines. In the United States, as more of the population have adopted this "anti-coronary life style", so has mortality from coronary artery disease declined. Though the link between these two events cannot be proved, the life style can certainly do you no harm:

1. Eat only small amounts of butter, cream, and fatty foods of all kinds.

2. Eat less meat, remove the fat, and grill the meat instead of frying it.

3. Eat no more than three eggs a week.

4. Eat plenty of fruit and vegetables.

5. Reduce your intake of salt. This advice is especially important for people with high blood pressure. A low-salt diet can reduce blood pressure – and the risk of coronary artery disease – considerably.

6. Take exercise regularly. There is good evidence that vigorous exercise two or more times a week diminishes the risk of heart disease. But exercise must be begun gradually and continued regularly. Sudden heavy exercise increases the risk.

Professional help: If you have high blood pressure, your doctor may prescribe *antihypertensive* drugs to lower it. If you are a woman taking the contraceptive pill and are over 35 or a heavy smoker or have a family history of coronary heart disease, the doctor will probably recommend a different form of contraception for you.

If a blood test shows a high level of *cholesterol* or other fats in your blood, you may be advised to start taking a drug that lowers the fat content. However, because such drugs may have unpleasant side-effects and must be taken constantly to be effective, most doctors prescribe them only for people with a very high cholesterol level or with a high level combined with dangerous factors such as *hypertension* (high blood pressure).

A diseased coronary artery can sometimes be replaced by a length of vein from the sufferer's leg; the graft usually takes well because it is the patient's own tissue. Such surgery is often advisable for active young people who have been seriously disabled by angina. The graft relieves the angina, but it does not control the underlying disease. And although the operation may be done on

Medical myth
Hard work and long hours bring on coronary artery disease.

Wrong. There is evidence, however, that emotional stress – the strain of a divorce, for example – increases the risk.

people of all ages, its success depends in part on your general health (see *Coronary artery bypass*, p.378, for details).

What are the long-term prospects?
Drugs and surgery can go some way toward alleviating any problems caused by coronary artery disease. However, the major responsibility for protecting your future health lies with you alone. If, despite your doctor's warnings, you persist with an unhealthy diet and an inactive life style, you will become increasingly at risk from serious, and possibly fatal, heart disease.

Angina
(also called angina pectoris)

Angina is not a disease in its own right but is the name given to pain arising when the muscular wall of the heart becomes temporarily short of oxygen. Normally, the coronary arteries supplying blood to the heart can cope with an increased demand, but this ability is restricted in a person who has *coronary artery disease* (p.374) or *high blood pressure* (p.382), or – more rarely – has a disease of the *heart valves* (p.392), or *anaemia* (p.419). In such a circumstance the oxygen supply to the heart may be adequate for some activities but become inadequate when exercise – or sometimes extremes of temperature or emotion – increases the demand above a certain threshold. When the person stops exercising, the oxygen requirement falls and the pain disappears.

What are the symptoms?
The main symptom is pain in the centre of the chest. The pain can spread to the throat and upper jaw, the back, and the arms (mainly the left one). It is a dull, heavy, constricting pain, which characteristically appears during exercise and fades when exercise stops. Less commonly, the pain may occur only in the arms, wrists, or neck, but you can recognize it as angina if you know that it arises whenever you are abnormally active or excited and disappears after the activity or excitement has stopped. Additional symptoms that can often accompany the pain are difficulty in breathing, sweating, nausea, and dizziness.

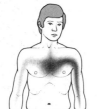

Site of the pain

How common is the problem?
Angina is a common condition – although accurate figures do not exist because many people do not report it to a doctor, and the sufferer does not usually need to be in hospital. In men it normally occurs after the age of 30 and is nearly always caused by coronary artery disease. The onset tends to be later in life for women; and although, as with the condition in men, the most usual cause is coronary artery disease, some of the other general causes are found to be more common among women than among men. People who smoke heavily or are overweight are more likely to suffer from angina.

What are the risks?
Since angina is a symptom rather than a disease, the risks are basically those of the condition that causes the angina. The heart may become so deprived of oxygen that there is risk of a heart attack (see *Coronary thrombosis*, p.379). The angina may occur with less provocation as time goes by, and it may last longer. If this happens, the sufferer is forced to become less and less active. Unfortunately there is evidence that a sedentary life style encourages the angina to occur even more easily during any activity or excitement, trapping the victim in a vicious circle.

What should be done?
If you think you are having attacks of angina, consult your doctor. Some of the causes are remediable, and the doctor can prescribe treatment to relieve the discomfort. *Consult the doctor as a matter of urgency* if the pain lasts longer than five minutes after exercise has ceased, or if attacks are increasing rapidly in frequency and length.

After examining you, the doctor may take a blood specimen for tests to identify thyroid disorder, anaemia, or other possible causes of chest pain. It may be advisable to find the level of *lipids* (fats) in your blood, in which case the blood must be taken in the morning before you have eaten. A urine test will determine whether or not you have diabetes (diabetics are more susceptible to heart disease). Hospital diagnostic tests that may also be required include a chest *X-ray*, *electrocardiogram (ECG)*, and coronary *arteriogram*. While an X-ray and an ECG are often given as part of the normal procedure for assessing a heart complaint, an arteriogram will not usually be given unless the doctor suspects (from the results of other, less involved tests) that any coronary artery disease is quite far advanced. The X-ray will look for signs of heart strain such as an enlarged heart. The ECG will measure the electrical impulses passing through your heart in order to confirm that the pain is indeed angina. The ECG will also help to show how much of the heart is affected by coronary artery disease. The arteriogram, which involves injecting a dye into the bloodstream and then taking X-rays of the coronary arteries, will show exactly where the arteries are narrowed or blocked.

What is the treatment?

Self-help: If you smoke, stop or cut down as much as you can. If you are overweight, go on a sensible diet (total intake of about 1,000 Calories a day is ideal); it might help if you join a slimming club. But do not use your angina as an excuse to vegetate; you should certainly not reduce your physical activity unless told to do so by your doctor. You will quickly come to know just what limits are imposed on your physical activities by your angina. Cultivate a more relaxed attitude to life, especially when driving a car.

Professional help: If and when the underlying cause of your angina is established, your doctor will treat the basic disease, and the angina will disappear if the treatment succeeds. Often, however, the underlying disorder is likely to be coronary artery disease, and the doctor will concentrate on preventing it from getting worse and on easing the discomfort and handicap of the angina itself.

There are many drugs that will temporarily increase the blood supply to the heart muscle. It is important to take them exactly as the doctor prescribes. One of the most commonly prescribed of these drugs comes in tablet form and you will probably be advised to dissolve one tablet under the tongue the moment an anginal attack starts. Or if you know that some activity such as climbing the stairs at your office always brings on your angina, you can take a tablet shortly beforehand rather than waiting for the pain to occur. If you are under stress, you may also need to take a tranquillizer.

An unfortunate side-effect of tablets that are dissolved under the tongue is that they often cause headaches. The headaches are usually mild, and are not normally a reason to discontinue the treatment. If you get severe headaches from taking a whole tablet, try crushing a tablet and putting only part of it under your tongue.

Among other drugs used for controlling angina, the most widely prescribed are a group called the beta-adrenergic blocking agents – *beta-blockers* for short. Beta-

Medical myth

A person with angina must avoid exercise and lead the life of an invalid.

Wrong. Regular exercise is good for you, provided you keep it within the limits imposed by the disorder. Experience will tell you how much you can do without pain. Do not be afraid, either, to enjoy sexual intercourse.

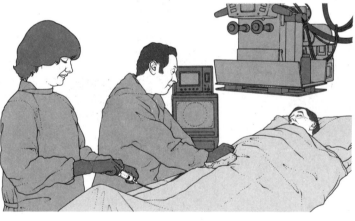

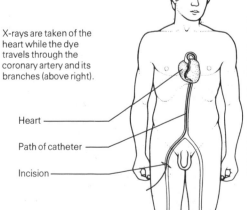

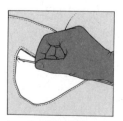

Coronary arteriography
A coronary arteriogram is done to discover where a coronary artery is narrowed or blocked. This procedure, for which you will be sedated but conscious, involves injecting dye into a coronary artery, so that it shows up on an X-ray. A narrow tube (catheter) is inserted into an accessible artery, usually in the groin (right) and then threaded up to the heart and into a coronary artery (far right). To do this, the radiologist is

guided by a picture on an X-ray screen. A special dye that shows up on X-rays is then injected along the catheter (above).

Inserting the catheter

X-rays are taken of the heart while the dye travels through the coronary artery and its branches (above right).

Heart

Path of catheter

Incision

What the X-ray shows
The heart can be seen as a shadowy outline on the X-ray. The coronary artery and its branches through which the dye flows show up on the screen as white lines (above). A narrowing of a line indicates the presence of plaque. Where a line stops abruptly, that part of the artery is completely blocked by atheroma or a blood clot.

blockers act to reduce the oxygen needs of the heart by reducing the heartbeat rate. One drawback of these drugs is that they must be taken exactly as prescribed, since an overdose can cause dizziness, fainting spells, and other side-effects. You should never stop taking such drugs abruptly – the dose should be lowered gradually. Under certain circumstances, too – for example, if you have had asthma – your doctor may not want to prescribe them. Follow the self-help advice recommended above, and you can reduce your need for treatment with drugs.

Most patients with angina do not need (and would not benefit from) surgery. If, however, the angina is due to *aortic stenosis* (p.398), surgical valve replacement may be recommended. If the cause is coronary artery disease, an operation may be advisable if many sections of the coronary network are blocked or if your angina cannot be controlled by drugs. The operation – *coronary artery bypass* (below) – usually produces a dramatic improvement in symptoms, although it does not cure the underlying causes of coronary artery disease which may affect other arteries later on in life.

What are the long-term prospects?
The outlook for people with angina is much better than is popularly supposed. If you have just been found to have angina and you are otherwise in good health, you have a 50 per cent chance of living for another 10 to 12 years with a good chance of remaining in reasonable health for much longer.

OPERATION: ## Coronary artery bypass

This operation is done to bypass diseased coronary artery by a length of vein taken from the thigh. This relieves the pain associated with coronary artery disease but does not cure the underlying cause of the disease. The long-term effects of the operation are still being evaluated.
During the operation You are under a general anaesthetic, and for part of the time your circulation and breathing are taken over by a heart-lung machine. An incision is made down the length of your breastbone, and your ribcage is opened to expose your heart. Meanwhile a small incision is made in your leg, from which a length of vein is removed. Wherever a blockage has been detected in the coronary arteries, a piece of this vein is grafted on to bypass the blockage. The usual operating time is about 4 to 5 hours.
After the operation You will spend a few days in an intensive-care unit, where your heartbeat will be constantly recorded on an ECG. You will be receiving fluid and blood though intravenous drips. There will be several drains from your chest. You may need to breathe oxygen through a tube leading into your throat and may also need the help of a respirator. You will probably have to stay in hospital for 2 weeks.
Convalescence You will need at least 3 months' convalescence. As you recover, your doctor will advise you to give up smoking and go on a low-fat diet.
See also information on operations, p.738.

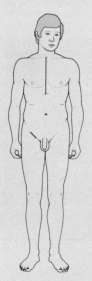

Sites of the incisions

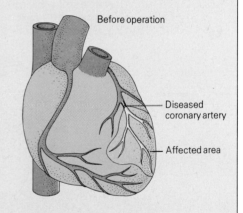

Before operation

Diseased coronary artery

Affected area

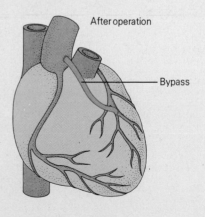

After operation

Bypass

Coronary thrombosis

(also called cardiac infarction, myo-cardial infarction, or heart attack)

Coronary thrombosis is the medical term for the most common variety of heart attack. The immediate cause is blockage of one of the coronary arteries by a blood clot (*thrombus*), which cuts off the blood supply to one region of the heart muscle, damaging the deprived tissue. Thrombosis generally occurs only in people with coronary arteries already narrowed by *coronary artery disease* (p.374). If the size of the damaged area (called an *infarct*) is small, and if the heart's electrical conducting system (see *Heart rate and rhythm*, p.388) is not thrown out of gear, the attack will not be fatal and the chances of recovery are good.

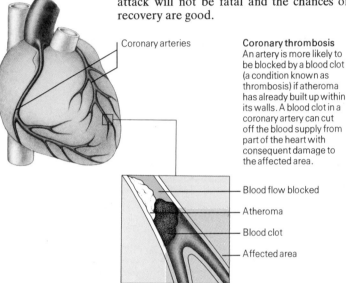

Coronary arteries

Coronary thrombosis
An artery is more likely to be blocked by a blood clot (a condition known as thrombosis) if atheroma has already built up within its walls. A blood clot in a coronary artery can cut off the blood supply from part of the heart with consequent damage to the affected area.

Blood flow blocked

Atheroma

Blood clot

Affected area

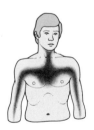

Site of the pain

What are the symptoms?

The main symptom is likely to be a crushing central-chest pain, which may radiate out to the neck, jaw, and arms. A heart attack can come on gradually – you may well have had *angina* (p.376) in the preceding weeks – but it can also happen with no prior warning. The pain may vary in degree from a feeling of tightness in the chest to an agonizing, bursting sensation. It may be continuous, or it may last for a few minutes, fade away, and then return. It may come on during exercise or emotional stress; but, unlike the pain of angina, it will not go away when exercise or stress ceases.

Among other possible symptoms of coronary thrombosis are dizziness, shortness of breath, sweating, chills, nausea, and fainting. In a few patients, mainly the elderly, these are the only symptoms. This condition, known as a "silent" infarct, can be confirmed only by hospital tests which also rule out other possible causes of the symptoms.

How common is the problem?

In the Western world there are more deaths from heart trouble – most of which are due to coronary thrombosis – than from any other disorder. For every fatal heart attack there are at least two that are not fatal ones; in Britain alone about half a million people have an attack every year. For most of this century the death rate from coronary thrombosis kept increasing in Western countries, but the rise stopped in the United States in the late 1960s and is now slowing down in Europe, probably because of the greater awareness of importance of life style.

What are the risks?

Two out of three people who have a heart attack recover, but the attack may be fatal if it interferes with the electrical impulses that regulate heartbeat, or if it severely damages the heart muscle. Most deaths occur within two hours of the onset of symptoms. About 10 per cent of patients admitted to hospital with heart attacks develop *shock* (p.386) which can be fatal. Somewhat less catastrophic is the possibility that *heart failure* (p.381) may develop.

Later complications of a heart attack can include the formation of a thrombus within one of the four chambers of the heart. If the thrombus becomes detached – it is then called an *embolus* – and is swept into the circulation, it can cause damage elsewhere in the body. Fortunately, emboli are rare and are often too small to do much damage.

Damage to the heart muscle may cause a weakening and stretching of one of the walls of the heart chambers. The resultant swellings (*aneurysms*) can lead to complications such as heart failure. And there is the added risk that an enforced rest in bed may result in thrombosis in the veins, especially in the legs.

What should be done?

A heart attack is a medical emergency. Get professional help if you or anyone in your family seems to be showing the symptoms. Even if the discomfort is mild, do not try to travel to the doctor; if your doctor is not immediately available, call an ambulance. While waiting for assistance, keep the sufferer as warm and calm as possible. Do not leave him or her alone; a comforting presence and reassurance are invaluable. If the affected person loses consciousness (see *Cardiac arrest*, p.388), do not give up. The heart rhythm may be only temporarily disturbed. So remove any loose false teeth from the mouth of the sufferer, and try mouth-to-mouth artificial respiration (see *Accidents and emergencies*, p.802) until help comes or the sufferer is breathing normally.

After a heart attack, most people are best off in hospital. A decision as to what is best in your case will depend on your doctor's assessment of the severity of the attack, how long you have had symptoms, and the facilities available both in hospital and in your home.

If you have had an attack, you may be put in an intensive- or coronary-care unit of a hospital. There you will need to undergo a number of diagnostic tests, including an *electrocardiogram (ECG)*. You may need several ECG recordings; in coronary-care units the ECG is continuously monitored. Blood specimens will also be taken at intervals to assess damage to the heart muscle. And the doctor will carry out other investigations to see whether a change in your way of life or drug treatment might help prevent another such heart attack.

What is the treatment?

Your doctor will probably try to control your pain with an *analgesic* such as morphine. Because morphine often causes vomiting, you may also be given an anti-emetic (anti-sickness) drug. To reduce the risk of blood clots forming in the veins (see *Deep-vein thrombosis*, p.405), you may have to take a regular dose of an oral *anticoagulant*. If your attack is a minor one, without complications, you may be allowed out of bed after 48 hours since a certain amount of mobility helps to ease the flow of blood and reduce the risk of blood clots developing.

What are the long-term prospects?

If you are reading these pages after having had a coronary thrombosis, the outlook is good. Mortality figures vary according to age and type of attack, but most deaths from coronary thrombosis occur within minutes or hours of an attack. This is why it is important for help to be summoned right away. If you show no sign of heart failure or disturbances of heart rhythm six hours after the pain disappears, you have a 90 per cent chance of full recovery from this particular attack. If you are alive one month after even a severe attack, you have an 85 per cent chance of surviving for at least a year and a 70 per cent chance of surviving for five years.

After a coronary thrombosis you will naturally be concerned about your heart. Because of the effects of stress and anxiety, it is important, though, not to be *too* concerned. For helpful comments about the best possible life style following a heart attack, see *After a heart attack* (below).

After a heart attack

Each year in Britain nearly half a million people recover from heart attacks and leave hospital to face life again. If you are one of this half million, the most important thing to remember is that you are not an invalid and that damaged hearts heal, just as fractured bones do. Every month that passes improves the prospects for future health; statistics show that 10 years after you had a coronary thrombosis your life expectation will be the same as if you had never had an attack.

You may find your activities limited by occasional pain in the chest (see *Angina*, p.376) or shortness of breath. If this is so, consult your doctor, who can probably give you medicines to relieve these symptoms; or, possibly, an operation may be advisable. More likely, you will find the only brake on your activities is your own anxiety. Make "Back to normal!" your motto. Whatever your job was before your heart attack, this is the job you should return to. Don't let well-meaning friends or colleagues persuade you to work part-time or take a less responsible job. There is not a shred of evidence that such a move will help your health.

But how can you prevent another attack? Surely, you will say, there must have been something about your way of life that brought on the coronary in the first place. If you have a condition, such as *high blood pressure* (p.382), which may predispose you to circulatory-system trouble, your doctor will deal with it. For the most part, however, nobody knows why some people are affected and others are not. There are some good rules of behaviour that most doctors believe will reduce the risk of further attacks:

1. Do not smoke.
2. Keep your weight down to normal and ensure that your diet is as fat-free as possible.
3. Take some regular exercise.
4. Avoid sexual intercourse for four or five weeks after your attack, but there should be no problem about resuming your normal sex life thereafter.

If you have not been accustomed to strenuous exercise, however, go gently. If you last played tennis 20 years ago, it would be unwise to take it up again; start with something gentler such as walking, swimming, or cycling. And try to find a physical recreation that you enjoy. You may be willing now to spend 20 minutes a day doing routine exercises before breakfast, but that enthusiasm is likely to fade. The anti-coronary life style can and should be fun.

Heart failure

(and congestive heart failure)

In a person suffering from heart failure, the pumping action of the heart has become inefficient, either because the muscle is weakened by disease or because there is a mechanical fault in the valves that control the flow of blood. If the heart is unable to maintain a normal output, blood accumulates in the veins leading to it.

Heart failure sometimes affects only one side of the heart, but more usually affects both sides. When the entire heart is affected in this way, the condition is known as *congestive* heart failure.

In left-sided heart failure the veins that carry blood from the lungs become engorged. As a result, the lungs become swollen and congested with fluid that passes from blood vessels into lung tissues (see *Pulmonary oedema*, p.368). In right-sided failure blood accumulates in the veins leading to the heart from other parts of the body, and waterlogging occurs in the affected parts – most obviously in the legs.

Despite its name, heart failure is not an immediate, life-threatening disease. Much of the outcome depends on the seriousness of the underlying trouble.

What are the symptoms?

Left-sided failure: The main symptom is breathlessness. At first you may feel breathless only after exercise, but the symptom becomes more and more apparent, especially in the evenings, when you are tired. Because it may be hard to breathe when you lie down, you may need to sleep with several pillows under your head or even sitting up. Severe attacks of breathlessness can become so bad that you want to lean out of a window in order to draw air into your lungs. Difficult breathing is likely to be accompanied by a wheeze. Bad attacks usually last no more than an hour, but the experience can be very disturbing while it lasts.

Sometimes the lungs become so congested that a bubbling sound occurs during breathing. There may also be chest pain, and frothy, blood-flecked sputum (phlegm). The fluid in the lungs decreases resistance to infection, and *pneumonia* (p.359) is a common additional disorder in sufferers from left-sided heart failure.

Right-sided failure: The most common symptom is weariness, but this symptom is a sign of so many illnesses that on its own it is not a dependable indication of heart failure. A more reliable symptom is the swelling of any part of the body in which fluid accumulates. If you are mobile, it usually shows up as swollen ankles. If you are bedridden, the swelling will be most noticeable in the lower part of your back. Internal organs such as the liver can also become swollen, and this can cause abdominal pain.

With congestive heart failure you are likely to have symptoms of both left-sided and right-sided failure. In addition there may be loss of appetite and even mental confusion. As the blood supply fails, arm and leg muscles waste away, but this may not immediately be apparent because of the swellings that accompany the condition.

How common is the problem?

Heart failure is quite a common condition; each year in Britain, about 1 person in 130 develops the condition. If you are already under a doctor's care for heart trouble, you probably know whether you are susceptible.

What are the risks?

Untreated heart failure imposes on the entire system a strain that can be fatal. If heart failure is successfully treated, the only dangers are those that are imposed by the underlying cause.

What should be done?

If you think you may have heart failure, see your doctor, who will check your blood pressure and will probably have your blood and urine analysed in order to find out whether the kidneys have been affected. Diagnostic tests will probably include a chest *X-ray* to look for lung trouble and check heart size. An *electrocardiogram (ECG)* will help determine whether your heart is under strain, and there may be other tests appropriate to the underlying cause.

What is the treatment?

Self help: Get plenty of rest in order to conserve energy; but although you should reduce your physical activities, do not let yourself become bedridden. A comfortable armchair is better than a bed. Moreover, heart failure need not mean lifetime restriction. Treatment of the failure and the underlying condition can result in eventual resumption of normal activities.

Even while resting, keep your legs on the move by frequently shifting your position or relaxing and contracting leg muscles. Since the circulation of a sufferer from heart failure is sluggish, blood tends to clot, especially in the legs and pelvis, unless speeded along by the pump action of leg muscles.

Because salt encourages fluid to stay in the body, cut down your daily intake.

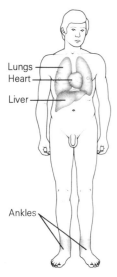

Lungs
Heart
Liver

Ankles

The effects of heart failure
If heart failure affects only the left side of your heart, your lungs become congested and you feel breathless. Symptoms of right-sided failure, however, can occur in any part of the body that easily accumulates fluid – for instance, in the liver or in the legs.

Back pressure from heart into veins

Reduced blood flow

Increased pressure in veins

Fluid forced into tissues

How heart failure causes excess fluid in tissues
When the heart fails, it is unable to maintain its normal output of blood. This, in turn, means that it can take in less blood from the veins leading to it. These become engorged with a backlog of blood, which passes back into the capillaries. Pressure then builds up in the capillaries, forcing some of the fluid into surrounding tissues.

Professional help: Apart from treating the underlying cause, your doctor can prescribe drugs that make life easier for you. Among these are *diuretics* which cause you to pass more urine than normal and thus lower the fluid content of your body. Such drugs are best taken in the morning because it is more convenient to urinate frequently during the day. Another drug may be prescribed to improve the strength of the heartbeat, especially if there is an irregularity of rhythm. Your doctor will carefully control the amounts and times of dosage, since too much can bring on nausea. It is important to follow the doctor's instructions and not to discontinue taking drugs until you are told to, even though you may feel you no longer need them.

If you must have a long period of bed rest, you may also need to take an oral *anticoagulant* to keep your blood from clotting. Blood samples must then be taken at intervals so that the doctor can make sure the dose is correct. An overdose of anticoagulant drugs can cause bleeding into the intestines, skin, or into the urine.

Acute (sudden) heart failure, with extremely severe breathlessness, is a medical emergency. The victim must go straight to hospital, where there are facilities for oxygen to be administered and drugs can be given by injection for immediate effect.

What are the long-term prospects?
With drug treatment your breathlessness should improve and swellings subside. If heart failure reaches a point where it no longer responds to rest and drugs, there is one other form of treatment that offers some hope: heart transplantation. Replacement of diseased hearts by healthy ones taken from accident or brain-disease victims has proved highly effective in certain cases, but the operation is still in an experimental stage and the risks must be balanced against the sufferer's prospects without such treatment. (See *Transplants*, p.402, for information about transplanting an organ from a donor whose blood and tissue types can only approximate to those of the recipient.)

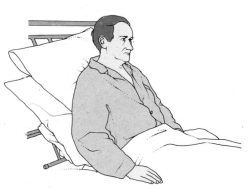

Coping with breathlessness
If you have left-sided heart failure, you may find it difficult to breathe when you lie down to go to sleep. Prop yourself up with several pillows, and this should ease your breathing.

High blood pressure
(hypertension)

As the heart pumps blood through the arteries, the force of the flow exerts pressure on the arterial walls, just as air pumped into a tyre exerts pressure on its lining and surface. And just as too much air pressure is bad for the life of a tyre, so too much blood pressure eventually damages the arteries. If the force with which your heart pumps blood through your circulatory system is much greater than necessary for maintaining a steady flow, you are suffering from what doctors call *hypertension* (high blood pressure). This puts the whole of your circulatory system under considerable strain.

Blood pressure is very variable. It varies from person to person and even in different parts of the body; it is, for example, higher in the legs than in the arms. For the sake of convenience, doctors normally measure it in one of the large arteries of an arm (see the box entitled *Testing blood pressure* on p.384). Two types of pressure, *systolic* and *diastolic*, are measured. Systolic pressure is the pressure at a moment when the heart contracts in the process of pumping out blood; diastolic pressure is the pressure at a moment when the heart relaxes to permit the inflow of blood. Thus the systolic figure, representing the moment of greatest pressure, is always higher than the diastolic figure. Doctors tend to speak of a patient's blood pressure as being, say, "110 over 75". This means that the systolic pressure is 110, the diastolic 75. And those figures are roughly normal for a healthy young adult. (For *Low blood pressure*, see the article on p.417.)

Whether or not a person is suffering from hypertension depends largely on medical judgement of the individual case. An elderly person, for instance, with a reading of 140/90 may well be judged to have normal pressure, since it tends to rise with age. But if your pressure when you are in a relatively calm emotional and physical state exceeds about 150/100, there is probably cause for concern. Even if only one of the two figures is high (this applies especially to the diastolic figure), you may be said to be suffering from at least some degree of hypertension.

There are two different types of hypertension; they are known as "essential" and "secondary" hypertension. Any person with essential hypertension has raised blood pressure for no obvious reason, whereas secondary hypertension results from one of a number of other conditions – for instance, kidney disease, hormonal disorders such as *Cushing's syndrome* (p.523) and *aldosteronism* (p.524), and changes in the body produced by taking oral contraceptives or becoming pregnant.

Essential hypertension is more common than the secondary kind. We do not know precisely why the essential kind develops, but a tendency towards the disorder seems to run in families. In other words, blood pressure appears to be influenced by heredity as well as by life style. It also seems likely that young fat people are more apt than their lean contemporaries to suffer from hypertension in middle age, and that there is a link between hypertension and high salt intake. It is certainly true that fat hypertensive people can lower their blood pressure by reducing the amount of salt in their diets, often just by not salting food at the table.

In most cases, the blood pressure rises steadily over the course of a number of years unless treated. Occasionally, however, an exceedingly high blood pressure develops very quickly. This dangerous condition (which can be either essential or secondary) is known as "malignant" hypertension; and it is significant that malignant hypertension is most often found among smokers.

What are the symptoms?

Hypertension is nearly always a symptomless disease; a hypertensive person can feel fine, without the slightest indication of inner trouble. Such symptoms as headaches, palpitations, and a general feeling of ill health usually occur only when the pressure is dangerously high. So it is risky to wait for treatment until symptoms develop. People who have malignant hypertension are more likely to suffer from these symptoms.

You should always be aware of the possibility that you may have high blood pressure, especially if you are over 40, if there is a history of hypertension in your family, and if you are overweight.

How common is the problem?

Hypertension is extremely common, especially in the Western world. In Scotland, for example, 15 per cent of all adults are thought to have some degree of high blood pressure. And one US study suggests that 1 in 10 Americans is hypertensive; the incidence rises steeply with age and appears to be twice as high among black people as among whites. The study also indicates that men are more at risk than women, whose chances of having high blood pressure are only about one-half to three-quarters as great. And around 95 per cent of all investigated cases, apart from those resulting from pregnancy or the use of oral contraceptives, turn out to be cases of essential rather than secondary hypertension. Malignant hypertension, fortunately, is a rare form of the disease.

What are the risks?

Even mild hypertension will, if untreated, lower your life expectancy to some degree, and severe hypertension will lower it considerably. In particular there are major risks to the heart and brain. Untreated malignant hypertension is serious and can be fatal within six to eight months.

Increased pressure in the circulatory system forces the heart to do more work to keep the circulation on the move, and this does damage to the inner lining of the coronary arteries. Over a period of years fatty tissue known as *atheroma* is likely to form where damage has occurred, and the coronary arteries may become narrowed or even close up completely. The result may be *coronary thrombosis* (p.379). Congestive *heart failure* (p.381) is also a possible consequence; hypertensive people are six times more likely to develop heart failure than are those with normal blood pressure.

Moreover, if you have high blood pressure, your chances of having a *stroke* (p.268) are four times greater than they might otherwise

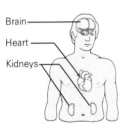

Brain
Heart
Kidneys

Organs affected by high blood pressure
High blood pressure forces the heart to work harder and may also damage blood vessels. If untreated, this disorder can lead to heart failure, a stroke in the brain, or kidney failure.

Testing blood pressure

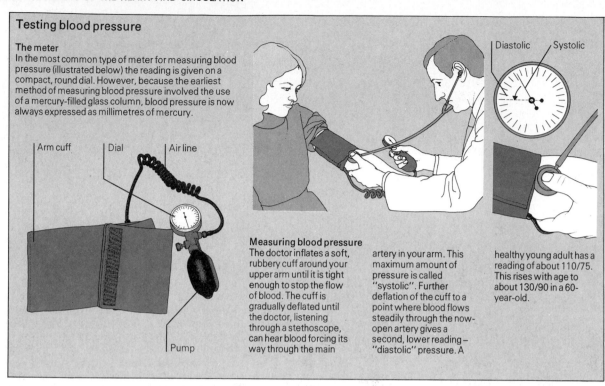

The meter
In the most common type of meter for measuring blood pressure (illustrated below) the reading is given on a compact, round dial. However, because the earliest method of measuring blood pressure involved the use of a mercury-filled glass column, blood pressure is now always expressed as millimetres of mercury.

Arm cuff Dial Air line

Pump

Diastolic Systolic

Measuring blood pressure
The doctor inflates a soft, rubbery cuff around your upper arm until it is tight enough to stop the flow of blood. The cuff is gradually deflated until the doctor, listening through a stethoscope, can hear blood forcing its way through the main artery in your arm. This maximum amount of pressure is called "systolic". Further deflation of the cuff to a point where blood flows steadily through the now-open artery gives a second, lower reading – "diastolic" pressure. A healthy young adult has a reading of about 110/75. This rises with age to about 130/90 in a 60-year-old.

be. As in the coronary circulation, increased blood pressure can lead to the formation of atheroma in an artery that supplies the brain. The kidneys may also be harmed, especially in certain cases of malignant hypertension. Damaged kidneys (see *Chronic kidney failure*, p.512) lead to a further rise in blood pressure, thus creating a vicious circle. And the brain, eyes, and other organs can be affected by damage to their blood vessels.

Hypertension during pregnancy should always be treated. If allowed to persist, it can decrease the efficiency of the placenta, thus depriving the fetus of adequate nourishment (see the article on *High blood pressure and pregnancy*, p.624).

What should be done?
Have your blood pressure checked once every three to five years. Some large shops and department stores now have do-it-yourself blood-pressure testing machines. But it is important to steer a middle course between ignoring the possibility of hypertension and worrying too much about it. If, however, you are taking the contraceptive pill or *oestrogens*, have your blood pressure checked more frequently.

Even if you show signs of hypertension at a first examination, your doctor may want to test your pressure again before beginning treatment. Because exertion, excitement, or some other physical or psychological factor can result in a misleading reading at a given moment, doctors prefer not to leap to conclusions. In a second examination the doctor will probably pay special attention to your chest and pulse rate and may well spend a few minutes looking into your eyes with an *ophthalmoscope*. The reason for this is that the blood vessels on the retina are the only blood vessels that can be seen without elaborate equipment, and their condition gives valuable information about the effects of an abnormally high blood pressure.

Further investigation varies according to age and the need to make sure that a given case is either essential or secondary hypertension. You may be given a chest *X-ray* to determine whether your heart has become enlarged, an *electrocardiogram (ECG)* tracing, and blood and urine tests to rule out kidney trouble. If your doctor needs further information, you may also have your kidneys X-rayed after a dye injection (this is called an *intravenous pyelogram* or *IVP*).

What is the treatment?
Self-help: The problem of secondary hypertension will generally be solved when and if the primary cause is satisfactorily dealt with. If the primary cause cannot be dealt with, the

Assessing the condition of blood vessels

Because blood vessels on the retina can easily be examined by a doctor shining a light from an ophthalmoscope onto the eyes, the eyes can be a window into the body's circulation. If vessels on the retina are damaged, others are likely to be in a similar condition.

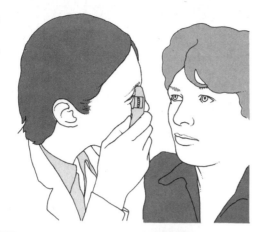

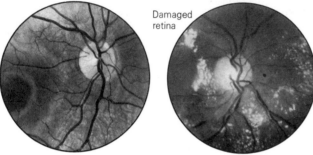

Healthy retina

Damaged retina

manner of treatment should be exactly the same as for essential hypertension, which although it is not curable, is controllable.

In many cases a thorough self-examination of your weight, diet, and life style can lead to satisfactory lowering of the blood pressure without the use of drugs. In particular:

1. If you smoke, give it up, or at least cut down as much as possible. A link between cigarette smoking and hypertension has not yet been firmly established, but there *is* a link between smoking and coronary artery disease. Since we know that the chances of heart trouble are increased by both cigarettes and high blood pressure, why not halve the risk instead of doubling it?

2. If you are overweight, choose a reducing diet to lose weight, stick to it until you reach a suitable weight for your age, sex, and height, and then try to stay there. Again there is no firm evidence that hypertension is kept under control by weight reduction alone, but we do know that slim people are hypertensive less often than those who are overweight, and slim people suffer less from certain serious diseases that are linked with hypertension. So there are convincing reasons for getting your weight down to a healthy norm (see the advice given under *Obesity*, p.492).

3. Salt your food less generously, and give up salt-rich foods such as salami, pickles, and salted fish. Use the minimum amount of salt when cooking.

4. Try to make your work schedule and recreation less demanding, avoid strenuous exercise, and learn to sidestep crises. A person who is always pressing ahead to the next objective, talks rather than listens, and constantly looks at his watch is at greater risk of all heart and circulatory disease.

5. Take alcoholic drinks in moderation. The optimists maintain that small quantities of alcohol help lower the blood pressure. There is no hard evidence that this is so, but small amounts of alcohol will do you no harm (see *The dangers of alcohol*, p.32).

Professional help: If self-help does not lower your blood pressure to a normal range, you will need some form of drug treatment. The drugs used in treating hypertension must always be administered under the supervision of a doctor. Continue your self-help measures, however, since all these drugs may have side-effects; and the lower the dose of drug you need, the better.

Since essential hypertension is usually a symptomless disease, you may resent having to take drugs when you do not feel ill. What may bother you even more is that because high blood pressure cannot be cured, you will probably have to go on taking regular doses of medicine for the rest of your life. This may mean subjecting yourself to the unwanted side-effects, though drugs are being developed that have fewer side-effects. Even so, some such drugs deaden the body's normal response to sudden changes in posture. Thus when you suddenly rise to your feet from a sitting position, there may be a slight delay before an adequate supply of blood for adjustment to the change is pumped to the brain. The result may be a temporary feeling of faintness or even an actual faint (a condition called postural hypotension). Other side-effects include a dry mouth, stuffy nose, and even headaches and drowsiness.

For these reasons your doctor will not put you on drugs unless satisfied that you really need treatment. Research has shown that it is best to prescribe a life-long course of drugs for any comparatively young person with a diastolic blood pressure of 105 or more. In some cases, though, it may be advisable to do so if the average reading for the diastolic pressure is above 90. Your doctor will decide your treatment on the basis of a number of medical considerations such as your age, general state of health, and sex (women appear to be less susceptible than men to the complications resulting from hypertension). When the decision has been made, the important thing is for you to accept it. The drugs most likely to be prescribed for your hypertension are members of the *beta-blocker* group, which lower blood pressure by reducing the force of the heartbeat. These drugs must be taken exactly as prescribed, and *you must never stop taking them abruptly* (as your doctor will warn you). They are generally not prescribed for people who are asthmatic or diabetic or for pregnant women. Beta-blockers may make your fingers and toes feel cold. And if they slow your pulse rate down too dramatically, your doctor will gradually take you off them and switch you to a different type of drug.

Beta-blockers are often used along with *diuretics* in treating hypertension. A diuretic helps by expelling fluid from your body, thus lowering the volume of the blood. To reduce the need to urinate frequently during the night, it is a good idea to take diuretics in the morning rather than at bedtime. Some diuretics also expel potassium, which needs to be replaced by tablets containing potassium.

If a beta-blocker or a beta-blocker in combination with a diuretic does not provide suitable treatment for high blood pressure, there are a number of other drugs that also reduce blood pressure.

What are the long-term prospects?
The prospects for future health depend chiefly on your own efforts to combat the problem. These efforts should include: adopting a healthier diet and life style; taking drugs exactly as prescribed; attending check-ups when they are advised; and reporting accurately and promptly any change in your condition so that the doctor can adjust drugs and drug doses accordingly.

Careful control of a formerly raised blood pressure will prevent nearly all risk of heart failure and will afford a 75 per cent chance of avoiding strokes. The effect of control on the chance of having a coronary thrombosis is less clear-cut, probably because many other factors are involved, and damage to the coronary circulation from high blood pressure is irreversible. Even so, it is logical to conclude that since your heart works under less strain when your blood pressure is lowered, you are less likely than you were to suffer from a heart attack.

Shock

The word "shock" has several possible meanings; but doctors define it for medical purposes as a condition in which the flow of blood throughout the body becomes suddenly inadequate, depriving vital organs of oxygen. This can happen for one of three reasons. First, the heart's pumping action may be drastically impaired, so that it pumps out an inadequate supply of blood – for example, after a *coronary thrombosis*, p.379 (*cardiogenic* shock). Secondly, following loss of blood or some other body fluid – for example, from a severed artery, a bad burn, prolonged diarrhoea, or a perforated ulcer – the volume of blood may be dangerously lowered (*hypovolaemic* shock). Thirdly, the diameter of the blood vessels may become so large – as a result, say, of an intense allergic reaction or an infection – that there is a relative shortage of blood even though the actual quantity has not diminished (*anaphylactic* or *septic* shock). There may be other factors involved, but these are the main physical causes.

If shock develops, the body's condition enters a vicious downward spiral. Lack of blood flowing to the brain means that the brain suffers from a lack of oxygen; this affects the nervous control of blood-vessel diameter, and so the vessels become over-dilated and floppy; the blood pressure drops even further; and so on. Once in the downward spiral, the body cannot recover of its own accord. Treatment must therefore be given as soon as possible.

What are the symptoms?
Symptoms, which may appear without warning, include sweating, faintness, nausea, panting, rapid pulse rate, and pale, cold, moist skin. Blood pressure plummets to levels far below those regarded as acceptably low (see *Low blood pressure*, p.417). As the blood supply to the brain fails, the person in shock becomes drowsy, confused, and even perhaps unconscious.

How common is the problem?
No statistics are available because, although persons in shock often die, the cause of death is recorded as the disorder or injury that has brought on the condition. Apart from accident victims, people most at risk of suffering shock are those with internal bleeding from any cause; with severe *blood poisoning* (p. 421); or with some type of heart or serious lung trouble, such as *asthma* (p. 355).

What happens during shock

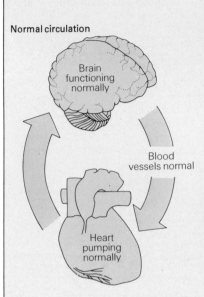

Normal circulation

Brain functioning normally

Blood vessels normal

Heart pumping normally

A person is in shock when, for some reason, blood pressure drops and body tissues and organs receive an inadequate supply of blood. The brain first tries to compensate by constricting the blood vessels in non-essential areas of the body, such as the skin, causing pallor. It also speeds up the heartbeat rate. However, if these measures fail and pressure remains low, the brain may not be able to function normally. Muscles in the blood-vessel walls relax and blood pressure drops even further. If this condition is untreated, the body's vital organs quickly die from lack of oxygen.

The effect of shock on the circulation

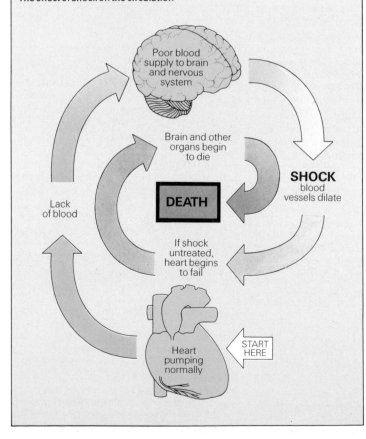

Poor blood supply to brain and nervous system

Brain and other organs begin to die

Lack of blood

DEATH

SHOCK blood vessels dilate

If shock untreated, heart begins to fail

START HERE

Heart pumping normally

What are the risks?

Untreated shock leads to death because the body cannot recover of its own accord. Even if recovery procedures begin within minutes shock can lead to brain and kidney damage.

The chances for recovery from hypovolaemic shock are fairly good if the underlying cause is swiftly dealt with. But other types of shock may be fatal.

What should be done?

If someone near you is in shock – an immediately recognizable condition – get professional medical aid immediately. For advice on what to do while awaiting help, see *Accidents and emergencies*, p.807. People in shock can do nothing for themselves.

As soon as possible, the victim should be taken to hospital, probably to an intensive-care unit. Here the medical staff use special equipment, for example a continuous blood-pressure recorder, and a continuous *ECG* recorder; such equipment gives immediate information on the victim's condition. The main tasks of the doctor are, first, to assess how deeply shocked the person is, and, secondly, to identify the underlying cause.

What is the treatment?

In most cases the priority is to restore blood pressure to normal, so that body organs get enough blood to stay alive. The doctor inserts a fine tube into a vein, usually in the arm, and connects the tube to a container of plasma or blood (see *What are blood groups?*, p.428, for information about blood transfusions). This raises the volume of blood and, thus, the blood pressure. If the brain is not already damaged, it responds by regaining control of blood-vessel tone and diameter. In many cases a special watch is kept on the kidneys to prevent the onset of kidney failure. *Diuretic* drugs will stimulate the kidneys to produce more urine, tiding them over a possible failing point until they can recover from the lack of oxygen.

When emergency procedures have restored blood pressure to something like normal levels, treatment for the underlying condition depends on the severity of the condition and its cause. For example, an operation may be carried out to repair a bleeding ulcer; or high doses of *antibiotics* may be injected into the bloodstream in order to combat an overwhelming infection. The prospects for full recovery depend partly on the underlying cause and partly on the swiftness of emergency treatment during the crucial minutes when the body is in the state of medical shock.

Heart rate and rhythm

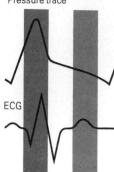

Pressure trace

ECG

Systole | Diastole

The upper trace (from a continuous pressure recorder) shows how blood pressure changes as the heart contracts (systole) and relaxes (diastole). The lower trace (from an ECG machine) shows the simultaneous electrical activity generated by the heart's pacemaker.

The muscle fibres of the heart must contract in unison if it is to function effectively as a pump. Electrical impulses from a group of cells in the right atrium – nature's own "pacemaker" – control the contractions of your heart, and these impulses flow along pathways that branch out to the muscle fibres in all its four chambers. Sometimes these electrical impulses are affected by signals transmitted to the heart from other parts of the body via an external nerve supply. Such signals can alter the impulses travelling along the conducting pathways and may also damage the pathways themselves, causing problems with the regularity of heartbeat. If, for this or any other reason, some portion of this complex conducting system goes wrong, the regular rhythmic pace of heartbeats is disturbed, and one of the following group of disorders may be the result.

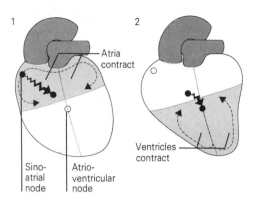

Atria contract

Sino-atrial node | Atrio-ventricular node

Ventricles contract

The electrical impulse that initiates a heartbeat originates from the sino-atrial node (the heart's natural pacemaker). The impulse passes through the walls of the atria (1) to the atrio-ventricular node, from where it is relayed to the ventricles, causing them to contract in turn (2).

Cardiac arrest
(and ventricular fibrillation)

Cardiac arrest is just what its name suggests: the heart stops beating. When the heart stops, blood supply to the brain ceases, and there is loss of consciousness within a few seconds. Cardiac arrest in someone who has seemed to be in good health is often due to unsuspected *coronary artery disease* (p.374). When coronary artery disease is not to blame, the cause of the arrest is sometimes a disorder of rhythm known as ventricular fibrillation, which occurs if the muscle fibres of the ventricles twitch without coordination.

What should be done?
If cardiac arrest happens when nobody else is present, it is fatal. But recovery is possible if the heartbeat can be restored within a minute or two. Obviously, specialist medical help should be summoned; meanwhile, the flow of blood should be maintained by *cardiac massage*. For instructions on what to do if someone near you loses consciousness suddenly and for no apparent reason, see *Accidents and emergencies*, p.805.

The prospects for recovery are good if treatment is given promptly and the circulation is kept going until the victim reaches the hospital. For a person suffering from ventricular fibrillation the heartbeat can often be restored by means of a defibrillator, an apparatus that passes a surge of electric current through the heart.

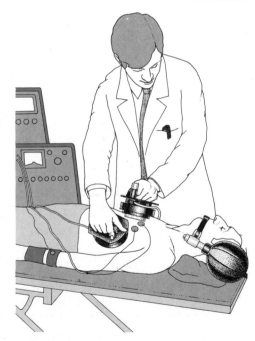

Using a defibrillator to restart the heart
Impulses from the right atrium spread throughout the heart muscle by a natural electrical process. If the heart stops, an electric shock may jolt it back into normal function. A defibrillator is a machine that sends electrical current through the chest via 2 metal plates placed on the chest wall at either side of the heart.

Atrial fibrillation
(and flutter)

If you suffer from atrial fibrillation, disordered muscular contractions in the two atria of your heart are making the atria beat much too fast – at a rate of about 400 pulsations a minute; and because the ventricles cannot beat faster than about 160 times a minute, they are unable to keep pace. Atrial fibrillation reduces the efficiency of the heart as a pump partly because rapid atrial contractions push out too little blood, and partly because the ventricles continue to beat at a much slower rate; the resultant lack of coordination between the atria and the ventricles reduces the volume of blood pumped out by the heart.

Atrial flutter differs from fibrillation only in that the muscle fibres contract at a somewhat slower rate (up to about 300 pulsations a minute). Both fibrillation and flutter tend to come and go, with periods of normal heart function between attacks.

What are the symptoms
Often there are no symptoms. The most common symptom is palpitations (an enhanced awareness of faster or more powerful heartbeats). If you have atrial fibrillation, you may also experience dizziness, occasional attacks of *angina* (p.376), and fainting spells. You may develop some of the symptoms of *heart failure* (p.381).

How common is the problem?
Atrial fibrillation and flutter are quite common. They usually occur as a consequence of *coronary artery disease* (p.374) or *rheumatic fever* (p.393). The fibrillation or flutter can also be caused by *thyrotoxicosis* (p.525) or high fever. In about 10 per cent of cases, especially among elderly persons, there is no obvious cause for the condition.

What are the risks?
The main danger is that the stagnant blood in the atria will clot, with a high risk of *embolism*. If a blood clot forms in an atrium, the clot may break into small pieces, which may travel through the circulation to a point where their size prevents them from going any further. An embolism can block all flow of blood beyond that point. The damage caused by such an embolism depends on its size and location in the circulation (see *Arterial embolism*, p.415, for further information).

A further possibility is heart failure. Normally, even though the atria are not functioning well, the ventricles alone can cope with the task of pumping blood. However, if the ventricles are also diseased they will not be able to cope with the load, and heart failure may follow atrial fibrillation.

What should be done?
If you suffer from symptoms associated with either of these disorders, consult your doctor, who will probably arrange for an *electrocardiogram* (*ECG*) to confirm the diagnosis. Since atrial fibrillation often comes on intermittently, you may require a continuous ECG recording for 48 hours. This is done by means of lightweight, portable equipment that is worn on a belt strapped to the chest or waist and that allows you to carry on normal activities while the recording is being made. The doctor may also order other diagnostic tests if there are any signs of an underlying heart disorder.

What is the treatment?
Treatment largely depends on the cause of the disorder. You may be prescribed a drug that improves the efficiency of ventricular contractions, upon which circulation must depend if atrial contractions are faulty. *Betablockers* are also particularly effective in controlling any atrial flutter or fibrillation associated with underlying thyroid disease. Your doctor may also prescribe an *anticoagulant* drug which will act to prevent the formation of an embolism.

If your heart is basically sound, or if the underlying cause of atrial fibrillation has been treated successfully, the doctor may consider a type of treatment called *electroversion*. This consists of an electric shock (administered under mild anaesthesia), which frequently restores normal heart rhythm. The shock is produced by a defibrillator (see *Cardiac arrest*, opposite).

Ectopic heartbeats

The word "ectopic" means "out of place", and ectopic heartbeats are simply small irregularities in the otherwise steady pulsation. If you feel that your heart has "missed a beat" or gained an "extra beat", you are experiencing this common and very minor disorder. Do not worry about it. Almost always the condition is harmless, and no treatment should be necessary. If you find the occasional irregularities troublesome, though, your doctor may prescribe an anti-arrhythmic drug to reduce their frequency. Since such heartbeats are often associated with excessive use of tobacco, alcohol, or caffeine, try cutting down on these (see for example, the article on *The dangers of smoking*, p.38).

Heart block

Under normal circumstances your heartbeat rate is controlled by a natural pacemaker, which consists of a group of specialized cells in the wall of the right atrium. Electrical impulses transmitted from the pacemaker to the two atria, and then to the ventricles, cause the rhythmic contractions of heart muscle that we call heartbeats. Heart block occurs when some abnormality within the conducting system results in a failure of transmission, so that the beating of the atria is not coordinated with the beating of the ventricles.

In first-degree block the slow conduction of the heartbeat causes no symptoms. In second-degree block some of the atrial beats fail to get through to the ventricle, and the pulse is irregular. In the disorder known as third-degree heart block, the failure is complete, and the ventricles go on beating independently of the pacemaker and the atria. Normally the heartbeat rate, which is really the ventricular rate, quickens in order to cope with the demands of exertion or emotion; but because of the heart block this no longer happens. As a result, the heart pumps too little oxygenated blood to the brain and other parts of the body at times when a greater supply is needed.

Heart block can occur for no obvious reason, but it is often associated with *coronary thrombosis* (p.379). An overdose of some drugs, particularly those affecting the heart, can also cause it.

What are the symptoms?
There are often no symptoms. If you take little exercise and are not subjected to emotional upsets, you may never know you have this disorder. On the other hand, complete (third-degree) heart block sometimes produces the symptoms of *heart failure* (p.381).

The most severe symptoms are experienced by sufferers from so-called Stokes-Adams attacks. The main symptom of a Stokes-Adams type of heart block is sudden loss of consciousness, and this is often accompanied by convulsions. Such attacks can occur if the ventricles, beating without any control from the pacemaker cells, slow down drastically or miss a few beats, so that for a few seconds the heart does not pump enough blood to keep the brain functioning normally.

How common is the problem?
In Britain each year about 1 person in 3,000 experiences heart block. It occurs just as commonly in men as in women.

What are the risks?
There is very little risk that a minor degree of heart block will have serious consequences. Before the advent of artificial pacemakers, you would have had only a 50 per cent chance of living for more than a year if you had third-degree heart block. The mortality rate for people who have Stokes-Adams attacks is still relatively high, but advances in the development of artificial pacemakers are constantly reducing it.

What should be done?
Attacks of extreme weakness and breathlessness are symptoms of many different types of heart disease, including heart block. If you experience these symptoms – and even more if you have episodes of loss of consciousness – consult your doctor without delay.

What is the treatment?
For many forms of heart block no treatment is necessary. Even complete heart block may not require treatment if you are fairly elderly and experiencing no symptoms. Heart block associated with coronary thrombosis or with Stokes-Adams attacks is generally treated with an artificial pacemaker, an electrical device that takes over from the faulty natural pacemaker and conducting system.

Paroxysmal tachycardia

The heart of a healthy adult beats at a rate of 50 to 80 pulsations a minute, rising to about 160 a minute during periods of exertion. If you have an attack of paroxysmal tachycardia (meaning "rapid heart"), your heartbeat suddenly speeds up to a rate of 160 or more. An attack of paroxysmal tachycardia can last for anything from a minute to several days.

What are the symptoms?
The main symptom is palpitations. You suddenly become aware of your rapid heartbeat rate, and you may be overcome by a feeling of anxiety. Some sufferers from paroxysmal tachycardia say it is accompanied by a deceptive premonition of impending death. Additional symptoms may include breathlessness, fainting spells, and chest pain.

How common is the problem?
This is a fairly common disorder, especially among young people. But despite any anxiety or fright, paroxysmal tachycardia is not normally a serious disorder. There is a slight risk of congestive *heart failure* (p.381) but virtually no danger of further complications.

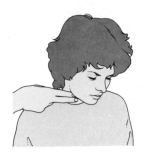

Massaging the carotid artery
Massage of the neck over the carotid artery may slow down a rapid heartbeat. It should never be done by anyone without medical training because excess pressure can lead to cardiac arrest.

What should be done?

When you get the pounding feeling in the chest that characterizes paroxysmal tachycardia, you may be alarmed, especially if this is your first attack. Although there is little cause for concern, you should see your doctor if symptoms last for more than a few minutes; you may have an underlying disorder such as *atrial fibrillation* (p.389), and it is easier to diagnose the basic trouble if the doctor examines you while an attack is going on.

If you are young to middle-aged, with no background of heart trouble, tachycardia is unlikely to be serious. Try to relax, and practise the self-help measures suggested below. If, however, you get recurrent attacks, they may be worrisome and exhausting, and you will do well to seek help. After examining you, the doctor may order an *electrocardiogram (ECG)* to confirm the diagnosis and rule out other possible causes of palpitations.

What is the treatment?

Self-help: Heartbeat rate can be slowed down by certain nerve impulses, which can be induced in several ways. Try holding your breath for a while, or take a slow drink of water, or bathe your face in cold water. If none of these measures works, hold your nostrils closed and then try to blow your nose, causing your eardrums to "pop".

If you have had an attack of paroxysmal tachycardia, preventive measures against further attacks are worth considering. Cigarettes, alcohol, tea, and coffee may all increase your susceptibility, so try cutting down on these. There also seems to be a link between anxiety and tachycardia, though there is doubt about whether anxiety leads to an attack or the other way round (see *Anxiety*, p.300). At any rate, if you can reduce your level of anxiety, you are bound to benefit your general state of health.

Professional help: Your doctor may massage an artery in your neck; a gentle pressure here will slow down the heart. (*But never let anyone not in the medical profession attempt this treatment! It can be dangerous!*) If the attack warrants further treatment, the doctor may inject into your bloodstream a drug that combats rapid heartbeat. In an extreme case, *electroversion* may be advisable.

As preventive medical treatment, the doctor may prescribe a drug such as a *betablocker*. Such drugs decrease the excitability of the heart muscle.

Pacemakers

A pacemaker is a device that provides an artificial electrical impulse to replace the irregular or absent impulse in the heart of a person with a disorder such as heart block. An electrode is placed in contact with the heart wall, either directly or by means of a thin tube pushed through the circulatory system from a convenient vein. This electrode is connected to a small generating unit powered by a battery with a life span of three to four years (nuclear-powered pacemakers now being tested will last much longer). The electrical impulse can come either at a regular pre-set rate or at a rate determined by existing electrical activity in the heart.

If a pacemaker is required for only a short time – as when a coronary thrombosis temporarily disturbs heart rhythm – the generating unit may be worn on a belt. Otherwise it is implanted under the skin, usually in the loose tissues of the chest wall. People with pacemakers are examined at intervals to make sure the device is working well. A fading battery is quickly and easily replaced. These days, pacemaker operations are relatively common. In Britain each year 1 in every 20,000 people has a pacemaker operation, and in the US, about 1 in every 4,000 people has one.

Modern pacemakers are remarkably resistant to outside interference. If you have a pacemaker, however, stay away from powerful radio or radar transmitters, and do not go through security screens at airports, shops, libraries, etc. If you undergo surgery, your surgeon may also need to take certain precautions since some *diathermy* techniques for controlling bleeding can affect pacemaker function. One final word: if you want to be cremated, tell your family to warn the undertaker that you have a pacemaker. These devices explode in extreme heat and must be removed before cremation.

Heart

Electrode from pacemaker to heart

Pacemaker

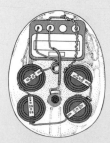

Positioning a pacemaker
The pacemaker (left) is connected to your heart by a wire fed along a vein that runs close to your collar bone (far left). If the pacemaker is to be permanent, the doctor will insert it under the skin on your chest wall.

Heart valves

The heart has four valves. The mitral valve controls the flow of blood from the atrium into the ventricle on the left side; and the tricuspid valve is the equivalent of the mitral on the right side. The aortic valve controls the output of blood from the left ventricle into the aorta; and the pulmonary valve controls the exit from the right ventricle into the pulmonary artery, which carries blood to the lungs for oxygenation. Inflammation of a valve can cause one (or sometimes both) of two kinds of damage: *stenosis* and *incompetence*. Stenosis is a thickening of the valve, with consequent narrowing of its opening; incompetence is a valvular distortion that prevents the valve from closing fully.

The diseases described below are, with two exceptions, disorders of valvular stenosis or incompetence. The exceptions are rheumatic fever and bacterial endocarditis, which are included in this group because of their close association with valvular heart disease.

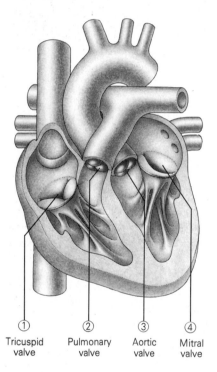

① Tricuspid valve   ② Pulmonary valve   ③ Aortic valve   ④ Mitral valve

How the valves work
With each heartbeat the ventricles contract (systolic pressure). These contractions force the blood out of the heart through the aortic and pulmonary valves into the circulation and the lungs. Between heartbeats the ventricles relax (diastolic pressure) and the aortic and pulmonary valves close. The mitral and tricuspid valves then open to allow blood to flow from the veins via the upper chambers to the ventricles.

Systolic (ventricles contract)

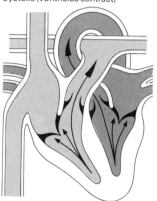

Valves ② and ③ open
Blood pumped out of heart to lungs and body tissues

Diastolic (ventricles relax)

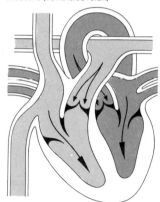

Valves ① and ④ open
Blood passes into the heart from the body tissues and the lungs

What can go wrong
When a valve is narrowed (stenosed), less blood flows through it, and the heart muscle must generate more pressure to pump through an adequate supply of blood. When a valve is incompetent, some of the blood that has flowed through it leaks back into the heart, which must pump it out again. Both conditions increase the heart's work load and can lead to heart failure.

Normal opening

Inadequate opening (stenosis)

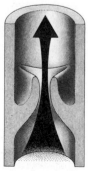

Normal closing

Inadequate closing (incompetence)

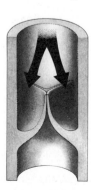

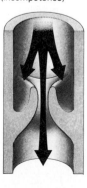

Rheumatic fever

Rheumatic fever is not technically a heart disease since it affects many other parts of the body. It is included here because the most important consequence of an attack may be some type of valvular heart disease. Rheumatic fever begins with a throat infection caused by certain kinds of streptococcus bacterium. The streptococcal infection is followed by general illness, the main symptoms of which are fever and joint aches, and this illness often causes various body tissues to become inflamed and damaged.

All heart tissues, including the pericardium (the membranous bag that encloses the heart), can be affected. But it is the valves and the endocardium (the inner lining of the heart) that are most often involved. Apart from the heart, the body tissues most likely to suffer as a result of rheumatic fever are those of the joints. Heart trouble used to be much more common than joint trouble in rheumatic-fever victims; until recently the heart was involved in about 75 per cent of all cases. Nowadays, though, the pattern is changing, perhaps because of the widespread use of *antibiotics*, and heart disease seems to have become less common than joint disease among people who have had rheumatic fever.

What are the symptoms?
Most commonly you have a sore throat that seems to clear up quickly; but you begin to feel out of sorts and feverish about a week – or up to six weeks – later. Thereafter your symptoms depend on the organ or organs mainly affected. Inflammation of the heart rarely provides symptoms that you can identify. Joint trouble, which usually affects the knees and ankles but may extend to fingers, wrists, and shoulders, is more readily recognized. Joints inflamed as a result of rheumatic fever are likely to be swollen, tender, hot, red, and extremely painful. More than one joint is normally involved.

In as many as 10 per cent of rheumatic-fever cases a complication known as *chorea* occurs about two to six months after the streptococcal infection. The main symptoms, which are due to the fact that chorea affects the brain, are involuntary jerky movements of hands, arms, and face. The speech may also be temporarily slurred. But there is no permanent damage.

If you have rheumatic fever, you may also develop a red, ring-shaped rash with a white centre. Such rashes (there may be several) usually appear somewhere on the torso; and as one fades away, another may arise. Similarly, rheumatic nodules (lumps) may appear on knuckles, wrists, elbows, or knees. The

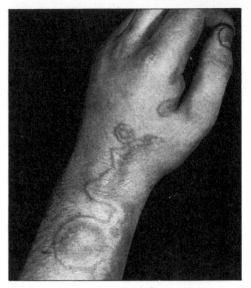

Visual symptoms
Symptoms of rheumatic fever include a ring-shaped rash that appears on the torso or limbs and tends to fade away after several days. This photograph also shows a swollen wrist joint. After a few days the swelling subsides and another joint somewhere else may begin to swell.

rashes are not itchy, the lumps are painless, and they all disappear in time.

How common is the problem?
Rheumatic fever used to be much more widespread than it is now; penicillin is an effective weapon against streptococcal throat infections. Children and adults under 30 are still fairly susceptible, however. Up to 1 per cent of teenage boys and girls show signs of having – or of having had – heart disease associated with rheumatic fever.

What are the risks?
Once you have had rheumatic fever, you are at risk of further attacks. Before preventive treatment was possible, one in every four children aged four to 13 who had had rheumatic fever suffered a recurrence. With antibiotic treatment the risk is much reduced. But about 60 per cent of rheumatic-fever cases are still apt to develop valvular heart disease The severity of the heart trouble is often proportional to the number of attacks of rheumatic fever. There is also a slight risk of *heart failure* (p.381) as the result of a very severe attack.

What should be done?
Always consult your doctor if any member of your family has aching, swollen joints along with a feverish illness. The doctor will suspect

rheumatic fever and will pay special attention to the heart, listening with a *stethoscope* for any indication of trouble. Diagnostic tests may include analysis of blood specimens to determine any changes that may have occurred as a consequence of rheumatic fever; a chest *X-ray* to look for signs of heart enlargement; and an *electrocardiogram* (*ECG*). If a joint is swollen, it may be necessary to withdraw some fluid, under local anaesthesia, in order to establish the cause.

What is the treatment?
If there are signs of heart involvement, your doctor will keep you in bed until satisfied with your condition. Bed rest may also be prescribed if the disease has attacked your joints.

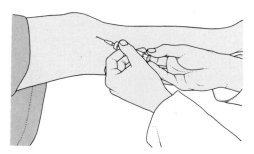

Removing fluid from an inflamed joint
The doctor may withdraw fluid from a swollen joint if there is a chance that you have rheumatic fever. This is done for 2 reasons. A small amount of fluid is needed for analysis, and as much as possible is withdrawn to relieve discomfort in the inflamed area.

While in bed, you will probably be given regular doses of aspirin to reduce inflammation and ease pain. If inflammation does not respond to this treatment, a *steroid anti-inflammatory* drug may then be prescribed as an alternative.

Long-term treatment with antibiotics (in the form of tablets) is almost always prescribed for people who have had an attack of rheumatic fever. By guarding against streptococcal infections this has greatly reduced the recurrence rate; only about 4 per cent of today's sufferers have more than one attack. Because heart trouble caused by rheumatic fever is more severe the more attacks you have, this reduction in the recurrence rate means that any resulting heart trouble is likely to be mild. The antibiotic must be taken regularly for many years – certainly, for a youngster, into adult life.

What are the long-term prospects?
Once an attack of rheumatic fever is over, there will be few, if any, symptoms, since the joints and skin generally heal completely. There remains the risk of damaged heart valves, especially in a person who has had more than one attack. With modern treatment for valve disorders, however, the prospects are good.

Bacterial endocarditis

The endocardium is the inner lining of the heart muscle. It lines the chambers of the heart and it also covers the heart valves. If it is damaged, for example in *mitral incompetence* (p.396), the damaged area can be colonized by bacteria – or, occasionally, fungi – that may have entered the bloodstream. Once a colony is formed, the bacteria multiply and further damage the place where they are growing. Sections of the colony may break off and be swept away in the circulation to other parts of the body as *emboli*, blocking small arteries and preventing blood from reaching tissues supplied by those arteries (see *Arterial embolism*, p.415). The pumping action of the heart remains largely unimpeded – but it is the heart valves themselves that are primarily affected by the disease. As the bacteria multiply, they eat into the tissues of the heart valves, which become weak and inefficient; as they are gradually destroyed, *heart failure* (p.381) develops.

What are the symptoms?
No single, main symptom will tell you that you are suffering from this disease. You may have a fever, but your temperature will rarely exceed 39°C (about 102°F). In addition, you may have sudden chills (especially when part of the bacterial colony breaks off and forms an embolus), headaches, aching joints, fatigue, and loss of appetite. If the valves have been affected, the symptoms of heart failure may eventually appear.

Other symptoms depend on the location of each embolus. The sufferer may have painful lumps in the pulp of the fingers or small bruises behind the nails. It is fairly common for emboli to lodge in the brain, and this may cause temporary weakness on one side of the body or loss of vision (see *Transient ischaemic attack*, p.270). Hardly any part of the human body is safe from attack by emboli from bacterial endocarditis.

How common is the problem?
Bacterial endocarditis is rare, especially among children and the elderly. Most cases occur in people between the ages of 15 and 55. It causes only 1 in 250,000 deaths. Men and women are affected equally.

Over 50 per cent of bacterial endocarditis cases are people with hearts damaged by *rheumatic fever* (p.393). Rheumatic fever has become much less common in recent years, leading to a significant fall in the number of cases of bacterial endocarditis. Other possible – but much rarer – causes are *congenital heart disorder* (p.656) and *syphilis* (p.612), and the bacterial infection sometimes occurs at the site of a heart-valve transplant (see the box on *Heart-valve replacement*, p.397, for information on what is involved if you have a heart-valve transplant). Bacteria can be introduced into the bloodstream during minor operations, dental extractions, and some diagnostic procedures, but this rarely results in endocarditis. A higher risk is associated with major heart surgery.

Susceptible people – those, chiefly, who already have heart trouble – are generally given a course of *antibiotics*, usually in tablet form, immediately before undergoing a medical or dental operation or when developing boils or other skin infections since it is vital to prevent infections from entering the endocardium via the bloodstream.

What are the risks?
There can be irreversible heart damage if bacterial endocarditis is not discovered and treated soon after the initial infection. Emboli may also do permanent damage to the brain and other parts of the body.

What should be done?
If you suspect that you may be suffering from this disease, do not delay in consulting your doctor. Because the symptoms of bacterial endocarditis are many and varied, the disease can be confused with a wide variety of complaints, and it will help a doctor who has not seen you recently if you point out that you have – or have had – any heart-valve disease or murmur, or any of the symptoms commonly associated with endocarditis.

If a diagnosis of bacterial endocarditis seems likely, your doctor will probably have you admitted to hospital for tests. Samples of your blood will be taken and tested to discover what kind of bacterium is causing your endocarditis.

What is the treatment?
The treatment depends largely on the bacterium responsible. Your doctor will choose the most suitable antibiotic as a weapon against it. If endocarditis is diagnosed and effectively treated within six weeks of the initial infection, you have a 90 per cent chance of complete cure. Your bacterial endocarditis may also cause you to be anaemic, in which case your doctor will prescribe a course of iron treatment, probably to be taken in tablet form.

Mitral stenosis

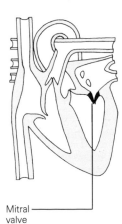

Mitral
valve

Mitral stenosis occurs when the mitral valve – the one between the left atrium and ventricle – becomes narrowed. In order to force blood through the narrow opening, the muscular wall of the atrium thickens and pressure within the chamber gradually rises. This pressure is transmitted back through the pulmonary veins to the lungs, making them congested. To keep blood flowing through the lungs at a normal rate, the right ventricle must pump more and more vigorously, and so it too becomes enlarged.

What are the symptoms?
The main symptom of mitral stenosis is breathlessness, which is caused by congestion in the lungs. It is most apparent after exercise, but it can occur whenever you are lying down. You may also cough up small amounts of blood; you may find yourself increasingly susceptible to attacks of *acute bronchitis* (p.353); and you may even have chest pain similar to *angina* (p.376).

As pressure builds up through the entire circulatory system, you may experience general fatigue, swollen ankles, and other symptoms that indicate *heart failure* (p.381). If this happens, chest symptoms usually become less troublesome because the heart failure causes fluid to accumulate in other parts of the body than the lungs.

How common is the problem?
About 60 per cent of all sufferers from *rheumatic fever* (p.393) develop some kind of heart disease following the illness. And almost 75 per cent of these people have some degree of mitral stenosis. But the number of rheumatic-fever cases has been declining in recent years, and so mitral stenosis is also less common than it used to be.

What are the risks?
Breathlessness and general weakness can be disabling, especially during pregnancy or for people who have a chest infection or overactive thyroid gland (see *Thyrotoxicosis*, p.525). But the main danger is of *atrial fibrillation* (p.389), with consequent formation of an *embolus*. Nearly half of all mitral-stenosis sufferers develop atrial fibrillation, and nearly half of these suffer from emboli. Your chance of avoiding this complication, however, is good if you are under 45.

What should be done?

Consult your doctor if you have any of the symptoms mentioned above. Sometimes mitral stenosis is discovered by accident – at a regular check-up, for example. After examining you, paying special attention to your heart and lungs, the doctor may be able to diagnose mitral stenosis by listening to the heart with a *stethoscope*, but will probably refer you to a heart specialist for further tests. These may include a chest *X-ray* and *electrocardiogram* (*ECG*) to see whether the left atrium is enlarged. The ECG will also show whether or not you have developed atrial fibrillation. The specialist may also want an *echocardiogram* test for further confirmation of the diagnosis.

What is the treatment?

Self-help: If you have no disabling symptoms, you can live a normal life and need no treatment for mitral stenosis. But always ask your doctor for *antibiotic* treatment before you undergo dental or medical surgery; this will help to protect you from the risk of *bacterial endocarditis* (p.394).

Professional help: If breathlessness is troubling you, your doctor may prescribe a *diuretic*, which can help by draining fluid from your body. However, certain diuretics also cause you to lose potassium, which needs to be replaced. For this reason your doctor may prescribe potassium tablets.

If you have developed atrial fibrillation, it can usually be controlled by *beta-blockers* or a drug that steadies the heartbeat, and you may be given *anticoagulants* to prevent the formation of emboli.

If your mitral stenosis is so severe that it restricts your daily activities, surgery may be advisable. It may be necessary, for example, if you become pregnant and your symptoms get worse as a consequence. The usual operation is called mitral *valvectomy* and involves widening the narrowed valve. Inevitably, such an operation carries a small risk; but if you are healthy, the chances of survival are extremely good, and your symptoms may not return for many years. If your symptoms do return, you may require a second valvectomy, or it may be wiser to replace the troublesome valve with an artificial one. About 80 per cent of those who have had the operation have survived for at least five years. (See *Mitral incompetence*, below, for more about mitral-valve replacement.)

Mitral incom- petence

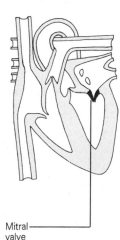

Mitral valve

If the mitral valve is incompetent (does not close properly), blood that has already passed from the left atrium into the left ventricle may leak back into the left atrium. As a result of the incompetence, your heart has to work harder to clear the backlog of blood collecting in the left atrium. The heart wall enlarges in an attempt to cope with the additional work-load. *Rheumatic fever* (p.393) is usually the cause of the disorder, but incompetence is sometimes present from birth (see *Congenital heart disorders*, p.656) or arises at a later date in connection with some other type of heart trouble.

What are the symptoms?

Often there are no symptoms, but mitral incompetence is usually indicated by shortness of breath, fatigue, and the symptoms of congestive *heart failure* (p.381). You may also have some difficulty in swallowing because the enlarged wall of the left atrium may actually put pressure on your oesophagus.

How common is the problem?

Mitral incompetence can be permanent if the valve is damaged, or it may be temporary, as in the acute phase of rheumatic fever. But because the number of rheumatic-fever cases has been declining in recent years, the resulting mitral incompetence is also less common than it used to be.

What are the risks?

The risks are similar to those of mitral stenosis. In fact the two disorders often occur together. If you are among the relatively few people who have incompetence without stenosis, however, you are less susceptible to *atrial fibrillation* (p.389). But *bacterial endocarditis* (p.394), which is more commonly associated with mitral incompetence than with stenosis is a possibility.

What should be done?

Consult your doctor if you have any of the symptoms mentioned, especially if you are finding swallowing difficult. The doctor will listen to your heart through a *stethoscope* and will probably arrange for further tests such as a chest *X-ray* and *electrocardiogram* (*ECG*).

What is the treatment?

As with mitral stenosis, no treatment is likely to be required if you have no symptoms. But if you have discovered that you have mitral incompetence, be sure to get *antibiotic* treatment before having any teeth extracted or

OPERATION: Heart-valve replacement

This is an operation to replace damaged heart valves either by specially designed plastic and metal valves or by valves made from some of your own tendinous tissues.

During the operation You are under a general anaesthetic and your circulation and breathing are taken over by a heart-lung machine. An incision is made either along your breastbone or along the line of a lower rib on your left side. Your ribs are pulled apart and the heart is opened up. Any damaged valves are cut out. The new valves are then sewn into place with dissolving stitches. The operation takes from 2 to 4 hours.

After the operation You will spend the first few days in the intensive-care unit, where you will have one or two drainage tubes in place at the bottom of the incision. You will breathe oxygen through a tube leading into your throat, and may need the help of a respirator. Your bladder will be drained by a catheter. You will be receiving fluid and blood through intravenous drips and your heart will be monitored constantly by an ECG machine. The usual hospital stay is 2 weeks.

Convalescence Convalescence takes several months. If you have had an artificial-valve replacement, you will have to take anticoagulant drugs for life. Artificial valves can sometimes be heard clicking in your chest – this is quite normal. See also information on operations, p.738.

Ball and cage valve

Tissue valve

Types of valve
A tissue valve is made from your own body tissues – usually tendons. There are several types of man-made valve, which work very much like tissue valves.

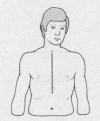

Site of the incision

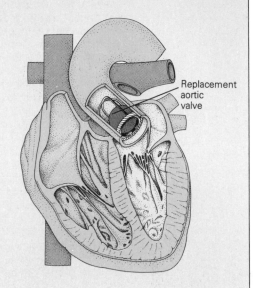

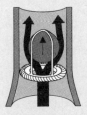 Replacement aortic valve

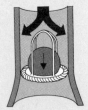

A ball-and-cage heart valve is an efficient and reliable design. Blood can pass in one direction by forcing the ball away from the ring into the cage (above left). If blood attempts to flow in the opposite direction, it forces the ball firmly against the ring and so closes the valve (above right).

---

undergoing any kind of surgery. This is a way of being reasonably armed against the threat of bacterial endocarditis.

Medical treatment for mitral incompetence is much the same as for mitral stenosis. If your symptoms are extremely severe, however, your doctor may advise surgery, which means replacement of the incompetent valve with an artificial one.

There are two possible types of replacement: a mechanical valve or a valve formed from grafted tissue. It is up to the surgeon to judge which of these is more appropriate for your special case. Mechanical replacements are efficient, but they cause clotting of blood in some people (from 5 to 10 per cent). If you have a mechanical valve replacement, you will need to take an *anticoagulant* drug to

guard against this complication. Anticoagulants are not suitable for anyone with a gastric or duodenal ulcer that is liable to bleed, or for anyone who lives far away from the laboratory facilities that are essential for monitoring this sort of treatment. Tissue-graft valves involve much less risk of clotting, but on the whole they seem to work less dependably than mechanical valves.

About 80 per cent of valve-replacement patients live active lives for at least five years afterwards. If, at any time after the operation, you suddenly become short of breath or dizzy, or if your urine looks abnormally dark or your chest begins to ache, see your doctor as soon as possible. Any of these symptoms may indicate a mechanical failure of the replacement valve.

Aortic stenosis

If the aortic valve is narrowed, less blood is pumped through from the left ventricle into the aorta. Consequently the quantity of blood that the heart can pump throughout the body is lowered. In an effort to squeeze more blood through the valve, the left ventricle then develops a thickened muscular wall. The ventricle wall then requires more and more blood to supply its larger area with oxygen.

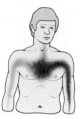

Site of the pain

What are the symptoms?
At first aortic stenosis may produce no symptoms at all. As the condition worsens, you will begin to feel breathless after physical activity. You may then develop *angina* (p.376) and have spells of dizzinesss or even fainting whenever you exert yourself. Eventually your symptoms may be those of left-sided *heart failure* (p.381). You will continue to feel breathless, especially whenever you lie down, and may have to sleep sitting up. Breathlessness is sometimes accompanied by wheezing and, in some cases, there may be a bubbling sound from the lungs.

How common is the problem?
Rheumatic fever (p.393), which is usually associated with other valve defects, is often the cause of aortic stenosis. The aortic valve is affected in about 40 per cent of people who get heart-valve trouble after an attack of rheumatic fever. A person who has this disorder alone, with no other valve defects, is likely to have been born with it (see *Congenital aortic stenosis*, p.658). The chances of having the problem are three times greater for a man than for a woman.

What are the risks?
Aortic stenosis often leads to inadequate blood flow in the coronary arteries, and there is an increased risk of sudden death from *cardiac arrest* (p.388). If your aortic stenosis continues untreated, fluid in the lungs will decrease your resistance to infection, and you may develop pneumonia.

What should be done?
As with *mitral stenosis* (p.395), you may first learn that you have a damaged heart valve following a routine medical examination. If you have any of the symptoms of aortic stenosis, do not delay in consulting your doctor, who will examine you, listen to your heart, and probably order diagnostic tests without delay. A chest *X-ray* should show whether or not the aortic valve is narrowed. An *electrocardiogram* (*ECG*) can help the doctor to determine the severity of the stenosis if there is one. And the diagnosis can

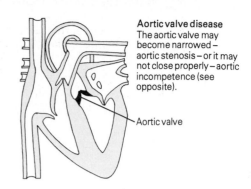

Aortic valve disease
The aortic valve may become narrowed – aortic stenosis – or it may not close properly – aortic incompetence (see opposite).

Aortic valve

be further confirmed by means of further tests such as *cardiac catheterization, coronary arteriography*, and scanning by *ultrasound*.

What is the treatment?
Self-help: If you know you have mild aortic stenosis, avoid strenuous activity; for example, play golf and go for walks, but do not play squash or run for buses. Do not be afraid of sexual intercourse, but take it at a relatively leisurely pace. Before undergoing surgery or dental extractions, ask your doctor to give you *antibiotics* to protect you from *bacterial endocarditis* (p.394). And have a heart examination at least once every 18 months.
Professional help: The only treatment for severe aortic stenosis is surgery, and the most common form of surgery involves valve replacement. As with *mitral incompetence* (p.396) you will be given either a mechanical valve or a valve formed from grafted tissue. If your doctor decides on a mechanical valve, you will have to take *anticoagulants* drugs for life. The prospects for full recovery are much the same for all heart-valve disorders.

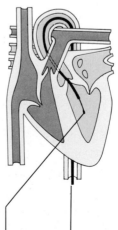

Cardiac catheterization
Aortic stenosis can be confirmed by cardiac catheterization. A catheter (thin tube) containing an electronic device to measure pressure is threaded along an accessible artery to the heart. There it measures the pressure in the left ventricle and in the aorta.

Catheter in left ventricle

Catheter passing up aorta

Aortic incompetence

If the aortic valve does not close properly, blood may leak back from the aorta to the left ventricle. The most likely cause of the disorder is *rheumatic fever* (p.393); the aortic valve can also be damaged by *syphilis* (p.612), but this now causes only about 1 per cent of all aortic-incompetence cases. Severe incompetence causes the left ventricle to enlarge and its walls to thicken as a result of the extra work required. Sometimes, too, part of the valve ruptures because of damage done by *bacterial endocarditis* (p.394).

What are the symptoms?
There are often no symptoms for years after aortic incompetence first occurs, but symptoms develop swiftly if the valve is ruptured. The main symptom is breathlessness. There may also be *angina* (p.376) and all the symptoms of *heart failure* (p.381).

With rheumatic fever and syphilis so much less widespread than they used to be, aortic incompetence is no longer a common disease. But if permitted to run its course, the disorder can lead to heart failure.

What should be done?
Consult your doctor if you have any of the symptoms. Examination and diagnostic tests are similar to those for other heart-valve disorders, except that the doctor may arrange for blood tests to find out whether you have an active or quiescent syphilitic infection. If aortic incompetence is suspected, you should limit your physical activities to more leisurely pursuits. After various diagnostic tests, your doctor may decide that a valve-replacement operation is advisable. In this case you will be given either a mechanical valve or a valve made from some of your own fibrous tissue.

Tricuspid stenosis and incompetence

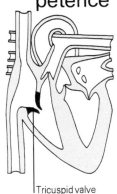

Tricuspid valve

Tricuspid stenosis and incompetence, which generally occur only in conjunction with other valvular disease account for less than 5 per cent of all valvular heart diseases. Both of these diseases may be due to *rheumatic fever* (p.393), although tricuspid incompetence is more often caused by the expansion of the right ventricle as a result of a condition such as mitral-valve disease.

What are the symptoms?
If the tricuspid valve is damaged, the heart is unable to pump blood to the lungs efficiently. Consequently your symptoms may be those of congestive *heart failure* (p.381).

What are the risks?
The symptoms of heart failure may gradually worsen, until you are eventually disabled by the disease. As with any other heart-valve

diseases, there is an additional risk of *bacterial endocarditis* (p.394) developing.

What should be done?
Consult your doctor if you feel unusually tired and are often breathless. Your doctor will arrange for diagnostic tests to confirm whether you have a tricuspid-valve disorder. These may include a chest *X-ray* and an *electrocardiogram* (*ECG*).

What is the treatment?
No treatment is required if the disease is mild. If it arises from other disorders, as it generally does, they must be treated of course. Otherwise treatment of a tricuspid-valve disorder will be similar to that for a mitral-valve disorder (see *Mitral stenosis*, p.395). If you are severely affected by the disease, your doctor may advise a valve-replacement operation.

Pulmonary stenosis and incompetence

Non-congenital pulmonary-valve disorders, usually caused by *rheumatic fever* (p.393), are rare, comprising 2 per cent of all heart-valve disorders resulting from rheumatic fever.

What is the treatment?
Pulmonary stenosis and incompetence may only be discovered during a routine medical examination. If the pulmonary valve is severely affected, your doctor may advise a valve-replacement operation (see *Mitral stenosis*, p.395).

(For information about *Congenital pulmonary stenosis*, see p.658.)

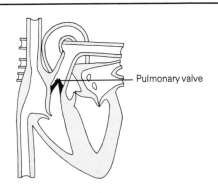

Pulmonary valve

Heart muscle and pericardium

The walls of your heart are made of muscle, which contracts rhythmically about 100,000 times a day. If this muscle becomes diseased, the result is a reduction in the force of heartbeats, with consequent impairment of circulation. There are many forms of heart-muscle disorder (cardiomyopathy). The tiny fibres of the muscle may become inflamed or swollen, or the muscle may be weakened by internal chemical change. In some cases the disease is confined to the heart; in others the heart is only one of the affected organs. Cardiomyopathies are generally less common than most other types of heart disease. The three most common kinds, along with two disorders of the pericardium (the membrane within which the heart is enclosed), are discussed in the following articles.

Myocarditis

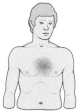

Site of the pain

Myocarditis (inflammation of the heart muscle) occurs as a rare complication of a generalized infection such as *mumps* (p.700) or *diphtheria* (p.703); of a parasitic infestation such as toxoplasmosis (see *Infestations*, p.567); or a respiratory viral infections. In mild cases the only symptoms may be slight chest pain and shortness of breath. In more serious cases, such as those caused by diphtheria, myocarditis can lead to *heart failure* (p.381).

If, while treating you for the underlying disease, your doctor suspects you may be suffering from myocarditis, you may need to have a chest *X-ray* and an *electrocardiogram* (*ECG*) in order to verify the diagnosis.

What is the treatment?
The primary aim is to eliminate underlying infection. In addition, you will be advised to rest completely. In some forms of myocarditis, treatment with *steroids* speeds healing.

Nutritional cardio-myopathy

Like any muscle, the heart muscle can be damaged by vitamin or mineral deficiency or by poisoning. The most important form of such nutritional cardiomyopathy in Western societies is found among alcoholics (see *Alcoholism*, p.304). Heart specialists attribute the damage to either the poisonous effects of alcohol or the lack of vitamin B_1 characteristic of the alcoholic's diet. In non-alcoholics, nutritional cardiomyopathy can also occur because of vitamin B_1 deficiency, or it may result from the lack of potassium in the bloodstream in some people who have persistent diarrhoea or who are under long-term treatment with *diuretic* drugs.

Symptoms of nutritional cardiomyopathy vary greatly. There may simply be palpitations and swollen hands and feet. Or, since the damage can cause a disorder of heart rhythm such as *atrial fibrillation* (p.389) or even *heart failure* (p.381), the sufferer may have the symptoms of those ailments.

What is the treatment?
Once nutritional cardiomyopathy has been diagnosed, treatment will probably consist of an attempt to correct any dietary fault. How this is done depends on the circumstances; but if your problem is alcoholism, only total abstinence can halt the disease.

Hypertrophic cardio-myopathy

If, for some reason, there are defective cells in the heart muscle, the walls of the heart may become thickened in an effort to compensate for the weakness. In severe cases the swollen walls may impede the flow of blood into and out of the heart. Symptoms of this disorder (known as hypertrophic cardiomyopathy) include fatigue, chest pain, shortness of breath, and palpitations. If you have any such symptom, see your doctor, who may order diagnostic tests such as *electrocardiogram* (*ECG*), chest *X-ray*, and perhaps *biopsy* (removal of a small piece of the muscle for microscopic examination).

What is the treatment?
There is no treatment for the disease, but the symptoms may be relieved by *beta-blocker* and *diuretic* drugs. A few people who have been in danger of heart failure as a result of hypertrophic cardiomyopathy have had heart transplants (see *Transplants*, p.402).

Acute pericarditis

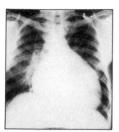

X-ray of pericardial effusion
The fluid that collects around the heart (pericardial effusion) is opaque to X-rays and makes the heart look much larger than normal (compare this X-ray with the one of a normal heart on p.740).

Pericarditis is an inflammation of the pericardium, which is a membranous bag enclosing the heart. When the pericardium becomes inflamed, fluid can collect in the space between it and the heart; this so-called pericardial *effusion* may cause further complications (see "What are the risks?" below). Acute pericarditis is a severe attack of pericarditis that comes on suddenly. It is usually caused by viral infection, but it may also be caused by *rheumatic fever* (p.393), diseases of the connective tissue (see, for instance, *Systemic lupus erythematosus*, p.556), or *chronic kidney failure* (p.512). Acute pericarditis can also – though very rarely – follow either *coronary thrombosis* (p.379) or a physical injury to the chest.

What are the symptoms?
The main symptom is pain, usually in the centre of the chest. The pain may radiate to the left shoulder and become worse if you breathe deeply, cough, or twist around. You may also be short of breath.

How common is the problem?
Mild pericarditis is probably a common feature of viral illnesses. But pericarditis severe enough to cause acute pain is unusual.

What are the risks?
The main risk is that a pericardial effusion will grow so rapidly as to cause dangerous pressure on the heart. This happens very seldom, however. In general, pericarditis is not a serious disorder, but it can be associated with more severe illness.

What should be done?
Chest pain, especially if associated with difficulty in breathing, can be a symptom of several serious illnesses, so if the pain is severe and lasts for more than a few minutes, call your doctor. After examining you, the doctor will probably order diagnostic tests such as a chest *X-ray*, *electrocardiogram* (*ECG*), and blood tests. These will help determine whether your symptoms are due to pericarditis and, if so, what has been the underlying cause of the inflammation.

What is the treatment?
Pericarditis due to a viral infection usually clears up without treatment; within 10 to 14 days the inflammation subsides, leaving no ill-effects. In some cases, especially if the pericarditis is associated with coronary thrombosis, the doctor may prescribe a *steroid* drug to speed up healing. When acute pericarditis is due to a connective-tissue or metabolic disorder, the underlying disease must be treated. If the pericardial effusion endangers your heart, some of the fluid may be removed by means of a needle and syringe. The needle is inserted into the pericardium via the chest. Such treatment is given in hospital and can be carried out under a local anaesthetic.

Constrictive pericarditis

When pericarditis (inflammation of the membranous bag that encloses the heart) is due to a chronic infection such as *tuberculosis* (p.563), the course of the illness is very different from that of *acute pericarditis* (above). Long-standing inflammation can thicken, scar, and contract the pericardium until it shrinks so much that the normal beating of the heart is affected. This disorder is termed constrictive pericarditis.

What are the symptoms?
The main symptom is a swelling of the legs and abdomen. This is caused by an accumulation of fluid due to sluggish blood flow. Any or all of the symptoms of *heart failure* (p.381) may also develop if the condition is not treated immediately.

How common is the problem?
Because tuberculosis is no longer widespread, constrictive pericarditis has become increasingly rare.

What are the risks?
Without surgical treatment, heart failure is virtually inevitable.

What should be done?
Whatever the cause, you should see your doctor now if you have any symptoms of heart failure. Recommended diagnostic tests will probably include chest *X-ray*, *electrocardiogram* (*ECG*), and perhaps further studies with *ultrasound* or *radioactive isotopes*. The doctor may also recommend *cardiac catheterization* in order to get a detailed assessment of the state of your heart. And your sputum will be tested for indications of tuberculosis.

What is the treatment?
No self-help or treatment by drugs is possible. But constrictive pericarditis can be cured by an operation to remove the thickened pericardium from the surface of the heart (*pericardectomy*). The prospects for full recovery after surgery are excellent.

Transplants

Surgery to replace damaged body organs by healthy ones is now routine; several thousand such operations are done every year around the world. Healthy replacements come either from people who have consented (or whose surviving relations consent) to the medical use of parts of the body after death, or from living donors who are usually related to the person needing a transplant. In Europe (including Britain) a surgeon who decides that someone would benefit from a kidney transplant feeds detailed requirements into a special computer, called Eurotransplant, in Holland. The computer matches the needs of individuals awaiting operations (particularly the *tissue type* of the required organ) with donated organs as they become available.

The system works well in many cases. For instance, a kidney must be removed within 30 minutes after the donor's death and can be kept in storage for no more than 24 hours before transplantation. With the help of Eurotransplant, doctors can single out suitable recipients for donated kidneys with little waste of time.

What are the difficulties?

With modern medical techniques the operation itself is straightforward. Yet most transplants performed so far have been replacements of kidneys (and corneas – see *Corneal ulcers and infections*, p.316). More than 30,000 of these have been done, whereas heart, lung, and liver transplants add up to fewer than 1,000 altogether. Why is there such a contrast?

To answer that question it must be understood that the body's defence system treats a "foreign" organ as if it were an infecting microbe and tries to destroy it through the action of white blood cells and *antibodies*. An ideal transplant would have tissues identical to those of the organ it replaces. But because a perfect match is impossible, the body's fight to reject a new organ must be counterbalanced by treatment with *immunosuppressive* drugs. Such treatment carries very great risks and must be given with a precision that is difficult to achieve. As a result, it is impossible to predict the success of most transplants.

There are two exceptions to this rule. First, an organ transplant between identical twins involves no risk of rejection, because the tissues of identical twins are a perfect match and do not provoke a response from the defence system. (Of course, this only applies to kidneys and other organs of which the twin has two.) Secondly, corneal transplants "take" easily because the cornea has no blood supply and therefore lacks the rejecting weapons of blood-borne white cells and antibodies. But in general there is a slightly stronger possibility of eventual failure than of success. And rejection of a transplanted heart, liver, or lung may mean sudden death.

Kidney transplants are far less risky. Failure is not necessarily fatal since the patient can be kept alive by means of an artificial kidney (*dialysis* – see *Artificial kidney aids*, p.513) until another transplant becomes available. It is because no similar safety net exists for other vital organs that surgeons tend to suggest transplantation only if the sole alternative is early death.

What are the long-term prospects?

Treatment with immunosuppressive drugs begins immediately after the operation and must continue for the rest of the patient's life. Unfortunately, such treatment reduces resistance to infection, may encourage the growth of *malignant* tumours, and may damage bones as well as other body organs. So the drug dosage must be meticulously calculated; too little can lead to rejection of the transplant at any time, and too much can have fatal side-effects.

In spite of the difficulties, though, some recipients of kidney transplants live for 15 years or more, and a few recipients of new hearts, lungs, or livers are today leading productive lives five or more years after the operation.

How a heart transplant is done

In many heart-transplant operations the surgeon does not remove the entire heart but cuts away only the two main pumping chambers (the ventricles), the main heart valves, and part of the two smaller chambers (the atria). Most of the connections to the major blood vessels are left intact, making it easier to connect up the donated heart tissues. This "partial" heart transplant is possible because it is usually only the main heart valves or the muscular walls of the ventricles that are damaged.

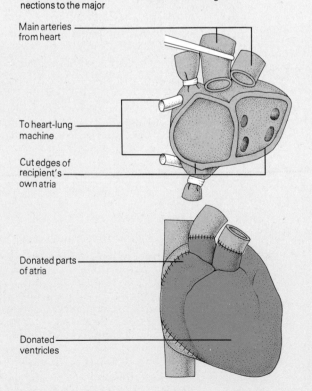

Main arteries from heart

To heart-lung machine

Cut edges of recipient's own atria

Donated parts of atria

Donated ventricles

Circulation

The blood makes two separate circuits from and to its central pump, the heart. In the shorter of these circuits (pulmonary circulation) "used" blood is pumped to the lungs where it takes in oxygen and expels carbon dioxide. It then returns to the heart. From there the oxygenated blood is pumped throughout the body (systemic circulation) in order to supply all tissues with nutrients and to pick up waste products before returning to the heart and then being re-oxygenated in the pulmonary circulation.

The arteries that carry blood away from the heart have thick, muscular walls to restrain and absorb the peaks of blood pressure resulting from heartbeats. The main artery (the aorta) has an internal diameter of about 30mm (1¼in). It branches into smaller arteries, then into arterioles, and finally into microscopic capillaries, whose thin, porous walls permit easy exchange of nutrients and oxygen for waste products between the blood and the tissues. Gradually the capillaries merge to form venules, and the venules merge to form soft-walled, flexible veins, which, aided by valves, carry oxygen-depleted blood back to the heart.

Blood does not flow at a constant rate to all parts of the body. The rate varies according to how much blood is needed by certain tissues at a given moment. Thus the womb of a pregnant woman makes greater demands on the circulation than the womb of a woman who is not pregnant. When you run, blood is diverted to the leg muscles at the expense of the abdominal organs (which need more blood to help your digestion after a meal). When you feel cold, less blood flows in vessels near the chilled skin (you turn pale) and more in deeper vessels, thus conserving heat. This pattern is reversed when you are overheated – more blood flows in the blood vessels near the surface of the skin, thus causing you to look flushed.

The highly complex circulatory system can go wrong not only if the central pump misfunctions, but if trouble arises within the blood vessels themselves. There can be a weakness in an artery wall – and in some cases the layers of which it is composed may even split – or the hardening of an artery that makes it incapable of absorbing increased blood pressure, or the formation of blood clots that cause blockages. The most common such conditions are described below.

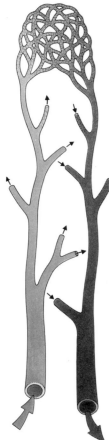

The blood vessels
The arteries carrying fresh blood (brown) away from the heart become smaller, branching into arterioles and then capillaries. An intricate network of tiny capillaries reaches every part of the body, and oxygen is exchanged for carbon dioxide. The capillaries then merge to become venules and these in turn become veins, which carry the "used" blood (grey) back to the heart.

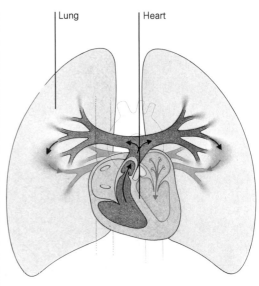

Lung　　Heart

Pulmonary circulation
"Used" blood (grey) is pumped from the right ventricle through the pulmonary artery into the lungs. Capillaries in the lungs surround air sacs (alveoli) from which the blood easily absorbs oxygen and into which it expels carbon dioxide. The capillaries merge to become pulmonary veins. These carry the freshly oxygenated blood (brown) into the left side of the heart.

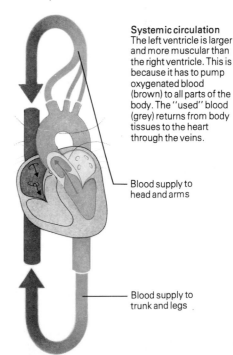

Systemic circulation
The left ventricle is larger and more muscular than the right ventricle. This is because it has to pump oxygenated blood (brown) to all parts of the body. The "used" blood (grey) returns from body tissues to the heart through the veins.

Blood supply to head and arms

Blood supply to trunk and legs

Arterio-
sclerosis

*(hardening of the
arteries)*

As people grow older, their arteries tend to harden, and so most adults have some degree of arteriosclerosis. But although gradual loss of elasticity in arterial walls is inescapable, the severity of the condition is directly linked with the extent of any additional *athero-sclerosis* (p.372). A combination of arterial ageing and narrowing from *atheroma* makes the arteries increasingly rigid, so that less blood can pass through.

Arteriosclerosis sometimes affects a major artery such as the aorta. More often, though, the arteries in which there is a serious diminution of blood supply are those that carry blood to the brain and legs.

What are the symptoms?
Arteriosclerosis that impairs the flow of blood to your legs can cause pain, most often in the calves. The pain is generally felt only when the legs are active; it increases with increased activity and disappears shortly after the activity is stopped. This is because working muscles make greater demands on the circulation. Another possible symptom is pain in the toes, and this persists even when you are resting. It tends to be worst at night; the best way to relieve it (at least in the early stages) is to sleep with your legs dangling over the edge of the bed as this encourages blood flow in the toes.

If your brain is affected, you may get dizzy when you move your head in a certain way, and you may have occasional attacks of temporary loss of vision (see *Transient ischaemic attack*, p.270).

How common is the problem?
Although nearly everyone has arterio-sclerosis to some extent, most people are unaware of it. Severe arteriosclerosis is mainly a disorder of men; the male to female ratio of sufferers is about 5 to 2 and this statistic supports the evidence that cigarette smokers are particularly at risk (see *Lung cancer*, p.366). The older you are, the more likely you are to be severely affected. The disease seems to run in families, and its effects are apt to be worsened if you already suffer from *anaemia* (p.419), *diabetes mellitus* (p.519), or *heart failure* (p.381).

What are the risks?
As with atherosclerosis, the risk depends on the part of the body affected. There is a very real danger that the condition may lead to *thrombosis* in a diseased artery, eventually causing the sufferer to have a *stroke* (p.268). Other possible serious complications include *coronary artery disease* (p.374), *dry gangrene*

(p.415), and formation of a dissecting or fusiform type of *aneurysm* (p.407).

What should be done?
Start now on self-help measures to slow down the development of atherosclerosis even if your feel fine. If you think you have symptoms of arteriosclerosis, consult your doctor, who, after examining you, may want to have an *electrocardiogram* (*ECG*), since coronary arteries may be affected by this disorder. A chest *X-ray* and blood and urine tests can also be helpful in diagnosing your condition.

What is the treatment?
Self-help: Recommendations for the treatment of atherosclerosis are generally applicable to arteriosclerosis. For example, reduce your intake of animal and dairy fats, and restrict yourself to three eggs a week. Since cigarette smokers are especially at risk, you should give up smoking at once. In addition, if your legs are affected, try to keep them warm and dry. When cutting toenails, avoid cutting the flesh; an open wound is highly susceptible to infection in anyone with arteriosclerosis. It may be advisable to put your feet into the care of a chiropodist.

Professional help: Your doctor can help you by treating any condition – for instance, anaemia, diabetes, or heart failure – that aggravates the effects of arteriosclerosis. Among medicines sometimes prescribed for arteriosclerosis are *vasodilators* (drugs that widen blood vessels) and *anticoagulants*. Any such medicine usually has to be taken on a long-term basis.

Surgery is a possible treatment if the disease is not extensive. It usually involves replacing a narrowed stretch of artery with either an artificial tube or a section of vein removed from another part of the body. The operation can be successful, but it cannot do anything to remove the factors that cause arteriosclerosis.

What are the long-term prospects?
Although arteriosclerosis is almost certain to become more severe as you grow older, symptoms such as pain in the legs sometimes become less troublesome. The reason for this is that when certain arteries or their branches no longer carry an adequate blood supply to a given part of the body, other arteries that supply the affected part often grow big enough to compensate for the loss. If you eat sensibly, do not smoke, are careful to avoid infection, and take moderate exercise regularly, you are likely to delay or even prevent the onset of complications.

Deep-vein thrombosis

A thrombosis is the formation of a blood clot (*thrombus*), which may partially or completely block a blood vessel. Thrombosis in an inflamed vein near the skin causes *thrombophlebitis* (p.407). If blood clots form in a vein deeper down, the result is known as deep-vein thrombosis. Among the many potential causes, the most important is immobility. Although the condition occurs most frequently in the legs, it can occur anywhere, especially in the lower abdomen.

What are the symptoms?
The area drained by the vein – usually the calf or thigh – becomes swollen and painful as the normal flow of blood is obstructed, raising the pressure in the veins and capillaries. In a leg this causes oedema (cushion-like swellings that remain indented if you press them with a finger). If the thrombosis is not in a leg, there may be no symptoms unless pieces of the clot break off, are swept away in the circulation, and cause embolism (see *Pulmonary embolism*, p.406).

How common is the problem?
Deep-vein thrombosis is fairly rare, affecting about 1 person in 1,700 in an average year. Particularly susceptible are old or overweight people, anyone with a blood disease such as *polycythaemia* (p.429), and women who are taking *oestrogens*, either in the form of the contraceptive pill or as post-menopausal therapy. There is a risk of venous thrombosis, too, if you have any condition causing prolonged immobility, especially during recovery from an illness, when blood flow can become sluggish.

What are the risks?
Deep-vein thrombosis can have dangerous complications such as pulmonary embolism, which may be fatal.

What should be done?
If you think you may have a deep-vein thrombosis, see your doctor, whose physical examination will concentrate on your heart, lungs, and circulation. To locate a deep-vein thrombosis in your leg, the doctor may require *venography*. Among the more special tests that are performed in certain cases are *ultrasound* and *radioactive fibrinogen* tests, both of which may be able to confirm the doctor's diagnosis and show the exact location and size of the thrombus.

What is the treatment?
Self-help: To prevent the development of deep-vein blood clots, keep your weight down and keep on the move. Cases of this disorder have become rarer now that people are encouraged to be up and about soon after surgery or childbirth. If you are a woman over 35 and taking the contraceptive pill, ask your doctor about alternative methods of contraception; the risks of thrombosis associated with the pill increase with age. If you smoke, you must give it up.

Professional help: If you are about to have surgery for another reason and the doctor believes you to be susceptible to deep-vein thrombosis, you may be given injections of an *anticoagulant* drug both before and after the operation. If you are bedridden for a long period, you will be encouraged to flex your leg muscles, wiggle your toes, and bend your ankles to keep the circulation active. The legs of an immobilized person are sometimes mechanically elevated and put in plastic bags, which are alternately filled with air and deflated; the resultant pumping effect keeps the blood flowing.

If deep-vein thrombosis has already occurred, you may be given high doses of an anticoagulant together with an *analgesic* such as aspirin to relieve any pain. Because these drugs, if wrongly used, can cause bleeding, they must be taken exactly as prescribed, usually for a period of several weeks. Most clots are gradually re-absorbed into the bloodstream. In obstinate cases a *thrombolytic* drug is sometimes used for dissolving the clots. But such cases are rare.

Surgical removal of blood clots is sometimes necessary. With the sufferer under general anaesthetic, a thrombosis can be mechanically sucked from a vein in an operation (*thrombectomy*) that is usually successful.

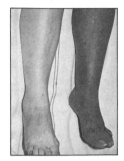

Thrombosis in the leg
The leg swells over the site of the blood clot and this stretches the skin taut. The leg is painful and the swollen area may look dark red (above right).

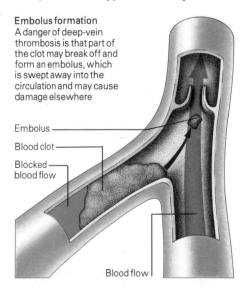

Embolus formation
A danger of deep-vein thrombosis is that part of the clot may break off and form an embolus, which is swept away into the circulation and may cause damage elsewhere

Embolus

Blood clot

Blocked blood flow

Blood flow

Pulmonary embolism

Pulmonary embolism nearly always occurs as a complication of *deep-vein thrombosis* (p.405). A blood clot detached from the wall of a deep vein is swept in the bloodstream through the heart and along the pulmonary artery towards the lung. If the loose clot (called an *embolus*) is fairly large, it may become lodged in an artery within the lungs, blocking off some of the blood destined for oxygenation and thus reducing the volume of

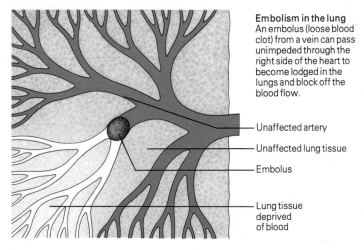

Embolism in the lung
An embolus (loose blood clot) from a vein can pass unimpeded through the right side of the heart to become lodged in the lungs and block off the blood flow.

— Unaffected artery

— Unaffected lung tissue

— Embolus

— Lung tissue deprived of blood

freshly oxygenated blood returning to the left side of the heart. Any such pulmonary embolism is apt to be a serious matter.

What are the symptoms?
Symptoms depend on the size of the embolism and its location within the lungs. Because the heart and body tissues are deprived of their full supply of oxygen, some degree of breathlessness is always present. The sufferer may also feel faint and have chest pain. There may be a cough, perhaps with blood-tinged sputum, and *cyanosis*. A massive pulmonary embolism can cause collapse and death within minutes.

How common is the problem?
Pulmonary embolisms are not common, but their effects are widely felt. In Britain only about 1 in 3,300 people has an attack during an average year. The disorder affects 3 females for every 2 males, and people who are in bed recovering from operations are particularly at risk. Massive pulmonary embolism (an attack in which at least half the blood flow in the lungs is blocked off) occurs in many cases and can be fatal. Deep-vein thrombosis and pulmonary embolism cause around 1 in every 20 deaths – usually as a complication of some other serious disease such as cancer.

What are the risks?
Any blockage of blood flow into the lungs can lead to right-sided *heart failure* (p.381). Your susceptibility to chest infection is increased by a small pulmonary embolism, and a massive pulmonary embolism can cause death.

What should be done?
Anything that predisposes you to deep-vein thrombosis also increases your chances of having a pulmonary embolism. See your doctor if you have symptoms of either disorder, especially if you have been confined to bed. The doctor will examine your lungs and heart with a *stethoscope* and, if pulmonary embolism is suspected, will want a chest *X-ray* and an *electrocardiogram* (*ECG*) to see if your heart – especially the right side – is under strain. A special *radioactive fibrinogen* test might be necessary to confirm the diagnosis.

If someone collapses with suspected massive pulmonary embolism, the doctor's first task is to revive the sufferer by giving emergency treatment (see "What is the treatment?" below). But collapse from pulmonary embolism resembles collapse from *coronary thrombosis* (p.379), and so the doctor will probably carry out further tests in order to determine the cause.

What is the treatment?
Self-help: To forestall pulmonary embolism, which is generally a consequence of deep-vein thrombosis, follow the self-help advice of that article. If an embolism occurs, you must get professional help.
Professional help: Admission to hospital is likely to be necessary. It may be thought advisable to give the sufferer an injection of a *thrombolytic* drug. More usually, however, treatment is by an *anticoagulant* drug given in tablet form.

If the embolism is severe, emergency treatment may be required. This will probably involve *cardiac massage* and the sufferer may also be given oxygen via a face mask or tube. The blockage will then be removed surgically under general anaesthetic.

What are the long-term prospects?
Massive pulmonary embolism is fatal in about 1 in 3 cases. Anyone who survives the critical first few days, however, stands a good chance of complete recovery. Chances are even better when the source of emboli is found and treated to forestall further trouble. Less severe embolism may damage part of the lung, but the sufferer will almost always make a satisfactory recovery if emboli are prevented from re-forming.

Thrombophlebitis

Phlebitis is inflammation of a vein, usually caused by infection or injury. When this happens, blood flow through the roughened, swollen vein may be disturbed, leading to the development of blood clots (*thrombi*), which adhere to the wall of the inflamed vein. The resultant disorder is called thrombophlebitis.

Thrombophlebitis generally occurs in superficial veins (those near the surface of the body) because they are the ones most at risk from infection and injury, and is particularly common in the legs.

What are the symptoms?
The main symptoms are pain, redness, tenderness, itching, and a hard, cord-like swelling along the length of the vein. If infection is present, you may also be feverish.

How common is the problem?
In Britain every year about 1 person in 300 consults a doctor about thrombophlebitis. Slightly more women than men have it. It is rarely a cause of death; only 1 out of 1,000 sufferers is apt to die as a direct result.

You are more likely to be thrombophlebitic if you have *varicose veins* (p.409) or if you are undergoing medical treatment that involves inserting tubes or needles into your veins. (Any such procedure can cause phlebitis through physical irritation.)

What are the risks?
If there is infection and it remains untreated, it can lead to *blood poisoning* (p.421). There is also a slight chance that blood clots may be carried away in the circulation to become lodged elsewhere – in a deeper vein, for example (see *Deep-vein thrombosis*, p.405).

What should be done?
If there is no prolonged infection, thrombophlebitis usually clears up in a week or so. You should in any case, consult your doctor, who will probably be able to diagnose your ailment by a physical examination and without special tests.

What is the treatment?
Self-help: To ease pain, take an aspirin or two every few hours. A zinc ointment, obtainable from a chemist's without a prescription, should relieve itching.

Professional help: If there is infection, the doctor may prescribe an *antibiotic*. It may also be advisable to compress the affected area within an elastic bandage; this is done to hasten recovery by speeding up blood flow in the vein, and thus sweeping away blood clots and preventing any further clots from forming. With treatment, thrombophlebitis nearly always clears up completely in a couple of weeks or so.

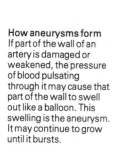

Thrombophlebitis usually affects the veins near the surface of the body and occurs most commonly in the legs.

Aneurysms

An aneurysm is a permanent swelling of an artery due to a weakness in its wall. Aneurysms can form anywhere, but they are most common and troublesome when they occur in arteries of the head or in the aorta. There are, basically, three reasons why an aneurysm might develop in an artery:

1. Of the four layers that comprise the arterial wall, the supportive strength resides chiefly in the muscle layer, and this layer may be congenitally defective. Some people, in fact, are born with part or all of this layer missing at some point in the arterial network; and the normal pressure of blood in the artery causes a balloon-like swelling to develop at that point. Aneurysms due to congenital defect are nearly always found in arteries at the base of the brain. Because of their shape and size, they are known as "berry" aneurysms.

2. Inflammation, whatever the cause, may weaken the arterial wall. *Syphilis* (p.612) used to be a common cause of arterial inflammation leading to aneurysms but no longer is, because of effective treatment with *antibiotics*. Most aneurysms due to inflammation ("saccular" aneurysms) are now caused by disorders such as *polyarteritis nodosa* (p.556) or *bacterial endocarditis* (p.394).

3. A portion of the layer of the arterial wall may slowly degenerate as the result of a chronic condition such as *atherosclerosis* (p.372) or *high blood pressure* (p.382). An aneurysm resulting from atherosclerosis is likely to be a sausage-shaped swelling along a

How aneurysms form
If part of the wall of an artery is damaged or weakened, the pressure of blood pulsating through it may cause that part of the wall to swell out like a balloon. This swelling is the aneurysm. It may continue to grow until it bursts.

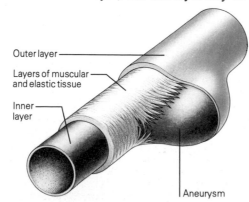

Outer layer

Layers of muscular and elastic tissue

Inner layer

Aneurysm

Types of aneurysm

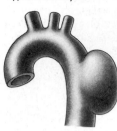

A saccular aneurysm develops when part of the muscular middle layer of the artery has been damaged.

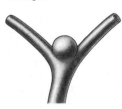

A berry aneurysm, due to a congenital defect, is found at the base of the brain, where an artery branches.

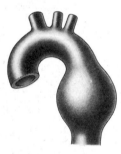

An aneurysm is described as fusiform when the swelling is due to weakness of the artery wall all the way round.

In a dissecting aneurysm, the inner and outer layers of an artery split apart. Blood is forced between the layers, causing the outer wall to swell. Sometimes a second split appears further along the artery and allows the blood back into the main flow. However, blood trapped in a dissecting aneurysm tends to form a clot, which may eventually seal off the aneurysm.

short length of the artery (called a "fusiform" aneurysm). A similar type of swelling may be caused by high blood pressure. The increased pressure of blood in an artery, however, can stretch the wall in any number of ways. It can even split the layers, forcing blood between them so as to form what is called a "dissecting" aneurysm.

Aneurysms can cause trouble in a number of ways. They can burst, leading to loss of blood supply for certain tissues, as well as to internal bleeding at the site of the aneurysm. Or they can swell so much that they press on and damage neighbouring organs, nerves, or even other blood vessels. Or they can disturb blood flow to such an extent that clots form.

What are the symptoms?

Symptoms vary, as suggested above, according to the type, size, and location of the swelling. Berry aneurysms are usually symptomless until they burst. A sudden severe headache at the back of the head or even unconsciousness may be the first sign of this trouble. If you have an aneurysm of the aorta, symptoms will depend on the section of the aorta that is affected and the type of aneurysm. Aneurysms in other parts of the body are rare and generally symptomless.

The most common symptoms of a saccular or fusiform aneurysm in the thoracic aorta (the portion that passes through the chest) are chest pain, hoarseness, difficulty in swallowing, and a persistent cough that is not helped by cough medicine. If the aneurysm is of the dissecting type, the sufferer is likely to have pain that can easily be mistaken for a *coronary thrombosis* (p.379).

A saccular or fusiform aneurysm in the abdominal portion of the aorta can usually be seen as a throbbing lump. Less specific indications that such an aneurysm has developed are loss of appetite and loss of weight. If the

aneurysm is located towards the back, it may press on the bones of the spine, causing severe backache. Dissecting aneurysms of the abdominal aorta are relatively rare. When they do occur, the abdominal pain is extremely severe.

How common is the problem?

Berry aneurysms, which stem from congenital defects, can give trouble at any age and are the most common aneurysms among people under 65. Your chances of having this type of aneurysm are slightly increased if any of your near relations has had the condition. Other types of aneurysm are rare in those under 65.

What are the risks?

The major risk is of the aneurysm bursting, with consequent internal bleeding. A burst aneurysm allows blood to flow into surrounding tissues, causing serious local damage. Moreover, the entire circulatory system may collapse if the leak drastically reduces the volume of blood in circulation. Unless expert medical help is at hand, a burst aneurysm in the aorta can be lethal. More than 40 per cent of people who suffer a burst berry aneurysm die as a result.

Even when it does not burst, an aneurysm of the aorta causes turbulence in the flow of blood that can result in the formation of a *thrombus*, with all the associated dangers. *Emboli* breaking away from the thrombus can block smaller arteries such as those that supply the kidneys, with resultant damage that can lead to *acute kidney failure* (p.511). Or the damage to the aorta can stretch the aortic valve of the heart and cause *aortic incompetence* (p.399).

Aneurysms sometimes occur in the arteries of the arms and legs. Such aneurysms are generally less hazardous than berry aneurysms or those in the aorta.

What should be done?

You can do nothing about berry aneurysms since you will probably be unaware that you have one unless it bursts. If you have any of the symptoms of an aneurysm of the aorta or if you inexplicably develop a lump anywhere on the body – but especially on the abdomen, and particularly if it throbs – consult your doctor without delay. Many of the symptoms can be caused by other, often trivial conditions, and so the doctor will probably want to give you a full examination before making a definite diagnosis. To find out the size, type, and location of an aneurysm, you may need to be extensively *X-rayed*, and may also have to undergo *arteriography* and *ultrasound* tests.

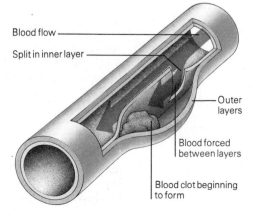

Blood flow

Split in inner layer

Outer layers

Blood forced between layers

Blood clot beginning to form

What is the treatment?
Self-help: Take steps to prevent or slow down the onset of atherosclerosis and to keep your blood pressure under control. If you have already developed an aneurysm, there is no effective self-help.
Professional help: Surgery is the usual treatment for an aneurysm, but the surgeon must consider its location, its size, and the state of the rest of your arteries before deciding whether to operate. The operation is difficult and risky. When an aneurysm of the aorta or a peripheral artery is removed, the two ends of the artery can sometimes be rejoined. More often, however, the missing portion must be replaced by a graft or by synthetic material such as teflon.

Berry aneurysms are almost always discovered during the investigations after one of them has burst. The remaining swellings are then isolated from the rest of the circulation by closing the neck of each with a metal or plastic clip. This is usually successful although blood from the burst aneurysm may already have escaped and caused damage.

What are the long-term prospects?
About 30 per cent of the people with ruptured berry aneurysms die very soon afterwards, and another 15 per cent die from further bleeding within a few weeks. The long-term outlook is better for anyone who survives for six months after the operation.

Surgery for aneurysms of the thoracic aorta is often not possible, and in such cases the long-term outlook is poor. With operable chest aneurysms there is an 80 to 90 per cent chance of survival. Abdominal aneurysms need to be removed only if very big, or if they are growing. With or without surgery, the outlook is good for most of these, as for aneurysms in peripheral arteries. It should be remembered, though, that many aneurysms are due to generalized disease such as atherosclerosis, which may also affect other blood vessels in other ways.

Varicose veins

Formation of varicose veins
Varicose veins are caused when the valves in the veins do not work efficiently, perhaps because the veins themselves have swollen as a result of pressure on them.

Varicose veins are twisted and swollen. This disfiguring and sometimes painful distortion usually occurs in the legs as a result of the strain imposed on leg veins by our upright posture. It is through the veins that blood returns to the heart from the tissues of the legs. The heart has no suction action, and the flow of blood in the veins is due partly to the pumping action of leg muscles.

Normally, blood is collected from the leg tissues in a network of "superficial" veins (those on the surface of the muscles), which are connected with "deep" veins (those embedded in the muscles) by means of "perforating" veins. As you move about, and your muscles contract and relax, the deep and perforating veins expand, sucking blood in from the superficial veins. All deep and perforating veins have one-way valves in order to prevent used blood from flowing back into superficial veins. So when the muscle contracts, blood is pumped up by the deep veins to the heart.

If, for some reason, the valves of the perforators do not work efficiently, blood may be squeezed the wrong way, back into the superficial veins, which respond to increased pressure by expanding and twisting to form varicose veins – generally visible because they lie on loose tissue just under the skin.

What are the symptoms?
The most common early symptom is the appearance of a prominent, bluish, swollen vein in your leg when you stand up. The most usual site is either at the back of the calf or up the inside of the leg at any place from ankle to groin. Varicose veins can also occur around the anus (see *Haemorrhoids*, p.483) or in the vagina if you are pregnant (see *Varicose veins during pregnancy*, p.623). As the vein grows more prominent, it may become tender to the touch, and the skin above it or at the ankle

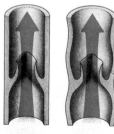
Normal vein   Varicose vein

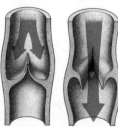

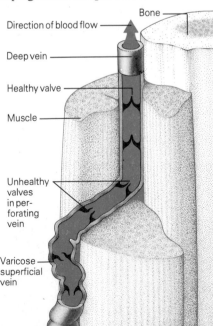

Bone

Direction of blood flow

Deep vein

Healthy valve

Muscle

Unhealthy valves in perforating vein

Varicose superficial vein

Appearance of varicose veins
When valves in the veins become inefficient, blood is forced from the deep veins into the veins lying just under the skin. The increased pressure of fluid in these superficial veins causes them to twist and bulge.

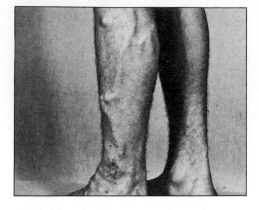

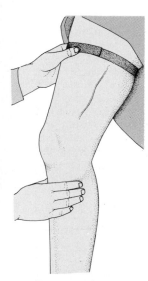

Using a tourniquet
To discover which valves are damaged, the doctor first applies a tourniquet to your leg while you are lying down. The tourniquet should stop the flow of blood through the vein but, if a valve is damaged at that point, some blood will leak past when you stand up, making the varicosed vein stand out below the tourniquet. This is repeated at various points down your leg.

may begin to itch. The whole leg aches, and you find that your feet become swollen after a short period of standing and your shoes seem too tight in the evening. Women usually find all these symptoms intensified for a few days before and during menstruation.

Your symptoms may not worsen beyond this stage. But some people with severe varicose veins find that impaired circulation causes brownish skin discoloration (varicose "eczema"), especially near the ankles.

How common is the problem?
Varicose veins are extremely common; about 1 person in 100 visits a doctor each year with this disorder. Women are three times more likely than men to have them, and the disorder tends to run in families; about half of all sufferers have parents with the same complaint. Some people are actually born with abnormal or fewer than normal valves in the veins, and although this usually causes no trouble at all, it does make such people more susceptible to varicose veins. You are also especially prone if you are very tall, very fat, or pregnant, or if you spend most of your working day on your feet, standing fairly still.

What are the risks?
Varicose veins are usually troublesome rather than disabling, but they occasionally have serious consequences. For example, a combination of the force of gravity and valve failure in perforating veins can give the tissues so little blood that the undernourished skin breaks down and an ulcer develops. Varicose ulcers will not heal as long as the veins that cause them remain under pressure (see *Varicose (venous) ulcers*, p.260).

Another, though rare, danger is that if you knock or cut the skin over a varicose vein, you may release a torrential flow of blood from the blood-swollen vein. This needs swift medical attention. The most common prob-

lem is inflammation of the wall of the vein; blood then tends to clot on the wall, leading to *thrombophlebitis* (p.407).

What should be done?
If you think you are susceptible to varicose veins, especially if you are pregnant, guard against them by adopting the self-help measures recommended below. If you already have varicose veins, the self-help measures will ease symptoms and slow the progress of the condition, but they will not cure it, and surgery may be advisable. So if discomfort increases, ask your doctor for advice and help. The doctor is unlikely to need special tests to confirm the diagnosis, and a simple procedure involving the use of elastic tourniquets on the leg should provide the doctor with a fair indication of which perforating veins have damaged valves.

If further investigation is required, the performance of leg veins can be observed by means of *venography* or *thermography*. The venographic process involves injecting dye into a varicose vein and *X-raying* its progress through the circulation. In thermography the temperatures of various parts of the leg are recorded in such a way as to give a heat map. The aim of both techniques is to discover the precise location of weak valves. Thermography has the advantage over venography in not requiring an injection.

What is the treatment?
Self-help: Try to keep off your feet as much as possible. Whenever you can, sit with your legs up on a footstool. If symptoms are very troublesome, lie or sit as often as you can, with your legs raised above the level of your chest; this ensures good drainage from your ankles and feet. Buy, or get a prescription from your doctor for, support tights or stockings, and put them on before you get out of bed every day. Some people prefer elastic bandages, but they are difficult to apply properly – you will need a nurse or doctor to show you how – and they can be uncomfortable, especially in hot weather.

If you break the skin and blood begins to flow from a varicose vein, lie down, raise the affected leg, and keep it raised. Do this no matter where you are, even in a public place. The bleeding will instantly slow down, and you can control it by moderate pressure with a clean handkerchief. Professional medical help is then needed to clean and dress the wound and ensure it is not infected.

Do not try to cope with varicose ulcers or eczema without professional advice. And never scratch an itch caused by varicose

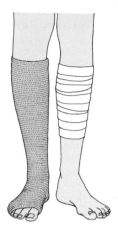

Simple self-help
If you have varicose veins, you can wear various types of support stockings (above) and should always try to sit with your feet up (right).

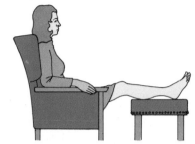

veins; scratching can further damage the vein and rapidly lead to ulceration.

Professional help: Your doctor can prescribe support tights and stockings as well as soothing dressings to relieve skin irritation.

The most satisfactory answer to the problem of varicose veins is provided by surgery. Every symptom of the disorder is immensely relieved when the veins are treated surgically; and the operation, whatever form it takes, has good results. In the most common form of surgery the affected veins are simply stripped from the leg. This does not leave a noticeable scar since a large section of vein can be removed through a tiny incision by means of special equipment. The incompetent valves of perforating veins are permanently closed by being tied up with thread. The remaining small veins rapidly enlarge to take over the function of collecting blood and channelling it to deep veins.

Varicose veins can sometimes be dealt with by injecting a small amount of a *sclerosant* chemical into them; the walls become inflamed and mat together so that the veins stop carrying blood. If you have such treatment, it will probably be as an out-patient and involve only two or three visits to the clinic or hospital. But because there are several drawbacks – for instance, injection is unlikely to succeed if the varicose vein is in the thigh – many doctors prefer stripping the veins. If, afterwards, there are minor recurrences of the complaint, they can usually be treated fairly easily by injection.

After varicose veins have been treated, either by surgery or injection, you will have to wear support stockings or elastic bandages for about six weeks. You should do as much walking as possible – but no standing, or sitting with your legs hanging down.

Varicose veins come back (usually in a different place) in about 10 per cent of treated cases. Even after successful surgery, varicose ulcers often remain troublesome.

OPERATION: ## Varicose-vein removal

Varicose veins can be removed by an operation and their work is gradually taken over by other smaller veins.

During the operation You are under a general anaesthetic. Incisions about 50mm (2in) long are made at the top of your inner thigh and at the ankle to reveal parts of the affected vein. Several very small cuts are also made down the leg where branches of the main vein go deeper into the leg. The branches are severed, then tied to stop them bleeding. A flexible wire is passed from the ankle to the thigh along the main vein. A hook is attached to the wire at the upper end. As the wire is withdrawn, the hook pulls the vein from beneath the skin. At the same time the leg is bandaged tightly to prevent bleeding. The operation usually takes 30 minutes for each leg.

After the operation Your legs will remain bandaged for several weeks and you will have to wear elasticated grips for some time after this. You will probably leave hospital about 3 or 4 days after the operation.

Convalescence Once you are at home you will be advised to walk up to several kilometres a day and always relax with your feet well up. You should take about a month away from work.
See also information on operations, p.738.

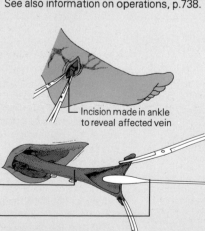

Incision made in ankle to reveal affected vein

Affected vein

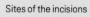

Sites of the incisions

Flexible stripping wire inserted into vein

Raynaud's disease

(and Raynaud's phenomenon)

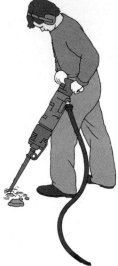

Possible cause of Raynaud's phenomenon
High-vibration machinery such as a pneumatic drill can, when used regularly, damage the blood vessels and lead to Raynaud's phenomenon.

This circulatory disorder affects fingers, and occasionally toes, when the small arteries that supply them become extra-sensitive to low temperatures and suddenly contract reducing the flow of blood to the affected area. At first the contraction is only a temporary spasm and is eased by warmth, but it may eventually become permanent. Lack of oxygenated blood makes the affected area pale, often with a bluish tinge. When a spasm ends, fresh blood returns and the pallor goes.

The problem may also occur as a secondary effect of conditions other than cold. It is an occasional occupational disorder of workers with chain saws, pneumatic drills, etc. It is sometimes caused by a disorder of the connective tissue such as *scleroderma* (p.557), by *pulmonary hypertension* (p.416), by *Buerger's disease* (opposite), by an emotional disturbance, or by a nerve disorder. And it can be triggered by sensitivity to *beta-blocker* drugs.

In all cases where it is secondary to another condition it is called Raynaud's phenomenon instead of Raynaud's disease.

What are the symptoms?
Change of colour in the fingers (or other affected areas) is the main symptom. There is generally no pain, but may be numbness or "pins and needles" in the affected area.

Raynaud's disease worsens very gradually. Raynaud's phenomenon, on the other hand, may worsen quickly. In late stages of the disorder the affected flesh may shrink, and small ulcers may form as the tissues suffer from an inadequate blood supply.

How common is the problem?
The condition is quite common, especially among women. It nearly always occurs for the

first time in young adulthood. In severe cases prolonged contraction of the arteries may result in *dry gangrene* (p.415), but this is rare. More often the blood supply eventually weakens the fingers and sometimes diminishes the sense of touch.

What is the treatment?
Self-help: Keep your hands and feet warm and dry. Wear loose-fitting gloves and socks and comfortable, roomy shoes. If you smoke, give it up; cigarettes do further damage to an inadequate circulation. Try to stay indoors in very cold weather.

Professional help: Medical treatment is based on attempts to encourage the small arteries to expand. Even when permanent damage has been done to arterial walls, *vasodilator* drugs improve the circulation. Alcohol is a vasodilator, and your doctor may suggest that you should drink small amounts of alcohol with your meals, because moderate quantities of alcohol seem to ease the symptoms of Raynaud's disease.

One type of surgery sometimes performed in cases of Raynaud's disease is an operation (*sympathectomy*) in which the nerves that govern the ability of the arteries to contract are cut. But although this often produces a dramatic improvement, the nerves tend to grow back; and if the condition has begun to be permanent, there may not even be temporary improvement. For some reason, too, sympathectomy is more successful when performed on the nerves to the toes than on those to the fingers.

Most people simply learn to live with Raynaud's disease. As for Raynaud's phenomenon, treatment depends on the underlying cause.

Chilblains

Prolonged exposure to low temperatures will normally cause the blood vessels in and just below the skin to constrict, thereby conserving heat (and turning you pale). A chilblain is a disordered version of this normal reaction. The delicate nervous control of blood vessels near the surface goes wrong, and the result is extreme pallor and numbness of the affected area, with patches of red, swollen, itchy, often broken skin. Repeated exposures to cold and damp intensify the problem. If the temperature is well below freezing, the skin and the tissues beneath may actually freeze (see *Frostbite*, opposite).

Although chilblains can occur anywhere on the body, the hands and feet are the most commonly affected parts. Some people –

especially children – seem to be particularly susceptible to the disorder.

What should be done?
Chilblains are a nuisance but are unlikely to have lasting ill-effects. To keep them under control in cold weather wear warm, dry clothes, including a hat that covers your ears; and change gloves, shoes, and socks whenever they are damp. If your skin is itchy, pat the affected areas with talcum powder. Try not to scratch since scratching can worsen skin damage, and avoid putting home ointments on the numb areas.

If chilblains cause insupportable discomfort, see your doctor, who may prescribe a *vasodilator* drug.

Frostbite

Medical myth

The best way to deal with frostbite is to rub the affected area with snow.
Wrong. Rapid rewarming is the right treatment. For complete instructions see Accidents and emergencies, p.809.

Frostbite – freezing of the skin and underlying body tissues – occurs when part of the body is severely affected by temperatures well below freezing (compare *Chilblains*, opposite). The flow of blood to the affected area stops, and skin cells may be permanently damaged in severe cases. Any part of the body may be affected, but hands, feet, nose, and ears are most at risk. Frostbitten skin is hard, pale, cold, and painless; when thawed out, it becomes red and painful. Anyone subjected to a couple of hours or more of extreme cold may become frostbitten, but people with *atherosclerosis* (p.372) or on *beta-blocker* drugs are most susceptible.

To guard against frostbite wear several layers of warm clothes under a waterproof, windproof outer garment. Make sure that your ears, hands, and feet (and nose, if possible) are protected. And remember that fatigue, alcohol, and lack of oxygen due to extreme heights can affect your judgement, causing you to disregard the bodily discomfort that indicates onset of frostbite.

Frostbite must be treated promptly. Every minute of delay lessens the chances of recovery. So memorize instructions for dealing with this problem (see *Accidents and emergencies*, p.809) before venturing into cold conditions, where professional help may not be available. If, after warming the frozen area, you do not fully recover, see your doctor as soon as possible. There is a risk of *dry gangrene* (p.415), which may necessitate amputation of the affected part, but frostbite usually has no ill-effects if treated speedily.

Acro-cyanosis

You have the condition known as acrocyanosis if the extremities of your body – fingers, toes, wrists, or ankles – sometimes look blue. The bluish tinge results from the sudden contraction of tiny arteries that supply the hands and feet; because of such spasms, these parts get less blood than they need, and waste products build up in local veins, giving the skin its abnormal colour. Nobody knows why acrocyanosis develops. It is intensified by cold, is present to an equal degree in both hands or both feet, and is not painful. The affected parts nearly always feel cold and may be sweaty, but acrocyanosis does not cause ulcers or other skin problems.

What should be done?
Do not worry about acrocyanosis. It is quite common, especially among women; it is not a sign of major disorder; and does not respond to treatment. Simply do what you can to protect your hands and feet from cold.

Buerger's disease

(thromboangiitis obliterans)

This disorder results from recurrent attacks of inflammation of the arteries or (more rarely) veins, which eventually cause *thrombosis* in the blood vessels and disruption of circulation. Thrombosis in an artery denies oxygenated blood to the tissues served by that artery, and the starved tissues may die as a consequence; thrombosis in a vein prevents blood from returning to the heart, with resultant swelling of the tissues from which the blood is not drained away.

Any blood vessels may be affected, but Buerger's disease most commonly affects the legs. The cause of these attacks of inflammation followed by thrombosis is not known. It may be that they are due to some disorder of the connective tissue within the walls of blood vessels – connective tissue composed chiefly of the substance collagen (for further information see *Collagen diseases*, p.556).

What are the symptoms?
The symptoms depend on the areas affected. Probably the most common symptoms are coldness and pain in the legs; the pain is felt after exercise and usually disappears with rest. The legs may also tingle and can become painfully hot and swollen if veins are mainly affected. If arteries are affected, there may be ulceration or even *dry gangrene* (p.415). Other possible symptoms are those of *Raynaud's phenomenon* (opposite), which is sometimes brought on by Buerger's disease.

How common is the problem?
This disorder is rare. Those who get it are nearly always male cigarette smokers from 25 to 45 years old.

What are the risks?
The major danger is that gangrene of the legs – or, occasionally, arms – may necessitate amputation. Otherwise the risks are those of *arteriosclerosis* (p.404). If veins are seriously affected, the disease called *thrombophlebitis* (p.407) may develop.

What should be done?
If you have any of the above symptoms, consult your doctor, who will probably

suspect the presence of this disease, especially if you are a man under 45, and will examine you with this diagnosis in mind. You may be given blood tests to determine, among other things, the level of *cholesterol* in your blood, which is usually normal or low with Buerger's disease; it would probably be high if your symptoms were caused by arteriosclerosis. To identify the site and nature of the circulatory obstruction, the doctor may also want you to undergo *arteriography*, a test which involves injecting a dye into the bloodstream.

What is the treatment?
Self-help: Since smoking increases the frequency and severity of attacks, do not smoke. Never expose your arms or legs to extreme cold, and put your feet into the care of a chiropodist, who will warn you to be careful not to wound the flesh when cutting your toenails. The reason for this is to minimize the risk of a wound becoming infected and the consequent risk of gangrene.

Professional help: Your doctor may prescribe *vasodilator* drugs for relief of pain, or an operation called *sympathectomy* to cut the nerves that are causing your blood vessels to constrict. But neither of these measures can be guaranteed to help the problem. If gangrene sets in, amputation of affected areas may be unavoidable.

The outlook, though, is not necessarily bleak. Even if each flare-up of Buerger's disease leaves some residual disability, it is quite common for the disease to burn itself out after several years.

Temporal arteritis
(also called cranial or giant-cell arteritis)

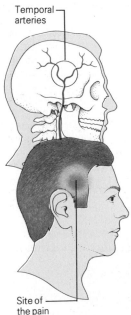

Temporal arteries

Site of the pain

If any of your arteries is chronically inflamed, with the inflammation causing a thickened lining and a reduction in the amount of blood that the arteries can carry, you have the disease known as arteritis. Temporal arteritis is so called because the arteries chiefly affected are the two that run behind the temples in the scalp. These temporal arteries are branches of the main arteries that supply your head (the carotids).

What are the symptoms?
The most common symptom is a dull, throbbing headache on one or both sides of the forehead. The artery that is the source of the headache may be swollen, red, and painful if touched. Among other possible symptoms are mild fever, loss of weight and appetite, and a generalized muscular ache in addition to the headache – though such muscle aches are more characteristic of a very similar disease called *polymyalgia rheumatica* (p.557).

How common is the problem?
Temporal arteritis mainly affects people over 55; your chances of having the disease rise steeply with age. About 1 in every 2,000 60-year-olds is likely to have the disease, compared with around 1 in 125 80-year-olds. Women are twice as susceptible as men.

What are the risks?
In severe cases, temporal arteritis can cause a *stroke* (p.268). But the eyes are most commonly affected. Half the sufferers from this disease have eye trouble, which leads, more often than not, to some loss of vision. Before modern drug treatment about 30 per cent of people with temporal arteritis went blind.

What should be done?
Anyone with persistent headaches should consult a doctor. If your headaches are accompanied by some of the other symptoms of temporal arteritis and if you are over 55, your doctor will suspect that you have this condition. A blood test will indicate whether temporal arteritis is causing your trouble. The doctor may also decide that a small piece of one of your temporal arteries should be removed (under a local anaesthetic) for microscopic examination; and more than one such *biopsy* is sometimes needed. To confirm the diagnosis or help determine which piece of artery to remove, the doctor may require an *arteriogram*, but this is rarely necessary.

What is the treatment?
Your doctor will probably prescribe an anti-inflammatory *steroid* drug. You may need to take the tablets for a long time; regular blood tests will show whether the steroid is suppressing the disease by damping down the inflammation of the affected arteries. There are several possible side-effects of steroids, but most of them are unlikely to occur as a result of the dose required for temporal arteritis. Once you start on the drug, however, you must continue to take it regularly until your doctor says you may cut down on the dosage and eventually stop.

What are the long-term prospects?
If you see your doctor early enough and cooperate in keeping the steroid treatment going, you have a 75 per cent chance of complete recovery. But good results are less likely if the disease is not diagnosed at a fairly early stage.

Arterial embolism

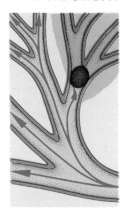

Blockage by an embolus
An embolus is carried along with the flow of blood in the arteries. It may become lodged at a point where the arteries branch or narrow. Any area of tissue that depends solely on the blocked artery for blood supply will die if the embolism is untreated.

An *embolus* is a solid particle – usually a fragment of clotted blood or a piece of *plaque* – that is swept along in the bloodstream. The embolus may be very small; but because arteries divide into successively smaller vessels, there comes a point where the embolus can go no further, and so it creates a blockage (*embolism*) that deprives certain tissues of an adequate blood supply. The embolus may originate in the heart (for example, after *mitral stenosis*, p.395); or it may be a fragment of bacterial growth resulting from *bacterial endocarditis* (p.394); or – rarely – it may be a tiny foreign object sucked into an artery through a wound.

The severity of an arterial embolism depends on its location. The brain and legs are most commonly affected. For the special type caused by a clot in a vein rather than an artery, see *Pulmonary embolism* (p.406).

What are the symptoms?
Embolism in internal organs usually goes unnoticed unless it affects a large area. It may cause loss of function in part of the intestine, however, with resultant symptoms of *ileus* (p.472). For the symptoms of embolisms in the brain, see *Stroke* (p.268) and *Transient ischaemic attack* (p.270). In other parts of the body – particularly the limbs – pain may be the earliest symptom. This is followed by a tingling or prickling sensation, and the affected area eventually becomes numb, weak, and cold. If the embolism is in an arm or leg, the skin is at first pale but turns bluish because of lack of oxygen. Both legs may be affected if a large embolus creates a blockage at the bottom of the back, where the aorta divides in two. Such "saddle" embolisms can cause severe pain in the abdomen and back as well as in the legs.

How common is the problem?
Arterial embolism, generally of a minor type, is common in people over 50. People already suffering from disorders that cause blood clots or bacterial colonies to form in the heart, or *atheroma* in the arteries, are especially susceptible.

What are the risks?
If a major artery is blocked, the tissues it supplies will die within hours if untreated (see *Dry gangrene*, below). In the brain the result can be a fatal stroke. People with blockage in the aorta (for example, of the saddle type) have only a 50 per cent chance of surviving.

What should be done?
Suspect arterial embolism if you have pain or inexplicable paleness, numbness, and tingling in an arm or leg. The worse and more extensive the symptoms, the less time you should waste before calling your doctor, who will probably make a swift diagnosis without special tests, but who may also want diagnostic *arteriography* to pinpoint the blockage.

What is the treatment?
Self-help: While waiting for medical help, keep the affected limb cool, and move it as little as possible; this reduces the need for oxygen. No self-help is possible for embolisms in any part of the body other than the arms and legs.
Professional help: Minor embolisms are normally treated with *vasodilators* or aspirin. In severe cases, powerful *analgesics* relieve the pain, and injections of an *anticoagulant* prevent further clotting. Additional treatment depends mainly on the location and extent of the trouble.

In most cases of arterial embolism severely affecting an arm or leg, surgery is urgently required in order to prevent gangrene from setting in. The operation (*embolectomy*) involves the insertion into the artery of a tube through which the embolus is mechanically sucked out. If this is done in time, complete recovery is likely.

Dry gangrene

Gangrene is dead, deoxygenated flesh; its characteristic black colour is a sign that the skin and (often) underlying muscle and bone are dead. There are two basic types of gangrene: dry and wet (for a description of *wet gangrene* see p.416). Dry gangrene does not involve bacterial infection; the flow of life-giving blood to certain tissues is simply stopped or reduced. This may be the result of *arterial embolism* (above), poor circulation due to *diabetes mellitus* (p.519), or *arteriosclerosis* (p.404), and it is occasionally caused by prolonged *frostbite* (p.413). The oxygen-deprived area dies, but the gangrene does not spread beyond that area.

As the flesh dies, it is painful. Once dead it becomes numb and slowly turns black. A visible line marks the border between the dead and living tissues.

How common is the problem?
In Britain only 1 person in 25,000 dies as a result of dry gangrene each year. But because dead tissues lack resistance to infection, there

is always a risk that the dry gangrene will lead to wet gangrene or *blood poisoning* (p.421).

What should be done?

If you have one of the disorders that can lead to dry gangrene, there are a number of precautions you can take. Do not smoke. Make sure your diabetes is kept under control. If you think you may be getting dry gangrene, consult your doctor without delay.

What is the treatment?

Your doctor will try various measures to improve circulation to the affected part before it is too late. *Anticoagulant* drugs or *vasodilators* may prove helpful, but surgery to unblock or bypass a clogged artery may also be advisable. If the gangrene appears to be becoming infected, you will be given *antibiotics* to prevent wet gangrene from setting in. If the dry gangrene does not respond to treatment, amputation of the affected part will be unavoidable. And it is usually necessary to remove some adjacent living tissue along with the gangrenous area; otherwise, the circulatory disorder that has brought on the gangrene may hinder complete recovery from the operation.

Wet gangrene

Wet gangrene may develop when either a wound or *dry gangrene* (p.415) becomes infected by bacteria. Some of the invading bacteria, which thrive only in an oxygen-free environment, produce poisons that break down the surrounding tissues, and so the gangrenous area spreads rapidly. A particularly virulent type of wet gangrene – generally called "gas gangrene" – is caused by certain strains of bacteria that not only spread rapidly but also produce a foul-smelling gas within the affected tissues. All such oxygen-hating organisms flourish in dirty conditions. Wet gangrene, therefore, usually results from a major injury in which a wound has not been thoroughly cleaned.

What are the symptoms?

The dying tissues are painful; when dead, they are numb and blackened. In mild cases there is redness and swelling around the blackened area, and thin pus oozes from it. There may also be an unpleasant smell. In more severe cases there is fever as well, and gas bubbles may occur in the dead tissue, making the skin and muscles crackle and pop if you press them.

If gas gangrene is not swiftly dealt with, it can cause *shock* (p.386), which in turn can quickly lead to the death of the sufferer if not treated immediately.

How common is the problem?

Mild forms of wet gangrene can complicate any case of dry gangrene. The more severe forms are now rare in countries such as Britain where standards of medical care and general hygiene are high.

What should be done?

If you are in danger of developing wet gangrene, see your doctor or go to a hospital without delay. A dirty injury must be properly cleansed as swiftly as possible. A doctor can recognize wet gangrene by sight, touch, and (often) smell and will arrange for immediate admission to hospital.

What is the treatment?

If you have wet gangrene, all the affected area must be removed surgically. You will also be given high doses of *antibiotics*. Severe cases are also treated with specially prepared *antiserum* for combating the invading bacteria. A modern technique for preventing further spread of severe wet gangrene is known as *hyperbaric* oxygen treatment. After removal of the dead tissue, the sufferer is placed inside a special chamber into which oxygen is pumped under high pressure. The oxygen permeates the flesh; and residual bacteria, if any, cannot survive since they live only in oxygen-free tissues.

Pulmonary hypertension

(cor pulmonale)

Pulmonary hypertension (raised blood pressure in the lungs) is a disorder of the circulation resulting from any disease that blocks the flow of blood through the lungs. Among the common causes are *chronic bronchitis* (p.354) and *emphysema* (p.358). People who live at high altitudes over a long period of time are especially susceptible to the problem. Whatever the cause, though the main result is a rise in pressure within the pulmonary arteries, which carry blood from the heart to the lungs. In time this leads to thickening of the arteries, further obstructing the flow of blood, and so creating a vicious circle. In its effort to compensate for poor circulation through the lungs, the right side of the heart becomes enlarged, but the extra work can lead to right-sided *heart failure* (p.381).

What are the symptoms?

There are often no symptoms until the condition is well advanced. Thereafter the main symptom is swollen ankles caused by a backlog of blood in the veins leading to the heart. If pulmonary hypertension is caused by chronic bronchitis and emphysema, the skin may have a bluish tinge because it contains less oxygen and more waste products than it should. If you already suffer from breathlessness because of the underlying lung disease, pulmonary hypertension is likely to make you even more breathless. And you may have certain symptoms of right-sided heart failure.

How common is the problem?

Pulmonary hypertension is a common disorder of people who have frequent chest infections, especially of middle-aged and elderly cigarette smokers.

What are the risks?

The main risks are from the lung disease that causes pulmonary hypertension; but the disorder may lead to heart failure.

What should be done?

You should already be getting treatment for the basic lung trouble. If you notice that your ankles are swelling at times when your chest condition seems particularly acute, tell your doctor, who will examine you and take a specimen of urine to test the health of your kidneys, which may be affected by prolonged heart failure. If there is evidence of heart failure, you may need to undergo further diagnostic tests for this disorder.

What is the treatment?

Self-help: If you are still smoking in spite of lung trouble, give it up NOW.

Professional help: Heart failure due to pulmonary hypertension can be relieved by bed rest and treatment with oxygen (to reduce *spasm* in the pulmonary arteries) and *diuretics* (to take excess fluid out of the system). Further attacks are likely, though, unless the underlying disorder is treated. Symptoms of chronic bronchitis are generally relieved, for example, by preventive measures against chest infection and by *bronchodilator* drugs to ease spasm in air passages. Prolonged treatment with oxygen sometimes helps to lower pulmonary blood pressure, and your doctor may arrange for you to do this at home.

If your pulmonary hypertension is due to chronic lung disease, long-term treatment will aim at halting further deterioration. The doctor may give you *antibiotics* and immunize you against influenza in order to prevent acute chest infection.

What are the long-term prospects?

Pulmonary hypertension is hard to reverse once it has developed, but with careful treatment can be kept under control.

Low blood pressure
(hypotension)

Chronic *high blood pressure* (p.382) is a serious problem, but chronic lower-than-average blood pressure hardly ever is. The type of low blood pressure that can give trouble is the kind that comes on abruptly and causes dizziness or faintness. The most common such condition is a phenomenon known as postural hypotension. When you spring up from a sitting or lying position, your blood vessels have to contract in order to maintain normal blood pressure in the new posture, and this process is carried out automatically by reflex action of the nervous system. But if you have postural hypotension, the reflex action is in some way defective; as a result, your blood pressure falls and the flow of blood to the brain is temporarily reduced by a sudden change of posture. The result is dizziness or even brief loss of consciousness.

Postural hypotension is usually due to overdosage with some types of drug for high blood pressure. These have an effect on the nervous system, which, if the dosage is too high, can cause postural hypotension. The simple treatment is a reduction of the dose. Occasionally, too, postural hypotension may occur as a complication of pregnancy or of certain conditions such as *diabetes mellitus* (p.519) or *arteriosclerosis* (p.404).

Sometimes low blood pressure causes such a diminished flow to a person's brain that he or she will faint. This can be due to an illness or to a physical reaction to something such as sudden emotion, undernourishment, or standing too long in the heat. Occasional fainting spells due to hypotension are seldom cause for concern.

What should be done?

If you have dizzy turns or feel rather faint when you stand up abruptly, make a habit of rising slowly from a sitting or lying position. If you have frequent fainting spells, consult your doctor, who will check your blood pressure and may arrange for further diagnostic tests to determine the underlying cause. No special treatment for long-standing hypotension is likely to be necessary.

Blood disorders

Introduction

The circulating blood is the means by which oxygen, nutrients, and chemical substances vital to the functioning of tissues and organs are carried around the body. It consists of two basic parts, the blood cells (sometimes called blood corpuscles) and the fluid in which they are suspended, the plasma. The blood disorders discussed in this section are principally concerned with the blood cells.

The red cells are by far the most numerous type of blood cell. Their function is to carry oxygen from the lungs to all parts of the body. They contain a red pigment called haemoglobin, which combines with oxygen in the lungs and releases it through the capillaries to the tissues as the blood circulates around the body.

The white cells, of which there are many varieties, are concerned with protecting the body from infection. The most numerous white cells are the neutrophils, which attack and engulf microbes. The next most numerous are the lymphocytes, whose functions include producing *antibodies* against invading microbes. Other, less numerous varieties of white cell also assist in protecting against the spread of infection.

A third type of blood cell is the platelet. These gather at the site of an injury to a blood vessel, and plug the hole as the first stage in the blood-clotting process. Other substances in the plasma then assist in sealing the wound.

Most blood cells are produced in the bone marrow, through which the blood circulates. However, the majority of lymphocytes are made in the lymph glands, which are found in the neck, armpits, groin, and many other parts of the body. The lymph glands, and the channels and ducts connecting them, are known as the lymphatic system. When the cells become old or defective they are filtered out of the bloodstream and broken down – mainly by the spleen, but also, to a lesser extent, they are dealt with by the liver and lymph glands.

Disorders of the blood are grouped as follows: lack of haemoglobin, causing anaemia; disorders of the clotting process, causing bleeding and bruising; cancerous changes in the white cells, causing leukaemia; disorders in the production of blood cells in the bone marrow; and disorders affecting the cells or glands of the lymphatic system.

Basic parts of the blood

Blood can easily be separated into its different parts (right) like cream from milk, because red blood cells are heavier than white blood cells and platelets, which in turn are heavier than the plasma in which they are suspended.

Plasma
Plasma is a yellowish fluid that contains salts, various proteins, antibodies, and blood-clotting factors.

White blood cells
White blood cells protect the body against infection by destroying bacteria and producing the antibodies that provide immunity.

Platelets
Platelets help plug a damaged blood-vessel wall and form the first stage of a blood clot.

Red blood cells
Red blood cells, which account for almost half of blood volume, contain a red pigment, haemoglobin, which carries oxygen throughout the body.

Plasma

White cells and platelets

Red cells

White blood cells
1 Neutrophil
2 Lymphocyte

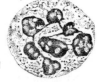
1

2

Platelets

Red blood cells

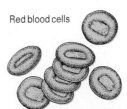

Anaemia

The most important component of red blood cells is the red pigment haemoglobin, which combines with oxygen in the lungs and carries it through the circulation to all tissues in the body. Anaemia occurs when the amount of haemoglobin in the blood falls below that needed to carry adequate amounts of oxygen to the tissues.

There are several reasons why too little haemoglobin may circulate throughout the body. The fault may be in the production of haemoglobin itself, or in the production of red blood cells. A supply of iron is needed to make haemoglobin, so lack of iron in the body means that not enough haemoglobin

can be made (this is called iron-deficiency anaemia). Lack of vitamin B_{12} causes too few and defective red blood cells to be produced (pernicious anaemia); and lack of folic acid has the same effect (folic-acid deficiency). If red blood cells are made at the normal rate, but are broken down too quickly, then their numbers in the circulation fall (haemolytic anaemia). And inherited defects (such as sickle-cell anaemia) cause the production of faulty haemoglobin.

The characteristic symptoms of anaemia include some or all of the following: paleness, tiredness, weakness, fainting, breathlessness, and palpitations.

Iron-deficiency anaemia

Iron is an essential component of haemoglobin, the red pigment in red blood cells. A deficiency of iron in the body causes inadequate production of haemoglobin, and therefore leads to anaemia.

Each day, the body requires a small amount of iron for the manufacture of new haemoglobin, to replace the haemoglobin lost in the continuous breakdown of red blood cells. This iron is obtained, in most people, from reserves found mainly in the bone marrow, liver, and spleen. These reserves are replenished by iron absorbed from the diet and by iron recycled from the breakdown of red blood cells. Some people – for a variety of reasons described below – have little or no iron stored in the body, but can stay healthy if they balance the iron they lose with the iron absorbed from their diet. If this is not possible, they become anaemic.

Lack of iron reserves are due to one or more of three main reasons. First, there may not be enough iron in the diet to replace the amount that is normally lost daily, or the body may need more iron during a period of growth. This problem occurs mainly in the very young (see *Iron-deficiency anaemia in children*, p.681), in pregnant women (see *Anaemia during pregnancy*, p.623), and in old people living on a restricted diet.

Secondly, there may be enough iron in the diet, but the digestive system is unable to absorb it. The most common cause of this failure is the absence of part of the stomach, as a result of an operation (see *Stomach ulcer*, p.465). Another cause of failure to absorb enough iron is *coeliac disease* (p.684).

Thirdly, the iron reserves may become depleted through the need to replace a large loss of blood. The loss may be through an injury, in which case, once the blood has been replaced the iron reserves will soon build up again. But in many women, heavy periods can drain their reserves over several months or years. In other cases blood loss may be unseen because it is internal. Common sites of internal loss include the stomach, where it may be caused by an ulcer or *cancer of the stomach* (p.466), and the intestine. Blood loss sufficient to cause anaemia may also result from *haemorrhoids* (p.483).

Finally, a person may have adequate iron reserves, but may not be able to use them due to the effects of a debilitating, long-term disease. Such diseases include *rheumatoid arthritis* (p.552) and *chronic kidney failure* (p.512); in these cases the anaemia responds only when the underlying disease is brought under control.

How common is the problem?

About 1 woman in 10 has a mild form of iron-deficiency anaemia, while another 3 in 10 are on the verge of having it through having virtually no reserves of iron (the problem is much less common in men). But only a small proportion of these people need medical treatment for the disorder.

What are the risks?

Iron-deficiency anaemia itself is very unlikely to be fatal. But it does weaken the body's resistance to the effects of illness or injury, especially if large amounts of blood are lost.

What should be done?

If you have the symptoms of anaemia, see your doctor. Do *not* attempt to treat the condition yourself with iron pills, tonics, or vitamin tablets. In treating your symptoms, you may well prevent diagnosis of a serious but treatable underlying disease.

The doctor diagnoses anaemia by taking a blood sample and having it tested. If the cause of the anaemia is not obvious, you may then have to visit your local hospital for further tests. These include more blood tests to measure the level of iron in the blood; an examination of a tiny sample of bone marrow (*biopsy*): tests on your faeces, for evidence of internal bleeding; and, if bleeding is detected, tests to determine its source, such as a *barium meal*, a *barium enema*, or *endoscopy*.

What is the treatment?

Self-help: Although the disorder must be treated by a doctor, you can help yourself by making sure your diet contains plenty of iron. Iron-rich foods include meat (especially beef and liver), wholemeal bread, dark green leafy vegetables, and dried fruits.

Professional help: Anaemia can only be cured by curing the underlying problem. If this involves an operation, you may be given a blood transfusion beforehand to make you fitter for the strains of the surgery.

If the anaemia is severe, and its underlying cause cannot be discovered or treated, you may be admitted to hospital for a day and given a blood transfusion or, in some circumstances, an infusion of iron into a vein, to stock up your iron reserves. If the anaemia is mild, then you will be given iron in the form of tablets or injections. Iron tablets have a reputation for causing indigestion and bowel upsets, but this should not happen if you do not take the tablets on an empty stomach and do not take more than the doctor has prescribed. In rare cases when a patient genuinely cannot tolerate taking iron tablets, he or she is given iron directly by injection in the buttock or thigh, or into a vein.

When a course of iron has cleared up the anaemia, the doctor will suggest that you continue taking iron for up to three months, to build up your iron reserves. If the cause of the anaemia was a poor diet, the doctor will advise you on what you should eat in the future to prevent the problem from recurring. The prospects for people with iron-deficiency anaemia are generally excellent. Treatment for the underlying problem or keeping to the right diet can clear up the problem for good in some cases; and in the other cases, repeated courses of iron tablets (or a blood transfusion if symptoms become severe) will keep the anaemia under control.

Pernicious anaemia and folic-acid deficiency

(including other megaloblastic anaemias)

The production of red blood cells, which takes place in the bone marrow, requires two vitamins – vitamin B_{12} and folic acid (sometimes called vitamin B_C). The body absorbs these vitamins from certain foods we eat (see *Vitamins*, p.494). If the bone marrow's supply of either vitamin is inadequate, the production of red cells falls and those that are formed are defective. The result is anaemia.

In the Western world, nearly everyone's diet contains sufficient quantities of B_{12}, so deficiency of the vitamin is nearly always caused by the body's failure to absorb it from the diet. In a healthy person the liver contains enough B_{12} to last for up to three years. A failure to absorb B_{12} will eventually deplete these reserves in the liver and when it does, anaemia develops.

There are various reasons why some people cannot absorb B_{12}. Before the vitamin can be absorbed from the last part of the small intestine, it must combine in the stomach with a special chemical known as intrinsic factor, secreted by the lining of the stomach. In some people, for reasons that are not fully understood, the stomach lining stops secreting enough intrinsic factor and sufficient quantities of the vitamin cannot be absorbed; the resulting disorder is pernicious anaemia.

Some forms of digestive-tract surgery may lead to poor absorption or non-absorption of B_{12}. If this happens, the resulting anaemia is called megaloblastic anaemia. In about 5 per cent of patients who have the lower part of their stomach removed as treatment for a *stomach ulcer* (p.465) or a *duodenal ulcer* (p.468), the stomach is unable to form enough intrinsic factor. In a small percentage of patients who have had an operation on the small intestine, bacteria multiply in a loop of the intestine and interfere with the absorption of B_{12}. All patients who have had an operation to remove the last part of the small intestine, the site of B_{12} absorption, are likely to suffer from a deficiency (see, for example, *Crohn's disease*, p.473).

Deficiency of folic acid is nearly always due to inadequate amounts in the diet – which usually means a lack of green vegetables. The body does not have large reserves of this vitamin, so any deficiency reveals itself within a few weeks in the form of anaemia known as folic-acid deficiency. People with *coeliac disease* (p.684) are also susceptible to folic-acid deficiency as they are unable to absorb sufficient amounts of the vitamin even if it is plentiful in their diet.

Both types of anaemia produce the general debility associated with all anaemias, but deficiency of B_{12} is the more serious, because besides being needed for the production of red blood cells, B_{12} is also vital to the maintenance of the nervous system. Deficiency of B_{12} can therefore damage various parts of the nervous system, particularly the spinal cord, causing additional symptoms.

What are the symptoms?

The main symptoms of anaemias due to deficiency of vitamin B_{12} or folic acid are those of other anaemias – paleness, fatigue, shortness of breath, and palpitations (particularly on exertion). In both disorders, the mouth and tongue are often sore.

Anaemia due to B_{12} deficiency also produces other symptoms – yellowing of the skin, indigestion, abdominal pain, and loss of appetite and weight. Because the spinal cord is often affected, the sufferer may not be able to walk or keep balance properly, and may experience continuous tingling in the hands and feet. In addition, there may be some loss of memory, confusion, and depression.

How common is the problem?

Anaemia due to B_{12} deficiency affects about 1 in every 2,500 persons. It is equally common in men and women, rare before the age of 40, and most common in those over 50. If you have a close relative in whom deficiency of intrinsic factor has caused the disease, you run a much greater than average risk of contracting this type of anaemia.

Folic-acid deficiency is slightly more common than B_{12} deficiency. It is found in 10 per cent of elderly people admitted to hospital, usually because they have been living on a poor diet. It also occurs in pregnant women, who need extra supplies for the developing baby. Up to 3 per cent of women having one child, and 10 per cent of women having twins, suffer from mild folic-acid deficiency.

What are the risks?

Pernicious anaemia and folic-acid deficiency present little danger to the health if treated promptly. Delay in treatment of pernicious anaemia can cause permanent damage to the nerves in the spinal cord, creating lasting difficulties with walking, the risk of falling, and perhaps mental disorders severe enough to demand psychiatric treatment.

What should be done?

If you have the symptoms of anaemia described, see your doctor. If your movement, balance, or memory are also affected, make the appointment without delay. Inform the doctor if you have a close relative with pernicious anaemia. Tests on a blood sample can rule out the possibility that you have either of the disorders, but an exact diagnosis can usually be made only by further tests in hospital. These will include a *biopsy* of your bone marrow, further blood tests, and perhaps a *barium meal* examination of the digestive tract. In addition, you may undergo a special test called a Schilling test. This involves taking vitamin B_{12} by mouth, then collecting urine over a 24-hour period.

What is the treatment?

Once the ability to absorb vitamin B_{12} through the digestive tract has been lost, it

---

Blood poisoning (septicaemia)

Blood poisoning is not one, single disease, but a condition brought on by the spread of a bacterial infection in the blood. The "poison" is either the bacteria causing the infection, or poisonous chemicals called *toxins* made by bacteria or released by them when they die.

Even a minor infection such as a *boil* (p.251) or a small contaminated wound releases a few bacteria into the bloodstream. In a healthy person, the white blood cells soon destroy the bacteria and remove the toxins without the person noticing. If you catch an infection such as *acute pyelonephritis* (p.502), there will be a substantial amount of bacteria or toxins in your blood. This makes you feverish and unwell – the symptoms of many infectious diseases. *Antibiotic* drugs aid the body's natural defences in combating the infection.

Large amounts of powerful toxins in the blood may cause *septic* shock in which the victim becomes pale, cold, and clammy. This condition is an emergency (see *Shock*, p.386). Such severe blood poisoning usually only occurs in people who are already seriously ill in hospital. Severe illness weakens a person's natural resistance to infection, so any bacteria which manage to enter the bloodstream can multiply unchecked.

may never be regained, and so treatment of B_{12} deficiency consists of a life-long course of vitamin injections (in the buttock or thigh). The injections are usually given at the doctor's surgery. For the first month, you will probably receive an injection once a week. Sore mouth, loss of memory and depression may disappear dramatically after the first injection. Problems with walking and balancing may take several months to improve – although if they existed for a long time before treatment began, it is possible they may never disappear completely.

After the first few weeks, the injections are reduced to one a month. It is vital that you do not miss an injection. If you do, your symptoms will almost certainly return.

Folic-acid deficiency caused by an inadequate diet can be cleared up completely – initially by a course of folic-acid tablets, and thereafter by a diet that contains adequate amounts of the vitamin. In cases of deficiency caused by a failure to absorb sufficient quantities, extra folic acid (in tablet form) may need to be given indefinitely unless the underlying fault in absorption can be corrected.

Sickle-cell anaemia

In the inherited disease called sickle-cell anaemia, the red blood cells contain an abnormal haemoglobin, called haemoglobin S. This defective haemoglobin causes the red cells to become deformed in shape – "sickled" – especially when short of oxygen. These sickled cells do not flow smoothly through the tiny blood vessels (capillaries) and may clog the vessels, preventing blood reaching the tissues. This causes *anoxia* (lack of oxygen), which makes the sickling worse. Such attacks are called sickle-cell "crises".

What are the symptoms?
In its severe form, sickle-cell disease produces all the symptoms of *anaemia* (p.419). In a sickle-cell crisis there is pain in the bones (usually the limb bones) or the abdomen. Such crises tend to occur during infections, and may complicate surgical operations.

How common is the problem?
Both the severe and the mild, symptomless forms of the disease are virtually unknown except in people of African descent. About 1 in every 1,000 black Americans has the severe form of sickle-cell disease; it is equally common in West Indians.

What are the risks?
Anyone with the severe form of the disease should take medical advice before flying or visiting high altitudes (over 2,000m). Severe sickle-cell crises may result in damage to vital organs by impairing blood flow to these organs and can in some cases lead to death from *heart failure* (p.381), *kidney failure* (p.511), or *stroke* (p.268).

What should be done?
If anyone in your family has sickle-cell anaemia, consult a *genetic counsellor* (p.619) before planning to have children.

If you or your child displays symptoms of anaemia accompanied by pain in the joints or abdomen, see your doctor, who will consider the possibility of sickle-cell anaemia especially if the disease is known to run in your family. Analysis of a blood sample will disclose whether the disease is present.

There is no cure for an inherited disease such as sickle-cell anaemia; only treatment for the symptoms. Crises of acute pain are the main problem; these are treated with *analgesics* (painkillers). If a crisis has been brought on by an infection, the infection is treated straight away with an *antibiotic*.

Thalass- aemia

An inherited defect prevents the formation of the normal blood pigment, called haemoglobin A, in the red blood cells. As partial compensation, the cells contain instead another form of haemoglobin, haemoglobin F, which is found usually only in newborn babies. But only a small amount of haemoglobin F is made in adults, so there are fewer red cells than normal. Also, cells containing haemoglobin F are destroyed more quickly than normal haemoglobin A cells. As a result, people with thalassaemia tend to suffer from profound anaemia.

Thalassaemia in its most severe form is seen only in those people who inherit the defect from both parents (see *Genetics*, p.704). When it is inherited from only one parent, the result is the thalassaemia "trait", which rarely causes any symptoms (except, perhaps, sometimes during pregnancy).

What are the symptoms?
The symptoms are similar to those of *haemolytic anaemia* (opposite): paleness, tiredness, weakness, breathlessness, and palpitations. A child who suffers from the dis-

ease tends to be inactive and you may notice that he or she is often unable to keep up with his or her playmates.

How common is the problem?
The thalassaemia trait is far more common than the severe form. But in people of Northern European ancestry the trait is rare; consequently the severe form is extremely rare. The disease occurs mainly in people from the Mediterranean and the Middle and Far East.

What are the risks?
People who have the trait are at little or no risk. For those with the severe form, repeated blood transfusions are needed to treat the anaemia; this treatment carries the risk of a build-up of iron in the body, which may damage the liver and the heart, and may lead to death from *heart failure* (p.381).

What should be done?
If you or your child displays any of the symptoms described, see your doctor, who will consider the possibility of thalassaemia, especially if this disease is known to run in your family. Initially the doctor will arrange for a blood sample to be taken for analysis.

If you have any form of the disease in your family – even as a trait – and you are considering having a child, then see your doctor about the possibility of your child being affected. The doctor may refer you to a *genetic counsellor* (p.619), a doctor with specialized knowledge of hereditary diseases. Nowadays, diagnosis is possible during pregnancy by the procedure called *fetoscopy*. If the unborn child is severely affected, the parents will be offered termination of pregnancy.

What is the treatment?
The underlying genetic defect that causes thalassaemia cannot be cured. Regular blood transfusions throughout life will relieve the symptoms of anaemia, but further drug treatment may have to be given to some sufferers, in order to avert the side-effects of these repeated transfusions.

Haemolytic anaemia

Haemolytic anaemia occurs when red blood cells are broken down more quickly than they are replaced. This eventually results in a shortage of red blood cells.

If the disease is *congenital*, it is usually due to an inherited fault in red-cell production. The fault results in abnormally shaped red cells that have a much shorter life than usual. One type of congenital haemolytic anaemia is known as hereditary spherocytosis; two other types – *thalassaemia* and *sickle-cell anaemia* (opposite) – are caused by a fault in production of haemoglobin, rather than a fault in the production of the red cell itself.

If the disease is acquired, it may be due to taking a particular drug for some other disorder – for example, *ulcerative colitis* (p.480), or certain skin disorders. The drug damages the red cells, thus shortening their life. Alternatively, a breakdown may occur in the body's normal ability to distinguish its own cells from foreign bodies such as bacteria and viruses (this is a so-called *autoimmune* disorder). The result is the formation of *antibodies* which attack and destroy the body's own blood cells, including red cells.

What are the symptoms?
The main symptoms are those of all anaemias. Occasionally attacks of weakness, raised temperature, and vomiting occur. In addition, the skin may be yellow, and, rarely, the urine is darker than normal.

How common is the problem?
All forms of haemolytic anaemia are rare; the disorder occurs in only 1 in 15,000 people. Your chances of having a congenital form of the disorder are increased if one or more of your close relatives suffer from it. The disease is rarely fatal.

What should be done?
If you have the symptoms described, see your doctor. If in addition your skin is yellow, or if you are being treated for another disease with drugs, then consult the doctor without delay. Tests on a blood sample will disclose if you have haemolytic anaemia; to determine the cause, further tests as a hospital out-patient may be needed.

What is the treatment?
The principal treatment for heriditary spherocytosis is to remove the spleen, the main site of destruction of the red cells. This considerably improves the condition, and the spleen's other functions are taken over by the liver and the lymph glands. Haemolytic anaemia caused by drugs is simply cured by discontinuing the drugs. If the cause is an autoimmune disorder, the condition usually improves naturally over the years. The doctor may prescribe treatment with *steroids*, to lessen symptoms and hasten the natural recovery. If this does not occur, then it may be necessary to remove the spleen.

Bleeding and bruising

Bleeding occurs when a blood vessel is cut or damaged. If blood from an internal wound seeps into the tissues, a bruise is formed. Where delicate blood vessels are near the surface – as, for example, in the nose – sometimes only very slight injury or irritation is necessary to set off bleeding.

In the majority of people, no harm results from minor bleeding because the body soon checks any blood loss. It does this by means of three mechanisms, which act in conjunction with one another. First, muscular contraction of the larger affected blood vessels narrows their calibre, so restricting the flow of blood to the area of the wound. Secondly, the platelets in the blood gather where the vessels are damaged, sticking to the vessel walls and to one another to form a plug at the site of the damage. And thirdly, chemicals in the blood plasma produce interlacing strands of a substance called *fibrin* in the damaged area; blood cells are trapped in the fibrin mesh and form a clot that seals the break.

In the rare bleeding diseases haemophilia and thrombocytopenia, one of the mechanisms to halt blood loss is faulty. Bleeding from a cut, which should normally stop within a few minutes, may carry on for hours, or even days. Extensive bruising may result from only minor injuries, and internal bleeding occur in the joints, perhaps causing crippling damage. These disorders therefore need prompt diagnosis and treatment.

Bruises
Blood from an internal injury collects in surrounding tissues to form a bruise. Once the internal bleeding has stopped, white blood cells called monocytes help to break down the leaked red blood cells that give the bruise its blue colour when seen through the skin surface.

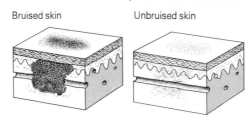

Bruised skin   Unbruised skin

Haemophilia

One of the best known and most common of the bleeding diseases (though it is still very rare) is haemophilia. In this disorder, which affects chiefly males, there is not enough of a chemical called anti-haemophilic globulin or Factor VIII, which is vital to the blood's clotting mechanism.

The way haemophilia is inherited (see *Genetics*, p.704) means that mainly men are affected by the disease, but it is passed on by female *carriers*.

What are the symptoms?
Symptoms usually appear when the baby boy becomes active. After some activities that would not normally be harmful, such as crawling, he gets bruises on his knees and elbows, and any cuts bleed for a long time. Internal bleeding caused by falls results in deep bruising, and may make a limb swollen and painful for several days. Repeated internal bleeding and accumulation of scarred tissue produce stiff joints that limit movement.

How common is the problem?
In Britain about 1 male in 50,000 has haemophilia. In about 75 per cent of cases, there is a family history of the disease, but in the remaining cases, the haemophiliac is the first of his line, probably because of a fault arising spontaneously in the mother's genes.

What are the risks?
Today the risks of being crippled or dying from the disease are greatly reduced because of effective and well-organized treatment. However, a major injury can still present a threat to life. Also, special precautions must be taken before any operation – even dental extraction – is carried out.

What should be done?
In families with a marked history of the disease, any member should seek *genetic counselling* (p.619) before starting a family. In general, the family and its doctor are usually alert to the problem and what measures to take. In all other cases, there is a risk, especially if the disease is mild, that it will not be recognized by the parents. If your baby son shows any of the symptoms described, see your doctor without delay.

If you are an adult male and you notice that you bruise or bleed in a seemingly abnormal way, you should also see your doctor. After questioning you at length, the doctor will probably refer you to a blood specialist (a *haematologist*) at a local hospital for blood tests. If haemophilia is diagnosed, you are given some form of identification (such as a bracelet or a card) containing details of the disease; you should carry the identification on you at all times.

·What is the treatment?

Self-help: The child must be protected against injury but not to the extent of banning all exercise. For example, while he must not play games like football, he should be encouraged to engage in running, swimming, and similar activities.

If a haemophiliac does get a wound that bleeds, it should be cleaned carefully. Firm pressure should then be applied to it with a clean pad. If the bleeding does not stop, the hospital that deals with his case should be contacted. If the haemophiliac receives an injury to a joint, such as a bruise on the knee, an ice pack should be applied to the joint, which should then be firmly bandaged; again, the hospital should be contacted because of the risk of permanent damage to the joint.

A haemophiliac should not take any drug without first consulting a doctor. Even aspirin should not be taken, as it may cause stomach bleeding. Special dental care will be necessary because of the bleeding involved.

Professional help: Recently, preventive treatment for haemophilia has become possible by regular transfusions into the bloodstream of Factor VIII, the deficient clotting chemical. Haemophiliacs can be taught to give these transfusions themselves, by injection. In the case of injury, any bleeding or bruising that does occur can be stopped by a further injection or transfusion of Factor VIII. Depending on the severity of the disease and the injury that has caused the bleeding or bruising, treatment may involve a short stay in hospital.

Thrombo-cytopenia

See p.239,
Visual aids to diagnosis, 29.

The blood cells known as platelets play a vital part in the body's mechanisms to stop bleeding. In thrombocytopenia, the blood contains only about one third (or even less) of the normal number of platelets, and, as a result, any bleeding takes longer to stop.

Thrombocytopenia is most commonly the result of the body forming *antibodies* against its own platelets; healthy platelets are damaged and are then broken down at an abnormally high rate. This disorder is known as ITP (idiopathic thrombocytopenic purpura) and often begins in children between the ages of two and six. Another main cause of thrombocytopenia is that the person is taking drugs such as *antibiotics*, *diuretics*, or anti-inflammatory agents that damage the bone marrow, so reducing the production of platelets or making them defective.

As well as being a disease in itself, thrombocytopenia can occur as a symptom of other blood disorders, including certain forms of *leukaemia* (p.426).

What are the symptoms?

The main symptom is a rash consisting of minute, purplish-red dots, which are tiny areas of bleeding just beneath the skin. The rash is extremely variable in size and can appear on any part of the body.

In serious cases there will be a tendency to bruise easily, and bleeding takes longer than usual to stop.

How common is the problem?

Although thrombocytopenia is one of the more common bleeding disorders, it is still fairly rare, affecting only 1 person in 10,000. ITP is roughly four times more common

in women than in men; the drug-induced form is equally common in both sexes. The main risk of the disorder is that of a bleed occurring in the brain and causing a *stroke* (p.268); bleeding into other internal organs may also cause serious complications.

What should be done?

Consult your doctor without delay if you notice the characteristic rash, or any abnormal bleeding. The doctor will check to see if you are taking any drugs for another disorder, and will take a blood sample for laboratory analysis. The result will show how low the platelet level is, and also whether the thrombocytopenia is a symptom of some underlying disease.

What is the treatment?

If a drug is identified as the cause of the disease, it will be stopped immediately. At the same time the doctor will probably prescribe *steroid* tablets, which act to reduce the risk of further bleeding. If the platelet count is very low and bleeding severe, transfusions of platelets are given.

Steroid tablets are also prescribed for ITP. The tablets prevent antibodies from destroying platelets, allowing the level of platelets in the blood to rise.

With suitable treatment, most cases of the disease clear up within a few weeks. But in a few cases ITP fails to clear up even after six months. Then the patient may be advised to have surgery to remove the spleen, which is the principal site of platelet destruction. The operation produces a complete cure in about 70 per cent of cases and a great improvement in the remainder.

Leukaemia

Leukaemia is a cancer affecting white blood cells. Normally, the number of white blood cells produced balances the number dying off, so that there are just enough white blood cells in the body to protect against infection. In leukaemia, one of the cells destined to develop into a white blood cell suddenly divides at an abnormally fast rate and produces other abnormal cells. The result of this over-production is that large numbers of abnormal white cells spread through the body, interfering with vital body functions.

There are two main types of leukaemia. Lymphatic leukaemia affects cells called lymphocytes, produced in lymph glands; and myeloid leukaemia affects the neutrophils, which are produced in the bone marrow. Both lymphatic and myeloid leukaemias can be acute or chronic. If untreated, acute leukaemia can lead to death within weeks, while chronic leukaemia may persist for as long as 15 years.

Acute lymphatic leukaemia primarily affects children and is described elsewhere (see *Leukaemia in children*, p.682). The three types of leukaemia discussed here – chronic lymphatic, and acute and chronic myeloid – mainly affect adults.

Acute myeloblastic leukaemia
(acute myeloid leukaemia)

The disease is caused by a cancerous change in a developing neutrophil, one type of white blood cell made in the bone marrow. The defective, or leukaemic, cell multiplies uncontrolledly, gradually producing large numbers of leukaemic cells, all of which continue to multiply in the same way. As their numbers increase, the cells start to take over the bone marrow, disrupting production not only of normal neutrophils but also of other cells made in the marrow – including red blood cells and platelets.

Eventually, the leukaemic neutrophils spill over into the bloodstream, where their level becomes progressively higher. They then invade various organs and tissues – particularly the lymph glands, spleen, and liver – which become enlarged.

What are the symptoms?
The main symptoms are lowered resistance to infections (especially of the mouth and throat), lip and mouth ulcers, an increased tendency to bruising and bleeding, and anaemia marked by paleness, tiredness, shortness of breath, and heart palpitations.

The disease often occurs suddenly, with the symptoms becoming pronounced over one or two weeks; less commonly they appear gradually over two or three months. Occasionally an elderly person may have "smouldering" leukaemia where the onset of the disease is very gradual.

How common is the problem?
Acute myeloblastic leukaemia is very rare. Only 1 person in 40,000 dies from it each year; most sufferers are over 60.

What are the risks?
There is a low cure rate for the disease, which, if untreated, can be fatal within weeks. In some cases, the leukaemia runs such a rapid course that death may occur within a few days, even before treatment can be started. But modern treatment gives a fair chance of relief from symptoms, sometimes for years.

What should be done?
Anyone with the symptoms described should see a doctor without delay. After examining you, the doctor will arrange for blood samples and perhaps a bone-marrow sample (*biopsy*) to be taken for analysis. Further blood tests may be required if acute myeloblastic leukaemia is suspected.

What is the treatment?
As soon as the diagnosis has been confirmed, the sufferer is admitted to hospital and given blood transfusions, including special transfusions of platelets to help prevent bleeding and bruising. Various combinations of drugs are the basis of treatment – firstly *steroid* drugs and large doses of powerful *antibiotics* to relieve the main symptoms.

Treatment of the leukaemia itself is by giving *cytotoxic* (anti-cancer) drugs. These drugs help clear the bone marrow of leukaemic cells, but as a side-effect they also destroy many of the marrow's already depleted store of healthy cells. Once the leukaemic cells in the marrow are destroyed, it takes at least two weeks before significant numbers of healthy cells start to repopulate the marrow and eventually enter the bloodstream. This period of very low *cell count* can be highly dangerous for the patient. If necessary, he or she will be placed in intensive care, including special precautions to prevent any infection, and will be given further transfusions of red cells and platelets.

When the danger period is over, the patient's condition improves dramatically. At some time between three and 12 weeks after the beginning of treatment, all signs of leukaemia will have disappeared and the disease is then said to have gone into remission. If in hospital, the patient is then usually fit enough to go home. Further drug treatment as an out-patient, at four- to six-week intervals, will then be needed for about a year, to keep the disease at bay. But the leukaemia almost always returns and further treatment usually proves ineffective.

Chronic lymphatic leukaemia

The disease begins with the abnormal development of a lymphocyte, a type of white blood cell present in the lymph glands. Instead of maturing in the normal way, the cell carries on multiplying and produces a vast excess of defective (leukaemic) cells. After some time – perhaps several years – the leukaemic cells gradually crowd out many of the normal white cells in the lymph glands, and reduce the ability of the healthy cells to produce antibodies against infections. The leukaemic cells also overflow from the lymph glands into the bloodstream, and then from the bloodstream into various parts of the body such as the spleen, the liver, and the bone marrow. As they invade more and more of the bone marrow, they interfere with the marrow's production of red cells, white cells, and platelets. Deficiencies of these cells, which occur in the advanced stages of the disease, cause *anaemia* (p.419), susceptibility to infections, and bleeding and bruising.

What are the symptoms?
It may be five years or more after the initial cell defect before symptoms appear – although occasionally the disease is detected before this, during a routine blood test. In some cases, the first signs of the illness are enlarged lymph glands – in the side of the neck, armpits, or groin – or an enlarged spleen, felt as a dragging or "full" sensation in the upper left abdomen. In other cases, the first symptoms are those of anaemia or recurrent attacks of a severe infection like *pneumonia* (p.359). In some cases, general ill health, loss of appetite and weight, raised temperature, and sweating at night are first indications of the disease.

In the very advanced stages of the disease, shortage of platelets will cause prolonged bleeding from cuts and possibly spontaneous bleeding from, for example, the fragile lining of nose or mouth.

How common is the problem?
Like other leukaemias, chronic lymphatic leukaemia is extremely rare; only 1 person in 20,000 develops the disease. It occurs almost exclusively in people over 60 years of age. The disease cannot be cured, but modern treatment allows the sufferer to live a normal life long after the diagnosis of the illness.

What are the risks?
Though chronic lymphatic leukaemia cannot be cured even without treatment some patients do not develop symptoms for up to five years after diagnosis. Modern treatment can do much to relieve symptoms and may add another 10 years to life expectancy.

What should be done?
Anyone who has persistent enlarged glands, persistent raised temperature, or recurrent infections should see a doctor, who will arrange for a blood sample to be taken. Laboratory analysis of the sample indicates whether the disease is present; sometimes before a definite diagnosis is made, a *biopsy* of bone marrow may be taken.

What is the treatment?
If the disease has been detected in its very early stages, the patient's own doctor will carry out six-monthly check-ups, at which a blood sample will be taken. As soon as symptoms appear, out-patient treatment is usually given. If severe anaemia is already present, a short initial stay in hospital may be needed for a blood transfusion.

The usual treatment for chronic lymphatic leukaemia is a *cytotoxic* (anti-cancer) drug. Tablets of this drug are taken for a minimum of several months and maybe up to a year to reduce the size of the glands and lessen the anaemia. If the glands are particularly enlarged, *steroids* may also be given, or *radiotherapy* may be used. Large doses of *antibiotics* are given to combat any infection, and anaemia is treated by blood transfusion.

With combined drug treatment, most sufferers are able to live a fairly normal life for five to 10 years after diagnosis of the leukaemia. But eventually the illness becomes resistant to all forms of treatment.

Chronic myeloid leukaemia

The disease begins in the same way as *acute myeloblastic leukaemia* (p.426), with a cancerous (leukaemic) change in the population of neutrophils – white blood cells made in the bone marrow. The abnormal cells multiply uncontrolledly, increasing in numbers and spilling over into the bloodstream, where their numbers can increase to 20 times the normal level. Some of the excess neutrophils can carry on with their job of protecting the body against infection, so lowered resistance is not a feature of the disease. But as the leukaemic cells spread throughout the marrow, they prevent the normal production of red cells. Often the neutrophils infiltrate and enlarge various organs, such as the spleen, lymph glands, and liver.

What are the symptoms?
A person suffering from the disease feels generally unwell, loses weight and appetite, and may sweat at night. In addition, the enlarged spleen may cause a dragging sensation in the left upper abdomen. The low level of red blood cells causes symptoms of *anaemia* (p.419), and in some cases, enlarged lymph glands are felt in the neck, armpits, and groin.

How common is the problem?
Chronic myeloid leukaemia is extremely rare – only 1 person in 100,000 dies from it each year. It affects men and women equally, and usually develops in middle or old age. The disease usually proves fatal within two to three years. A person with any of the symptoms described should see the doctor, who will carry out a full examination and arrange for a blood sample to be taken. Further tests may include a *biopsy* of bone marrow.

What is the treatment?
Treatment does not cure the disease but allows patients to lead a fairly normal life. Most people suffering from the disease can be treated as out-patients. However, if the anaemia is severe, a stay in hospital for blood transfusions will first be necessary.

The basic treatment is a course of *cytotoxic* tablets for four to six weeks. This restores bone-marrow production to normal and clears up the symptoms; the disease is then said to be in remission. However, careful watch is kept on the patient's condition, and further blood tests are carried out at intervals of two to four weeks. At some stage, between a few months and a year later, the level of white cells in the blood will start to rise again. As the rise becomes rapid, or if anaemia or other symptoms develop again, a further course of drugs is given. Eventually the disease may become resistant to a particular drug, in which case another, similar, drug is tried. But from about this time onwards, the patient usually suffers frequent relapses and may need to take drugs continuously. After a further period of time – up to about three years – drugs are no longer able to control the disease, and it will usually be only a matter of weeks before the disease proves fatal.

What are blood groups?

On the surface of every red blood cell is an identical pattern of molecules called *antigens*. These are important in matching blood for transfusions and have been classified in several ways. The best-known antigens belong to what is called the ABO blood-group system. This means that you have A, B, or a combination of A and B antigens on each red cell, or alternatively you have no antigens from this system and are said to be blood group O.

As well as belonging to the ABO system, you are also either Rhesus positive or Rhesus negative from the Rhesus system. In addition you have antigens from other, less well-known blood-group systems, such as the MN system and the P system. So in fact everyone has a blood group from each of the many systems, depending on which antigens are present on the red blood cells. Your blood groups are inherited from your parents by means of a complex system of *genes* carried by egg and sperm.

Why are blood groups important?
If blood from different groups is mixed, *antibodies* in the plasma of one type may react with antigens on the red cells of the other causing the cells to clump together, clogging blood vessels and perhaps causing *shock* (p.366) or acute *kidney failure* (p.511). So if you need a blood transfusion the medical staff must select the correct "matched" blood. Mismatched ABO or Rhesus groups are the most likely to cause clumping, which is partly the reason why these two groups are the best known. The Rhesus blood-group system may also be important in pregnancy (see *Rhesus incompatibility*, p.626).

How common are your blood groups?
You can find out how common your ABO and Rhesus blood groups are in Britain by looking at the table. If you do not know your blood groups, the easiest way to find out is to donate blood.

Percentage of population in each blood group

ABO blood-group system	Rhesus blood-group system	
	Rhesus positive	Rhesus negative
A	34.9	5.5
B	6.6	1.4
AB	2.5	0.4
O	37.6	7.8

Bone marrow

The marrow inside the bones is an active tissue with a rich blood supply since it is responsible for producing the vast majority of blood cells – all of the red cells and platelets, and most of the white cells.

In an adult, active blood-forming marrow is confined to the bones of the trunk, chiefly the ribs, breastbone, shoulder blades, and pelvis. The limb bones contain fatty (non-active) marrow which, however, can convert to active, blood-forming marrow if there is ever a need for increased blood-cell production. In young children, active blood-forming marrow is found in all bones.

Polycy-thaemia

Normally a precise control mechanism in the body adjusts the production of red blood cells in the bone marrow, so that the number of red cells made equals the number that die. In polycythaemia the mechanism becomes faulty and the marrow produces too many red cells whereas the numbers that die remain constant. The result is that the number of red cells in the blood rises.

There are three main types of the disorder. Primary polycythaemia (sometimes called polycythaemia rubra vera), an over-production of red cells, is the most serious form of the disease.

Secondary polycythaemia occurs as a symptom of another, underlying disease, such as severe *chronic bronchitis* (p.354). The underlying disease prevents the blood's red cells from obtaining enough oxygen to pass on to the body's tissues, and consequently the bone marrow responds by producing many more red cells. The outcome depends on the success in treating the underlying disease.

The third type of the disorder, pseudo-polycythaemia, as its name implies, is not a true polycythaemia, because it is not caused by a fault in the bone marrow. The high density of red cells is, instead, a result of a deficiency of plasma, the fluid in which blood cells are suspended. The cause of the plasma deficiency is unknown, but there is an association of the disease with being overweight, under stress, and drinking too much alcohol. Although pseudopolycythaemia itself does not present any risks to health, and seldom needs treatment, the life style associated with it is unhealthy and can lead to other disorders. Sufferers are well advised to cut down on their intake of food and alcohol.

The remainder of this article deals with primary polycythaemia, the most serious form of the disease. The red cells that are produced are healthy but they are so numerous and so concentrated that they have adverse effects on the body.

What are the symptoms?
Typical symptoms of primary polycythaemia include recurrent headaches, dizziness, a feeling of fullness in the head, and a high colour. Sometimes there is skin itching – often severe and made worse by a hot bath. Examination by the doctor may reveal an enlarged spleen, felt as a swelling just under the ribs on the left side of the abdomen.

How common is the problem?
Primary polycythaemia is a very rare disorder. Only 1 person in 50,000 is found to have it each year. The disease is equally common in men and women, and occurs mainly in those over 40 years of age.

What are the risks?
Although primary polycythaemia cannot be cured, it takes many years to develop, and once it is controlled by treatment, many patients survive for up to 20 years. The abnormal concentration of red cells can lead to *coronary thrombosis* (p.379), *deep-vein thrombosis* (p.405), *stroke* (p.268), *gout* (p.498), or kidney damage.

What should be done?
Anyone with the symptoms of polycythaemia should see a doctor, who will arrange for analysis of a blood sample. If polycythaemia is disclosed, a special test called a *blood-volume estimation* will be necessary to discover which of the three types of the disorder is present. If the test is positive, other procedures such as *IVP X-rays* of the kidneys may then be arranged.

What is the treatment?
In most cases of primary polycythaemia, out-patient treatment is given. The first aim of treatment is to lower the number of red cells in the blood, to remove the risk of thrombosis. To do this, half a litre of blood is regularly taken from the body, via a vein in

the arm, to remove excess blood cells. In mild cases, removal of blood once every three to four weeks may be the only treatment necessary. Drugs such as *radioactive phosphorus* (injected into a vein) or tablets of a *cytotoxic* drug will usually be successful in controlling the over-production of red cells. A course of treatment may be effective for a period anywhere between three months and several years. When symptoms recur, a further course is given, but eventually the disease becomes resistant to all forms of treatment.

Myeloma

Among the less common types of white blood cell in the bone marrow are the plasma cells (not to be confused with the fluid in which all blood cells are suspended, also called plasma). Their job is to produce *antibodies* that neutralize the invading microbes of any disease you have already had, or have been inoculated or vaccinated against. Normally, plasma cells make up only a minute fraction of the cells in the marrow, but in myeloma, one plasma cell undergoes a cancerous change and begins to multiply slowly but steadily, in an uncontrolled fashion. In some cases the defective plasma cells come to occupy more than half the marrow. This has three serious effects. First, production of other blood cells in the marrow is disrupted. Secondly, the excess plasma cells cause a build-up of pressure within the marrow, which weakens the surrounding bone. Thirdly, the remaining normal plasma cells are hampered in their job of protecting the body against infection.

What are the symptoms?
The first symptom is an increased susceptibility to infections, especially chest infections. There may also be symptoms of *anaemia* (p.419). But the most characteristic symptom of the disease is pain in the bones – particularly in the vertebrae (the backbones) – caused by the pressure of the excess plasma cells. Sometimes, this causes one or more vertebrae to split and cave in, producing acute back pain. If this happens to several vertebrae, the spine will become permanently deformed and the person will be unable to stand up straight. Occasionally, a limb bone may become so weak that it is easily fractured.

How common is the problem?
Myeloma is rare, occurring in only 1 person in 10,000. It affects mainly those over 50 and is twice as common in men as in women.

What should be done?
Anyone over 50 who has developed bone pain, especially in the back, should see a doctor. Laboratory analysis of blood and urine samples and *X-rays* of the skeleton will confirm the diagnosis and show what damage has been done to the bones.

What is the treatment?
Myeloma is rarely cured, but treatment can allow several more years of fairly normal life. In the early stages of the disease, the usual treatment is by tablets of a *cytotoxic* (anticancer) drug. Often *steroids* are also given in the form of tablets.

This treatment steadily destroys the cancerous plasma cells in the bone marrow, quickly relieving bone pain and allowing the damaged bone to thicken and heal. Bone pain can also be relieved by *radiotherapy*; if a fracture occurs, it will be treated first by radiotherapy, and then set in the normal way (see *Fracture*, p.534), and any anaemia is treated by blood transfusion.

Drug treatment usually lasts for up to one year. Most patients stay reasonably healthy for at least two years; some are advised to lose weight, to reduce strain on the spine. A close check is kept on the patient, and when a relapse occurs, the same treatment is given as before. This may bring the illness under control again, but at some stage it will become resistant to drugs and the patient is likely to succumb to an infection.

Aplasia
(also called aplastic anaemia)

In aplasia, the marrow's production of all blood cells falls drastically. The most common form of the disease is secondary aplasia, which occurs as a result of damage to the bone marrow by a drug taken for some other disorder, for example, accidentally drinking some poisonous substance, or exposure to a chemical or radiation. The marrow is then unable to function normally.

The other form of the disease is primary aplasia. Its causes and exact nature are unknown, and consequently it is more difficult to treat than secondary aplasia.

What are the symptoms?
There are three main groups of symptoms. Shortage of red cells causes the symptoms of *anaemia* (p.419); shortage of white cells

causes susceptibility to infection, especially of the mouth and throat; and shortage of platelets leads to spontaneous bruising and bleeding – often from the nose or mouth.

How common is the problem?
Secondary aplasia is far more common than primary aplasia, though the disease in either form is rare. Each year, 1 person in 25,000 is found to have secondary aplasia.

What are the risks?
Mild aplasia usually clears up completely after treatment. Severe aplasia, on the other hand, is a dangerous condition: in about 50 per cent of cases diagnosed as severe, the patient dies of an infection or serious bleeding within a year.

What should be done?
If you develop any of the symptoms described, see your doctor, who will arrange for a blood sample and bone-marrow sample (*biopsy*) to be taken for diagnosis.

What is the treatment?
In mild cases of secondary aplasia, the person often recovers without treatment if the cause of the disease is removed. People suffering from the primary form of the disease may also recover spontaneously, though this natural recovery is less likely.

In all cases where symptoms are pronounced, anaemia and bleeding problems are treated by blood transfusions, which involve a short hospital stay; and infections are treated by *antibiotics*. If there is no improvement within a few weeks, drugs to stimulate the functioning of the bone marrow are given. Drug treatment allows many patients to stay relatively healthy and active for a number of years, and may even produce a cure in a proportion of sufferers.

If drugs do not bring about normal production of cells in the bone marrow, then a bone-marrow graft may be attempted in a young and otherwise fit person. Bone marrow from a donor (who must usually be a brother or sister) is injected into the patient's vein, and the cells make their way to the bone marrow. The procedure is successful if the healthy, new marrow produces increasing quantities of blood cells. Unfortunately the procedure, which is complex and can be carried out only at a special hospital, is sometimes unsuccessful.

Agranulo-cytosis

The white blood cells known as neutrophils act as the body's first defence against infections. Normally the neutrophils develop in the bone marrow and are then released into the bloodstream. In agranulocytosis the formation of neutrophils in the bone marrow is slowed or even stopped. The result is that the blood contains too few neutrophils, which leads to a weakening of the body's resistance to infections.

Most cases of the disease are mild; often they are caused by a drug that is being taken for some other disorder. In a few cases, the disease follows infection – exactly why this should happen is unknown.

What are the symptoms?
The characteristic symptom of the disease is susceptibility to infection. The mouth and throat are particularly vulnerable, and ulcers often occur on them.

What are the risks?
In a small proportion of sufferers, infections such as *pneumonia* (p.359) can progress unusually rapidly and be extremely severe, or even fatal. Such cases are extremely rare, however, as statistics show that the disease itself occurs in only 1 person in 100,000.

What should be done?
If you have been suffering from a series of minor infections – even ordinary colds – then see your doctor, particularly if you are on a course of drugs. Some drugs are known to carry the risk of damaging the bone marrow, and the doctor will be alert to this possibility.

Following a physical examination, the doctor will arrange for a sample of your blood to be sent for analysis. Even if the results indicate agranulocytosis, a bone marrow sample must be examined for a definite diagnosis.

What is the treatment?
Some cases are so mild that they require no treatment other than discontinuing the drug causing the disease. Recovery then occurs naturally. Any infection will be treated with a course of *antibiotics*.

In rare cases, when the cause of the disease cannot be detected, or when withdrawal of the drug thought to be responsible for the disease does not bring about any improvement, drugs that stimulate the bone-marrow tissue are given. Sometimes the disease recurs periodically in a mild form, but in the majority of sufferers it clears up completely. If this happens, there are usually no long-term problems.

Lymphatic system

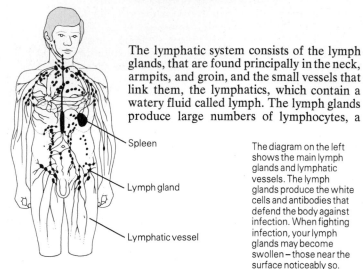

Spleen

Lymph gland

Lymphatic vessel

The lymphatic system consists of the lymph glands, that are found principally in the neck, armpits, and groin, and the small vessels that link them, the lymphatics, which contain a watery fluid called lymph. The lymph glands produce large numbers of lymphocytes, a

The diagram on the left shows the main lymph glands and lymphatic vessels. The lymph glands produce the white cells and antibodies that defend the body against infection. When fighting infection, your lymph glands may become swollen – those near the surface noticeably so.

type of white blood cell, which produce *antibodies* against recurrent infections. The glands act as barriers to the spread of infection through the lymphatics, by trapping the microbes travelling along them. Thus, when you suffer from an infection, the lymph glands often become swollen. The lymph carries nutrients and oxygen from the blood to every cell in the body, and eventually drains back into the bloodstream through the lymphatic system.

The spleen is essentially a very large lymph gland lying on the upper left side of the abdomen. In addition to producing lymphocytes, the spleen also removes old and malformed red cells from the bloodstream and breaks them down.

Lymphoma

This disease occurs when a lymphocyte in a lymph gland begins to multiply uncontrolledly, producing many malformed lymphocytes that cause swelling of the gland. The swollen, cancerous tissue is a form of *malignant* tumour called a lymphoma. Lymphocytes are mobile cells, and cancerous lymphocytes usually spread to the spleen and to lymph glands in other parts of the body, producing further tumours in these organs.

What are the symptoms?
The first symptom is usually a swollen gland, in the neck (the most common site), or in the armpit or groin. Occasionally several glands become swollen at the same time. If the spleen is affected, a fullness or dragging sensation in the upper left abdomen may be felt. Other symptoms include feeling generally unwell, loss of appetite and weight, raised temperature, night sweats, itching of the skin, and susceptibility to infection, since malformed lymphocytes cannot protect the body against infection.

How common is the problem?
Lymphomas are rare; they affect only about 1 person in 10,000. They occur most often in the middle-aged and elderly, and twice as many men as women are affected.

What are the risks?
If untreated, all types of lymphomas are ultimately fatal. In general, slowly growing tumours are difficult to treat, but because they grow so slowly, will allow many years of

fairly normal life. Fast-growing lymphomas that develop over a period of weeks usually respond well, and some can be cured.

What should be done?
If you have a swelling that persists for no obvious reason for more than two weeks, see your doctor. If the swelling is an enlarged gland, the doctor will take a blood sample and arrange for you to have the gland examined, and probably removed, in hospital. Tests on the blood sample and gland tissue will enable an exact diagnosis to be made.

If the disease is present, its extent is determined by more hospital tests, such as a chest *X-ray* and a *lymphangiogram*.

What is the treatment?
If only the glands in a single part of the body are affected, treatment may consist simply of *radiotherapy*. If the disease is more widespread, *steroid* and *cytotoxic* (anti-cancer) drugs are used. Treatment usually consists of giving a combination of drugs during a short stay in hospital, then repeating this course at intervals of a few weeks.

Patients in whom the disease has developed rapidly may be cured. If the tumours develop slowly, or if treatment arrests but does not cure the disease, symptoms eventually recur and the patient is then given further courses of drugs. At some stage, however, the disease will become resistant to treatment, and the patient will have a progressively weaker resistance to infections, one of which will eventually prove fatal.

Hodgkin's disease

Hodgkin's disease is superficially identical to the development of *lymphoma* (opposite). Cells in one of the lymph glands multiply in an uncontrolled manner and spread to other lymph glands in the body. One important difference is that Hodgkin's disease cells are less *malignant* than lymphoma cells, and the rate of cure is much higher.

What are the symptoms?

The main symptoms are persistent swollen glands, usually in the neck. The skin may be itchy, and there may be pain in the enlarged glands after taking alcohol.

Hodgkin's disease is rare – it occurs in only 1 person in 10,000 – and affects mainly those between the ages of 20 and 40. Three times as many men as women have the disease. Treated early, the rate of cure is high. Analysis of a blood sample and a *biopsy* of the gland will enable a diagnosis to be made.

Further hospital tests, such as a chest *X-ray* and a *lymphangiogram*, are necessary to determine the extent of the disease.

What is the treatment?

Radiotherapy is used if the disease is caught early, and brings about a cure in up to 90 per cent of such cases.

If the disease is at an advanced stage when discovered, treatment with drugs is given, sometimes in combination with sessions of radiotherapy. About 20 per cent of patients with advanced Hodgkin's disease are cured by this intensive drug therapy.

If no signs of the disease have reappeared after five years, the patient almost certainly has been cured. Those who have advanced Hodgkin's disease and are not cured by the treatment will eventually become resistant to drugs, and finally lose all resistance to infections, one of which will prove fatal.

Immuno-deficiencies

Immunodeficiency is a breakdown in the body's ability to defend itself against infection. It is nearly always brought about as a result of some other disease.

The most common type of immunodeficiency is a failure of the lymphocytes to produce sufficient *antibodies* as a protection against invading microbes. This failure is often caused by a disease such as *lymphoma* (opposite), *myeloma* (p.430), *Hodgkin's disease* (above), and some types of *leukaemia* (p.426). A reduction in antibody production may also be caused by certain types of *immunosupressive* drugs. Much more rarely, immunodeficiency can be a disease in its own right. In such cases, it is caused by an inherited disorder.

What is the treatment?

If the immunodeficiency is a condition brought on by another disease, or by the effects of a drug which cannot be discontinued, then treatment consists of giving injections of a concentrated solution of the missing antibodies, prepared from donated blood. The effects of each injection last for only a few weeks, because the introduced antibodies slowly break up. Injections are continued until the underlying disease has been cured, or the immunosuppressive drug has been discontinued.

The treatment for the inherited types of immunodeficiency is a bone-marrow graft from someone with the same *tissue type*. The success of the operation is unpredictable.

Enlarged spleen

The spleen, an organ about the size of your fist, is situated in the upper left abdomen. It acts as a large lymph gland whose main functions are to remove damaged red blood cells from the blood and to fight infection.

The spleen may become enlarged, nearly always as a symptom of another disorder, such as *malaria* (p.567), *cirrhosis of the liver* (p.487), or one of many blood disorders.

An enlarged spleen sometimes becomes overactive in removing various types of cell from the blood. Also, it is prone to rupture as a result of injury. For these reasons, and because the

spleen is not an essential organ, you may be advised to have your enlarged spleen removed (*splenectomy*). A splenectomy may also be done as part of the diagnostic procedure in some blood disorders.

Spleen removal is a fairly major, but relatively safe, operation. The absence of the organ causes no problems, since most of its functions are taken over by lymph glands elsewhere in the body. The operation is usually avoided in small children, however, as children who do have it seem to become generally less resistant to infections of all sorts.

Disorders of digestion and nutrition

Introduction

Your body needs a regular supply of nutrients for several reasons. They provide the molecular building blocks needed to make new body tissue as you grow. You need a constant supply of nutrients to replace old, worn-out tissue. You also need energy-rich nutrients such as glucose and other sugars to supply energy for the thousands of chemical reactions (called *metabolic* reactions) occurring in your body all the time.

Nutrients are extracted from the food you eat as it passes through your digestive system. The digestive system consists partly of the digestive tract, and partly of the digestive glands. The digestive tract is basically a long tube running from mouth to anus. The digestive glands, the liver and pancreas, make various chemicals needed to attack and break down the pieces of food you swallow. The tract and glands work together as a system, the function of which is to take in food and break it down into minute pieces (molecules) small enough to be absorbed into the bloodstream.

The first part of the tract is your mouth. Your front teeth tear or bite off pieces of food, then your back teeth crush and chew the food into small pieces and mix it with saliva. The saliva lubricates the food so that it can be easily chewed and swallowed. Your tongue moves the food around the mouth and holds it in position as it is chewed, then forms it into a ball (a *bolus*) and pushes it to the back of the mouth, ready for swallowing.

The second region of the tract is a muscular tube, the oesophagus (gullet). When you swallow, food is propelled down this tube by a progressive wave of contraction of the muscles in its wall. At the base of the oesophagus is a ring of muscles – the oesophageal *sphincter* – which relaxes to allow the food to pass into the third region of the tract, the stomach. When food enters the stomach, powerful muscles in the stomach wall start to crush and pummel it into a pulp. In addition, the stomach wall manufactures powerful digestive juices, one of which is hydrochloric acid. These juices start to break the food chemically into yet smaller pieces. The semi-digested food then passes through another ring of muscles – the pyloric sphincter – and along a short tube, the duodenum, into the fourth

region of the tract. This is the long, tightly-coiled small intestine, the region where most of the nutrients are absorbed into the bloodstream.

Just beneath the liver lies the gallbladder, a pear-shaped sac about 75mm (3in) long. The gallbladder stores and concentrates bile, a fluid produced by the liver which contains mainly waste products of metabolic reactions. After a meal, bile is released into the small intestine via the bile duct, where it aids the digestion of fats. More digestive juices (*enzymes*) are released from the pancreas through a duct which joins the bile duct just before it enters the small intestine. As the food is pushed along the intestine by waves of contraction of the muscles in its wall, enzymes and other chemicals reduce it to molecules which are small enough to seep through the wall of the small intestine into the bloodstream. Nutrients are then carried to the liver for storage and distribution.

Following the small intestine, the next-to-last region of the tract is the large intestine. Here, water is absorbed from undigested and indigestible remains; the result is semi-solid faeces. The faeces are stored in the end of the large intestine, chiefly in the part called the rectum. Finally, the wastes are expelled at convenient intervals through the last region of the tract, another muscular sphincter called the anus.

Most disorders of the digestive tract affect only one region of the tract. In this section of the book, such disorders are grouped together, along with a general description of what that particular region of the tract looks like and how it works. Some digestive disorders are more generalized and affect two or more regions of the tract; these also are grouped together.

Finally, there is a group of articles describing disorders of nutrition. These are problems concerning the amount or type of food eaten, or the ability of the digestive system to absorb certain chemicals in the food. Some nutritional disorders are rare, inherited diseases that require the sufferer to eat a life long special diet or take daily doses of specific drugs. Other nutritional problems can affect anyone – for example, any person who eats too much will suffer from obesity.

The digestive system

The digestive system is divided into a number of regions (shown on the right), each of which has its own part to play, either in the breakdown and absorption of food or in the expulsion of waste matter. Digestive enzymes (special substances which speed up chemical reactions) assist in the process of breaking food down into molecules small enough to pass through the wall of the small intestine and into the bloodstream.

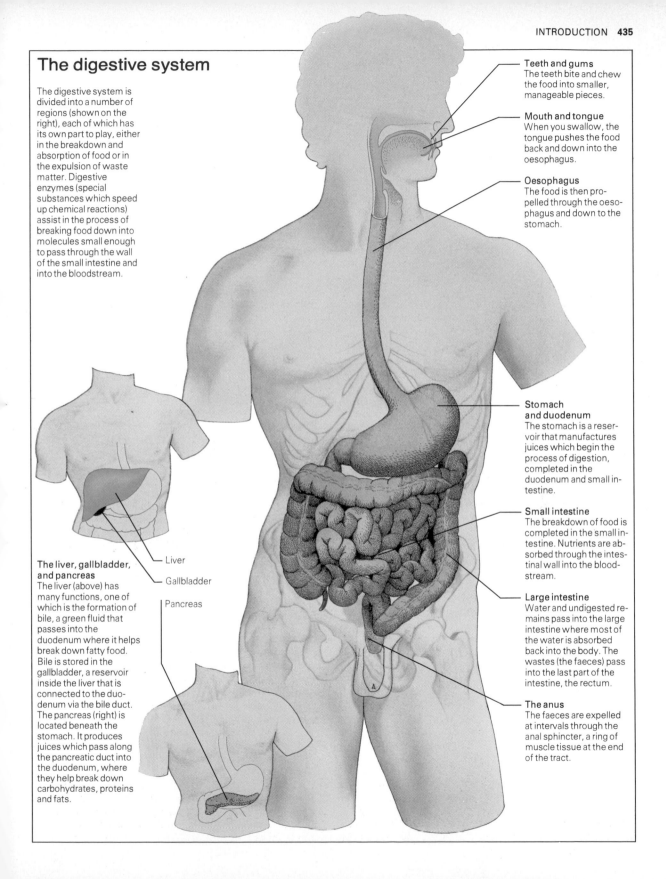

Teeth and gums
The teeth bite and chew the food into smaller, manageable pieces.

Mouth and tongue
When you swallow, the tongue pushes the food back and down into the oesophagus.

Oesophagus
The food is then propelled through the oesophagus and down to the stomach.

Stomach and duodenum
The stomach is a reservoir that manufactures juices which begin the process of digestion, completed in the duodenum and small intestine.

Small intestine
The breakdown of food is completed in the small intestine. Nutrients are absorbed through the intestinal wall into the bloodstream.

Large intestine
Water and undigested remains pass into the large intestine where most of the water is absorbed back into the body. The wastes (the faeces) pass into the last part of the intestine, the rectum.

The anus
The faeces are expelled at intervals through the anal sphincter, a ring of muscle tissue at the end of the tract.

Liver

Gallbladder

Pancreas

The liver, gallbladder, and pancreas
The liver (above) has many functions, one of which is the formation of bile, a green fluid that passes into the duodenum where it helps break down fatty food. Bile is stored in the gallbladder, a reservoir inside the liver that is connected to the duodenum via the bile duct. The pancreas (right) is located beneath the stomach. It produces juices which pass along the pancreatic duct into the duodenum, where they help break down carbohydrates, proteins and fats.

Teeth and gums

The main function of your teeth is to break up the food you eat into manageable pieces which can be easily swallowed. Despite their appearance, teeth are just as much living structures as any other part of the body.

The pulp in the middle of each tooth receives a rich supply of blood vessels and has nerves that sense heat, cold, pressure, and pain. A hard substance called dentine surrounds the pulp. On the crown of the tooth (the part above the gum), the dentine is covered by an even harder substance, enamel.

The root of the tooth (the part buried in the gum) is covered by a sensitive bone-like material called cementum. Shock-absorbent periodontal tissue lines the bony socket of each tooth, preventing the skull and jawbone from being jarred by biting and chewing.

Enamel is the hardest substance in the body. Even so, acids produced by the action of bacteria on sugar erode the enamel and cause dental decay. Good oral hygiene and limited intake of sugary foods will minimize decay and other tooth and gum disorders.

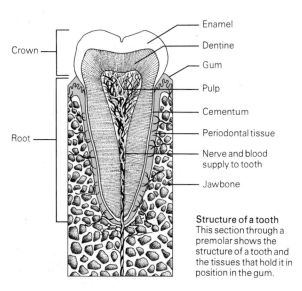

Enamel
Dentine
Gum
Pulp
Cementum
Periodontal tissue
Nerve and blood supply to tooth
Jawbone

Crown
Root

Structure of a tooth
This section through a premolar shows the structure of a tooth and the tissues that hold it in position in the gum.

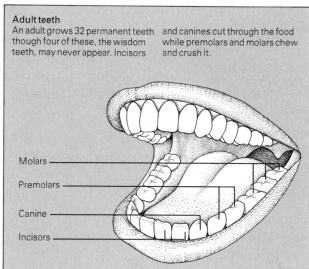

Adult teeth
An adult grows 32 permanent teeth though four of these, the wisdom teeth, may never appear. Incisors and canines cut through the food while premolars and molars chew and crush it.

Molars
Premolars
Canine
Incisors

Dental decay
(caries)

If you pass the tip of your tongue over your teeth some hours after brushing them, you can feel patches of a slightly rough, sticky substance. This substance, called *dental*

plaque, consists of mucus, food particles, and bacteria, and forms mainly between the teeth and where the teeth meet the gums. The bacteria in the plaque break down the sugar in food, and in the process form acid. The acid erodes the tooth's enamel, forming a minute cavity – the beginnings of dental decay.

If the decay is not treated, the acid eats slowly through the enamel into the dentine beneath. Dentine contains minute canals leading to the pulp, and bacteria pass through the canals and inflame the pulp. The body responds by sending more white blood cells to the pulp to combat the bacteria. As the blood vessels enlarge to accommodate the extra white cells, they press on the nerves within the tooth, causing toothache. If decay is untreated the infected pulp will eventually die (see *Dead teeth*, opposite). This will end

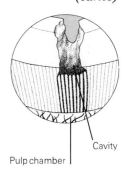

Cavity
Pulp chamber

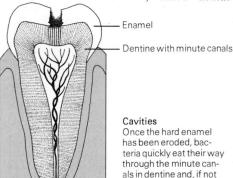

Enamel
Dentine with minute canals

Cavities
Once the hard enamel has been eroded, bacteria quickly eat their way through the minute canals in dentine and, if not treated, eventually reach the pulp chamber.

the toothache but may lead to formation of an *abscess* (see *Abscesses in teeth*, p.439).

What are the symptoms?

In the early stages of decay the main symptom is mild toothache when you eat something sweet, or very hot or cold. If the decay continues you may experience an unpleasant taste coming from the tooth – a result of stagnant food and bacteria in the cavity.

If the later stages of decay are reached, the pulp becomes inflamed, and you may suffer persistent pain after eating sweet, hot, or cold food. You may also have a sharp stabbing pain, especially when you lie down. Sometimes it is difficult to locate the painful tooth.

How common is the problem?

Dental decay is one of the most common ailments of mankind, particularly in countries where people consume large amounts of sugar. In Britain, by the time a child is 5 he or she has had on average 3 teeth decayed, filled, or extracted. Among the adult population about 30 per cent of people have no natural teeth – in contrast with the figure of only 14 per cent in the United States.

What are the risks?

Tooth decay generally presents no serious danger to health. But there is a risk for people suffering from a heart disease; this could be worsened if bacteria from a dead tooth entered the bloodstream (see *Bacterial endocarditis*, p.394). Also, if you suffer from a disease that affects blood clotting, such as *haemophilia* (p.424), you should have a tooth extracted only in hospital.

What should be done?

Keep dental decay to a minimum by taking good care of your teeth (see *Keeping your teeth and gums healthy*, p.438). Brush them regularly, reduce your sugar intake, use fluoride toothpaste, and pay regular visits to your dentist. *X-rays* taken every year or so will reveal any small cavities under fillings.

What is the treatment?

Self-help: Prevention of decay is of paramount importance. By the time that symptoms cause distress, little self-help is possible. Pain-relieving tablets such as aspirin may provide some relief until you can arrange an urgent visit to the dentist.

Professional help: The dentist may place in the cavity a temporary sedative dressing or filling containing oil of cloves and zinc oxide. When the inflammation has subsided, the temporary filling is replaced by a permanent one. If the decay is advanced it may be necessary to clean out the pulp cavity and put in a filling, or even extract the tooth (see *Going to the dentist*, p.447).

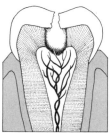

Acid erodes cavity

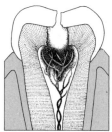

Acid eats through to pulp

Pulp becomes inflamed

Dead teeth

At the heart of every healthy tooth is the pulp, a living tissue that makes the tooth sensitive to heat, cold, pressure, and pain. When the pulp dies, the tooth dies.

The pulp may die after *dental decay* (opposite) has penetrated to it, or sometimes after a blow to the tooth. But occasionally it can die for no apparent reason. No symptoms signal the death of a tooth (other than the ceasing of pain in a decayed tooth); and you may not know you have a dead tooth until your dentist tells you at a check-up. Eventually, most dead teeth turn slightly grey.

What should be done?

Once a dead tooth has been detected, your dentist may decide to treat it. There is a risk, especially after dental decay, that poisonous substances and bacteria from the dead pulp will seep out through the root and cause an *abscess* (see *Abscesses in teeth*, p.439).

What is the treatment?

As a dead tooth can continue to function efficiently, there is usually no reason for it to be extracted unless it is badly decayed. The dentist usually drills a hole into the tooth, cleans it out, disinfects it, and fills the pulp chamber and the canal in the root – a process called root-canal treatment. Any cavities in the crown of the tooth are filled in the normal way. For details of these various treatments see *Going to the dentist*, p.447.

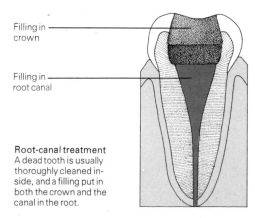

Filling in crown

Filling in root canal

Root-canal treatment
A dead tooth is usually thoroughly cleaned inside, and a filling put in both the crown and the canal in the root.

Keeping your teeth and gums healthy

Anyone who eats a normal Western diet will find it almost impossible to prevent tooth decay completely. This is due mainly to the enormous quantities of sugar that are part of Western food. You can, however, cut decay to a minimum and keep your teeth in a healthy condition until old age if you take the steps illustrated here. Regular brushing, the use of dental floss, and a reduction in the sugar content of your diet will all prove worthwhile.

Brushing your teeth

Brush your teeth from side to side (right) and up and down (far right) in a circular movement. Use a small toothbrush so that you can get into all the crevices. There are no hard and fast rules on exactly how you brush so

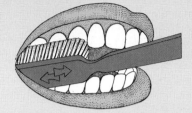

long as you clean your teeth thoroughly and remove all plaque. Disclosing tablets (see below) will reveal any plaque. Do not stop brushing your gums if they bleed; regular brushing will improve this.

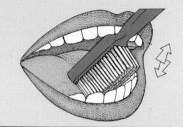

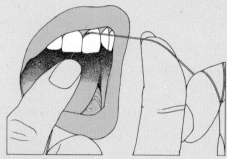

Using wooden points

Wooden points can be used for removing plaque (below). If you are not careful, however, you may damage your gums. Take advice from your dentist or dental hygienist.

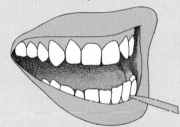

Sugar consumption

After you have eaten something sweet, your teeth are attacked for up to an hour by acid. Try to limit sweet foods to mealtimes and finish a meal with cheese. Cheese is particularly effective in neutralizing acid formation. Crisp foods, like celery and apples (below), may help keep your teeth clean but are not as effective as was once supposed.

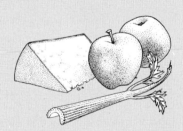

Using dental floss

Dental floss is thread which is drawn through the gaps between teeth (above) to remove plaque and food particles. Take about 500mm (18in) of dental floss and wind most of it around the first or second fingers on each hand. Draw the floss between the teeth and, with a sawing action, rub the sides of each tooth one by one.

Fluoride

Fluoride, which hardens the enamel and reduces tooth decay, occurs in certain water supplies. Most dentists believe that the level of fluoride in the water should be at least 1.0 part per million. If the level is lower than this, fluoride tablets or drops might be recommended, especially for children under 12, as their teeth are still forming. However, keep tablets away from children as they are pleasantly flavoured and a large dose could make a child seriously ill. Your dentist will advise you on fluoridization. He or she may apply a fluoride jelly or prescribe a mouth wash as well as advising fluoride toothpaste.

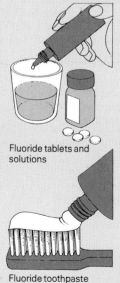

Fluoride tablets and solutions

Fluoride toothpaste

Regular dental visits

See your dentist regularly from an early age (below). An inspection every 6 months will ensure that any cavity is filled before decay can spread, and that gum disease is treated before it becomes serious.

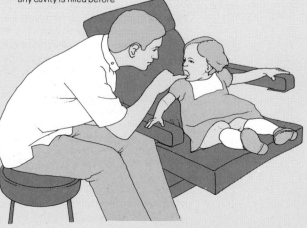

Disclosing tablets

These tablets contain a dye which stains plaque. Chew a tablet to colour the plaque, then remove the stains with floss and a toothbrush.

Abscesses in teeth

A tooth *abscess* is a pus-filled cavity in the tissue around the tip of the root, which is embedded in the jawbone. The abscess usually forms when a tooth is decaying or dead; poisonous products of the tooth's dead pulp, together with bacteria, are present in the pulp chamber and the root canal and can easily infect the surrounding jawbone.

If the abscess is not treated it eats into the jawbone until it has eroded a small canal, or sinus, through the bone and its overlying gum. Just before the canal reaches the surface of the gum, it forms a swelling – a gumboil.

What are the symptoms?

The abscess aches persistently or throbs, and the tooth usually feels extremely painful when you bite or chew. If the gumboil bursts, foul-tasting pus drains into the mouth and the pain may lessen. The glands in your neck may swell and become tender, and the side of the face may swell. Often your temperature rises and you feel generally unwell.

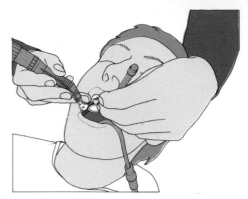

Treating an abscess
When you have a tooth abscess, your dentist will try to save the tooth. A small hole will be drilled through the crown (above) so that the pus is released. The dentist will then clean out the pulp chamber, disinfect it, and put in a temporary filling.

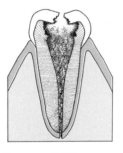 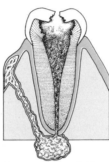

How a gumboil forms
If dental decay is not treated, the pulp may become infected and pus forms (above left). Pus in the base of the tooth develops into an abscess and seeps out through the root of the tooth. The pus then eats through the jawbone, eroding a channel called a sinus, to emerge in the gum as a painful swelling known as a gumboil (above right).

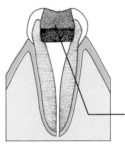

Filling the pulp chamber
At a later visit your dentist will fill the pulp chamber and the drilled hole with a permanent filling (left).

Filling

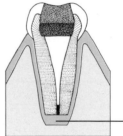

Apicectomy
Occasionally a dentist will perform an apicectomy. This is a small operation by which the infected tissue at the base of the tooth is removed (left).

Infected tissue removed

How common is the problem?

Anyone who does not visit the dentist regularly is likely to have a tooth abscess at some time; a decayed tooth that is not treated will die (see *Dead teeth*, p.437), and some dead teeth eventually cause abscesses.

What are the risks?

If the abscess is not treated by a dentist or doctor, there is a slight risk that the infection could spread via the bloodstream and cause generalized *blood poisoning* (p.421).

What should be done?

See a dentist as soon as possible. If it is past dental-surgery hours and the abscess is extremely painful or enlarging rapidly, see your doctor, who may prescribe an *antibiotic* to prevent the infection from spreading further; visit the dentist at the earliest opportunity.

What is the treatment?

Self-help: Take aspirins to provide some relief from the pain. Rinse your mouth every hour with salt water; this may hasten the bursting of the gumboil and helps to wash away any pus.

Professional help: The dentist will probably extract a badly affected back tooth or a milk tooth. To save a front tooth, the dentist drills a small hole through the crown and into the pulp chamber. This releases the pressurized pus, and, therefore, the pain. The dentist cleans out, disinfects, and fills the pulp chamber with a temporary filling. At a later visit, if the infection has not returned, the dentist fills the pulp chamber and the drilled hole. About six months later *X-rays* of the area are taken to make sure that new bone and tissue are growing into the abscess cavity.

In a few cases the abscess does not clear up and a small infected cavity remains, and your dentist may have to carry out a small operation called an *apicectomy*. After deadening the gum with a local anaesthetic, the dentist cuts away the bone covering the tip of the root, removes the infected tissue, and fills the root canal. In rare cases even this treatment fails to clear up the trouble, and the tooth may have to be extracted.

Discoloured teeth

Teeth may become discoloured – as distinct from the slight yellowing that occurs with age – for a variety of reasons. Smoking can cause brown surface staining; the death of a tooth can turn it grey throughout. Certain drugs, such as tetracycline, can cause faulty enamel formation if taken in large doses during childhood. Severe attacks of certain childhood infections, such as whooping cough or measles, can produce patches of discoloration. And grossly excessive amounts of fluoride in the water, as found in some parts of Africa, can cause *fluorosis* – white or brown markings in the teeth; this does not happen, of course, in areas where a controlled amount of fluoride is added to the water supply to reduce tooth decay.

What is the treatment?
If the discoloration is superficial, the dentist will clean the tooth with a rotary polisher and polishing paste. Deeper discoloration is treated by bonding a tough white plastic facing or porcelain crown to the tooth. If a grey dead tooth is brittle, often because it has been root-filled, the crown may be ground down to gum level and replaced with a post crown (for details of all these procedures see *Going to the dentist*, p.447).

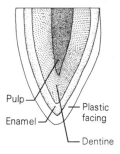

Treating a discoloured tooth
One possible treatment for a discoloured tooth is to cover it with either a plastic facing or a porcelain crown. The covering of the tooth is closely matched to that of the neighbouring teeth.

Pulp — Enamel — Plastic facing — Dentine

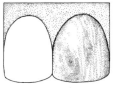
Discoloured tooth

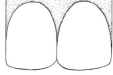
Treated discoloured tooth

Crowded and badly occluded teeth

In the ideal set of teeth, the teeth are straight, regularly spaced, and exactly the right size for the jaws. The ideal relationship of the upper and lower teeth when closed (which is called the *occlusion*) is that the upper teeth slightly overlap the lower, with the points of the molars alternating. However, very few people have perfect teeth. One reason for this is that we inherit different characteristics from each parent, and sometimes the two do not match. For example, if the teeth are too big for the jaws, the result is crowding of the teeth; they can develop only by sloping backwards or forwards or by overlapping their neighbours. If the teeth are too small for the jaws, the result is gapped teeth. If the lower

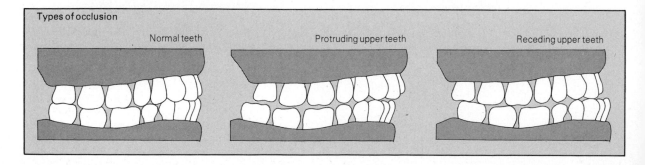

Types of occlusion

Normal teeth   Protruding upper teeth   Receding upper teeth jaw is smaller than the upper, and the lips are also too small, the teeth in the upper jaw protrude (this is sometimes called a faulty occlusion or *malocclusion*).

It is not only heredity that causes irregularity of teeth. Crowding is sometimes the result of premature loss of milk teeth through decay. For example, when milk molar teeth are lost early, the permanent molar teeth move along the jawbone to fill the gaps. As a result, when the permanent premolars and canines appear, between the ages of 11 and 13, they are crowded out of the natural arch of the teeth. And in some cases, teeth fail to appear at all (see *Problems of missing teeth*, p.442). Sometimes the crowding that takes place when the second teeth appear is only temporary. This is particularly so with the lower front teeth; the jaw will often grow enough to relieve the crowding.

In the normal cases of crowding described, there is a slightly increased risk of dental decay and gum disease because it is more difficult to keep crowded teeth clean.

How common is the problem?

At least 30 per cent of young teenagers would benefit from treatment of crowded teeth; it would help them to keep their teeth and gums' cleaner and chew food more efficiently, and improve the appearance of the mouth.

What should be done?

If you are an adult with a minor problem such as a few teeth crowded or twisted, the dentist will probably tell you that the condition can be corrected only with much time and trouble. If the problem is severe, you will have to accept that there is no easy remedy. If the appearance of your teeth causes you psychological problems, you may wish to undergo one or more major operations to correct the condition. On the other hand, you may simply learn to live with the condition, gaining encouragement from the way that people with more severe problems have come to terms with them.

If your children are developing crowded or badly occluded teeth, they should see a dentist. Treatment is most effective during childhood and early adolescence, when teeth and jaws are still growing and developing.

What is the treatment?

In the case of children, help them to help themselves. As always, all the family should guard against dental decay by following the rules for *Keeping your teeth and gums healthy* (p.438). Your own dentist may be able to treat minor crowding, but major treatment is best carried out by an *orthodontist*, who specializes in correcting various irregularities of the teeth.

The orthodontist will take *X-rays* to check that all the second teeth are forming and are likely to emerge. If crowding seems likely, one treatment is to extract a neighbouring tooth that has already appeared, to provide space for the new tooth.

The basic treatment for irregular teeth is to use an appliance on them over a period of months. The appliance (often called a "plate" or "brace") is anchored by fitting it round several teeth. It often has springs that exert continuous force on a tooth, twisting it, or pushing it backwards or forwards, or

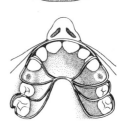

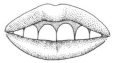

Treatment for crowded teeth The treatment for crowded teeth takes time and will involve the use of a plate. Careful cleaning of the teeth is essential as food and bacteria are easily trapped underneath the plate. If the front teeth protrude to such an extent that the lips cannot be closed in the ordinary way (top right), the premolars are removed to make room for the front teeth which are pulled back by a plate (middle right). When the treatment is complete the lips and teeth are able to come together normally (bottom right). An improvement in speech may also be noticeable.

moving it sideways through the jaw, as the case demands, so that it becomes regularly aligned. This process is most effective during childhood and adolescence, before the jawbone matures and hardens.

An appliance can trap *plaque*, so any person who wears one must take especial care to clean both teeth and appliance thoroughly after every meal.

Appliances are often used when a child's upper incisors are protruding and the canines are prominent and crowded. In such cases, the orthodontist will take casts of the teeth and X-rays to look for teeth that have not emerged. The child may first need some premolars extracted; then an appliance is fitted to move the canines into the correct position. Later, a new appliance will be made, to pull back the upper incisors so there is no gap between them and the canines. Such treatment starts about the age of 10 to 13, lasts up to 24 months, and calls for perseverance

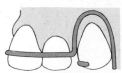

Retainer plate in position
This device holds the teeth in their new position.

by both child and parent. The final part of the treatment is to fit another appliance, called a "retainer plate", for 6 to 18 months, to hold all the teeth in their new positions while the jawbone hardens around them.

For an adult with a minor problem, extractions and/or an appliance are used. However, whereas a child quickly adjusts to wearing an appliance, most adults are embarrassed by wearing one and the treatment takes much longer in a mature, hardened jawbone.

If, as an adult, you suffer psychological stress because of crowded or badly occluded teeth, it is possible to have corrective surgery, in which pieces of the jawbone and some teeth are repositioned.

Problems of missing teeth

Permanent (second) teeth that are missing from a child's mouth can cause dental trouble in later life unless steps are taken to prevent or treat the condition.

A child's second teeth may be missing for one of three reasons:

1. The most common reason is that they may have been lost through early decay or an accident. Molars and premolars are the teeth most susceptible to early decay.

2. They may have failed to develop. This happens most commonly with the upper side incisors and the premolars.

3. They may have developed but have been *impacted* – prevented from emerging above

Problems caused by missing teeth
If teeth are missing (in this case from the lower jaw) the corresponding tooth in the upper jaw tends to move downwards to fill the gap, and the teeth around the gap tilt. Chewing becomes difficult and decay is likely to set in as the teeth are difficult to clean.

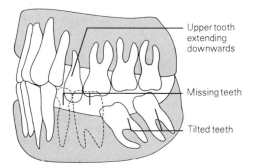

Upper tooth extending downwards

Missing teeth

Tilted teeth

the gum by the root of an adjacent tooth. Among the teeth most commonly impacted are the upper canines, the premolars, and the wisdom teeth.

Even if a child loses only one molar through decay, this can cause several problems in later life. One is that the corresponding molar in the other jaw will have too much space into which to emerge and may interfere with chewing. When you chew, your jaw moves from side to side as well as up and down, and if a molar slots into a space in the row of teeth above or below it, it checks the sideways motion of the jaw. As this results in food not being chewed thoroughly, the molar will probably have to be extracted.

Another common problem is that, because the teeth on either side of the missing molar are robbed of their supporting pressure, they gradually twist or tilt in the gum. Sometimes the missing molar and twisted teeth make the child avoid eating on that side of the mouth. Very rarely, the extra chewing on one side of the mouth may strain the joints of the jaw and make eating painful.

Other teeth naturally tend to grow into the spaces left by missing teeth. To do so, they will emerge too much from the gum or grow at an angle. This can produce *crowded or badly occluded teeth* (p.440). In biting or chewing, the teeth do not close together correctly, placing stresses on the teeth and jaw.

A more common danger that can result from teeth growing into gaps at an angle is that cleaning these areas may be difficult and food may become wedged in the spaces that are formed and go bad; this can lead to *dental decay* (p.436) and *gingivitis* (p.445).

What should be done?
Regular dental check-ups will enable the dentist to detect and treat any problems caused by missing teeth. If your child has lost a second tooth, consult the dentist. If you suffer from any of the long-term troubles described, you should also see the dentist.

What is the treatment?
The dentist may fill the gaps by fitting false teeth (see *Going to the dentist*, p.447). Or you may be sent to an *orthodontist*, a dentist who specializes in treating irregularly positioned teeth. The orthodontist uses the person's own teeth to fill any gaps – for example, by fitting appliances to other teeth to make them move into the gap; or by arranging for an operation to remove certain teeth and replace them in their correct position. The operation, known as a *transplantation*, requires a general anaesthetic and usually involves a hospital stay of 2 or 3 days.

To treat pain in the jaw caused by a bad occlusion, the dentist may fit an appliance known as a bite-plane or bite-raiser over the upper teeth and gums.

Problems with wisdom teeth

The rearmost teeth in each side of the jaw are the wisdom teeth (see diagram below). In most people the four wisdom teeth appear between the ages of 17 and 21, but in some people one or more never develop. This is nothing to worry about. In fact, it may well be an advantage, as the emergence of wisdom teeth often causes problems; and, even when they form normally, they are more difficult to clean, and are therefore prone to decay. Sometimes the wisdom tooth emerges at an angle, and the space between it and the next tooth becomes a place where food particles are trapped and stagnate. Quite often, the wisdom tooth fails to emerge properly because it becomes *impacted* – trapped by the tooth next to it. Around an impacted tooth, the gum forms a pocket in which food tends to gather and go bad. Bacteria then produce a painful infection, called *pericoronitis*, in the area around the tooth.

If a wisdom tooth simply fails to appear, there will normally not be any symptoms. If it emerges at an angle and forms a stagnation area for food particles, you may have an unpleasant taste in the mouth and bad breath.

The main symptoms of pericoronitis are pain when you bite on the area, and an unpleasant taste. There will probably also be swelling around the tooth. If you have any of these symptoms, see your dentist or doctor as soon as possible.

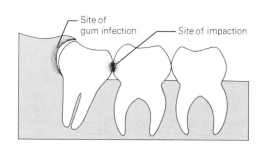

Position of wisdom teeth
Wisdom teeth are the back teeth, located behind the first two molars in both the upper and the lower jaw (left).

Molars

Wisdom teeth

Impacted wisdom tooth
A wisdom tooth can become impacted when it grows at an angle against the adjacent tooth (right). This tooth may be removed to allow the wisdom tooth to grow unimpeded (far right).

Impacted wisdom tooth

Adjacent tooth removed

Gum infection caused by an impacted wisdom tooth
If an impacted wisdom tooth is partially erupted (right), food and bacteria can become trapped under the gum flap causing decay and bad breath.

Site of gum infection

Site of impaction

What is the treatment?
Self-help: You can obtain relief from the pain by taking aspirin, or rinsing the area round the tooth with salt water.

Professional help: Your dentist or doctor will prescribe an *antibiotic* to clear up the infection but this will usually give only temporary relief, and the long-term solution is to have the wisdom tooth extracted. Your dentist will take *X-rays* to determine the position of the tooth. If it lies at a difficult angle, or if other wisdom teeth are affected, you will probably go into hospital and have the extraction done under a general anaesthetic.

Denture problems

Most modern dentures look natural and fit well; but no denture can be as efficient and comfortable as your own teeth. With natural teeth, the forces of biting and chewing are absorbed by the teeth, the roots of the teeth, and the special shock-absorbent material called periodontal tissue lining the sockets in the jawbone. But with dentures, the forces are absorbed in unnatural ways. The most critical of these is the pressure that a baseplate (false gums) places on the ridges of the natural gums, especially if the dentures are worn day and night. This pressure can produce inflammation of the gums and eventually cause *mouth ulcers* (p.450).

The baseplate of a partial denture also puts an abnormal sideways load on the natural teeth round which the baseplate fits. Partial dentures, especially badly-fitting ones, have the further disadvantage of trapping food particles, which can cause *dental decay* (p.436) and often lead to *gingivitis* (p.445) or even *destructive gum disease* (p.446).

The mouth fungus that causes *oral thrush* (p.451) can also lead to a condition known as denture sore mouth, particularly if you have been taking *antibiotics* or if an illness has lowered your resistance to infection.

What are the symptoms?
Early symptoms of excessive pressure on the ridges of the gums are pain when the dentures are in place, especially when you are eating, and red, inflamed gums. If the inflammation persists, the gums become deep red and soft, and bleed easily – after scratching by a toothbrush, for example. If the denture rubs the gums, a mouth ulcer may form on that spot.

Biting and chewing with false teeth
With the loss of your teeth you lose periodontal tissue, a shock-absorbent material that lines the sockets of the jawbones (upper diagram). Dentures can press against your gums (lower diagram), leading to soreness, inflammation of the gums, and mouth ulcers. Regular visits to the dentist and proper care of your dentures will minimize the problems.

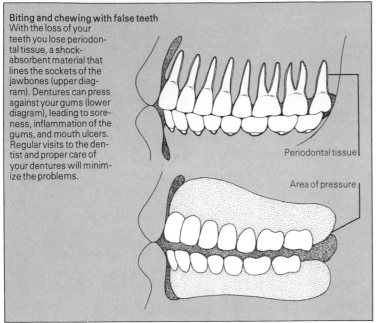

Periodontal tissue

Area of pressure

Looking after your dentures
Always remove your dentures at night and keep them in a glass of water containing a cleansing agent so that they do not dry out and warp (top right). Clean your dentures daily, making sure that all food and plaque is removed (middle right). Your dentist will show you the best method. It is vital to remember to clean any natural teeth thoroughly (bottom right), especially where teeth and gums meet.

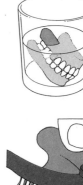

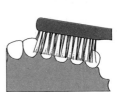

After an old denture has been worn for many years, hard, pale pads (*denture granulomas*) form at the main pressure points, especially those under the edges of the denture.

Further symptoms arise when the gums and jawbone shrink – which is bound to happen after a few years of continuous pressure, even if the denture has caused no other problems. You then have to close your mouth further to bite properly – and even further if the false teeth are worn down. Symptoms of gum and jawbone shrinkage include a loose denture, sunken cheeks, and a protruding lower jaw. Much more rarely, there are pains in the jawbone joints due to the extra movement needed to bite.

The symptoms of denture sore mouth are redness, softness of the part of the palate normally covered by your denture, and inflammation or cracked skin at the corners of the mouth.

What are the risks?
A long-term risk is that if your jaw and mouth movements change a great deal to cope with the slow shrinkage of jawbone and gums, you will find it difficult to adapt to new dentures when you eventually need them.

What should be done?
You should have full dentures checked by a dentist at least every two years. If you have a partial denture or other false teeth, go to the dentist more often – once every six months –

to safeguard your natural teeth. If you have pain, ulcers, bleeding in your mouth, or denture sore mouth, consult your dentist within a few days.

What is the treatment?
Self-help: Remove dentures at night to give the gum tissues a regular rest period, and keep them in a glass of water so that they do not dry out and warp. Partial dentures may feel a little tight when inserted in the morning, but this is normal and the feeling disappears after a few minutes. Clean dentures daily – your dentist will tell you how – and clean natural teeth and gums thoroughly.

If you have denture sore mouth, ensure you keep your dentures scrupulously clean, and soak them overnight in a solution of proprietary *antiseptic* made for the purpose.
Professional help: The useful life of dentures varies greatly – from six months to five years or more – depending on how well your gums and jaws keep their shape. When your dentures become worn or ill-fitting, the dentist will make new ones or, in cases when the false teeth are not too worn, will adapt the existing baseplate to your new gum shape.

To treat denture sore mouth, your dentist will prescribe antifungal lozenges which should clear up the problem in 10 days or so.

A few people have persistent problems coping with dentures, and never really adapt to them. It also becomes difficult to adapt to new dentures as you grow older.

Gingivitis

Gingivitis is the medical name for inflamed and swollen gums. It is caused by *dental plaque* (a sticky deposit of food particles and bacteria) forming at the base of the teeth.

Bacterial poisons from the plaque create microscopic ulcers at the edge of the gum, which becomes infected and swollen. As the gum margin swells, a pocket forms between the gum and tooth. This becomes a trap for more plaque, the gum swells even more, the pocket deepens, and if not treated the condition gradually worsens.

Plaque and calculus formation
An underlying cause of gingivitis is plaque and calculus formation. If plaque is not removed from the teeth it builds up. The bacteria in the deeper layers die, and mineralization and hardening occur. The hard mass which results is called calculus and it can only be removed by a dentist. If you visit your dentist regularly and clean your teeth properly, calculus will not form.

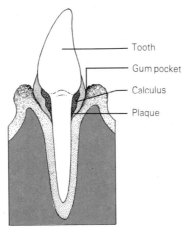

Tooth

Gum pocket

Calculus

Plaque

What are the symptoms?
Healthy gums are pale pink and firm, and have a stippled appearance. They should not bleed, or bleed only slightly, when cleaned with a toothbrush. In gingivitis, the gums become red, soft, and shiny, as well as swollen. They bleed easily at the slightest damage – by a toothbrush, for example.

How common is the problem?
Gingivitis is extremely common. About 9 out of 10 adults have it, though usually in a mild form. Pregnant women and diabetics are particularly susceptible. The disorder is less common in children.

What are the risks?
The main risk is that, unless checked, gingivitis will almost certainly lead to *destructive gum disease* (p.446). *Vincent's disease* (p.452) is another possibility.

Nothing more than mild gingivitis is likely to develop if you keep your teeth and gums clean and have regular dental check-ups. If you have not taken this care and gingivitis has developed, see your dentist.

What is the treatment?
Self-help: Brush your teeth regularly and use dental floss at least once a day, to remove all plaque. To see how successfully you are doing this, use a disclosing tablet (see *Keeping your teeth and gums healthy*, p.438).

Professional help: In serious cases, the dentist or dental hygienist may advise an antibacterial mouthwash and remove plaque and *calculus* – a hard chalky deposit which traps plaque – from the base of your teeth. Calculus is removed with a scaler (see *Going to the dentist*, p.447). The dentist or hygienist will also show you the most effective way to use a toothbrush and floss.

Virtually all cases of gingivitis respond to treatment, and the gums return to normal. It is then up to you to keep your teeth and gums clean if you wish to avoid further attacks and the risk of destructive gum disease.

How gum disease progresses from neglect

Gum disease may occur as a direct result of inadequate cleaning. Once plaque builds up on your teeth, gum disease will probably set in. Gums may become inflamed and sore and will remain so until the plaque is removed. If this is not done, irreparable damage may leave only one course of action; extraction of teeth. Proper cleaning will prevent damage from plaque.

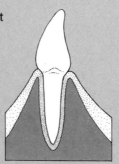

When the gums are healthy, they fit firmly around the base of the tooth. They are pink and will not normally bleed.

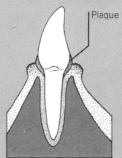

Plaque

If plaque is allowed to build up between the teeth and gums, painful inflammation may result.

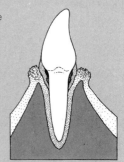

The plaque finds its way between teeth and gums, and the bone and fibres holding the tooth in position are gradually destroyed.

Destructive gum disease

Destructive gum disease is the end result of *gingivitis* (p.445) that has been neglected. In gingivitis, *dental plaque* and a hard substance called *calculus* collect in the pockets between the swollen gums and the base of the teeth. The plaque contains bacteria that over the years eat into the bone surrounding and supporting the teeth. Eventually, the bony sockets can become so eroded that the teeth become loose.

Damage caused by gum disease
If the process of gum disease is not checked, the bacteria in the plaque will eat into the bone and tissue that surrounds and supports the tooth. Eventually the tooth will become loose in its socket. When gum disease has reached this stage, there may be no other alternative than extraction.

Loose tooth
Gum pocket
Calculus
Plaque

What are the symptoms?

The pockets between gums and teeth gradually deepen. The plaque in the pockets tastes foul and causes bad breath. As the disease progresses, the teeth loosen in their sockets and tapping them produces a dull thud, instead of the sharp noise of firmly-set teeth. More and more cementum (the sensitive tissue covering the root of the tooth) is exposed. The cementum aches when very hot, very cold, or sweet food is eaten. Sometimes an *abscess* forms deep inside a pocket and erodes its way into the jawbone.

Treatment of gum disease
With severe gum disease a deep pocket may develop where the gum meets the tooth (upper diagram). One type of treatment for this problem involves cutting the pocket away (lower diagram) so that the area around the tooth can be kept clean and free from plaque. The gum usually grows back so long as the area is kept clean.

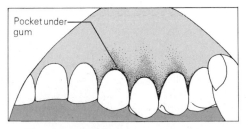
Pocket under gum

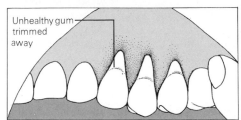
Unhealthy gum trimmed away

How common is the problem?

Adults lose more teeth from destructive gum disease than from dental decay. Statistics show that in Britain among adults aged 16 to 35, 2 out of 3 have some degree of destructive gum disease; it is even more common among the middle-aged.

What are the risks?

Without great care, you can lose all your teeth and will need dentures; you may then have *denture problems* (p.443). A spreading abscess can cause problems of its own (see *Abscesses in teeth*, p.439).

What should be done?

Destructive gum disease can be halted at any time before the advanced stage – so see a dentist as soon as you notice any of the symptoms described. To discover how advanced the disease is, the dentist usually assesses the depth of the pockets by a dental examination and takes *X-rays* to discover the condition of the underlying bone.

What is the treatment?

Self-help: Follow the measures described in *Keeping your teeth and gums healthy* (p.438), paying special attention to the gums and bases of the teeth.

Professional help: If the disease is at an early stage, the dentist can keep it under control (provided you clean your teeth thoroughly) simply by treating any dental disorders that encourage plaque to form or persist.

If the pockets have become very deep, other treatment will be required. The usual treatment is some form of surgery on the gums. In a *gingivectomy*, a minor operation performed in a dental surgery or in a dental hospital, the gums are trimmed to reduce the depth of the pockets. After a gingivectomy, the gums are given a protective coating – usually of oil of cloves, zinc oxide, and cotton wool – which must stay in place for one or two weeks until the gums heal. The temporary coating should not prevent you from eating and drinking normally.

Other treatment is done at the dentist's. Sensitive parts of the teeth exposed by repeatedly brushing them in only one direction can be covered by plastic bonded on to the tooth to protect the underlying cementum. As an alternative, very sensitive cementum can be given a protective layer of fluoride varnish, or your dentist will prescribe a toothpaste that does the same job. Very loose teeth can be anchored with a device called a periodontal splint – a continuous plastic or gold backing along several teeth.

Going to the dentist: the examination

(continued overleaf)

How often should you go?

You should visit a dentist every six months or so. Regular inspections are necessary not only to minimize tooth decay but to check the health of your whole mouth. A neglected mouth, besides being vulnerable to the disorders described in this section, can create the risk of infections entering the bloodstream and so endanger general health. Dentures, like natural teeth, need regular inspection and all dentures eventually wear down and need replacing. If you have a full set of dentures, you should visit a dentist about once every two years.

(For details of how to find and sign on with a dentist, see *Dental care*, p.742.)

What happens at the examination?

The dentist first examines your mouth for signs of any disorders which are not confined to the teeth. Red, puffy gums indicate gingivitis or destructive gum disease; a white discoloration of the inside of the mouth can signify oral thrush, leukoplakia, or oral lichen planus.

The dentist then inspects your teeth with a mirror and a needle-shaped probe, looking for any colour changes that indicate decay or any crack that indicates the beginning of a cavity. Existing fillings are examined to see if any parts have been chipped off or if any fresh cavities are developing round the edge of a filling. The dentist may give you a disclosing mouthwash containing dye. This colours *dental plaque* – a film of food particles, mucus, and bacteria, that causes dental decay.

If you have dentures, they will be checked for fit and their effects on the supporting gums and any natural teeth will be examined.

During the examination, the dentist asks about your general health. Have you had a heart or chest condition, diabetes, or jaundice? Do you suffer from any allergies? Are you pregnant, or taking any tablets? The dentist must take certain precautions; a person with a heart condition who has a tooth extracted, or any other treatment that causes bleeding, runs the risk of contracting *bacterial endocarditis* (p.394). Diabetics who do not control their disease carefully can fall into a coma if they undergo stress in the dentist's chair; and if treatment of diabetics requires a general anaesthetic, it may have to be carried out in hospital. People who have had some types of jaundice may be symptomless carriers of hepatitis and need a blood test before the dentist decides how to treat them. Those with allergies often react to *antibiotic* drugs. If a woman is pregnant, the dentist will examine her gums with particular care for signs of gingivitis. And if you are taking any drugs, the dentist must ensure there can be no harmful reaction between them and a drug the dentist may want to give you.

Why are X-rays taken?

Every year or two, "bite-wing" *X-rays* will be taken to check for dental faults undetected during normal inspections. X-rays are also taken of dead teeth whose roots have been filled, to check that an *abscess* is not forming at the base. They are also used to assess the progress of any wisdom teeth and to show how much bone is supporting the teeth in destructive gum disease.

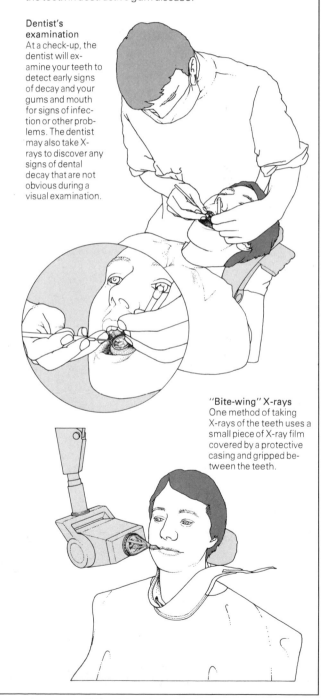

Dentist's examination
At a check-up, the dentist will examine your teeth to detect early signs of decay and your gums and mouth for signs of infection or other problems. The dentist may also take X-rays to discover any signs of dental decay that are not obvious during a visual examination.

"Bite-wing" X-rays
One method of taking X-rays of the teeth uses a small piece of X-ray film covered by a protective casing and gripped between the teeth.

Going to the dentist: scaling, polishing, fillings, and crowns

Scaling

Scaling is the process by which calculus is removed from the teeth. Here, an ultrasonic scaler is being used (right). The tip of the instrument vibrates 25,000 times a second and breaks up the calculus into thousands of tiny pieces.

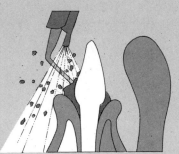

Polishing

Your dentist may polish your teeth with a specially adapted drill (right) when you go for an examination. This process will remove all the plaque as well as surface stains.

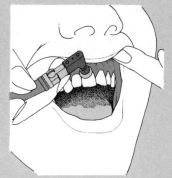

Fillings

When a tooth is partly decayed or chipped, the dentist replaces the damaged area with a filling. White plastic fillings are used on front teeth; silver amalgam (a mixture of silver, tin, and mercury) is generally used on back teeth. If the treatment is likely to cause pain, the dentist injects your gum with local anaesthetic. The decayed area is drilled away, and the hole is shaped to retain the filling securely. With a broken front tooth, the surface is roughened and the filling bonded to it. After you have had a local anaesthetic, you must take care when eating to avoid biting your lip and tongue if they are still numb.

Filling a tooth

The dentist will fill a tooth if the enamel has been damaged (right). This is because bacteria can destroy the dentine within and, if not checked, will finally attack the pulp.

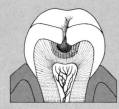

The dentist drills out a hole, removing all traces of decay or other damage (right). The hole is shaped so that the filling will not fall out.

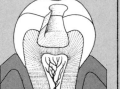

The hole is filled with an amalgam of silver, tin, and mercury (right). If the filling is to be easily visible, it will be made of a white filling of quartz in a plastic resin.

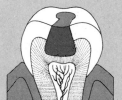

Fitting a post crown

Because of excessive decay or weakness, a tooth may not be strong enough to hold a crown. In such a case a post crown can be fitted.

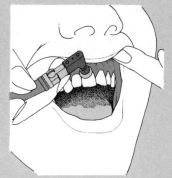

Tooth root (in gum)

Damaged portion

The tooth is trimmed down to the gum margin and the pulp is removed from the root canal which is then filled with antiseptic material.

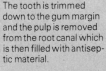

Cleaned-out root canal

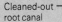

Trimmed tooth

A gold post is then fitted into the root. Once the post is secure a crown can be cemented onto it.

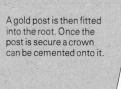

Post in root canal

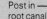

Crown

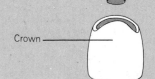

Crowns

When a tooth is severely decayed, broken, discoloured, or brittle, the dentist will usually make an artificial crown for it if the base of the tooth and the root are sound. Generally, a white porcelain crown is fitted on a tooth that can be seen. On back teeth, gold or a gold-platinum alloy is used, because of its strength. The treatment usually requires two or three visits, the first one or two to prepare the tooth. Between visits a temporary plastic or aluminium crown is worn.

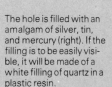

Fitting a crown

A cracked, heavily filled, or broken tooth (above) can be replaced by a crown. The remaining part of the tooth is shaped to receive the crown (above right). The crown, a hollow shell, is fitted over the shaped tooth and cemented in place (right).

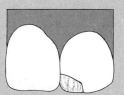

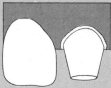

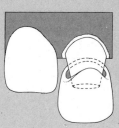

Going to the dentist: bridges, extractions, and dentures

Bridges

If you have a gap (or gaps) of anything up to about four teeth, flanked by sound natural teeth, you may need a bridge – an artificial tooth (or teeth) that bridges the gap. A space is left between the base of the bridge and the gum ridge so that you can clean the base of the bridge and the gum properly. Bridges at the front of the mouth are made of platinum alloy faced with porcelain; those at the back are usually made of gold or a gold-platinum alloy.

Extractions

There are several reasons for extracting a tooth. It may be too decayed or badly broken to be filled or crowned; it may be causing crowding or faulty occlusion; it may be loose because of advanced gum disease; or it may be preventing another tooth from emerging above the gum. Two injections of local anaesthetic are given before most extractions. A general anaesthetic may be used when the patient is a small child, when wisdom teeth are badly impacted, or for multiple extractions.

After an extraction you must not take alcohol, rinse out your mouth, take violent exercise, or probe the empty socket. If the socket bleeds persistently, use a clean, tightly folded handkerchief as a compress. Keep it in place for half an hour by clenching the teeth, and sit upright. If bleeding persists, contact your dentist.

Dentures

To replace many missing teeth, a partial denture is required. A full denture replaces all natural teeth. Dentures are made of tough plastic or are partly plastic and partly metal. Full dentures stay in place by resting on the gum ridges and also by suction in the case of upper dentures. On a partial denture, the baseplate (artificial gum) often has clasps that fit round natural teeth to help keep it in place.

Fitting a denture normally requires up to five visits. Impressions of the gums are taken; then wax bite blocks are fitted into the mouth, one for each jaw, and are adjusted to show the correct depth for the denture. The dentist discusses with you the size and colour of the false teeth. In most cases, a preliminary denture is made with a wax baseplate, and the dentist makes any necessary adjustments; after the denture is made, it is fitted and adjusted so that you bite evenly. At the final visit the dentist checks that your new teeth are working satisfactorily, and not causing soreness or ulcers.

Fitting a bridge

If a complete tooth is missing, the gap can be filled by building a bridge.

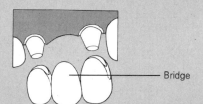

Missing tooth

The two teeth on either side of the gap are shaped so that they can receive a bridge holding the false tooth.

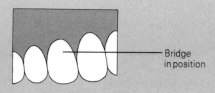

Bridge

The bridge is cemented to the two shaped teeth so that it is held firmly in position.

Bridge in position

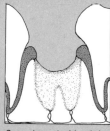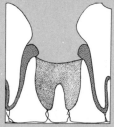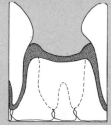

After a tooth extraction After a tooth is extracted (above), a blood clot forms in the socket.

Sometimes the blood clot may break down and this leaves what is known as a dry socket.

Eventually new bone will grow to fill the gap and gum will grow over this.

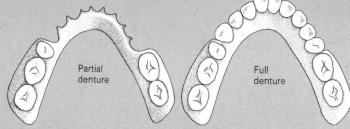

Partial denture

Full denture

Taking impressions of the teeth

To help with the making of dentures, impressions of the teeth are made in trays filled with a putty-like substance. The tray with a recess (right) is used for the lower teeth, while the other one is used for the upper teeth.

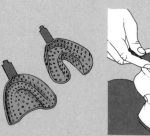

Mouth and tongue

The inside of your mouth is covered by a delicate elastic lining of mucous membrane. It is kept moist and lubricated by saliva, which is produced by three pairs of glands in the mouth. These are the sublingual glands (under the tongue), the submandibular glands (in the floor of the mouth), and the parotid glands (above the angle of the jaw).

The saliva runs along the salivary gland ducts into the mouth; production of saliva rises when you are about to eat and when you are actually eating.

The tongue has a complex system of muscles which enables it to move food around as it is chewed, and then to mould chewed food into a ball (*bolus*), ready for swallowing. The upper surface of the tongue is covered with hair-like projections called papillae, among which are clustered groups of cells sensitive to taste – the tastebuds. These distinguish four main types of flavour; sweet, salt, sour and bitter. Changes in the shape of the mouth, tongue and lips, in association with the vocal cords in the larynx, form the large variety of sounds necessary for speech.

The majority of disorders that affect the mouth and tongue are not serious and are simply treated. However, because of the faint possibility that an apparently harmless lump, ulcer, or sore spot may be a *malignant* tumour, any condition of the mouth or tongue that persists for more than three weeks should be seen by your doctor or dentist. As with teeth and gums, good oral hygiene will minimize mouth problems (see *Keeping your teeth and gums healthy*, p.438).

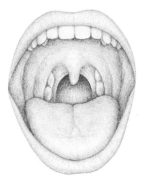

The mouth
The mouth is the first region of the digestive tract. The teeth crush the food into small pieces while saliva from the salivary glands lubricates it, making it easier to swallow. Food that is gulped down without adequate chewing takes longer to digest.

Mouth ulcers

See p.248, **Visual aids to diagnosis, 64**.

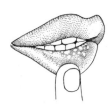

Mouth ulcers
Aphthous ulcers are the most common type of mouth ulcer. They are white, often painful, and may appear as clusters on the lower lip.

A mouth ulcer is a break in the lining of the mouth that uncovers the sensitive tissue beneath. All mouth ulcers look very much the same, but they vary considerably in their cause and seriousness. The two most common and painful types of ulcer are aphthous ulcers, which tend to occur when you are under stress, run down, or ill, and traumatic ulcers, which result from an injury to the lining of the mouth by, for example, a toothbrush, a rough denture, hot food, or biting the mouth or tongue.

Some ulcers are caused by infection, such as *cold sores* (opposite) in which blisters in the mouth eventually turn into ulcers. Rarely, an ulcer may be the first sign of a *tumour of the mouth or tongue* (p.454), or even of a more generalized disease such as *anaemia* (p.419) or *leukaemia* (p.426).

What are the symptoms?
You usually first become aware of an aphthous or traumatic ulcer when eating something spicy or acidic (such as a grapefruit) makes it smart. All ulcers look much the same; they can usually be seen in a mirror as pale yellow spots with red borders. Aphthous ulcers are small (2 or 3mm, roughly $\frac{1}{10}$ in, across), sometimes appear in clusters on the sides of the mouth, are painful, and last for up to 10 days. A traumatic ulcer is usually larger and lasts for a week or more. When a traumatic ulcer is caused by a rough tooth or denture, it will not heal until the cause is dealt with.

How common is the problem?
Mouth ulcers are very common; at any particular time, 1 person in 10 has one or more. Aphthous ulcers occur most often in adolescents and young adults, and they tend to appear more often in women (especially just before a period) compared to men.

What should be done?
The vast majority of mouth ulcers do not signify any major health problem and usually heal by themselves or with your own self-help. If you suspect that a jagged tooth or

rough denture is causing traumatic ulcers, consult your dentist. But if an ulcer fails to heal within three weeks, or if ulcers keep recurring, then see your doctor, who will examine you to detect any underlying condition. The doctor may take a blood sample for laboratory analysis, and you may have to enter hospital for a morning or afternoon to have a *biopsy* of the ulcer under a local anaesthetic. Laboratory examination of the ulcer tissue will show whether it signifies an underlying disorder, which will then be dealt with as necessary.

What is the treatment?
Self-help: Chemists sell various applications and lozenges that numb and protect the exposed tissue in the ulcer, thereby relieving the pain and healing the ulcer more quickly. An antiseptic mouthwash or warm, salt mouth rinses also help. Avoid eating spices (such as chilli) or sharp-tasting acidic food until the ulcer has healed over.
Professional help: To deal with troublesome and persistent aphthous ulcers, your doctor or dentist may prescribe a mouthwash or cream containing a *steroid* drug.

Cold sores
(herpes simplex)

See p.238,
Visual aids to diagnosis, 24.

Cold sores are caused by the virus herpes simplex. The infection occurs in two stages. In the first stage blisters form on the inside of the mouth, then develop into painful ulcers. The gums become swollen and deep red, and often the tongue is furred. You may have a raised temperature and feel generally unwell. The older you are, the more severe the infection; in young children, an attack is usually so mild it may pass unnoticed.

After the infection has cleared up, the virus lies dormant. Later, another infection (commonly a cold), or exposure to sunshine or wind, reactivates it. This is the second stage of the infection. A blister forms on the edge of the lip or nearby, and then bursts to become the typical encrusted cold sore.

Cold sores are very common and present no serious risks. The main danger is that, during the first infection when the body has no immunity or resistance to the virus, touching the ulcers and then your eye could cause formation of a *corneal ulcer* (p.316). Another risk is the development of the sores of *herpes genitalis* (p.613).

What is the treatment?
Mild cases of the first infection need no treatment. In severe cases the doctor will advise you to rest, take aspirins if you have a temperature, and paint the blisters with a prescribed antiviral agent. Cold sores always clear up naturally but if the blisters are painful or persist for more than three weeks, consult your doctor, who may prescribe the same ointment used for the initial blisters.

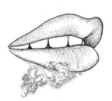

Site of cold sores
Most cold sores appear around the mouth. They may be accompanied by sensations of tingling and numbness which can precede or even follow their presence.

Oral thrush

Oral thrush is an outbreak of the fungus candida albicans, one of the many microbes which are usually present in small numbers in the mouth. If your natural resistance to infection is low through illness, or if a course of *antibiotics* has upset the natural balance between the microbes in the mouth, this fungus may multiply out of control. As it does so, it produces sore patches in the mouth and sometimes in the throat as well. The patches are creamy-yellow and slightly raised. If they are rubbed off, for example, when eating or cleaning your teeth, they leave a painful raw area. The fungus can also contribute to *denture problems* (p.443).

How common is the problem?
Many people have an attack of oral thrush at some time in their lives. It is most prevalent in very young children and elderly people. The same fungus can, in women, cause *vaginal thrush* (p.602). If you have the symptoms described, see your doctor within a day or so.

What is the treatment?
The doctor will examine you and may take a smear of the patch for laboratory analysis, or perhaps arrange for you to have blood tests as a hospital out-patient, to rule out the possibility of any serious underlying disease. Meanwhile the thrush will be treated by a course of antifungal lozenges, taken for up to 10 days. Oral thrush in itself is not serious and is quickly cleared by the above treatment, though it has a tendency to recur.

If you are a man, take care not to transfer the fungus to the vaginal area of your partner while you have an outbreak.

Leukoplakia

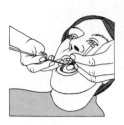

Taking a biopsy
Your dentist or doctor may remove a small piece of tissue from the area affected by leukoplakia, for laboratory analysis.

In leukoplakia, a part of the soft, delicate lining of the mouth or tongue thickens and hardens. This sometimes occurs to protect an area made sore by the repeated rubbing of a rough tooth or denture – or sometimes it appears as a protective reaction to the heat of inhaled tobacco smoke (when the condition is known as smoker's *keratosis*). In most cases, though, there is no obvious cause.

What are the symptoms?
The patch, which develops over a period of weeks, is white or grey and may be of any size. At first it causes no discomfort, but when it is well-formed it feels rough and stiff and may be sensitive to hot or spicy foods.

People of any age can develop the problem, but it is most common in the elderly. If you develop what appears to be leukoplakia, you should consult your dentist or doctor.

What is the treatment?
The treatment is to deal with any source of irritation that has caused the patch to form. This means a rough tooth or denture will be filed smooth, or, in the case of smoker's keratosis, you will be advised to give up smoking. This may be all that is needed to make the patch disappear.

If the problem has not cleared up within three weeks, your doctor may cut away the patch and arrange for it to be examined in a laboratory (*biopsy*) because in about 3 per cent of cases such patches are a sign of a tumour of the mouth (see *Tumours of the mouth and tongue*, p.454).

Oral lichen planus

Oral lichen planus is a change in the lining of the mouth. The actual nature of the change is variable. Most commonly the disorder starts as a number of small, pale pimples which gradually join to form a fine, white, lacy network of slightly raised tissue. In other cases the disorder takes the form of shiny, red, slightly raised patches. The changes occur most commonly on the insides of the cheeks and the sides of the tongue. Some sufferers complain of a sore mouth, and some have a dry, metallic taste; but a few remain unaware of the condition.

Oral lichen planus can be brought on by emotional stress, by patches of irritation in the mouth – such as those caused by ill-fitting dentures – or by poor oral hygiene; often, though, the cause is unclear.

How common is the problem?
Oral lichen planus is rare. It can affect any adult but occurs most often in middle-aged and elderly women. Half of those who suffer from it also have lichen planus on the skin (see *Lichen planus*, p.261).

What should be done?
Any colour or texture changes to the inside of the mouth that do not clear up within three weeks should be seen by your doctor, who by examining you will determine whether you have oral lichen planus. The best way to treat the disorder is to keep your mouth healthy by brushing your teeth and gums twice each day. If brushing is painful, try a very soft toothbrush, and use it gently. Ask your dentist to check that any dentures fit properly and have no rough spots. If the condition is irritating, the doctor will prescribe tablets or a mouthwash containing an anti-inflammatory *steroid* drug, to be sucked or used every few hours. This treatment usually causes the patches to shrink and they should eventually disappear within a few days.

Vincent's disease

Vincent's disease, sometimes called acute ulcerative gingivitis, is a painful bacterial infection and ulceration of the gums – usually the parts of the gum between the teeth. It can spread to other parts of the lining of the mouth if left untreated. The infection results from a combination of factors that include failure to clean the teeth and gums properly, throat infections, and smoking. It is often preceded by *gingivitis* (p.445).

What are the symptoms?
The symptoms appear over the course of a day or two. The gums become red, swollen, and sometimes so painful that eating is impossible. After a while, ulcers appear on the gums, which bleed. You may have a metallic taste in your mouth, and bad breath.

How common is the problem?
Vincent's disease is uncommon; it mainly affects young adults. If you have the symptoms of Vincent's disease, see your dentist or doctor as soon as possible.

What is the treatment?
A mouthwash is usually prescribed to relieve the pain and inflammation in the gums. After

Development of Vincent's disease
Vincent's disease may develop from gingivitis, when the gums become inflamed and painful (upper diagram). As Vincent's disease progresses ulcers appear in the mouth, especially on the gums and around the roots of teeth (lower diagram).

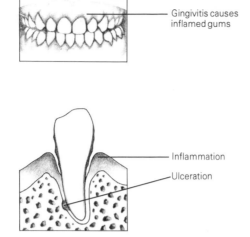

Gingivitis causes inflamed gums

Inflammation

Ulceration

a few days, when the inflammation has receded, the dentist can clean your teeth and gums with a scaler (see *Going to the dentist*, p.447, for further details). You may be put on a course of *antibiotics* to clear up the infection. Regular follow-up visits every two weeks or so – often to a dental hygienist – may be necessary in some cases.

When the disease has been eradicated, your dentist may advise minor surgery on the gums. This is because Vincent's disease causes scarring of the gums where they meet the teeth. The scarred tissue encourages trapped food and *dental plaque* to build up and this may lead to a recurrence of the problem. Trimming the gums to a smooth shape makes them easier to keep clean and also improves their appearance.

Salivary gland infections

A salivary gland becomes infected and swollen most commonly as a symptom of *mumps* (p.700). Rarely, an infection can also be caused by bacteria, especially if you are run down or if one of your glands has been damaged by a *salivary duct stone* (below). When infected, the gland becomes swollen and painful, and the lymph glands in the neck beneath the angle of the jaw may also feel enlarged and tender. Pus from the infected gland trickles into the mouth and causes an unpleasant taste. If the infection is neglected the gland may become scarred so badly that it ceases to function. If you have any swelling in your mouth, under the chin, or around the jaw, consult your doctor for an examination.

What is the treatment?
The doctor will treat any infection of the salivary glands with an *antibiotic*; this usually clears up the trouble. However, if the infection persists you may be advised to attend a hospital as an out-patient and undergo *sialography*, to show whether the gland has been damaged. If it has, you will probably be advised to have the damaged area or the entire gland removed by surgery; the other salivary glands will compensate for the loss.

Salivary duct stones

A stone forms in the duct of a salivary gland when chemicals in the saliva encrust a minute particle in the duct. The stone partially blocks the duct, and when you eat a meal most of the large quantity of saliva produced cannot pass the stone. The gland therefore becomes swollen with saliva. The submandibular glands in the floor of the mouth are most susceptible to this uncommon disorder.

What should be done?
If you have any swelling under your chin or behind or under the angle of your jaw, particularly if the swelling increases at meal times, consult your doctor or dentist, who will arrange for an *X-ray* of the mouth. If the cause of the swelling is not clear from this, you may also be given a *sialogram*.

If you have a salivary duct stone it will be removed under local anaesthetic. Sometimes the trouble recurs, in which case you will be advised to have a minor operation during which a permanent opening is made near the duct. The opening permits saliva to bypass the duct and drain into the mouth almost directly from the gland. In this way, the possibility of further stones and subsequent scarring of the duct is avoided.

Salivary duct stones
The ducts from the submandibular glands, which open under the tongue, are most commonly affected by stone formation.

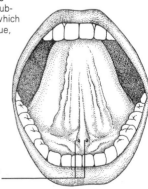

Openings of salivary ducts under tongue

Salivary gland tumours

Certain cells in a salivary gland may multiply to form a tumour. Why this happens is not known. Most tumours form in the parotid gland, the one above the angle of the jaw, and most are *benign*. They generally develop slowly over a number of years, causing the gland gradually to swell. It remains swollen, but there are no other symptoms.

In a few cases, there is a risk that the growth may be, or may turn, *malignant*. Cancerous tumours of the salivary glands are very rare – they account for less than 1 per cent of all cancers.

If one of your salivary glands is swollen or you have any pain or discomfort in your mouth, you should see your doctor. You may have to go to a hospital as an out-patient for a *sialogram*, a test which will help to disclose whether it is a tumour or a *salivary duct stone* (p.453) that is causing the problem.

What is the treatment?

If the diagnosis is a tumour, you may be advised to have it removed by surgery (a small, slowly-growing tumour may be left in place but kept under supervision). If the tumour is found to be malignant and its cells have started to spread, *radiotherapy* may be used to destroy them.

In operations on the parotid gland there is a risk of damage to an adjacent nerve that controls the movements of the lower face. This damage is often unavoidable in the case of a large tumour; however, further surgery at a later date can often help to restore the appearance of the face.

Tumours of the mouth and tongue

Tumours can occur anywhere in or on the mouth, except on the teeth. There are two types – *benign* and *malignant*. The causes of both are unknown. A benign tumour is usually a slowly growing lump and does not affect the surrounding areas. A malignant tumour is a form of cancer. Its cells do not remain in one place but spread to the surrounding area, then further afield. Malignant tumours of the tongue tend to spread within a few months, those in other parts of the mouth usually do so over a period of years.

One form of slowly-growing malignant tumour which occurs on or near the upper lip is known as a rodent ulcer; this is a form of skin cancer, and is described in detail elsewhere (see *Rodent ulcer*, p.258. See also *Salivary gland tumours*, above.)

What are the symptoms?

Benign tumours of the mouth usually occur singly. The tumour starts as a small pale lump, which then grows slowly over a period of many years. If it grows very large (more than about 10mm – roughly $\frac{3}{8}$in – across), it may cause fitting problems with dentures, and even some slight distortion of the appearance of the face.

A malignant tumour also occurs singly, as a small pale lump, but then turns into an ulcer with a hard, raised rim and a fragile centre that bleeds easily. The ulcer grows and erodes the surrounding area of the mouth. As the ulcer enlarges, the cancerous cells spread into the tongue and make the tongue muscles stiff and fixed; this leads to difficulty in eating, swallowing, and speaking. Malignant tumours are not usually painful until they reach an advanced stage.

How common is the problem?

Malignant tumours of the mouth are very rare, affecting only 1 person in 25,000 each year. They are extremely rare in people under 40, and most common in those over 60. Tumours of the mouth tend to occur more frequently in men than they do in women. Benign tumours of the mouth are probably about as rare as malignant tumours.

What are the risks?

Benign tumours usually present no risk. Malignant tumours carry the risk of spreading (*metastasizing*); the later they are diagnosed and treated, the poorer the outlook.

What should be done?

Consult your doctor or dentist if you have any lump, ulcer, or unexplained colour change in your mouth that does not clear up within three weeks, or if your dentures have begun to fit badly, or your tongue has become stiff and awkward to control.

If the trouble is caused by a tumour, a small sample of the tissue will be taken for laboratory examination (*biopsy*) to find out whether it is benign or malignant. This is a painless procedure, easily done in a few minutes using a local anaesthetic.

What is the treatment?

Most benign tumours cause no problems and are usually just kept under observation at half-yearly or yearly check-ups, to ensure that they have not become malignant.

Large benign tumours on the lips can be removed and the facial features restored by one or more sessions of *plastic surgery* (p.260). The appearance of the gums can usually be improved by the fitting of special dentures or plates.

The treatment for malignant tumours, and its success, depends on the stage the disease has reached. When the diagnosis is made at an early stage and the tumour has not spread, it is removed by surgery. If the tumour has spread, *radiotherapy* is used to destroy the cancerous cells. In some cases, *cytotoxic* drugs are used in addition to radiotherapy. Up to 75 per cent of mouth and tongue tumours diagnosed early are completely cured.

Tongue troubles

See p.248, **Visual aids to diagnosis, 65 and 66.**

The upper surface of the tongue is covered by papillae, tiny hair-like projections of tissue that contain taste buds. Normally, the papillae are pink and velvety and are crossed by fissures. The deep-red muscular body of the tongue lies beneath. Occasionally, various alterations take place to this normal colour and texture. Most tongue troubles are minor and heal quickly. If, however, you have any tongue trouble that persists for more than three weeks, consult your doctor or dentist.

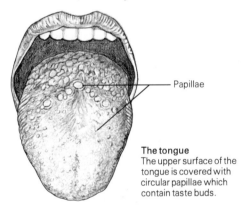

Papillae

The tongue
The upper surface of the tongue is covered with circular papillae which contain taste buds.

Glossitis
In glossitis, papillae that were previously normal no longer form properly and the body of the tongue is exposed. The surface of the tongue becomes smooth and dark red, and often feels sore, especially if you eat spicy foods. Glossitis is sometimes a symptom of another condition, such as *iron-deficiency anaemia* (p.419) or *pernicious anaemia* (p.420); so if you have the symptoms described, see your doctor, who will find out whether you have such an underlying disorder. If you do, treatment of it will also quickly clear up the glossitis. If there is no underlying cause, glossitis is no cause for concern, and should heal rapidly. Avoiding hot, spicy or hard foods will relieve the soreness.

Fissured tongue
Some people have tongues that are fissured more deeply or extensively than usual. This is a natural occurrence and does not signify any disease. Sometimes bacteria – which are always present in the mouth – accumulate in these cracks, perhaps staining them black or brown. Neither the fissures nor the discoloration are any cause for concern. To restore the tongue to its normal colour, all that is necessary is to brush it twice daily with a toothbrush dipped in a diluted antiseptic, such as a mouth rinse.

Black hairy tongue
In rare cases, the papillae on the tongue become unusually long and hair-like. Why this happens is unknown, but fungal or bacterial mouth infections, smoking, and *antibiotic* drugs are all possible causes. Bacteria in the mouth sometimes stain the elongated papillae black or dark brown. The disorder is harmless, and should be treated in the same way as a stained fissured tongue (above).

Geographical tongue
In some people, the papillae on the tongue fail to form properly – not over the entire surface of the tongue, as in glossitis, but in patches. The patches, which come and go, reveal the smooth, deep-red body of the tongue beneath. They are often sore, and, as in glossitis, spicy foods make the soreness worse. The disorder is harmless. What causes geographical tongue is unknown, and no treatment for it has proved effective.

Furred tongue
People who are ill, especially with a fever, often have a whitish or yellowish, furry coating on the surface of the tongue. This is because people who are ill tend to talk and eat less than usual, their tongue becomes less active, and a film of bacteria, food particles, and excess cells accumulates on it.

Also, during illness the mouth is often dry and lacks saliva to wash away this film. The tongue should return to normal as soon as the illness clears up.

Lumps or ulcers on the tongue
If a lump or ulcer on your tongue fails to heal in three weeks, see your doctor without delay, even if the affected area is painless. The lump or ulcer may be harmless, but it could be a *malignant* tumour (see *Tumours of the mouth and tongue*, opposite).

Oesophagus

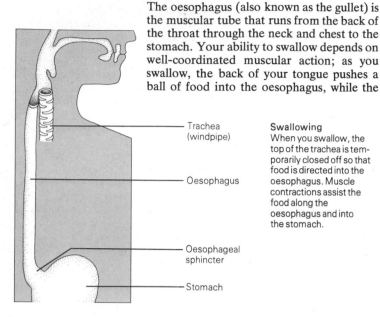

Trachea
(windpipe)

Oesophagus

Oesophageal
sphincter

Stomach

Swallowing
When you swallow, the top of the trachea is temporarily closed off so that food is directed into the oesophagus. Muscle contractions assist the food along the oesophagus and into the stomach.

The oesophagus (also known as the gullet) is the muscular tube that runs from the back of the throat through the neck and chest to the stomach. Your ability to swallow depends on well-coordinated muscular action; as you swallow, the back of your tongue pushes a ball of food into the oesophagus, while the soft palate closes off the passage to your nose, and the top of the windpipe tightens so that food cannot get into your lungs. Rhythmic contractions of the oesophageal muscles (*peristaltic* contractions) send the food down through the chest to the base of the oesophagus, where the muscular valve (or *sphincter*) at the entrance to the stomach relaxes to let the food pass through.

Difficulty in, or pain while, swallowing (*dysphagia*) is not in itself a disease; it is a symptom of nearly all diseases of the oesophagus. And since it is the major symptom of a *malignant* growth somewhere in the oesophagus, always consult your doctor without delay if you begin to have trouble swallowing. Chances of a serious disorder are slight, but if the condition is serious, an early diagnosis is essential.

With the exception of hiatus hernia, disorders of the oesophagus are rare. Oesophageal cancer, for example, accounts for only 2 per cent of all cancer deaths.

Hiatus hernia

A hiatus hernia
The stomach sits below the diaphragm. The oesophagus passes through a hole in the diaphragm and enters the stomach. A hiatus hernia (below) occurs when part of the stomach squeezes back through this hole and into the chest.

A domed sheet of muscle, the diaphragm, separates the chest from the abdomen, and the oesophagus has to pass through a hole (or hiatus) in the diaphragm to reach the stomach. A hiatus hernia occurs when the muscular tissue around the hole weakens and the abdominal portion of the oesophagus – often along with part of the stomach – protrudes upwards through the hiatus into the chest. The protrusion (or hernia) forms a bell-shaped swelling at the base of the oesophagus. Most people who have this type of hernia are not troubled by it. In some cases, however, it affects the efficiency of the muscular valve (the oesophageal *sphincter*) that maintains a one-way flow from the oesophagus to the stomach; the result is *acid reflux*, when acid fluid from the stomach wells up into the oesophagus.

(For information on hernias in general see *Hernias*, p.537.)

What are the symptoms?
The main symptom is usually heartburn (a painful burning sensation in the chest). Very rarely, the pain extends into the neck and arms; if severe, it can be mistaken for the pain of *coronary thrombosis* (p.379). If you bend forward or lie down, stomach acid can easily run into the oesophagus – that is why heartburn can often be particularly troublesome after you have gone to bed.

Another possible symptom is the sudden regurgitation of acid fluid into the mouth. Belching is also common, but this often happens because the sufferer has swallowed air in an attempt to relieve the discomfort.

How common is the problem?
Hiatus hernia is quite common, especially among overweight, elderly people. By no means everyone with hiatus hernia has symptoms, however. Some degree of hiatus hernia often occurs in pregnancy (see *Heartburn during pregnancy*, p.622).

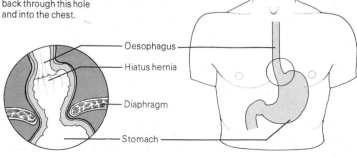

Oesophagus

Hiatus hernia

Diaphragm

Stomach

What are the risks?

Hiatus hernia is not in itself a severe or dangerous condition. But persistent acid reflux caused by hiatus hernia can lead to inflammation or even ulceration of the oesophagus. Inflammation can lead in turn to *stricture of the oesophagus* (p.458). If oesophageal ulcers bleed – a rare but possible development – *anaemia* (p.419) may result.

What should be done?

If symptoms are troublesome, adopt the self-help measures suggested below; consult your doctor only if symptoms persist. It may then be advisable for you to attend a local hospital to undergo diagnostic tests such as *electrocardiography (ECG)*, a *barium meal*, an *X-ray*, and perhaps *endoscopy*.

What is the treatment?

Self-help: The most effective self-help measure is to lose weight, which almost always cures hiatus hernia. For advice on how to do this see *Obesity*, p.492. Avoid stooping, particularly after a meal. Do not wear tight corsets or belts. Raise the head of your bed about 100mm (4in) in order to prevent acid reflux at night. Avoid alcoholic drinks, which tend to aggravate the symptoms; and do not smoke, since smoking aggravates stomach and digestive disorders. Try taking one of the antacids easily available over-the-counter at the chemist. This will provide relief by neutralizing stomach acid and protecting the lining of the oesophagus. As with a *duodenal ulcer* (p.468), the symptoms can often be relieved by eating several small meals each day instead of two or three large ones.

Professional help: If over-the-counter antacid tablets are ineffective, your doctor may prescribe another type as a liquid mixture to be taken after meals. To reduce the backflow of acid from stomach to oesophagus, the doctor may also prescribe a drug to increase the speed with which food passes through the stomach. The above measures usually cure hiatus hernia, but if it persists then you may need surgery to repair it. The operation is relatively simple and results are usually good (see *Hernia repair*, p.539). But whatever the treatment, hiatus hernia will probably recur in anyone who remains overweight.

Cancer of the oesophagus

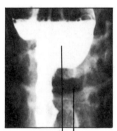

Oesophagus |

Tumour |

When the sufferer swallows a dye that shows up white on X-ray, the dye builds up in front of the tumour and outlines it where it projects into the oesophagus.

Cells in the lining of the oesophagus start to multiply rapidly and form a *malignant* tumour, which eventually results in narrowing and constriction of the passageway to the stomach. The cause is unknown, though cancer of the oesophagus has been linked with prolonged exposure to such irritants as cigarette smoke and alcohol.

What are the symptoms?

The main symptom is difficulty or pain when swallowing, which worsens rapidly. At first only solids are hard to swallow, but liquids also become troublesome later on. An additional symptom is rapid, progressive loss of weight. Occasionally, a belch may bring up blood-stained mucus.

How common is the problem?

Cancer of the oesophagus is very rare, occurring in only 1 person in 15,000. Men are twice as susceptible as women, and the risk seems to be greatest for heavy smokers and drinkers in the 50–60 age group. If the condition is detected in an early stage, chances for successful treatment are fair.

What should be done?

If food seems to stick in your throat when you try to swallow it, see your doctor right away. Even though the chance of a cancerous tumour is slight, the doctor will order diagnostic tests – a *barium swallow*, an *X-ray*, and a thorough examination of the oesophagus by *endoscopy*, and *biopsy*.

If cancer of the oesophagus is diagnosed, the usual treatment is to remove the affected part by surgery. *Radiotherapy* is then used to ensure that any remaining cancer cells are completely destroyed. If an operation is not possible, radiotherapy will be used to slow down the progress of the disease.

Achalasia

In normal swallowing, food is guided down the oesophagus by rhythmic *peristaltic* contractions of the muscles in its wall. In the rare disorder known as achalasia, the nerves that control the muscles at the lower end of the oesophagus become defective and contractions become irregular and uncoordinated. Why this should happen is not known, but as a result the lower part of the oesophagus becomes distorted and swollen with food.

What are the symptoms?

The main symptoms of achalasia are discomfort and pain on swallowing and, usually, chest pains. Because food accumulates in the oesophagus, there is likely to be a foul taste in the mouth and bad breath. Occasionally, too, food may be regurgitated into the mouth. The sufferer is likely to find only liquids hard to swallow at first, but will eventually have problems with solids as well.

As achalasia worsens, the oesophagus is never properly emptied, and there is always a chance that the sufferer might inhale food particles while asleep. These can cause chest infections such as *pneumonia* (p.359). Because of the difficulty in eating, loss of weight and other signs of malnutrition are usual.

What should be done?
If you suspect you may have achalasia, consult your doctor, who will examine you and probably arrange a *barium swallow*. Visual examination of the oesophagus by *endoscopy* may be used to confirm the diagnosis. To relieve pain, the doctor may prescribe an *antispasmodic* (a drug that prevents muscle spasms). One form of treatment for achalasia involves passing a slender rubber bag (called a *bougie*) down the oesophagus and filling the bag with water, in order to stretch the muscles at the bottom. This procedure allows food to pass into the stomach more easily, but is not permanent and must be repeated every few weeks. The only permanently effective treatment for the condition is surgery – an operation (*cardiomyotomy*) in which some of the muscles at the stomach entrance are cut to widen the passageway for food. About 80 per cent of such operations are successful.

Pharyngeal pouch

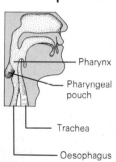

Pharynx

Pharyngeal pouch

Trachea

Oesophagus

In this rare disorder, which occurs most often in elderly men, a small bulge or sac develops at the back of the throat (the pharynx) just at the top of the oesophagus. It usually happens as a result of muscular incoordination during swallowing. Food enters the sac as you swallow, enlarging it downward to a baglike pouch. Over the years the pouch gradually grows bigger, and swallowing becomes increasingly difficult. The pouch itself may show up as a swelling in your neck, probably on the left side, and especially after drinking. Other symptoms are regurgitation of fluid or undigested food from the pouch into your mouth (this generally happens several hours after eating), an irritating cough, and a metallic taste in your mouth.

The only risk of a pharyngeal pouch is that fluid from the pouch may enter your lungs during sleep, causing an infection.

What should be done?
Consult your doctor if you have any difficulty in swallowing. The doctor will usually be able to diagnose pharyngeal pouch from a physical examination, but a *barium swallow* may be needed to confirm this. Often the disorder needs no treatment, but in some cases surgical removal of the pouch – a relatively simple operation – will be recommended.

Diffuse spasm of the oesophagus

This is an exceedingly rare condition. There is no known cause for diffuse spasm of the oesophagus. The sufferer experiences irregular, repeated spasms of the muscles of the oesophageal wall, and these can result in chest pains, difficulty in swallowing, and *acid reflux* (see *Hiatus hernia*, p.456). The condition develops gradually, with intermittent attacks over a period of years, and those who suffer from it usually learn to live with it. To help relieve the spasms, an *antispasmodic* drug may be prescribed.

Stricture of the oesophagus

This is a rare disorder that usually occurs in elderly people. It is the result of an accumulation of scar tissue in the oesophagus, often caused by persistent *acid reflux* (see *Hiatus hernia*, p.456). Because of the gradual enlargement of the scarred portions of the oesophageal wall, the passageway for food becomes increasingly constricted.

What are the symptoms?
The main symptom is difficulty in swallowing; you should always consult your doctor if you have this symptom. There may also be bouts of heartburn (see *Indigestion*, p.463).

What is the treatment?
The usual treatment for stricture is dilation of the passageway by means of either a waterfilled rubber bag or a flexible metal rod called a *bougie* (see *Achalasia*, p.457). This procedure must be repeated every few weeks or so and some people find it unduly distressing. Surgery to remove the scar tissue may be feasible in such cases.

Infections of the digestive tract

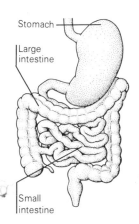

Stomach

Large intestine

Small intestine

A gastrointestinal infection occurs when certain microbes multiply rapidly in the stomach and intestines, causing disorders of various kinds in the digestive tract. The intestines normally contain many bacteria that are harmless: in fact, some are essential because they manufacture vitamins you need but cannot make yourself. The presence of such organisms is not considered to be an "infection". This term generally applies to invasion of the digestive tract by foreign, dangerous microbes (usually bacteria) such as those that cause salmonellosis or typhoid fever. The unchecked multiplication of such microbes will cause symptoms such as diarrhoea and/or vomiting, along with more generalized illness if the organisms enter the bloodstream and are thus able to spread to infect other parts of the body.

Gastroenteritis is a general term for a minor infection of the digestive tract; but the disorder may also have non-microbial causes – for example, it may occur after eating a food to which you are allergic, or after consuming poisonous chemicals. In such cases the symptoms may be indistinguishable from those caused by minor infections of the tract – which is why this disorder is included in a group of articles dealing primarily with infections of the digestive tract.

Gastro-enteritis

Gastroenteritis is irritation and inflammation of the digestive tract which produces the symptoms of an "upset stomach". It is most commonly caused by viruses (see *General infections and infestations*, p.558), which can easily be passed from one person to another by personal contact, without direct reference to food or drink. Such infections are the most common cause of the 24- or 36-hour attacks of vomiting and/or diarrhoea often identified as cases of "gastric flu".

Gastroenteritis can also result from eating or drinking something contaminated by microbes. A different kind of "food poisoning" can occur if you eat something containing a toxic substance – a non-edible mushroom, for example, or a rhubarb leaf. And some foods – shellfish, strawberries, eggs, pork, and many others are "poisonous" to individuals who are allergic to them. Such kinds of food poisoning, though not caused by microbial infection, may bring on attacks of gastroenteritis which can be very serious indeed (see *Food poisoning*, p.462).

Another possible cause of gastroenteritis is a change in the natural bacterial population of the digestive tract. If you have an illness that weakens you, or if you suddenly make drastic changes in your diet (for example, when visiting a foreign country), the balance may be disturbed so that certain bacterial strains strengthen at the expense of others and upset your bowel functions. *Antibiotic* drugs can have a similar effect by acting selectively on the bacterial population in the digestive tract and disrupting their natural equilibrium.

What are the symptoms?

The symptoms of gastroenteritis range from a mild attack of nausea followed by diarrhoea – which happens to nearly everybody from time to time – to a severe illness. There may be one or two bouts of vomiting and a few disagreeably soft bowel movements that hardly interfere with your routine. Or you may vomit repeatedly and have recurrent attacks of watery diarrhoea with abdominal pains and cramp, accompanied by fever and extreme weakness. In an occasional severe case, total prostration follows a very bad attack of gastroenteritis. Usually, though, whatever the symptoms of gastroenteritis, they fade away within 48 hours.

How common is the problem?

Gastroenteritis is such a widespread condition that it accounts for nearly 10 per cent of visits to general practitioners. The viral form, like many viral illnesses, is most prevalent in winter and usually occurs in small epidemics. Schoolchildren, for instance, who bring the disorder home from a local epidemic at school, may infect other members of their family, who pass the disorder on to neighbours, and so on.

What are the risks?

Risks depend on the cause – for example, the type and number of infecting microbes, or the amount and virulence of the poisonous food substances – and on the age and general health of the sufferer. The danger of debilitation leading to prostration is greatest for newborn babies and infants less than about

18 months old, and the elderly. The result of repeated attacks of diarrhoea is apt to be *dehydration*, which upsets body chemistry and, if unchecked, can lead to *shock* (p.386). In a normally healthy person a few bouts of vomiting and diarrhoea are no more significant than the runny nose and cough of a common cold. But if there is also severe pain in the abdomen (not just the occasional spasm of *colic*), there is a possibility that the symptoms may be due to some other abdominal disorder such as *appendicitis* (p.476) which requires urgent treatment.

What should be done?

If the self-help measures recommended below do not effect a cure (or at least great improvement) within two or, at most, three days, consult your doctor. (Note that this time should be reduced for babies and young children – see *Gastroenteritis in infants*, p.649.) After examining you and asking questions about what and where you have recently eaten or drunk, and whether any of your family or other associates have been complaining of upset stomachs, the doctor may decide to send a sample of your faeces to a laboratory for analysis. More probably, your answers to questions and the doctor's observations of the state of your health (often along with knowledge of a local epidemic of this disorder) will confirm the diagnosis. Analysis of faeces may be necessary, however, if diarrhoea is prolonged, to make sure that your gastroenteritis is not due to an unusual type of gastrointestinal infection such as *amoebic dysentery* (opposite).

What is the treatment?

Self-help: If you have an attack of gastroenteritis, stay at home, resting and taking in plenty of fluids, until the attack subsides; to avoid dehydration because of diarrhoea, you may need to drink at least an extra half-litre (about a pint) or so per day. Do not eat at all, and drink only water for the first 24 hours (a few sips every 15 minutes or so if you are having bad spells of vomiting). Then start drinking diluted fruit juices. Do not sweeten them; sugar sometimes prolongs diarrhoea. If you are producing a lot of watery faeces, try adding a level teaspoon of salt to every litre (about two pints) of diluted fruit juice. This prevents dehydration by helping to keep your blood chemistry balanced. After about two days following the advice given above you should be able to resume your normal diet.

Do not take aspirins or other painkillers. Such drugs are likely to aggravate the condition (as are antibiotics, which tend to upset the equilibrium of intestinal bacteria, thus worsening the diarrhoea). Remember, too, that gastroenteritis is often caused by poor hygiene and is easily passed on to others. So, to avoid contaminating food, be sure to wash your hands after going to the lavatory and before preparing a meal.

Professional help: There is no specific treatment for viral gastroenteritis. If there is no doubt about the diagnosis and your nausea and diarrhoea are not due to some other disorder such as a generalized infection or appendicitis, your doctor will probably advise you to continue the self-help measures recommended above. If your vomiting is severe, you may also be given an injection (or tablets) of an *anti-emetic* drug. Persistent diarrhoea is sometimes helped by doses of kaolin, which hardens the faeces, or of a drug that slows down bowel activity. Any such treatment is stopped as soon as the bowels begin to function normally again.

Salmonellosis

Bacteria known as salmonellae are often present in the bodies of farm animals and birds, which may not suffer symptoms as a result of the infection. A human being who eats salmonella-infected meat, however, may have various unpleasant symptoms in addition to *gastroenteritis* (p.459). Salmonellae are not killed by deep freezing, and even fresh, apparently safe meats can contain them. They are killed, however, by being thoroughly cooked. One cause of infection in people is failure to unfreeze food sufficiently before it is heated, so that it does not get cooked all the way through. It sometimes happens, too, that meat is not frozen swiftly enough after an animal is slaughtered; the delay permits a small number of bacteria naturally present in the meat to breed into a multitude, infecting the meat.

You need not eat infected food in order to get salmonellosis. The bacteria can spread from person to person on the fingers of anyone who handles infected meats or has recently recovered from the disease.

What are the symptoms?

The main symptom is diarrhoea. It is often accompanied by abdominal pain, vomiting, and fever; and occasionally there is blood in the faeces. The type and degree of diarrhoea vary enormously. There may be only one or two loose bowel movements a day, or the

Foods likely to
cause salmonellosis

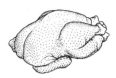

Insufficiently
thawed poultry

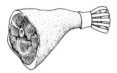

Insufficiently
cooked meat

Cooked meat
poorly reheated

sufferer may have an acute attack of watery diarrhoea every 10 to 15 minutes. If this continues for several hours, it can culminate in total prostration and *dehydration* (see "What are the risks?" below). A relatively mild attack of salmonellosis can easily be mistaken for an attack of gastroenteritis.

How common is the problem?

Apart from an occasional small epidemic, salmonellosis is not often specifically identified since the faeces of most people with "upset stomachs" are not analysed. Nobody, therefore, knows how many cases of this disorder are diagnosed as gastroenteritis.

What are the risks?

If the offending bacteria spread from the digestive tract into the bloodstream, they may settle in other organs such as the kidneys, gallbladder, heart, or joints, causing inflammation and perhaps even *abscesses* in various organs. This seldom happens, however. Most salmonella infections are mild and cure themselves without treatment. In a severe attack, excessive loss of body fluid resulting from repeated bouts of diarrhoea can cause death from *dehydration*.

What should be done?

If you have diarrhoea that lasts for more than three days, or if you have a combination of fever, diarrhoea, vomiting, and abdominal pain, consult your doctor. The diagnostic procedures are summarized in the article on gastroenteritis. Note that a baby or young child who is vomiting badly or has severe diarrhoea should receive medical attention within several hours – see *Gastroenteritis in infants*, p.649.

What is the treatment?

If salmonella infection spreads from the digestive tract, treatment will depend upon the resultant disorder, whether specific or generalized. Otherwise, treatment is exactly as for gastroenteritis, and complete recovery can be expected.

Very rarely, after the diarrhoea has gone and the sufferer is fit and well, a few live salmonellae remain in the digestive tract and are excreted from time to time in the faeces. These residual bacteria seldom last for more than three months, but they pose a continuing danger of spreading the infection to others. *Antibiotic* treatment may be prescribed by your doctor to combat this "carrier" state. If you know that you have had salmonellosis, you should not only be particularly careful to wash your hands after every bowel movement but should check with your doctor from time to time over the next few months to ascertain whether you are still excreting the living organisms.

Bacillary dysentery

This is a rare disease in developed countries, affecting only 1,000 to 2,000 people in Britain a year. It is caused by the shigella bacillus, a bacterium which invades the lining of the colon, and is spread from person to person in unhygienic conditions. The main symptoms of bacillary dysentry – abdominal pain and diarrhoea – are similar to those of *gastroenteritis* (p.459), but in some cases the diarrhoea may also be blood-stained.

Preventive measures and treatment are much the same as for most other gastrointestinal infections. In severe cases *antibiotics* may be prescribed since their benefits then outweigh the drawbacks of using them for most gastrointestinal infections.

Amoebic dysentery

Amoebic dysentery, caused by a minute single-celled animal, is so rare in developed countries that only 100 to 200 cases are reported in Britain each year. The main symptom is blood-stained diarrhoea, which may persist for a few weeks and may then recur from time to time. Occasionally the microbes spread from the digestive tract into the bloodstream and settle in the liver, where they form areas of pus called *abscesses*.

What is the treatment?

Your doctor, who will suspect amoebic dysentery if you have recently been abroad – particularly in a tropical area – will make arrangements to have your faeces analysed at a tropical-medicine laboratory. Treatment involves taking a combination of drugs three times a day for 10 days. This may result in vomiting. In such cases daily injections of an *anti-emetic* drug may be given as well. After diarrhoea has ceased, faeces are examined monthly until it appears certain that no offending organisms remain in the digestive tract. Meanwhile, you should be careful to wash both hands thoroughly after every bowel movement and before handling food to avoid spreading the infection.

Typhoid
(typhoid fever)

Typhoid is a *contagious* disease spread under insanitary conditions, either from person to person or through contaminated food, drink, or plumbing facilities. Some people who are not themselves susceptible are nonetheless "carriers"; that is, they harbour the offending bacteria in their bodies and are a constant source of infection to others. The bacteria not only inflame intestinal walls but spread via the bloodstream throughout the body. Symptoms begin like those of severe *influenza* (p.559), but these are followed by persistent fever of around 40°C (104°F), increasing weakness, diarrhoea (usually blood-stained), and often delirium. For a few days there may also be a pink abdominal rash, which fades as the disease progresses. Recovery comes slowly – after two or three weeks if there are no complications. But this is a life-threatening disease because there are often complications – for instance, extensive bleeding or rupture of the intestines.

Typhoid has, fortunately, become so rare in Western countries that only 100 to 200 cases occur in Britain each year, and nearly all can be traced back to recent travel or residence in a less developed part of the world. If you are in such an area, or have returned within the past month or so and developed what seems to be a particularly bad attack of flu, see a doctor without delay.

What is the treatment?
If you are somewhere where medical help is not swiftly available, stay in bed, drinking nourishing fluids such as milk or soup, and try to reduce your temperature by sponging your body with tepid water. Despite persistent fever, do not take *analgesics* such as aspirin or paracetamol; a typhoid-weakened body is especially sensitive to such drugs.

If you develop typhoid in this country, you will be treated in an isolation hospital. A two-week course of *antibiotics* will reduce the severity of the attack and speed recovery. After three or four weeks, or whenever your faeces are free of infectious bacteria, it will be safe for you to go home.

Cholera

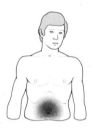

Site of the pain

Cholera is caused by a type of bacterium that damages the intestinal lining, causing the loss of up to 15 litres (about 25 pints) of fluid a day. The bacteria are spread through polluted water or raw fruits and vegetables in places where hygiene is poor. Thus most cases in Britain (there are about 1,000 a year) can be traced back to visits or temporary residence in less developed areas of the world. The symptoms of the disease are abdominal pain and diarrhoea; faecal matter resembles murky water and, in severe cases, is excreted almost continuously. The sufferer becomes extremely thirsty, has no fever, but vomits intermittently and may have muscle cramps. If cholera is untreated, *dehydration* can lead to death.

If you are abroad or have recently been abroad and have an attack of extremely watery diarrhoea that becomes increasingly severe instead of clearing up within a few hours, get medical help without delay. Until such help arrives, drink as much non-alcoholic fluid as you can. If your illness is diagnosed as cholera in this country (an easy diagnosis for the doctor to make if you let him or her know you have recently been abroad), you will be admitted to hospital. The main treatment is simply to replenish the body's supply of fluid by means of an *intravenous drip*. To destroy the cholera bacteria you will also be given an *antibiotic* drug. Full recovery in one to two weeks is probable, and there are no long-term after-effects.

Food poisoning

"Food poisoning" is a term with a number of meanings. It may refer to eating food that, growing in its natural state, contains poisonous chemicals. It can refer to food contaminated with microbes which multiply and produce poisonous substances called *toxins*. (An extremely rare but very serious disease, *botulism*, is an example of this kind of food poisoning.) The term food poisoning can also apply to chemical pollutants such as mercury which have found their way into the food, or to food which causes an allergic reaction in the digestive tract of a susceptible person. In Britain, 90 per cent of food poisoning outbreaks notified to doctors are caused by staphylococcus or salmonella bacteria. The former often come from a cut or *boil* (p.251) on a food-handler's skin; salmonella are usually in the food already (see *Salmonellosis*, p.460). Either kind of bacteria thrives in poorly cooked food or food left warm for a few hours. As they multiply staphylococci produce toxins which are not destroyed when the food is reheated before serving. If you suspect you have food poisoning, turn to the articles concerned with *infections of the digestive tract* (p.459) for further information on symptoms and treatment; for urgent cases turn to *Accidents and emergencies*, p.812.

Stomach and duodenum

The stomach acts as a food reservoir and processor, transforming the bulk of a chewed and swallowed meal into a slow trickle of pulp. Food enters the stomach through a muscular one-way valve, the oesophageal *sphincter*. Once inside, rhythmical contractions of the powerful muscles in the stomach wall crush the food, which is further broken down by the chemical action of acid and *enzymes* made in the stomach lining. All this activity goes on as long as food remains in your stomach; in an empty stomach there is little muscular activity and virtually no release of acid or enzymes.

The processed matter trickles out of the stomach through another muscular valve, the pyloric sphincter, into the duodenum. This is a tube about 250mm (10in) long in which more enzymes are secreted to further the digestive process before the pulp passes into the small intestine. It takes up to five hours for the contents of a meal to reach the small intestine, leaving the stomach and duodenum empty. Over-production of the powerful acids and enzymes at work in the stomach and duodenum can damage the mucous membrane that lines the stomach. Also, this membrane is easily irritated in some people by certain foods, drugs, or fluids. In most cases the irritation results only in the familiar symptoms of indigestion. But sometimes, more seriously, the action of powerful stomach chemicals can lead to development of an ulcer in the lining of either the stomach or the duodenum.

Oesophageal sphincter

Pyloric sphincter

Stomach

Duodenum

Duodenum

Duodenum

Muscles of the stomach wall

Indigestion
(dyspepsia)

Indigestion is not a disease but a collection of symptoms, which usually occur during or soon after eating or drinking. A variety of disorders, only a few of them serious, can cause indigestion, but often the cause is impossible to identify.

What are the symptoms?
Different people have different symptoms and tend to describe them in different terms. What one person calls heartburn another will speak of as pain in the chest. What one person thinks of as a belch may be someone else's hiccup. If you are suffering from indigestion, you probably feel a general sense of discomfort or distension in the abdomen; or there may be sharp, dull, or gnawing pain in the chest; or you may complain of heartburn, nausea, or the regurgitation into the mouth of acid fluid; or you may need to belch or break wind; or you may have more than one of these conditions. But most bouts of indigestion have one thing in common: they are in some way related to food or drink (although in some cases, symptoms of indigestion are caused by swallowing air while eating or chewing gum). The discomfort of indigestion is aggravated by wearing tight clothes.

How common is the problem?
Indigestion is so common as to be virtually universal. Some people get one or more of the symptoms after eating particular foods such as cabbage, beans, onions, cucumbers, or pork, or after drinking wine or carbonated drinks like soda or tonic water. Others suffer if they eat too fast or have an especially rich or big meal. And others feel pangs of indigestion whenever they are anxious, nervous, or depressed. Pregnant women are particularly prone to indigestion, as are heavy smokers, people who suffer from constipation, the obese, and the elderly.

What are the risks?
Indigestion is troublesome and may even be painful, but it is not in itself dangerous. Many people have indigestion on and off throughout their life without further complications. You probably know how your stomach behaves in given situations, and you either use self-prescribed remedies for indigestion or

try to prevent it by avoiding the things that cause it. Perhaps you even take the occasional calculated risk of eating or drinking unwisely (for you) simply because the fun of temporary pleasure outweighs the near-certainty of consequent discomfort. There are no serious risks in such behaviour. What you ought to watch out for, however, is a change in symptoms. There is always a chance that the change may be caused by a more serious illness. If the character or timing of your "indigestion" alters, or if it becomes more frequent or severe, something else may be happening: it may indicate a *hiatus hernia* (p.456), *gallstones* (p.489), a *duodenal ulcer* (p.468), or even, very rarely, *cancer of the stomach* (p.466).

What should be done?
Familiarize yourself with your particular symptoms, and deal with the trouble by the self-help methods recommended below. If the pattern of symptoms changes – if, for example, a feeling of nausea after eating becomes actual vomiting; or if you begin to have indigestion every day instead of occasionally; or, in particular, if you lose weight or lose your appetite – consult your doctor without delay. If your doctor suspects an underlying disease is causing the new type of symptom, he or she will arrange for diagnostic tests, usually including *X-rays* of the stomach and duodenum, for which you will need to have a *barium meal*. Other possible tests may include X-ray of the gallbladder, *endoscopy*, and analysis of your blood and faeces.

What is the treatment?
Self-help: Spend some time thinking about the nature of your indigestion. Does it usually follow a particular kind of food? If you can, avoid that food in the future. Does it occur if you eat late at night? If you drink alcohol after a meal? Try to adjust your eating and drinking habits to your stomach's idiosyncrasies. In addition, there are several general steps you can take to lessen the chances of getting indigestion. Do not smoke. Make a habit of never losing your temper or becoming over-excited during meals. Do not "bolt" your food or eat standing up. Try to relax for half an hour after a meal. Some sufferers from indigestion find that certain commercially available antacids help relieve the symptoms. If you take any such preparation be sure to follow the instructions printed on the label. (If you are pregnant, be sure to ask your doctor for an antacid suitable for pregnant women; some antacids cause problems with vitamin absorption and should not be taken during pregnancy.)

Professional help: The doctor's first task is to find out whether your indigestion is caused by an underlying disease. The more accurately you can describe your symptoms and their relationship to food and drink, the easier it will be for your doctor to discover the probable cause. Do not neglect to point out all recent developments that do not conform to the familiar pattern. Your doctor will probably want to know whether you have been subjected to any recent emotional stresses or tensions or changes in life style.

If, after a physical examination and appropriate diagnostic tests, no serious disorder appears to be responsible for the symptoms, your doctor will no doubt suggest a routine of eating, drinking, and sleeping that seems likely to relieve your symptoms. He or she may also prescribe a tranquillizer if stress or tension seems to play a part in the pattern of your indigestion.

Gastritis

Gastritis – inflammation of the mucous membrane that lines the stomach – may sometimes be caused by a viral infection or may be a side-effect of certain drugs such as aspirin and other antirheumatic medicines. But in most cases this disorder is the direct result of a bout of heavy drinking, smoking, or overeating, or of eating a food that "disagrees" with the sufferer.

What are the symptoms?
The symptoms of viral gastritis are similar to those of *gastroenteritis* (p.459). If the disorder is due to excessive drinking, smoking, or eating, or to irritation by a drug, the symptoms resemble those of *indigestion* (p.463).

How common is the problem?
Nearly everyone has an occasional mild attack of gastritis. Only rarely do pain and/or vomiting caused entirely by gastritis persist for more than a day or two. You are more likely to suffer if you smoke heavily or drink large quantities of alcohol.

What are the risks?
There is virtually no danger of lasting damage to health from occasional attacks of gastritis. If you have recurrent severe attacks – those in which vomiting and pain continue for more than 24 hours – you run an increasing risk of damaging the lining of the stomach and developing *gastric erosion* (p.467).

What should be done?

If you often have gastritis, examine your lifestyle. You will probably find that you smoke, eat, or drink either too much or too carelessly. Once you have found the likely cause, try moderation and prudence as a way of avoiding further attacks. If, then, you still have symptoms of digestive-tract illness, consult your doctor.

To ease an attack adopt the self-help measures suggested below; but see your doctor without delay if you begin to vomit blood or if the attack lasts longer than 48 hours. After considering the general state of your health and the possible side-effects of any drugs that you have been taking, the doctor may arrange for you to undergo a series of diagnostic tests at a hospital to make sure that your trouble is simply gastritis. The tests will be those usually given to people with a suspected *stomach ulcer* (below).

What is the treatment?

Self-help: Eat nothing during the first full day of an attack. Instead, take frequent small amounts of non-alcoholic fluid – preferably milk or water. After 24 hours begin eating; have only foods that you know "agree" with you, and have only a little at a time. If your abdominal pain is troublesome, take an antacid. If your gastritis is apparently related to your alcohol consumption or smoking, try giving these up for a month; if this stops the attacks, the rest is up to you.

Professional help: If the diagnosis of your disorder is clearly gastritis, the doctor will probably prescribe a sedative antacid. For severe nausea and vomiting you may be given an injection of an *anti-emetic* drug. If a drug seems to be causing the gastritis, a change of medicines – along with clear instructions about the best timing for taking regular doses – may be advised.

Stomach ulcer

(also called gastric or peptic ulcer)

A stomach ulcer is a raw spot (often about 30mm – a little more than 1in – across) that develops in the lining of the stomach. The exact cause of such ulcers is not known; they do not seem to be closely associated with over-production of stomach acid (compare *Duodenal ulcer*, p.468). There is evidence, however, that irritation of the stomach lining from bile regurgitation into the stomach from the duodenum is sometimes a factor. (Note that an alternative name for stomach *or* duodenal ulcer is peptic ulcer; an alternative name for stomach ulcer is gastric ulcer.)

What are the symptoms?

The major symptom is a burning, gnawing pain – usually diffused through the upper part of the abdomen but occasionally confined to the chest – which lasts for from 30 minutes to three hours. Bouts of pain come and go, weeks of intermittent pain alternating with short pain-free periods. Although there is usually a relationship between pain and eating, the nature of the relationship is unpredictable; pain may begin right after you have eaten something, or it may not occur until hours afterwards. Other possible symptoms are loss of appetite and, consequently, of weight, and occasional vomiting of acid fluid (which almost always relieves the pain).

How common is the problem?

It has been estimated that about 1 in 5 men and 1 in 10 women in the Western world get a peptic (stomach or duodenal) ulcer at some time. Stomach (gastric) ulcers, on the other hand, are about equally common in both sexes. You are especially likely to develop one if you smoke or drink heavily, if you have irregular or hurried meals, if you consume large amounts of aspirin-containing painkillers, if you are elderly, or if you are a manual rather than sedentary worker.

What are the risks?

Bleeding from a stomach ulcer is not common but can be dangerous, particularly in the elderly. A sudden severe bleed can cause *shock* (p.386); less severe bleeding, if it continues undetected for several months, may cause *anaemia* (p.419). Another risk, though only a slight one, is that the ulcer may erode right through the stomach wall (*perforation*).

If a stomach ulcer remains untreated, there may be serious loss of weight, and poor nutrition caused by lack of appetite predisposes the body to infections. There is a slight chance, too, that a recurrent stomach ulcer may cause *pyloric stenosis* (p.468), or that it may undergo *malignant* change and eventually become a cancer (see the article on *Cancer of the stomach*, p.466).

What should be done?

If pain persists for more than two to three weeks, consult your doctor. To determine whether there is an ulcer and whether it is in the stomach or duodenum, your doctor will arrange for you to undergo *endoscopy* and/or a *barium meal*. Other possible procedures include a blood test, taking a sample of stomach fluid for a check on acidity, and laboratory analysis of your faeces to see whether there is any internal bleeding.

What is the treatment?

Self-help: A stomach ulcer will often heal completely if you stay in bed for about two weeks, eating small, frequent meals, taking antacid tablets (which can be purchased without a doctor's prescription) to relieve pain, and avoid all temptation to smoke. If your symptoms are not severe enough to justify two weeks in bed, try at any rate to eat little but often, avoiding alcohol, caffeine (in coffee and tea), and tobacco, and resting or sleeping as much as possible. If pain stops and does not recur, there are no grounds for concern. If it persists – even though antacids temporarily ease it – do not rely on self-treatment; see your doctor.

Professional help: The doctor will probably supplement the self-help measures recommended above by prescribing a drug to speed up the normal healing process. Since around 40 per cent of all peptic ulcers recover without being treated or simply with self-help measures, no further treatment may be required. But because about 45 per cent of apparently cured ulcers recur within a couple of years, the doctor is likely to want to examine you again. If healing does not occur after six to eight weeks of drug treatment or is only temporary, surgery may be advisable. Removal of the small portion of the stomach that contains the ulcer will generally effect a cure – see *Stomach removal*, opposite.

What are the long-term prospects?

Prospects for a cure without surgery are excellent if treatment is begun early, if drugs are used exactly as prescribed, and if the sufferer continues to eat and drink moderately and does not smoke. Surgery, whether for perforation, bleeding, or a stubbornly persistent ulcer, involves little risk except for the elderly. In most cases treated surgically the cure is complete and permanent.

Cancer of the stomach

A stomach cancer usually starts as an ulcer in the lining of the stomach. But this does *not* mean that if you have a *stomach ulcer* (p.465) it will inevitably lead to cancer; the chances of this happening are very slim. Why a small proportion of ulcers become cancerous is not known. As in all cancers, the *malignant* cells may *metastasize*, spreading to other organs such as the lungs or liver.

What are the symptoms?

The first symptoms are so insidious that the sufferer often ignores them: vague indigestion – discomfort and occasional vomiting – is combined with loss of appetite. As the disease progresses there may be severe pain in the upper abdomen, loss of weight, frequent vomiting, and indications of prolonged bleeding from the cancer – for instance, *anaemia* (p.419), or perhaps blood in the vomit and faeces.

How common is the problem?

Cancer of the stomach is one of the most common cancers in Britain; each year 1 person in 3,000 is found to have the condition. It is twice as common in men as in women, and the chances of getting it increase with age.

What are the risks?

If, when a stomach cancer is discovered, it is too far advanced to be removed, no treatment can cure it, but drug treatment may alleviate the symptoms for many years.

What should be done?

If you develop the symptoms of *indigestion* (p.463) for the first time in your life – or if your usual indigestion changes in character – consult your doctor without delay. A long-standing stomach ulcer – but not a *duodenal ulcer* (p.468) – sometimes leads to stomach cancer, which is one reason why doctors advise surgery for a stomach ulcer that fails to heal or keeps recurring. If, along with your indigestion, you find that you have lost your appetite and that this persists for more than two or three days, be sure to tell the doctor, who will consider the possibility of stomach cancer and will arrange for you to have a *barium meal* and *endoscopy* as a hospital outpatient. The diagnostic procedure will probably also involve a stomach *biopsy*.

What is the treatment?

Self-help: The only possible self-help is to reject the notion of putting up stoically with an extensive bout of indigestion combined with appetite loss. Get yourself to the doctor if this happens to you.

Professional help: If the condition is discovered in a sufficiently early stage, the cancer, along with a small part of the stomach surrounding it, will be removed by surgery – see *Stomach removal*, opposite.

If surgery is not feasible, it is sometimes possible to slow down the development of cancer by means of *radiotherapy* and/or the use of *cytotoxic* drugs.

OPERATION:
Stomach removal
Gastrectomy

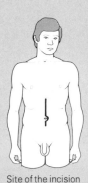

Site of the incision

An operation to remove part of the stomach (partial gastrectomy) or all of it (total gastrectomy) is carried out when stomach ulcers fail to heal despite drug treatment or dietary changes, when an ulcer bleeds badly or perforates, or for cancer of the stomach.

During the operation You are given a general anaesthetic and your stomach is sucked clean by a tube passed into your nose and down your oesophagus. The surgeon makes an incision in the upper abdomen and removes part or all of the stomach, then sews together the remaining cut edges to maintain a passageway for food. The operation usually takes 2 hours.

After the operation You will be connected to a drip feed, and one or more tubes will drain off excess fluid that collects at the operation site. After a few days your digestive tract should have recovered sufficiently for you to resume eating and drinking. The usual hospital stay is about 10 to 14 days.

Convalescence Your doctor may prescribe drugs to control after-effects such as nausea and

diarrhoea. Eating small, frequent meals is often advised. Most patients make a full recovery in roughly 1 to 2 months.

See also information on operations, p.738.

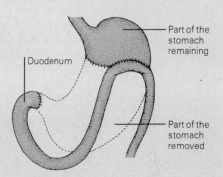

Duodenum — Part of the stomach remaining

Part of the stomach removed

In one form of partial gastrectomy (illustrated), the remaining part of the stomach is attached to the area of the small intestine between the duodenum and the ileum. In another method, the duodenum is re-attached to the stomach.

What are the long-term prospects?
Your chances of a complete cure are higher if the tumour can be removed surgically at an early stage. Even if it recurs, symptoms can often be relieved by drugs and radiotherapy for many years. If you are determined to fight the cancer, it is thought that you are likely to respond better to treatment.

Gastric erosion

Gastric erosion – an area of inflammation in the mucous membrane that lines the stomach – is usually caused by certain drugs that can irritate the membrane when taken in tablet form. Aspirin is the most familiar of these, particularly if taken regularly in the large doses often prescribed for sufferers from *rheumatoid arthritis* (p.552). Other anti-rheumatic drugs and *steroids* used in treating severe *asthma* (p.355) and such conditions as *temporal arteritis* (p.414) and *Addison's disease* (p.524) can also cause gastric erosion.

What are the symptoms?
This disorder is distinguished from *gastritis* (p.464) in that the main (and often only) symptom is bleeding of the inflamed area. If there is also vomiting, there may be blood in the vomit; it may be red but is more likely to be black and to resemble coffee grounds because it has been partly digested. The faeces may be streaked dark or black with blood. If

bleeding is gradual you may not be aware of it, but you may eventually have symptoms of *iron-deficiency anaemia* (p.419).

How common is the problem?
Gastric erosion is not common; and cases severe enough to produce blood in vomit are rare. Those people taking large amounts of aspirin or other antirheumatic pills are, however, particularly at risk.

What are the risks?
If persistent internal bleeding is not detected and treated, a large amount of blood will be lost, and anaemia will result. There is a slight risk, too, of sudden severe bleeding, which will be vomited as red blood and/or passed as black faeces. To minimize the risks, many doctors recommend paracetamol as a safer alternative to aspirin. New antirheumatic drugs are now available which are less irritating to the stomach lining than those

currently prescribed. If you are regularly taking a painkiller (including antirheumatics) consult the doctor if you have any of the following symptoms: vomiting blood; feeling abnormally fatigued (one symptom of anaemia); persistent indigestion; or passing dark or black faeces.

What is the treatment?
Self-help: No self-help is possible if you already have gastric erosion. To guard against the disorder, anyone taking regular doses of a drug that may cause the condition should make a habit of swallowing the pills with or immediately after food, never on an empty stomach. If you do take aspirin, choose the soluble variety of this drug.

Professional help: If you have been vomiting blood, you will be admitted to hospital as a matter of urgency, and given a blood transfusion, if necessary, plus any necessary treatment for anaemia. In other cases, your doctor will take you off the offending drug and will prescribe one that is less irritating to your stomach lining. *Endoscopy* may be carried out in order to observe the inside of your stomach. If there is no serious underlying disease, and if you avoid taking the drug that has irritated your stomach lining, your gastric erosion should not recur.

Pyloric stenosis

Pyloric stenosis is a rare disorder which occurs when the outlet from the stomach to the duodenum (the pylorus) becomes partly or completely blocked. This most commonly happens as a result of a *stomach ulcer* (p.465) or *duodenal ulcer* (below), but occasionally is caused by *cancer of the stomach* (p.466). It results in an uncomfortable, swollen abdomen; copious vomiting; and the repeated belching of foul-smelling gas. (For details of *Congenital pyloric stenosis* – a different disorder – see p.660.)

What are the risks?
If the pylorus becomes totally blocked, repeated vomiting may eventually result in loss of weight, *dehydration*, malnutrition, and disturbance in the body's chemical balance.

What should be done?
If you repeatedly belch foul-smelling gas and/or vomit recognizable bits of food, consult your doctor. If pyloric stenosis is suspected, you will need to undergo *endoscopy* to confirm the diagnosis and to determine the best course of treatment.

If an ulcer is causing the problem, it may respond to treatment by drugs and/or a change in diet. If this proves ineffective, or if the stenosis is a result of cancer, surgery will be necessary. (For details of this operation, see *Stomach removal*, p.467.)

Duodenal ulcer
(also called peptic ulcer)

A duodenal ulcer is a raw area in the lining of the duodenum, which is the exit tube from the stomach to the rest of the digestive tract. The ulcer, which is usually less than 15mm (about ⅓in) wide, is caused by erosion of the surface of the duodenum by acid secreted by the stomach. The pain of a duodenal ulcer is due to the action of stomach acid on the exposed surface of the ulcer. Duodenal ulcers are one type of peptic ulcer; the other type is the *stomach ulcer* (p.465).

Medical myth

Peptic ulcers are caused by the stresses and strains of a demanding job.

Wrong. If a hard-working person has an ulcer, it is probably the result of smoking, along with frequent – and frequently alcoholic – business lunches.

What are the symptoms?
The sufferer has recurrent bouts of abdominal pain which is characteristically gnawing and is usually localized in a small spot somewhere in the upper abdomen; sometimes though, when the ulcerated area is on the back wall of the duodenum, it is felt in the back. Typically, the pain (which resembles a "hunger pain") occurs several hours after a meal. It can generally be relieved by antacid tablets, a glass of milk, or a couple of biscuits. There may be a sensation of being bloated after eating, and vomiting may also occur.

How common is the problem?
More than 10 per cent of people in the Western world develop a duodenal ulcer at some time. The disorder is four times as common in men than in women, and occurs most frequently in young and middle-aged adults.

Heavy smokers are particularly susceptible to duodenal ulcers, as are people who naturally produce stomach acid in large quantities. Your chances of developing a duodenal ulcer are greater, too, if you often take painkillers that contain aspirin or similar substances, antirheumatics, or *steroids*.

What are the risks?
Although duodenal ulcers are painful, the risk of severe or permanent damage from complications is low, and the ulcers often disappear in time even if untreated. In some cases a duodenal ulcer may begin to bleed,

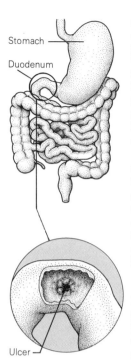

Stomach

Duodenum

Ulcer

Duodenal ulcer
The exact cause of a duodenal ulcer is not clear. It may result from an excess of acid flowing from the stomach into the duodenum. An additional factor may be an abnormality in the protective mucous lining of the duodenum.

and even slight bleeding can result in *iron-deficiency anaemia* (p.419) if the bleeding persists. Sudden, heavy bleeding may lead to the vomiting of blood or the passing of black, tarry faeces. The loss of a large amount of blood is an emergency requiring immediate medical attention. A further possible complication is persistent scarring from the ulcer leading to obstruction of the entrance to the duodenum (see *Pyloric stenosis*, opposite).

In a few cases – perhaps 1 to 2 per cent of all duodenal ulcers – the ulcer erodes through the duodenal wall into the abdominal cavity and *peritonitis* (p.470) will result unless surgical treatment is swiftly carried out. The *perforation* causes sudden, intense pain, which may be followed by *shock* (p.386) and collapse. Any such emergency requires immediate treatment.

What should be done?

If you think you might have a duodenal ulcer, try the self-help measures recommended below. If the symptoms do not disappear within two weeks, see your doctor, who may order the same hospital diagnostic tests as for a stomach ulcer.

What is the treatment?

Self-help: If you smoke, stop. Reduce your intake of alcohol, particularly of wine and spirits. In general, you may eat whatever you like; but eat slowly and try to rest for half an hour after meals. It is also wise to eat several small meals regularly spaced through the day, instead of two or three large ones; food in the stomach tends to neutralize the stomach acid that causes pain. Missing meals or eating irregularly is likely to make symptoms worse. Antacid tablets or medicines taken regularly will also help. Such simple measures may well be enough to cure your ulcer without the need for any further treatment.

Professional help: At first your doctor may simply give you further advice on diet and eating habits, and prescribe a more suitable antacid. If this does not help, the probable alternative is a drug which reduces production of stomach acid. It is important to follow instructions strictly when taking such a drug; there is a risk of the ulcer recurring if drug treatment is stopped suddenly.

Surgery is seldom necessary for duodenal ulcers; operations are performed only in rare cases where an ulcer fails to respond to a long period of treatment or where complications occur. The type of operation varies, but the general aim is to reduce the acid-producing capacity of the stomach. This can be done either by cutting away a section of the stomach (see *Stomach removal*, p.467) or by cutting the nerves that control acid production in the stomach – an operation called vagotomy. Such operations are safe and usually successful, but occasionally there are troublesome after-effects. Among these may be: faintness, drowsiness, or trembling and sweating soon after eating; loss of weight, with diarrhoea; anaemia; or vitamin D deficiency (see *Vitamins*, p.494). These after-effects should, however, respond quickly to further drug treatment.

Swallowed foreign body

Normally, air goes down the trachea (windpipe) into the lungs, and food goes down the oesophagus into the stomach. If solid matter is accidentally "breathed in", it may get stuck in the throat (in which case it is generally coughed up) or it may slip into the respiratory tract, causing choking. If this happens, prompt first aid is essential – see *Accidents and emergencies*, p.803, for advice on what to do for someone who is choking.

Most foreign bodies that go down the oesophagus – even, amazingly enough, sharp and awkwardly shaped ones – are carried through the digestive tract and excreted without trouble. To be on the safe side, though, consult your doctor if you have swallowed anything sharp (like a fish bone or needle) or something with a diameter of more than 10mm (⅜in).

If you find it difficult to swallow, have abdominal pain, or are feverish, you may need to have your digestive tract X-rayed; this technique nearly always locates and identifies the foreign body, which can usually be removed by an *endoscope* with a claw-like attachment. Only rarely is surgery required to remove a large, firmly stuck, pointed foreign body.

Blood in vomit

Blood in vomit should never be disregarded – it could indicate a serious digestive-tract disorder such as bleeding *stomach ulcer* (p.465) or an area of *gastric erosion* (p.467).

Fresh blood in the vomit is recognizable as such; it is bright red, and may occur in streaks or may be virtually the only substance you bring up. Blood that has been in the stomach for some hours will have gone dark red or black and may look like coffee grounds.

Consult your doctor without delay if you suspect there is blood in your vomit, unless you *know* that it came from a recent nosebleed. If possible, take with you a sample of the vomit to aid the doctor's diagnosis. If you have blood in your vomit *and* your skin is cold, you are sweating, and you feel weak, you may be suffering from *shock* (p.386). Get to hospital *now*.

Generalized intestinal problems

The intestines – the section of the digestive tract between the duodenum and the anus – consist of a long, thin, coiled tube (the *small intestine*, p.473) leading to a shorter, wider tube (the colon) that leads into a final, short tube (the rectum). When both the colon and rectum are mentioned together, they are often termed the *large intestine* (p.476).

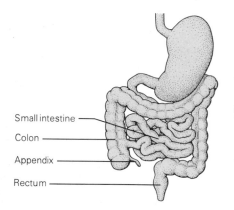

Small intestine

Colon

Appendix

Rectum

The intestines
The intestines are made up of the small intestine, the appendix, and the large intestine (colon and rectum). They form a long coil which fits into the abdominal cavity. Nutrients from the food which passes along the small intestine are absorbed into the bloodstream. Most of the water in the intestinal contents is absorbed into the bloodstream in the large intestine.

Food passes from the stomach through the duodenum into the small intestine, where it is further broken down by *enzymes* in the various digestive juices. As it travels along the small intestine, propelled by rhythmic muscular contractions, nutrients are absorbed into the bloodstream through the thin intestinal walls. Most of the fluid is removed from the intestinal contents as they pass through the colon; and what remains is a mixture of undigested and indigestible food – largely vegetable fibres ("roughage") – along with bacteria, mucus, and dead cells from the lining of the digestive tract. This material (the faeces) passes into the rectum, where it remains until excreted through the anus. In general, the entire digestive process, from food entering the mouth to being excreted from the anus, takes about 24 hours.

Problems that are not specifically related to one section of the intestinal tract but that may occur anywhere within it are discussed in the following group of articles. Also included is peritonitis, a serious disease that affects the peritoneum. The peritoneum is the thin membrane within which many abdominal organs (including the intestines) are enclosed.

Peritonitis

Peritonitis is inflammation of the peritoneum, the two-layered membrane that lines the abdominal cavity and covers the stomach, intestines, and other abdominal organs. This condition almost always is the result of an underlying disease rather than a disease itself. It may occur as a complication of a disorder in which the digestive tract is irritated or ruptured – for instance, a perforated *stomach ulcer* (p.465) or *duodenal ulcer* (p.468), *diverticular disease* (p.479), or *appendicitis* (p.476). It may also be a complication of a *pelvic infection* (p.596), in which a woman has inflammation of the fallopian tubes and/or uterus within the lower abdomen. Another possible cause is infection from an injury that pierces the abdominal wall. Peritonitis may occasionally be a complication of abdominal surgery.

What are the symptoms?
Symptoms vary, depending on the source of irritation or infection, but there is always severe abdominal pain. It is most severe near the site of the original problem; for example,

it is worst in the right side of the abdomen if caused by appendicitis. The pain increases when you move about. If you press the most tender spot, it hurts. There is often a feeling of nausea, followed by vomiting, and there is also likely to be some fever. After two or three hours your abdomen may swell up as the pain becomes less severe and less localized. Decrease of pain, however, does not indicate an easing of the trouble; it is a danger sign (see "What are the risks?" below).

How common is the problem?
Peritonitis is rare in countries with a high standard of medical care. However, if treatment for an abdominal emergency such as a perforated duodenal ulcer or appendicitis is delayed, peritonitis is almost inevitable.

What are the risks?
If peritonitis is neglected, the sufferer can become *dehydrated* from repeated vomiting. Decrease of severe pain indicates paralysis of the intestines, and death will follow without emergency treatment.

What should be done?

Peritonitis is a serious disorder. Call your doctor or an ambulance immediately if you get severe abdominal pain lasting for more than 10 to 20 minutes, especially when accompanied by any of the other symptoms mentioned above. To establish the underlying cause of the attack, the doctor will question you and examine your abdomen, pressing here and there in order to locate the inflamed area. You may also have diagnostic tests such as *X-rays*. (For further information on urgent diagnostic procedures in such cases see *Acute abdomen*, p.477.)

What is the treatment?

Prompt surgery to correct the underlying cause of peritoneal inflammation is generally the only possible treatment. After you have been admitted to hospital, the contents of your intestines will be removed through a tube passed down through the oesophagus and stomach. To treat the inflammation and strengthen you for the operation if you are weak and dehydrated, you will be given *antibiotics*, often along with nutrients and fluids in an *intravenous drip*. Your abdomen will then be opened, and the organ that is causing the trouble will be either removed (as in appendicitis) or repaired (as in the case of a perforated ulcer).

Prospects for full recovery are excellent. With the help of antibiotics, few people today die of peritonitis.

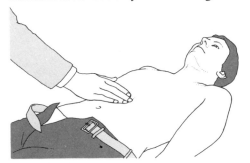

Doctor's examination for peritonitis
If your doctor suspects that you have peritonitis, he or she will "palpate" your abdomen to check whether the characteristic hardness of peritonitis is present. You can help the doctor by relaxing your abdominal muscles.

Intestinal obstruction

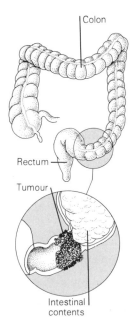

Colon

Rectum

Tumour

Intestinal contents

Blockage by a tumour
Part of the intestine has become completely blocked by a cancerous tumour, preventing the intestinal contents from passing down into the rectum.

An intestinal obstruction is a partial or complete blockage of the intestines, making it impossible for the digestive process to run its full course. Any one of several factors can cause an intestinal obstruction. The most common causes include strangulated *hernia* (p.537) or blockage of the intestine by a band of tissue, usually caused by a prior inflammatory disease or resulting from an operation on the abdomen; but passage through the intestinal tubes can also be impeded by a growth such as *cancer of the large intestine* (p.481) or *carcinoids* (p.472). Sometimes part of a healthy intestine can become knotted or twisted (a condition known as volvulus). Rarely, the cause of intestinal obstruction is partial or total blockage by a non-digestible object, such as a large coin or key, that has been swallowed accidentally (see *Swallowed foreign body*, p.469).

What are the symptoms?

Symptoms depend on the location of the obstruction and on whether it is complete or partial. An obstruction in the small intestine causes intermittent cramp-like pains in the middle of the abdomen along with increasingly frequent bouts of vomiting. But if blockage is in the large intestine there may be little or no vomiting. Complete blockage anywhere in the digestive tract naturally results in constipation; if the large intestine is blocked, this may be so extreme that you cannot even pass wind. Partial obstruction is more likely to cause diarrhoea than constipation because only the liquid portion of the faeces can pass the obstruction. In an obstruction resulting from volvulus the twisted portion of the intestine sometimes relaxes, with consequent relief from pain and the passing of large amounts of wind and watery faeces. The relaxation is usually only temporary, however, and should not deter you from seeking advice and treatment from your doctor.

How common is the problem?

Intestinal obstruction is not common. Fortunately, the underlying cause is usually discovered and dealt with before blockage becomes complete.

What are the risks?

Any disruption of the normal functioning of the intestines can lead to muscular paralysis (see *Ileus*, p.472). Persistent vomiting can cause *dehydration* and, eventually, *shock* (p.386). If the blockage is not relieved, there is also a danger that the intestine will rupture, producing *peritonitis* (opposite). If the obstruction is due to cancer, there is the additional risk that the disease may spread.

What should be done?

If you have a combination of symptoms that suggests the possibility of intestinal obstruction, call your doctor or an ambulance as a matter of urgency. The doctor will suspect this disorder from a clear account of the symptoms along with an examination of the abdomen. You will then be admitted to hospital without delay in order to determine the cause and exact site of the obstruction. *X-rays* will probably provide sufficient information for treatment to be started immediately, but a quick exploratory operation called a *laparotomy* (see *Acute abdomen*, p.477) is sometimes necessary. You will probably be given fluids in an *intravenous drip* to prevent dehydration and shock, and the dammed-up contents of your digestive tract will be removed by means of a tube passed down through the stomach into the intestines.

What is the treatment?

Surgery to relieve the blockage is virtually inevitable; it can usually be carried out at the same time as the laparotomy. If the source of the trouble is a volvulus, the surgeon may be able to untwist the intestine in such a way as to prevent recurrence of the problem. Often, though, to eliminate any risk of recurrence, the preferred procedure is to remove the part of the intestine in which a blockage of this type has occurred. Prospects for full recovery from an intestinal obstruction are excellent after surgery unless the underlying disorder does not respond to treatment.

Ileus

In a healthy intestine, rhythmic muscular contractions of the intestinal wall coax food through the digestive tract. Ileus is a serious disorder in which the intestines become paralysed. It sometimes follows a serious abdominal condition such as an *intestinal obstruction* (p.471), or a perforated *stomach ulcer* (p.465) or *duodenal ulcer* (p.468). Bacteria stagnate in the trapped, partly digested food, producing gas that distends the intestines and abdomen. The swollen abdomen presses on the chest, impairing breathing; and in addition to being badly constipated, the sufferer may become feverish and may repeatedly vomit foul-smelling fluid. At the outset of an attack of ileus there is dull, persistent pain in the abdomen. This may soon disappear, but relief from pain does not signify an improvement and the condition may be fatal unless the underlying cause is successfully treated.

Some degree of ileus follows many abdominal operations and is so routinely dealt with in hospital that you are unlikely to know you have had it. Otherwise, the condition arises from a serious disorder such as a perforated ulcer and so you are likely to be extremely ill already and in need of urgent treatment. Successful treatment for the underlying disorder should also cure the ileus.

Carcinoids

(and the carcinoid syndrome)

A carcinoid is a special type of intestinal-wall growth that, although *malignant*, develops so slowly that over half of the people who have it never know about it. The growths are usually only discovered during a diagnostic test or surgery for some other, unrelated disorder. They can become big enough, however, to cause *intestinal obstruction* (p.471).

In about 10 per cent of all cases, carcinoid cells *metastasize* – that is, they spread through the bloodstream to the liver, where they multiply, forming *hormone-producing tumours* (p.518). These tumours manufacture hormones that are carried in the bloodstream and have widespread effects on the body. The result is a characteristic group of symptoms called the carcinoid syndrome.

What are the symptoms?

The main symptom of the carcinoid syndrome is flushing of the skin on the face and neck, which is triggered off by some activity such as taking exercise or drinking alcohol. It looks like a blush, but it lasts for much longer – up to several hours. Other symptoms include watering and swelling of the eyes; explosive diarrhoea, often with abdominal cramp; wheezing and other symptoms of *asthma* (p.355); and the symptoms of *heart failure* (p.381), including breathlessness.

What should be done?

If you have a combination of symptoms suggesting you might be suffering from the carcinoid syndrome, your doctor will arrange for various tests to confirm the diagnosis. Tests include an abdominal *X-ray*, and *endoscopy* to view the inside of your digestive tract along with a *biopsy* of any growth present.

What is the treatment?

Carcinoids discovered in their early stages can often be surgically removed, but surgical cure of the carcinoid syndrome is not possible. Treatment is therefore mainly by drugs and is aimed at easing symptoms – reducing flushing attacks and keeping diarrhoea under control; and asthma is relieved by *bronchodilators*. In some cases a *cytotoxic* drug may slow the progress of the disease.

Small intestine

The small intestine is a tube about 35mm (1½in) in diameter and about 5m (16ft) long. It runs between the duodenum and the colon (the first part of the large intestine), and is the main site for the absorption of nutrients into the bloodstream.

Like the stomach and the large intestine, the small intestine is constantly in motion, controlled automatically by a network of nerves, to push the food along its length by *peristaltic* waves of contractions of the muscles in its wall.

In the small intestine the process of breaking down the food into small particles, already begun in the stomach and duodenum, continues aided by the secretion of additional *enzymes* from the small-intestine wall. Once food molecules are small enough, they pass through the thin lining of the intestine into

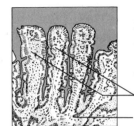

Microscopic structure of the small intestine
The inside surface of the small intestine is made up of finger-like projections called villi, through which food is absorbed.

Villi

Wall of small intestine

the bloodstream, and then on to the liver for storage and distribution.

To make sure that as much of the food as possible is absorbed from the small intestine, the inside of its wall is covered with minute finger-like projections called villi. The villi present a very large surface area for maximum absorption of nutrients into the body.

Crohn's disease

(also called terminal ileitis)

Crohn's disease is a chronic (long-term) inflammation of part of the digestive tract. The part most commonly affected is the terminal section of the small intestine (the ileum) although patchy inflammation can occur anywhere in the intestines. What causes the disease is a mystery; it is neither hereditary nor infectious. It begins with the development in the intestinal wall of patches of inflammation, which may or may not grow or spread from one part of the system to another. For no known reason some of the spots heal, but they may leave scar tissue that thickens intestinal walls and narrows the passageway.

What are the symptoms?
Crohn's disease normally manifests itself in periodic attacks of cramps, abdominal pain (especially after eating), diarrhoea, and a general sense of feeling ill; often there may be slight fever. Attacks tend to begin when you are in your twenties and to recur (sometimes every few months, sometimes every few years) for the rest of your life. About one-quarter of sufferers have only one or two attacks, which never again recur.

How common is the problem?
This has been a rare disorder in the Western world, with only 1 case per 5,000 people, but it is gradually becoming more common. There are about twice as many sufferers today as there were 20 years ago.

What are the risks?
If the condition endures for years, there is a gradual deterioration in bowel functioning. Sometimes the inflamed intestinal wall may leak, causing *peritonitis* (p.470). There is a risk of poor absorption of nutrients, with consequent loss of appetite and weight (see *Malabsorption*, p.475), or of *intestinal obstruction* (p.471). Severe bleeding, resulting in *iron-deficiency anaemia* (p.419), can also occur. There is also a faint chance that Crohn's disease, if untreated, can increase susceptibility to cancer of the intestine (see *Tumours of the small intestine*, p.474).

What should be done?
If your symptoms suggest the possibility of Crohn's disease, consult your doctor, who, after examining you, will probably want *X-rays* of your digestive tract (for which you will need a *barium meal* and perhaps a *barium enema*). You may also have to undergo *endoscopy* of the intestines in order to locate the inflamed areas. Blood samples may be taken to see whether you are anaemic.

What is the treatment?
Self-help: Follow the doctor's advice about diet and rest during an attack. In general, milky foods are most suitable because they provide you with energy and body-building materials without producing the bulk that might irritate the intestines.

Professional help: In most cases treatment by drugs eases attacks of Crohn's disease. Among the drugs used are *analgesics*, anti-inflammatory agents, and antidiarrhoea tablets. The doctor will also recommend certain foods and warn you against others, and may suggest a modification of your daily routine to relieve pressure on your digestive system.

To guard against further attacks, a long-term course of anti-inflammatory *steroids* or other drugs is generally prescribed. At first you will take high doses of such drugs, but the dosage will be gradually decreased. Such treatment may not effect a full cure, but should reduce severity of attacks.

If repeated attacks have scarred and narrowed your intestines so badly that the inflammation does not respond to drug treatment, you will probably need an operation to remove the worst-affected length of intestine. Occasionally a *colostomy or ileostomy* (p.482) is necessary. Surgery can provide dramatic improvement and postpone further attacks of Crohn's disease for many years.

Coeliac disease in adults

In a person suffering from coeliac disease, the lining of the small intestine reacts adversely to gluten, a protein present in wheat and other grains. It is very rare for coeliac disease to appear for the first time in adulthood; it nearly always reveals itself in infancy. For this reason it is dealt with fully in the children's section (see *Coeliac disease*, p.684).

What are the symptoms?
If coeliac disease does appear for the first time in an adult, the symptoms are abdominal pain and swelling, diarrhoea, weight loss, and a general lack of energy. If you develop these symptoms, then see your doctor. Diagnosis and treatment of the disease is basically the same for adults as for children.

Tumours of the small intestine

Like those in other parts of the body, tumours of the small intestine can be *benign* or *malignant*. Most are benign, symptom-free, and usually remain undetected unless tests or treatment for some other disorder reveal their presence. But in about 1 out of 10 cases, the growths are malignant. Very rarely they are *carcinoids* (p.472).

What are the symptoms?
Malignant tumours in the small intestine may cause loss of weight; the symptoms of *anaemia* (p.419) – paleness, tiredness, and palpitations on exertion; and, occasionally, blood in the faeces.

How common is the problem?
Tumours of the small intestine are extremely rare, comprising fewer than 5 per cent of all digestive-tract tumours, even though the small intestine is the most extensive part of the tract. If you have *Crohn's disease* (p.473) or *coeliac disease* (above), your chances of developing cancerous small-intestinal growths appear to be slightly increased.

What are the risks?
There is the risk of *intestinal obstruction* (p.471) from any large growth. A malignant tumour, of course, is life-threatening unless discovered and treated at an early stage. So the main risk is that the rather generalized symptoms of cancerous small-intestine tumours may be ignored until it is too late for effective treatment.

What should be done?
If you lose weight for no clear reason, if you have abdominal pain, if you notice any

---

Constipation and diarrhoea

There is no uniform pattern of bowel action. Most people have about one movement a day, but some have four or five a day, and at the other extreme there are people who regularly open their bowels only once a week. In general, the more frequent the bowel actions the more liquid the faeces. Consider yourself constipated only if your normal pattern changes and you begin to have irregular, unusually infrequent, or difficult movements. Similarly, you have diarrhoea only if you are passing abnormal, excessive quantities of mostly liquid faecal matter.

Constipation and diarrhoea are not in themselves disorders; they are symptoms of disorders. Some people are constipated largely because they have become dependent on laxatives, over-use of which may lead to natural inactivity. Others lose their normal bowel reflexes because they tend to be too busy to take time off for a regular few minutes in the lavatory. Other possible causes include diet (especially a diet low in *fibre*), the use of certain medicines (especially cough mixtures), haemorrhoids or an anal fissure (which can inhibit bowel activity through fear of pain), or even a psychological disorder such as severe depression. And diarrhoea can be brought on by, for example, stress, by certain foods such as prunes or beans, and by medicines such as antacids or *antibiotics*.

If constipation persists for more than two weeks or diarrhoea for more than 48 hours, or if you notice any other change in your bowel habits, always seek medical advice.

change in your bowel habits, and/or if your faeces are dark, consult your doctor, who will examine your abdomen and will probably arrange for in-hospital diagnostic tests. A *barium meal* will reveal tumours, if any. To determine whether they are benign or malignant, you may also be subjected to an *endoscopic* examination and *biopsy*.

What is the treatment?

Once detected, small-intestine tumours are usually best removed by surgery even if they are benign. Sometimes malignant growths are either too numerous or widespread for surgical removal; in such cases *steroid* drugs and *radiotherapy* are given to help keep the growths under control.

Meckel's diverticulum

Meckel's diverticulum – a pouch near the lower end of the small intestine – is a *congenital* disorder (one that is present at birth). About 1 person in 50 has such a pouch, but well over half of all such cases are symptom-free. A Meckel's diverticulum is like an appendix, in that it becomes significant only when inflamed (see *Appendicitis*, p.476). Symptoms of this disorder are severe bleeding from the rectum, sometimes preceded by pain and vomiting.

Inflammation of the diverticulum may be diagnosed as appendicitis (with or without the added complication of *peritonitis*, p.470), or even perforated *duodenal ulcer* (p.468). But this does not matter because the initial move in all such conditions is to open up the abdomen (see *Acute abdomen*, p.477). The surgeon then discovers the true source of the symptoms, and removal of Meckel's diverticulum (along with treatment for peritonitis, if necessary) cures the condition.

Malab- sorption

Intestinal wall

Flattened villi

Flattened villi
Serious symptoms of malabsorption may indicate a need for biopsy of the small intestine, to determine whether the villi have become flattened. Flattening of the villi causes a reduction in the surface area of the small intestine, and this in turn reduces the small intestine's ability to absorb nutrients.

A healthy body requires a constant supply of nutrients for energy and for building body tissues. The small intestine is the major site for absorption into the bloodstream of these nutrients. If there is something wrong with the structure of your small intestine, or if the chemicals and *enzymes* within it are not properly assisting the digestive process, certain elements of the diet may not be fully absorbed. Malabsorption, therefore, is basically a symptom of a disease that affects the functioning of the small intestine.

There is a long list of diseases that can cause malabsorption. A physical change in the absorptive inner surface of the small intestine (as in *Crohn's disease*, p.473) or reaction to one element in the diet – for example, to gluten (see *Coeliac disease*, opposite) can cause it. In a rare inherited disease called alactasia, lack of one of the digestive enzymes results in an inability to digest and absorb various sugars present in milk. Other diseases that may be linked with malabsorption are *iron-deficiency anaemia* (p.419), *pernicious anaemia* (p.419) and *chronic pancreatitis* (p.491). It may also be an occasional complication of *diabetes mellitus* (p.519), thyroid disease (see *Thyroid and parathyroid glands*, p.525), or *cystic fibrosis* (p.685).

Another cause is digestive-tract surgery. One form of *stomach removal* (p.467), for instance, changes the "climate" of the small intestine, although the effects of this change are unlikely to be noticed until several months or even years afterwards.

What are the symptoms?

The usual symptoms are occasional abdominal discomfort, generally loose bowels, and yellowish-grey, greasy-looking faeces, which have a peculiarly strong odour and tend to float because of a high fat content. Over a period of months or years, unchecked malabsorption leads to loss of weight and energy, breathlessness, and various symptoms of particular vitamin or mineral deficiency such as a sore tongue, prickling sensations, and numbness in arms and legs (see *Vitamins*, p.494).

How common is the problem?

Severe, generalized malabsorption is extremely rare in the Western world. Up to one-third of all individuals who undergo digestive-tract surgery show signs of the condition during the post-operative period, but the signs are mild and with hospital care they usually disappear soon afterwards.

What should be done?

If you believe that you may be suffering from malabsorption, see your doctor. After giving you a full physical examination, the doctor may want several samples of blood and faecal material for analysis, in order to estimate the levels of various proteins, fats, and minerals.

Once the condition is diagnosed, the main task of the doctor is to discover the underlying cause of malabsorption and treat it accordingly. A high-protein, high-calorie diet supplemented by vitamin and mineral extracts might help in certain cases.

Large intestine

The large intestine, which is about 1.5m (5ft) long and about 50mm (2in) in diameter, consists of two main sections: the colon and the rectum. The small intestine opens into a pouch-like chamber called the caecum, which is the first part of the colon. The rest of the colon then runs up the right side of the body, across under the ribcage, and down the left side, thus forming a frame for the highly convoluted small intestine. The rectum is a short tube – about 120mm (5in) long – leading downwards from the end of the colon to the anus. Fluid and various mineral salts from the intestinal contents are absorbed into the bloodstream through the membranous wall of the colon, while indigestible solids are compacted and propelled towards the rectum, where they are stored as faecal matter until ready for releasing through the anus.

The large intestine is especially subject to inflammation because of infection, and it is more susceptible than other sections of the digestive tract to develop tumours and *polyps*. Moreover, the large intestine, like the teeth, appears to be adversely affected by the kind of food most Europeans and North Americans now eat: colonic and rectal disorders are far more common in the Western world than they are in Africa and Asia.

The large intestine
Undigested food in the form of liquid faeces flows from the small intestine into the colon (the first part of large intestine), where most of the water content is absorbed back into the body. The semi-solid faeces that remain move down into the second part of the large intestine, the rectum, from where they are eventually excreted as stools.

Colon

Appendix

Rectum

Appendicitis

The appendix is a thin, worm-shaped pouch, around 90mm (3½in) long, that projects from the first part of the colon. In herbivorous animals such as rabbits, the appendix is relatively large and plays an important role in the digestive process. But in human beings, the relatively small appendix seems to be an evolutionary relic – any function that it might have is still obscure.

Like the rest of the intestines, your appendix contains bacteria that are harmless as long as they remain in balance. Some doctors believe that appendicitis may result from the entrance to the appendix becoming partially or completely blocked. Such a blockage may be caused by an unusually hardened piece of intestinal matter (a "faecolith"), a swollen lymph gland, more rarely a tumour, or even a tapeworm. Whatever the cause of the blockage, it could lead to an increase in the bacterial population in the stagnant contents of the pouch, which becomes swollen, inflamed, and pus-filled.

However, appendicitis may be caused by any of a number of factors, and very often the actual cause of an attack is never discovered. There is no way to predict or prevent the onset of this condition.

What are the symptoms?
The symptoms of appendicitis are variable enough to make diagnosis difficult at times, even for the most experienced of doctors. Usually the symptoms come on quite quickly, often within 24 hours of the onset of inflammation of the appendix.

The principal symptom is severe abdominal pain, which usually starts as vague discomfort around the navel, but becomes sharper and more localized during the course

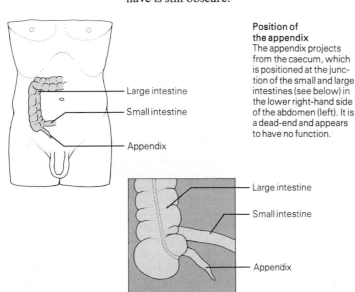

Position of the appendix
The appendix projects from the caecum, which is positioned at the junction of the small and large intestines (see below) in the lower right-hand side of the abdomen (left). It is a dead-end and appears to have no function.

Large intestine

Small intestine

Appendix

Large intestine

Small intestine

Appendix

OPERATION: **Appendix removal**
Appendicectomy

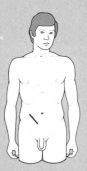

Site of the incision

Removal of the appendix is usually carried out for appendicitis, when the organ becomes inflamed and may burst. However, the surgeon may not be able to confirm the diagnosis of appendicitis until your abdomen has been opened up and examined inside – a procedure called *laparotomy*. Both the laparotomy and the following appendicectomy are usually carried out as a matter of urgency.

During the operation The appendix is cut away and removed through an incision in the lower right side of your abdomen. Provided there are no further abdominal problems, the operation should take less than one hour.

After the operation You should be able to resume eating and drinking within 24 hours, and be ready to leave hospital about 5 days after the operation.

Convalescence You will probably be back to normal 2 or 3 weeks after leaving hospital. Lack of an appendix has no effect on future health.

See also information on operations, p.738.

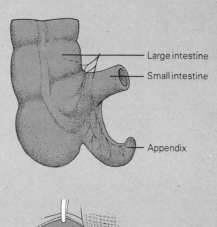

Large intestine

Small intestine

Appendix

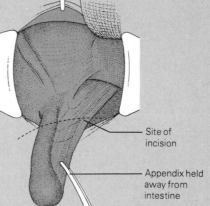

Site of incision

Appendix held away from intestine

Appendix removal is a relatively simple operation. The appendix is simply pulled away from the surrounding tissue and cut off at its base (right). The resulting hole in the intestine is stitched. Because a burst appendix can be dangerous, the appendix may well be removed during any other operation on a nearby area in the abdomen – for example, on the uterus or gallbladder.

Acute abdomen

If your intestines and the interior lining of your abdominal cavity become inflamed (see *Peritonitis*, p.470), the result will be pain, vomiting, and fever. As the inflammation worsens these symptoms become more marked, and the muscles of your abdominal wall will probably go into *spasm*, making your abdomen feel hard and board-like. The picture will be much the same whether the cause of your inflammation is leakage of acid from a burst *duodenal ulcer* (p.468), *appendicitis* (opposite), *Crohn's disease* (p.473), an inflamed diverticulum in the colon (see *Diverticular disease*, p.479), bleeding from an injury, etc. If you have the above symptoms, you will of course call your doctor or an ambulance immediately; this is an obvious emergency.

When no certain diagnosis can be made immediately, your doctor may use "acute abdomen" as a working diagnosis; and the best course of action may then be for the surgeon to "take a look inside" – an operation termed an exploratory *laparotomy* (see the operation *Appendix removal*, above).

The term "laparotomy" means simply an incision through the abdominal wall. The surgeon would not usually perform this exploratory operation unless he or she suspected a disorder which would need to be treated by surgery anyway. The site of the incision might be in different parts of the abdomen, depending on the tentative diagnosis.

Once your abdomen is open, the surgeon will be able to locate the source of the trouble and carry out the specific treatment, such as removal of the inflamed appendix or closing a perforated duodenal ulcer.

of a few hours. If you have appendicitis, you will probably feel pain in a small spot in the lower right part of your abdomen (the site of the inflamed appendix). Even slight pressure on the spot will increase the pain. You will also feel feverish and nauseated and may actually vomit; you will lose your appetite; and you may either be constipated or – less likely – have diarrhoea. If you have a dull, recurrent pain in the lower part of your abdomen, this may lead you to suspect that you have what is sometimes called a "grumbling appendix". However, most doctors would agree that there is no such condition (see the box on *Grumbling appendix*, below).

How common is the problem?
Every year, about 1 person in 500 has an attack of appendicitis. Anybody of any age may be affected, but the disease is rare among children less than two years old.

What are the risks?
Appendicitis presents very little risk as long as the condition is diagnosed early. One risk is that the sufferer may think, in the early stages of the problem, that the pain is caused by *gastroenteritis* (p.459) and take a laxative; purgative medicines can cause an inflamed appendix to burst (*perforate*). There is also a chance that the swollen appendix will burst if treatment is delayed. When the appendix bursts, the contents are discharged into the abdomen and the likely result is *peritonitis* (p.470). But it is possible that the *omentum*, a flap of tissue that covers the intestines, will envelop the inflamed appendix, cordoning off the area and preventing the spread of infection. When infection is localized in this way, the result is an appendix *abscess*.

What should be done?
If you have a pain in the lower right side of your abdomen along with any of the other symptoms of appendicitis, consult a doctor without delay. For the reasons mentioned in "What are the risks?" above, do not take a laxative. Your doctor will question you about the nature and onset of symptoms and will carefully examine your abdomen to test the location and severity of pain.

If the doctor decides that you are probably suffering from appendicitis, you will be admitted to hospital as soon as possible. If there is some doubt about the diagnosis and if your symptoms do not indicate an urgent need for surgery, you may undergo further diagnostic procedures such as blood tests and an abdominal *X-ray*. Alternatively, an exploratory operation – *laparotomy* – will be done immediately (see *Acute abdomen*, p.477). If the cause of the trouble is found to be appendicitis, your appendix will almost certainly be removed there and then.

What is the treatment?
The cure for appendicitis is swift surgical removal of the offending organ. The operation, known as *appendicectomy* (p.477), is straightforward and there is very little risk of complications. Usually, the appendicectomy can be started as soon as laparotomy has revealed the cause of the problem.

Removal of the appendix does not affect general health and, of course, prevents any recurrence of appendicitis.

If diagnostic tests or laparotomy reveal an appendix abscess then it is unlikely that removal of the appendix will be attempted there and then – the omentum adhering to the inflamed organ complicates this operation. The sufferer will receive large doses of *antibiotics* to settle the problem, and will probably be allowed to go home after a few days, though the antibiotics will be continued for some weeks. Because appendicitis is likely to flare up again, the sufferer will eventually be readmitted to hospital for appendicectomy, but only when tests show that the abscess has disappeared completely.

"Grumbling appendix"

Most doctors would agree there is no medical condition equivalent to the complaint popularly called "grumbling appendix". The only major recognized disorder of the appendix is appendicitis, which is an acute condition – that is, its onset is usually swift (within hours) and very painful.

If you have recurrent mild pain in the lower abdomen, perhaps accompanied by a slight upset in bowel habits, you should not expect to receive the emergency care given for appendicitis or a similarly serious abdominal condition (see *Acute abdomen*, p.477). It is far more likely that you have a less serious, chronic (long-term) problem such as *irritable colon* (opposite). Your doctor is unlikely to order sophisticated diagnostic tests unless your symptoms become troublesome, or your bowel habits undergo a marked, prolonged change.

Irritable colon

(also called spastic colon or mucous colitis)

Normally, the intestinal contents are propelled along by regular, coordinated waves of muscular contraction (known as *peristalsis*). In an irritable colon the waves are irregular and uncoordinated, and this interferes with the progress of faecal matter through the intestines. The cause of the disorder is not fully understood; like indigestion, it is most likely the result of a number of factors. Some doctors believe that the cause is mainly psychological since the disorder appears to be most prevalent among people under stress.

What are the symptoms?
The predominant symptoms may be either diarrhoea or constipation – in other words the faeces may either be excessively liquid or too hard. Sometimes, constipation with hard, dry, pellet-like faeces may alternate with the diarrhoea, which is usually worse in the morning. Some pain on defecation is also common. The most consistent symptoms are cramp-like, spasmodic pains, usually felt in one side of the lower abdomen; these are usually relieved by defecation.

If you have an irritable colon, you will occasionally feel mildly nauseated, bloated, flatulent, and without much appetite.

How common is the problem?
The condition appears to be twice as common in women as in men in Britain; about 1 person in 1,500 consults a doctor because of irritable colon in an average year, but many people simply learn to live with it. Although the condition may cause abdominal discomfort over many years, there is virtually no danger of further complications.

What should be done?
Because some of the symptoms of irritable colon are similar to those of *cancer of the large intestine* (p.481), *ulcerative colitis* (p.480), and *Crohn's disease* (p.473), all of which are potentially dangerous, you should consult your doctor. A series of tests such as *X-ray*, *sigmoidoscopy*, *barium meal*, and examination of the faeces for blood should enable the doctors to make a diagnosis.

What is the treatment?
Self-help: Anyone with an irritable colon should try to discover the factors that make the symptoms worse. Emotional stress may be important, in which case you will need to try to maintain a calm, orderly life style. If you discover that fried foods, for instance, or raw vegetables seem to aggravate your symptoms, try to avoid them. It may be helpful to cut out alcohol and tobacco. Often a dramatic improvement results from a diet high in *fibre*.
Professional help: The various symptoms of an irritable colon can often be lessened by drugs. If constipation is your predominant symptom, your doctor may recommend a mild laxative; if, however, your main problem is diarrhoea, you may be prescribed a drug to combat this. If you have severe abdominal pain, the doctor may also prescribe an *antispasmodic*; and if you are extremely tense, anxious, or under unusual stress, it may help to take tranquillizers for a while.

Such drugs can mitigate the symptoms of an irritable colon. They cannot cure the disorder, however. In most cases it persists through life, with symptoms alternately easing and worsening at irregular intervals.

Diverticular disease

(diverticulosis and diverticulitis)

Small, sac-like swellings known as diverticula (singular: diverticulum) sometimes develop in the walls of the last part of the colon. The presence of diverticula in the colon is called diverticulosis. Many older people develop the diverticula without ever knowing, since diverticulosis is often symptom-free. Occasionally, however, for no known reason, one or more of the diverticula becomes inflamed. If this happens, the condition is no longer called diverticulosis but diverticulitis. There seems to be some connection between diverticular disease (that is, diverticulosis or diverticulitis) and the conventional Western diet, which is low in *fibre* content.

What are the symptoms?
If you have diverticulosis (the presence of diverticula) you may have no symptoms at all.

Or you may experience cramping pains and sometimes tenderness in the left side of the abdomen. The symptoms may be temporarily relieved by the passage of wind or faeces. The faeces are often small and hard and there may be occasional attacks of diarrhoea. Occasionally the diverticula bleed; such bleeding may not be noticeable until you pass bright red blood in the faeces.

If diverticulitis (the inflammation of diverticula) occurs, you will have severe abdominal pain, often spasmodic at first but becoming more constant, and localized in the lower left side of your abdomen. You may also feel nauseated and have a fever. The abdominal pain is aggravated if you touch the sore spot. In some people diverticulitis flares up and causes disabling pain within a few hours. In other people the symptoms may linger on in a mild form for several days or more before becoming severe.

How common is the problem?
About 1 person in 3 past the age of 60 in the Western world has diverticulosis, but only a few suffer from troublesome symptoms. And only a minority of these – of whom two-thirds are women – develop diverticulitis.

What are the risks?
Untreated diverticulitis can lead to serious complications, for example, the formation of an *abscess* in the colon around an inflamed diverticulum. If the abscess *perforates* the intestinal wall, *peritonitis* (p.470) can develop.

What should be done?
Always consult a doctor if your bowels behave in an unusual manner for more than a week or two, or if you have a persistent pain in the lower part of the abdomen. After examining you physically, your doctor will probably arrange for blood tests, a *sigmoidoscopic* examination of your lower bowel, and a *barium enema*, to make sure that *cancer of the large intestine* (opposite), which has similar symptoms, is not causing your trouble.

What is the treatment?
Self-help: It may be possible to prevent the formation of diverticula by modifying your diet *now*. Eat wholemeal rather than white bread, breakfast on rough oatmeal or bran-containing cereals, and eat plenty of *fibre* – found in most fruits and vegetables. Many individuals with mild symptoms of diverticulosis have found that the symptoms disappear within one or two weeks of beginning to take such measures. A high-fibre diet of this kind can, however, cause your abdomen to become distended, and you may pass a lot of wind. It may be necessary to adjust the amount of fibre in your diet until you find what suits you. If diverticulitis develops, no self-help measures are possible.

Professional help: If your trouble is diagnosed as diverticulitis, you will be admitted to hospital, where the contents of your stomach will be sucked out through a *nasogastric* tube. You will be unable to eat or drink at first, and will be given the fluids you need via an *intravenous drip*. This will free your diverticula of solid matter and allow them to recover. To clear up any infection, you will be given injections of *antibiotics* and, if necessary, of pain-killers. After a few days, when symptoms have subsided, you will gradually be able to resume normal eating and drinking. If, though, your doctors feel that diverticulitis is likely to recur, they may advise an operation to remove the affected section of the colon – see *Colostomy and ileostomy*, p.482.

Prospects of full recovery from even a severe attack of diverticulitis are excellent if treatment is given rapidly.

Diverticulum

Diverticulosis
In diverticulosis, small out-pouchings (diverticula) form in the wall of the colon and project into the abdominal cavity.

Ulcerative colitis

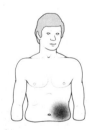

Site of the pain

Ulcerative colitis is a long-term condition in which raw, inflamed areas called ulcers develop in places along the lining of the large intestine. These ulcers may originate in the rectum, when the disorder is known as proctitis, and gradually spread upwards into the colon. In many cases the entire large intestine may ultimately be affected. Nobody knows why some people are more susceptible to this disorder than others.

What are the symptoms?
Symptoms usually recur over a period of years. You may have an attack of ulcerative colitis without any warning, or it may come on gradually. A characteristic early symptom is left-sided abdominal pain, which is relieved by a bowel movement; but the act of moving the bowels is itself painful, and you will probably have diarrhoea which is stained dark red or black with blood, and may have streaks of mucus in it. In a severe attack, there may also be sweating, nausea, loss of appetite, and a fever of up to 40°C (104°F).

How common is the problem?
Ulcerative colitis is a relatively rare condition, which is found in only about 1 of every 2,500 people in this country. It is more common in women and is most likely to affect young and middle-aged adults.

What are the risks?
In a severe attack of the disease there is the danger that large amounts of blood may be lost, and that *toxins* from the ulcerated area will cause *blood poisoning* (p.421). People who have suffered from ulcerative colitis for 10 years or longer are slightly more at risk from *cancer of the large intestine* (opposite).

What should be done?
If you have an attack of painful diarrhoea, with blood and mucus in the faeces, consult your doctor. A severe attack should alert you to call a doctor without delay. If laboratory analysis of blood samples and faecal matter show no evidence of an infection (the most usual cause of such symptoms) the next step is

to arrange for hospital tests that will help the doctor make a firm diagnosis. (If you are in great pain or bleeding profusely, these tests will be carried out right away.) Your large intestine will be examined with a *sigmoidoscope*, and perhaps with a *colonoscope* as well; and a *biopsy* from the intestinal wall will probably be taken during one of these viewing tests. You may also have *barium enema*.

What is the treatment?

Self-help: If your condition is diagnosed as ulcerative colitis, you will probably be under a doctor's care for several weeks. During that period and thereafter, you can help prevent further attacks by changing to a high-*fibre* diet as described in *diverticular disease* (p.479). It may help, too, to cut down on your intake of milk and other dairy products.

This disease can be aggravated by certain *broad-spectrum antibiotics* that often cause diarrhoea as a side-effect. If you have had earlier attacks of ulcerative colitis, be sure to point this out to any doctor unacquainted with your history – especially if you are consulting him or her about some sort of infection for which antibiotics might, under normal circumstances, be prescribed.

Professional help: The usual treatment is a four- to six-week course of drugs aimed at healing the ulcers. The main drugs used are *steroids*. They may be given as tablets, enemas, or rectal suppositories.

Treatment for a severe attack of ulcerative colitis is generally carried out – at least for the first two weeks – in hospital. Nutrients and steroid drugs may be administered via an *intravenous drip*, or orally in concentrated liquid form. To prevent future attacks of ulcerative colitis, further drugs are often prescribed in tablet form to be taken indefinitely.

If you have recurrent attacks of ulcerative colitis, your doctor may advise you to have an operation to remove the colon (see *Colostomy and ileostomy*, p.482). Apart from preventing further attacks of the disease, this would also eliminate the risk of cancer of the colon developing.

Benign tumours of the large intestine
(including polyps)

Some tumours of the large intestine are *malignant* (see *Cancer of the large intestine*, below), but *benign* growths are more common. They occur singly or in groups, for no known reason; and most are small, grape-shaped growths known as *polyps*, though an occasional benign tumour can grow large enough to create an *intestinal obstruction* (p.471). Since about 1 out of 100 benign tumours becomes malignant, they are routinely removed if discovered.

Many people have symptom-free growths without knowing. Often they are discovered only as a result of *X-rays* performed for another reason. Sometimes, though, benign tumours signal their presence by producing streaks of dark blood in the faeces, or a mucous discharge from the anus that stains underclothing. They are frequently both diagnosed and simultaneously removed by means of *colonoscopy*, *sigmoidoscopy*, or *proctoscopy*. If this is not feasible in your case, you may need a relatively simple *laparotomy* (see *Acute abdomen*, p.477) to cut away the tumours, thus avoiding the slight risk of obstruction or malignancy.

Cancer of the large intestine
(cancer of the colon and cancer of the rectum)

In cancer of the large intestine (colon and rectum) abnormal cells multiply and form either an ulcerous area that bleeds easily or a constriction that hinders passage of faeces. If allowed to progress, the disease spreads along the intestinal wall and through it to adjacent abdominal organs; it may also enter the bloodstream and affect other parts of the body. The cause of *malignancy* in the large intestine is not known, but a highly refined, low-*fibre* diet may be an important factor.

What are the symptoms?

The main symptom that should not be ignored if it lasts for more than about 10 days is a change in type of bowel movements – either increased constipation or diarrhoea. Blood in the faeces, too, should always be reported to your doctor; never assume that it is merely caused by *haemorrhoids* (p.483).

There may also be vague indications of *indigestion* (p.463) and pain along with tenderness in the lower part of the abdomen. Sometimes the major symptom is simply a lump somewhere in the lower right-hand quarter of the abdomen. And sometimes there are no symptoms at all until the cancer makes itself known via an *intestinal obstruction* (p.471) or *peritonitis* (p.470) resulting from a ruptured colon.

How common is the problem?

Cancers of the large intestine are the third most common form of cancer in Britain. They account for 14 per cent of all cancer deaths in this country. Each year 1 person in 1,200 is diagnosed as suffering from the condition.

Men and women are equally susceptible to cancer of the large intestine. It can occur at any age, but is more prevalent among people who suffer from *ulcerative colitis* (p.480) and those over 40, but especially among those in their 60s and 70s.

What are the risks?

Because most cancers of the large intestine develop and *metastasize* rather slowly, you have an 80 per cent chance of complete cure if your condition is diagnosed early. If the malignancy has already spread beyond the intestine the outlook is much less favourable.

What should be done?

If you have any of the symptoms mentioned above, consult your doctor, who will examine your abdomen and will then insert a gloved finger into your rectum to test the possibility of a rectal growth. You may also need to provide samples of faecal matter for laboratory analysis. If the doctor suspects the presence of cancer – or, for that matter, of a *benign tumour of the large intestine* (p.481) –

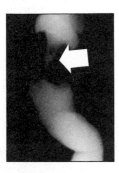

Cancer of the colon appears on an X-ray as a dark mass (arrow) on the inside wall of the colon.

you will need to undergo such in-hospital diagnostic procedures as a *barium enema*, *sigmoidoscopy*, and possibly *colonoscopy*.

What is the treatment?

Surgery is the best possible treatment for this type of cancer if it has not progressed too far. If the cancer is in the colon, the cancerous tissue is removed along with part of the healthy colon on each side, and the two ends of the intestine are then sewn together. This operation is called an intestinal *resection*. If the cancer is in the rectum, a colostomy is usually necessary (see the box on *Colostomy and ileostomy*, below).

If the cancer has become too widespread for surgery, its progress can often be arrested by *radiotherapy* and/or *cytotoxic* drugs.

What are the long-term prospects?

The outlook is very good for people with cancer of the large intestine if the condition is discovered early enough for surgery.

Most people who have operations for cancer of the large intestine survive in good health for five or more years. The success rate for cure among sufferers given only radiotherapy and drug treatment is lower.

OPERATION: ## Colostomy and ileostomy

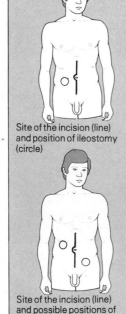

Site of the incision (line) and position of ileostomy (circle)

Site of the incision (line) and possible positions of colostomy (circles)

In the treatment of certain digestive-tract diseases such as cancer of the large intestine, diverticulitis, and ulcerative colitis, it may be necessary to remove part of the tract (intestinal *resection*). If possible the two cut ends are sewn together to maintain a passageway for food. When this is not feasible, an artificial opening (a "stoma") is made in the abdominal wall, through which undigested material can pass into a bag. This is called a colostomy when the colon opens through the stoma, and an ileostomy when the lower part of the small intestine (the ileum) opens through the stoma. In some cases a temporary colostomy is performed to allow a diseased colon to heal, or to prevent it bursting because of an obstruction in the intestine.

Before the operation you will probably be given laxatives, an enema, and perhaps drugs to temporarily reduce the natural population of microbes in your intestines.

During the operation You are given a general anaesthetic, and the diseased part of the digestive tract is removed through an incision in the abdominal wall. The free upper end of the tract is

joined to the lower end if possible; otherwise it is stitched into a second incision to form the stoma. The operation takes about 2 to 3 hours.

After the operation You will receive nutrients through a drip, and one or more drains will draw off fluid from the abdomen. Within 2 or 3 days you will be given a special diet, and begin to pass waste materials and gases into the bag. The usual hospital stay is 2 weeks.

Convalescence You will need about 2 months to recover from the operation, and you should gradually become adept at emptying and cleaning the bag. People with colostomies can eventually return to an almost normal bowel routine, emptying their bag at regular intervals. Sometimes bowel control becomes so good that the wearer needs only a pad over the stoma for most of the day, which is exchanged for the bag when a bowel movement is expected. Patients with ileostomies usually need to keep the bag in place all the time.

See also information on operations, p.738.

The anus

The anus consists of a tube 40mm (1½in) long leading from the rectum through a ring of muscles (the *sphincter*) to the anal orifice. If you are a healthy individual past early childhood, you normally control the sphincter, keeping the orifice closed, or letting it open for the passage of faeces. This part of the digestive tract is relatively simple in structure and function and rarely presents any problem. In fact, the only common anal disorder is haemorrhoids (piles).

One factor in anal disorders is that waste products of low-*fibre* foods create small, hard faeces, which can injure the sphincter walls as they pass through. And because they do not pass easily, nearly every act of defecation can put a damaging strain on the anus. And a factor in the prevalence of haemorrhoids is that many of us worry so much about our "bowels" and work too hard at forcing sphincter muscles to do what they would do naturally if we let them.

Haemorrhoids
(piles)

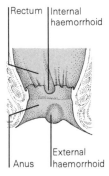

Different types of haemorrhoid
An internal haemorrhoid forms inside the lower part of the rectum and may not be visible from the outside. An external haemorrhoid appears at or just inside the anal orifice and may become visible if it prolapses (protrudes through the anal orifice).

Haemorrhoids are anal *varicose veins* (p.409). The affected veins lie just under the mucous-membrane lining of the lowest part of the rectum and anus. They become swollen because of repeatedly raised pressure within them, usually as a result of persistent straining during the act of defecation. The need to strain results in most cases from constipation. Haemorrhoid problems often occur during pregnancy (see *Varicose veins during pregnancy*, p.623), or if you are overweight (see *Obesity*, p.492). If you suffer from haemorrhoids, the veins in your anus become swollen, twisted, and thin-walled, and are easily ruptured by the passage of faeces. An internal haemorrhoid is one that occurs near the beginning of the anal canal. If the bulging vein is farther down, virtually at the anal orifice, it is considered to be external.

External haemorrhoids sometimes *prolapse* (that is, protrude outside the orifice). This may happen only during defecation, after which the prolapsed vein usually springs back into place. But occasionally one or more prolapsed haemorrhoids can persist, and they will remain prolapsed until replaced manually. *Thrombosis* may also occur; that is, the blood in the haemorrhoid clots.

What are the symptoms?
Bleeding is the main, and in many people the only, symptom. The blood is bright red and appears when you defecate. You may notice it as streaks on toilet paper or on faecal matter, or for a minute or so there may be an actual flow of blood. In addition, bowel movements may become increasingly uncomfortable and even painful. Prolapsed haemorrhoids often produce a mucous discharge and itching around the anal orifice. Moreover, severe haemorrhoids sometimes

prolapse unexpectedly even when you are not attempting to defecate. If there is thrombosis, there may be severe pain.

How common is the problem?
Haemorrhoids are quite common, and most sufferers have occasional bleeding from them. Serious trouble is less common. In Britain about 1 person in 100 requires treatment for the disorder each year.

What are the risks?
Haemorrhoids themselves are not dangerous, though they can cause discomfort. The great risk is that bleeding thought to be from haemorrhoids may actually be caused by *cancer of the large intestine* (p.481), especially in people over 40. That is why you should always see a doctor at the first sign of anal bleeding. Too much loss of blood may result in *iron-deficiency anaemia* (p.419).

What should be done?
Consult your doctor if you detect signs of anal bleeding. He or she will examine your rectum and anus with a gloved finger and may scrutinize the area through a *proctoscope*. To exclude the possibility of cancer, you may also need to have a *barium enema X-ray* and possibly *sigmoidoscopy*.

What is the treatment?
Self-help: To produce soft, easily passed faeces eat plenty of fresh fruit, vegetables, and whole-grain cereals or bran. If you already have haemorrhoids, clean yourself thoroughly but gently after every bowel movement, using soft toilet paper and soapy water, and dry yourself carefully afterwards. A sensible diet and good hygiene will generally keep haemorrhoids under control and

OPERATION: **Piles removal**
Haemorrhoidectomy

There are several different methods for removing painful or bleeding piles. The traditional method is to cut them out during an operation; you may need painkillers for the first few bowel movements following the operation. Alternatively your anal opening may be manually stretched, or a small cut made in it. The idea behind these methods is to weaken the anus, thus diminishing the abdominal straining that often contributes to piles. All the above methods require a general anaesthetic and a 3- or 4-day stay in hospital.

Another method is to place a tight rubber band over the base of each pile, which then withers painlessly over the next few days. This process,

called ligation, can be done during a brief visit to an out-patient clinic and in many cases may not even require a local anaesthetic.

See also information on operations, p.738.

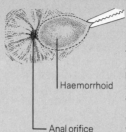

Haemorrhoid

Anal orifice

Surgical removal
The traditional surgical method of removing haemorrhoids – by stretching the area taut and cutting out the haemorrhoids – is rarely done unless the condition is very severe.

may even clear up a mild case. You can also buy astringents in the form of rectal suppositories that may shrink painful haemorrhoids if inserted nightly for a week or two.

For a particularly painful attack (generally caused by a prolapsed and/or thrombosed vein), stay in bed for a full day, taking four-hourly doses of a painkiller such as paracetamol. An ice compress or a pad soaked in witch-hazel may relieve the swelling enough for the exposed haemorrhoid to withdraw, and a warm salt bath may also help. If pain persists for more than 12 hours, then see your doctor.

Professional help: Doctors usually treat haemorrhoids by prescribing soothing and/or painkilling ointments or suppositories

containing various *steroid* drugs. Some suppositories also contain a local anaesthetic to numb the area and allow you to move your bowels with less discomfort. Additional measures, if constipation persists, consist of a combination of bulk-additives in the diet and laxative medicines.

If your case is a stubborn one, a more active type of treatment may be necessary. Two possible procedures – neither of which need involve an overnight hospital stay – might be either injection into a haemorrhoid of a special shrinking agent or else *cryosurgery*, which is a method of destroying body tissue by freezing it. Occasionally, though, surgery to remove the piles (haemorrhoidectomy) may be the only answer.

Anal fissure

A fissure is an elongated ulcer that extends upwards into the anal canal from the anal *sphincter*. When the sufferer defecates, irritation of the ulcer causes *spasm* (contraction) of the sphincter, with consequent severe pain and, sometimes, bleeding. This rare condition, which occurs most often in women, can

sometimes be cured by adding roughage to the diet, and taking a laxative such as liquid paraffin. If the fissure is persistent or recurs, though, the sufferer may need a minor operation to stop spasms and relieve irritation. The ulcer nearly always heals without further treatment in a few days.

Anal fistula

This is a rare disorder in which erosion of tissues caused by a spreading *abscess* within the anus results in the development of an anal fistula. The fistula itself is a tiny tube leading directly from the anal canal to a pin-hole-sized opening in the skin near the anal orifice. The continual discharge of watery pus through this small hole irritates the skin and may cause discomfort and itching; in some

cases, too, the underlying abscess is painful. There is a very slight possibility that an anal fistula indicates the presence of *Crohn's disease* (p.473) or even perhaps *cancer of the large intestine* (p.481).

The usual treatment is a minor operation to open up the fistula, thoroughly clean out the abscess, and dress the wound so that the hole will heal and close up.

Liver, gallbladder, and pancreas

The liver, gallbladder, and pancreas work together with the digestive tract as the digestive system. The liver is the largest single organ in the body. It fills the top right-hand part of the abdomen and plays a crucial and complex role in regulating the composition of various chemicals and cells in the blood. Nutrients that are absorbed into the bloodstream from the small intestine are transported to the liver for processing, storage, and eventual distribution via the bloodstream.

Many old, worn-out red blood cells, which contain the red oxygen-carrying pigment haemoglobin, are broken down in the liver. The haemoglobin is converted into another pigment, bilirubin. Fluid containing bilirubin and various other substances – among them *cholesterol* – trickles along tiny tubes to the gallbladder, a collecting bag lying on the surface of the liver. After a meal the gallbladder empties its contents, called bile, along the bile duct into the duodenum.

The pancreas lies just below the liver and behind the stomach. It has two distinct functions, one of which is to make certain hormones (hormonal disorders of the pancreas are dealt with elsewhere – see *Pancreas*, p.519). Its other function is to make *enzymes* and other chemicals that periodically pour down the pancreatic duct to the duodenum, where they set to work breaking food into particles that are small enough to be absorbed into the body.

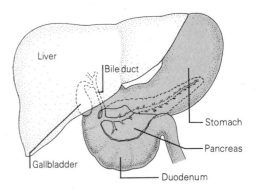

Liver and stomach (seen from front)

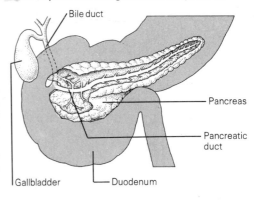

Liver displaced to show gallbladder and pancreas

Jaundice

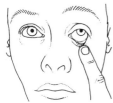

Visual symptoms
In jaundice, the whites of the eyes turn yellow; this is usually a more reliable sign that the yellowing of the skin, which is often difficult to detect.

See p.244,
Visual aids to diagnosis, 47.

Jaundice is not a disease but a sign of disease. Many diseases can cause jaundice – including gallstones, various forms of hepatitis, tumours of the liver or pancreas, and – rarely – cirrhosis of the liver (all of these diseases are described on the following pages). Occasionally, jaundice may be brought on when taking certain drugs – for example, some major tranquillizers.

If you have jaundice, your skin and the whites of your eyes turn yellow, due to a build-up of the yellowish-brown substance bilirubin in the blood. Bilirubin is a waste product formed when old red blood cells are broken down. Normally it is extracted from the bloodstream by the liver, collects in the gallbladder as bile, passes down the bile duct into the intestines, and is excreted in the faeces (bilirubin colours the faeces brown).

If the liver fails to function properly – because of an infection such as hepatitis, for example – bilirubin cannot be extracted and builds up in the bloodstream, causing the skin and the whites of eyes to turn yellow. It may also cause severe itching. The faeces are no longer brown but chalky grey. In addition, bilirubin may darken the urine.

Jaundice can also appear if the exit for bile is obstructed – for example, by a *gallstone* (p.489). Bilirubin accumulates in the bile and then overflows back into the bloodstream. Another form of jaundice is haemolytic jaundice – a symptom of *haemolytic anaemia* (p.423) or a side-effect of a drug.

If you develop jaundice for any reason, you should visit a doctor without delay for a full examination. Treatment will depend on the underlying cause of the jaundice.

Acute hepatitis A

Acute hepatitis A is a sudden liver infection caused by the hepatitis A virus. The virus spreads from person to person when food or water is contaminated by sewage.

What are the symptoms?
In the early stages of the infection you develop flu-like symptoms – a raised temperature, generalized aching, and weakness. You may also have nausea, loss of appetite, and tenderness in the upper abdomen.

After a few days, as the flu symptoms subside, *jaundice* (p.485) may appear, because the inflamed liver cannot remove the pigment bilirubin from the blood. In two or three weeks the jaundice and other symptoms start to gradually fade, but you may feel depressed and run-down for several weeks, or even months, after.

How common is the problem?
Isolated cases of acute hepatitis A occur each year in Britain but epidemics are extremely rare. As the disorder can easily be mistaken for influenza if jaundice does not appear, many cases go undiagnosed. In less developed areas of the world, the disease is common and spreads via insanitary toilet facilities and contaminated food or water.

What should be done?
Virtually all sufferers recover completely, though in some cases this takes many weeks or months and attacks of the disease can recur for up to a year. If you develop flu-like symptoms and then jaundice, see your doctor without delay. After questioning and examining you, the doctor may well take a blood sample for laboratory analysis to identify the causative virus – the early symptoms of hepatitis A are similar to those of the more serious *acute hepatitis B* (below).

What is the treatment?
Self-help: Acute hepatitis A leaves the sufferer feeling extremely weak and debilitated. Rest or stay in bed for as long as you feel weak. Avoid large fatty meals. Do not drink alcohol for at least six months as it can prolong the illness or cause it to recur. To prevent spread of the infection you should have your own crockery, cutlery, and towels, and if possible use a separate, heavily disinfected lavatory and washbasin. Such precautions are important, because you may remain infectious for weeks or months.
Professional help: *Antibiotics* are not effective against viral infections, so there is little specific treatment the doctor can give. If you yourself have not had the disease, but you have been in contact with someone who has since developed it, or you are considering visiting a part of the world where it is common, your doctor may give you an injection of *gammaglobulin* to increase your resistance to the disease for up to six months.

Acute hepatitis B

This viral infection produces symptoms which are similar to those of *acute hepatitis A* (above), but it is less easily transmitted and has more serious risks attached (see "What are the risks?" below). The hepatitis B virus is usually spread by contact with infected blood. In countries such as Britain and the USA this usually means it spreads via inadequately sterilized needles that may be used in acupuncture, tattooing, or unsupervised drug injections. In addition, certain people are symptomless carriers of the disease, so it is possible that a blood donor may be a carrier and infect other people following a blood transfusion. In Britain, only 1 person in 1,000 is a carrier of hepatitis B (far fewer people actually suffer from it) and no one who is known to have had the disease is permitted to donate blood. The risk of infection under such conditions is virtually nil.

Finally, acute hepatitis B can be spread by sexual or intimate contact because a carrier has the virus present in saliva and seminal fluid or vaginal discharge.

What are the risks?
The majority of cases of acute hepatitis B clear up without any long-term effects. In some cases, the patient may have such a rapidly progressing illness that it ends in death. But in a small proportion of cases the disease may lead to *chronic hepatitis* or *cirrhosis of the liver* (opposite).

What should be done?
If you develop *jaundice* (p.485) along with flu-like symptoms, consult your doctor without delay. Diagnosis and treatment of acute hepatitis B are the same as for acute hepatitis A, though your doctor will advise you to attend regular check-ups so that if you develop any further liver problems they can be detected at an early stage. The doctor may also want to examine your partner to see if he or she is a symptomless carrier.

If you have had acute hepatitis B, you should never donate blood. Also, take particular care over your personal hygiene to avoid infecting others.

Chronic hepatitis

Chronic hepatitis is a very rare disease in which inflammation of the liver smoulders on for many months or years. The inflammation is thought to be a result of an *autoimmune* reaction in which the body makes *antibodies* against its own tissues. Chronic hepatitis is usually preceded by an infection such as *acute hepatitis B* (opposite), but occasionally it may be associated with a digestive-tract condition such as *ulcerative colitis* (p.480) or *Crohn's disease* (p.473).

Rarely, chronic hepatitis can be caused by excessive doses of certain drugs which include alcohol and paracetamol. In some cases the cause of the disease is unknown.

What are the symptoms?
Symptoms tend to come and go in the early stages, but they gradually worsen and become more persistent over the years.

The main symptoms are tiredness, loss of appetite, yellowing of the skin and the whites of the eyes (see *Jaundice*, p.485), and indigestion after eating fatty foods or drinking alcohol. There may also be some aching or pain in the joints.

Sometimes, chronic hepatitis develops so slowly there are no symptoms at all in the early stages (though the liver is suffering damage); in such cases the condition may be discovered by a routine blood test – for example, at a regular check-up following an attack of acute hepatitis B.

What are the risks?
Chronic hepatitis is a serious disease because it gradually impairs liver functioning over many years. The main risk of the disease is that the sufferer will eventually develop *cirrhosis of the liver* (below).

What should be done?
Consult a doctor if you get jaundice, especially if you have previously had acute hepatitis B. A physical examination followed by blood tests, and perhaps a liver *biopsy* in hospital, will enable the doctor to diagnose the disease if it is present.

What is the treatment?
The main treatment is to avoid all substances that may further inflame the liver. In particular, cut out alcohol and paracetamol completely. Many patent medicines contain paracetamol in small amounts, so you must never take a tablet without being certain there is no paracetamol in it or checking with your doctor first.

Although liver damage may not be reversible, drug treatment can relieve symptoms and slow down further damage. Your doctor will probably prescribe *steroid* and other drugs to combat the disease. Frequent check-ups and blood samples will ensure that symptoms are kept to a minimum, and that complications such as cirrhosis of the liver are detected and treated should they arise.

Cirrhosis of the liver

Cirrhosis is the slow deterioration of the liver due to gradual internal scarring (*fibrosis*) of its tissues. These changes make the liver progressively less able to carry out its numerous and vital functions. There are many causes of the disease. The commonest by far in the Western world is *alcoholism* (p.304). Malnutrition, *chronic hepatitis* (above), congestive *heart failure* (p.381), and biliary cirrhosis (an *autoimmune* problem) are other causes; in some cases the cause of cirrhosis cannot be identified.

What are the symptoms?
The liver's central role in the functioning of the body is reflected by the number and variety of symptoms that appear as cirrhosis gradually develops.

In the very early stages, while there are still plenty of healthy liver cells, there are only very mild symptoms. As the disease progresses loss of appetite and weight, nausea, vomiting, general malaise and weakness, and indigestion and abdominal distension all become increasingly pronounced. There is a tendency to bruise and bleed easily, leading to nosebleeds. Small, red, spidery marks (*spider naevi*) may appear on the face, arms, and upper trunk.

In the later states, *jaundice* (p.485) may occur. Men lose their sex drive, their breasts swell, and they become impotent. Women usually stop having periods (see *Amenorrhoea*, p.583). Eventually, *liver failure* may develop, in which fluid retention in the abdomen and ankles, irritability, and lack of concentration are the main symptoms. Memory is impaired and there is marked trembling of the hands, confusion, and drowsiness.

How common is the problem?
Cirrhosis is a rare condition except among heavy drinkers, both men and women. It is, therefore, most common in countries with a high alcohol-consumption rate, such as France. Rarely, certain drugs that are safe in recommended doses can damage the liver if taken in excessive amounts.

What are the risks?

The speed at which cirrhosis progresses is variable. If the disease is detected at an early stage, strict adherence to the treatment described below can halt its progress. But those who are unable to give up alcohol completely may eventually suffer fatal liver failure.

Cirrhosis of the liver makes severe bleeding in the digestive tract much more likely; if this happens, it is usually difficult to control and may precipitate liver failure. If you are at risk from cirrhosis and you vomit up blood you should get medical help without delay. Admission to hospital for an emergency blood transfusion will be necessary.

Very rarely, a tumour develops in the liver as a result of cirrhosis (see *Tumours of the liver*, below).

What should be done?

If you suspect that you have cirrhosis – and it is a distinct possibility if you drink heavily and regularly – you should consult your doctor. A physical examination is usually sufficient for a preliminary diagnosis, though you will have to attend hospital for specific blood tests and a liver *biopsy* to assess the exact nature and extent of the damage.

What is the treatment?

Self-help: Whatever the underlying cause of the cirrhosis, you should stop drinking alcohol immediately. If you continue to drink, the disease is certain to get worse. When you do stop your liver will remain particularly sensitive to alcohol, and amounts of alcohol that would have no effect on a healthy person may kill a cirrhotic.

Never take any drugs unless the type of drug and the dosage has been approved by your doctor. Try to follow a nutritious diet which contains plenty of protein, carbohydrates, and vitamins, but which is low in fats and salt (see *Eating and drinking sensibly*, p.24, for further details).

Professional help: Your doctor will give you advice on diet, and may prescribe various drugs to counteract the symptoms of cirrhosis. For example, *diuretics* act to cut down the amount of fluid in the body.

To guard against malnutrition, your doctor may advise or prescribe various dietary and vitamin supplements. And depending on the cause of the cirrhosis and the stage it has reached, *corticosteroids* or *cytoxic* drugs may also be prescribed.

What are the long-term prospects?

The prospects for cirrhosis sufferers vary enormously. The heavy drinker who develops early cirrhosis but who then cuts out alcohol completely and eats a nutritious diet should be able to lead a fairly normal life. But the alcoholic who will not (and often cannot) abstain will eventually develop liver failure. Hospital treatment by an *intravenous drip* containing various drugs and nutrients can usually bring about some improvement, but repeated episodes of liver failure make this treatment progressively less effective.

Tumours of the liver

Like tumours elsewhere in the body, liver tumours may be either *benign* or *malignant*. Benign tumours are very rare, and are usually discovered during a routine medical examination, or by tests for some other problem. If they grow very large and burst they can cause the serious condition *acute abdomen* (p.477). If and when they are discovered, benign liver tumours can usually be removed by surgery.

There are two types of malignant (cancerous) tumour. The majority are *metastases*, seedlings of cancers which have started in other parts of the body and have spread via the bloodstream to the liver. About one third of all cancers that have started to metastasize spread to the liver in this way, and in some cases it is the symptoms of the secondary liver cancer that draw attention to a primary cancer elsewhere (see, for example, *Lung cancer*, p.366). Cancer may start in the liver (primary liver cancer) but, like benign liver tumours, this is very rare indeed.

What are the symptoms?

If the liver tumour is a secondary tumour, there may be symptoms of the primary cancer, which is already receiving treatment of its own. As liver cancer develops, it causes further loss of weight and appetite, indigestion and abdominal discomfort, and general ill-health. *Jaundice* (p.485) – in which the skin and the whites of the eyes take on a yellowish tinge – commonly appears.

What should be done?

You should inform your doctor if you have the symptoms described above (always consult your doctor if jaundice develops).

What is the treatment?

Unfortunately the outlook is poor once cancer has spread to the liver; and similar prospects apply for primary malignant tumours of the organ. In some cases *cytotoxic* drugs help to slow the progress of the disease.

Gallstones

(including biliary colic)

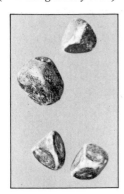

Appearance of gallstones
Gallstones appear in different guises. They may be large and fairly smooth (as shown above) or small, sharp and crystalline.

Gallstones are stones which form in the gallbladder, the collecting bag for bile. Bile is a liquid rich in fatty substances – particularly *cholesterol* – which are extracted from the blood by the liver. Bile also contains bilirubin, a pigment formed by the breakdown of old red blood cells. A gallstone starts as a tiny solid particle in the gallbladder, which grows as more material solidifies around it. Why the stone develops, or why some people have one and others more than one, is not clear. There is no firm evidence for a direct connection between gallstones and *atherosclerosis* (p.372), a condition in which the level of cholesterol in the blood is higher than normal; but it is known that gallstones occur most commonly in people with unusually high levels of cholesterol in their blood.

What are the symptoms?

Between one-third and one-half of gallstones do not produce any symptoms; they just lie in the gallbladder. But some gallstones travel with the bile along the bile duct, where they may get stuck. If this happens, the result is *biliary colic* – an intense pain in the upper right-hand abdomen (or sometimes between the shoulder blades). Over a period of a few hours pain builds to a peak and then fades; it makes you feel sick and you may actually

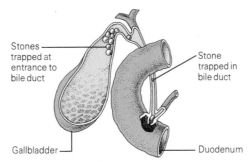

Gallstone sites
Gallstones that remain in the gallbladder or pass through the bile duct into the duodenum do not usually cause any symptoms. Problems arise if the gallstones become trapped in the bile duct or its entrance, as shown above.

vomit. Biliary colic is a result of the gallbladder trying to force its bile past the stone and into the duodenum. If the stone falls back into the gallbladder, or is forced along the bile duct and passes into the duodenum, then the pain relents.

Additional symptoms of gallstones include flatulence and abdominal discomfort following a heavy, fatty meal. These symptoms are often termed gallstone dyspepsia.

How common is the problem?

About 1 Briton in 10 has one or more gallstones. The older you are, the more likely you are to have them – up to 1 in 3 elderly people have gallstones. And women are four times more likely than men to get them.

What are the risks?

If a gallstone remains lodged in the bile duct for any length of time, it may block the exit for bile and cause the yellowing of the skin and the whites of the eyes characteristic of *jaundice* (p.485).

Another risk is inflammation and perhaps infection of the gallbladder as the trapped bile stagnates; this will require special treatment (see *Cholecystitis*, p.490). People with gallstones are also more susceptible than others to *acute pancreatitis* (p.490).

What should be done?

If you have a severe pain resembling the biliary colic described above, consult your doctor, who will examine you and question you as to the exact nature of the pain. If he or she suspects gallstones, you will be asked to provide blood samples for analysis. You may also be advised to undergo a hospital diagnostic test called a *cholecystogram* in which your abdomen is *X-rayed* several hours after you swallow a special pill to show up the gallbladder. Sometimes an *ultrasound scan* can detect gallstones.

What is the treatment?

Self-help: Eat sensibly. Avoid overeating and eating any foods (particularly rich and fatty things) that bring on the pain of biliary colic. Take proprietary antacids to combat any indigestion or flatulence.

If biliary colic develops, go to bed, take two *analgesic* (painkilling) tablets, and do not eat but take occasional sips of water. If the pain persists for more than about three hours, you should call your doctor.

Professional help: To relieve the colic the doctor may prescribe a strong painkiller. However, if tests show that the stones have passed into the duodenum (and hence out of the body) but that you are likely to suffer a recurrence of the problem, then the doctor may recommend surgery to remove any remaining gallstones and the gallbladder (see *Gallbladder removal*, p.490).

Surgery is also recommended for people whose gallstones recur. Gallstones can sometimes be dissolved by an acid called chenodeoxycholic acid (which occurs naturally in bile) taken in tablet form. However, this method of treatment is rare.

OPERATION: **Gallbladder removal**
Cholecystectomy

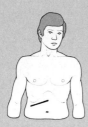

Site of the incision

This operation is done when gallstones or some other gallbladder problem causes serious symptoms. It has little, if any, effect on the functioning of your digestive system.

During the operation Under a general anaesthetic, the gallbladder is cut away and removed through an incision in the upper right abdomen. During the operation, which usually takes 1½ hours, the surgeon may explore the bile duct and remove any stones found there.

After the operation You will have one or more tubes draining excess fluid from the operation site. There may also be a tube draining bile from the bile duct; this may stay in position for up to 10 days. You will be on a drip feed at first, but after a few days you will be able to eat and drink, and 10 to 14 days after the operation you should be well enough to go home.

Convalescence The usual recovery period is 2 months, during which time you may gradually resume normal eating and drinking habits unless advised otherwise by your doctor.

See also information on operations, p.738.

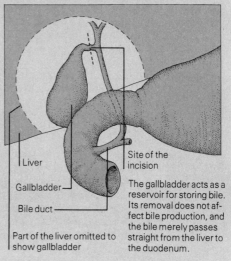

Liver

Gallbladder

Bile duct

Part of the liver omitted to show gallbladder

Site of the incision

The gallbladder acts as a reservoir for storing bile. Its removal does not affect bile production, and the bile merely passes straight from the liver to the duodenum.

Cholecystitis

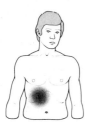

Site of the pain

In cholecystitis, the gallbladder becomes inflamed and swollen. This is usually a result of a *gallstone* (p.489) blocking the flow of bile from the gallbladder into the intestine. Occasionally, the inflammation is a result of infection spreading from the intestine.

The symptoms of cholecystitis itself may be preceded by severe pain in the upper part of your abdomen, usually on the right-hand side. This pain is called *biliary colic*. As cholecystitis develops your temperature rises, and nausea and vomiting follow.

If the condition is not treated you may develop *jaundice* (p.485). In rare cases when the gallbladder swells so much that it bursts, a particularly severe form of *peritonitis* (p.470) may develop.

Each year in Britain 1 person in 1,000 is seen by a doctor because of cholecystitis.

Three-quarters of these sufferers have already had previous gallbladder trouble.

What should be done?
If you think you might have cholecystitis, and especially if you have already had gallbladder trouble, consult your doctor immediately. You will probably be admitted to hospital and given an *intravenous drip* to provide you with nutrients and fluids; you may be given painkillers, and broad-spectrum *antibiotics* to combat any infection. Once the infection and inflammation have subsided, tests to find the underlying cause will be carried out.

People who have cholecystitis are usually advised to undergo surgery for *gallbladder removal* (above). In severe cases of cholecystitis, this may be done as soon as the sufferer is admitted to hospital.

Acute pancreatitis

Why the pancreas suddenly becomes inflamed, as it does in this rare disease, is not fully understood. The inflammation is thought to be due to pancreatic juices, which contain powerful *enzymes*, leaking into and irritating certain areas of the pancreas.

In Britain about half the people who develop acute pancreatitis already suffer from *gallstones* (p.489). The gallstone may block the duct carrying pancreatic juices into the intestine. Factors that contribute to the development of acute pancreatitis include excessive consumption of alcohol, *hyperparathyroidism* (p.528), or an abdominal injury. Very rarely it is a complication of an attack of *mumps* (p.700).

The main symptom of acute pancreatitis is agonizing pain in the upper abdomen. It comes on around 12 or 24 hours after a large meal or a heavy bout of drinking. The pain bores through to the back and the chest, and over several hours it rises to a peak, accompanied by vomiting and retching. In severe cases the sufferer is obviously very ill, has bruising over the abdomen, and may even have the symptoms of *shock* (p.386). If this happens, get the person to hospital at once.

What are the risks?
The main danger of acute pancreatitis is that shock, if it develops, may lead to death. There is also a long-term risk of *chronic pancreatitis* (below). However, the majority of people who have the disease make a full recovery.

What is the treatment?
If the doctor who attends you suspects acute pancreatitis (or some other serious abdominal complaint – see *Acute abdomen*, p.477) you will be admitted to hospital immediately. The diagnosis is made by taking *X-rays* of the abdomen and blood samples for analysis.

The immediate treatment is to give fluids and nutrients via an *intravenous drip*, and to relieve pain by injections of *analgesics*. As the sufferer recovers, he or she will gradually be able to resume eating and drinking, but should never again drink alcohol. After a few weeks, tests are carried out to see if gallstones are present; if they are, arrangements will be made to remove them.

Chronic pancreatitis

Chronic pancreatitis is a rare disease that takes many years to develop. It sometimes follows recurrent attacks of *acute pancreatitis* (opposite). The sufferer does not recover fully between attacks, and gradually the inflamed pancreas becomes less able to supply its digestive juices and hormones (see *Pancreas*, p.519, for information on pancreatic hormones). But most chronic-pancreatitis sufferers have not had a previous acute attack. They do, however, consume alcohol to excess and/or suffer from *gallstones* (p.489).

What are the symptoms?
Pain is the main symptom (although 1 sufferer in 10 has no pain at all). It is a dull, cramping, boring pain, aggravated by food and alcohol and relieved by sitting down and leaning forward. As the disease progresses the attacks of pain last longer and come more frequently. Some sufferers complain of indigestion between attacks. Additional symptoms (which do not occur in all cases) are mild *jaundice* (p.485) and loss of weight. In addition, the pancreas may become unable to make the hormone insulin, so *diabetes mellitus* (p.519) may develop.

What should be done?
Symptoms such as jaundice, severe abdominal pain, or unexplained loss of weight certainly indicate a visit to the doctor. If your doctor suspects a pancreatic disorder, you will undergo a number of hospital tests to disclose the exact problem.

What is the treatment?
Self-help: Give up alcohol at once and completely, and adhere strictly to the low-fat diet advised by your doctor.
Professional help: Your doctor may prescribe one of several *analgesic* drugs if your pain is particularly severe. You will also need to take tablets with each meal; they contain *enzymes* which you need to digest your food but which your damaged pancreas can no longer manufacture.

In some cases, bouts of abdominal pain become almost unbearable, and sufferers are advised to undergo surgery to remove the damaged pancreatic tissue. Provided you stick rigidly to your no-alcohol, low-fat diet plus additional tablets of pancreatic enzymes, and attend for check-ups when advised, your chances of improvement are good.

Cancer of the pancreas

Why certain cells in the pancreas should become *malignant* is not known. The main symptoms of pancreatic cancer are loss of appetite and weight, nausea, vomiting, *jaundice* (p.485), and upper abdominal pain, often spreading into the back and relieved by sitting up and leaning forward.

The disease is rare in Britain but is becoming less so; recent research has shown a possible link between pancreatic cancer and the consumption of large amounts of coffee.

If you develop the symptoms described above, consult your doctor without delay. If cancer is suspected there are a number of diagnostic tests that may be carried out to confirm the diagnosis. Cancer detected early can sometimes be cured by surgery to remove the pancreas, though the sufferer will then be diabetic and will receive appropriate treatment. Various drugs and *radiotherapy* may also be used, but if the malignancy is established when diagnosed, the outlook is poor.

Nutrition and metabolism

Disorders caused by intrinsic flaws in body chemistry are known as "inborn errors of *metabolism*". Metabolism – the chemical processes that keep bodily functions going – is controlled ultimately by the genes; and some individuals inherit a fault or faults in metabolism that leads to disease. Some of the diseases covered here, such as porphyria, are examples of inborn errors.

A related type of disorder is one in which body chemistry is disturbed not by an innate flaw, but by poor nutrition – eating the wrong kinds or amounts of food. Many diseases (for example, coronary artery disease) are linked to diet and in this sense are nutritional disorders. The disorders of nutrition discussed here (obesity, for instance) are defined as those that stem directly from what you eat.

Between the clear-cut classes of (1) disease due to faulty metabolism and (2) disease due to poor nutrition, there lies a broad twilight zone. If you have an inborn error of metabolism, you are less well adapted to your environment than others, but your flawed metabolism may do little harm if the environment is in some way modified. Thus people with the genes for porphyria do not necessarily suffer if the problem is recognized and their diet and environment controlled. Conversely, a condition such as obesity, which seems to be caused entirely by eating too much, has a strong genetic basis; many people who eat just as much do not get fat. Thus fat people can slim down by adjusting their diets, but many must also accept the fact that they have a predisposition to obesity.

All the disorders discussed below have a genetic basis, sometimes identifiable (as in porphyria) and sometimes rather vague (as in obesity or gout). But they are also influenced strongly by environment. Once a person is born, we can as yet do nothing to make good any defects in his or her genes. But we can often counter flaws in metabolism with drugs, or change the environment so that the flaws do not become apparent.

Obesity

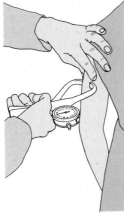

Skin callipers
Callipers are used to measure the thickness of a fold of skin. This gives an indication of the degree of obesity.

Your body needs food for warmth, for building and repairing tissues, and for providing energy to maintain vital chemical and physical functions. Energy requirements vary, even among individuals of similar height, build, age, and sex. But the basic needs of most people are quite close to an average: about 2,300 Calories a day for women, 2,800 for men (though a professional athlete or manual worker may need around 4,000 – see *Counting calories*, p.27). If you eat more than you need for the energy you expend, your body stores the surplus as fat. And if the fatty tissues become conspicuous, you may be considered "obese".

What are the symptoms?

The most obvious symptom is an increase in weight. Not all people who put on weight are necessarily obese; for instance, a pregnant woman or a weight-lifter gets heavier for other reasons. But an increased amount of fat in the body tissues is the commonest reason for an increase in weight. The only other notable symptoms of obesity may be a general feeling of heaviness and a tendency to become overheated. Obesity is associated, however, with a wide range of serious disorders (see "What are the risks?" below).

How common is the problem?

This question cannot be answered precisely because obesity cannot be precisely defined. Some experts on the subject suggest as a general rule that anyone who exceeds the "desirable" weight (see the *Weight chart* on p.28) for a person of his or her height, build, and age by more than 20 per cent may be considered fat – perhaps unhealthily so. By this definition one in every 5 men and almost one in every 3 women in our society are, to some extent, obese.

What are the risks?

Statistics compiled by insurance companies and health organizations indicate that obesity is associated with dangerous conditions such as diabetes, stroke, coronary artery disease, kidney and gallbladder trouble, and certain forms of cancer (cancer of the colon or rectum, for example). Moreover, the fatter you are, the stronger the association. The statistics suggest that someone who is more than 40 per cent over his or her desirable weight runs twice the risk of dying from coronary artery disease, and a person who is 20 to 30 per cent overweight may be three times more likely to die from diabetes than those people of desirable weight.

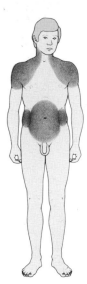

Where fat builds
up in men

There are also some more direct drawbacks to obesity. It seems to contribute directly to *high blood pressure* (p.382), which is itself a risk factor in both coronary artery disease and stroke. If you have high blood pressure, you may be able to reduce your blood pressure simply by losing weight. Similarly, *diabetes mellitus* (p.519) sometimes seems to develop as a direct consequence of obesity and to disappear when the sufferer slims down. Finally, a very fat person in need of surgery presents both the surgeon and anaesthetist with a potentially grave problem; and childbirth can be especially difficult for a grossly overweight woman.

What should be done?

Most people can cope with this problem themselves; to lose your excess store of fat and remain healthily slim, follow the self-help measures recommended below. Consult your doctor only if you are among the minority of obese people who cannot lose weight by sensible dieting and moderate, regular exercise (see *How to lose weight*, p.28).

What is the treatment?

Self-help: If you are fat, it is because your body is not using all the energy you feed it. This may be for any of several reasons, psychological as well as physical. Whatever the reason, it applies to you alone; so do not begin by making unhelpful comparisons between your moderate intake of food and your slender neighbour's gluttony. In order to lose weight, *you* must somehow consume more energy than you take in. In other words, you must create an energy deficit. There are two ways in which to do this. First, change your diet; secondly, take more exercise.

Any such recipe for slimming is almost too obvious to be worth repeating. There are pitfalls, however – and the watchword is realism. To begin with, crash diets or a few days at a "health farm" do not work. There is a sound biological reason for this. If you lose weight swiftly by nearly starving yourself, most of the dramatic fall in weight is due to your having used up the body's store of glycogen (a substance similar to starch) and the water that accompanies it. Glycogen is stored up for precisely that purpose: to tide the body over a period of food shortage. When, as the result of a nearly total fast, you have depleted your store of glycogen and water, you have indeed lost weight, but you have lost very little of the unwanted fatty tissue. After a crash diet, the food you eat simply replenishes the depleted store of glycogen and water – and back comes the weight.

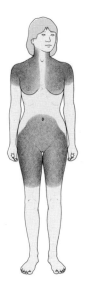

Where fat builds
up in women

So do not try to achieve massive weight losses in a few days. Aim instead at a food-and-exercise programme that gives you an energy deficit of around 500 Calories a day. This will use up half a kilogram (about one pound) of fatty tissue a week – a seemingly modest goal; but at this rate you will lose 25 kilograms (more than 50 pounds) in a year.

In working out a diet for yourself, remember that you will be well on the way to the recommended weight loss if you eat an average of 1,500 to 2,000 Calories per day. Make sure that the diet is balanced (see *What is a balanced diet*, p.26); within the balanced diet, choose foods you like, for you need to establish eating patterns that you can adhere to indefinitely. Avoid foods with a high calorific content relative to bulk – for instance, most things fatty or sugary – and stick to watery, fibrous, low-fat, low-carbohydrate foods. Thus, potatoes should be boiled, and bread (preferably wholemeal) should be used as a "mopper-up" of (low-fat) sauces, not as a vehicle for butter.

Almost as important as the kind and amount of food you eat is the timing of meals. One of the most effective slimming aids is to monitor everything you eat, ensuring that all food is consumed only at set intervals, ritualistically. Many obese people are fat partly because they eat almost unconsciously, hardly noticing what they pop into their mouths. Dieticians and therapists have found that such people are greatly helped by following simple rules that ban all casual snacks and turn eating into a formal ritual. If you need to lose weight, make it a rule never to eat anything except at mealtimes; always eat with a knife, fork, and/or spoon; and never finish a plateful of food without an occasional pause for slow and thorough chewing.

As for the second element in your slimming programme – exercise – "slow but steady" is again the watchword. An hour's moderate cycling will burn off around 350 Calories (almost a whole day's target deficit). There is good evidence that the old belief that exercise is self-defeating because it simply increases appetite is untrue. In fact, heavy exercise temporarily raises body temperature and is therefore likely to make you feel that the last thing you want to do is eat.

Finally, many obese people find it easier to follow a sensible diet-and-exercise regime if they do not have to go it alone. It may help if you join a recognized slimming club such as Weight Watchers. This can be a very positive step since it formalizes your intention to lose weight in addition to putting you in touch with people who share your problem.

If your reasonable efforts to slim down do not succeed, you may be one of the unfortunate few who are constitutionally unable to lose weight. An occasional individual finds that he or she adapts to a low energy intake by an actual reduction in basic energy requirement, so that the more such persons fast, the less they need. If this is the case with you, you will have to consult your doctor.

Professional help: There are anti-obesity drugs, but many physicians prefer not to prescribe them because some of them can have major side-effects. Moreover, such drugs are appetite suppressors, but most obese people do not suffer specifically from excess appetite. Some have low energy requirements, and many simply eat whether hungry or not. Newly developed drugs designed not to suppress appetite but to increase the body's energy requirements are being tested but are still largely in the experimental stage.

For many people who cannot lose weight in any other way, doctors sometimes try more drastic forms of treatment. For example, teeth can be wired together so that patients cannot open their jaws to eat and have to exist on specially prepared soups. The wiring may be kept in place for several weeks, with resultant dramatic loss of weight. In addition to its discomfort, this treatment has obvious drawbacks. If it produces no fundamental change in eating habits, fat returns when teeth are unwired; and mouth infections and dental decay can occur because teeth cannot be properly cleaned while wires are in place.

A more complex – and more risky – procedure is digestive-tract surgery to bypass part of the small intestine. This reduces the area of gut through which food can be absorbed, and it also diminishes appetite. Such operations are done only in specialist centres – and only rarely even there since there is a mortality risk. Cosmetic surgery, in which deposits of fat are literally sliced away, is another possible treatment, sometimes done in conjunction with one of the other procedures.

About 60 per cent of fat people treated in one of these drastic fashions do manage to slim down. But, apart from the risks, the rewards are highly uncertain

---

Vitamins

The body needs food for energy and for building up the tissues; it also needs a variety of complex organic compounds that, like oil and grease in a car, provide neither fuel nor structural material but are essential for smooth running. These compounds are called vitamins. Although human beings can manufacture some vitamins for themselves (notably vitamin D, which the skin can make from sunlight, and vitamin K, made by bacterial action in the intestines) most of these compounds are present in one or more of the foods we eat (see the table on p.496).

The precise function of some vitamins is not yet fully understood. But they are known to be involved in basic *metabolic* activities – for example, in controlling absorption of calcium (which is needed for strong bones and for the functioning of nerves and muscles), and in regulating the supply of energy to body tissues. Thus a lack of any one vitamin can lead to widespread disorder. If the deficiency is severe or prolonged, it may be fatal.

Although extreme vitamin deficiency is uncommon in the West, there is some evidence of marginal deficiency. In many cases the consequences are trivial; a lack of vitamin B in children, for instance, may lead to chapped lips. But some medical authorities believe that the mental confusion common in old people is often partly due to a low intake of B vitamins. And it may also be true that a low intake of some vitamins (including folic acid) during a woman's early pregnancy can lead to certain problems (see *Pernicious anaemia and folic-acid deficiency*, p.420). So there are no grounds for complacency even in the well-fed Western world.

Who lacks vitamins?

In the so-called "developed" countries, unmistakable vitamin-deficiency disease such as scurvy or pellagra is virtually non-existent. It can occur, however, in special circumstances. Vagrants often show signs of vitamin C and B deficiency; and *alcoholism* (p.304), which is sometimes associated with vagrancy, seems to exaggerate the effects of a low B intake. Neglected, undernourished children may also fall victim to the effects of vitamin C or D deficiency. Moreover, some people who are neither vagrant nor deprived suffer from vitamin deficiency because of defects in metabolism. For instance, one form of mental defectiveness in infancy seems to be caused by an inability to utilize vitamin B_6. And there are occasional individuals who, because they are unable to absorb vitamin B_{12}, suffer from pernicious anaemia.

For similar reasons, you may be at risk from deficiency disease after an operation on, say, the stomach or the bile duct of the liver. Or you may put yourself at risk by adhering to a special diet (no doubt for "health reasons")

that denies you an essential vitamin. Vegans (strict vegetarians, who reject all animal products such as eggs or cheese) may be exposing themselves to B_{12} deficiency, since conventional plant foods lack B_{12}. Finally, the children of many dark-skinned immigrants to northern countries may be getting insufficient vitamin D, which is chiefly synthesized from sunshine (as well as being present in foods such as milk and oily fish). These children are often swaddled as babies and wear too much clothing to get adequate sunlight, and their traditional diet may contain too little vitamin D to compensate for this lack.

All the above examples are of cases in which the end result is unmistakable vitamin-deficiency disease. But marginal deficiency – not disease directly due to severe lack of vitamins, but relatively minor trouble, probably due to some degree of insufficiency – is far more widespread. For instance, old people who do not eat properly because they live alone or in institutions commonly have the sores, the raw, red tongue, and the coarse skin associated with vitamin B and possible C deficiency. Of course, there can be many other causes of such disorders, but the condition sometimes grows less noticeable when B and C vitamins are added to the diet. Some people with fractured bones – especially the elderly – are also often found to be deficient in vitamin D (see *Osteomalacia*, p.543).

Marginal deficiency of C and B vitamins is reportedly common among school children, as evidenced by innumerable cases of chapped lips and sores at the corners of the mouth. Examination of school meals suggests that diet is partly to blame. School meals are often low in fresh vegetables, and such vegetables as there are tend to be left lying about on warming tables – a process that destroys much of their vitamin content.

Pregnant mothers and their fetuses are particularly at risk, not least because a fetus can be severely damaged by even marginal vitamin deficiency. Folic-acid deficiency often occurs during pregnancy because of the woman's increased need for this vitamin.

Should you eat differently?

The chances of your becoming deficient in any one vitamin depend mainly on two factors: first, how available it is in food; and, secondly, how effectively your body can store it. Nature has equipped us pretty well to avoid vitamin deficiency. However, we are not good at retaining vitamin C in the body, and so we can show signs of deficiency within a few weeks if deprived. Luckily, though, vitamin C is present in many foods, and there is no good reason for deprivation. Vitamin A is much less widespread in our everyday diet (the richest sources are fish-liver oils), but our bodies are extremely efficient at building up reserves of it. By and large the solutions balance out the problems.

Three guidelines should keep you on the right track. First, have a varied diet. Eat a limited quantity of meat, fish, or dairy products, but make sure that the quantities are balanced (see *What is a balanced diet?*, p.26). Do not spurn offal, especially liver. A good way to eat is the Chinese way – bits of varied meats serving as garnish for piles of cereal and vegetables.

Secondly, eat plenty of fresh vegetables and fruit. You will then be sure to get enough C and most of the B vitamins. Wholemeal bread (or other whole grains) can provide vitamin E and some B vitamins.

Thirdly, prepare your food with care. This is especially important for making the most of vitamin C, which dissolves in water and is destroyed by prolonged boiling. Potatoes are not outstandingly rich in vitamin C, but most of us eat a lot of them, and so they are our most important single source. They should therefore be cooked carefully. Because the main concentration of vitamin C lies just under the skin, it is sensible to cook and eat potatoes in their jackets. Frying has certain drawbacks, but it conserves more of the C than boiling. Mashing reduces the C content by introducing air, which oxidizes the vitamin. And do not rely for C on potatoes that have been stored for several months, since the C content falls drastically with storage. Oranges, watercress, and beansprouts are more dependable sources – although they are usually eaten in small quantities, and so in practice are not so important as potatoes.

Finally, never boil green vegetables in water with sodium bicarbonate in it. The sodium bicarbonate preserves colour but destroys most of the vitamins.

Are vitamin pills effective?

Should you take vitamin pills to avoid marginal deficiency? The answer is "No" – not a categorical no, perhaps, but a fairly decided no. A varied diet of fresh food, along with exposure of the skin to plenty of sunlight to top up vitamin D reserves, should provide all your vitamin requirements (assuming that there are no defects in your metabolism). Pills may not harm you, but you are unlikely to need the extra-large doses of vitamins that they provide; and in some cases a high dose *can* be harmful. This is particularly true of vitamins that the body can store efficiently,

How vitamins got their names

The plethora of names and confusion of classifications for vitamins are an accident of history. They were assigned letters of the alphabet (nobody knows why) roughly according to the order in which they were discovered. As research continued, the chemical composition of each vitamin was determined, and each was given a chemical name (in a few cases, more than one name). To add to the confusion, some vitamins that were at first thought to be a single substance were later discovered to comprise a group, or "complex", of different chemicals. Vitamin B provides the best-known example of this. And – even more baffling to people who are not biochemists – vitamin PP is included in the "B complex" group. The reason: PP – whose initials stand for "Pellagra-Preventing" – was discovered separately and named independently, but is now considered to belong chemically among the Bs.

such as A and D. Too much vitamin A dries out the skin and enlarges the liver and spleen. Too much D leads to excess calcium in the blood, which can cause certain gastrointestinal and nervous disorders.

Mothers have been known to endanger their children's health by giving them overdoses of cod-liver or halibut-liver oil. It is more sensible to rely on a good, varied diet and to supplement it with oil and/or pills only as your doctor instructs you to. To be sure, extra doses of some vitamins do sometimes have a therapeutic value. In particular, vitamin A (or certain derivatives) may prove useful against certain skin disorders. But this does not mean that extra-large doses of vitamin A – or any other vitamin – will necessarily prevent disease.

There seems to be no danger of overdosing yourself with vitamin C pills, which some people believe provide protection against the common cold. Surplus C is rapidly excreted in the urine, and there are no known ill-effects. Are vitamin C pills, then, likely to reduce the number or severity of colds? There is no dependable answer to this question. Various research projects have resulted in conflicting evidence. Most authorities would hesitate to recommend big doses of C, but they would also be unwilling to dismiss the idea high-handedly. If you want to take vitamin C tablets, go ahead; at least they do no harm.

NAME OF VITAMIN		FOODS RICH IN IT
A (retinol)		Oily fish, cod- or halibut-liver oil, milk, butter, eggs, spinach, carrots.
The B complex		
B_1 (thiamine)		Pork, liver, wholemeal cereals, green vegetables.
B_2 (riboflavine)		Liver, kidney, milk, cheese, eggs, green vegetables.
PP (niacin or nicotinic acid)		Fish, meat, wholemeal cereals.
B_6 (pyridoxine)		Most foods.
B_{12} (cobalamin)		Animal products only, especially liver.
B_c (folic acid)		Liver, fresh vegetables.
C (ascorbic acid)		Fresh vegetables and fruit, especially citrus fruits.
D (calciferol)		Oily fish and fish oils, butter, eggs. (The skin also manufactures it from sunlight.)
E (tocopherol)		In most foods, especially wheatgerm and dark-green, leafy vegetables.
K (phytomenadione)		Green, leafy vegetables.

ITS ROLE IN METABOLISM	RESULTS OF DEFICIENCY	PEOPLE AT RISK
Essential for good vision, particularly at night; and for growth generally.	Coarse, dry skin; clouded vision. (But excess amounts can lead to headaches, vomiting, enlarged liver and spleen.)	People with *cystic fibrosis* (p.685) or severe liver disease.
Assists the functioning of brain, nerves, and muscles.	*Nutritional cardiomyopathy* (p.400); numbness of hands and feet (in the severe form called "beriberi"); mental confusion.	Old people and others who do not eat enough fresh vegetables and fruit.
Helps break down food to provide energy.	Chapped lips, sore tongue, clogged skin pores.	Anyone who relies on canteen-style food (excessive boiling or steaming removes it).
As in B$_2$ (PP = Pellagra-Preventing).	Sore, red, cracked skin (in the severe form called "pellagra"); swollen tongue; general digestive upsets; diarrhoea; anxiety, or even dementia.	Alcoholics and vagrants.
As in B$_2$.	Irritation of the skin and dry lips; mild convulsions in babies.	Babies fed on dried milk; women on the contraceptive pill.
Helps produce red blood cells; essential for healthy nerves.	*Pernicious anaemia* (p.420).	People with *Crohn's disease* (p.473); strict vegetarians.
Helps produce red blood cells.	As in B$_{12}$.	Pregnant women.
Many, varied roles in respiration, growth, and response to infection and stress.	Coarse skin; internal bleeding; stiff limbs; bleeding gums (in the severe form called "scurvy").	Old people who do not eat a varied diet, and alcoholics.
Essential for good bone structure.	In children, *rickets* (p.687); in adults, *osteomalacia* (p.543); in old people, a tendency to bone fracture. (But excess amounts can lead to digestive upsets, impaired kidney function, and depressed mental states.)	Some dark-skinned immigrant children and mothers. Old people.
Probably helps to protect cells from damage and degeneration.	Deficiency is unlikely.	None.
Essential for proper clotting of blood.	Internal and external bleeding.	People with severe *jaundice* (p.485) or *cirrhosis of the liver* (p.487); newborn babies of women who have been deficient in the vitamin.

Gout

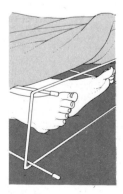

Sites of the pain

Among the body's waste products is uric acid. It normally passes out through the kidneys; but if, for some reason, there is more than the kidneys can deal with, it accumulates, forming crystals. When uric-acid crystals are caught in the spaces between joints, the tissue surrounding an affected joint becomes inflamed, and the inflammation irritates the nerve endings that supply the joint, producing extreme pain. This is what happens in gout. Sometimes the crystals also accumulate within the kidneys themselves, and *kidney failure* (p.511) may result.

Since all human beings produce about as much uric acid as the kidneys can handle, everyone is to some extent susceptible to gout. Some people develop the disease for no apparent reason other than inborn predisposition. In many sufferers, however, gout develops because of an environmental factor that upsets the uric-acid balance. Such factors include lead poisoning, which impairs kidney function, and diseases such as *psoriasis* (p.254) or *leukaemia* (p.426).

What are the symptoms?

The main symptom is severe pain, sometimes in an elbow or knee but more often in a hand or foot, frequently at the base of the big toe. The pain usually comes without warning (though experienced sufferers may note some early twinges). Within a few hours the joint is so tender that the sufferer cannot endure even the weight of bedsheets. There is often fever of up to 38.5°C (about 101°F). Inflamed skin over the joint is likely to be red, shiny, and dry.

The first attack involves only one joint and lasts only a few days. Sometimes there will be no more attacks, but there is normally a second, though perhaps not for months or years, followed by another, then another, and so on. They occur at shorter intervals, last longer, and involve more and more joints. If the disease is not treated, the inflammation of soft tissues around the joint and the irritation to bone can lead to joint deformity; the overlying skin may degenerate; and there may be symptoms of kidney damage, such as *renal colic* (see *Kidney stones*, p.509).

How common is the problem?

Gout is one of the commonest forms of joint disease. It affects males most commonly, usually after puberty, and women mainly after the menopause. A genetic basis for susceptibility is suggested by the fact that certain races seem more prone than others to gout. For instance, it is widespread among Polynesians but relatively rare among Scots.

Gout aid
A bed cradle prevents bedclothes from pressing on a painful, gouty toe.

What are the risks?

Gout is one of the most curable of metabolic disorders. If untreated, though, it can lead to *high blood pressure* (p.382) or kidney disease.

What should be done?

Even though your first attack may subside in a few days and there is no early recurrence, consult your doctor. Do not try to ease the pain with aspirin, which can slow down the excretion of uric acid; the doctor may prescribe an appropriate painkiller. Because the disease sometimes passes away forever after a single attack, no further treatment is normally advisable at this point. But the doctor needs to keep track of subsequent attacks if specific therapy must eventually be begun.

After you have had your first attack, you may be advised to make some changes in your eating and drinking habits. In particular, the doctor may suggest cutting down on rich foods and alcohol.

What is the treatment?

Self-help: To ease the pain, apply a hot compress or ice to the affected joint. To relieve the weight of bedclothes use a protective bed cage. Take no painkilling drugs other than those prescribed by your doctor.

Professional help: There are three lines of treatment (of which, with luck, only the first two will be necessary). The first is simply control of pain, for which the doctor may prescribe an *analgesic* (but not aspirin). The second line of attack is control of the inflammation. For this most doctors prescribe drugs, taken either by mouth, injection, or rectal suppository.

Since the symptoms of gout may disappear after the first attack, or the disease may lie dormant for months or years, your doctor will not at first take further measures. If symptoms recur, however, the disease must be attacked at its metabolic roots, and this will require the third line of treatment. Unfortunately, once third-line drugs are begun, they must be continued for the rest of your life.

Third-line drugs work in one of two ways. The first way is to increase the excretion of uric acid via the kidneys; your doctor may advise you to help this process by increasing your intake of non-alcoholic fluids, and perhaps by taking regular doses of sodium bicarbonate, which helps to neutralize uric acid. The second way is to reduce the amount of uric acid produced by the body. The choice of drug will depend on a number of factors, including your body chemistry. If you use the drugs exactly as prescribed, you can look forward to a normal life.

Hyper-lipidaemia

Hyperlipidaemia is the name of a wide range of disorders in which the blood contains too much fat. The body needs various kinds of fat (also called *lipid*) as fuel, as structural components, and – in the case of *cholesterol* – as raw material for making hormones and other vital chemicals. Necessary fats are carried through the body by the blood; but a fault or faults in the transport system can lead to excessive amounts of lipids in the blood. The cause of hyperlipidaemia is sometimes an inherited chemical defect. More often the disorder is associated with a generalized disease such as *diabetes mellitus* (p.519).

What are the symptoms?
In most types of hyperlipidaemia there are no specific symptoms. In extreme types, such as a rare, inherited disease called familial hypercholesterolaemia (FH), an accumulation of lipids will, in the worst cases, form yellowish weals beneath the skin. These tend to be particularly prominent around the elbows, the webs of fingers, and the Achilles tendon.

How common is the problem?
Because most cases show no symptoms until the consequences become apparent, it is difficult to assess the frequency with which hyperlipidaemia occurs. Worldwide research indicates that a "safe" blood level of cholesterol, one of the most important lipids, is around 120 milligrams (mg) per 100 millilitres (ml), and that 280mg per 100ml in middle-aged people poses a high risk of *coronary thrombosis* (p.379). Since the average level among British adults is 200 to 230mg per 100ml, we are all on the way to being hyperlipidaemic. In a country such as Britain, about 1 adult in 20 has blood levels of cholesterol above 280mg per 100ml.

What are the risks?
High levels of fat in the blood are probably an important cause of *atheroma*, the condition in which fatty *plaques* build up on artery walls. These plaques, in conjunction with clotted blood, may eventually block blood vessels. Thus, a hyperlipidaemic person is highly susceptible to diseases such as atherosclerosis, coronary thrombosis, and stroke.

You are unlikely to know you are hyperlipidaemic unless you have a medical checkup. If your health is good and your weight and blood pressure normal, do not worry about the chemical content of your blood unless you have reason to believe that FH runs in your family. In that case consult your doctor.

What is the treatment?
Self-help: Some doctors believe that a diet low in saturated fats will lower the levels of fats – particularly of cholesterol – in the blood (see *Cholesterol*, p.27). Other experts disagree with this, but even so, a low-fat diet will stop you becoming obese.

Professional help: In extreme cases, doctors sometimes prescribe drugs that reduce blood concentration of cholesterol by increasing excretion of it. Since cholesterol is excreted by means of the bile, however, and since a surplus of cholesterol in the bile may lead to *gallstones* (p.489), your doctor may prefer to avoid this type of treatment.

Porphyria

Porphyria is an inherited disease caused by a flaw in the complex series of chemical reactions involved in the body's manufacture of haemoglobin (the red blood pigment). As a result of this flaw in metabolism, certain chemicals called porphyrins accumulate injuriously in some part of the body – usually in the liver and digestive system, the brain and nervous system, or the skin. Symptoms of the disease are unlikely to appear before early adulthood; even then, they may not become apparent unless triggered off by some factor such as the taking of certain drugs (including alcohol), becoming pregnant, or even exposing one's body to sunlight. The symptoms vary enormously, depending on body parts affected. There may be vomiting, abdominal pain, muscle cramps and weakness, psychological disorders such as depression or mania, or skin conditions such as blistering and itching. Attacks normally subside after a few days, but some extremely rare forms of the disease may threaten sanity or even life.

All forms of porphyria are notably rare in Britain, where only about 500 cases are treated in an average year. Your doctor is unlikely to suspect that you have the disease unless there are known cases among other members of your family. Chemical tests on urine or faeces can generally determine whether you are a sufferer. Treatment is based on avoiding trigger factors and easing symptoms; the underlying genetic fault cannot be corrected. Certain drugs, foods, or even climates may be banned; psychiatric effects may be minimized by means of tranquillizers; female sufferers will need special advice on contraceptive methods and appropriate specialist care during and immediately after pregnancy.

Disorders of the urinary tract

Introduction

In many ways your body is like a factory containing a number of machines, all of which need energy in order to work together smoothly. The energy is contained in the food you eat. Energy-containing nutrients pass from the bloodstream into body cells, where various chemicals called *enzymes* act to release the energy. During this process, chemical waste products are produced in the cells, and must be removed because they would poison the cells if allowed to accumulate. The waste products pass out of the cells and are carried in the bloodstream to the two kidneys, where they are filtered out, along with any excess water, in the form of urine. Thus normal production and excretion of urine are essential to life.

The kidneys are situated just above the waist on either side of the spinal column. Each kidney contains over one million tiny filtering units, called glomeruli, which remove waste chemicals and excess water from the blood travelling through them. The urine so formed is channelled to the middle of the kidneys. A narrow pipe (the ureter) carries the urine from each kidney down to a temporary storage place in the lower abdomen, the bladder. From time to time the urine, released by the bladder, passes out of the body through a tube (the urethra). This whole system, from kidneys to urethra, is known as the urinary tract, and it is subject to a number of disorders. Infection may reach the kidneys via the bloodstream, or travel up the urinary tract from the opening of the urethra. Infection or inflammation of the kidneys, or even damage caused by external injury, can cause scarring of the filtering tissue which may not only reduce the efficiency of the kidneys but can ultimately lead to their failure. Stones can form in one or both kidneys and cause great pain as they pass down the ureters. This pain is commonly known as renal colic. As in other parts of the body, tumours – both *benign* and *malignant* – can occur in the urinary tract.

The structure of the urinary tract is slightly different in men and women, partly because of its close links with the reproductive system. The disorders described in this section apply to both sexes. Problems related specifically to men, women, or children are discussed in the appropriate special sections of the book.

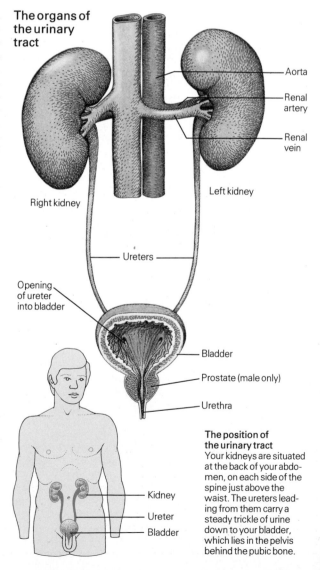

The organs of the urinary tract

Aorta

Renal artery

Renal vein

Left kidney

Right kidney

Ureters

Opening of ureter into bladder

Bladder

Prostate (male only)

Urethra

Kidney

Ureter

Bladder

The position of the urinary tract
Your kidneys are situated at the back of your abdomen, on each side of the spine just above the waist. The ureters leading from them carry a steady trickle of urine down to your bladder, which lies in the pelvis behind the pubic bone.

How the urinary tract works

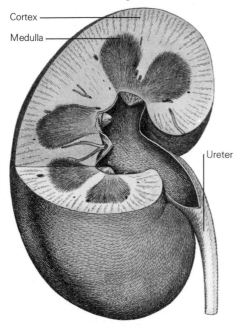

Cortex
Medulla
Ureter

How the kidneys function

When blood from the renal artery reaches the outer part of the kidney (the cortex), left, it passes through minute globular structures (glomeruli), right, which filter off liquid containing nutrients and waste products from the blood. The filtered liquid passes from each glomerulus into the central section of the kidney (the medulla) along a long, thin tubule surrounded by blood vessels which reabsorb the nutrients from the liquid. Blood leaves the kidneys via the renal vein and returns to the general circulation. The remaining liquid continues along the tubule into the ureter and is collected in the bladder as urine.

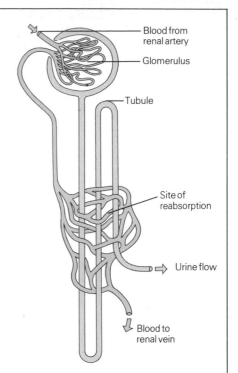

Blood from renal artery
Glomerulus
Tubule
Site of reabsorption
Urine flow
Blood to renal vein

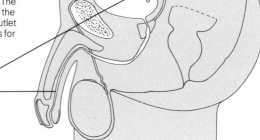

Ureters
Bladder
Openings of ureters into bladder
Sphincter muscle
Urethra

Male urinary tract (right)

The male urethra is about 250mm (10in) long. The opening at the tip of the penis provides an outlet for semen as well as for urine.

Bladder
Urethra

The bladder

Urine trickles down the ureters from the kidneys to the bladder. The bladder has elastic, flexible walls, which allow it to expand as it fills and then contract to expel urine through the relaxed sphincter when you urinate. The urine is prevented from flowing back up into the ureters when the bladder contracts by valves that link the ureters to the bladder. In a healthy person, urination is determined more by habit than necessity; although in general, women tend to empty their bladders more frequently than men.

Female urinary tract (right)

A woman's urethra – only 25mm (1in) long – and bladder lie just in front of her reproductive organs. Because of its position close to the anus and entrance to the vagina, a woman's urinary tract is more susceptible than a man's to infection.

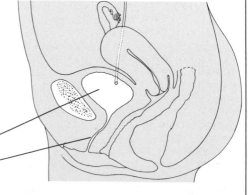

Bladder
Urethra

Infections, inflammation, and injury

In a healthy urinary tract there are no microbes, and the urine itself is sterile. But although the waste products in the urine may be harmful to us if allowed to accumulate, they provide conditions that certain microbes, especially bacteria, thrive in. Usually the microbes gain access from the outside by coming up the urethra and into the bladder. Or they may travel to the kidneys from another part of the body via the bloodstream. Either way, once in the urinary tract they multiply and may spread along it, disrupting normal working and causing swelling and inflammation – the typical effects of any infection. Infection of the kidney itself is called pyelonephritis; this can come on quickly (acute) or can persist in a mild form over many years (chronic). Inflammation of the bladder (often caused by infection) is cystitis; inflammation of the urethra is urethritis.

Sometimes swelling and inflammation of the kidney can occur even though there are no microbes present. Glomerulonephritis, which affects the minute filtering units of the kidney (the glomeruli), is an example of this type of inflammation. (Two forms of the disorder which most commonly affect children are described separately – see *Nephritis*, p.690, and *Nephrotic syndrome*, p.691.)

Injury to the kidneys from a knock or wound is not common as they are protected by the ribcage. Similarly the bladder lies well protected within the pelvic (hip) bones. So your urinary tract is only likely to be damaged by a major injury that requires expert medical attention in hospital.

Acute pyelonephritis

Acute pyelonephritis (sometimes called acute pyelitis) is a kidney infection that comes on suddenly. The infection and resultant inflammation affect chiefly the supporting tissue within which the tiny filtering units, the glomeruli, are embedded (compare *Glomerulonephritis*, p.504). This occasionally occurs when microbes from another part of the body are carried to the kidneys in the bloodstream. In most cases, however, infecting bacteria come from the skin around the urethral opening. In women poor hygiene in this area, especially when wiping the area after a bowel movement, can allow bacteria to enter the urethra and spread, in the urine, up through the bladder and ureter to the kidney. This is especially likely if, for one of a variety of reasons, there is a partial blockage of the normal flow of urine; bacteria flourish in the resultant stagnant pool and cannot be washed out of the tract as easily as when the urine is flowing freely. Though this explains some cases of acute pyelonephritis, it can sometimes occur for no apparent reason in an otherwise healthy person.

What are the symptoms?

In most cases the symptoms start with sudden intense pain in the back just above the waist. Although both kidneys may be affected, the pain is usually worse on one side of your body, and it spreads around that side down into the groin. Your temperature rises rapidly, often reaching 40°C (104°F) and you may feel cold and shivery. There may also be nausea and vomiting. You may experience *dysuria* (difficulty or pain in urinating), and you are likely to have the feeling of constantly needing to urinate although your bladder is empty. The urine usually contains traces of blood and this may make it appear cloudy or, occasionally, light red.

How common is the problem?

Acute pyelonephritis is a common condition at all ages; on average about 1 person in 250 consults a doctor about it each year. It is four time more common in women than in men because the potential entry tube for bacteria – the urethra – is so much shorter in women. Various conditions that affect the flow of urine make you more susceptible; these include pregnancy (pressure on the ureters from the swollen uterus reduces the flow of urine), *kidney stones* (p.509), a *tumour of the bladder* (p.508), or (if you are a man) an *enlarged prostate* (p.574). In addition, a flaw in the urinary tract increases the risk of developing the disorder.

What are the risks?

With prompt treatment, complications are highly unlikely. In extremely young or frail people the infection occasionally spreads into the blood and leads to *blood poisoning* (p.421). Repeated attacks may indicate that there is a basic flaw in the urinary tract that needs to be corrected.

What should be done?

If you have symptoms of this disorder, consult your doctor. In many cases no treatment will be required other than *antibiotics* and bed rest (as outlined below); the attack will then subside in a day or two. But after your recovery the doctor may want you to have blood and urine tests, and perhaps a special *X-ray* of the kidneys known as an *intravenous pyelogram* (*IVP*). You may also need to undergo *cystoscopy* to examine your bladder.

If you are a healthy adult, such diagnostic tests are seldom required after a single attack of acute pyelonephritis. If you have had previous attacks, though, or if the sufferer is a child, tests are advisable in order to disclose any underlying problems and so prevent long-term damage to the kidneys (see *Urinary infections in children*, p.689).

What is the treatment?

The treatment for acute pyelonephritis is bed rest and a light, bland diet including extra fluids such as fruit juice or water. In addition, your doctor will prescribe antibiotics, which can usually be taken by mouth. In some cases – very young and old people, for example – admission to hospital may be necessary so that drugs and extra fluids can be given by *intravenous drip*. Antibiotics generally bring the infection under control in 24 to 48 hours, but treatment may continue for up to 10 days.

Chronic pyelonephritis

Chronic pyelonephritis is a condition in which, over the course of many years, the kidneys become increasingly damaged as a result of repeated (but usually unnoticed) infections of the urine. In most cases the condition starts in infancy and persists unsuspected until, years later, symptoms of kidney trouble begin to occur (see also *Urinary infections in children*, p.689).

The infecting bacteria usually gain access to the urinary tract through the open end of the urethra (the tube that leads from the bladder to the outside), as explained in the article on *acute pyelonephritis* (opposite). Normally, such invasions are confined to the lower parts of the tract (see *Cystitis*, p.505) since the outflow of urine keeps the infection from spreading upwards. In the act of urinating, the bladder contracts, squeezing urine out and down the urethra while, at the same time, valves operate to close off the two ureters where they enter the bladder; this prevents urine from being simultaneously forced back into the kidneys. Sometimes, however, the valves do not work properly, and urine squirts upwards as well as downwards. If this happens with infected urine, the infection may reach the kidneys. And a combination of recurring infections and faulty valves probably causes most cases of chronic

Intravenous pyelogram
An intravenous pyelogram (also known as an excretion urogram) provides a series of X-rays of the whole urinary tract. A special liquid that shows up on X-ray pictures is injected into your bloodstream. It travels round your body until it reaches the kidneys, where it is excreted as waste matter. The process takes several hours and X-ray pictures (one of which is shown on the right) are taken at regular intervals.

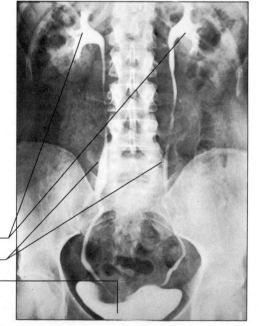

Kidneys
Ureters
Bladder

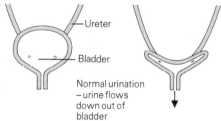

Ureter
Bladder

Normal urination – urine flows down out of bladder

Infected urine in the kidneys
A possible cause of infection in the kidneys is inefficiency of the valves that connect the ureters to the bladder. Normally the valves prevent urine from flowing upwards when you urinate (see diagram above). If the valves do not close properly when you urinate, urine may be squeezed back up the ureters (see diagram right). Any infection in the urine can then travel up to the kidneys.

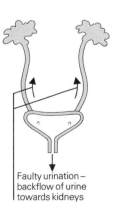

Faulty urination – backflow of urine towards kidneys

pyelonephritis. *Kidney stones* (p.509) may also cause the disorder. Only rarely is chronic pyelonephritis preceded by repeated attacks of other urinary-tract infections such as acute pyelonephritis or cystitis.

What are the symptoms?

Chronic pyelonephritis seldom produces symptoms until the condition is well-established. Eventually, though, early signs of *chronic kidney failure* (p.512) such as increased urination and tiredness may appear. As the disorder progresses, nausea or itching skin may also be noticed.

In many cases the condition is discovered at a much earlier stage when someone is given a blood or urine test for some other reason.

How common is the problem?

Each year in Britain, about 500 people are diagnosed as having chronic kidney failure due to chronic pyelonephritis. Most of these are women. There are many more people who are known to have the condition but in whom it has not led to kidney failure. And because it progresses so slowly, there are yet others with the disease who live to a ripe old age without learning that they have it.

What are the risks?

The main risk is that the condition will develop undetected until the kidneys are so damaged that chronic kidney failure develops. This does not often happen nowadays, however, since increasing awareness of the dangers of urinary infections in young children has resulted in better preventive treatment at an early stage.

What should be done?

If you have repeated mild urinary infections or any of the symptoms of chronic kidney failure, be sure to consult your doctor. The diagnostic tests are generally the same as those arranged for acute pyelonephritis.

What is the treatment?

Self-help: If you are found to have chronic pyelonephritis with no symptoms, your doctor may advise you to forestall its progression by such simple measures as drinking plenty of fluids (up to three litres – about five pints – daily), and avoiding too much protein and salt in your food. The doctor may also arrange blood tests at regular six- or 12-month intervals to check on the progress of the disorder.
Professional help: Treatment depends on the stage at which the disease is discovered. Although surgery to repair faulty valves is sometimes necessary in children, it is not generally helpful for adults. Any other cause of repeated infections – kidney stones, for example – may respond to appropriate treatment for that condition. Otherwise, the usual treatment is *antibiotics*. These are usually given for only a short period whenever a urinary-tract infection does occur. But a prolonged course of low-dose antibiotics (for, say, six months to two years) is sometimes advisable in order to make sure that the urine remains free of bacteria. Because of the normally slow progress of chronic pyelonephritis, many doctors who discover the condition in middle-aged patients do not attempt special treatment but simply advise such people to look out for signs of kidney failure and to have regular check-ups.

Glomerulo-nephritis

Glomerulonephritis is the term used for several related diseases in which the essential fault is damage to the glomeruli, the tiny filtering units in the kidneys. The damage is usually the result of inflammation caused by abnormal proteins that become trapped in the glomeruli.

In a healthy kidney, the blood passes through the glomeruli, and certain chemicals – not all of them waste – are filtered out. Most of the water, and some chemicals that are useful to the body (such as glucose), are then returned to the bloodstream. The remaining waste materials are collected as urine and pass down the ureter to the bladder.

In glomerulonephritis, this process is adversely affected by the damaged glomeruli. Usually the most obvious disturbance is that red blood cells somehow leak through the glomeruli into the urine. Some proteins also pass from the blood into the urine; and if this loss is excessive – as most often happens in children – the result is an illness called *nephrotic syndrome* (p.691). If more and more of the glomeruli are damaged, the kidney becomes less and less efficient as a filter and regulator of the chemical content of the blood. Waste products accumulate in the body, producing the condition known as *kidney failure* (p.511).

Glomerulonephritis can occur in mild or severe forms. It may be acute, flaring up over a few days, or it may be chronic, taking months or years to develop.

What are the symptoms?

The mildest forms of glomerulonephritis produce no symptoms at all. The condition may be noticed only when a urine sample is tested for some other reason. In other cases the urine may have a smoky appearance (caused by the presence of small amounts of blood cells) or be bright red (indicating larger amounts of blood cells).

In severe forms of acute glomerulonephritis you may feel generally unwell, with drowsiness, nausea, and vomiting (which are symptoms of a form of kidney failure). You will probably produce very small amounts of urine, and there will be an accumulation of fluid in your body tissues (*oedema*), which you notice as puffiness under the skin, particularly around the ankles. If fluid accumulates in your chest, you may also become short of breath.

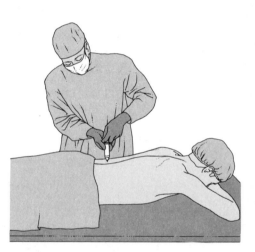

Kidney biopsy
In a kidney biopsy, a small area of skin and muscle overlying the kidney is first numbed with a local anaesthetic. The doctor then passes a hollow needle through the numbed area into the kidney, and withdraws a tiny sample of kidney tissue for laboratory analysis.

How common is the problem?
Glomerulonephritis is not common. In Britain only about 1 person in 7,000 is treated in hospital for the disorder. The acute form of glomerulonephritis most commonly occurs in children (see *Nephritis*, p.690).

What are the risks?
The main risk of all forms of glomerulonephritis is that they may lead to kidney failure. The disorder can also lead to *high blood pressure* (p.382) and *anaemia* (p.419), since the kidneys play a part in regulating the chemicals that control blood pressure and the production of red blood cells.

What should be done?
If you have any of the symptoms of glomerulonephritis, consult your doctor, who will arrange for a urine sample to be tested. If this suggests that you have glomerulonephritis, you will be admitted to hospital for a few days for further tests. These may include an *intravenous pyelogram* (*IVP*) and a *biopsy* of the kidney tissue.

What is the treatment?
Many forms of glomerulonephritis are so mild that they require no specific treatment. Other forms can be treated with *steroids* or *cytotoxic* drugs.

If you have oedema, a *diuretic* drug may help. Any high blood pressure must also be treated, and you may need iron and vitamin tablets and perhaps blood transfusions if you have become anaemic as a result of this disorder. If glomerulonephritis leads to kidney failure, appropriate treatment will be given.

Urethritis

Inflammation of the urethra (the tube that leads from the bladder to the outside) is known as urethritis. In women, it is usually the result of bruising without infection during sexual intercourse (see *Chronic urethritis*, p.601). Urethritis in men is generally the result of infection caused by a sexually transmitted disease (see *Urethritis in men*, p.578, *Non-specific urethritis*, p.612, and *Gonorrhoea*, p.611).

Cystitis

Cystitis is inflammation of the bladder, usually caused by infection entering the bladder via the urethra from outside. The major symptom is a frequent urge to urinate, with only a small amount of strong-smelling, possibly blood-stained, urine being passed each time. The urine is likely to burn or sting as you pass it and you may have a feeling of discomfort just below the navel (the location of the bladder). You may also have a slightly raised temperature.

The disorder is far more common in women than in men, because the entrance to a woman's urethra is nearer the anus, making it easier for microbes to reach the bladder. Cystitis rarely occurs in a man unless an underlying disorder such as an *enlarged prostate* (p.574) or a urinary-tract abnormality is also present.

For further information see *Cystitis in men*, p.577, *Cystitis in women*, p.600, and *Urinary infections in children*, p.689.

Injury to kidneys or ureters

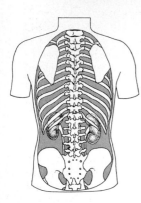

Your kidneys are well protected by your ribcage and the muscles that support your back.

The most likely cause of injury to a kidney is either a direct blow to the side of the body just under the ribs (from a football boot, for example) or a crushing force such as occurs in a road accident or when someone is trapped under heavy masonry. In any of these events a kidney may be bruised, or its membranous outer covering and the ureter torn. Sometimes a large blood clot forms under the covering and produces a lump over the kidney that can be felt through the skin if it develops on the lower part of the kidney, below the ribcage. There is also a danger that blood or urine may leak into the abdomen through a tear, causing *peritonitis* (p.470). If the inside of the kidney is damaged, blood will pass into the urine.

What are the symptoms?
A mild injury to a kidney or ureter may cause pain and tenderness in the lower part of the back. There may also be a slight fever; and there may well be intermittent traces of blood in the urine, though you may not notice the blood until a day or two after the injury has occurred. If you suffer such an injury and develop severe back pain or notice blood in the urine, one or both of your kidneys – and perhaps the ureters, too – may have been seriously injured. In either event, consult your doctor. In particular, blood in the urine is a symptom of potentially serious conditions and should never be ignored. You will probably need to undergo an *X-ray* of the kidneys – *intravenous pyelogram* (*IVP*) – to help the doctor assess the damage and determine what kind of treatment is necessary.

What is the treatment?
The ability of the kidneys and ureters to heal themselves is remarkable; even major tears and injuries seldom require treatment other than a seven- to 10-day period of rest. Unless the IVP shows the injury to have been very slight, however, it is normally advisable for the sufferer to rest in a hospital bed, where painkillers can be administered and the pulse and blood pressure checked frequently to ascertain whether there is serious internal bleeding. After an interval of about three months it will be advisable to have another IVP to make sure there has been no permanent damage to the kidneys or ureters.

In the unlikely event that a week of so of bed rest does not cure the trouble, an operation to remove the kidney or repair the torn ureter may be necessary. Removal of a kidney is not usually a complicated operation; and people with only one kidney are able to lead quite healthy, normal lives.

Injury to bladder or urethra

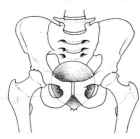

Your bladder lies in a protected position within the circle of bones that form your pelvis.

Because the bladder lies protected within the abdomen, injuries to it are uncommon. When damage occurs, it is generally due to a direct blow to the pelvis that causes a fracture of a pelvic bone, with a sharp fragment of the bone piercing the bladder wall. Any such rupture is bound to have serious consequences because it allows urine to leak into the abdominal cavity (see "What are the risks?" below). In males rupture of the urethra is more common, but less dangerous; it can be caused by a fall or a kick in the groin. Because the female urethra is very short, urethral damage in women almost never occurs.

What are the symptoms?
Rupture of the bladder produces severe pain in the abdomen, and there may also be signs of *shock* (p.386). A urethral injury is also extremely painful and is generally followed by an inability to urinate; sometimes there is a blood-stained discharge from the penis (or the urethral orifice in a woman).

What are the risks?
Rupture of the bladder is dangerous because leakage of urine into the abdominal cavity causes *peritonitis* (p.470) – a condition that requires prompt and specialized hospital treatment. Damage to the urethra, on the other hand, is unlikely to lead to peritonitis; the chief risk in a man is that the healed urethra will be scarred, causing a poor outflow of urine due to *urethral stricture* (p.578).

What should be done?
If, following an accident, you have any of the symptoms of a ruptured bladder or urethra, consult your doctor without delay. Physical examination, followed perhaps by a special *X-ray* of the bladder and *cystoscopy*, should allow a diagnosis to be made promptly.

What is the treatment?
Injury to the bladder or urethra requires admission to hospital. You will be given *antibiotics* to prevent infection; and if your bladder is ruptured, you will need an urgent operation to repair the leak and clean out the abdominal cavity. If your urethra is damaged, you will probably have to be *catheterized* for several days in order to drain out urine while the urethra heals. Occasionally, however, surgery is necessary.

Cysts, tumours, and stones

A growth or swelling in the body should be investigated by a doctor, and the urinary tract is no exception to this rule. The tract can be affected by *cysts*, tumours, or the formation of stones. Cysts are usually soft, fluid-filled sacs; tumours are more solid. Both cysts and tumours may be either *benign* or – much less often – *malignant*. However, such growths are relatively uncommon in this part of the body. More common are the pebble-like stones (calculi) that sometimes form in the kidneys or bladder. Although such stones may cause a lot of discomfort, they are rarely a serious threat to health.

Kidney cysts

There are two types of kidney cyst. The first is a single fluid-filled sac that develops in a kidney for no known reason; over a period of years the cyst may slowly grow bigger, but it is unlikely to cause trouble unless – as rarely happens – a cancer forms in its wall. The other type of cyst is the result of an inherited disorder called polycystic disease, a *congenital* condition in which many cysts of varying sizes develop in both kidneys. Nobody knows why cysts grow swiftly in some people and slowly or hardly at all in others. Many people suffer no ill-effects, although in some there may be progressive damage leading to a form of *kidney failure* (p.511).

What are the symptoms?
A single cyst produces no symptoms unless it becomes large enough to cause pain in the lower part of your back. In any such event, you may be able to feel the soft lump with your fingers. Polycystic disease occasionally causes blood in urine (*haematuria*) or repeated attacks of *chronic pyelonephritis* (p.503). Most often, though, it is symptomless unless cysts eventually replace so much normal kidney substance that the sufferer develops *chronic kidney failure* (p.512), at which point symptoms of the latter disorder – such as tiredness and increased frequency of urination begin to appear.

How common is the problem?
It is impossible to estimate the number of people with kidney cysts since so many have one of the two kinds of condition without knowing it. The presence of cysts is often discovered only because some other problem necessitates an examination of the kidneys. We know, however, that severe polycystic disease is extremely rare. In Britain it causes about 3 per cent of all cases of chronic kidney failure; in other words, fewer than 100 new cases of advanced polycystic disease come to light in an average year.

What are the risks?
The only possible risk of a solitary cyst is that *malignancy* may develop, and this rarely happens. Polycystic disease, as pointed out above, may lead to chronic kidney failure, but this is also a rare occurrence.

What should be done?
If you have a single kidney cyst, it will probably be discovered only when tests are done for another reason. Because of the slight possibility of cancerous cells in the cyst, your doctor will probably want a further test, cyst *aspiration*, which involves piercing the cyst with a needle to withdraw some fluid for examination. Aspiration of a kidney cyst can usually be done painlessly with a local anaesthetic, and occasionally the cyst disappears altogether. If the cells in the fluid are normal, nothing further need be done.

Your doctor may discover that you have polycystic disease by chance when testing you for a different disorder. But if you know that the disease runs in your family, you will do well to consult the doctor about it, not only for your own sake but also to find out if the condition is likely to affect your children. Whether or not your kidneys are affected, you should have annual check-ups.

What is the treatment?
No treatment is required for a painless benign kidney cyst. If it becomes big enough to hurt, however, or in the unlikely event that it is found to be malignant, surgery to remove the affected kidney will probably be necessary (for further information about this procedure see *Tumours of the kidney*, p.508).

There is no specific treatment for polycystic disease. If the presence of cysts is discovered at an early stage, and you have regular check-ups thereafter, your doctor may be able to help you slow down the progressive damage to the kidneys in the same way as for chronic kidney failure.

Tumours of the kidney

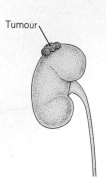

Tumour

Growths on the kidney tend to be situated near the top, where they are hidden within the ribcage.

There are two major types of tumour of the kidney, both of which are *malignant* but only one of which occurs in adults. This type, known as a hypernephroma, forms on the edge of the kidney as a result of the uncontrolled multiplication of abnormal cells. As the tumour grows, it eats into healthy kidney tissue; but because the efficiency of the kidney as a filter is affected only at a very late stage in the development of the disease, eventual *kidney failure* (p.511) is very rare. The tumour more often makes itself known by causing generalized symptoms such as persistent fever and loss of appetite and weight. There may also be vomiting and mild, generalized abdominal pain, and the urine may be red or smoky because of bleeding from the tumour.

Hypernephromas are rare; they occur most often in men over 40, and they account for only 3 per cent of all deaths from cancer. (For information about the other main type of kidney tumour, which affects only children, see *Wilm's tumour*, p.692.)

What are the risks?
The main risk of a hypernephroma is that some of the tumour cells may break off into the bloodstream and spread to other parts of the body, particularly the lungs or bones. However, hypernephromas spread less readily and are more amenable to treatment than many other types of cancerous growth.

What should be done?
If you have symptoms suggesting that you may have a kidney tumour – especially if your urine looks reddish or abnormally cloudy – consult your doctor, who will probably want samples of your urine for laboratory analysis. If a tumour is suspected, you will then need to undergo a series of diagnostic tests, among them an *intravenous pyelogram* (*IVP*), an *ultrasound scan*, and an *arteriogram* of the kidney. These tests are usually carried out during a short stay in hospital.

What is the treatment?
If tests show the presence of a hypernephroma, surgery to remove the affected kidney will be necessary; a single healthy kidney can readily compensate for the loss of the other. *Radiotherapy* and anti-cancer (*cytotoxic*) drugs may also be advisable to kill off any remaining cancer cells. Following this treatment you will need regular check-ups for up to five years, in order to make sure that cancer has not recurred.

Tumours of the bladder

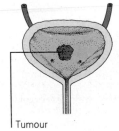

Tumour

Most bladder tumours are warty, cauliflower-shaped growths that project from the inside wall of the bladder.

Tumours of the bladder, like those in many other parts of the body, can be either *benign* or *malignant*. Both types originate from cells lining the bladder and tend to produce a growth (or, in some cases, more than one) that projects inwards, into the space reserved for urine. In addition, malignant (cancerous) tumours spread within the walls of the bladder and may spread to other parts of the body. If any type of tumour occurs near the place where the ureter enters the bladder, it can block the flow of urine from the kidney, causing the kidney to become swollen with urine (a condition known as hydronephrosis). This damages the kidney and makes it prone to infection (see *Acute pyelonephritis*, p.502).

What are the symptoms?
The characteristic symptom of a bladder tumour is blood in the urine (*haematuria*). The act of urinating is not usually painful, but there may be a burning feeling; and the sufferer tends to pass small amounts of urine at frequent intervals. If hydronephrosis has developed, you may also have pain in the small of your back. And since a bladder with a tumour is especially susceptible to infection, there may be symptoms of *cystitis* (p.505).

How common is the problem?
Tumours of the bladder are not common. In an average year in Britain, 1 person in 2,500 is diagnosed as having the disorder; it is most common in men over 50.

What are the risks?
All benign tumours and many small malignant ones respond well to treatment. Occasionally, though, the cancerous cells spread (*metastasize*) to other parts of the body, and, once this has happened, prospects for successful treatment are poor.

What should be done?
Always consult your doctor if you see blood in your urine. The doctor will take urine and blood samples for analysis, and, depending on the results, you may need to undergo such diagnostic tests as *cystoscopy* and an *intravenous pyelogram* (*IVP*) or a *cystogram*. If a growth is discovered, a sample of it will be taken by *biopsy* in order to determine whether it is benign or malignant.

What is the treatment?
The usual treatment for all bladder tumours is to try to destroy them by burning them

away with a special probe attached to a cystoscope (a process known as *fulguration*). The surgeon views the bladder through the cystoscope and manipulates the probe to destroy the cells. This usually clears up the problem, but you will need six-monthly check-ups for at least three years to make sure there is no recurrence of the trouble.

If a tumour has affected a large area of the bladder, abdominal surgery may then be

necessary. In severe cases the whole bladder may have to be removed, and the ureters will then be connected to a specially made opening in the abdominal wall. Thereafter, the urine will flow into a bag (an "external bladder"), which must be emptied every day or so. Modern techniques have made this a safe, efficient, and unobtrusive process. After surgery, *radiotherapy* may be used to destroy any remaining abnormal cells.

Kidney stones
(renal calculi)

The kidneys are among several organs in which stones are apt to form. A kidney stone normally begins as a tiny speck of solid material deposited in the middle of the kidney, where urine collects before flowing into the ureter. As further bits of material cling to the first speck, it gradually builds into a solid mass. This process can occur in one or both kidneys; and, over a period of years, a stone with a diameter of 25mm (1in) or even more can develop. Since most kidney stones contain the mineral calcium, it seems likely that stone formation is caused by an excessive amount of calcium in the urine. (For several possible reasons for the development of kidney stones and for their prevalence in tropical climates, see "How common is the problem?" below.)

A stone with a diameter of more than about 5mm (1/5in) is likely to remain in the kidney, unable to pass into the ureter; and such trapped stones may not be a problem if

Pain from kidney stones
A kidney stone can cause severe pain (renal colic) as it travels from the kidney to the bladder. This may take 2 or 3 days, and the pain follows the stone's progress.

Kidney
Urethra
Stone travelling along ureter
Bladder

Site of the pain

not many are formed. Very small stones, too, seldom give trouble since they are easily carried away and passed in the urine. A larger stone, however, may cause pain and other problems (see "What are the risks?" p.510) if and when it passes into the ureter and as it moves towards the bladder.

What are the symptoms?
If stones are too big to pass from the kidney into the ureter, there may be no symptoms or – at most – occasional mild pain as little "chips" break off and are carried down the ureter. The most common symptom of troublesome kidney stones is *colic* (a stabbing pain that tends to come in waves, often a few minutes apart). Colic can result from disorders in various parts of the body (see, for example, *Gallstones*, p.489, or *Intestinal obstruction*, p.471), and, typically, it makes you double up with pain. Kidney pain of this type (renal colic), which can occur when a stone passes from a kidney down one of the ureters, will subside whenever the stone stops moving or is discharged in the urine. The pain almost always occurs on one side of the body at a time – though, of course, if you have stones in both kidneys, a subsequent attack may be on the other side.

Renal colic is usually felt first in the back, just below the ribs on either side of the spinal column. Over a period of hours or days, the pain follows the course of the stone as it travels along the ureter around to the front of the body and down towards the groin. It may make you feel nauseated, and there may be traces of blood in your urine. After the stone reaches the bladder, passage through the remainder of the urinary tract is likely to be painless or nearly so. (See also *Bladder stones*, p.510.)

How common is the problem?
About 1 person in 1,000 in Britain has the disorder. Because passage of a stone often produces severe pain, kidney stones are a frequent cause of hospital admissions (the current figure is about 12,000 a year in England and Wales alone). Nevertheless, the incidence in the Western world is declining; this may be partly because of changes in diet and life style, but nobody knows the precise reasons for the decline, or why some people are particularly liable to develop stones. It *is* known that the problem runs in families, and

it is prevalent in tropical countries, probably because of an over-concentration of calcium in the urine; the reason for this is that people in hot climates lose so much body water in sweat that they tend to produce less urine. It is an interesting fact that World War II troops serving in desert areas suffered more frequently from kidney stones than did those in temperate climates.

Males are more prone than females to the disorder, and so are people over 30. On rare occasions children may develop a form of kidney stone that is due to a chemical abnormality in the blood.

What are the risks?
Although most kidney stones either remain harmlessly in the kidneys or are eventually passed in the urine, an occasional stone may get stuck in a ureter, blocking the flow of urine on one side. Surgery is then required. Kidney stones also make you more liable to infections in the urine and, consequently, to attacks of *acute pyelonephritis* (p.502). As a result of repeated infections and (sometimes) scarring from large stones, *chronic kidney failure* (p.512) may follow long-standing trouble from kidney stones, but this very rarely happens.

What should be done?
If you tend to suffer from kidney stones, see your doctor at six-month intervals to make sure there is no permanent damage to the kidneys. If you get an attack of renal colic, your doctor will probably refer you to a hospital for blood and urine tests, an *intravenous pyelogram* (*IVP*) and possibly *cystoscopy*.

Such diagnostic tests help locate stones in the urinary tract if there are any, and indicate whether further treatment is necessary.

What is the treatment?
Self-help: It is always wisest to consult your doctor if you have an attack of renal colic. But you will also do well to drink large quantities of water (at least five litres – about eight pints – each day), which will help flush the stone through the urinary tract. To relieve pain, take a mild *analgesic* such as soluble aspirin or paracetamol.

Professional help: There is no satisfactory medical treatment for kidney stones that do not pass out of the body of their own accord. If you are particularly susceptible to this disorder, though, your doctor may prescribe a drug which can, in certain cases, prevent stones from forming. If a stone obstructs the lower part of the ureter, it can sometimes be removed during cystoscopy (for which you will be fully anaesthetized). The doctor puts a slim pair of tweezers through the cystoscope into the bladder and up into the ureter where the stone is trapped. The tweezers grasp it and draw it out. If this is not possible, a more major abdominal operation to remove the stone, requiring a hospital stay of about 10 days, may be necessary.

In the unlikely event that stones or related infections have done extensive and irreparable damage to one of your kidneys, the entire kidney may need to be removed. In such cases the remaining healthy kidney can adequately compensate for the loss of the other. In general, however, kidney stones are merely a painful inconvenience.

Bladder stones
(Vesical calculi)

A *kidney stone* (p.509) that has come, perhaps painfully, through the ureter into the bladder is relatively small, and it can pass out of the body in the urine with comparative ease. Stones that form within the bladder itself, however, tend to be bigger than kidney stones and to remain lodged in the bladder. They may cause troublesome symptoms such as an over-frequent urge to urinate, pain on passing urine, and blood in the urine (often blood seems to be "squeezed out" in the last few drops). Nowadays, bladder stones are not a common problem, and they are becoming increasingly uncommon; nobody knows why.

If you have bladder stones that are too large to pass naturally through the urethra, they must be removed. This can sometimes be done (under general anaesthetic) by inserting a *cystoscope* up the urethra into the

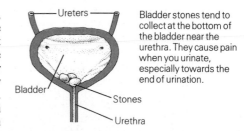

Bladder stones tend to collect at the bottom of the bladder near the urethra. They cause pain when you urinate, especially towards the end of urination.

bladder. The cystoscope is equipped with a device that can either draw out the stones or crush them into tiny pieces that can be washed out. An alternative minor operation involves opening the bladder in order to get at the stone or stones. Another treatment is to pulverize the stones by bombarding them with high-powered *ultrasound* waves so that they can easily be flushed out.

Kidney failure

Kidney (renal) failure occurs in one of three forms. Acute failure is an illness in which kidneys suddenly (during the course of days or even hours) stop functioning. Chronic failure is more accurately termed chronic impairment since this condition develops over many years and may not result in severe renal problems. End-stage failure, resulting from chronic failure, is the most severe renal disorder, in which the kidneys function so poorly that they can no longer sustain life without the assistance of modern technology.

Acute kidney failure

The kidneys may suddenly stop working for any number of reasons; but, broadly speaking, there are three main causes. A disease such as *glomerulonephritis* (p.504), can abruptly damage the kidneys enough to cause their failure. Or a sudden drop in blood pressure such as occurs after severe bleeding or a major heart attack can mean an inadequate supply of blood to the kidneys, which are particularly susceptible to such deprivation. Or, finally, the flow of urine may be suddenly and completely obstructed by a blockage in the ureters, bladder, or urethra.

As a consequence of any of these events, waste products and water build up in the body because they can no longer be effectively removed, and the chemicals normally regulated by the kidneys become unbalanced.

What are the symptoms?
The most notable symptom is that you pass an abnormally small amount of urine something under 0.5 litres (less than a pint) a day. Within a short time you lose your appetite, feel increasingly nauseated, and begin to vomit. If treatment is delayed, drowsiness, confusion, convulsions, and coma may develop. In most cases, though, symptoms of the condition that has caused acute kidney failure are at first more apparent than those due to the failure itself.

How common is the problem?
Mild attacks of acute kidney failure are not uncommon, but the more serious forms (those due to glomerulonephritis, for instance) are extremely rare. A busy general hospital is likely to have no more than one or two such cases in a year.

What are the risks?
Much depends on the severity of the underlying problem; but acute kidney failure is a potentially dangerous condition and in some cases treatment with artificial kidney aids may have to continue for life.

What should be done?
The sufferer urgently requires hospital treatment and there may well be an intensive series of diagnostic tests involving blood and urine samples, an *intravenous pyelogram* (*IVP*), and possibly a kidney *biopsy*.

What is the treatment?
When the cause of acute failure is heavy bleeding or a heart attack, emergency treatment is usually required; its form depends on the circumstances. When diagnostic tests show that the cause is an obstruction, the sufferer is likely to need an abdominal operation to relieve the blockage. If, however, the underlying cause of failure is a disease of the kidneys themselves – or if, as often happens, the kidneys remain severely affected even though the basic cause of failure is successfully treated – treatment procedures are less clearly defined.

An *intravenous drip* of blood or plasma, possibly with a *diuretic* drug included in it, may be all that is needed to restore the kidneys. But your doctor may have to use an artificial device for performing the functions of your kidneys until they recover of their own accord. This type of treatment is called dialysis and is painless (for a full account see *Artificial kidney aids*, p.512). Sufferers from acute kidney failure must sometimes remain in hospital for six weeks or more before the kidneys function normally again.

While under treatment you may need a special diet which is high in calories but low in protein, and which includes no more than perhaps 600ml (one pint) of fluid a day. This type of diet gives the kidneys (or the substitute apparatus) a minimal amount of work to do by providing plenty of usable energy – glucose in the form of jam or honey – with few of the waste materials produced by protein-rich foods such as meat and eggs. As your kidneys recover, you will be gradually weaned away from dialysis and permitted to resume a normal diet.

Chronic kidney failure

Chronic kidney failure is a condition in which mild, repeated attacks of inflammation over a period of years injure and scar the kidneys so as to damage their efficiency without necessarily destroying it. The inflammation may be caused by various diseases – chiefly *chronic pyelonephritis* (p.503) or *glomerulonephritis* (p.504), but also such persistent conditions as *kidney stones* (p.509), *kidney cysts* (p.507), *high blood pressure* (p.382), or it may occasionally be caused by excessive consumption of painkilling drugs (opposite). If you suffer from chronic kidney failure, there is a gradual build-up of waste products and chemicals in your blood, your kidneys become increasingly unable to limit the amount of water in your urine, and you are likely to have high blood pressure. (One function of the kidneys is control of blood pressure; high blood pressure can therefore be both a cause and a result of chronic failure.)

What are the symptoms?
Symptoms appear gradually, and there may be none for many years. Then you may notice that you are urinating more often than you used to. You may also feel progressively more tired and lethargic. If your chronic kidney failure continues to worsen, you will begin to have the symptoms of *end-stage kidney failure* (opposite).

How common is the problem?
About 2,000 new cases of this condition are diagnosed in Britain every year. The older you are, the greater your chances of having it.

Artificial kidney aids

A person whose kidneys are either temporarily unable to function or have become badly damaged by long-standing inflammation is likely to receive a type of treatment called dialysis. In dialysis the functions of the kidneys – removing waste products and regulating chemical and water balance – are taken over by a machine.

There are two forms of dialysis, both of which are painless. The first, peritoneal dialysis, is usually carried out in hospital. The doctor makes a small incision in the abdominal wall and threads a thin plastic tube through into the abdomen. A special fluid flows slowly through the tube and fills the peritoneal space (the space between the inner layer and outer layer of the peritoneal membrane, which covers the abdominal organs). Waste products seep from the abdomen into the fluid, which is continuously sucked out along with excess water. The process may last for several hours.

Recently, a new type of peritoneal dialysis has been developed in which the fluid is left in the peritoneum for up to 12 hours at a time. Chronic ambulatory peritoneal dialysis, as it is called, allows you to carry out the regular changes of fluid at home, when convenient.

The second form of dialysis – haemodialysis – is carried out by means of what is popularly called a "kidney machine". In Britain there are about 2,500 people who regularly use such machines on a long-term basis. The machine filters waste products from the patient's blood. To do this, blood from an arm or leg artery is led along a thin tube to the machine, through a filter, and back along another tube into an adjacent vein. A slow flow of blood trickling through the machine for a six- to eight-hour period, repeated two or three times every week, is enough to keep waste products and water in the body within safe limits. Many people have a kidney machine at home and connect themselves up in the late evening, sleep through the night while being dialysed, and disconnect themselves in the morning. This routine permits them to have full freedom during the day.

People are naturally worried at first when realizing that their lives depend on an artificial aid. But they quickly learn how to operate the machinery and insert needles; and relief from symptoms of kidney failure is frequently quick, impressive, and long-lasting.

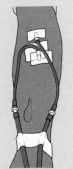

If you have to use a kidney machine regularly, a suitable artery and vein in an arm or leg will be stitched together or linked by a short piece of blood vessel to form what is called an arteriovenous shunt, so making it easier for you to insert the needles that connect you to the machine (above).

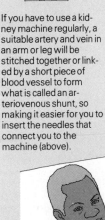

What are the risks?

Obviously, the main risk is that the scarring will become progressively worse, leading to end-stage kidney failure. This happens in three out of four cases. There are also the risks associated with high blood pressure and with *anaemia* (p.419), *osteomalacia* (p.543), and *hyperparathyroidism* (p.528). These diseases sometimes occur as a result of the kidneys' inability to control blood chemicals.

What should be done?

If you find that you have to urinate with abnormal frequency and that the problem persists for more than a week without apparent cause, consult your doctor, whose first move will probably be to check your blood pressure. The combination of frequent urination and high blood pressure will suggest the need for further investigation, especially if there is a history of kidney trouble in your family. You will also probably need to undergo blood and urine tests, an *intravenous pyelogram* (*IVP*), and possibly a *biopsy* to allow analysis of kidney tissue.

What is the treatment?

Self-help: Be sure to follow your doctor's advice about diet; people with kidney failure are generally advised to eat low-protein foods (see *Acute kidney failure*, p.511) and to drink several litres of fluid per day. Take no medicines at all without first consulting the doctor. And – most important – have regular medical check-ups even if you feel completely well. This will allow problems to be discussed at an early stage, and treatment can then be modified as necessary.

Professional help: No treatment can repair the scarred kidney tissue, but close medical supervision can slow the progress of chronic kidney failure and counteract troublesome symptoms. Your doctor may prescribe iron and vitamin pills along with drugs to control your blood pressure. To stave off the development of osteomalacia, you may also need to take an aluminium hydroxide preparation. With regular check-ups, a carefully guided diet, and such drugs as seem advisable for your special problems, you should be able to lead a comfortable life for years to come.

End-stage kidney failure

This is the name given to the most advanced form of kidney failure. What usually happens is that, despite treatment, *chronic kidney failure* (opposite) progresses to a stage in which the kidneys can no longer sustain life. It is often something minor such as urinary infection that tips the balance from chronic failure to end-stage failure.

What are the symptoms?

The importance of the kidneys in maintaining health is revealed by the veritable galaxy of symptoms that occur when end-stage kidney failure eventually develops. The symptoms include many or all of the following: lethargy, weakness, headache, a furred tongue and unpleasant breath, *oral thrush* (p.451), nausea, vomiting, diarrhoea, an accumulation of water (*oedema*) in the lungs (producing shortness of breath) and just under the skin (producing generalized swelling), pain in the chest and perhaps in the bones, and intensely itchy (though rash-free) skin. Women may stop having periods.

End-stage kidney failure is rare: on average there are only 1,300 new cases in Britain in an average year.

What is the treatment?

A person who develops end-stage failure will already be receiving treatment for the preceding chronic failure. He or she will have instructions to report any illness or change in condition to the doctor.

The various aspects of any one patient's treatment programme will be tailor-made to his or her individual case. Many of the symptoms of end-stage failure can be alleviated by drugs, but only for a short while. Because the kidney damage is irreversible, the only satisfactory form of treatment is one that will take over from the kidneys' functions. This means either dialysis (see *Artificial kidney aids*, opposite) or an operation to transplant a healthy, donated kidney into the body (one kidney can always do the work of two if necessary). About 1,000 kidney transplantations are carried out annually in Britain (see *Transplants*, p.402, for further details).

It must be remembered that dialysis and transplantation are not suitable treatments for all patients; for example, they are rarely offered to people over 60.

What are the long-term prospects?

End-stage kidney failure is no longer the swiftly fatal disease it once was. Statistics show that well over half of today's patients who have had end-stage failure are able to live comparatively normal lives five years after the onset of the condition. A good proportion of transplant recipients are still alive and well up to 10 years after receiving their new kidney.

Hormonal disorders

Introduction

Hormones are chemicals made in special glands called endocrine glands. These glands are composed of hormone-producing cells clustered around blood vessels. Together with the brain and nervous system, hormones coordinate and control various organs and tissues so that all parts of the body work together smoothly and efficiently. Hormones do not act on the body as quickly as nerves; the latter are responsible for coordinating second-by-second activities such as walking or talking, whereas hormones control intermediate and more lengthy processes such as the level of sugar in the blood, growth, and sexual development.

Each hormone (and there are dozens of them in your body) circulates in the bloodstream to all parts of the body, but it affects only certain organs and tissues. The more there is of a hormone circulating in the blood, the more effect it has. The amount of hormone released into the bloodstream by an endocrine gland is in turn affected by any of a number of factors – an infection, stress, or a change in the chemical composition of the blood, including a change in the level of some other hormone in the blood. The pituitary gland, in particular, produces several hormones whose specific jobs are to regulate the activity of various other endocrine glands. The pituitary, therefore, has a wide-ranging control of the hormonal system and is sometimes called the body's "master" gland.

Only the more common hormonal problems are discussed in this book. The ones dealt with in this section affect both men and women – that is, they occur in endocrine glands found in both sexes. They comprise disorders of the pituitary gland, pancreas, adrenal glands, and thyroid and parathyroid glands. There are several other endocrine glands which are possessed exclusively by one sex – the ovaries and placenta in women, and the testicles (testes) in men. Disorders of these glands are discussed in other sections of the book (see *Special problems of men*, p.570; *Special problems of women*, p.582; and *Pregnancy and childbirth*, p.616).

Many hormonal disorders require the expert diagnosis and treatment of an *endocrinologist*, a doctor who specializes in such problems.

Hormone-producing glands

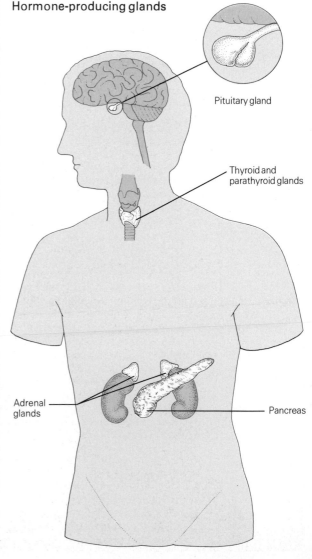

Pituitary gland

Thyroid and parathyroid glands

Adrenal glands

Pancreas

Pituitary gland

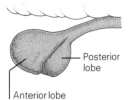

Posterior lobe

Anterior lobe

The pituitary gland is made up of 2 parts, the anterior and posterior lobes. Both lobes produce hormones which control many processes within the body.

The pituitary gland, a peanut-sized organ situated just beneath the brain, is the most important endocrine (hormone-producing) gland in the body. Sometimes called the "master" gland, it is like a control centre, regulating many aspects of growth, development, and everyday running of the body.

The gland consists of two parts, the anterior (front) lobe and the posterior (rear) lobe.

The anterior lobe produces six hormones. Growth hormone, as its name implies, regulates the physical growth of most parts of the body. Prolactin stimulates the breasts to produce milk. The four other hormones made by the anterior lobe stimulate four other hormone-producing glands – the thyroid, adrenals, ovaries in women, and testes in men – which then produce hormones of their own.

The posterior lobe of the pituitary gland produces two hormones. Antidiuretic hormone (ADH) acts on the kidneys and plays a large part in regulating the volume of urine. The other hormone, oxytocin, stimulates uterine contractions in childbirth and milk ejection during breast-feeding.

Disorders of the pituitary gland are rare. Each year about 1 person in 30,000 receives hospital treatment for such a disorder.

Acromegaly

In this rare condition an adult's pituitary gland produces an excessive amount of growth hormone. This results in excessive growth, but in an adult it cannot lead to greater height, since vertical growth ceases once the main bones of the body have finished forming at the end of adolescence (compare *Gigantism*, p.516). Instead the excess growth hormone produces acromegaly, in which the bones thicken and all other structures and organs enlarge. The cause of this hormone over-production is a *pituitary tumour* (p.518).

What are the symptoms?
Acromegaly generally does not become apparent until middle age. The first symptom you notice is usually gradual enlargement of your hands and feet, typically revealed by the tightening of a ring on your finger, or an increase in your shoe size. Your head and neck grow broader, and your lower jaw, brows, nose, and ears become prominent. Your skin and tongue thicken, and your features become coarser. You may develop a deeper voice, and suffer from tingling in the hands, fatigue, increased sweating, stiffness, and generalized aches. In women there may be an increase of hair on the body and limbs.

In some cases of acromegaly, *diabetes mellitus* (p.519) develops, so you may also have symptoms of this disorder. And if the pituitary tumour is large, it may also cause you to have symptoms from pressure on adjacent parts of the brain.

What are the risks?
The longer acromegaly is left untreated, the greater the risks become. If the heart continues to enlarge, *heart failure* (p.381) may develop. In addition, *high blood pressure* (p.382) may appear, and a large pituitary tumour can cause visual problems or damage the rest of the pituitary gland, causing *hypopituitarism* (p.517), which, if left untreated, can lead to death.

What should be done?
Anyone who develops the symptoms described should see a doctor. If the doctor suspects acromegaly, he or she will refer the person to a specialist for tests to be carried out. A blood sample will be taken to assess the amount of growth hormone in the body and an *X-ray* of the skull plus a *CAT brain scan* will reveal any abnormal growth in the pituitary gland.

Visual symptoms
The woman shown below has the typical prominent jaw, square head and large hands of a person suffering from acromegaly.

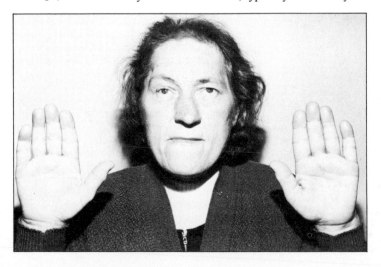

What is the treatment?

If tests show that there is a pituitary tumour, but it is no longer active and the disease has halted, then no treatment may be necessary.

If an active tumour is causing problems because of its size, it will be removed or destroyed. Otherwise, a drug can be given in tablet form to lower the level of the growth hormone. The best form of treatment depends on a number of factors, and you should be guided by your specialist. You will also require treatment for any other disorder resulting from acromegaly.

What are the long-term prospects?

Surgical removal of a pituitary tumour is effective in improving any visual defects. You may not make a complete recovery, though, since the changes in your bones and your appearance are largely irreversible. However, treatment halts the progress of the disease and relieves many of the symptoms.

Gigantism

Gigantism is the counterpart in children and adolescents of *acromegaly* (p.515) in adults. Over-production of growth hormone, usually caused by a *pituitary tumour* (p.518), leads to excessive growth of all parts of the body. However, whereas acromegaly occurs when the limb bones have stopped growing, in gigantism this is not the case, and heights of over 2.2m (7ft) can be reached.

What should be done?

If a young person grows at an excessive rate, even if he or she has tall parents (see the *Growth charts* on p.645, and also *Growth disorders*, p.687), then a doctor must be consulted without delay. Treatment to slow down the sufferer's rate of growth is as for acromegaly, and in most cases is successful in halting the disorder.

Dwarfism

In rare cases, children fail to grow properly because of a failure by the pituitary gland to produce enough growth hormone. (There are other causes of stunted growth more common than growth-hormone deficiency – see *Growth disorders*, p.687.)

Deficiency of growth hormone may be present from birth or develop at any age during childhood or adolescence (adults are not affected because they have stopped growing anyway). Except when it is due to a *pituitary tumour* (p.518), the cause of the deficiency is unknown. In some cases, deficiency of growth hormone is accompanied by under-production of other hormones; this leads to retarded sexual development (see *Special problems of adolescents*, p.706, and *Hypopituitarism*, opposite).

What should be done?

Dwarfism in an infant is often detected at the regular check-ups all babies are given after birth. If you are worried that your child seems small for his or her age, then consult the *Growth charts* on p.645. If there is a problem, medical examinations and blood tests will be carried out to determine whether it is due to any of the causes that are more common than growth-hormone deficiency – which is usually the last cause to be considered. Deficiency is detected by measuring the amount of growth hormone in blood samples, both before and after stimulation of the pituitary gland by drugs or exercise. Tests will also be carried out to detect a pituitary tumour.

Treatment, other than when the disorder is caused by a tumour, consists of giving the baby or child injections of human growth hormone twice each week. This is done until the end of adolescence, which is when normal growth stops. In most children the response to treatment is excellent and they grow into normal adults.

Shown below are 3 girls each aged 10. Only 1 is at a normal stage of physical development for her age.

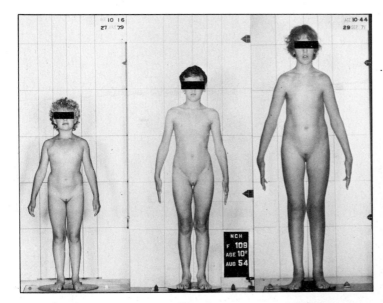

| Dwarfism | Normal | Gigantism |

Diabetes insipidus

In the normal production of urine, the kidneys first filter water, salts, and other substances from the blood. They then absorb some of the salts and much of the water from this fluid, leaving concentrated urine ready to be passed from the body. The absorbed water and salts are returned to the bloodstream, to maintain the correct concentration of blood and body fluids. What stimulates the kidneys to absorb water from the urine is antidiuretic hormone (ADH), produced by the posterior lobe of the *pituitary gland* (p.515). In diabetes insipidus, there is a deficiency of ADH and the body passes large quantities of dilute (watery) urine.

The most common cause of the disorder is damage to the pituitary gland resulting from a severe head injury. Some cases are caused by an operation on the pituitary gland, or *radiotherapy* treatment of the gland or surrounding area. Another cause is pressure on the gland from a *pituitary tumour* (p.518). In some cases, however, investigations are unable to reveal any obvious cause.

Diabetes insipidus should not be confused with *diabetes mellitus* (p.519), commonly known as sugar diabetes.

What are the symptoms?

You pass large quantities of colourless urine – as much as 20 litres (35 pints) every 24 hours. This great fluid loss causes an unquenchable thirst; you will be constantly interrupted by day and woken at night by the need to urinate and drink. Other symptoms, also resulting from the unusually frequent need to pass urine, are dry hands, and constipation.

What should be done?

As soon as symptoms appear, see your doctor, who will arrange for you to visit hospital to have a water-deprivation test. You will be deprived of all fluid while the volume of water in your urine is measured on several occasions. In a normal person deprived of fluid for several hours, ADH would absorb water from the urine to help conserve water in the body; if the volume of water in your urine remains high, this shows you have a deficiency of ADH. The effect on your urination following an injection of artificial ADH confirms the diagnosis.

What is the treatment?

Drink as much water as you need. In some cases, when the degree of urination is not excessive, restriction of salt in the diet and taking *diuretic* tablets may be all that is necessary; both these measures make the kidneys conserve water. A causative pituitary tumour will have to be removed.

In many cases, the most effective treatment is with an artificial form of ADH called desmopressin, taken as nasal drops. Initially, you visit the doctor daily for one or two weeks to establish the correct dosage. Once this has been done, you take drops twice a day. How long you have to go on taking them is very much determined by what has caused the disorder. When this has been a head injury, surgery, or radiotherapy, the defective gland often rights itself within a year or so, resulting in a complete cure. If this fails to happen, and in other cases, treatment with artificial ADH or diuretic tablets will be for life.

Hypopituitarism

(also called Simmond's disease)

The pituitary gland plays a vital role in regulating growth, sexual development, and basic *metabolism*, chiefly through the activities of its anterior (front) lobe. It does this by producing six hormones which affect various parts of the body (see *Pituitary gland*, p.515). In hypopituitarism, the anterior lobe of the gland fails to produce any of the six hormones. The effects of this deficiency are wide-ranging and include sexual underdevelopment or infertility, a prematurely aged appearance, weakness, pallor, and general ill-health.

The most common causes of hypopituitarism are serious head injury, a *pituitary tumour* (p.518), or side-effects of treatment for such a tumour. Occasionally the disease develops in a woman following severe blood loss during childbirth, but some cases occur for no known reason.

Hypopituitarism is usually a chronic (long-term) illness. It cannot be cured, but modern treatment can counteract many of its effects.

What are the symptoms?

Because the pituitary gland stimulates several other endocrine (hormone-producing) glands, the symptoms of hypopituitarism are a combination of the symptoms of several other hormonal disorders. These include *hypothyroidism* (p.526), *Addison's disease* (p.524), *amenorrhoea* (p.583), *dwarfism* (opposite), and infertility.

What are the risks?

If hypopituitarism is not treated promptly, it can be fatal. This is mainly because the disease makes the *adrenal glands* (p.523) unable to respond to stress or infection. Rarely, it can bring on *hypoglycaemia* (p.522).

What should be done?
Hospital tests on blood samples will show whether you have hypopituitarism and, if so, whether a pituitary tumour is the cause.

What is the treatment?
A person with hypopituitarism will need lifelong treatment with tablets and injections of natural hormones to replace those missing because of the disease. Thyroxine tablets replace hormones normally produced by the thyroid gland and thus correct hypothyroidism; hydrocortisone tablets replace the hormones manufactured by the adrenal gland; and injections of testosterone are given to men to make up for underproduction of this sex hormone by the testes.

In women, various hormone treatments restore sex drive and periods (and young women can be treated with oestrogen to promote breast development). A man or woman who has become infertile but who wishes to have children can often be made fertile again by injections of indirectly acting pituitary hormones that stimulate the sex glands (the testes or ovaries).

Pituitary tumours

There are two types of pituitary-gland tumour; both always occur in the anterior (front) lobe and never in the posterior (rear) lobe. Why they occur is unknown.

One type is an adenoma, a *benign* tumour that causes excess production of one of several hormones and leads to *acromegaly* (p.515) or *gigantism* (p.516), *galactorrhoea* (below) or *Cushing's syndrome* (p.523). It may also press on surrounding areas and cause other disorders, as described below.

The other type of tumour is a craniopharyngioma, a growth that does not increase production of any hormones but that enlarges and exerts pressure either on the rest of the anterior lobe, causing *dwarfism* (p.516) or *hypopituitarism* (p.517), or on the posterior lobe, causing *diabetes insipidus* (p.517). Some craniopharyngiomas are *malignant*.

Both types of tumour, if they grow large enough, may press on the nerves to the eyes, progressively causing headaches, a *squint* (p.327), and deteriorating sight.

A doctor treating any of the disorders described will arrange for blood tests to measure the levels of various hormones, *X-rays* of the skull, and perhaps a *CAT brain scan* to be taken to disclose whether the disorder is being caused by a pituitary tumour.

What is the treatment?
Whenever possible, a pituitary tumour is removed or destroyed by surgery and/or *radiotherapy* and the results of such treatment are now usually excellent.

Surgery to remove the tumour is a delicate procedure, involving the use of extremely fine instruments. The tumour is usually reached via a nostril, or a hole made in the bridge of the nose. If the tumour is large and pressing on the nerves to the eyes, *open-brain surgery* may be necessary. Recovery from the actual operation is rapid, but there is always a risk that the rest of the small, delicate pituitary gland will have been damaged during the operation, and that as a result hypopituitarism or diabetes insipidus will develop. However, this is an acceptable risk, because both these diseases can be treated by lifelong *hormone-replacement therapy*.

Instead of cutting out the tumour, the surgeon may destroy it by *cauterizing* (burning) it, freezing it, or placing a tiny *radioactive implant* in it.

If the tumour has spread or is difficult to pinpoint, radiotherapy of the whole gland may be necessary. Like surgery, radiotherapy may damage the rest of the gland.

Hormone-producing tumours

Normally, only the endocrine glands or a tumour in an endocrine gland produce hormones. But, rarely, hormones can be manufactured by a tumour in an organ not normally concerned with hormone production. When this happens, the excess hormone in the body causes the same symptoms as those brought on by an overactive endocrine gland. For example, a tumour of the kidney, lung, or breast can produce parathyroid hormone. This brings on the symptoms of overactive parathyroid glands (hyperparathyroidism) causing indigestion and making the sufferer depressed, though the parathyroids themselves are working normally. Symptoms clear up only through treatment of the tumour.

Abnormal milk production (galactorrhoea)

Galactorrhoea is production of breast milk at times when it is not supposed to be produced. Milk production under control of a hormone, prolactin, normally occurs in a woman a few days before, and in the months following, the birth of a baby. Production at any other time in a woman – and at any time in a man – constitutes galactorrhoea. The problem is not a serious threat to health, though it may be irritating; however, the underlying cause of galactorrhoea may be a prolactin-producing pituitary tumour, which is more serious and may lead to other symptoms. Because the majority of sufferers are female, the disorder is dealt with as a special problem of women – see *Galactorrhoea*, p.590.

Pancreas

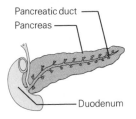

Pancreatic duct
Pancreas
Duodenum

The pancreas is a gland about 150mm (6in) long. Its head lies within the curve of the duodenum, to which it is linked by the pancreatic duct.

The pancreas is a long, thin·gland that lies crosswise just behind the stomach. It has two major functions. The first is to produce *enzymes* which flow through the pancreatic duct into the duodenum, where they help to digest food (see *Liver, gallbladder, and pancreas,* p.485, for digestive disorders of the pancreas). The second major function of the pancreas is to produce the hormones insulin and glucagon, which play an important part in regulating the glucose level in the blood.

Glucose is contained in many foods we eat (not only in sweet things) and is the main source of energy for all cells in the body. Insulin stimulates cells to absorb from the blood enough glucose for the energy they need, and stimulates the liver to absorb and store the rest; insulin therefore acts to lower the glucose level in the blood. Glucagon (along with hormones produced by other glands) stimulates the liver to release glucose, and thus raises its level in the blood.

Diabetes mellitus

Diabetes mellitus is a common disorder caused by a deficiency or total lack of insulin production by the pancreas. This results in a low absorption of glucose – both by the cells that need it for energy and by the liver that stores it – and consequently in a high level of glucose in the blood. (Diabetes mellitus should not be confused with the much rarer disorder *diabetes insipidus,* p.517.)

There are two main forms of diabetes mellitus – insulin-independent (commonly called maturity-onset diabetes) and insulin-dependent (juvenile diabetes).

Insulin-independent diabetes: In this form, which chiefly affects people over 40, the insulin-producing cells in the pancreas function, but the output of insulin is inadequate for the body's needs. Sufferers are usually overweight, and insufficient insulin is produced to cope with the excess blood glucose and increased body size that their overeating brings about. Heredity is also an important factor; nearly a third of insulin-independent diabetics have a family history of the disease. Like many body organs, the pancreas becomes decreasingly efficient with age.

Insulin-dependent diabetes: In this form of the illness, which occurs mainly in young people, the pancreas produces very little or no insulin, and sufferers depend on insulin injections for treatment. The reason for the defect is not fully known but is believed to be an *autoimmune* problem which permanently damages or destroys the insulin-producing cells. The body is unable to use glucose because of the lack or absence of insulin, and is forced to obtain energy from fat instead – which leads to fresh problems (see "What are the risks?" below).

Either form of diabetes may be brought on by another disease – for example *acromegaly*

(p.515), *thyrotoxicosis* (p.525), or *Cushing's syndrome* (p.523). When diabetes is caused in this way, it is known as secondary diabetes. Some people with secondary diabetes remain diabetic even after successful treatment of the causative disease.

What are the symptoms?

Both forms of diabetes cause the same main symptoms. You may need to urinate as often as every hour or so, throughout the day and night. This is because the excess glucose in the blood overflows into the urine, and, to carry it, the volume of urine has to be increased. Some people notice white "sugar spots", dried splashes of glucose-filled urine, on their underwear or shoes. Microbes multiply in the sugary urine and can cause such urinary-tract problems as *cystitis* (p.505), *balanitis* (p.578) and *pruritis vulvae* (p.603).

The excess loss of fluid makes you perpetually thirsty, and taking sweetened drinks increases the amount of urination and makes the thirst worse.

The glucose-starvation of the body's cells causes extreme tiredness, weakness, and apathy – so much so that you may feel unable to get up in the morning. Some diabetics (especially insulin-dependent diabetics) lose a lot of weight, since fat and muscle are burned up to provide energy. Other possible symptoms include: tingling in the hands and feet; leg cramps; reduced resistance to infections (boils and urinary-tract infections are sometimes the first signs of diabetes); blurred vision due to excess glucose in the fluid of the eye; and *impotence* (p.614) in men or *amenorrhoea* (p.583) in women.

The symptoms of insulin-dependent diabetes usually develop rapidly, over weeks or months; but those of the insulin-independent form often do not appear until many years after the actual onset of the disease, which is sometimes detected only by chance at a routine medical examination.

How common is the problem?

In Britain, diabetes mellitus affects about 1 person in 70; but up to one quarter of diabetics have a form of the disease that does not produce noticeable symptoms. It becomes increasingly common with age: 0.5 per cent of children have it, compared to 3 per cent of elderly people. Insulin-dependent diabetes is most common among boys and young men; the insulin-independent form occurs most often among those who are overweight, especially middle-aged and elderly women.

Diabetes is known to run in families. However, even if both parents of a child are diabetic, there is only a 1 in 20 risk that their child will develop the illness.

What are the risks?

The efficiency of modern treatment has transformed what was once an often fatal disease in early life into one from which such deaths are extremely rare. However, there are still risks attached to the disease. Diabetic *hyperglycaemic* coma (drowsiness accompanied by incessant urination and intense thirst, or even unconsciousness) may occur in insulin-dependent diabetics. This is the result of the body using fat as a substitute for glucose to provide energy, and poisonous acids – ketones – forming as a by-product. A coma may happen before treatment starts, after an infection such as *influenza* (p.559), or if the diabetic neglects his or her treatment. Fortunately, prompt hospital treatment usually brings about a full recovery from the coma.

Other complications, which can affect both types of diabetic, occur only in a minority of cases and usually 15 to 20 years after the onset of the disease. Such risks include *diabetic retinopathy* (p.323), *peripheral neuropathy* (p.283), and *chronic kidney failure* (p.512).

Diabetics also run a higher than average risk of developing *atherosclerosis* (p.372), a disease of the arteries, with its attendant risks of strokes, heart attacks, and high blood pressure. The blood vessels to the legs become narrowed, causing cramp, cold feet, pain on walking ("intermittent claudication"), and even ulcers or *dry gangrene* (p.415). To avoid sores or cuts that may lead to gangrene, you should try not to cut your nails too short, shoes should be well-fitting, and a chiropodist should treat corns or ingrowing toe nails. If any cut fails to heal within 10 days, you should consult your doctor.

What should be done?

If you suspect you have diabetes mellitus, see your doctor, who will ask you to provide a urine sample to be tested for the presence of glucose and ketones. The presence of large quantities of both will show that you have the disease. If only glucose is present, a blood sample will be taken to measure the amount of glucose in your bloodstream, because occasionally people have some glucose in their urine without being diabetic. If there is still no clear result, you will need to undergo a glucose-tolerance test. A series of blood samples are taken before and after you swallow a glucose drink; if the level of glucose in the later samples is abnormally high, this shows that you are not producing enough insulin and that you have the disease. Following a firm diagnosis, you will be given a full physical examination before treatment starts.

Diabetics are encouraged to join the *British Diabetic Association* (p.768), which can provide them with valuable support and guidance. Your doctor will give you a card to carry at all times, giving your name and address, the fact that you are diabetic, and instructions on how you can be helped if you are unwell. You can buy a bracelet or neck pendant with the same information. Finally, you must declare your diabetes to insurance companies and car-licensing authorities. If you fail to do this, your insurance cover or licence may be invalid.

What is the treatment?

No cure has yet been found for diabetes mellitus, and you will require lifelong treatment. This is largely self-administered so its effectiveness depends mainly on you.

Insulin-independent diabetes: Diet alone can control this form of the disease in a third of all cases. The diet restricts the amount of carbohydrates you eat and in overweight sufferers brings about considerable weight loss. The amount of calories allowed each day will vary between 800 and 1500, depending on your weight (see *Obesity*, p.492). Generally you should have only small, regular intakes of carbohydrates, so that there are no large peaks and troughs in the glucose content of the blood; do not eat sugar, sweets, cakes, jam, and so on. Make sure your diet contains enough *fibre* by eating wholemeal bread and plenty of salads, fruit, and vegetables; avoid beer and sweet drinks at all times (once your diabetes is under control you can drink lager, dry wines, and spirits in moderation); take regular, moderate exercise, and do not smoke cigarettes, which can further damage blood vessels and lead to atherosclerosis.

In mild cases, merely avoiding the concentrated sugar of sweets, cakes, biscuits, and sweet drinks can be enough to bring the blood-glucose level down to normal. This is particularly the case if you can reduce your weight, because then the insulin that your pancreas does produce may be sufficient for your reduced body size.

Your progress in keeping your blood glucose down will need to be checked, and your doctor will take blood samples or arrange for you to attend a clinic at regular intervals. You will be encouraged to check your own progress with a urine-testing or blood-testing kit. Tests should be carried out daily until the effects of your diet start producing a normal level of blood glucose. It is easy, once you get normal results, to slip back into old habits – especially if your are only a mild diabetic – and you must guard against this by using the

test as a check once or twice a week and keeping all your medical appointments.

Despite keeping strictly to their diet, many diabetics find sooner or later that their urine or blood tests are failing to show normal results. Then, in addition to the dietary measures, the doctor will prescribe *hypoglycaemic* tablets, which lower the blood glucose. There are several different tablets available, and if you suffer from side-effects on one type, your doctor will transfer you to another. In rare cases, when too high a dosage is taken, *hypoglycaemia* (p.522) can result. If this happens, eat something sweet at once (otherwise you may lose consciousness), and see your doctor within a day or two about an adjustment of the dosage. To deal with such an attack if you are out, you should always carry sugar lumps or glucose tablets.

In the same way that diet alone may start failing to control the disease, so hypoglycaemic tablets in conjunction with diet may also gradually cease to be effective. When this happens, insulin injections will be needed, and the insulin-independent diabetic will then have become insulin-dependent.

Insulin-dependent diabetes: This form of the disorder is treated by a controlled diet and by daily or twice-daily injections of insulin (extracted from beef or pig pancreas or synthesized by microbes following *genetic engineering*) to make up for the deficiency or lack of the body's own insulin.

Insulin can be taken only by injection; any insulin taken by mouth is destroyed by digestive juices before it is absorbed into the bloodstream. You will be shown how to use a syringe to inject yourself just under the skin of your thigh, arm, or abdomen. Most people learn how to do this efficiently within a few days. Parents of diabetic children will need to administer the injections until the child is about 10 years old.

You must keep rigorously to the timetable of meals and snacks advised by your doctor. This keeps the supply of glucose to the blood steady, so that regular doses of insulin always have approximately the same amount of glucose to act on. Insulin is available in various types and strengths, and the one that your doctor prescribes will depend on many factors including your age and the severity of your diabetes. Always make sure that you obtain the same type and strength of insulin each time you renew your prescribed supply.

Your doctor will advise you to check the effectiveness of your treatment by means of the same urine or blood tests that insulin-dependent diabetics use. You may have to carry out the test several times each day.

Some urine tests are not very satisfactory because they give only a positive or negative result, and the amount of glucose in your urine is only an approximate reflection of the amount of glucose in your blood. So nowadays more diabetics are using a specially treated plastic strip or a small battery-operated meter to measure the actual level of glucose in the blood. Because blood tests give an accurate blood-glucose measurement, they enable you to maintain more accurate control of your diabetes.

Self-discipline is essential for the successful control of diabetes. Check with your doctor whether you can engage in such strenuous exercises as squash or heavy digging in the garden. Exercise burns up glucose and may bring on hypoglycaemia, so you may need to eat extra food beforehand.

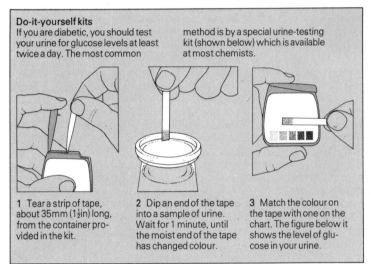

Do-it-yourself kits
If you are diabetic, you should test your urine for glucose levels at least twice a day. The most common method is by a special urine-testing kit (shown below) which is available at most chemists.

1 Tear a strip of tape, about 35mm (1½in) long, from the container provided in the kit.

2 Dip an end of the tape into a sample of urine. Wait for 1 minute, until the moist end of the tape has changed colour.

3 Match the colour on the tape with one on the chart. The figure below it shows the level of glucose in your urine.

Any illness, from a cold to a heart attack, will cause stress and thus increase the body's demand for insulin. If you are unable to eat normally, take glucose drinks (but do *not* reduce your dose of insulin) and consult a doctor as soon as possible.

Diabetes can cause additional problems during pregnancy (see *Diabetes and pregnancy*, p.626) and in children. Young children may find it difficult to understand why they must diet and not have sweets and lemonade; but you must be firm in enforcing the diet.

If you are a diabetic, make sure that you always tell doctors or dentists about your condition before any treatment, so that they can take any necessary precautions.

What are the long-term prospects?
Provided you treat your diabetes sensibly, you can expect to lead a full and healthy life. You should have few problems with employment; diabetics are found in most walks of life. However, if you are on insulin, you should try to avoid shift work, which can interrupt the regularity of diet and injections. Also you must not work at heights, or drive public-service or heavy-goods vehicles, because of the risk that you might have an attack of hypoglycaemia.

Even if you are among the small minority who develop complications, these can be minimized by regular medical check-ups and strict control of your diabetes.

Hypo-glycaemia

Hypoglycaemia is a low level of glucose in the blood – the opposite of the *hyperglycaemia* found in untreated *diabetes mellitus* (p.519). The cells in the body are therefore deprived of energy-providing glucose. The condition is almost entirely confined to sufferers from diabetes mellitus who are on insulin injections (and some on hypoglycaemic tablets). Taking too much insulin, not keeping to the prescribed meal timetable, or taking unusually strenuous or prolonged exercise can all bring on an attack. In rare cases, hypoglycaemia can sometimes be caused by *Addison's disease* (p.524), *hypopituitarism* (p.517), or a growth in the pancreas that causes over-production of insulin.

What are the symptoms?
Symptoms vary considerably from person to person but often start with a feeling of being uncomfortable, followed by profuse sweating. Other symptoms include dizziness, weakness, trembling, unsteadiness, hunger, blurred vision, slurred speech, tingling in the lips or hands, and headache. You may, unknown to yourself, become aggressive or uncooperative (conditions sometimes mistakenly attributed to drunkenness). In extreme cases you may lose consciousness; in younger sufferers, convulsions may occur (see *Convulsions in children*, p.667).

What should be done?
If you are a diabetic on insulin, an attack of hypoglycaemia will be artificially induced under medical supervision so that you can recognize exactly what form it takes in your particular case.

If you do have an attack, reflect on its cause, and try to prevent the possibility of another one. If you have attacks as often as once every three or four days, see your doctor, since you may need a reduction in your dose of insulin or hypoglycaemic tablets.

What is the treatment?
Self-help: If you are at risk from hypoglycaemia, then you should always carry glucose tablets, sugar lumps, or sweets. At the first sign of an attack, eat some until you feel normal again – which will be within a few minutes. Make sure your relatives and friends know about the symptoms, so that if you become confused or uncooperative, they can give you something sweet. Tell them that a small drink of milk, or syrup smeared inside your mouth, may bring you round sufficiently to eat properly. However, they should never try to feed you if you become unconscious, because this could choke you.

An increasingly used alternative to glucose tablets and sugar is an injection of glucagon, a hormone that helps raise the blood-glucose level. Many sufferers ensure that their relatives and friends know how to inject the hormone into an arm or leg muscle if they become unconscious. If the measures described do not work, or are unavailable, see *Accidents and emergencies* (p.805) and summon medical assistance right away.

Professional help: The doctor who attends you will give you an injection of glucose into an arm vein. This works so quickly that you may even come round while the injection is being given. You may then be admitted to hospital for a check-up, and the doctors will discuss with you the cause of your hypoglycaemia attack. If Addison's disease or hypopituitarism, rather than diabetes, is the problem underlying your hypoglycaemia, then you will receive appropriate treatment to prevent further attacks.

Adrenal glands

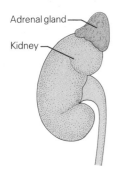

Adrenal gland

Kidney

The adrenal glands – one on top of each kidney – secrete hormones to help the body cope with physical and mental stresses.

The adrenal glands (sometimes called the suprarenal glands) are two grape-sized organs that lie one on top of each kidney. Each adrenal gland consists of two parts – the medulla (core) and the cortex (outer layer).

The adrenal medulla produces two hormones, adrenaline and noradrenaline, which play an important part in controlling heart rate and blood pressure. Production of the hormones is stimulated by the brain.

The adrenal cortex produces three groups of *steroid* hormones. One group, the most important of which is aldosterone, controls the concentration and balance of various chemicals, such as sodium and potassium, in the body. The second group has a number of functions, among them helping to convert carbohydrates into the energy-providing glycogen in the liver. Hydrocortisone is the main hormone in this group. The third group consists of the male hormones androgens and the female hormones oestrogen and progesterone, which influence sexual development (sex hormones are also produced by the testes and ovaries). Each sex produces both male and female hormones, but androgens predominate in a man, oestrogen and progesterone in a woman. Production of all steroid hormones except aldosterone is controlled by the *pituitary gland* (p.515); aldosterone production is stimulated by another hormone, renin, produced by the kidneys.

Cushing's syndrome

(including Cushing's disease)

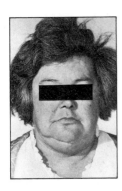

Visual symptoms
Someone with Cushing's syndrome or Cushing's disease gradually grows fatter and the face becomes red and usually moon-shaped.

In Cushing's syndrome, there is an excess of *steroid* hormones in the blood. In the majority of cases it is caused by large doses of steroid drugs taken for another illness, such as *rheumatoid arthritis* (p.552) or *asthma* (p.355). Rarely, the condition is due to the cortex (outer layer) of one or both adrenal glands producing extra amounts of steroid hormones. This can be caused by a tumour in an adrenal gland itself, or a tumour elsewhere in the body over-stimulating the adrenal glands. If the tumour is in the pituitary gland (see *Pituitary tumours*, p.518), then the condition is called Cushing's disease rather than Cushing's syndrome.

What are the symptoms?
Symptoms usually appear over several months. The first is a fattening of your face, which becomes round and red. Your body also becomes fatter, and there may be a pad of fat between your shoulder blades which makes you look round-shouldered. This is accompanied by a contrasting loss of muscle from your arms and legs. You feel weak, tired, and depressed. Your skin may become spotty, and purple streaks (like stretch marks) sometimes appear spontaneously on your abdomen or buttocks, and bruises come up on your arms and legs. Your bones become thin (see *Osteoporosis*, p.543) and are easily fractured. And you may develop *diabetes mellitus* (p.519), *high blood pressure* (p.382), or *heart failure* (p.381).

A woman with the disease has a deep voice, masculine body hair, and *amenorrhoea* (p.583). Men may become impotent and lose their hair; both sexes lose their sex-drive.

How common is the problem?
Cushing's syndrome is uncommon. It affects only a very small proportion of people on long-term steroid treatment. Cushing's disease is rare; it tends to affect chiefly young to middle-aged women.

What should be done?
See your doctor if you have several of the symptoms described above. If the doctor suspects Cushing's disease, you will be admitted to hospital for specialized tests.

If steroid drugs taken for another disorder are the cause, your doctor will gradually reduce your dosage and provide alternative treatment if necessary. *Never* stop taking steroid drugs without the advice of a doctor – you could develop *acute adrenal failure*.

When a pituitary tumour is the cause, either the tumour is removed by surgery or *radiotherapy* or the adrenal glands are removed and you are put on a lifelong course of hydrocortisone tablets (see *Addison's disease*, p.524). If a tumour of one adrenal gland is responsible, the entire gland will be taken out; you should be able to function adequately on the other gland.

Your doctors will discuss with you the best treatment in your particular case. All forms of treatment should bring about a return to normal or near-normal health, although in some cases this will be dependent on a lifelong course of drugs.

Addison's disease

In Addison's disease, the production of *steroid* hormones by the cortex (outer layer) of the adrenal glands progressively decreases over the years. The body can compensate for the deficiency of all these steroid hormones except hydrocortisone, deficiency of which leads among other things to low levels of energy-providing glucose in the blood. The most common cause of Addison's disease is destruction of the cortex by the body itself, due to an *autoimmune* problem.

What are the symptoms?
Symptoms usually develop very gradually. There is loss of appetite and weight, a feeling of increasing tiredness and weakness, and *anaemia* (p.419). You may also have bouts of diarrhoea or constipation, and mild indigestion with nausea or vomiting. Your skin will become, and remain, strikingly darker as though you have a permanent suntan.

Addison's disease is extremely rare. It affects mainly people between the ages of 30 and 50, and sometimes occurs in conjunction with another autoimmune disorder, such as *pernicious anaemia* (p.420) or Hashimoto's disease (see *Hypothyroidism* p.526).

What are the risks?
If the disease is not treated, you run the risk of suffering from *acute adrenal failure*, which always requires emergency treatment in hospital. You also risk *hypoglycaemia* (p.522).

What should be done?
If you believe you might have Addison's disease, discuss the matter with your doctor, who may be misled by your "tan" and vague symptoms. Analysis of blood samples for low levels of steroid hormones will reveal whether you have the disorder. If Addison's disease is diagnosed, you will need to take hydrocortisone tablets twice daily for life, to replace the hydrocortisone your adrenal glands are not making. The tablets will clear up all your symptoms. You will be given a card, detailing the treatment you need should you suffer acute adrenal failure; always carry this on you. If you have any illness or infection, however minor, tell your doctor, who may increase your dose of hydrocortisone to prevent acute adrenal failure.

By taking the tablets prescribed and following the advice above, you should be able to lead a normal, healthy life.

Phaeochro-mocytoma

The hormones adrenaline and noradrenaline, produced by the medulla (core) of each adrenal gland, work together with your nervous system to control your heart rate and blood pressure. Very rarely, a tumour (usually *benign*) develops in the medulla of one adrenal gland and causes it to produce an excessive amount of its hormones. The result is that slight exercise, exposure to cold, or a minor emotional upset produce in you the racing heart, paleness, and sweating normally brought on only by intense fear or over-excitement. In addition, you may feel faint and have a bad headache. The symptoms usually last for several hours. During an attack your blood pressure is very high (see *High blood pressure*, p.382).

What should be done?
If you have attacks of the kind described, see your doctor, who will probably arrange for you to have blood and urine tests (before which you go on to a special diet for a few days), and an *angiogram* of the adrenal glands. In the meantime, you will be given a course of *antihypertensive* tablets to prevent any further attacks.

If an adrenal tumour is diagnosed, it will be removed surgically, and in the great majority of cases this cures the disorder.

Aldo-steronism
(including Conn's syndrome)

Aldosteronism is a rare illness in which an over-production of the hormone aldosterone by the adrenal cortex leads to high blood pressure. Usually the condition is brought on by and accompanies congestive *heart failure* (p.381), *cirrhosis of the liver* (p.487), or one of certain other long-term diseases. In rare cases it is due to a tumour (usually *benign*) in one adrenal gland – then the condition is known as Conn's syndrome.

The main symptoms are those of *high blood pressure* (p.382). Other symptoms include a tingling and weakness in the limbs, muscle *spasms* of the hands and feet, and increased thirst coupled with excessive urination. Your doctor will arrange for blood tests to show whether you have aldosteronism and, if so, an *angiogram* of the adrenal glands to show whether it is caused by an adrenal tumour. If it is, then surgical removal usually cures the disorder. When the condition has been brought about by another disease, it is kept under control by a lifetime course of *diuretic* tablets.

Thyroid and parathyroid glands

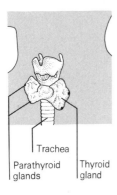

Trachea

Parathyroid
glands

Thyroid
gland

The thyroid is an H-shaped gland consisting of two lobes in the lower neck, one on each side of the trachea (windpipe), joined by a thin strand of thyroid tissue. It makes a hormone – thyroxine (often called T_4) – under the control of thyroid-stimulating hormone from the *pituitary gland* (p.515). Thyroxine controls the rates at which chemical reactions occur in the body; the more thyroxine there is, the faster the body works.

An essential constituent of thyroxine is the chemical iodine. Most people get sufficient iodine to make thyroxine from their diet – from fish and fish products, and from drinking water. Some countries also add iodine to

table salt or bread, to ensure that everyone receives a plentiful and regular supply.

Embedded in each of the four corners of the thyroid gland is a parathyroid gland, which is about the size of a pea. The four parathyroid glands produce parathyroid hormone which, together with vitamin D (see *Vitamins*, p.494), controls the level of calcium in the blood of a healthy person by causing the intestine to absorb more calcium from food, and by making the kidney excrete less calcium into urine. The body requires calcium for many purposes – the strengthening of bones and teeth, the clotting of blood, and the functioning of nerves and muscles.

Thyrotoxicosis

Thyrotoxicosis is overactivity of the thyroid gland. It is also called hyperthyroidism, toxic goitre, or Graves' disease depending on what has caused the disorder.

Activity of the thyroid gland is normally controlled by thyroid-stimulating hormone made in the *pituitary gland* (p.515). In thyrotoxicosis the control mechanism goes wrong and the thyroid becomes overactive and continuously produces large quantities of its own hormone, thyroxine. Sometimes the whole gland is overactive; in other cases a *thyroid nodule* (p.527) causes the trouble. Increased amounts of thyroxine cause a generalized speeding-up of all chemical reactions in the body, which affects mental as well as physical processes.

What are the symptoms?

As your mental processes speed up, you become fidgety, anxious, and tired but unable to relax or sleep. You feel shaky and your hands may tremble; this is especially noticeable when you are trying to perform delicate movements such as writing.

You begin to ignore the cold, and feel comfortable in summer clothes even on a cold day. You perspire most of the time, and you may have disagreements with other people about the level of heating.

Your heartbeats become faster and may be irregular (see *Atrial fibrillation*, p.389), even when you are trying to relax. This may cause a fluttering or racing feeling (palpitations) in your chest. You easily become breathless and as contractions of your intestinal muscles speed up, you get diarrhoea.

Because speeded-up body processes require more energy, you eat more yet still lose weight. Your muscles waste away and you may become so weak that you find it difficult to walk or lift your arms above your head. Women may have scanty or absent periods, and some people with thyrotoxicosis notice a swelling in the front of their neck (a goitre – an enlarged thyroid gland).

The final group of symptoms concerns the eyes. Not all people who suffer the disease have eye problems, and in only a small proportion of those who do are the eye problems serious. The eyes feel gritty and uncomfortable, and appear staring and protruding (see *Exophthalmos*, p.326). This can cause double or blurred vision, and perhaps redness and puffiness of the eyelids.

How common is the problem?

Thyrotoxicosis is a fairly rare disorder, affecting about 1 in every 3,000 adults each year. It can occur at any age, but is very rare in children. For reasons that are not known, it is about five times more common in women than it is in men.

What are the risks?

Like the symptoms, the risks of thyrotoxicosis are variable. You may recover completely, although some people have recurrent bouts of the disorder; in others it can be fatal if left untreated.

Elderly sufferers who already have *high blood pressure* (p.382) or *arteriosclerosis* (p.404) are at greatest risk. Additional strain placed on your heart and circulation by untreated thyrotoxicosis may well lead to atrial fibrillation, *angina* (p.376) or *heart failure* (p.381).

What should be done?

Some symptoms of thyrotoxicosis may be similar to those occurring in certain psychological disturbances such as *anxiety* (p.300). So, if you have several of the symptoms described above, you should visit your doctor and mention that you suspect thyrotoxicosis may be responsible. After examining you, the doctor may take a blood sample and have it analysed for increased levels of thyroxine. If a diagnosis of thyrotoxicosis is made, you will be put in touch with a specialist, who will probably order a thyroid *scan* to see if your whole gland is overactive, or whether the overactivity is in a distinct nodule within it.

What is the treatment?

Your specialist will discuss with you the various aspects of treatment. Thyrotoxicosis itself can be treated in one of three ways; in addition, any complications that have arisen will also be treated.

The first form of treatment that most sufferers receive is tablets containing an antithyroid drug. In most cases the drug brings the disorder under control in about eight weeks, though tablets may have to be continued for up to a year. The drug cures some people, but in others (about 20 to 30 per cent of sufferers) the problem returns, and so they need some other type of treatment.

The second form of treatment is an operation to remove any nodule in the thyroid gland, or most of the gland if it is generally overactive. Surgery cures the trouble in about 90 per cent of people who have it. In 5 per cent, the disease recurs and in the other 5 per cent (as a result of the operation), the remnant of the gland produces too little thyroxine (see *Hypothyroidism*, below, and *Hypoparathyroidism*, p.528). The third form of treatment is *radioactive* iodine, taken as a clear, slightly salty drink. Iodine is an essential constituent of thyroxine and as the radioactivity is concentrated in the thyroid gland, it slowly destroys part of it.

Each form of treatment has its advantages and disadvantages, and your specialist will advise which is the most suitable form in your particular case.

Despite the wide-ranging effects of thyrotoxicosis, most sufferers are restored to normal health – though treatment may last some years. A very small proportion are left with a reminder of their illness, in the form of parathyroid problems, hypothyroidism, or minor eye trouble.

Hypo-thyroidism

(including cretinism and Hashimoto's disease)

Hypothyroidism is the name for underactivity of the thyroid gland (compare hyperthyroidism, more commonly called *thyrotoxicosis*, p.525). When it occurs, only small amounts of the thyroid hormone thyroxine are produced, and all chemical processes in the body slow down as a result.

Underactivity of the thyroid gland can be due to any one of a number of causes, or it can occur for no apparent reason. It can occasionally be caused by treatment for thyrotoxicosis or by the lack of thyroid-stimulating hormone due to a disorder of the pituitary gland (see *Hypopituitarism*, p.517). Hypothyroidism can also occur if for some reason there is a lack of iodine in the diet.

Hypothyroidism also occurs in Hashimoto's disease, a rare disorder that is caused by an *autoimmune* destruction of the body's thyroid by *antibodies* circulating in the blood.

Very rarely, a baby is born with a defective thyroid gland, or even with no gland at all. The result is little or no thyroxine in the baby's body; a condition which, untreated, can lead to cretinism (see "What are the risks?" opposite).

What are the symptoms?

Symptoms come on over a period of months or even years. Someone who has not seen you for some time will be struck by the deterioration in your physical and mental health.

If you have hypothyroidism, your whole body slows down. You feel continually tired and worn out. Even simple mental tasks, like adding up a shopping bill, take longer. You may have general aches and pains and be able to move only slowly. Your heart slows to 50 beats per minute or less, and contractions of your intestinal muscles slow down, leading to bouts of constipation.

Because slowed-down body processes need less energy, you eat less, yet still gain weight. You begin to feel the cold, and wear far more clothing compared to people around you. Your hair tends to become thin, dry, and lifeless. One marked symptom of hypothyroidism is that your skin becomes dry, thickened, and swollen due to a mucuslike substance that collects in it. It makes your face look rather puffy; hypothyroidism is sometimes known as *myxoedema* because of this puffy, swollen appearance. Swollen, myxoedematous tissue also forms on your vocal chords, making your voice deeper and hoarse; in your ears, causing hearing loss; and in your wrists, where it presses on the nerves going to the hands and causes numbness and tingling in them (see *Carpal tunnel syndrome*, p.281). Women have heavy, prolonged periods, and both women and men lose their interest in sex.

In more severe cases of hypothyroidism the sufferer becomes very cold and drowsy, and eventually unconscious. This "myxoedema coma" may be brought on by cold weather or certain drugs, especially *sedatives.*

Babies born with hypothyroidism are lethargic and difficult to feed, have large tongues, and in some cases an umbilical hernia (see *Hernias*, p.537), and may develop prolonged jaundice (see *Neonatal jaundice*, p.647) soon after birth.

How common is the problem?
In Britain in an average year 1 person in 500 is seen by a doctor because of hypothyroidism. It can affect anyone, but is commonest in middle-aged women.

What are the risks?
Left untreated, a baby with hypothyroidism will become dwarfed and mentally retarded (a cretin), and an adult will suffer much general ill-health. The disease is unlikely to be fatal unless myxoedema coma develops.

What should be done?
Many people feel jaded and fatigued at some time or other. It does not mean that they have all got hypothyroidism. But if you notice that several of the symptoms described above occur together, visit your doctor. After examining you, the doctor will arrange for blood samples to be taken for analysis. If they contain a low level of thyroxine, hypothyroidism is the diagnosis. If, in addition, the samples contain antibodies active against the thyroid gland, the diagnosis is Hashimoto's disease.

The condition in babies is usually detected at the examination of every baby carried out just after birth.

What is the treatment?
Whatever its cause, the treatment of hypothyroidism is straightforward. You have to take tablets of artificially made thyroxine every day for the rest of your life. After a few days of the treatment you feel much better, and after a few months you should have returned to normal health.

Babies are started on the tablets as soon as possible. If treatment is started before the baby is about three months old, he or she has a very good chance of growing and developing normally without further symptoms. Parents must ensure that the child always takes the tablets as prescribed by the doctor.

Myxoedema coma is a medical emergency that demands immediate hospital care.

Non-toxic goitre
(also called simple goitre)

If you have a non-toxic goitre, then your thyroid gland is still functioning normally but is generally enlarged and can be seen and felt as a lump in the front of your neck. There are several causes of non-toxic goitre too rare to be dealt with here. The most common cause is lack of iodine in your diet. The chain of events runs so: if there is a deficiency of iodine, the thyroid gland cannot make enough thyroxine; the *pituitary gland* (p.515) detects a low level of thyroxine in the blood; in an attempt to raise the level, it releases more thyroid-stimulating hormone; this stimulates growth of the thyroid gland in a vain attempt to produce more thyroxine.

If you have a swelling in the front of your neck, see your doctor. You may have to give a blood sample or undergo certain hospital tests to rule out other thyroid disorders, but once the diagnosis of non-toxic goitre is confirmed, the cure is simple. Eat more iodine – found in fish, fish products, and sea salt.

Thyroid nodules
(including thyroid cancer)

A thyroid nodule is a distinct lump growing in an otherwise normal thyroid gland. One or more nodules may be present at any one time. There are four types of nodule: a *cyst* (a soft, fluid-filled sac); an area of bleeding called a haemorrhage; a *benign* growth known as an adenoma; and a *malignant* growth called a carcinoma (thyroid cancer). Why thyroid nodules develop, or why some people have more than one, is not known. A thyroid nodule usually shows up as a swelling in the front part of the neck. Only rarely is it painful or big enough to cause breathing or swallowing difficulties. If you suspect you have a thyroid nodule, consult your doctor, who will probably refer you to a specialist for tests.

What should be done?
All nodules except carcinomas are fairly common, and, in the main, harmless. If a

nodule is small and not growing, the specialist may advise that it be left alone. A large, unsightly cyst can be *aspirated*. If a thyroid *scan* shows that a nodule may possibly be a carcinoma or an adenoma, part or all of the gland will be surgically removed or destroyed (see *Thyrotoxicosis*, p.525, for details). Such treatment may be followed by lifelong thyroxine tablets because the thyroid may no longer be able to make this hormone (see *Hypothyroidism*, p.526).

The outlook for thyroid cancer is generally good; with treatment many sufferers can be completely cured.

Hyperpara-thyroidism

In hyperparathyroidism, excessive amounts of parathyroid hormone are produced – in most cases because of a small, usually *benign* growth (adenoma) in one or more parathyroid glands. Occasionally it occurs because of a generalized enlargement of all four glands. It is not known what causes the growth(s) or enlargement. The abnormally high level of hormones creates a high level of calcium in the blood, mainly by removing calcium from bones. Meanwhile, in attempts to lower the blood-calcium level, the kidneys pass calcium into the urine, but the effects of this are limited, and over the years the calcium level gradually builds up.

What are the symptoms?

Most people do not have any symptoms until the disorder is well advanced – that is, until middle age in most cases. However, some cases are detected earlier as the result of a routine blood test, or tests for some other disorder. The excess calcium in the blood upsets the body's *metabolism*, resulting in indigestion and depression. Loss of calcium from the bones makes them soft and liable to fracture more easily than normal. After several years, the excessive amounts of calcium passing through the kidneys into the urine can cause *kidney stones* (p.509).

If you suspect that you are suffering from the disease, see your doctor, who will arrange for you to have samples of your blood analysed. If analysis shows that you have the disorder, you will be given *angiogram X-rays* and *ultrasound* or *isotope scans* to show which glands are affected.

What is the treatment?

Surgery to remove either the adenoma or three out of four generally enlarged glands completely cures the disorder in most cases. There is a risk that after the operation the amount of parathyroid hormone produced will not be enough to maintain a normal level of calcium in the blood (see *Hypoparathyroidism*, below). Any kidney stones that have formed may require treatment.

Hypopara-thyroidism

Hypoparathyroidism is the failure of the parathyroid glands to produce sufficient hormone. This results in the level of calcium in the blood falling below normal. The disorder can occur either as part of the failure of several hormone-producing glands or by itself; in both cases, the cause of the defect is unknown. The disease, which is rare, affects children more commonly than adults.

Hypoparathyroidism can also be the result of an operation on the thyroid gland (see *Thyrotoxicosis*, p.525) or parathyroid glands (see *Hyperparathyroidism*, above).

What are the symptoms?

The main symptoms are painful cramp-like spasms of the hands, feet, and throat, known as *tetany* (not to be confused with the infection called *tetanus*, p.564). Other symptoms include tingling and numbness of the face and hands, *cataracts* (p.319) on the eyes, dry skin, thin hair, and often *oral thrush* (p.451) or, in women, *vaginal thrush* (p.602). If the disease is not detected in a child, he or she may suffer from vomiting, headaches, mental retardation, convulsions (see *Convulsions in children*, p.667), and poor tooth development.

If you suspect that you have the disorder, see your doctor, who will arrange for you to provide blood samples for laboratory analysis; the results will disclose whether you have the disease.

What is the treatment?

Once the illness has been diagnosed, you will require lifelong treatment with vitamin D tablets, which raise your blood calcium to a normal level. If you are suffering from an attack of tetany, your doctor will send you to hospital, to receive an injection of calcium into a vein; this provides relief within minutes. The correct dose of vitamin D will restore you almost to normal health. To check on the dose, you will need to see your doctor every few months for tests on the level of calcium in your blood.

Disorders of the muscles, bones, and joints

Introduction

Muscles, bones, and joints provide your body with a supportive framework that allows flexibility of movement. All movement – of organs within the body as well as of the body itself – is carried out by muscles, each of which is composed of contractible fibrous tissues. *Voluntary* muscles, such as those in the limbs, are under conscious control and are usually arranged in pairs. For example, if you want to bend your elbow, you contract the biceps muscle in your upper arm; to straighten the arm you permit the biceps muscle to relax, and your brain "orders" the triceps muscle to contract. *Involuntary* muscles, such as those in the heart and digestive tract, work and are regulated without conscious control.

Articles in this section of the book deal only with voluntary muscles – mainly those of the limbs, neck, and trunk. Disorders affecting the involuntary muscles – chiefly heart problems, and digestive-tract disorders such as irritable colon, for instance – are discussed in sections that deal with the organs or systems whose movements they control.

Most of the 200-odd bones of your skeleton serve mainly as an internal framework for the various parts of the body. In addition, some bones also encase and protect certain organs. The skull, for example, protects the brain, and the ribcage and backbone shield the heart, lungs, and, to some extent, upper-abdominal organs such as the stomach, liver, and kidneys.

Bones are not rigid, lifeless structures. They are composed of living cells embedded in a hard framework of minerals (mostly calcium and phosphate). And inside some bones is a soft core called the marrow, a very active tissue with a rich blood supply that manufactures most types of blood cells (see *Blood disorders*, p.418, for further information).

Some bones – those of the skull, for instance – are joined closely together by means of almost immovable connective fibres (*sutures*). But when we speak of a "joint", we are generally referring to a special structure between certain neighbouring bones that permits them to move in relation to one another. There are several different types of joint. Each of your vertebrae (backbones) can

move only slightly in relation to its neighbours, but this provides enough flexibility over the whole spinal column to allow you to bend your back almost double. The fingers have "hinge" joints, which permit movement in only one plane. The shoulder, a "ball-and-socket" type of joint, has a greater range of movement; it allows the arm to move in almost any direction.

Joints are complicated structures. Where the two bones touch, each has a covering of smooth, flexible, shock-absorbing cartilage, and the cartilage-covered bone ends are encased in a flexible, watertight membrane called the joint *capsule*. In addition, some joints have another thin membrane inside the capsule. This extra *synovial* membrane secretes small amounts of a fluid to lubricate the joint. The whole joint structure is bound together and prevented from over-free movement by tough bands of elastic tissue called ligaments.

Bone tissue
Viewed under a microscope, bone is seen to be composed of tiny cylinders made of organic material impregnated with minerals, mainly calcium and phosphorus. These cylinders are formed by special cells called osteoblasts living inside the bones.

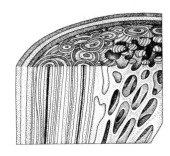

Muscle tissue
A muscle is composed of millions of microscopic filaments of two types – called actin and myosin – that slide past each other when stimulated by a nerve impulse. It is this movement that makes the muscle contract, often to about two-thirds its original length.

Relaxed

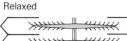

Contracted

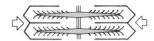

The musculoskeletal system

How the skeleton and muscles work together

Skeletal muscles are attached to 2 or more bones. When a muscle contracts, the bones to which it is attached move. Muscles nearly always work in coordinated groups; contraction of one muscle is accompanied by relaxation of another, while other muscles stabilize nearby joints.

Head and neck muscles
Contraction of these muscles produces facial expressions and head movements. They are also responsible for speech and swallowing.

Involuntary muscles

Involuntary muscles are those that are not under conscious control – that is, you cannot mentally "order" them to contract or relax; they work of their own accord. They include the muscles that propel food through the intestine and those in the heart and blood vessels that control blood pressure.

Heart   Intestine

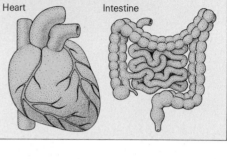

Abdominal muscles
Bands of muscle at the front of the abdomen assist in the regular movements of respiration, balance the muscles of the spine during lifting movements, and keep the intestines and other abdominal organs firmly in place.

Arm muscles
The bulk of the arm muscles is concentrated at the shoulder and just below the elbow. Long tendons connect the muscles in the forearm to the wrist and fingers.

The male and female pelvis

Most bones in the female skeleton are the same shape as (though usually a little smaller than) the bones in the male skeleton. One exception is the pelvis (hip bone). A woman's pelvis is usually broader than a man's, and has a larger space in the middle. This is to accommodate the head of the baby as it passes from the uterus (womb) through the pelvis to the outside world during childbirth.

Leg muscles
The leg muscles are among the most powerful in the body, and have strong, broad anchorage points, especially at the pelvis (hip bone).

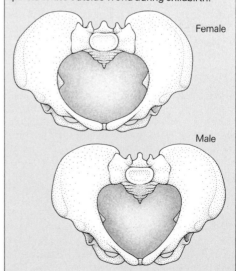

Female

Male

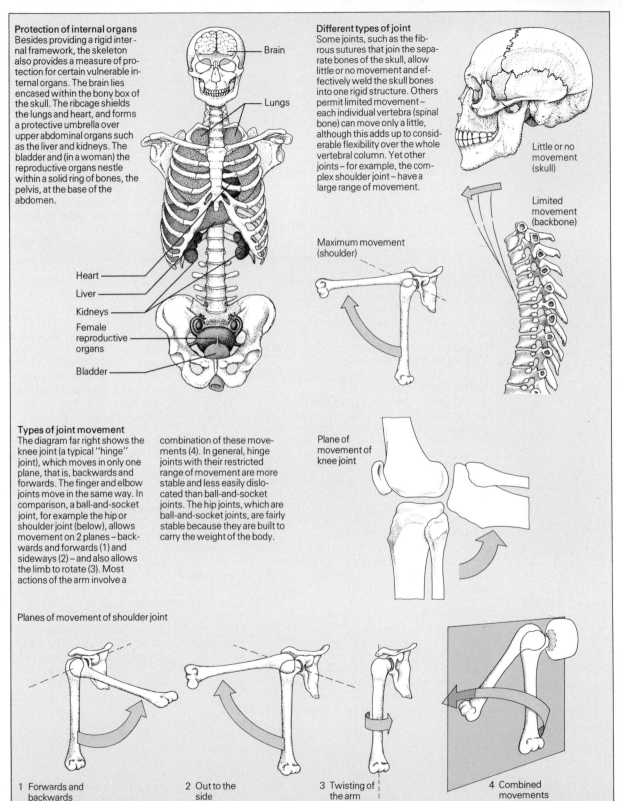

Protection of internal organs

Besides providing a rigid internal framework, the skeleton also provides a measure of protection for certain vulnerable internal organs. The brain lies encased within the bony box of the skull. The ribcage shields the lungs and heart, and forms a protective umbrella over upper abdominal organs such as the liver and kidneys. The bladder and (in a woman) the reproductive organs nestle within a solid ring of bones, the pelvis, at the base of the abdomen.

Brain

Lungs

Heart

Liver

Kidneys

Female reproductive organs

Bladder

Different types of joint

Some joints, such as the fibrous sutures that join the separate bones of the skull, allow little or no movement and effectively weld the skull bones into one rigid structure. Others permit limited movement – each individual vertebra (spinal bone) can move only a little, although this adds up to considerable flexibility over the whole vertebral column. Yet other joints – for example, the complex shoulder joint – have a large range of movement.

Little or no movement (skull)

Limited movement (backbone)

Maximum movement (shoulder)

Plane of movement of knee joint

Types of joint movement

The diagram far right shows the knee joint (a typical "hinge" joint), which moves in only one plane, that is, backwards and forwards. The finger and elbow joints move in the same way. In comparison, a ball-and-socket joint, for example the hip or shoulder joint (below), allows movement on 2 planes – backwards and forwards (1) and sideways (2) – and also allows the limb to rotate (3). Most actions of the arm involve a combination of these movements (4). In general, hinge joints with their restricted range of movement are more stable and less easily dislocated than ball-and-socket joints. The hip joints, which are ball-and-socket joints, are fairly stable because they are built to carry the weight of the body.

Planes of movement of shoulder joint

1 Forwards and backwards

2 Out to the side

3 Twisting of the arm

4 Combined movements

Injuries

Muscles, bones, and joints are more susceptible to damage from injury than most other parts of the body. Because every muscle has a limited pulling strength, it will be torn or otherwise damaged if required to overcome a force too powerful for it – a weight too heavy to be lifted, for example. Similarly, bones cannot change shape to accommodate extreme physical pressures, so they split or snap if subjected to too much stress. Finally, each joint in the body is designed to allow a particular range of movements. If overflexed or forced to move in an unnatural direction, the ligaments or other tissues that bind neighbouring bones will be damaged.

Some of the injuries discussed in the following group of articles (for instance, pulled muscles and sprains) are minor and may be self-inflicted on the sports field, in the gymnasium, or even in the garden. More serious injuries – especially fractures and dislocated joints – are usually the result of powerful external forces such as those suffered during road traffic accidents.

Pulled muscle

If a muscle is over-stretched – for example, by being forced to do violent, unaccustomed exercise – some of its fibres may tear. When this happens, the muscle contracts and may also become swollen because of internal bleeding. Occasionally, the muscle may be ruptured (completely torn through).

What are the symptoms?
The chief symptom is pain when the injury occurs. The pulled muscle feels tender, may become swollen, and will not function efficiently until the torn fibres have healed. Only if ruptured, however, will the muscle be entirely unable to function. A muscle that gradually becomes stiff, painful, and tender (often overnight) has not necessarily been pulled; it may be simply strained.

How common is the problem?
Almost everybody pulls a muscle at some time. People active in sports are particularly susceptible to this injury. Ruptured muscles are much less common.

What are the risks?
In most cases recovery is quick and complete, and there is no danger of permanent loss of mobility. The older you are, the greater the damage you can do and the slower your recovery. A ruptured muscle, on the other hand, may become permanently useless unless it is successfully treated.

What should be done?
If you have a pulled muscle that does not seem severely damaged, apply the self-help measures suggested below. If you are in great pain or the affected area becomes badly swollen, consult your doctor, who will probably be able to assess the extent of damage by a careful examination of the injury.

What is the treatment?
Self-help: Try to use the pulled muscle as little as possible while the pain persists. Bandaging or strapping the affected area will give it support, but be careful not to bind it too tightly; further swelling might interfere with blood circulation. You may also want to take a painkiller such as paracetamol. As the pain dies away, you should start to exercise again to prevent joints from becoming stiff.
Professional help: Treatment depends on the severity of the injury. Your doctor may well prescribe a stronger painkiller than paracetamol, along with a muscle-relaxant drug. You may be advised to use crutches for a leg injury or a sling for an arm. The doctor may also recommend *physiotherapy*. If the muscle is ruptured, the only possible treatment may be surgery.

Thigh strain
This is a common injury, especially among people playing sports. An ordinary crêpe bandage around the affected area gives some support.

Sprain

A sprain occurs when, because excessive demands are made upon a joint, the ligaments that bind the neighbouring bones and keep the joint in position are torn. The severity of the sprain depends on how badly the ligaments are torn. Any joint can be sprained, but the knees, ankles, wrists, and fingers are especially prone to such damage.

What are the symptoms?
Pain and tenderness in the injured area range from mild to severe depending on the extent

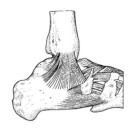

of damage. A sprained joint will still function, but only at the cost of further pain. There may also be swelling and, later, skin discoloration. In a sprain so bad that all supporting ligaments are torn through, the joint will be misshapen as well as swollen.

How common is the problem?
Sprains are common. In an average year in Britain 1 person in 30 consults a doctor about this type of injury.

What are the risks?
There is no danger in a minor sprain. Repeated stretching and tearing of the ligaments, however, will weaken any joint. This is particularly true of the ankle, which, if often twisted, may begin to give way from time to time without apparent cause.

What should be done?
For a mild sprain try the self-help measures recommended below. If the pain is severe or persists for more than two or three days, see your doctor, who will examine the joint and will probably have it *X-rayed* since a bad sprain is often impossible to distinguish from a fracture by simple visual examination.

What is the treatment?
Self-help: If you have a mild sprain, support the joint with a crêpe bandage and rest it. An

Sprained ankle
The tough, fibrous ligaments of the ankle are vital in holding the ankle bones firmly in place. If you fall with your ankle in an abnormal position, you may put the weight of your whole body on those ligaments, causing them to tear. The result is the familiar sprained ankle.

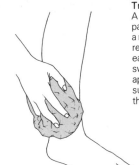

Treating a sprain
A cold compress or ice pack applied to the site of a recent sprain will help to reduce the swelling and ease the pain. When the swelling has lessened, apply a firm bandage to support the joint while the ligaments heal.

ice pack helps keep down any swelling. After a day or so, start to exercise the joint as much as possible, but without forcing it to bear weight. When not exercising the damaged joint, rest it in an elevated position (place your leg up on a chair when you sit, for example) to help drain away the swelling.
Professional help: If you have a severe sprain, your doctor may encase the affected portion of the injured limb or finger in plaster. Occasionally, surgical repair of badly torn ligaments is necessary. After any such operation you must undergo a period of several weeks in plaster. When the cast is removed, you will probably need to wear a supportive bandage and have *physiotherapy* to strengthen the joint for normal use.

Severed tendon

If you cut or badly injure your forearm, hand, calf, or foot, the cut may go partly or completely through one or more tendons. Tendons are long, fibrous cords that connect some bones – particularly those of the fingers and toes – to the muscles that move them. The muscles controlling fingers are situated in the forearms, and those controlling toes are in the calves. So, apart from the obvious damage of a cut or injury, a severed tendon will make you unable to move one or more of your fingers or toes properly. Because the

damage will not heal of its own accord and may worsen, it is essential for you to seek medical help for any such injury.

What should be done?
Get to a hospital as soon as possible if you think you have severed one or more tendons. Depending upon the nature of the injury, the surgeon may try to sew the cut ends together immediately. This will probably be done under a general anaesthetic because of the necessity to make a large incision in order to find the severed ends of the tendon. In some cases it is best to wait for the wound to heal before attempting to retrieve and rejoin the cut ends. It is occasionally necessary to transfer a piece of less essential tendon from elsewhere in the body to patch the damaged one.

The results of tendon repair are usually good for tendons that flex the toes. Those responsible for finger movements are more difficult to repair surgically, and the results are often disappointing; in many cases the affected fingers may be less manoeuvrable than they were before the injury.

Locating the severed ends
When a tendon is severed, the muscle to which it is attached contracts, causing the tendon to spring away from the site of the injury. In such cases, surgery is required to locate the severed ends before they can be rejoined.

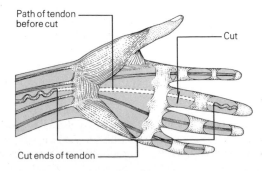

Path of tendon before cut

Cut

Cut ends of tendon

Dislocation

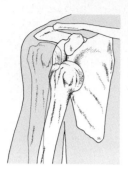

Dislocation of the shoulder
The shoulder joint is a ball-and-socket joint. The ball of the upper-arm bone fits into a cup-shaped socket in the shoulder blade. (The normal position of the arm bone is shown in brown in the illustration above.) The shoulder is a very manoeuvrable joint and as a result tends to become dislocated fairly easily.

A joint is dislocated if the bones that should be in contact are torn apart so that the joint no longer functions. The cause is usually a severe injury, which exerts a force great enough to tear the joint ligaments. In addition to displaced bones, there is likely to be serious damage to the joint capsule, surrounding muscles, blood vessels, and nerves. And the dislocating force sometimes produces a *fracture* (below) in one or both of the affected bones.

Dislocations not caused by injury may be *congenital* (see *Congenital dislocation of the hip*, p.644) or may occur as a complication of *rheumatoid arthritis* (p.552). Finally, a dislocation can happen repeatedly, without apparent cause, to someone with a joint already weakened by earlier injury. The jaw and shoulder joints are especially susceptible to this "spontaneous" type of dislocation.

What are the symptoms?
A dislocated joint looks misshapen, is extremely painful, and becomes rapidly swollen, discoloured, and immovable. Other possible symptoms depend on the extent of damage to surrounding tissues.

How common is the problem?
Dislocations are less common than other kinds of injury to muscles, bones, and joints. In Britain only 1 person in 2,500 dislocates a joint in an average year.

What are the risks?
Dislocation of spinal vertebrae can damage the entire spinal cord, sometimes causing paralysis in the body below the level of injury (see *Spinal-cord injury*, p.278). Similarly, dislocation of a shoulder or hip can damage the main nerves to the affected arm or leg, with resultant paralysis. Less dramatically, any joint that has been dislocated tends to become susceptible to the development of *osteoarthritis* (p.550).

What should be done?
Do not let anyone try to replace your dislocated joint in its normal position unless you are sure he or she knows how; there may be a fracture or other damage that can be worsened if not correctly handled. Simply protect the damaged area by the best means at hand (see *Accidents and emergencies*, p.810), and get to a doctor or hospital speedily.

Do not eat or drink in the meantime since you may need to have a general anaesthetic in order to undergo *reduction* (the technical term for re-positioning) of the dislocation. The doctor will examine and *X-ray* the joint and surrounding areas to determine the extent of the damage.

What is the treatment?
Self-help: None is feasible in most situations, but reduction without an anaesthetic is possible in uncomplicated cases provided it is done within a few minutes of dislocation, and as long as you know exactly what you are doing. For instance, people who have recurrent spontaneous dislocations often learn how to re-position the joint by themselves. Even in such cases, though, a doctor should be seen promptly to make sure there are no more serious problems.
Professional help: After 15 to 30 minutes a dislocated joint normally becomes so swollen and painful that reduction must be done under a general anaesthetic. Following reduction – assuming that your blood vessels, nerves, and bones are in order – the joint will be immobilized and splinted for two or three weeks so that damaged tissues can heal. Obey the instructions of your *physiotherapist* when beginning to use the joint again.

Sometimes surgery is necessary to achieve satisfactory re-positioning. Or if one of your joints has become very weak because of repeated dislocation, the doctor may recommend an operation to tighten the ligaments that bind the adjoining bones.

Fracture

A fractured bone is a broken bone. The break occurs as a result of physical forces greater than the structure of the bone can withstand. For purposes of diagnosis and treatment, doctors describe different kinds of fracture in the following ways:

A "simple" fracture is one in which the bone itself is broken, but neighbouring muscles and other tissues remain largely undamaged. In a "compound" fracture, on the other hand, there is considerable damage to surrounding tissues, including overlying skin.

A "complete" fracture is one in which the break is total and the pieces of bone part company. In an "incomplete" fracture the break is more like a crack and does not extend right across the bone.

A fracture is usually caused by severe stresses imposed during some form of injury, but this is not always the case. Any bone weakened by old age or disease – by, for example, *osteoporosis* (p.543) – may break with little or no provocation. This is called a "pathological" fracture. Such fractures are

Types of fracture

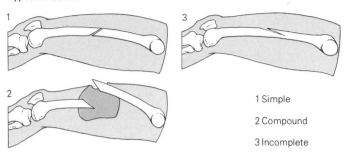

1 Simple

2 Compound

3 Incomplete

common in the hips of elderly people, whose bones are weakened by a combination of disuse, the changes in the composition of bone associated with ageing, and (sometimes) disease. Another type of fracture, a "fatigue" fracture, may occur in a normal, healthy bone that has been subjected to prolonged periods of abnormally high stress.

What are the symptoms?

A fracture makes the area look swollen, bruised, and possibly deformed. You will probably be in severe pain, which is worsened by any pressure on the area or attempted movement of that part of the body.

A minor fracture – of a wrist bone, say – may cause only minor symptoms, and can be mistaken for a *sprain* (p.532).

How common is the problem?

Few people go through life without breaking a bone. The bones most likely to break are those in the wrists, hands, and feet, which are often damaged during a fall. Fractures of other bones – the arm and leg bones, and the spine and hip – are usually the result of much more powerful forces, such as those encountered in road traffic accidents.

The older you get the more likely you are to break a bone. This is because children, although very active and prone to injury, have springy, resilient bones that tend to bend rather than snap. At the other end of the scale, the bones of elderly people are fragile and brittle, and problems with balance and coordination make falls more likely (see *Accidental falls*, p.719, for further information).

What are the risks?

There are two main risk areas if you suffer a fracture. The first is concerned with the bone itself. If a fracture is not treated, or if treatment is delayed, the broken pieces of bone may begin to rejoin out of alignment, and surgery may be needed to re-separate and realign the fragments in the correct position. In a bad compound fracture where the skin is broken, infection may get into the bones and complicate the healing process (see *Osteomyelitis*, p.695). And it is possible (but uncommon) for a fragment of broken bone, cut off from its blood supply, to gradually die.

The second risk area associated with fractures is damage to neighbouring tissues. Sharp bone fragments may compress or sever nearby blood vessels or nerves. Fractures of the skull or spine can damage the brain or spinal cord (see *Brain injury*, p.276, and *Spinal-cord injury*, p.278). Occasionally, other internal organs are damaged by a fractured bone: for example, a broken rib can puncture a lung (see *Pneumothorax*, p.362). If you have been badly injured in an accident, any damage to soft tissues will be repaired surgically, often at the same time as the fracture is dealt with.

What should be done?

If you or someone near you suffers a possible fracture, follow the first-aid instructions in *Accidents and emergencies* (p.810) and send for medical help immediately. Do not give an injured person anything to eat or drink. This may delay treatment by making doctors wait for several hours before they can give a general anaesthetic.

Any presumed sprain that has not improved after two or three days may be a fracture. In such cases, see your doctor, who will probably want an *X-ray* to confirm the suspicion that you have a fracture.

What is the treatment?

The first task in treating a fracture is to realign broken pieces of bone if they are in the wrong position. The technical term for this process is *reduction*. It usually needs to be done under general anaesthetic, and may

The use of traction
When you break your thigh bone, the powerful muscles connecting it to the lower leg contract. This causes the 2 broken ends of the bone to ride over each other. Treatment aims to overcome the contracted thigh muscles, stretching them and so pulling the broken bone back into the correct position. This can be achieved by putting the leg in traction – applying heavy weights to the lower leg.

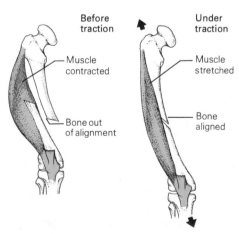

Before traction

Muscle contracted

Bone out of alignment

Under traction

Muscle stretched

Bone aligned

Top ten fractures

Here is a list of the broken bones most often treated by British doctors in an average year:

1. Forearm bones (ulna and/or radius), broken near the wrist.
2. Bones in the hands (carpals and metacarpals) or feet (tarsals and metatarsals).
3. Collar bone (clavicle).
4. Ribs.
5. Fingers and thumbs (phalanges).
6. Shin bones (tibia and/or fibula).
7. Thigh bone (femur), often broken at the hip.
8. Skull.
9. Upper arm bone (humerus).
10. Backbones (spinal bones or vertebrae).

involve cutting open the tissues around the fracture in order to reposition the bones correctly. To keep infection from developing in the bone or neighbouring tissues, the sufferer will be given *antibiotic* drugs.

The second part of treatment is *immobilization*: the holding together of various bone fragments in the correct alignment until they are completely reunited. By no means all fractures are put in plaster of Paris or even in one of the more modern light-weight plastic or resin coverings. There are many ways to secure a bone during the weeks it needs to knit together. In fact, some bones are held together naturally and require no plaster or splint. A broken rib, for example, is held by numerous chest muscles to nearby unbroken ribs; a fractured finger can be bandaged to a neighbour to stabilize it while it heals.

The thigh bone is so deeply buried beneath large muscles that a fracture in it cannot be held immobilized by plaster or a splint. Instead such fractures are often held in position by means of *traction* (the attachment of weights to the leg in order to pull apart two overlapping pieces of bone).

In some cases a fracture is held in position internally. An operation is performed to hold the broken ends in place by means of one or more metal screws, nails, or plates. Immobilization by an internal method has a big advantage in that you can begin to use your injured limb after a few days rather than weeks or months. This contributes much to

the third main part of the treatment, *rehabilitation* of joints or muscles that you have not been using during the immobilization phase.

From the earliest possible moment a *physiotherapist* will advise you how to exercise the part containing the fractured bone and how to keep nearby joints active. This helps to prevent swelling and stimulates the development of a good blood supply, which aids healing. In addition, activity of joints stops muscles and bones from wasting. And, above all, it prevents the joints themselves from becoming stiff from disuse. *Osteoarthritis* (p.550) is a very real risk in a joint immobilized for several weeks or longer.

How long will it take your fracture to heal? The answer depends on many factors. These include the type of bone affected, the nature of the fracture, and your age. A child's broken finger may heal completely in two weeks; an adult's shin bone may take longer than three months.

An occasional fracture fails to heal in spite of prompt, efficient treatment. If your doctor suspects that this is happening in your case, he or she may order additional X-rays and may take special measures to encourage healing. The commonest procedure is a *bone graft*, which involves taking small pieces of bone (only a few millimetres long) from some other site in your body (often the hip bone) and packing them around the break. The fresh bone encourages the area to reunite and become healthy once again.

Sports injuries

Footballers, athletes, and others who take vigorous exercise regularly run a high risk of injuring muscles, ligaments, bones, or joints (see *Pulled muscle* and *Sprain*, p.532). Such injuries are most common early in the season, when the training sessions begin.

If you are injured during a game you may be eager to return to the action as quickly as possible, but treatment to allow you to do this may have long-term dangers. If the injury is a cut or bruise without serious damage to muscles or ligaments, it is reasonable for your coach or trainer to relieve pain with an ice-pack or an anaesthetic spray and bandage the area; but if there is any possibility of muscle or ligament injury, relief of pain may permit you to sustain further damage without realizing it. Whenever the extent of your injury is uncertain – or whenever you have become unconscious, even for only a few seconds – you should take no further part in the day's play.

What should be done?

Many injuries require no treatment other than rest, and possibly *physiotherapy* to strengthen muscles and increase the circulation of blood to damaged tissues. But some injuries – for example, recurrent damage to the footballer's knee cartilage – are best treated by surgery.

A recurrent injury presents you with the difficult decision of whether or not to retire from your sport. It is an unfortunate fact that once an injury to a ligament or bone recurs you stand a high chance of having sustained permanent damage, and the price of not retiring may be early development of *osteoarthritis* (p.550) or some other joint problem. Before reaching a decision, get an accurate diagnosis of the extent of the damage. This may involve diagnostic tests such as *X-rays*, *endoscopy* of the joint interior, or perhaps an exploratory operation.

For first-aid treatment of injuries see *Accidents and emergencies*, p.801.

Hernias

A hernia is a bulge or protrusion of soft tissue that forces its way through or between muscles. Normally, body muscles are taut and firm; they press on various tissues and organs, helping to restrain them and keep them in the correct position. However, muscles sometimes are, or become, weak or slack – because of overstrain or *congenital* weakness, for example. When this happens, the soft tissues force their way through the weak point and create the bulge or sac known as a hernia.

Hernias can occur in many parts of the body, but they are most common in the abdominal wall. The abdominal wall is made up of flat sheets of muscle that encase the abdominal organs – the stomach, intestines, liver, kidneys, and reproductive organs. Normally, these abdominal organs are held in by the firm muscles of the abdominal wall, even

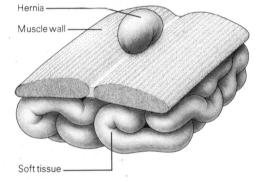

Hernia

Muscle wall

Soft tissue

when the pressure inside rises – for example, during coughing, sneezing, lifting a heavy weight, or straining to pass urine or faeces. But if a weak point appears in the wall, pressure inside the abdomen may force the muscles to part at that point. Some portion of abdominal contents – frequently intestinal tissue – is then pushed through the muscles and becomes an often visible bulge.

One quite common type of hernia is hiatus hernia, which occurs in the diaphragm (the sheet of muscle that separates the chest from the abdomen). *Hiatus hernias* are fully described on p.456. For descriptions of the several kinds of hernia that are most likely to occur in the abdominal wall, see the illustrations on the next two pages.

What are the symptoms?
The main symptom of an abdominal hernia is likely to be a bulge or swelling. The bulge usually appears slowly over weeks, but it may sometimes form suddenly – during the strain of lifting a heavy weight, for example. You may have a feeling of heaviness or tenderness at the site of the bulge.

Most hernias can simply be pushed back into place (in which case they are called *reducible*). A hernia that cannot be replaced is called *irreducible*, and such hernias can normally be cured only by surgery. In fact, surgery is generally advisable even for reducible hernias since they frequently recur and may occasionally cause pain.

What are the risks?
If an abdominal hernia contains a length of intestine, the contents of the intestine may be prevented from moving through. This is an *obstructed* hernia. If you have a hernia that becomes obstructed, you will suffer from increasing abdominal pains, nausea, and vomiting. Another risk of abdominal hernias is known as *strangulation*. A strangulated hernia is one that has swollen, cutting off the blood supply to the tissues within it. The strangulated hernia becomes enlarged, red, and very painful. Obstructed or strangulated hernias need urgent attention.

What is the treatment?
Always consult your doctor about a bulge or swelling that inexplicably persists for more than a week. If a physical examination confirms that you have a hernia, the doctor will probably recommend an operation. In general, surgery is the best treatment, even for reducible hernias. You may be advised to try wearing a supportive corset or truss for a while, but in the young this is usually only a stop-gap measure. Most hernias tend to get slowly worse, not better, and there are always the twin dangers of obstruction and strangulation. An obstructed or strangulated hernia often necessitates an emergency operation.

Hernias are repaired by pushing the protruding tissue back into place, after which the loose muscles are tightened or sewn together. You must obey your doctor's orders carefully while you are convalescing after the operation, because any sudden activity that strains the abdomen can cause a recurrence of the hernia. The word "convalesce" as used on the next two pages means a period during which all physical activity should be first avoided, then very gradually resumed.

What is a hernia?
A hernia is a bulge of soft tissue that protrudes through a weak point in a muscle wall. Injury and lack of use of the muscle are two possible causes of a weak point. The hernia usually appears because of raised pressure in the soft tissues beneath the muscle wall.

Where hernias occur
The abdominal wall is a large sheet of muscle at the front and sides of the abdomen which keeps the abdominal organs in place. Most hernias occur in the abdominal wall.

Different types of hernia

Here are the commonest types of abdominal hernia, along with some specific facts about each. For information about hernias in general see the previous page.

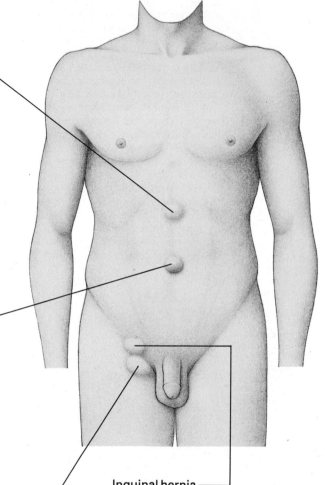

Epigastric hernia

A weak point in central abdominal muscles allows protrusion of fatty material covering the intestines somewhere on the line between the navel and the breastbone.

Symptoms The hernia is usually small and may not cause noticeable swelling, but can sometimes cause indigestion, belching, and even vomiting.

How common Very rare, totalling only about 2 per cent of all hernias.

Risks Painful strangulation is possible but extremely unlikely.

Treatment If the hernia causes no problems, it may not need surgery. Average hospital stay, if surgery is required, is 2 to 5 days; convalescence is 2 to 4 weeks.

Para-umbilical hernia

A weakness develops, for some reason, in the abdominal-wall muscles at a point just above or below the navel.

Symptoms A general feeling of heaviness in the abdomen, sometimes along with abdominal pain. There may or may not be noticeable swelling at the navel.

How common Fairly common, but 5 times more so in women than in men. Overweight women who have borne many children are especially prone to para-umbilical hernia.

Risks Obstruction and/or strangulation are possible risks.

Treatment Surgery is usually recommended. Average hospital stay is 2 to 5 days; convalescence 4 to 6 weeks.

Femoral hernia

This occurs in a similar position to a direct inguinal hernia (opposite), but slightly lower down.

Symptoms There are sometimes none, not even a swelling; many such hernias are discovered only if they become obstructed or strangulated.

How common 1 person in 250 has one (or two) femoral hernias. Overweight women who have borne many children are most prone.

Risks Because the hole through which a femoral hernia protrudes is small, risk of obstruction or strangulation is high.

Treatment As for inguinal hernia.

Inguinal hernia

There are two types of inguinal hernia. In a *direct* inguinal hernia the abdominal organs push aside weak abdominal-wall muscles lining the groin. An *indirect* inguinal hernia, which occurs 20 times more often in males than females, protrudes down the inguinal canal (one of the tubes through which, in men, the testicles descend from the abdomen to the scrotum just before birth).

Symptoms A bulge, or perhaps just a feeling of heaviness, in the groin area.

How common 1 person in 60 has one or, quite often, two inguinal hernias. Both types are more common in men than in women (see above).

Risks Obstruction and strangulation are possible complications.

Treatment An operation is performed to replace the protrusion and strengthen the weak muscles. Average hospital stay is 2 days; convalescence about 4 weeks.

Umbilical hernia

This hernia appears as a soft bulge of tissue around the navel of a newborn baby whose abdominal wall is not fully developed.

Symptoms The hernia rarely causes discomfort to the baby. A small swelling is likely to show up most when the baby cries.

How common No statistics are available because, although quite common, umbilical hernias are likely to be self-healing within a year of birth.

Risks Because the opening is wide, there is virtually no risk of strangulation or obstruction.

Treatment If an umbilical hernia persists or causes problems, surgery is usually done when the child is 3 to 5 years old. Average hospital stay is 2 to 5 days; convalescence 2 weeks.

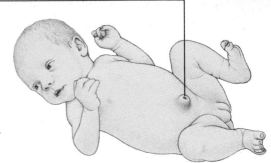

Incisional hernia

This is an occasional result of abdominal surgery. The cut abdominal-wall muscles heal but are weakened, and the intestines may protrude through a weak point.

Symptoms Incisional hernias almost always cause noticeable bulges, often along with some abdominal pain.

How common Overweight people who remain inactive after an abdominal operation often develop incisional hernias; they are also fairly common among elderly or thin patients.

Risks Strangulation and obstruction are unlikely.

Treatment A supportive corset may relieve the problem, but further surgery is generally necessary. Average hospital stay is 2 days; convalescence about 4 weeks. Strenuous exercise should be avoided for about 3 months, after which normal activities can be resumed. Some 15 per cent of the repaired hernias eventually recur.

OPERATION: ## Hernia repair

An operation to repair a weakened muscle through which soft tissue protrudes is usually carried out if the resulting hernia causes pain, or if there is a possibility that the hernia may become strangulated or obstructed.

During the operation Depending on the position and severity of your hernia, you will be given either a local or a general anaesthetic. A small incision is made over the hernia and the bulging tissue is pushed back into place. The muscles are then sewn firmly together. The operation usually takes less than one hour.

After the operation You will be encouraged to get out of bed the same day or the day after the operation. The area of the repair will be painful, so you may need to take painkillers. You should be able to leave hospital within 2 to 5 days.

Convalescence You should be able to return to work and continue with your normal everyday activities within a few days, but will be advised not to lift any heavy weights for up to 3 months.

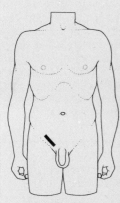

Site of incision
for inguinal hernia

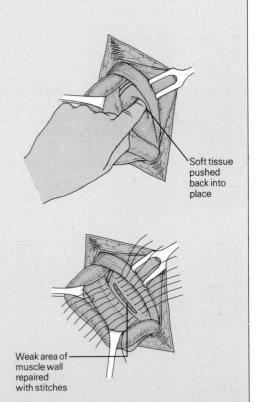

Soft tissue pushed back into place

Weak area of muscle wall repaired with stitches

Muscle and tendon disorders

A muscle is composed of special elongated cells which contract to produce movement. At each end of most muscles there is a band of fibrous tissue that connects the muscle to a bone. In some parts of the body these bands of tissue are very short or their fibres are inextricably mixed with the muscle tissue to which they are joined. But in other areas – especially in the hands and feet – the tissue forms long, tough cords known as tendons.

Both muscles and tendons are subject to damage from injury or disease. Diseases are discussed here; damage from injury is discussed elsewhere (see *Injuries*, p.532).

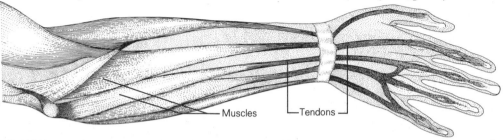

Tendons
Tendons are tough, fibrous bands or cords that join some muscles to the bones they move.

Muscles — Tendons —

Cramp

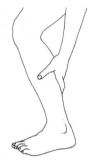

To ease cramp, massage the affected muscle.

Cramp is *spasm* in a muscle. It happens occasionally to almost everybody, and there is usually no underlying cause other than unaccustomed exercise or a prolonged period of sitting, standing, or lying in an uncomfortable position. Some people are roused from sleep quite regularly by sudden, severe cramp. In most cases there is no reason for concern; but occasionally recurrent cramps are a symptom of a more serious disorder such as *atherosclerosis* (p.372). Consult the self-diagnosis chart on cramp in Part II of this book to discover a possible cause of your attack.

As you try to move the cramped muscle, it contracts violently. There is usually visible distortion of the affected area along with sudden pain. The muscle feels hard and tense, and you cannot control it.

What should be done?
An ordinary cramp lasts no longer than a few minutes and will quickly clear up of its own accord. You can hasten the clearing-up process by massaging the muscle and gradually forcing it to function. If you are bothered by recurrent night-time attacks of cramp in the legs, try raising the foot of your bed about 100mm (4in). A milky drink just before you go to bed may also help. If you continue to have troublesome attacks, consult your doctor, who may be able to discover the cause and prescribe an appropriate drug.

Myaesthenia gravis

This rare disease affects only about 1 in 50,000 people, mostly women. It occurs when, because of faulty transmission of nerve impulses to the muscles they control, certain muscles become weak. The cause of the fault is unclear but is thought to be due to an *autoimmune* problem; in about 20 per cent of cases there is a growth in the thymus, a gland in the upper part of the chest.

Symptoms of muscular weakness usually appear first and most notably in the face. Your eyelids droop, and you may see double and find difficulty in talking and swallowing. If your arms or legs are affected, you may at times be almost unable to stand up or walk, and simple tasks such as combing your hair become almost impossible. The degree of weakness varies considerably from day to day, and even from year to year.

What should be done?
If you think you may have myaesthenia gravis, consult your doctor, who, after examining you, may want blood tests and chest *X-rays* in order to make a diagnosis. If you have the disease, treatment with special drugs that restore transmission of nerve impulses to the affected muscles should greatly improve your condition. Surgical removal of any thymus growth present often results in an improvement. Although myaesthenia gravis cannot usually be cured, treatment should minimize the symptoms of the disease so that you can lead a virtually normal life.

Muscle tumours

Growths in muscles are exceedingly rare. When they do occur, they are nearly always *benign*. *Malignancy* in a muscle is a rare but serious matter, since malignant muscle tumours grow and spread rapidly and are difficult to treat.

The first sign of a growth in a muscle is a visible lump in the affected area, and usually there are no further developments. If the growth is malignant, however, it enlarges rapidly and may be painful.

What should be done?

See your doctor within a week if you develop an inexplicable lump anywhere on your body. The doctor will examine you and, if the lump indicates the presence of a muscle tumour, will probably want *X-rays* and a *biopsy* to make sure the growth is not malignant. No treatment is necessary for a benign tumour. In the unlikely event of malignancy, possible treatments include injections of *cytotoxic* drugs, *radiotherapy*, and, if feasible, surgery.

Tendonitis

For some reason – possibly a minor injury – the fibrous tissues of a tendon become torn and inflamed. A painful tenderness develops over the affected area, and the tendon is usually slow to heal because the muscle is constantly in use. When it does heal, the inflamed fibres may leave a painful scar in the tendon. The pain will generally disappear after a few weeks or months, but it can persist and even worsen, especially in older people.

How common is the problem?

Tendonitis may occur in any place where a tendon joins muscle to bone, but it is most common at the shoulders or heels, on the outside of elbows (where it is known as tennis elbow, though you need not play tennis to get

it), or on the inside of elbows (where it is called golfer's elbow).

What is the treatment?

Rest the painful part for a few days, using a sling if necessary. A firm bandage and an *analgesic* such as paracetamol should help relieve the pain. After a few days start to exercise the joint gradually, to prevent it from stiffening. If pain persists or worsens, your doctor may want an *X-ray* in order to make sure you have no underlying bone or joint disease, and may then decide to inject the tender area with a *steroid* drug and perhaps a local anaesthetic. This is a slightly painful procedure that may need to be repeated, but it often effects a dramatic cure.

Tenosynovitis

Some tendons, particularly those that work fingers and thumbs, are sheathed in a membrane (the *synovium*) that assists freedom of movement. This synovium may become inflamed and swollen, especially if you constantly use your fingers in repetitive fashion such as typing or assembly-line work. In time the synovium heals, but it may become overtight or narrow as it does so. A tight synovium restricts movement of the tendon it covers, and the result is the disorder known as tenosynovitis. One example of what happens is the minor disability called "trigger finger" in which a tight synovium makes it hard for you to straighten your finger once you have

bent it. The straightening mechanism is jammed for a few moments before the tendon suddenly overcomes the obstruction and the finger completes its movement with a sudden jerk. In any such case the area over the tendon will become painful and tender, and an affected finger will hurt and make a soft, crackling sound whenever you move it.

Tenosynovitis is occasionally caused not by mechanical factors but by an infection. In such cases the sore finger or thumb becomes extremely painful and almost impossible to use, and you are also likely to have other symptoms and feel generally ill.

What should be done?

If your symptoms suggest the possibility of infection, see your doctor immediately. You will require treatment with *antibiotics*, and you may also need surgery to release pus produced by the invading bacteria. Troublesome non-infectious tenosynovitis is sometimes cured by injections of *steroids*. If the condition persists, a simple operation to slit open the constricting synovium will allow the tendon within to move freely again.

The synovium
The synovium is a membrane that covers a tendon and permits smooth movement. (Synovial membranes are also found inside joints – see p.550.)

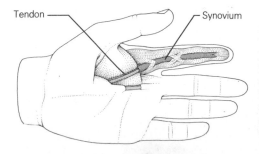

Tendon — Synovium

Dupuytren's contracture

You suffer from Dupuytren's contracture if, for some reason, the layer of tough fibrous tissue that lies under the skin on the palm of your hand has thickened and shrunk. This shrinkage eventually causes your ring finger and little finger to be permanently bent at the knuckles. Although not painful, the condition weakens your grasp. One or both hands may be affected, and some sufferers also have thickened skin pads over their other knuckles and on the balls of their feet. Dupuytren's contracture is a common condition in men over 40 and tends to run in families. For some reason, alcoholics and epileptics are particularly susceptible.

What should be done?
Because Dupuytren's contracture can make fingers permanently useless, you should see your doctor if you begin to develop it.

What is the treatment?
If treated early enough, stiff fingers can be unbent by an operation that either removes or cuts through the thickened tissue. With the aid of *physiotherapy* you can then regain full use of your hand. In some cases, though, the condition recurs.

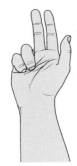

Dupuytren's contracture is a thickening of a sheet of tendon-like tissue in the palm of the hand, which causes your ring finger and little finger to bend involuntarily at the knuckles.

Ganglia

Ganglia are swellings under the skin, generally in the wrist or upper surface of the foot. A ganglion develops when, for some reason, a small amount of jelly-like substance accumulates in a joint capsule or tendon sheath, causing it to balloon out.

The size of ganglia varies, but they are usually small lumps no bigger than peas. They may be soft to the touch or quite hard, and they are usually either painless or merely cause a certain amount of discomfort.

What should be done?
Although ganglia are harmless, you should not ignore them. Always consult your doctor about an inexplicable swelling so that the possibility of *malignancy* can be excluded.

What is the treatment?
In addition to giving reassurance that your swelling is merely a ganglion, the doctor may be able to burst it by pressing on it. Ganglia that are especially obtrusive or uncomfortable can be cut away. But since they sometimes recur and frequently disappear of their own accord, surgery is rarely advisable.

Common site for ganglia
The wrist is one of the most common sites for the formation of ganglia.

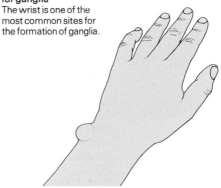

Fibrositis

Fibrositis is the medical term for stiffness and pain felt deep within the muscles. It may be caused by any of a number of factors, ranging from the physical straining of a muscle or joint to emotional tension reflected in the tensing up of muscular tissues. If you have an attack of fibrositis, there is nothing basically wrong with your muscles. Yet you are likely to have sharply localized pain, and you may even feel slight swellings in the area of the affected muscles.

Fibrositis often affects the back, causing an apparent non-specific *backache* (p.546). It is a common condition, especially in people past middle age, and it usually clears up in three or four days.

What is the treatment?
Relaxing hot baths and *analgesics* such as paracetamol should help to relieve the pain. If it persists for more than a couple of days see your doctor, who – after making sure that your symptoms are not those of a more serious disease such as *rheumatoid arthritis* (p.552) – may prescribe stronger painkillers or some type of muscle-relaxant drug.

Bone diseases

The bones that make up your skeleton are active, living structures. They are composed of several different types of cell embedded in a hard framework made of calcium and various proteins. The cells are constantly breaking down old bone and replacing it with new material, so that your skeleton is gradually but continuously renewed. If this system goes wrong, the result may well be one (or more than one) of the bone diseases included here. Inside some bones are spaces occupied by marrow, a tissue that manufactures many of the body's blood cells. Diseases of the bone marrow therefore have their main effects on the blood, and are considered elsewhere (see *Bone marrow*, p.429).

Osteoporosis

Osteoporosis is the wasting away of bone. The balance between the breakdown of old bone tissue and the manufacture of replacement material is disrupted; although the size of the bone remains the same, its structure becomes weak and fragile.

There are several possible causes of osteoporosis. It may occur in one or a few bones following prolonged *immobilization* of part of the body – as, for instance, in the treatment of *fractures* (p.534) or *prolapsed disc* (p.548). Some hormonal disorders – for example, *Cushing's syndrome* (p.523) – can cause a degree of generalized osteoporosis. It may also result from a diet containing too little protein or calcium, which limits the amount of basic ingredients required to maintain healthy bones (see *Osteomalacia*, below). However, by far the commonest cause is ageing. All bones suffer from osteoporosis if they become old enough.

What are the symptoms?
Osteoporosis does not usually produce symptoms unless it occurs in the vertebrae (backbones). If this happens, you have backache, and you may become shorter and round-shouldered because of the gradual compression of weakened vertebrae. In rare cases, one or a few vertebrae collapse and cause a sudden, severe attack of back pain.

How common is the problem?
Osteoporosis is a comparatively rare disease among young people in Britain. A significant proportion of those who suffer from it, however, have troublesome symptoms. It is much more common among the elderly. *X-rays* reveal some degree of the disease in at least half of all people over 60. Elderly women are most likely to be affected. This may be at least partly because of hormonal changes at the *menopause* (p.586). But although many older people have osteoporosis, most of them are not troubled by severe symptoms (though osteoporosis does account for loss of height in the elderly). A bone weakened by osteoporosis is much more likely than are healthy bones to fracture if you fall. The fracture is called a "pathological" fracture.

If you develop backache or sudden severe back pain, see your doctor. If he or she suspects osteoporosis, an X-ray of your spine will confirm the diagnosis.

What is the treatment?
Self-help: Be sure to have a good mixed diet rich in calcium (milk and cheese are good sources). Keep as active as possible; exercise keeps your bones and muscles strong and healthy. Paracetamol tablets will relieve any pain, and take sensible precautions to avoid falls (see *How to guard against falls*, p.720).
Professional help: There is no treatment that can reverse the effects of osteoporosis. Your doctor may prescribe calcium tablets to slow down the wasting process, and, if you are a woman past the menopause, you may also be given *hormone replacement therapy* to minimize subsequent bone wasting.

Osteomalacia

Osteomalacia is a softening and weakening of the bones because of vitamin D deficiency. If you lack vitamin D, you cannot absorb calcium and phosphorus from your food; both these chemicals are required for the growth, hardening, and maintenance of healthy bone. Lack of vitamin D in a child produces the disease called *rickets* (p.687); osteomalacia is the name for a similar problem in adults.

A healthy person obtains vitamin D from two sources – from food, and also by the action of sunlight on chemicals found in the skin. Therefore, a poor diet and/or lack of sunlight can cause vitamin D deficiency. More rarely, vitamin D deficiency is caused by a specific disease such as *chronic kidney failure* (p.512) or *coeliac disease* (p.684). Other rare causes are prolonged drug treatment for *epilepsy* (p.287) and some forms of digestive-tract surgery. In all these situations the absorption or handling of vitamin D is disrupted (see also *Vitamins*, p.494).

What are the symptoms?

Your bones become tender and painful, causing symptoms often mistaken for *rheumatoid arthritis* (p.552). You feel generally tired and stiff, you may have difficulty standing up, and you may suffer from muscular cramps.

Osteomalacia (like rickets) is common in less developed countries, but in the Western world it is a rare disease. Pregnant women are especially susceptible because of their increased need for calcium. Immigrants to Britain from hotter countries are also particularly at risk since the lack of sunshine causes a deficiency of D, which is not compensated for in their traditional diet. Bones weakened by osteomalacia tend to break under slight stress (see *Fractures*, p.534).

What should be done?

A normal Western diet provides ample vitamin D, even if you are pregnant. But if you suspect you have developed osteomalacia, see your doctor. If he or she shares your suspicion, you will be given blood and urine tests, along with *X-rays* of the bones. In some cases a *biopsy* of bone tissue will be taken.

What is the treatment?

Self-help: To prevent and treat osteomalacia, make sure your diet contains plenty of vitamin D and calcium. Milk, eggs, and liver are rich sources. Exposure to sunlight will also boost supplies of the vitamin.

Professional help: If your doctor finds you have osteomalacia, the remedy is to prescribe regular amounts of vitamin D and treat any underlying disease as necessary. If you are able to absorb vitamins from your digestive system you will receive tablets; if not, you will have vitamin D injections. This treatment generally cures the problem.

Paget's disease

In this disease the normal maintenance system that keeps your bones healthy and strong is disrupted, and new bone is produced faster than old bone is broken down. The disease occurs in two stages. In the first or "vascular" stage, bone tissue is broken down but the spaces left are filled with blood vessels and fibrous tissues instead of new, strong bone. In the second or "sclerotic" phase the blood-filled fibrous tissue becomes hardened and bone-like, but it is weaker and more fragile than healthy bone.

Paget's disease is extremely variable; it can occur in part or all of one or many bones. The hip bone (pelvis) and shin bone (tibia) are the commonest sites; the thigh bone (femur), skull, spinal bones (vertebrae), and collar bone (clavicle) are also frequently affected. The cause of the disease is unknown.

What are the symptoms?

Paget's disease does not always produce symptoms. When it does, bone pain is the most common problem. The aching discomfort is virtually continuous and is often worse at night. The affected bones become enlarged and misshapen, and they feel warm and tender. Depending on which bones are diseased, your legs may become bent, your skull may be misshapen, and your spine may develop a sideways curve.

How common is the problem?

In Britain, about 1 person in 100 over the age of 50 has Paget's disease, but it causes problems in only one-tenth of those affected.

One puzzling fact is that the disease has a clearly defined geographical distribution. For example, it is extremely rare in Norway, Japan, and South Africa. It is more common in Britain, especially in the north of England. The significance of this uneven distribution is not yet understood.

What are the risks?

Bones weakened by Paget's disease are more likely to break (see *Fractures*, p.534). Very occasionally, Paget's disease of the skull can compress the auditory nerve (which carries signals from ear to brain) as it passes through the skull. This can result in deafness. Another possible risk is *heart failure* (p.381) because the heart becomes over-strained in trying to cope with the greatly increased flow of blood through the diseased bones. In rare cases, a *bone tumour* (opposite) may develop.

What should be done?

If you think you may have Paget's disease, consult your doctor, who, after a physical examination, will probably order *X-rays* and various blood tests which will enable a firm diagnosis to be made.

What is the treatment?

There is at present no cure for Paget's disease, but the major symptom – pain – can be relieved by an *analgesic* drug such as paracetamol. If the pain is severe, your doctor may advise regular injections of a hormone called calcitonin, made naturally in the parathyroid glands (see *Thyroid and parathyroid glands*, p.525). Extra calcitonin seems to act to reduce the pain, but occasional sufferers develop an allergic reaction to the injections and others feel extremely nauseated by them. For these people, stronger analgesics are usually prescribed.

Bone tumours

Most bone tumours are secondary tumours – that is, they develop from cancer cells that have spread (*metastasized*) from a primary *malignant* tumour elsewhere in the body. Cancer of the lung, breast, prostate, kidney, or thyroid is particularly likely to spread to bone tissue. In some cases it is the secondary bone tumour that draws attention to the primary tumour; any bone tumour so weakens the bone that it breaks under a slight strain (see *Fractures*, p.534). Once cancer has spread to bone, the outlook is poor, and treatment is aimed at relieving the symptoms. Primary bone tumours – those which start in bone – are very rare. Most are *benign*, but a few are malignant and spread swiftly.

All bone tumours generally appear as hard, painless lumps on the bone. If you develop any such lump, see your doctor, who will examine it and order one or more *X-rays*. If the growth is found to be benign, nothing more needs to be done. If it is a primary malignant tumour, then amputation of the part of the body around the growth will be necessary. In addition, injections of *cytotoxic* drugs and/or *radiotherapy* may be advisable. If the cancer is in an arm or leg, an *artificial limb* (below) can be fitted.

Artificial limbs

An artificial limb is fitted whenever someone loses part or all of an arm or leg. The loss may be the result of an accident, if microsurgery to repair the damaged limb was not possible, or the result of a disease such as *dry gangrene* (p.415) or *wet gangrene* (p.416).

After you have lost a limb, a *physiotherapist* will first teach you exercises to keep your remaining muscles strong. Then you will be given a temporary artificial limb to use for short periods until you become accustomed to it and can wear it all day. Once you are active again, specialists at an artificial limb centre will make a limb specifically designed for you.

Ideally, an artificial limb should fulfil two requirements: mobility, enabling you to carry on your normal life; and naturalness, restoring your normal appearance. It is difficult to incorporate both functions in one limb, so you must discuss your needs with experts at the centre and arrive at a suitable compromise.

Once you have your new limb, your physiotherapist will teach you how to use it. Most people – even those with more than one artificial limb – learn to cope remarkably quickly. Although a great deal depends on your age and the state of your general health, the main factor is your attitude. If you have perseverance and enthusiasm, your artificial limb will soon help you return to an active life.

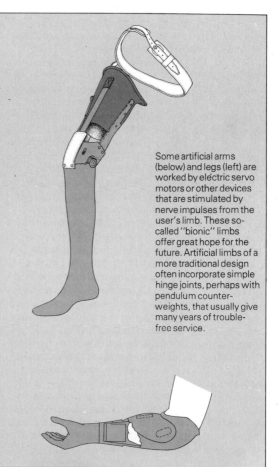

Some artificial arms (below) and legs (left) are worked by electric servo motors or other devices that are stimulated by nerve impulses from the user's limb. These so-called "bionic" limbs offer great hope for the future. Artificial limbs of a more traditional design often incorporate simple hinge joints, perhaps with pendulum counter-weights, that usually give many years of trouble-free service.

Backaches

The spinal column (backbone) stretches from the base of the skull to the bottom of the buttocks and consists of more than 30 separate bones called vertebrae. The vertebrae are linked by strong ligaments and have flexible, washer-like discs lying between them. Each disc is constructed of a tough, fibrous outer covering wrapped around a jelly-like inner substance, and this construction provides enough elasticity to permit some movement over the entire spinal column. It is partly the restrictions imposed by this limited flexibility that are responsible for most back troubles. A wrong-way twist or over-strain on one link in the chain can have a painful effect on the spinal column itself, and on the numerous muscles and ligaments that tie the vertebrae together.

Susceptibility to pain is increased by the fact that the spinal cord, which is a major part of the central nervous system, runs through a channel penetrating the length of the spinal column; and there are also narrow side channels through which *peripheral* nerves pass on their way to and from the rest of the body. Because of this, any trouble with a vertebra, ligament, or disc may put pressure on some element of the nervous system. As a result, a backache can lead to symptoms such as pain or weakness in almost any part of the body.

Non-specific backache
The vast majority of backaches are often termed "non-specific" because they have no obvious cause (and there are no obvious, easy cures). Most non-specific backaches are probably due to a strained ligament or vertebral joint that causes surrounding muscles to go into painful *spasm*. In other cases, pain is due to *fibrositis* (p.542) affecting the back muscles. In addition, some people tend to develop back pain when under stress, just as others develop tension headaches.

Symptoms of non-specific backache
Pain, generally along with stiffness, may develop slowly or suddenly. It may be a continuous ache or it may occur only when you are in a certain position. Coughing and sneezing as well as bending and twisting the back are likely to aggravate the pain. Sometimes the pain seems to be localized in one spot. Three of the most common sites for localized back pains – lumbago, coccydynia, and sciatica – are shown opposite.

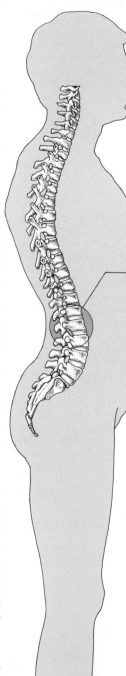

Standing correctly
To avoid back trouble, try not to slouch, but stand with your head up, your shoulders straight, and your chest forward. Balance your weight evenly on both feet.

How common is the problem?
In Britain, non-specific back disorders affect at least 1 out of every 50 people. Men and women are equally susceptible. Backaches of all kinds are a major health problem; they are the largest single cause of working days lost through illness in this country.

The spinal column
The spinal column is made up of over 30 separate bones – vertebrae – which form a protective casing for the spinal cord.

The spinal cord
Running through a continuous tunnel in the spinal column is the spinal cord, which transmits nerve signals between brain and body.

Although non-specific backaches are often so painful that it is difficult for sufferers to carry on with their daily routine, there is virtually no risk of complications. Such backaches are generally self-healing, but unfortunately they tend to recur.

What should be done?
Always follow the suggestions on *How to protect your back* (opposite). If you get what appears to be a non-specific backache, begin by trying the self-help treatment recommended under *Treatments for backache* (p.548). If pain persists for more than three or four days, or if you begin to have bowel or bladder trouble, consult your doctor.

Because of its nature, a non-specific backache is difficult to diagnose. After examining your back, the doctor may arrange for *X-rays* of your spine to make sure that you do not have a *prolapsed disc* (p.548) or *spondylosis* (p.549). But in most cases of suspected non-specific backache, sufferers are advised to continue with self-help measures for a few days. Your doctor may prescribe stronger painkillers or a muscle-relaxant drug, or perhaps injection of a *steroid* if you have a definable sensitive spot. *Massage* or *osteopathic* manipulation can sometimes give dramatic results.

Types of back pain

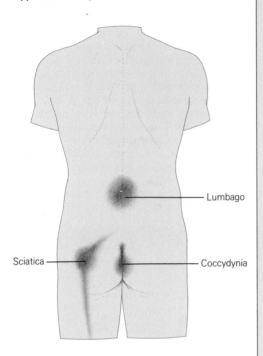

Lumbago

Sciatica

Coccydynia

Whatever the type of back pain, you should consult your doctor if it persists for more than 3 or 4 days. Consult the doctor as an emergency if you develop signs of spinal-cord injury, such as inability to control your bowels or bladder, or weakness, numbness or tingling in a limb.

Lumbago: The pain of lumbago is centred in the small of the back. It is often the result of unusual exertion such as moving furniture or unaccustomed heavy digging in the garden. It may develop suddenly, or come on overnight; it tends to be a severe pain and sometimes the sufferer is completely unable to move his or her back. It may be caused by a mixture of pulled muscles, muscle *spasm*, and sprained muscles or ligaments.

Coccydynia: This is a non-specific backache (see opposite) localized in the area of the coccyx, at the very base of the spinal column. It is a continuous ache that is worse when the sufferer is seated. It may be caused by a heavy fall on the buttocks or an injury from a blow, and women occasionally have pain in this area after childbirth. Some relief can be obtained by sitting on a rubber ring.

Sciatica: Sciatica is a type of *neuralgia* (p.290). It is pain caused by pressure on the sciatic nerve where it leaves the spinal cord. The pressure is often caused by either spondylosis or a prolapsed disc. You feel a burning pain shooting through your buttocks and along the back of your thigh down towards your ankle. If you cough, sneeze, or try to bend your back, the pain worsens.

How to protect your back

Lifting heavy objects (right)
Keep your back straight. Bend your knees and let your legs do the work; they are stronger than your back. Test the heaviness of a load before you lift it, and when in doubt get help.

WRONG

RIGHT

Footwear
Avoid high heels. The higher they are, the more they force your stance into an unnatural position that strains your back. Wear low-heeled, comfortable shoes, and try to stand correctly (see opposite).

Sitting properly (below)
Select a firm, high-backed chair whenever possible. If you want to slump, do not slump in a chair; lie down. If you must sit for hours on end, as in a long drive, use a cushion to support the small of your back.

WRONG

RIGHT

Back support in bed (right)
Sleep on a fairly hard ("orthopaedic") bed and mattress, or put a stiff board under the mattress you already have. The bed should give you constant support all the way down your back, so that it keeps your spine straight. To aid this, use only a single, relatively flat pillow.

WRONG

RIGHT

Weight control
If you are overweight, try to slim down. Fat people often have backaches because of the added burden their backs must carry.

Prolapsed disc
(slipped disc)

The term "slipped disc" is generally used rather loosely. If you believe you have "slipped a disc", you are more likely than not to be experiencing what is generally known as *nonspecific backache* (see *Backaches*, p.546). From a medical standpoint a slipped disc – more correctly called a prolapsed disc – is a specific disorder. Every flexible intervertebral disc consists of a fibrous outer layer surrounding a jelly-like inner substance. If a disc begins to degenerate and become less supple – because you are growing older, perhaps, or because you have been over-straining your back – the disc may *prolapse*. In other words, the pressure squeezes some of the softer central material out through a weak point in the harder outer layer. The result is a loss of cushioning effect of the disc and painful pressure on a nerve from the squeezed-out portion. In extreme cases discs may rupture.

What are the symptoms?

If you have a prolapsed disc in your neck, you are likely to wake up next day with an aching, twisted neck, which you cannot straighten out without extreme pain. You may also have weakness or tingling in your arms and hands.

Symptoms of a prolapsed disc anywhere below the neck may start abruptly or develop gradually. On attempting to lift something, for example, you may suddenly feel intense pain in your back or in one of your limbs – this is because the sudden strain has caused the prolapsed part of the disc to press painfully

---

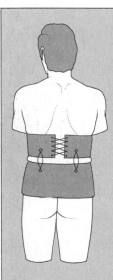

Two common treatments
For some types of backache, the doctor may advise wearing a special kind of corset (above) which supports the back. However, for other types of backache, complete bed rest on a firm mattress (below) that gives overall support may be the only answer.

Treatments for backache

The exact causes of back pain are often difficult to pinpoint. Consequently, if you develop backache, it may be difficult for your doctor to make an accurate diagnosis and prescribe immediate, precise treatment. Most doctors know that the average backache sufferer will recover in a few days provided he or she carries out the few simple self-help measures described below. But if your backache is severe, persistent, or recurrent, your doctor may order *X-rays* and other diagnostic tests to discover its underlying cause and permit more specialized types of treatment.

Self-help for backache

Whatever the cause of your backache, there are measures you can take to ease pain and speed healing. Take simple painkillers such as aspirin or paracetamol every four hours, as instructed on the container. Apply local heat to ease pain – for instance, by means of a hot water bottle wrapped in a towel. Lie on your back (or whichever position is most comfortable) for as long as you can, on a bed with a fairly hard ("orthopaedic") mattress or on an ordinary bed with a stiff board under the mattress. Rest allows the intervertebral discs and ligaments to soften, and thus increases the chances of recovery. So stay in bed as long as you can. If your backache persists for more than three or four days consult your doctor.

Professional help for backache

Much depends on your history of back trouble and your doctor's assessment of the situation. The doctor may prescribe stronger painkillers, or a muscle-relaxant drug. If you have a definable sensitive spot in the back muscles one or more *steroid* injections may relieve it rapidly. Some doctors may consider *physiotherapy*, some form of *massage, osteopathic* manipulation, a supportive belt or corset, or special exercises to stretch the spine. However, the most widely used and generally most successful treatment – especially for a suspected prolapsed disc – is to lie on a firm bed for two weeks. This means taking meals in bed, using a bed pan, and having bed baths. If you become bored and get up to sit with your family – at mealtimes, for example – this negates the treatment. It must be *complete* bed rest.

Occasionally, backache is not relieved by the above measures. If this happens, your doctor may refer you to an *orthopaedic* surgeon or a *neurosurgeon* for further examination and treatment. A few weeks in hospital may be advisable. Here, bed rest can be complete and your legs or neck put into *traction*. Surgical removal of a portion of prolapsed disc is usually recommended only after all other treatments have been tried; the operation is a major procedure, and the results cannot be guaranteed.

As you gradually recover from your backache and cautiously resume your normal routine, the doctor may arrange for specific physiotherapy exercises to strengthen your back muscles and joints. It is during the first few months that you are most likely to have a recurrence, but remember that throughout your life your back is always at risk.

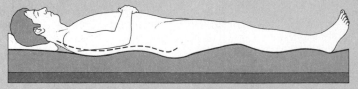

How a prolapsed disc causes pain

Flexible intervertebral discs act as shock absorbers to cushion the vertebrae from each other as you move your spine. Each disc is composed of a hard outer layer and a soft, jelly-like core. When your back is strained, pressure may push some of the soft substance through a weak point in the hard outer layer to press against a nerve where it leaves the spinal cord, and so cause pain.

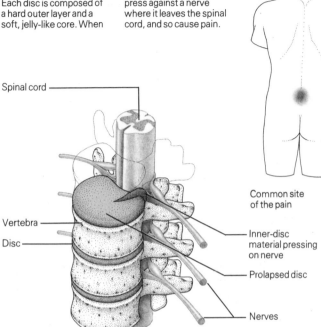

Spinal cord

Vertebra
Disc

Common site of the pain

Inner-disc material pressing on nerve

Prolapsed disc

Nerves

on a nerve. Alternatively, you may have back pains that build up slowly over a period of weeks. If the prolapsed disc is in the lower part of your back, you may develop sciatica (see *Types of back pain*, p.547).

How common is the problem?

Prolapsed discs are common. In Britain about 1 person in 200 is diagnosed as having this problem in an average year, and it affects twice as many men as women. Discs in the lower back are most likely to prolapse. Except in the neck, prolapsed discs tend to recur, but the most serious risk is of *spinal-cord injury* (p.278).

What should be done?

If you have the symptoms of a prolapsed disc, see your doctor. Do this as a matter of urgency if you have weakness, numbness, or tingling in your limbs, or if you lose bowel or bladder control. The doctor will carefully examine your back and legs and may arrange for an *X-ray* of your spine, or even *myelography* to discover the exact site of the disc.

Recommended treatments for prolapsed disc vary enormously. If the prolapsed disc is in your neck, you may simply need to wear a supportive collar for about two weeks. But much depends on your medical history, and your doctor's experience of the problem (see *Treatments for backache*, opposite).

Spondylosis

Spondylosis is a hardening and stiffening of the spinal column that results in a loss of flexibility. This happens if some of the spaces between vertebrae are narrowed because the intervertebral discs have degenerated and lost their elasticity through age, over-use, or injury. Sometimes bony outgrowths develop on the vertebrae or along the edges of degenerating discs, and these may press painfully on various nerves where they join the spinal cord. The narrowing and stiffening of intervertebral joints puts additional strain on the backbone and its supporting structures (muscles, ligaments, and other vertebral discs); and every new stress makes the back more susceptible to injury.

What are the symptoms?

Mild cases are usually symptomless. Often, however, you get intermittent pains in the part of your back most severely affected (see, for example, *Cervical spondylosis*, p.280, which affects the neck). Your back may become increasingly tender and difficult to bend or twist; and if the lower part of the back

is affected you may have the shooting pains in your buttocks and legs characteristic of sciatica (see *Types of back pain*, p.547).

How common is the problem?

Spondylosis is common, particularly in people over 40. About 1 person in 150 consults a doctor because of this problem in an average year. If you have had frequent trouble from a *prolapsed disc* (opposite), you may be especially susceptible to the condition. Very rarely, a severe attack of spondylosis in the lower regions can affect your ability to urinate, move your bowels, or walk.

What should be done?

If you think you may be suffering from spondylosis, try self-help measures recommended under *Treatments for backache* (opposite).

If symptoms persist for more than three or four days, consult your doctor, who, after examining you, may arrange for back *X-rays* and other diagnostic tests to help diagnose your problem and suggest further, specialized forms of treatment.

Joint disorders

Because you use one or more joints every time you move, you soon notice any problems with them. It is perhaps not surprising that they sometimes go wrong. A highly manoeuvrable joint such as the hip is a complicated structure. The whole joint is bound together by fibrous bands called ligaments. Inside the ligaments is a fibrous joint capsule lined on the inside by the *synovium*, a thin membrane that continuously produces tiny amounts of fluid to lubricate the joint. Where the bone ends are in contact, their surfaces are covered by a smooth, firm substance called articular cartilage.

Most joint disorders are dealt with in the following pages, but there are two main exceptions. Certain problems affecting the spinal column, which has a somewhat different

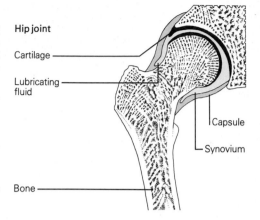

Hip joint
Cartilage
Lubricating fluid
Capsule
Synovium
Bone

jointed construction, are dealt with under *Backaches*, p.546. And for sprained or dislocated joints see *Injuries*, p.532.

Osteoarthritis

(osteoarthrosis)

Osteoarthritis is a condition that normally occurs as a result of wear and tear on the joints. Whether you suffer (or will suffer) from osteoarthritis depends on several factors – your age, for instance, and whether you have overused one or several joints during a particular sport or pastime.

Osteoarthritis develops most commonly in the larger weight-bearing joints – chiefly the hips, knees, or spine – of older people. Many doctors prefer to call the disease osteoarthrosis because the suffix "itis" means "inflammation", and the joints of a sufferer from this disease are not necessarily inflamed. What happens is that the smooth lining of the bones where they come into contact (known as articular cartilage) begins to flake and crack because of overuse, injury, or some other reason. As the cartilage deteriorates, the underlying bone is affected, and may become thickened and distorted. Movement becomes painful and restricted, and as it does so the disused muscles that work the joint gradually waste away.

Osteoarthritis should not be confused with *rheumatoid arthritis* (p.552). Also, the terms "arthritis" and "rheumatism", though extensively used, have no precise medical meanings and are best avoided.

What are the symptoms?
Episodes of pain, swelling, and stiffness in the affected joint occur at intervals over a period of months or years. Although it often affects several joints, osteoarthritis is rarely severe enough at any one time to cause symptoms in more than one or two joints. In a few cases, pain that begins as a minor discomfort may slowly become bad enough to disturb sleep and interfere with everyday life. Eventually, the joint degenerates and as it becomes stiff it may also become less painful.

Amount of swelling of the affected joint varies. You may scarcely notice it, or the joint may become extremely knobbly and swollen. And the pain itself is frequently deceptive. You may feel it directly in the area of the joint, or it can be "transmitted" so that it appears to come from other parts of the body. For example, osteoarthritis of the hip is sometimes felt most painfully in the knee.

How common is the problem?
Osteoarthritis is the commonest joint disorder, chiefly because it is a natural part of the ageing process. If you live long enough, you are certain to get it in some joints (though you may be unaware that you have it). *X-rays* show some degree of osteoarthritis in one or more of the joints of 9 out of 10 people past the age of 40. It seldom becomes a serious problem, however, and in nearly all cases poses no life-threatening risks.

Certain occupations and sports are closely associated with the eventual development of osteoarthritis. For example, many ballet dancers get it in their feet after years of standing on points. And soccer and rugby players are

Replacing damaged joints

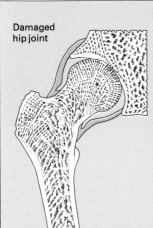

Damaged
hip joint

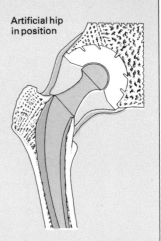

Artificial hip
in position

The replacement of natural joints by artificial ones made of metal or a combination of metal and plastic is a constantly developing and improving form of treatment for people who have one or more joints badly crippled by an arthritic condition. If the replacement is successful, it improves movement and relieves pain. The most common and generally satisfactory replacements are of hip joints; more than 90 per cent of these are successful.

Other joint replacements are more susceptible, during or after the operation, to setbacks such as infection or even the working loose of the joint. But even so most such operations are successful.

Replacement joints are advised only for people with severe arthritis for whom the small but real risk of failure is a reasonable gamble. Other factors that have to be taken into account include age, general health, and whether other joints are affected.

notorious for their knee problems (commonly termed "cartilage trouble").

What should be done?

If you have occasional mild attacks of pain and stiffness in a joint, there is no cause for concern. If symptoms become troublesome, try the self-help measures recommended below. Then, if necessary, consult your doctor, who, after examining you, may want blood tests along with X-rays of the affected joint or joints. If blood tests indicate nothing out of the ordinary, the chances are good that your problem is osteoarthritis and not a more serious disease such as rheumatoid arthritis.

What is the treatment?

Self-help: For obvious reasons the wear and tear on weight-bearing joints is greatest in obese people. Take off some of the strain by losing weight. If you are overweight, use a walking stick or cane, take frequent rests, and sleep on a firm bed. Keep warm, since heat generally helps to ease joint pains. It is important not to let the muscles around your osteoarthritic joints become weak through disuse. Regular exercise will strengthen the muscles and, in the long run, minimize symptoms. Apart from an occasional dose of aspirin or paracetamol, do not use painkilling drugs other than those prescribed by your doctor. Over-the-counter preparations advertised as doing wonders for "arthritis" should be avoided unless the doctor recommends them.

Professional help: Your doctor may prescribe a stronger painkiller than aspirin. Some anti-inflammatory drugs seem to ease symptoms, though why this is so is unknown.

If pain becomes severe, an injection of a *steroid* drug into the painful joint may help, but this type of treatment can do further damage to the joint cartilage if tried too often. The doctor may also arrange for a course of *physiotherapy*, which usually involves exercises and heat treatments.

Surgery is sometimes both feasible and advisable. The most common operation – chiefly for people with osteoarthritis of the hip – is joint replacement (see *Replacing damaged joints*, above). Hip-joint replacement has proved successful in about 90 per cent of the cases in which the procedure has been attempted.

If you wonder whether a change in your diet might have a healing effect on arthritic symptoms, the answer is simple: there is only one kind of diet that helps – a diet that makes you lose weight. Various "fad" diets that omit certain foods or chemicals are unlikely to ease the problem. Other possible treatments, none of which can be guaranteed to help, include *acupuncture*, special kinds of heated clothing (so-called thermal wear), and swimming regularly in heated pools. The fact is, of course, that there are no magic cures. If you have arthritic pains caused by natural degeneration of joints, ordinary painkillers such as aspirin should give you some relief.

Do not forget that there are many household gadgets and other aids available for those disabled by chronic diseases such as osteoarthritis. These include handrails for the bathroom and bedroom, cutlery, various cooking aids, and specially designed chairs. Your doctor, or one of many self-help organizations such as the *Disabled Living Foundation* (p.768), will be able to advise you.

Rheumatoid arthritis

Rheumatoid arthritis is a long-term disease of the joints. Its exact cause is not clear, but it is known to be an *autoimmune* disease. The *synovial* membrane of a joint gradually becomes inflamed and swollen, and this leads to inflammation of other parts of the joint. If the problem persists, the bones linked by the joint are slowly weakened; and in severe cases, bone tissue may eventually be destroyed. Joints usually affected are the small ones in hands and feet (chiefly the knuckles and toe joints), but rheumatoid arthritis can also affect wrists, knees, ankles, neck, etc. It occurs less often in the spine or hips, which are much more susceptible to *osteoarthritis* (p.550). In many cases the disease is not limited to joints, but also causes a degree of generalized inflammation – for instance, in heart muscle, blood-vessel tissues, and the tissues just beneath the skin.

What are the symptoms?

This disease may begin without obvious symptoms of joint trouble. Over a period of several weeks or even months you may feel generally off-colour, listless, and without appetite. You are likely to lose weight and to have vague muscular pains. Only later do you develop the joint problems characteristic of rheumatoid arthritis. In other cases, though, the joint symptoms appear suddenly, without the slow general build-up. Sooner or later the affected joints become red, swollen, tender to the touch, painful to move, and stiff. The stiffness is usually most noticeable first thing in the morning; with exercise, as you gradually begin to move about, the pain and stiffness tend to disappear.

Some sufferers get occasional attacks of *bursitis* (p.555). Some people become anaemic (see *Anaemia*, p.419) as well as arthritic. But symptoms and degrees of severity vary widely; only one or two joints may be affected, or the disease may rapidly become widespread. Some people suffer only one mild attack. Other sufferers have several episodes, which may or may not leave them increasingly disabled.

In a few cases – and it should be emphasized that these are relatively rare – the continuous deterioration of joint and bone tissues produces deformities and makes it difficult to live an active life.

How common is the problem?

In this country about 1 person in 200 suffers to some extent from rheumatoid arthritis. Most of these sufferers are between 40 and 60 years of age, but the disease can attack people in any age group.

What are the risks?

In severe cases swollen, deformed joints may become partly or completely dislocated. This can cause great discomfort and problems with walking if knee or foot joints are affected. Tendons may also become so weak that they snap, making it impossible for the sufferer to control certain movements. If the neck is involved, the interlocking mechanism of the top two vertebrae may be badly weakened, with consequent risk of paralysis or death from serious damage to the spinal cord. And because the disease can affect small arteries, there is a slight chance of development of a circulatory disorder (see *Circulation*, p.403).

What should be done?

If you develop apparent symptoms of rheumatoid arthritis, consult your doctor, who will examine your joints and may want *X-rays* and special blood tests. Rheumatoid arthritis can usually be identified from the results of these tests, but occasionally the only way to make a firm diagnosis is to observe the patient's progress over the course of several weeks or even months.

Knee problems

The hard-working knee joint is susceptible to most of the common joint disorders such as *osteoarthritis* (p.550) and *rheumatoid arthritis* (above). *Bursitis* (p.555) is also common in the knee, producing the familiar complaints of housemaid's knee, parson's (clergyman's) knee, and water-on-the-knee. In addition, there are several specific disorders that affect only the knee, largely as a result of this joint's unusual structure. Unlike the other joints in the arm and leg, each knee has two extra pieces of cartilage "floating" between the opposing surfaces of the upper and lower leg bones, one piece on either side of the kneecap. (This is in addition to the normal areas of cartilage that cover the ends of the bones – see *Joint disorders*, p.550, for the structure of a typical joint.) The extra cartilages, called menisci, generally turn out to be the source of knee trouble. They may be torn or crushed by sudden twisting of the knee; they may gradually disintegrate over many years of hard use; or, occasionally, the knee may suddenly lock in position because a loose fragment of meniscus has become jammed in the joint. Such problems are generally termed "cartilage trouble", and when the trouble becomes recurrent, an operation on the joint may be the only satisfactory form of treatment.

Before deciding on surgery, the doctor may make a preliminary visual examination of the inside of the knee using an *endoscopic* device called an arthroscope. If surgery is the answer, it is likely that both menisci will be removed. The coverings of cartilage at the ends of the leg bones within the knee are left in place, and should keep the joint working smoothly provided that the knee is used with caution from then on.

What is the treatment?

Self-help: The best thing you can do is to come to terms with what may be a permanent condition. Do not brood about it. Instead, follow the advice of your doctor and *physiotherapist*, take plenty of rest, and have regular, moderate exercise. Swimming in a heated pool is good for stiff joints. And a firm mattress and warm but lightweight covers help you to sleep comfortably without putting too much pressure on your joints. Some of the many aids available for the disabled may be useful in your home (for valuable help and guidance contact the *Disabled Living Foundation* – see p.768 for address).

Professional help: If you have a bad attack of rheumatoid arthritis, your doctor may arrange for you to be admitted to hospital under the care of a *rheumatologist*. The major element in treatment for severe cases is complete rest. You will remain in bed, probably with the affected joints encased in soft-moulded splints, until symptoms have subsided. Thereafter you will be put in the care of physiotherapists, who will teach you helpful exercises and may also provide you with removable splints that can be strapped onto painful joints when they need rest.

Whether or not your condition is severe enough to require a temporary stay in hospital, your doctor will also prescribe the regular use of pain-relieving drugs. The basic drug is likely to be aspirin in high doses (the equivalent of 15 or 16 ordinary-sized tablets a day). But the doctor may have to experiment for a while before finding the best possible pain-killing and/or anti-inflammatory drugs for you. The reason for this is that all the many possible drugs, including aspirin, used against rheumatoid arthritis can have unpleasant side-effects, particularly on the digestive and/or urinary systems.

Occasionally, surgery may help sufferers from this disease. In the early stages of rheumatoid arthritis, *synovectomy* (the removal of a badly inflamed joint synovium) is effective if only a single joint is badly affected. In later stages it is sometimes possible to replace a severely damaged joint with an artificial substitute. But because of the risks of surgery in such cases, most doctors tend to advise an operation only in severe cases where other treatment has failed.

What are the long-term prospects?

As has been pointed out, rheumatoid arthritis is variable in severity, duration, and outlook. Statistics currently available indicate that about 45 per cent of all sufferers recover completely after one or more episodes of painful joint inflammation. Another 45 per cent remain arthritic, but to a bearable extent, after their attacks. Only about 1 sufferer in 10 is severely disabled by the disease.

Infectious arthritis

Many infections – for example, rheumatic fever, German measles, mumps, and chickenpox – can cause joints to become swollen and painful. These arthritic symptoms will invariably clear up when the causative infection is dealt with. They are not infectious arthritis. True infectious arthritis is a rare disease caused by bacterial invasion of a joint. The bacteria may enter through a wound, or be carried via the bloodstream from a distant infection, or spread directly from an infection nearby. Once in the joint, they multiply and cause redness, pain, and swelling due to inflammation and accumulation of pus. It is unlikely that more than one joint will be affected by the disease, but the sufferer will have a raised temperature – as high as 40°C (104°F).

What should be done?

If you have symptoms of infectious arthritis, see your doctor without delay. Untreated, the joint may become stiff and almost useless. Your doctor will examine the swollen joint and may use a needle and syringe to suck out some of the accumulated fluid. Examination of the fluid should confirm the diagnosis, and *antibiotic* drugs (taken as tablets and/or injected directly into the joint) are used to treat the problem. As the joint heals, you will be taught how to exercise it in order to keep it from becoming permanently stiff.

Ankylosing spondylitis

Spondylitis is inflammation of the joints linking the vertebrae (backbones). In ankylosing spondylitis, the inflammation recedes but leaves behind hardened, damaged joints that effectively fuse together the separate bones of the spinal column.

The cause of this disease is as yet undiscovered. The first joints to be affected are the sacro-iliac joints that link the base of the spine to the hip bone (pelvis). Bony growths fuse together the formerly separate bones, and the resultant stiffness may slowly creep up your spine until eventually it affects many (if not all) of your intervertebral joints.

What are the symptoms?

Ankylosing spondylitis often starts with a low backache, which may spread into the buttocks. Pain and stiffness are generally at their worst in the morning. You may also have stiff, painful hips and a general feeling of stiffness in your spine. Some sufferers have vague chest pains and, oddly, tenderness over their heels. More generally, you will feel off-colour, with loss of energy and weight, a poor appetite, and a slightly raised temperature. And, for reasons that are not clear, your eyes may become red and painful.

How common is the problem?

Only about 1 person in 2,000 suffers from this disease. It is 10 times more prevalent in men than in women and occurs mainly in the 20-to-40 age group. It also seems to run (though to a limited extent) in families.

What are the risks?

Although the disease does not usually progress very far up the spine, it can sometimes do so, leaving the sufferer with a stiff spinal column that may cause the head to be permanently bent down onto the chest. The ribs can also become involved at the point where they join the spine, and this reduces the sufferer's ability to breathe because of constriction of the lungs. Chest infection is then an ever-present possibility. The jaw may be affected, causing difficulty in eating and speaking.

What should be done?

If you have symptoms of ankylosing spondylitis, consult your doctor, who, in examining you, will pay special attention to the extent of your back movements and chest expansion. You will also probably need to have diagnostic blood tests and *X-rays* of your back and pelvic area.

What is the treatment?

Self-help: Regular daily exercise – especially swimming, if possible – is essential (see *Keeping physically fit*, p.14).

Get in the habit of breathing deeply, sleep on a hard mattress, and do not use a pillow. Try to teach yourself to sleep on your front rather than on your back or side. All these self-help measures assist in keeping your back muscles strong and prevent your spine from becoming permanently stiffened into a bent position.

Professional help: Your doctor may refer you to a *physiotherapist*, who will probably teach you special exercises to improve your posture. The doctor may prescribe one or more of the several types of painkilling and anti-inflammatory tablets.

A very badly bent spine can be corrected by *osteotomy*, a surgical procedure for straightening bent, fused bones. But any such operation puts the spinal cord at risk and is therefore undertaken only in extreme cases. If your hips are badly damaged by ankylosing spondylitis you may be advised to have the joints replaced by artificial ones (see *Replacing damaged joints*, p.551).

Bunions

A bunion is an inflamed bursa (bag of fluid) overlying a bony protrusion from the outside edge of the joint (on the inside of the foot), at the base of the big toe.

Bunions are usually caused by a minor foot disorder known as hallux valgus. The technical name for the big toe is "hallux"; and if your big toe has grown or been forced into a position where it overlaps one or more other toes, you have a so-called hallux valgus. This tends to happen in people with an inherited weakness in toe joints, and badly fitting shoes (especially those with very high heels and pointed toes) make it worse. One result of the deformity is that the bony base of the twisted big toe is pushed out beyond the normal outline of the foot and forms the unsightly bump known as a bunion. As this rubs the inside of your footwear, the overlying skin toughens and thickens into a callus (see *Corns and calluses*, p.253).

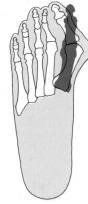

Normal position of big toe shown in brown

How common is the problem?

Bunions are common but not normally troublesome. In Britain only about 1 person in 1,000 consults a doctor about a bunion in an average year. Three times as many women as men suffer from the problem, and it tends to run in families.

What are the risks?

Sometimes the persistent pressure of a tight shoe causes painful *bursitis* (opposite) under the pressure point.

In addition, the affected joint is likely to develop *osteoarthritis* (p.550) sooner than it normally would.

What should be done?

If you have a bunion that has become troublesome, consult your doctor, who, after examining your feet, will probably refer you to a *chiropodist*.

What is the treatment?

Self-help: Always make sure your shoes fit comfortably and leave plenty of room for your toes. If you have developed bursitis, you can relieve pressure on the bunion and give it a chance to heal by cutting a hole in the top of an old shoe and wearing it exclusively until the inflammation clears up.

Professional help: The chiropodist will treat a bunion in much the same way as a corn or callus. If you have a severe hallux valgus, you may be advised to have an operation to straighten your big toe.

Most bunion operations require keeping the affected foot in a plaster cast for up to two months following surgery. Because of the pain and inconvenience after the operation, your doctor is not likely to recommend this type of surgery unless your bunion is causing you unbearable discomfort.

Bursitis

A bursa is a soft, lubricating pad that is present to minimize friction between body tissues that must constantly move over and under each other. Bursas are found near joints, either between the skin and underlying bones or between tendons and bones. If a bursa is irritated by pressure over it or by injury to the nearby joint, the little pad may become inflamed and fill with fluid. This is bursitis. The condition generally known as housemaid's knee is a familiar example of bursitis around the patella (kneecap). Other joints particularly susceptible to bursitis include the elbows, heels, base of the big toe (see *Bunions*, opposite), and shoulders.

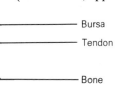

Bursa

Tendon

Bone

The knee bursa
An inflamed bursa in the knee is responsible for knee problems such as housemaid's knee.

What should be done?

Bursitis is not a serious disorder. It usually clears up of its own accord in a week or two, especially if you are careful to keep pressure off the tender spot while it remains swollen. If your trouble persists, consult your doctor, who will examine the joint to make the diagnosis. To bring down any swelling, the doctor may draw off fluid by means of a needle and syringe and then bandage the joint firmly.

What is the treatment?

Bursitis in a given position has a tendency to recur. If yours keeps coming back, it may be wise to have the offending bursa removed. This type of surgery can be done under either a local or general anaesthetic and seldom requires more than 24 hours in hospital. Where surgery is not feasible, as for a painful bursa lying deep in the tissues around a shoulder, the best treatment may be an injection into the most painful area of a *corticosteroid* drug and a local anaesthetic.

Frozen shoulder

A frozen shoulder is one in which the normal range of movement is impossible because of stiffness and pain. It normally starts with a trivial injury or minor problem such as *tendonitis* (p.541) or *bursitis* (above). This provokes disuse of the joint, leading to more stiffness and pain, followed by more disuse, and so on. Finally you can hardly move your arm at all, and the pain is often severe enough to disturb your sleep. The pain may be localized in the shoulder, or (more frequently) it may spread to your upper arm and/or neck.

If untreated, the condition runs a slow course. Symptoms gradually worsen over several months; they then tend to remain static for a few months, followed by a slow period of gradual improvement. Thereafter you usually feel no more pain, but your shoulder mobility often remains permanently impaired. This is why it is important to seek professional help for frozen shoulder.

What is the treatment?

A mild frozen shoulder should be kept in motion as much as possible; use painkillers such as aspirin or paracetamol to ease any pain. A severe case may require several days' rest before movement is attempted. Your doctor will probably give you antirheumatic drugs to try to damp down the inflammatory process and may also refer you to a *physiotherapist* for treatment. Injection of *steroids* into the shoulder may help mobility; but repeated injections may damage the joint, and so this type of treatment has to be given judiciously.

If your trouble is severe and persistent, there is another possible treatment; you may need to have your shoulder manipulated to its very limits under a general anaesthetic.

With prompt treatment, your frozen shoulder should thaw out and chances for recovery of pain-free mobility are good.

Collagen diseases

Connective tissue forms an essential part of every structure in the body. The main component of such tissue is a protein called collagen. In collagen diseases, which are rare, damage to the collagen in certain areas of connective tissue causes inflammation. Collagen diseases are regarded as *autoimmune* disorders in which the body's defence system starts working abnormally and constantly damages some of its own connective tissue.

There are no specific cures for collagen diseases, though treatment can relieve some of their symptoms. They sometimes "burn themselves out" – clear up of their own accord – but this usually takes many years. In a minority of cases they prove fatal.

Polyarteritis nodosa

Polyarteritis nodosa is an extremely rare disease that affects only about 1 person in 150,000; three out of four sufferers are male. What happens is that – for some reason not yet fully understood – the connective tissue in an arterial wall becomes damaged, with resultant inflammation of the artery. This can happen to almost any artery in the body at almost any time. Because of the inflammation, the affected artery becomes swollen and weakened, causing damage to any body organ that it serves. The symptoms, which may be severe, are those associated with trouble in the specific organ or organs that this collagen disease affects. For example, anyone with polyarteritis nodosa of the heart is likely to have symptoms of left or right *heart failure* (p.381). Similarly, lung damage from PAN (the commonly used, shortened form of the rather over-long name of the disease) may cause breathlessness; kidney damage may lead to *haematuria*; and so on. In addition, the sufferer usually has such general symptoms as persistent raised temperature, poor appetite, loss of weight, and an overall sense of lethargic ill-health.

What should be done?
This disorder is extremely difficult to diagnose. You will probably consult your doctor because of symptoms that suggest a vaguely defined organic problem, and you will have to undergo a number of diagnostic tests before the trouble can be identified as polyarteritis nodosa. Once the source of the problem is established, major treatment will be according to the site and extent of the damage. There is no cure for the basic arterial inflammation and weakness. The disease does not normally progress rapidly, though, and it can often be kept under control by means of *corticosteroid* and *immunosuppressive* drugs.

Systemic lupus erythematosus

This disease (often called SLE) inflames and damages connective tissue in any part of the body. The disease varies considerably in the areas it affects and in its intensity. Most commonly, it causes inflammation of various membranes that surround the kidneys, joints, lungs, and other organs. In many cases the skin is affected. A red rash appears on the cheeks of some sufferers and may spread to the entire upper body; exposure to sunlight aggravates the rash. If joints are attacked, there is likely to be stiffness and pain that can be mistaken for *rheumatoid arthritis* (p.552). But kidney inflammation, possibly leading to *kidney failure* (p.511), is apt to be the most common and severe symptom of SLE. Sufferers may also feel generally out of sorts, with loss of appetite and weight and slight but persistent raised temperature. Systemic lupus erythematosus is a serious disorder and most of the people who develop it will succumb after a number of years. Fortunately, it is rare, affecting only about 1 person in 20,000. Most of those affected are women between 30 and 50 years of age.

What should be done?
Anyone with this disease is likely to feel so ill that he or she will consult a doctor as a matter of course. A firm diagnosis of SLE can generally be based on the results of a series of blood tests. The progress of the disease can then be slowed down or even halted by vigorous treatment with various drugs such as *steroids, immunosuppressives,* and antirheumatics. *Physiotherapy* and *plasmaphoresis* may also prove helpful. In addition, if you have systemic lupus erythematosus, your doctor will want regular check-ups to monitor the course of the disease. Serious as it is, about 9 in 10

sufferers can expect to live relatively normal lives for at least 10 years following the onset of this disease.

Because SLE tends to reduce the efficiency of the body's defence system, however, the sufferer must be wary of infection, no matter how minor. Always get prompt medical treatment for even slight scratches. And before being given any type of immunization injection, be sure to point out that you have this collagen problem (see, for example, injections needed for *Going abroad*, p.566).

Scleroderma

Scleroderma is inflammation of the connective tissue in and around tiny blood vessels known as capillaries. As the inflammation heals, the resultant scars cause capillary tissue to shrink and stiffen. Most commonly affected by this very rare condition – which occurs in only about 1 person in 100,000 – are the skin and oesophagus. Patches of skin are likely to become shiny and uncomfortably tight, and a stiffening of the oesophagus may lead to increasing difficulty in swallowing (*dysphagia*). Like most other collagen disorders, scleroderma may also affect almost any body organ such as the heart, kidneys, or lungs, and it is usually accompanied by a general feeling of being out of sorts, with additional signs being a slightly raised temperature and loss of appetite and weight.

What should be done?

If you have any of the symptoms of this condition, you will naturally consult your doctor, who will probably arrange for blood tests and may also want to have an *X-ray* of your oesophagus (which involves a *barium meal*). If the diagnosis of scleroderma is confirmed, many of the symptoms can be kept under control by regular use of specific drugs. You may also be put in touch with a *physiotherapist*, who can often suggest exercises that help prevent the skin from becoming uncomfortably tight.

Polymyositis and dermato-myositis

Polymyositis is a connective-tissue disease in which the muscles – especially those of the shoulder and pelvis – become inflamed and gradually lose their strength. In one form of the disease (known as dermatomyositis) the skin also becomes inflamed. This usually happens, curiously enough, in areas of the body where the muscles are not affected. A red or violet rash is likely to appear on the face, shoulders, arms, knuckles, or any other bony place on the body of a sufferer from dermatomyositis. People with either form of the disease feel generally unwell, and they occasionally have bouts of muscular pain as well as weakness.

Polymyositis and dermatomyositis are rare; about 1 person in 17,000 suffers from one or the other form of this collagen disorder. Two-thirds of those affected are women.

What should be done?

Always consult your doctor if you have persistent and increasing muscular trouble and/or an inexplicable rash. Blood tests along with *electromyography* will confirm the diagnosis. Your chances of recovering from either polymyositis or dermatomyositis are good; the disease often clears up of its own accord within a few years. Meanwhile, treatment is aimed at relieving symptoms. High doses of *steroids* are usually prescribed to suppress muscular inflammation, and *immunosuppressive* drugs may also help. In addition, *physiotherapy* helps to minimize weakness.

Polymyalgia rheumatica

This connective-tissue disease causes inflammation of many of the body's muscles, particularly those of the shoulders and buttocks. Unlike *polymyositis* (above), polymyalgia rheumatica is much more likely to cause muscular pain than weakness. The affected muscles become tender, and associated joints feel stiff, particularly in the morning. In some cases a similar condition, *temporal arteritis* (p.414), may also develop. Polymyalgia rheumatica generally clears up of its own accord after a period that may be as short as a few months or as long as several years. While it lasts, however, it can be extremely painful.

To confirm the diagnosis your doctor will probably arrange for blood tests, and he or she may also want a *biopsy* of one of your temporal arteries to discover whether temporal arteritis is developing. If you have only a mild form of polymyalgia rheumatica, ordinary painkillers and anti-inflammatory drugs such as aspirin should be sufficient to control your symptoms. In severe cases *steroid* drugs may be prescribed.

General infections and infestations

Introduction

The articles in this section deal with diseases caused by identifiable organisms that live in or on the human body. Infections are caused by microbes – minute bacteria, viruses, or fungi invisible to the naked eye – that invade and multiply within the body. As they multiply, they use nutrients and oxygen meant for the body's own cells; they may clog up blood vessels and ducts; and they produce waste materials that are harmful to body tissues.

Not all microbes cause disease. Those that do are described as "pathogenic". Many other microbes live harmlessly in the human body; in fact the non-pathogenic microbes (chiefly bacteria) that normally reside in the human digestive tract are necessary to help break down certain foods for digestion.

The infectious diseases discussed in the following pages have generalized effects on the body. Infections that attack specific organs or parts of the body – for example,

the brain, the lungs, or the kidneys – are discussed in the relevant sections. Similarly, infections that are primarily diseases of children (mumps, chickenpox, measles, and others) are dealt with under the separate heading *Childhood infectious diseases* (p.698).

Infestations are caused by larger organisms – parasites – that invade or colonize the body. Infestations differ somewhat from infections in that the body has certain natural defences against microbes but generally lacks effective natural means to combat infestation. Many infestations are to a great extent diseases of tropical countries and areas with poor standards of hygiene.

Many of these organisms are *contagious* – that is, they spread between people in close contact. Why some infections and infestations spread more rapidly than others, and why some people are prone to certain infections or infestations, is not yet fully understood.

The main types of microbe

Viruses
Viruses are the smallest type of microbe. A virus reproduces by invading a cell and taking over the cell's own reproductive machinery, which it uses to produce hundreds of new viruses, often in less than an hour. The invaded cell (which is killed in the process) bursts and releases the viruses, which go on to invade other cells. Viruses can attack almost all living things – plants, animals, and even bacteria.

A type of virus magnified 225,000 times

Different shapes of virus

Bacteria
Bacteria are many times larger than viruses, yet far smaller than cells in the human body. They live virtually everywhere, and many are harmless – nearly everyone's intestine contains a large population of bacteria, which does not usually cause problems. Unlike viruses, bacteria can be controlled by antibiotic drugs. Since the advent of antibiotics, many human bacterial diseases have become less common and much more easily treated.

A typical bacterium magnified 30,000 times

Streptococci (spherical, joined in chains)

Bacilli (rod-shaped)

Infections

The microbes that invade your body and cause infections are spread in various ways. Some are coughed or sneezed into the air (droplet infection); others are transferred by direct (for example, hand-to-hand) contact; others are encountered by handling animals or animal products.

Once microbes enter your body, it takes a while for them to become numerous enough to cause symptoms. The time that elapses between invasion by the organism and the appearance of symptoms is known as the *incubation period*. This varies from disease to disease. In influenza, for example, it is a few days; in brucellosis it can be months. So if you develop an infectious disease of which the incubation period is known, it may well be possible to work back and discover when, where, and how you caught it, and who else is at risk from the disease.

The symptoms of an infection are caused not only by damage to body tissue from microbes but also by the body's own mechanisms for fighting infection. White blood cells engulf or destroy invading microbes, and produce *antibodies* against the invaders. You feel the effects of the combat within your body as some of the symptoms of your illness. (Headache and fever, so common in infectious diseases, are probably due to substances produced by the body's defences.)

The procedure of *immunization* (p.701) and *antibiotic* drugs give powerful assistance to the body's natural defences. Unfortunately, though, antibiotics do not work against most viruses. Drugs may relieve some of the symptoms of a viral infection, but the infection itself must run its course until – as usually happens in an otherwise healthy person – natural recovery takes place.

Influenza

Influenza, usually called flu, is caused by a virus that spreads from one person to another in the spray from coughs and sneezes (this is called droplet infection). The virus enters the upper part of the respiratory tract through the nose or mouth, and it may spread to the lungs. Symptoms begin to occur after an *incubation period* of one or two days. Influenza is normally an epidemic disease; that is, it affects many people within a community during a certain period of time, usually in winter or early spring. Some people wrongly call a mild infection of the upper respiratory tract "flu".

What are the symptoms?
Among early symptoms are chills and fever (sometimes as high as 39°C – about 102°F), sneezing, headache, muscular pains, and a sore throat. These are usually followed by a dry, hacking cough and, often, chest pains. Later the cough becomes looser, and you get a runny nose. Fever generally lasts for two to three days, after which you feel weak and lacking in energy for another few days. Barring complications, which very seldom occur, you should be fully recovered within about one or two weeks.

How common is the problem?
Epidemics occur at unpredictable intervals. Sometimes there may be as many as five or six successive winters without a notable epidemic; sometimes two or three different epidemics affect the same community in a single year. In a bad outbreak most people in an affected area are likely to have at least a mild attack of the disease. It can affect all age groups and both sexes. In a non-epidemic winter only about 1 person in 40 consults a doctor because of flu, but at least 10 times as many will seek medical help during an epidemic year.

Epidemics die out because everybody who has been attacked by a given type of virus becomes immune to further attack by the same organism. There are several strains of influenza virus, however, and new strains are constantly developing and spreading as sufferers travel from one area to another. The new viruses are usually identified by their place of origin; that is why you hear about Hong Kong flu, Russian flu, and so on.

What are the risks?
The chief risk of influenza is that the infection may spread from the upper respiratory tract down to the lungs, causing *acute bronchitis* (p.353) or even *pneumonia* (p.359). Such complications are rare, though. They are most likely to occur in very young children, elderly people, heavy smokers, diabetics, or people with chronic chest trouble. Only about 1 in 1,000 cases (chiefly in the elderly and ailing) ends in death.

How flu affects you
The flu virus enters your nose or mouth, infecting the nose and throat. It then spreads down into the trachea (windpipe) and may carry on into the lungs.

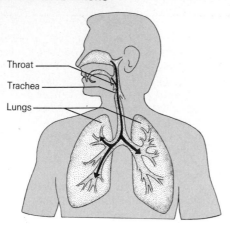

Throat
Trachea
Lungs

What should be done?

Influenza must run its course, but you can ease the symptoms by means of self-help measures recommended below. You need not see your doctor unless you are among the groups most susceptible to complications, or if you seem to be the only person in your area with the illness. In an apparently isolated case of flu the symptoms are perhaps deceptive, and you may be suffering from a different disease (see, for instance, *Glandular fever*, p.562). The doctor may therefore want a blood test in order to determine the exact cause of your symptoms.

What is the treatment?

Self-help: Go to bed as soon as symptoms begin, and stay there until your temperature returns to normal. Take paracetamol or aspirin, and drink as much water or fruit juice as you can. If your fever lasts for more than three or four days, or if you become short of breath while resting, call your doctor. In any event, you must expect to feel weakened and perhaps depressed for a week or so after your temperature drops, and you should rest as much as possible, gradually increasing your daily exercise until fully recovered.

Professional help: There is no specific treatment for flu since *antibiotics* are powerless against viruses. If a complication such as bacterial pneumonia develops, however, antibiotics will be prescribed, and you may be admitted to hospital.

Some doctors advise people most at risk from complications – diabetics and the elderly, for example – to have annual injections of an anti-influenza vaccine. Because of the many kinds of virus, however, it is extremely difficult to predict which strain will set off an epidemic, and so inoculation cannot guarantee protection. At best, the vaccine is effective for only one winter.

Rare diseases that start like flu

DISEASE	HOW CAUGHT
Brucellosis	By working with or drinking milk from infected farm animals.
Legionnaire's disease	Uncertain. Probably spreads through air-conditioning systems or water supplies.
Q Fever	By inhaling dust contaminated by infected animals, or drinking infected milk.
Psittacosis	By constantly handling birds, especially parrots and parakeets.
Weil's disease	By swimming or working in streams polluted by rats, whose urine carries the disease.

This table shows five rare diseases, each one causing flu-like symptoms in the early stages. Legionnaire's disease and brucellosis are bacterial infections; the others are caused by microbes that are neither viruses nor true bacteria, but that have some bacterial characteristics and are midway between bacteria and viruses in size.

EFFECTS	SYMPTOMS	TREATMENT	OTHER COMMENTS
Gets into the bloodstream and can cause inflammation anywhere in the body.	A few days to a few months after exposure, either a flu-like illness lasting 2 weeks develops, or a more severe illness (deep depression, fever, and joint pains) develops and lasts several months. Either may recur in the short term.	Antibiotics or steroids may ease symptoms. Within a year the disease burns itself out and is unlikely to return.	Farmers and vets are most at risk. But an extensive eradication programme is gradually bringing the disease under control.
Damages the lungs, kidneys, and nervous system.	Incubation period is not known. Symptoms resemble flu for 3 to 4 days, along with diarrhoea, vomiting, and drowsiness. In some cases the illness resembles pneumonia. It usually worsens and respiratory and/or kidney failure or shock may occur. Full recovery occurs in most cases, and takes 3 weeks.	Treatment in hospital is essential. Antibiotic drugs help.	This is a recently discovered disease and treatments for it are still being evaluated.
Damages the lungs, causing pneumonia.	9 to 20 days after exposure, a flu-like illness develops, sometimes with symptoms of mild pneumonia. Recovery takes 2 to 3 weeks. Thereafter the sufferer is immune for life.	Treatment as for flu, but antibiotics also help ease symptoms.	This is a widespread animal disease. There is a vaccine available for people in high-risk jobs in affected areas.
Spreads through the lymphatic system and affects the lungs, causing them to become inflamed.	7 to 15 days after exposure, a flu-like illness develops. Mild cases last a week. Severe cases last 2 to 3 weeks and may cause nosebleeds and shortness of breath that can lead to respiratory failure.	The disease usually clears up without treatment, but high doses of antibiotics help in some cases. An oxygen mask or artificial ventilation may be needed if shortness of breath becomes severe.	The disease is difficult to avoid where large numbers of birds are kept together. Solitary pets are unlikely sources.
Enters the bloodstream through a break in the skin and can damage any organs, especially the kidneys and liver.	3 to 15 days after exposure, a severe flu-like disease develops. This lasts a week. Some people then recover; others develop jaundice and/or acute kidney or liver failure.	Flu-like symptoms are treated as for flu. Further treatment depends on possible complications.	Do not swim in stagnant water. Wear rubber boots and gloves if you work in rat-infested areas.

Glandular fever

(infectious mononucleosis)

This type of viral infection is sometimes called "the kissing disease" because of a common belief that it is passed from one person to another through oral contact. Exactly how it does spread is not known, but it is not normally an epidemic disease such as *influenza* (p.559). If you get glandular fever, the virus is likely to spread through your bloodstream into almost any body organ. This accounts for the variety of symptoms, which include swollen lymph glands along with high temperature – hence the name glandular fever.

What are the symptoms?
You may assume at first that you have influenza since the early symptoms of glandular fever are similar to those of flu: fever, headache, sore throat, and a general sense of feeling out of sorts. After a day or two you may also become aware of having swollen, painful glands in your neck, armpits, and groin. In addition, you may also develop *jaundice* (p.485) or a rash similar to that of *German measles* (p.699). All major symptoms usually disappear within two to three weeks, but for a further period of at least two weeks you will probably feel weak, lacking in energy, and depressed.

How common is the problem?
Only about 1 person in 1,000 is likely to see a doctor because of glandular fever in an average year. However, the disease is probably more common than this, with many cases going undiagnosed or being mistaken for flu. Children and young adults are those most likely to catch glandular fever.

What are the risks?
Glandular fever is not a dangerous disease, but it tends to recur, sometimes several times, during the course of the next year or so. Succeeding attacks are usually milder than the first, however, and once the infection has

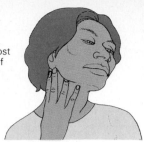

Visual symptom
Swollen glands in the neck are one of the most common symptoms of glandular fever.

disappeared altogether, there are no after-effects. Unfortunately, you do not gain immunity against re-infection from having once had the disease. This is probably because glandular fever is caused by more than one type of virus.

What should be done?
If symptoms of what you believe to be influenza persist for more than a week, and especially if your glands are swollen, consult your doctor. He or she will examine you, paying special attention to any lumps or swellings. If glandular fever is suspected, the doctor will probably take a sample of blood, analysis of which will determine whether you have the disease.

What is the treatment?
Self-help: Drink plenty of water and fruit juice, especially while you have a fever, and stay indoors. To relieve discomfort or pain, take aspirin or paracetamol. Rest is essential; do not attempt to return to your normal daily routine until advised to do so by your doctor; this is usually at least a month after the onset of the illness.

Professional help: Because glandular fever is a viral disease, *antibiotics* will not help; the disease must simply run its course. Some sufferers get bouts of depression during the convalescent period because they feel so tired and lethargic. If depression is a problem in your case, your doctor may be able to help.

Shingles

(herpes zoster)

See p.238,
Visual aids to diagnosis, 25.

Shingles is the result of infection by the same virus – herpes zoster – that causes *chickenpox* (p.700). During an attack of chickenpox the virus may find its way to the root of a nerve in the brain or spinal cord. Here it lies dormant, often for many years, until reactivated by some physical or emotional stress. For this reason it is difficult to assess the length of the infection's *incubation period*. When reactivated, the virus multiplies and produces intense, knife-like pain in the affected nerve. It also causes groups of blisters to form on the skin that lies above the nerve.

What are the symptoms?
Severe burning pain in an affected area often precedes the rash by several days. Almost any part of the body may be involved, but the disease is especially common on one side of the trunk, and most troublesome if it affects the face (especially near the eyes). The pain does not stop when the rashes erupt; in fact, it often lasts for several weeks after the blisters have disappeared.

Blisters caused by shingles are itchy and gradually become encrusted. They generally disappear after about seven days, but they leave scars like those caused by chickenpox. If your facial nerve is affected, you may suffer temporary facial paralysis. If your eyes are affected, there is a risk of painful and dangerous damage to the cornea (see *Corneal ulcers and infections*, p.316).

How common is the problem?

Shingles occurs unpredictably, but there are always several cases among children during a chickenpox epidemic. The disease is more common, and usually more painful, when it appears in adults.

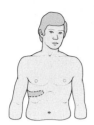

Common site of shingles

What should be done?

If you have shingles, you can do little apart from applying soothing calamine to the rash and taking tablets of an *analgesic* such as aspirin to ease the pain.

However, you should always see your doctor if you have shingles. Make an appointment without delay if your face is affected. The doctor may prescribe a more effective analgesic and may be able to hasten healing of rashes by painting them with an antiviral agent. In addition, you may need professional advice on how to protect your eyes.

Tuberculosis

Tuberculosis (often called TB) is a slowly-developing disease that can lead to chronic ill-health and may, if untreated, prove fatal. It is caused by bacteria, which are usually transmitted from one person to another through the air; but since cattle are also susceptible to a form of the disease, it can be carried in cows' milk and enter the body via the tonsils or intestine. The bacteria usually attack the lungs, but they can also spread to other parts of the body, especially the brain, kidneys, or bones. As they multiply, the bacteria create a small area of inflammation from which they then spread into the nearest lymph nodes.

The first (or primary) phase of the infection usually lasts for several months. During this period the body resists the disease by means of natural defences, and most or all of the bacteria are either destroyed or walled in by a fibrous capsule that develops around the inflamed area. Before the initial attack is overcome, however, a few bacteria may escape into the bloodstream and be carried elsewhere in the body, where they are again walled in. In many cases the disease never develops beyond this primary stage, and the affected person has good immunity against another attack. Sometimes, though, natural resistance cannot subdue the invading microbes, and the progress of the disease is not blocked (see "What are the risks?" below). Or the primary battle may be won, but the disease flares up again. This can happen – often after a lapse of many years – because, since the walling-in process does not actually kill the bacteria, they can become active again at a time when the sufferer is weak, ill, or undernourished.

This secondary phase of TB (sometimes called consumption) most commonly affects the lungs. As the bacterial population grows, the resulting lung damage reduces the sufferer's ability to breathe. Similarly, little pockets of trapped bacteria elsewhere in the body may become active again. Such secondary outbreaks of tuberculosis can usually be stopped if adequately treated, but they may leave disabling scar tissue wherever healthy tissues have been damaged.

What are the symptoms?

There are often either no symptoms or a flu-like illness as a result of primary infection; you may never even discover that you have had TB. If the disease progresses to the secondary stage, you are likely to develop a slight fever, lose some weight, feel fatigued without obvious cause, and develop various other symptoms, depending on which parts of the body are affected. Tuberculosis of the lungs (the most common type) may cause a dry cough, which eventually produces blood and pus-filled sputum. Sometimes shortness of breath and chest pain also develop. If any other body organ is affected, the symptoms of an infection of that organ will become apparent, but very gradually.

How common is the problem?

Having become a rare disease in Britain, tuberculosis is again on the increase, especially among immigrants. About 1 person in 5,000 is found to be tubercular in an average year, and many of the sufferers are relatively recent immigrants. Because all cattle in Britain are routinely checked for TB, milk is no longer a source of infection.

What are the risks?

Very rarely – generally in someone whose natural resistance is abnormally low – primary tuberculosis spreads so swiftly that it is fatal unless treatment is begun early. This occurs today almost exclusively among very young or very old people. Untreated secondary TB can also be fatal, but the health of the sufferer tends to deteriorate quite slowly;

even with successful treatment, affected organs may be left with severe scar damage.

What should be done?

If a baby is born into a family with a history of tuberculosis or is at risk from the disease for some other reason, he or she should be vaccinated against it. In Britain the school health service arranges a routine tuberculosis test (the "tuberculin" test) for children aged 12 or 13. If the child is considered susceptible, he or she will be vaccinated with the so-called BCG vaccine (see *Immunization*, p.701). Even if you have been vaccinated, however, always consult your doctor if you begin to lose weight, become generally unwell, or develop a fever with a persistent cough. The doctor may do a *Heaf* or *Mantoux* test and sputum tests, and arrange for a chest *X-ray*.

What is the treatment?

Self-help: If you are found to have tuberculosis, you must take prescribed drugs regularly and eat the nourishing foods that your doctor recommends. You must also be prepared to stay away from work and to rest for several months. Rest is essential for full recovery from the disease.

Professional help: Admission to hospital may be necessary. Special *antibiotics* are now available that will cure TB. Two or three types of antibiotic are used together, and they must be taken continuously for some time – usually from nine to 18 months.

After having had successful treatment for tuberculosis, you will be given periodic check-ups for at least two years to make sure that the disease does not flare up again. After this time you should be cured.

Tetanus
(lockjaw)

Tetanus is a serious, sometimes fatal disease caused by a type of bacterium (called clostridium tetani) that lives in the soil and can invade the human body through a wound from an infected object. This object can be anything from a nail to a thorn. The risks are greatest in wounds contaminated by soil and those in muscle or other tissues having a poor blood supply. The bacteria can multiply rapidly in dead skin or muscle, under low-oxygen conditions. *Toxin* produced by these bacteria attacks the spinal-cord nerves that control muscle activity.

What are the symptoms?

After an *incubation period* that may be as short as two days or as long as several months, the sufferer's limb, abdominal, and spinal muscles become rigid and subject to extremely painful *spasms*. These symptoms may take a week to develop in adults, the muscle rigidity preceding bouts of cramp.

How common is the problem?

As a result of immunization procedures (see *Immunization*, p.701), tetanus is extremely rare in Britain, where less than 50 cases are treated in an average year. Infants are immunized against the disease as a matter of course during their first year, and booster injections are normally given at intervals of about five years.

What are the risks?

In spite of specialist treatment, about 10 per cent of all tetanus cases end in death, often because of interference with breathing due to spasms of the throat and chest.

What should be done?

If anyone in your family has not been immunized against tetanus, have it done without delay. And make sure that you have booster shots every few years. (It is wise to keep a record of dates since some people react badly to these injections if given too frequently.) Even if you believe yourself immune, always clean out small wounds with soap and water and apply an *antiseptic*. This is especially important with cuts that occur out of doors.

If you have never had a tetanus injection and receive an obviously dirty wound, do not delay in getting to your doctor, who will probably start you immediately on a course of injections. If the wound has been swiftly and thoroughly cleansed, it is highly unlikely that the disease will develop.

If tetanus does develop, however, hospital treatment should start immediately.

What is the treatment?

Treatment for tetanus includes a course of *antibiotics*, along with three injections of an *antitoxin* to counteract the toxin produced by the invading bacteria. It is likely that treatment will take place in an intensive-care unit, where specialized equipment can be used to take over body systems affected by the paralysing effects of the toxin. For example, you may be given *muscle-relaxant* drugs, and your breathing will be aided or taken over by an artificial *respirator*.

The aim of treatment is to keep the body functioning for the three weeks or so that the disease takes to run its course; but, despite the most advanced treatment, the disease still proves fatal in a few cases.

Rabies
(hydrophobia)

Rabies is a viral disease of animals that can be passed on to people through a bite or scratch. If the virus reaches a person's central nervous system, it causes inflammation of the brain and is always fatal. The earliest symptom is a fever and general sense of being ill, as in any viral infection. After two or three days the infected person becomes irrational and has violent mouth and throat *spasms*, which are made worse by the sight of water ("hydrophobia" means "fear of water"). Death is likely to occur within a few days.

The *incubation period* for rabies varies from two weeks to two years, but is usually a month or two. Fortunately, the disease is not easily transmitted. In fact, only about 1 person in 10 who have been bitten by a rabid animal will develop rabies. To date the native animal population of Britain is rabies-free, and there are stringent laws specifically designed to keep the virus away from these shores. Rabies does occur, however, on the European Continent and elsewhere.

What should be done?
Take no risks. If you have been bitten or scratched by a possibly rabid animal (one that is acting aggressively and perhaps foaming at the mouth), see a doctor without delay. The animal should be captured, if possible, but not destroyed. If it survives for more than ten days, it is certainly not rabid. Meanwhile, you will probably be given a series of vaccinations to help prevent the disease developing.

Anthrax

Anthrax, caused by bacteria that infect farm animals, usually spreads to human beings via contaminated animal products. In Britain this extremely rare disease is largely confined to dock workers who unload infected pelts from abroad. The bacteria may invade only the skin, or can enter the lungs (causing severe pneumonia) or intestines by being inhaled or swallowed. Anthrax of the respiratory or digestive system is almost unknown in this country; both types result in serious, usually fatal illness and are almost impossible to diagnose until after the sufferer dies.

Cutaneous (skin) anthrax is slightly more common, and much easier to recognize. Its earliest symptom is a small pimple, which grows to 50mm (2in) or more across, with a black centre and swollen, itchy surrounding skin. The sufferer then develops a fever and feels increasingly ill.

If treated early, anthrax can be rapidly cured by injections of *antibiotic* drugs.

Bornholm's disease
(Coxsackie B virus, also called devil's grippe)

This viral infection is not common, and normally occurs in isolated incidents. We do not know how it spreads, but the symptoms are unmistakable. If you catch Bornholm's disease, you will suddenly begin to have severe, stabbing pains in either the chest or the abdomen. Each paroxysm of pain lasts for up to 30 minutes and there is complete relief between attacks, but there may be four or five such attacks every day. In addition you will develop a fever – up to 40°C (104°F) – often accompanied by headache, nausea, loss of appetite, and a dry cough.

There is no cure for Bornholm's disease, which, in spite of the pain and discomfort, is not a dangerous illness. It generally runs its course in three or four days, but it may be as long as two weeks before you feel completely well. To ease the sharp pains, your doctor will prescribe *analgesics*. You need not try to eat if you have no appetite, but you should drink plenty of fluids while you have a fever.

Leprosy

Leprosy (Hansen's disease) is a bacterial disease which, in spite of its reputation, can be caught only through prolonged, constant contact with a person who already has the disease. Though it does not kill, it can be disfiguring and even crippling because it causes permanent damage to skin and nerves. Among the symptoms are discoloured patches of hardened skin, lumps under the skin caused by a thickening around affected nerves, and paralysis of muscles controlled by the diseased nerves. The nerve damage numbs the hands and feet; as a result, fingers and toes can be damaged or even lost without the sufferer feeling any sensation.

Leprosy is a disease of tropical areas. About 15 million people throughout the world suffer from it; but there are only a few lepers in Britain, and nearly all of them are immigrants. The disease is curable by modern drugs. Treatment is slow, however, and may need to be continued for many years to prevent relapse. Sadly, the sufferer may well be left with permanent deformities.

Going abroad

If you are planning a trip abroad, make sure you are adequately protected against any dangerous diseases that may occur in your country of destination. About six weeks before you leave find out from your travel agent, airline, transport office, or the embassy concerned which vaccinations are compulsory for entry into the country, and which are sensible precautions in that area. Then, at least a month before you travel, consult your doctor. Discuss both official and advisable immunizations; do this in plenty of time because many vaccines have to be ordered in advance.

If you are going to a tropical or sub-tropical country, ask your doctor about tablets to protect you against malaria (opposite). You will probably have to start taking tablets before you set off, and continue throughout your visit and for one month after your return.

Some immunizations are not quite 100 per cent effective. In addition, there are many minor infections that you may catch, especially in tropical areas. So, while you are abroad, take the following precautions. Boil water and milk unless you are certain they are safe to drink; avoid eating salads, unpeeled fruits, and reheated foods; and *always* wash your hands before handling or eating any food.

Table of vaccinations for travel abroad

DISEASE	VACCINATION PROCEDURE	WHEN PROTECTION STARTS	HOW LONG PROTECTION LASTS	GEOGRAPHICAL AREA
Yellow fever	1 injection (there must be a 2-week gap between this injection and a polio vaccination)	10 days after injection	10 years	Compulsory for Africa, Central and South America
Cholera	1 injection	6 days after injection	6 months	Compulsory for most of Africa and tropical Asia
Polio	1 sugar cube (as a booster; see note below)	Immediately	3 years	Advisable for most tropical and sub-tropical countries, and all developing countries
Typhoid (and paratyphoid)	2 injections, 10 to 28 days apart	Immediately after 2nd injection	3 years	As for polio
Tetanus	1 booster injection (if 5 years since last booster; see note below)	Immediately	5 years	Everywhere
Hepatitis A	1 injection	Immediately	3 to 6 months	Advisable for most tropical and sub-tropical countries

Note: For infant and child immunizations see *Immunization*, p.701. If a booster is indicated on the above chart and you have not received any previous vaccinations for that particular disease, you will need to undergo the full course of treatment. A few countries still insist on smallpox vaccination.

Yellow fever

This viral illness, which usually attacks the liver, is carried by mosquitoes (and is also suffered by certain monkeys). It only occurs in Central and South America, and in parts of Africa. However, immunization is very effective and will usually be necessary for anyone who intends visiting those regions (see *Going Abroad*, above).

Attacks of yellow fever range from mild to fatal. A mild attack has symptoms similar to those of *influenza* (p.559). However, the symptoms of more severe cases include nausea, vomiting, bleeding, abdominal pains, and yellowing of the skin due to *jaundice* (p.485). The sufferer may feel very depressed and confused, and may even go into a coma. As with many viral illnesses, there is no really effective treatment for yellow fever, but a person who has recovered from the disease is immune for life.

Smallpox

Smallpox was a severe, highly infectious disease that often proved fatal. It began with flu-like symptoms that died down as the characteristic rash appeared. As the rash erupted, fever returned. People who survived the disease were left with varying degrees of scarring caused by the smallpox rash. The disease has now been eliminated, however, as the result of a successful worldwide vaccination campaign. Vaccination against smallpox is no longer necessary in most countries, and in 1980 the World Health Organization declared the disease officially extinct.

Smallpox viruses now exist only in medical laboratories, where they are controlled and maintained for research purposes.

Infestations

Infestations are invasions by parasites, which live either on the body (for example, lice) or in the body (for example, tapeworms). Parasites that live only on the skin usually cause no symptoms other than discomfort. Those that infest the inside of the body sometimes cause vague, ill-defined symptoms virtually unnoticed by the "host", and so they may remain undetected. If, however, they lodge in a vital place or become extremely numerous, they can cause severe problems.

It is almost impossible to get rid of parasites without treatment. The body does not normally have adequate natural defences against them. Fortunately, most types of dangerous infestation are rare in Britain, and parasite-killing drugs are highly effective in the few cases that do occur.

Malaria

Malaria is caused by minute one-celled parasites called plasmodia, which are transferred from one person to another by the female anopheles mosquito. There is no other carrier of the disease, and so plasmodia cannot enter your bloodstream unless you are bitten by a female anopheles mosquito that has sucked blood from someone who has malaria. (Very rarely the disease may be transmitted by a blood transfusion.)

Once in the bloodstream, the parasites travel to the liver, where they multiply rapidly. After several days, thousands of them flow back into the bloodstream, where they destroy red blood cells. In most cases, however, many parasites remain and multiply in the liver, and some of these are released into the bloodstream at intervals. This is why people with certain types of malaria have repeated attacks unless given proper treatment.

A particularly dangerous type of malaria is caused by plasmodium falciparum, one of the four species of plasmodia that affect human beings. In a person with falciparum malaria all the organisms are released from the liver into the bloodstream at the same time. Thus there is only one bout of the disease, but that bout is exceedingly severe.

Malaria-carrying mosquito
The tiny one-celled parasite that causes malaria is carried only by the female anopheles mosquito. When the mosquito bites a malaria sufferer, it sucks blood containing a few malaria parasites. The parasites multiply in the mosquito and, when this mosquito then bites another person, it injects thousands of parasites into the bloodstream.

What are the symptoms?
There are no symptoms at first. About nine to 30 days after the bite (depending on the type of plasmodium) a full day of headache, weariness, and nausea is followed by what is termed "the classical febrile paroxysm" of malaria. This lasts 12 to 24 hours. It consists of a sudden chill; then follows a feverish stage with no sweating and with rapid breathing; and a sweating stage accompanied by a fall in temperature. Similar bouts occur whenever more parasites are liberated into the bloodstream (generally every two or three days).

If malaria is untreated, attacks can continue to occur for years, but the sufferer slowly builds up a defence against the disease and the attacks come less often. Falciparum malaria is different in that its febrile paroxysm is likely to last for two or three days, to be exceptionally severe, and not to recur.

Children with malaria are apt to have prolonged high fever without chills; the effect of the fever on the brain sometimes causes unconsciousness or convulsions (*febrile* fits).

How common is the problem?
The anopheles mosquito does not live in northern Europe, but it is widespread in tropical and sub-tropical countries. However, the number of malaria cases in Britain rose sharply during the 1970s due to the rise in the number of immigrant sufferers and increased travel to equatorial regions.

What are the risks?
Since the malaria parasites destroy red blood cells, *anaemia* (p.419) may develop. Also the damaged cells clump together in small groups, which may block blood vessels and lead to brain or kidney damage. The chief threat comes from untreated falciparum malaria, which may block vessels in the brain or other vital organs and so prove fatal.

What should be done?
If you develop symptoms of malaria after a visit to a tropical or sub-tropical country, consult your doctor without delay. Be sure to tell the doctor where you have been and for how long. The doctor will probably arrange for blood tests at a local hospital or at a Tropical Disease Centre. Because it is not

always easy to detect the presence of parasites, you may need to stay in hospital so that blood tests can be taken at intervals.

What is the treatment?
Self-help: To guard against the infection, if you are going to visit a malarial area, ask your doctor to prescribe anti-malarial drugs to protect you. You must begin taking them before you travel, and continue to take them for one month after you have returned.

Professional help: Your doctor will prescribe a course of drugs to prevent malaria if you expect to be at risk.

If blood tests show that you have caught malaria, you will immediately start taking a drug to treat the disease. New and more efficient drugs to combat malaria are constantly being developed. With proper treatment, symptoms are relieved within a few hours, but the treatment must be continued for several weeks if the disease is not to recur.

Tapeworm

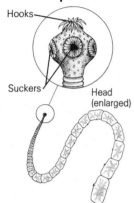

Hooks

Suckers

Head (enlarged)

Tapeworms are parasites that sometimes infest pigs and cattle. They can be passed into the human digestive system if a person eats infested pork or beef that has not been adequately cooked to kill the tapeworm. Within the human intestines a tapeworm anchors itself by attaching its head to the gut wall, and is nourished by absorbing food through its body walls. It may grow up to 10 metres (more than 30 feet) long. Segments break off and are excreted in the faeces, where they can be seen as short pieces of white ribbon.

What are the symptoms?
If the worm remains in the intestines, it does no great harm, but it often causes mild symptoms such as slight loss of weight, occasional abdominal pain, loss of appetite, and irritation around the anus.

What should be done?
Despite strict regulation of slaughterhouse procedures in Britain, occasional cases of tapeworm occur. Thorough cooking kills any worms that do exist, however. If you think you may have a worm, consult your doctor, who will probably want to examine a specimen of your faeces.

What is the treatment?
If necessary, the doctor will prescribe a drug to kill the worm. It will have effected a cure when you excrete the tapeworm's head, which may take several days.

Scabies

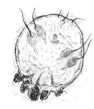

Scabies mite (greatly enlarged)

See p.248, **Visual aids to diagnosis, 67.**

Scabies is caused by a parasite, the itch mite, that burrows into the skin, laying eggs from which further mites emerge. The result is intense but relatively harmless irritation. Scabies rarely occurs on the head or face; it most often affects the hands, wrists, armpits, buttocks, or genital area. The mites are spread through close personal contact or through contact with infested clothes or bedding. Whole families sometimes have scabies. Spread of the mite is encouraged by several factors, among them overcrowding, poor hygiene, and sexual promiscuity.

What are the symptoms?
The main symptom is intense itching, which forces the sufferer to scratch affected areas in order to obtain relief. Continual scratching causes sores and scabs to form.

What should be done?
Although scabies occurs most commonly in unhygienic conditions, anyone can catch it. If your doctor diagnoses scabies, you will need to scrub all affected areas and then apply a prescribed *insecticide* to your whole body below the neck. You should repeat this procedure after a couple of days.

Itch mites that cause scabies do not live long if removed from human skin. Clothes and bedding are best treated as well, but items that for some reason cannot be laundered will be free of contamination if left isolated and unused for at least four days.

Lice

Lice are tiny but visible insects that live in the hair and suck blood from the skin. Infestation is often spread among children at school. Crab lice (see *Pubic lice,* p.613) live in the pubic hair and are usually spread by sexual intercourse. The eggs of lice are known as nits, and they too are visible as tiny white grains clinging to the hair. The bites of lice cause itching in affected areas, and there is a slight possibility of infection; but for the most part these parasites simply irritate rather than harm their hosts. The infestation is most

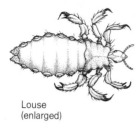

Louse
(enlarged)

common among those people who have poor and overcrowded living conditions.

What should be done?

If you find that your child has lice, report the fact to the school authorities; lice infestation is considered a public health hazard, and steps are always taken to trace sources and prevent further spreading.

What is the treatment?

For treatment, whether for a child or an adult, consult your doctor, who will prescribe a suitable shampoo or lotion. Two or three applications of this are necessary; although the first application may kill the lice, the nits are more difficult to remove. Headgear and any other clothing within which nits may be lodged should be burned.

Fleas

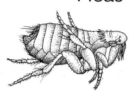

Flea
(enlarged)

See p.248,
**Visual aids to
diagnosis, 68.**

There are many species of flea, each parasitic on a different animal. With two exceptions – the sticktight and the jigger fleas, found in Africa, the West Indies, and the southern USA – animal fleas do not stay long on human skin. Fleas can leap great distances, and isolated flea bites on human skin are usually caused by animal (usually cat or dog) fleas temporarily leaving their hosts. Flea eggs hatch in bedding about seven days after they have been laid. The fleas may then live in the bedding, feeding off their animal hosts and, occasionally, humans. Their bites, made as they suck blood for nourishment, cause intense irritation for up to two days.

Flea infestations occur in all parts of the world, but are most common where there is close contact with domestic animals and where hygienic conditions are poor.

What should be done?

To avoid infestation, use anti-flea spray, powder, or shampoo on your pets' skin, and spray their bedding regularly as well. If you suspect infestation in your own bedding, furniture, or carpets you should apply a flea repellent to your skin and also spray the affected items. In severe cases it may be advisable to call in a professional fumigator to get rid of fleas in your home.

Some rare diseases caused by animal parasites

DISEASE	HOW CAUGHT	EFFECTS	SYMPTOMS	TREATMENT
Toxoplasmosis	By swallowing any substance containing the single-celled organism toxoplasma, which normally lives in the intestines of dogs and cats and is excreted in their faeces.	It invades the intestinal tract and may burrow into other parts of the body. It can enter the nervous system of young children or pass into the fetus of a pregnant woman. But serious complications are rare.	Usually symptomless but may cause vague abdominal pains and swollen lymph glands. It is a possible cause of meningitis in children or a fetal abnormality such as hydrocephalus (p.655) or, sometimes, brain malformation.	Prevention: Always wash animal and human eating utensils separately. Do not let dogs lick you. Cure: A 10-day course of a combination of drugs.
Hydatid disease	By swallowing eggs of a type of tapeworm that infests dogs and sheep. The tapeworm eggs are excreted in their faeces.	The tapeworm burrows into the body, where it grows into a cyst full of larvae. Cysts may form in almost any organ but take years to grow big enough to cause trouble.	A cyst in the liver may enlarge it. A cyst in the lung leads to shortness of breath. A cyst in the brain can cause fits.	Prevention: Wash hands before eating, especially if you work with sheep. Cure: Troublesome cysts must be removed surgically.
Toxocariasis	By swallowing eggs of toxocara, a small threadlike worm that lives in the intestines of dogs and cats.	The worm burrows into the body, where it may lodge in any organ. Children are more likely to be affected than adults.	There may be a slight fever and some respiratory difficulties. If a worm invades the eye, it can cause blindness. But usually there are no symptoms.	Prevention: Worm your pets regularly. Discourage them from licking children. Cure: If a child has the disease, remove all possible sources of infestation for about 6 months. If necessary, a special anti-parasite drug may be prescribed.

Special problems of men

Introduction

Male reproductive organs – the two testicles suspended in a sac (the scrotum) and the penis – are so intimately connected with organs of the urinary tract that disorders affecting one system often cause symptoms in the other. Each testicle consists of two elements: a gland (the testis) that produces sperm and the male sex hormone testosterone; and a long, tightly coiled tube called the epididymis, which lies behind the gland. Sperm are continually manufactured in each testis; they then pass into the epididymis, where they mature over a period of two to three weeks before being propelled into a duct known as the vas deferens, and then into the seminal vesicles, which produce seminal fluid. When you have an orgasm, your sperm pass into the urethra and are ejaculated in the seminal fluid. Thus your urethra, which runs from the bladder along the length of the penis, is a common passage for both seminal fluid and urine. (The muscular action of urination automatically closes the way into the urethra for seminal fluid, and vice versa.)

Sperm comprise only a small part of the seminal fluid, which is composed mainly of secretions from a number of glands. The various secretions probably act to mobilize the sperm and provide them with nutrients for their journey through the male and female reproductive tracts. The largest gland is the prostate, which encircles the top section of the narrow urethral channel at the point where the urethra leaves the bladder. Prostatic disease, therefore, can seriously affect both the reproductive and urinary systems. And, finally, the long urethra – very much longer than it is in women – can be affected because it is surrounded in the penis by the spongy, heavily veined tissues that make erections possible. Generally speaking, though, the length of the male urethra provides an effective barrier against invasion of the reproductive and urinary tracts by microbes. Infections of these tracts are, therefore, less common in men than in women.

The disorders discussed in the following articles are grouped according to the region of the urinary or reproductive system in which trouble can occur. A final grouping deals with sexual problems such as homosexuality and loss of sexual desire, which are primarily psychological.

The male reproductive organs

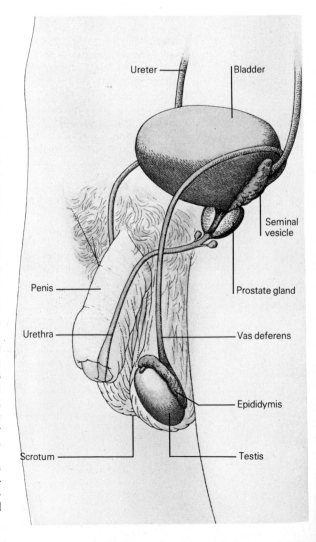

Ureter

Bladder

Seminal vesicle

Penis

Prostate gland

Urethra

Vas deferens

Epididymis

Scrotum

Testis

Testicles and scrotum

The paired male sex glands (testes) develop inside the abdomen of a male fetus; by the time of birth they will normally have descended through the abdominal wall to the familiar external position, where they hang suspended in a pouch of skin called the scrotum. (For a discussion of the problem of *undescended testes* see p.692.) Each gland is attached to the body by a single spermatic cord, which is composed of the sperm duct (vas deferens) and a number of nerves and blood vessels. The sperm that each testicle produces remain in the epididymis (a coiled tube lying behind the testis) for about three weeks, during which time they mature. They then pass into the vas deferens and seminal vesicles for storage; and, if not eventually ejaculated, they gradually disintegrate and are reabsorbed into the body. The following group of articles deals with disorders of the testis and epididymis (which, combined, form the testicle) and scrotum. The spermatic cord is not normally affected by disease.

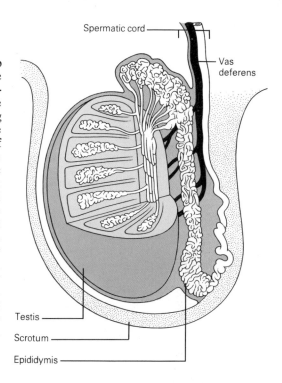

Spermatic cord

Vas deferens

Testis

Scrotum

Epididymis

Cancer of the testicle

Cancer occurs in the testicle when abnormal cells form and multiply uncontrolledly, producing a *malignant* tumour. Why this sometimes happens is not known. Unless the disease is treated at an early stage, the cancerous cells can spread (*metastasize*) via the *lymphatic system* (p.432) to lymph nodes in the abdomen, chest, and neck, and eventually to the lungs. Because there is no direct lymphatic connection between the two testicles, the disease is very unlikely to spread from one testicle to the other.

What are the symptoms?
The main symptom is a lump in the affected testicle. The lump grows slowly, and you may not be aware of it for some time since in 9 out of 10 cases there is no associated pain. You may well notice the swelling for the first time only when a minor injury to your scrotum forces you to examine the area closely. Alternatively, cancer may be discovered during a routine check-up.

How common is the problem?
Cancer of the testicle is rare. In an average year there are only about 600 new cases in Britain. It is, however, the most common type of cancer in younger men – those between the ages of 20 and 35. Three out of every four cases occur in men under 50.

What are the risks?
If cancer of the testicle remains undetected long enough to spread, it may reach vital parts of the body, particularly the lungs. With early detection and treatment, the chances for complete recovery are excellent.

What should be done?
As a preventive measure, get into the habit of examining your testicles at least once a week. If you notice a lump, no matter how trivial it seems, consult your doctor, who will probably refer you to a *urologist*. The swelling may well be harmless; there are often small swellings in the epididymis (see *Cysts of the epididymis*, p.573), and these are generally of no significance. A lump in the testis itself, however, is almost never harmless, and every such swelling must be explored surgically.

What is the treatment?
If your trouble is diagnosed as cancer, the only possible treatment is surgical removal of the affected gland.

The operation normally leaves one testicle intact, and so it is unlikely to have a marked effect on either potency or fertility. To make sure that all cancerous cells have been removed, you will probably be given a course of *radiotherapy* and perhaps some *cytotoxic* drugs for a short period after the operation. In rare cases in which neither radiotherapy nor drugs succeed in halting the spread of malignancy, certain lymph nodes may need to be removed. Unfortunately, such surgery (lymphadenectomy) involves cutting the nerves that control ejaculation; and so the sufferer is likely to become infertile – though not impotent since he can still have an erection and a "dry" orgasm.

Torsion of the testicle

Each testicle is enclosed in a fibrous double-layered sheath. A small amount of lubricating fluid lies between the two layers, thus permitting some movement of the contents. The sheathed testicle is attached to the spermatic cord in a way that prevents it from twisting out of its natural position. (Note that the normally close-fitting sheath is not to be confused with the scrotum, which is simply a loose pouch of skin in which the testicles hang.) In some males, though, the sheath is abnormally loose and baggy rather than firm. As a result, the testicle may become twisted. An extreme twist (torsion) can cause veins that lead from the testicle to be kinked, preventing blood from draining out of the organ, which then becomes swollen and painful. Such torsion can happen at any time, even when the sufferer is asleep.

What are the symptoms?
You feel a sudden pain in the testicle, and your scrotum soon becomes swollen, red, and tender. Intensity of pain varies; but it can be so severe that you feel nauseated and may vomit. In many cases the twisting comes undone of its own accord, resulting in immediate relief from pain.

How common is the problem?
Torsion of this type is very rare. Only about 1 male in 5,000 is likely to see a doctor about it in an average year. The problem occurs most often in adolescence, but it can happen at any age, even in infancy.

What are the risks?
If the twist does not come undone spontaneously and you do not see a doctor at once, arteries supplying the affected testicle will become blocked as well as veins, and the gland may die and shrivel away.

What should be done?
Even if the twist seems to have cured itself, see your doctor without delay. The doctor may try to undo the twist by gentle manipulation of the testicle. Even if this procedure relieves pain, however, there remains a probability of further torsion. Surgery is necessary in every case of torsion of the testicle, and it is usually done within hours of the attack. The operation effects a complete untwisting of the organ, if necessary, and the surgeon stitches the testicle in position so that the problem cannot recur. Because the bagginess of the sheath that permits torsion is likely to affect both testicles, however, the second one will probably be dealt with at the same time.

Injury to the testicles

An injury to the testicles usually causes severe pain, but you can assume there is no serious damage if the pain subsides within an hour or so and your scrotum is not bruised or swollen. Continued pain, bruising, or swelling is an indication of internal bleeding; go to your doctor or nearest hospital casualty unit without delay. If untreated, a blood clot may form and damage healthy testicular tissue. Surgery should allow full recovery within a few weeks.

Epididymitis

Inflammation of the epididymis (epididymitis) is caused by bacterial infection that has spread from the urinary tract into the sperm duct. The first sign that you are suffering from epididymitis is likely to be a sausage-shaped swelling – hot, tender, and very painful – lying in the back portion of one of your testicles. The swelling, which develops over the course of a few hours, is followed by a painful swelling and stiffening of the scrotum. The testis itself will be affected by the bacteria only if epididymitis is untreated.

How common is the problem?
Epididymitis is quite rare, chiefly because the kind of urinary-tract infection that can lead to the disorder rarely develops. When infection does occur, it normally produces symptoms that send the sufferer to his doctor before the infection has a chance to spread to the reproductive organs.

What should be done?
If you think you have epididymitis, consult your doctor without delay. Treatment with an

appropriate *antibiotic* almost always cures the disorder, but it is important to discover the cause of the urinary-tract infection that has led to your epididymitis. Such trouble in men usually is the result of some underlying structural abnormality in the bladder or kidneys. Your doctor will probably want you to have a series of diagnostic tests as soon as possible (for further details see *Cystitis in men*, p.577).

Cysts of the epididymis

Sometimes the tubes through which sperm pass from a testis to its epididymis develop *cysts* (fluid-filled out-pouchings). Although the cysts tend to grow because sperm accumulate within them, they are harmless. Cysts of the epididymis are very common; many men have at least one or two after the age of 40. The usual indication of their presence is a painless swelling in the upper rear portion of one or both testicles.

Your doctor is unlikely to recommend treatment unless your cysts grow too big for comfort (an extremely rare occurrence). When this happens, the cysts generally need to be cut away. Such surgery often results in sterilization of the affected testicle, so there may be a reduction in fertility.

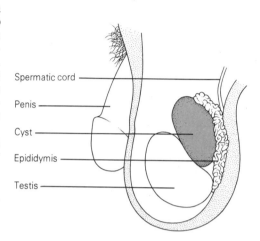

Spermatic cord

Penis

Cyst

Epididymis

Testis

Hydrocele

The normal double-layered sheath around each testicle (see *Torsion of the testicle*, opposite) contains just enough fluid for good lubrication. Sometimes, however, an excessive amount may be produced, forming what is known as a hydrocele – a soft, usually painless swelling around the testicle. Hydroceles are occasionally caused by inflammation or injury, but there is usually no obvious cause. They are harmless and quite common, especially in elderly men.

If you think you have a hydrocele, consult your doctor. Treatment is rarely necessary, but if the hydrocele becomes very large or painful, the fluid can be drawn off with a needle. This minor operation can be done in a few minutes with a local anaesthetic. Unfortunately, the problem tends to recur. If you have a troublesome recurring hydrocele, your doctor may advise surgery to remove part of the fibrous sheath so that fluid can no longer accumulate within it.

Hydrocele
A swelling caused by the accumulation of a clear, thin fluid between the outer and inner layers covering the testis may affect only 1 testis. Consult your doctor no matter how small and painless such a scrotal swelling may be.

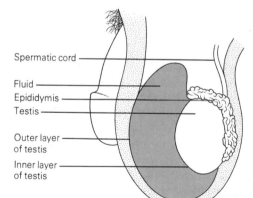

Spermatic cord

Fluid
Epididymis
Testis

Outer layer of testis

Inner layer of testis

Varicocele

If the veins that drain one of your testicles become abnormally distended, like varicose veins in the legs, you have a mild disorder called varicocele. There is usually no obvious cause for the condition, which produces a swelling around the testicle. The swelling tends to disappear when you lie down, but it is sometimes accompanied by an uncomfortable, dragging pain, especially in hot weather or after you have been exercising. The problem is most common in adolescents. Your doctor will probably recommend that you wear tight-fitting underwear or a jockstrap to relieve any pain. No other treatment is usually necessary unless the varicocele seems to be affecting your fertility (a rare but possible complication). In such a case your doctor may suggest an operation to remove the distended veins. Unfortunately the results of this surgery may be disappointing.

Prostate gland

The prostate gland is a cluster of little glands surrounding the urethra at the point where it leaves the bladder. The glands are tubular, with muscles that squeeze their secretions into the urethra. The exact function of the prostate gland is unclear; it is thought likely that the addition of secretions produced by the gland to the seminal fluid somehow stimulates active movement of the sperm after they have been ejaculated. The main disorders that can affect the prostate are infections and growths, which are seldom *malignant*. Because the prostate encircles the urethra, any prostate trouble is likely to hamper the free flow of urine from the bladder to the outside.

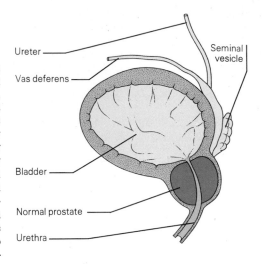

Ureter
Seminal vesicle
Vas deferens
Bladder
Normal prostate
Urethra

Enlarged prostate
(*benign prostatic hypertrophy*)

Routine tests show that nearly every man over 45 has some degree of enlargement of the prostate gland; harmless growths of normal prostate tissue are a natural result of the ageing process. What happens is that little gristly nodules gradually develop, and their accumulation changes the size of the gland. The change may cause no trouble even if the prostate becomes quite swollen. The size of a *benign* enlargement matters less than the consistency of the tissues. In some men the prostate gland, which normally relaxes to permit free flow of urine from the bladder through the urethra, becomes stiff and inflexible. Even stiffened prostates do not necessarily cause problems, however. As the gland grows more rigid, constricting the urethra that it surrounds, the muscles of the bladder tend to compensate by becoming more powerful. This extra strength is often enough to keep the urethral exit open. Serious trouble occurs only when the bladder muscles are unable to overcome resistance caused by the rigid prostatic tissue and the flow of urine is badly obstructed.

What are the symptoms?
Symptoms of severe prostate enlargement vary widely, but one symptom experienced by every sufferer is a weak urinary stream. You are likely to have a frequent urge to urinate (an urge so strong that it may wake you several times a night), yet manage to pass only a dribble whenever you try. You may also find that, no matter how strong the urge, it is difficult to start the sluggish stream; this is apt to be particularly noticeable first thing in

the morning. There is hardly ever any pain, and there is no surface swelling or lump since the prostate gland is deep within the lower abdomen. Occasionally, though, there may be blood in the urine (*haematuria*).

How common is the problem?
Prostate enlargement, though extremely common in men over 45, rarely becomes troublesome before the age of 55. Serious urinary trouble due to this disorder affects 1 in 10 elderly males.

What are the risks?
The condition is not dangerous in itself, but there are three main risks. First, if the bladder is never entirely emptied, pools of stagnant urine within it can become infected (see *Cystitis in men*, p.577). Secondly, as the muscular wall of the bladder strengthens in order to force urine through the narrowed urethra, the wall may become so thick that it pinches the ureters (the tubes that carry urine to the bladder from the kidneys). This can lead to *acute pyelonephritis* (p.502). Finally, if severe enlargement of the prostate remains untreated, the muscles of the bladder may no longer be able to overcome the resistance to urine flow and may suddenly or gradually fail to function.

Sudden failure occurs when, all at once, the bladder ceases to expel its contents. This condition is called acute *retention*. It is rare, but very painful, and requires emergency treatment. Gradual failure, which is more common, occurs when the amount of urine that can be expelled decreases little by little.

The effect of an enlarged prostate
When an enlarged prostate obstructs the urethra, and so reduces the flow of urine, the muscular wall of the bladder gradually thickens and strengthens as it works harder to force urine through the urethra.

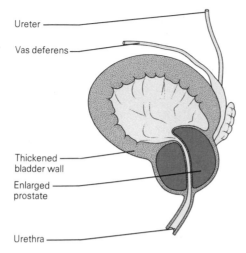

Ureter

Vas deferens

Thickened bladder wall

Enlarged prostate

Urethra

If the condition is allowed to persist, the quantity of residual urine in the bladder may become so great that the abdomen swells as if with pregnancy. More often than not, some of the accumulated urine dribbles away whenever the sufferer coughs, sneezes, or strains. If the condition is allowed to persist without treatment, sufferers will eventually develop acute retention or possibly even *kidney failure* (p.511).

What should be done?

If you have symptoms of an enlarged prostate, consult your doctor, who will examine the gland by means of a gloved finger inserted in the rectum and may then refer you to a *urologist* for tests. The urologist will observe your urinary stream, perhaps recording it with a gadget called a urine-flow meter. You may also be given an *intravenous pyelogram (IVP)* to rule out the possibility that your symptoms may be due to urinary-tract disease rather than to an enlarged prostate and to find out whether your bladder, ureters, or kidneys have been damaged in any way by pressure from the enlargement.

If you have the symptoms of acute retention, see your doctor or go to your local hospital without delay. Your bladder will need to be emptied by means of a *catheter* before the basic trouble can be first diagnosed and then treated.

What is the treatment?

If your symptoms are mild, and diagnostic tests indicate that urgent treatment is unnecessary, your doctor will probably take no action. In at least one in three mild cases the symptoms clear up without treatment, and so it is sensible to wait for a while. But if the problem does not go away or worsens, or if tests reveal serious obstruction to the flow of urine, the tissue that is causing the enlargement of your prostate must be removed.

The operation – called prostatectomy – can be done by traditional surgery or by a more modern method known as transurethral resection (TUR). Surgery to cut away the excess tissue involves an incision in the lower part of the abdomen.

In transurethral resection a thin tube is passed up the urethra to the prostate. In the tip of the tube is a loop of wire that can be heated by an electric current and manipulated with the help of a miniature telescope to slice away the troublesome nodules. This procedure requires a hospital stay of only four or five days (as compared with 10 to 14 days for surgery), and there is less postoperative pain. For one reason or another, however, TUR is not feasible in some cases.

What are the long-term prospects?

Regardless of the technique, most prostatectomies are successful; they relieve urinary difficulties, and prostate trouble seldom recurs. There may be some damage to the nerve supply of the penis, however, especially from traditional surgery. As a result, some sufferers lose their potency after the operation, and others remain potent but sterile because their semen is expelled backwards into the bladder instead of being ejaculated. Fortunately, the age of most men who need prostatectomy is such that they are not concerned about their loss of fertility. Seminal fluid in the bladder does no harm; it is expelled in the urine.

Cancer of the prostate

Cancer of the prostate does not normally progress in the manner typical of most cancers. Instead of spreading, this *malignancy* tends to lie dormant, seldom causing symptoms or giving rise to health problems. When – rarely – there are noticeable symptoms, they are indistinguishable from those of a *benign* enlargement of the prostate (see *Enlarged prostate,* opposite). Indeed, the fact that the growths on the gland are malignant is often discovered only during an operation for apparently benign prostate trouble.

There is a risk, however, that if the cancer is not discovered, it may *metastasize,* usually to the bones. This does not happen in most cases; but when it does, the sufferer will have symptoms of cancer of the bone (see *Bone tumours,* p.545), and in some cases it is these secondary symptoms that eventually indicate the presence of the primary malignant growth in the prostate gland.

How common is the problem?

Cancer of the prostate is rare in the young, but becomes increasingly common with age. About 15 per cent of all 40-year-old men have this relatively low-risk form of cancer. At the age of 80 virtually every male has it. But it causes the deaths of fewer than 1 man in 1,000. If you are over 50 when you discover you have developed the disorder, you will most probably die from some other, unconnected, cause.

What should be done?

If you have the characteristic symptoms of an enlarged prostate, your doctor will refer you to a *urologist*, who will begin by assuming that the affected tissues are benign. If, however, a rectal examination raises a suspicion that the tissues may be malignant, you will be advised to undergo a prostate *biopsy*. If cancer cells are found, you will then be given a *radio-isotope bone scan* to determine whether the cancer has spread to your bones.

What is the treatment?

Malignancy that has spread to the bones or any other part of the body will be treated in the appropriate way. In addition, any malignant tissues that remain in the prostate gland after you have had an operation for enlargement may be treated with *radiotherapy* in order to prevent further metastasis.

Most doctors agree that it is generally best not to attempt special treatment for cancer that remains confined to the prostate gland and gives you no trouble. Your urologist is likely to advise doing nothing apart from having regular check-ups to make sure that the malignancy has not spread. There are two good reasons for doing nothing. First, as stated above, this type of cancer seldom spreads and rarely gives serious trouble. Secondly, the traditional treatment – removal of the entire prostate – is a serious operation, with inevitable risks, that does not guarantee a cure for the basic disease.

Prostatitis

Prostatitis (inflammation of the prostate gland) is usually the result of a urinary-tract infection (see, for example, *Cystitis in men*, opposite) that has spread to the prostate. As with infection and inflammation anywhere in the body, prostatitis may get better of its own accord, may fester and form pus, or may linger indefinitely, becoming chronic.

What are the symptoms?

An acute attack of prostatitis (one that comes on suddenly) makes you feel generally ill, with a high fever, chills, and pain in and around the base of your penis. Later, as the prostate becomes increasingly swollen and tender, you may find it difficult and painful to pass urine through the narrowed urethra. Chronic prostatitis and mild attacks that clear up on their own may be symptom-free.

How common is the problem?

Prostatitis is not common; roughly 1 male in 2,000 sees a doctor about it in an average year. Elderly men with *enlarged prostates* (p.574) are most susceptible to this type of infection, and the disease tends to recur once you have had an initial attack.

What are the risks?

If prostatitis is untreated, or if, as sometimes happens, treatment by drugs is unsuccessful, the gland may fester, become pus-filled, and burst open, releasing pus into the urethra. This is not only painful, but the bursting can form a *fistula* (abnormal channel) through which pus continues to flow into the urethra. The result may well be severe infection anywhere in the urinary tract.

What should be done?

If you suspect you have prostatitis, consult your doctor, who, after listening to an account of your symptoms, will probably feel your prostate gland (by inserting a gloved finger into your rectum) to determine whether it is swollen and tender. The doctor will also want a sample of urine for analysis in order to identify the microbes that may be causing the inflammation.

What is the treatment?

If your trouble is clearly due to bacterial infection, your doctor will prescribe a course of *antibiotics*, which usually clears up the problem. In most cases, there is no need to abstain from sexual intercourse during treatment; in fact, it is often thought to be beneficial. Occasionally, drugs do not entirely cure prostatitis. If your disorder resists antibiotic treatment and if pus accumulates in your prostate, the doctor may need to perform an operation to drain it out. Such an operation means only a few days in hospital, and usually clears up the infection completely.

Bladder, urethra, and penis

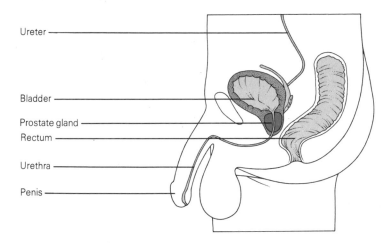

Ureter

Bladder

Prostate gland

Rectum

Urethra

Penis

For a full discussion of the structure of the bladder and urethra, as well as their structural relationships to the rest of the urinary tract, see *Disorders of the urinary tract* (p.500). In males the urethra is joined near the point where it leaves the bladder by several ducts that carry seminal fluid to the outside during ejaculation. And the many small glands that

we call the *prostate gland* (see p.574) surround the whole complex passageway.

The urethra runs for most of its length within the penis. The penis itself is composed mainly of spongy tissues full of tiny blood vessels. In an erect penis the spongy tissues are engorged with blood. In a relaxed penis the slightly bulbous end (known as the glans) is covered by a loose flap of skin (the foreskin or prepuce). In some religions or cultures, foreskins are traditionally removed, often just after birth. Apart from considerations of religion and ritual, such surgery (circumcision) is not advised routinely by British doctors. (For a discussion of the advantages and disadvantages see *Should I have my son circumcised?* p.644.)

In general the male bladder, urethra, and penis are not in themselves particularly susceptible to disease. The disorders discussed below are, in the main, rare. For conditions that affect, but do not originate in, these parts of the body consult appropriate articles in other sections of the book such as *Disorders of the urinary tract* (p.500) and *Special problems of couples* (p.606).

Cystitis in men

Cystitis (inflammation of the bladder) is a common and relatively harmless condition in women (see *Cystitis in women*, p.600). It is rare in males, but potentially more serious because it is usually caused by either an underlying urinary-tract disorder (such as a structural abnormality or a tumour) or an infection that has spread from elsewhere in the tract. The symptoms of the inflammation itself are similar to those of cystitis in women; but because such symptoms are probably secondary, indicating existence of a primary problem, you should see your doctor without delay. Although *antibiotic* drugs may well cure your inflamed bladder, the doctor will almost certainly want you to undergo tests in hospital to discover the underlying cause of the trouble. Such tests will probably include *cystoscopy* and an *intravenous pyelogram (IVP)*. Once the underlying problem has been identified, further treatment will be the appropriate one for that disorder.

Penile warts

Warts on the penis are similar to warts elsewhere on the skin (for full information on *warts* in general see p.252). Do not assume, however, that any wart-like growths on your penis – or just inside the urethral opening, where they sometimes appear – are necessarily true, harmless warts. Occasionally, a growth that resembles a wart may be an early symptom of either *cancer of the penis* (p.579) or *syphilis* (p.612). So always consult your doctor if you develop what looks like a penile wart or warts. If the doctor confirms the diagnosis of warts, he or she will probably prescribe a specific type of paint for removing them. Be sure to follow carefully the doctor's directions for applying the paint. Never try to treat warts on the penis with an over-the-counter preparation for warts elsewhere on the skin. The sensitive skin of the penis can be easily damaged by the powerful chemicals in ordinary wart paint.

Like all warts, those on the penis are caused by localized areas of viral infection and are therefore to some extent *contagious*;

in fact, warts on the genital area can sometimes be transmitted by intercourse. So if you have (or have had) penile warts, it is a good idea for your sexual partner to consult her doctor to make sure she does not have *vulval warts* (p.603), which might cause you to become reinfected when your own warts have been successfully treated.

Urethritis in men

Urethritis (inflammation of the urethra) in men is usually caused by an infection transmitted through sexual intercourse with an infected partner. The major symptoms are a copious, thick, yellow discharge from the tip of the penis, a scalding pain on passing urine (*dysuria*), and pain on ejaculation. Among the many forms of male urethritis the most common are *non-specific urethritis* (p.612) – generally known as NSU – and *gonorrhoea* (p.611). Because these diseases can become a problem for both sexual partners, they are discussed in the section of the book dealing with *Special problems of couples* (p.606).

Urethral stricture

Urethral stricture is a rare condition in which the urethra becomes shortened and narrowed as a result of the gradual shrinkage of scar tissue within its walls. The scar or scars are likely to have been caused by some sort of injury in the genital area; a common cause of urethral scar tissue used to be persistent *urethritis in men* (above) due to infection, but modern treatment of diseases such as *gonorrhoea* (p.611) has virtually eliminated them as causes. The narrowed tube of a sufferer from urethral stricture may make it increasingly difficult for him to pass urine, and ejaculation may also be painful. And the lengthwise contraction may force his erect penis into an awkwardly bent position.

Urethral scar tissue
A urethra that has been damaged by an accident or disease will usually heal readily. However, the healing tissue may become scarred, making that part of the urethra narrower and less pliable. Severe scarring of the urethra can, in some cases, completely block the flow of urine.

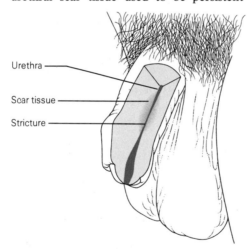

Urethra

Scar tissue

Stricture

What should be done?
If you have an increasingly troublesome urethral stricture, your doctor will probably refer you to a *urologist*, who may try to stretch the tube by means of a long, flexible instrument called a bougie or sound. This is inserted gently through the opening in the penis after you have been given a local anaesthetic. You will need a series of such treatments (*dilatations*) during the course of several weeks and will require follow-up treatments at intervals thereafter. If they do not cure the stricture, the urologist may recommend surgery to cut the scarred tissue or to remove it and replace it with grafted tissue.

Balanitis

Balanitis is the general term for several types of inflammation of the foreskin and underlying glans (another name for which is the balanus). The cause of this common complaint may be infection (see *Herpes genitalis*, p.613), friction with damp garments, or irritation from chemical substances in clothing or contraceptive sheaths or creams. Diabetics are especially susceptible because the excess sugar in their urine permits microbes to multiply. In some cases of balanitis the soreness and swelling at the end of the penis are increased because it becomes difficult to draw the foreskin back in order to clean the area. One rare form of the condition (called balanitis xerotica obliterans) has no known cause and does not itself cause the familiar redness and soreness of most kinds of inflammation. Instead the foreskin and/or glans become abnormally pale and shrivelled. Although painless, this condition may not only make the foreskin irretractable but may narrow the opening of the urethra, obstructing the easy passage of urine.

What is the treatment?
If you have balanitis, it is important to keep the area both clean and dry. Most kinds of balanitis will clear up – if you discover the cause and remove it – with the aid of a

soothing ointment; your local chemist can recommend an appropriate one. If the problem persists or if it is painful or difficult to draw back your foreskin, consult your doctor, who may prescribe *antibiotic* cream or tablets to relieve the inflammation. In stubborn cases the only answer may be either surgical loosening of the foreskin or circumcision (see *Should I have my son circumcised?*, p.644). If your trouble is balanitis xerotica obliterans, you may also need a minor operation to widen the opening of the urethra.

Priapism

An erection that persists in the absence of sexual arousal and cannot be made to subside is known as priapism. This is a rare and painful condition. It is usually caused by a sudden, inexplicable obstruction to the outflow of engorging blood from the erect penis. Occasionally, however, it may be due to disease or injury of nerves in the spinal cord that control erection.

What are the risks?
Whatever the cause, priapism is a serious matter; if the abnormal erection lasts for three or four hours, the spongy tissues of the penis may be permanently damaged, with erection never again possible.

What should be done?
If you have a painful erection that persists for no apparent reason, do not waste time trying to get it down with cold compresses or other home remedies. You should go to the nearest hospital at once.

What is the treatment?
Priapism is an emergency, and surgery to bypass the blockage and allow blood to drain out of the penis and back into the general circulation is the only possible treatment. The wound from the operation usually heals in a few days and, if treatment has been carried out in time, you should eventually be able to have normal erections again.

Cancer of the penis

This is a relatively rare form of *malignancy*: in Britain only about 15 men die of cancer of the penis in an average year. The cause of the disease is not known, but there is a high correlation between its development and many years of poor hygiene. Circumcised males are less susceptible than uncircumcised males to this problem – though if you wash your foreskin and glans regularly you run hardly any risk of developing the disease. The disease is most common in the elderly.

What are the symptoms?
The major symptom is a sore spot, an ulcer, or a warty lump that slowly spreads across the skin of the penis and down into deeper tissues. If untreated, the malignancy will *metastasize* (spread to other parts of the body, most often via the lymphatic system or the bloodstream). Cancer of the penis tends to spread first to the lymph glands in the groin, causing them to become swollen.

What should be done?
If you have a sore that discharges pus, or any type of growth on your penis, consult your doctor, who will probably want to have a *biopsy* taken for laboratory examination before diagnosing your trouble as cancer of the penis rather than *syphilis* (p.612) or merely harmless *penile warts* (p.577).

When cancer of the penis is discovered at an early stage of development, it can almost always be cured by *radiotherapy*. Only in late, neglected cases does surgical removal of the penis become necessary.

Haemospermia

"Haemospermia" means blood in the semen; the blood usually appears as pinkish, reddish, or brownish streaks in the seminal fluid. The cause of haemospermia is the rupture of little veins in the upper part of the urethra. This can happen during an erection, is quite common, and usually goes unnoticed.

What should be done?
If you or your sexual partner do notice your haemospermia, do not be concerned. Tiny holes in the veins always close up within a few minutes (although your semen may remain discoloured for several days).

There is no need to consult a doctor if you are sure that the blood was actually in the semen. However, if you think it may have come from the urethra *after* ejaculation, you should see a doctor so that the possibility of bladder trouble can be ruled out. Remember that whereas haemospermia is harmless, *haematuria* (blood in the urine) may be a symptom of serious trouble (see, for example, *Tumours of the bladder*, p.508).

Sexual problems of men

Sexuality depends on psychological as well as physical factors. By the sixth week of life inside the uterus, a male child has developed internal sex glands that secrete the male hormone testosterone, which almost certainly affects not only the body but the brain. Then, after birth, the child's sense of masculine identity and behaviour is reinforced by those around him who consider certain clothes, toys, and character traits – physical courage, for instance – appropriate for a boy. By the age of five the sense of belonging to the male sex has probably become firmly fixed in his mind; and this sense is confirmed at puberty, with the development of secondary sexual characteristics (for further details see *Special problems of adolescents*, p.706).

If this developmental pattern does not occur or fails to progress throughout life, the result is a departure from the norm, and our society has tended to view any such "deviation" – which may be physical, psychological, or both – as a social problem. The variations discussed in the following pages are probably the most common: homosexuality, transvestism, transsexualism, and the loss of normal sexual desire. Such variations are not necessarily disorders in themselves, and the increasingly enlightened approach of Western societies has begun to improve the self-respect of men who used to dread the humiliation of being discovered to be "different". However, traditional social prejudices can still create problems for them, and special advice may be needed.

(For articles dealing with problems especially affecting one-to-one relationships see *Sexual problems*, p.614.)

Male homosexuality

Myths about male homosexuality

All homosexual men are effeminate.

Wrong. Many homosexual males are as masculine in behaviour as are most heterosexuals. Some apparently effeminate men, in fact, are entirely heterosexual in tastes and practice.

All homosexuals are paedophiles.

Wrong. A paedophile is sexually aroused by children. Some homosexual men are indeed attracted to little boys, but most are not – just as most heterosexuals are not aroused by little girls.

Although homosexuality is sometimes a problem, it is not a disease. Apart from the fact that a homosexual male is erotically attracted to other males rather than females, he does not necessarily differ from heterosexuals. He may be just as masculine in behaviour and just as stable in sexual relationships. Social discrimination against homosexuals is largely based on prejudice; but because of it many homosexuals find it difficult to lead happy lives. Fortunately, Western societies are becoming more tolerant of what used to be called "perversion", and so homosexual men are likely to have easier lives in the future.

Nobody knows precisely why the homosexual is as he is. The most important factors, however, seem to be psychological rather than physical. (For information about *female homosexuality* see p.604.)

How common is the problem?

Nearly everybody has had some slight homosexual experience, especially in adolescence. Such experiences are common among men deprived of female company – for example, in single-sex institutions such as boys' boarding schools. But most adult males in a mixed society are not sexually attracted to other males. Only about 1 man in 20 leads an exclusively homosexual life in this country; the ratio becomes higher – perhaps 1 in 10 – if bisexuals (males who respond sexually to both men and women) are included.

What should be done?

You are likely to discover, rather than choose, your sexual orientation. If you feel homosexual impulses in adolescence, this is of little significance as long as you eventually become aroused by girls. If, when you reach manhood, you find that only males arouse you, you may be right to consider yourself homosexual. And if you can accept this fact, you do not need to seek help – unless, however, you are attracted to boys below the legal age of consent; in that case you should discuss the problem openly with your doctor or with a *psychiatrist* without delay.

If you find your homosexuality disturbing, you can seek guidance from a number of agencies that assist people with anxieties about sexual orientation. The *Albany Trust* (p.768) is one such agency. Others generally advertise their services in telephone directories. Psychological treatment is also available for homosexuals who wish they could become heterosexual; your doctor can probably refer you to a helpful clinic. *Psychotherapy* usually aims at investigating the underlying causes of your problem, at reducing anxiety brought on by heterosexual encounters, and at making you responsive to heterosexual stimulation. You will also be helped to improve your social skills with women. Although such treatment tends to be effective mainly with men who have not led wholly homosexual lives, do not hesitate to seek this type of help.

Transvestism

A transvestite male is addicted to "cross-dressing" – that is, wearing women's clothes. Although many transvestites can become sexually aroused only if dressed as women, they are not necessarily attracted to other men. *Male homosexuality* (opposite) and transvestism are different types of sexual behaviour, though both may occur together.

What should be done?

Transvestism is harmless and need not distress a tolerant sexual partner. But there are occasional males who lean towards transvestism without being entirely dependent on it for sexual arousal, and they sometimes feel that it adversely affects their sex life. Any such individual should have a frank talk with his sexual partner, who may well turn out to be quite understanding. If your transvestism worries you, consult your doctor or a *psychotherapist.* Professional counselling may help you either to live with the problem or to find new and perhaps more rewarding types of sexual behaviour.

Male transsexualism

A male transsexual is convinced that he is female despite his masculine body.

Transsexualism in a man should not be confused with *male homosexuality* (opposite); the transsexual generally wishes he could change his sex so as to have a heterosexual relationship with a man. And although the transsexual may wear women's clothes, he differs from transvestites (see *Transvestism*, above) in that transvestites do not usually wish they had female bodies. Transsexualism is very rare.

If you are transsexual, consult your doctor, who will probably refer you to a psychiatrist.

Some transsexuals are helped by being given female sex hormones (oestrogens), which reduce facial hair and cause breasts to develop. This treatment, along with counselling and training in accepted female skills, can help the transsexual to assume a female role, if not all the bodily features.

Sometimes the only answer is surgery to convert male sexual organs to female ones. There are limits, however, to what such a "sex-change" operation can achieve. Many transsexuals are dissatisfied with the results, and continuing psychological counselling is often necessary.

Loss of sexual desire in men

The male sex hormone testosterone is responsible for sexual drive. If, therefore, your testosterone level is lowered, your *libido* (sexual interest and capacity for arousal) is likely to diminish. The underlying cause of the drop in testosterone level may be a physical complaint such as liver, kidney, or pituitary disease or a side-effect of certain drugs. Or the cause may be fatigue, stress, or pain. Most often, though, the root of the problem is mainly psychological.

Some sufferers lose their desire for sex in general, but loss of sexual interest in a familiar partner is the most common complaint. This is apt to happen when there are other problems (which may or may not be sexual) in the relationship. A complaint such as *impotence* or *premature ejaculation* (p.614) that tends to interfere with the enjoyment of lovemaking can cause a man to shun sex instead of wanting it. And sometimes a particular problem with one partner is repeated with successive partners until sex in general loses its attractions.

How common is the problem?

Generalized loss of sexual desire is not a common complaint. However, loss of interest in a sexual relationship in which the excitement of novelty has worn off is a common cause of loss of sexual desire.

What should be done?

If self-help measures recommended below do not help you to regain sexual desire, consult your doctor, who will probably examine you to find out if there is a physical cause. If none seems likely, you may be referred to a specialist in sexual or marital problems.

What is the treatment?

Self-help: It may help to discuss the problem openly with your partner in a straightforward effort to clear up possible misunderstandings. If you are bored with a long-standing relationship, try to freshen it up by experimenting with new approaches to making love.

Professional help: Treatment depends on the underlying cause, which is often difficult to determine. *Psychotherapy* can be particularly valuable for those men worried about problems such as impotence or premature ejaculation. Treatment may include self-help exercises, discussion of relaxation techniques, and a review of some facts about sexual arousal that you may have forgotten.

Special problems of women

Introduction

The problems dealt with in this section are mainly exclusive to women. Aspects of female health not discussed here are covered in other sections of the book. They include *pregnancy and childbirth* (p.616), problems of adolescent girls, *special problems of the elderly* (p.716), *special problems of couples* (p.606) (including sexually transmitted diseases), and general problems that affect women in much the same way as they affect men.

The first group of articles in this section deals with problems connected with the menstrual cycle – the four-weekly cycle of egg ripening, egg release, and shedding of the lining of the uterus (womb) as a period. The menstrual cycle is controlled by a complex system of hormones, and the cycle is disturbed if the hormonal balance is upset by any one of a number of factors, some of them emotional.

The second group of articles concerns breast problems. Although men can also have such problems, particularly nipple disorders, these are extremely rare in comparison with the high number of breast problems among women. Breast *abscess*, which is more common shortly after childbirth, is included here because it can also occur at other times, but other post-natal breast problems are discussed under *post-natal problems for the mother* (p.641).

Another group of articles deals specifically with disorders of the female reproductive organs – the ovaries, uterus, and cervix – which are more likely to occur as a woman approaches middle age and which may also be affected by the hormonal changes associated with middle age. The group of articles on diseases of the bladder and urethra is included here because such disorders in women tend to be different from those in men. Disorders of the vagina and vulva (the canal leading from the uterus and cervix to the outside and the area around the opening of this canal, respectively) are discussed in a separate group of articles from those that deal with the reproductive organs. This is because such problems are generally less serious and more easily treated than problems of the reproductive organs. Finally, female sexual problems are covered at the end of the section.

If you suffer from one of the disorders in this section, you may need to consult your family doctor. In some

The female lower-abdominal organs

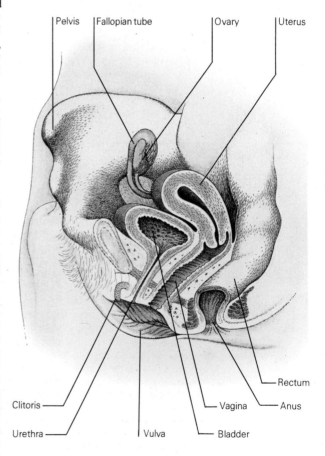

cases, the doctor will refer you to a gynaecologist for expert diagnosis and treatment. If no serious underlying disorder is found, the gynaecologist will usually relieve your problem by treating your symptoms and this may be enough to prevent recurrence of the trouble.

Menstruation and the menopause

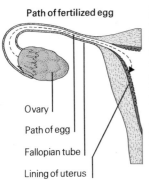

Path of fertilized egg

Ovary

Path of egg

Fallopian tube

Lining of uterus

The menstrual cycle (28 days)

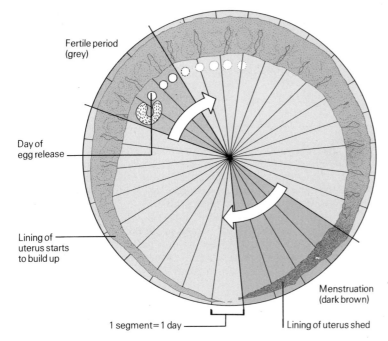

Fertile period
(grey)

Day of
egg release

Lining of
uterus starts
to build up

1 segment = 1 day

Menstruation
(dark brown)

Lining of uterus shed

Each month, if you are a woman of fertile years, ovulation (egg production) occurs. One of your two ovaries releases an egg (ovum). The egg is a single cell, barely visible to the naked eye, that is drawn into the fallopian tube with the help of the tentacle-like hairs at its mouth and then travels down the fallopian tube to the uterus (womb). This journey takes about five days. After sexual intercourse, male sperm make their way up to the fallopian tubes. If you have sexual intercourse within a day or two before or after the release of the egg, a sperm may fertilize the egg. It is to prepare for the possibility of fertilization that, during the nine days or so preceding ovulation, the lining of your uterus thickens and becomes engorged with blood. It is then in a suitable condition for a fertilized egg that reaches the uterus to burrow into it and start developing into an embryo. When this happens, you are pregnant.

If the egg is not fertilized, the thickened, blood-filled lining of the uterus is not required. Both the unfertilized egg and the lining are shed about 14 days after the start of ovulation (even if ovulation occurs irregularly), and pass through the cervix (the neck of the uterus) into the vagina, and then out of your body. This discharge, called menstruation or a period, lasts on average for five days. During the next nine days a new lining grows in the uterus, after which ovulation starts again. The entire cycle lasts on average 28 days. But in most women, the cycle fluctuates in length – sometimes by a day or two, sometimes by longer.

Each stage in the menstrual cycle is controlled by a system of interrelated hormones and other chemicals produced in the hypothalamus (part of the brain), the pituitary gland, and the ovaries.

Menstruation usually starts between the ages of 11 and 14. The first period is called the *menarche*. Periods are irregular for the first year or two because ovulation often fails to occur. Periods also become irregular, for the same reason, after the age of 45, as the years of fertility draw to a close. Finally, periods cease altogether – the last period is known as the menopause.

The various problems relating to the length, frequency, and effect of periods are covered in the following articles.

Amenorrhoea

Amenorrhoea is the medical term for the temporary or permanent absence of periods. In some girls, periods fail to start at the normal age, which is usually between 11 and 14. This is known as primary amenorrhoea. It is generally the result of natural late onset of puberty (see *Early or late development*, p.706), but rarely it is due to some abnormality in the reproductive or hormonal system.

In a woman who has had regular periods, a delay or absence of periods is called secondary amenorrhoea. It is due to a change in the balance of hormones that control the release of an egg from the ovary. Such a change occurs with the onset of pregnancy. The hormones may also be disrupted by emotional factors (for example, a quarrel or a new job), by a rapid weight change (see *Anorexia nervosa*, p.709), by illness, or by certain drugs. Women who have just stopped taking the oral contraceptive pill may experience secondary amenorrhoea for a few months.

Less commonly, absence of periods is the result of a disorder that has an effect on egg production – for example, a *hypothalamic-pituitary abnormality* (p.587) can occasionally produce secondary amenorrhoea.

Periods normally stop permanently at the *menopause* (p.586) or when both ovaries have been removed or destroyed as treatment for some other disorder.

How common is the problem?
Amenorrhoea is common; each year 1 woman in 100 is concerned enough to consult a doctor about this condition. Secondary amenorrhoea occurs much more often than does primary amenorrhoea.

What are the risks?
Amenorrhoea in itself presents no risk to health, except in rare cases when it is a symptom of a more serious disorder. However, a woman with amenorrhoea may find it difficult or impossible to have a child while the condition persists.

What should be done?
If you are over 16 and have never had a period, you should consult your doctor, who will examine you to make sure that no underlying disorder is causing your amenorrhoea.

In most cases, the examination will reveal that there is nothing wrong and no treatment will be necessary; you can wait confidently for your periods to start naturally.

If your periods have already started and a period is delayed for two weeks or more, consult your doctor, who will examine you. If there is a possibility of pregnancy, carry out a pregnancy test, or ask your doctor to arrange one. If you are not pregnant and are otherwise well, your doctor will probably advise you to wait for a few months, during which time periods may start again naturally. It is important to realize that amenorrhoea is no safeguard against becoming pregnant. An egg could be released at any time; so if you do not wish to get pregnant, you must use some form of contraception.

What is the treatment?
If your periods have not restarted within nine months, your doctor may arrange for you to have diagnostic tests to look for some underlying problem. If no problem is found, no treatment will be given unless you wish to get pregnant – in which case your doctor may prescribe a fertility drug to restart egg production (see *Infertility*, p.607).

Oligo-menorrhoea

Oligomenorrhoea means infrequent periods. It occurs when a woman has fewer periods than the usual 11 to 13 a year. The periods that do occur are normal and are generally preceded by ovulation in the usual way.

How common is the problem?
Oligomenorrhoea occurs most commonly – as a natural development – in those women who are approaching the *menopause* (p.586), but some women have the condition throughout adult life, as a result of their particular hormone cycle (see *Hypothalamic-pituitary abnormalities*, p. 587). It rarely indicates any underlying problem.

What should be done?
Oligomenorrhoea presents no risks and does not require treatment unless you wish to become pregnant (see *Infertility*, p.607).

Dys-menorrhoea

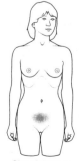

Site of the pain

Dysmenorrhoea is the medical term for painful periods. If these start within about three years of the onset of menstruation, the condition is known as primary dysmenorrhoea. The pain in most cases is thought to be a result of normal hormonal changes during menstruation. It often persists throughout the child-bearing years.

If periods become painful in a woman who has been menstruating longer than three years, the condition is known as secondary dysmenorrhoea. This is far more likely than primary dysmenorrhoea to be caused by an underlying gynaecological disorder, such as *fibroids* (p.593), *endometriosis* (p.595), or a *pelvic infection* (p.596).

What are the symptoms?
Period pains vary considerably. Some women have a dull pain in their abdomen or back, others have severe cramping abdominal pain. Typically, the pain is worse at the beginning of the period. In some cases there is also nausea and vomiting.

Dysmenorrhoea is very common, but the majority of cases are mild and do not require medical attention. There is no risk attached to the condition unless it is a symptom of an underlying disorder.

What is the treatment?
Take paracetamol tablets to relieve the pain, and if it is severe, rest in bed. You should

consult your doctor if the pain worsens or if you develop period pain following three or more years of relatively pain-free periods. The doctor will probably examine you to find out what is causing the dysmenorrhoea, and any underlying disorder will be treated accordingly. Several drugs are available that relieve pain; your doctor may prescribe one of them, or recommend that you start taking the contraceptive pill or some other drug that affects your hormone balance in such a way as to lessen period pains. Often primary dysmenorrhoea disappears after you have a child, or as you get older.

Menorrhagia

Menorrhagia means unusually heavy periods. You have menorrhagia if your periods are prolonged (lasting for more than seven days), or if large clots of blood are passed, or if flooding occurs. Menorrhagia is often brought on by disturbance of the hormones that control the menstrual cycle. It can also be caused by *fibroids* (p.593), *endometriosis* (p.595), or a *pelvic infection* (p.596). The presence in the uterus of an intra-uterine contraceptive device such as the coil may also produce the condition (see *The IUD*, p.609).

How common is the problem?
Menorrhagia is a common complaint. An estimated 5 to 10 per cent of women suffer from it, either regularly or occasionally. It is especially common in women approaching the menopause.

Apart from being inconvenient, menorrhagia can be distressing. One general risk is that if you regularly have heavy periods you may be in danger of developing *iron-deficiency anaemia* (p.419) because of the regular loss of blood; so make sure your diet contains sufficient iron.

What should be done?
If you have been having heavy periods for some time, consult your doctor. If you have a single unusually heavy period, follow the self-help measures recommended below. But if such a period was exceptionally late as well as heavy and there is a chance you may have been pregnant, you may be having an early *miscarriage* (p.628). In this case, you should consult your doctor immediately.

The doctor will question and examine you to discover the extent of the bleeding and to see if there is any abnormality of your uterus. You may need to have a blood test to find out if menorrhagia has made you anaemic.

What is the treatment?
Self-help: If you are having a single unusually heavy period and you are sure you are not pregnant, go to bed and take paracetamol for any pain. If the bleeding does not lessen within 24 hours, call your doctor.
Professional help: If your doctor discovers no abnormality of the uterus, you will probably be given the oestrogen-progestogen contraceptive pill to reduce the bleeding. If you are already on the pill, or if the pill is unsuitable in your case, your doctor can prescribe another drug that will lessen the bleeding. If you are using the coil, your doctor will probably recommend that you change to another method of contraception. And if a blood test shows that you are anaemic, you may have to take iron tablets.

If this treatment does not work after a few months, your doctor will probably arrange for you to have a *D and C* (p.593) to show if an underlying disorder is causing the menorrhagia. Even if nothing is found, the D and C itself sometimes clears up the problem. Finally, *removal of the uterus* (p.594) may be the only answer for menorrhagia that persists despite the above treatments.

Premenstrual tension

Each month various glands in your body release hormones into the bloodstream. The two main sex hormones are oestrogen and progesterone, both of which are made in the ovaries. They control various physical changes in your body – the changes of the menstrual cycle itself (see *Menstruation and the menopause*, p.583), along with associated physical changes such as increased breast tenderness. In addition, the monthly cycle of hormonal changes may affect your mood and produce certain mental or emotional changes. This combination of physical and emotional changes that occurs in most women in the few days before a period is known as premenstrual tension.

What are the symptoms?
Changes of mood usually take the form of increased irritability, aggressiveness, and possibly depression. Physical changes include a slight increase in weight (due to fluid retention), slightly enlarged and tender breasts, bloated stomach, lower abdominal pain, and

swollen ankles. The degree of these symptoms varies enormously. Usually they are either unnoticeable or moderate enough not to cause any problem. But occasionally the symptoms are so pronounced that they adversely affect personal relationships or performance at work. Pronounced premenstrual tension is more common in women who tend to suffer from *depression* (p.297).

What should be done?
If you have pronounced premenstrual tension, it helps if you can understand the problem and discuss it with a sympathetic friend. Try to avoid any situations that are likely to cause stress or irritation during the days when you are affected. Keep your weight down to a reasonable level to help discourage fluid retention. If the symptoms continue to be distressing, or if they are severe, consult your doctor. He or she may prescribe hormones to change your natural hormone balance and so relieve your symptoms. The commonest preparations are either the oestrogen-progestogen contraceptive pill or just progestogen, which is taken as tablets or vaginal suppositories (pessaries) during the 10 days before a period. If fluid retention is a particular problem in your case, a *diuretic* drug may be given. If your psychological symptoms are not relieved by this treatment, your doctor may prescribe *analgesics* (painkillers) or tranquillizers for you to take on the days when the problem is at its worst.

Menopause

The menopause is the technical term for your last period. It is, however, often used in a broader sense to mean the months or even years before and after the last period – a time known medically as the *climacteric*. The last period occurs at an average age of 51, but can happen as early as 40 or as late as 58. In the years leading up to the menopause, the regular monthly pattern of hormone production and egg release by the ovaries is upset. As a result, your menstrual cycle is disrupted and periods become irregular. Finally, when the ovaries stop working altogether, your periods cease completely.

The menopause is a natural stage of life and does not signify any disease or disorder.

What are the symptoms?
About 25 per cent of women do not notice any changes at the menopause, apart from the cessation of periods. Another 50 per cent notice slight physical or mental changes. The remaining 25 per cent suffer inconvenient or even distressing symptoms. Physical symptoms include hot flushes, sweating, dryness of the vagina (sometimes causing soreness during sexual intercourse), palpitations, joint pains, and headaches. Among the nonphysical symptoms often associated with the menopause are depression, anxiety, irritability, lack of concentration and confidence, and sleeping difficulties. The length of time over which symptoms occur varies considerably. They may continue for anything from a few weeks to five years.

What should be done?
If you have troublesome symptoms, bear in mind that they present no risks to health; and remember also that some emotional and physical problems are common to your time of life and that they may be accentuated by the menopause. Accept the menopause as a natural fact of life and not something to be embarrassed about.

Discuss your symptoms with your partner or an understanding friend. If, however, you still feel you cannot cope, see your doctor. He or she will examine you to make sure that there is no other condition causing your problems, and may prescribe drugs to relieve the symptoms. However, see your doctor immediately if you have any spotting of blood between periods, or prolonged bleeding or another period six months after what appeared to be the last. Any of these symptoms could indicate a *malignant* growth. The earlier such growths are detected, the higher the chance of complete cure.

What is the treatment?
Self-help: Do not add avoidable difficulties to those that may occur as natural symptoms of the menopause. For example, do not neglect your health or personal appearance. Most people need to eat less as they grow older, and it is better to control your weight by eating sensibly than allowing yourself to become depressed by what you wrongly believe to be an inevitable weight gain. Try not to let any hot flushes and sweating embarrass you. Usually, you will be the only person who is aware of them. If sweating is a nuisance at night, wear an absorbent cotton nightdress and keep a spare one beside the bed. If you find that intercourse makes your vagina sore, use a proprietary vaginal lubricant. You may be worried about when you can safely stop contraception. This depends on your age. If you are under 50, you should continue with

contraception for 24 months after the date of your last period; if you are over 50, for 12 months after the last period.

Professional help: The treatment you receive will depend on a variety of factors. If you are troubled by irregular or prolonged periods, hot flushes, or excessive sweating, your doctor may prescribe a hormone preparation to alter your hormonal balance and so lessen symptoms. This type of treatment is often called *hormone-replacement therapy.* The hormones may be oestrogen and progestogen combined in the form of the contraceptive pill, or administered separately in the form of tablets, vaginal cream, or little pellets implanted under the skin. They will make your periods regular, but will not restore fertility. Usually your doctor will prescribe the hormones for several months, then gradually reduce the dose, and eventually stop the treatment. By this time the menopausal changes should be complete, and symptoms should not return. If they do, you may need a further short course of treatment. In some cases, treatment has to be continued for many years and you need regular checkups to monitor its effects.

There are various drugs besides hormones that lessen menopausal symptoms. These may be prescribed for women who are well over 50, or who have a heart or circulatory condition, or who for some other reason are considered unsuitable for hormone therapy. If you have mainly emotional or psychological symptoms, your doctor may decide to prescribe tranquillizers, antidepressants, or sleeping pills.

Treatment for menopausal problems will not slow down or stop the changes of the menopause itself.

Hypo-thalamic-pituitary abnormalities

These are problems that are characterized by some disturbance in the production of various female sex hormones.

The menstrual cycle is the result of interaction between hormones and similar chemicals produced in the hypothalamus (a part of the brain), the pituitary gland (just below the brain), and the ovaries. This delicately balanced system can be upset in a number of ways. The hypothalamus may be disturbed by emotional factors, drug abuse, weight changes (see *Anorexia nervosa,* p.709), severe illness, and, occasionally, stopping the contraceptive pill. In some cases the pituitary gland acts abnormally for no apparent reason; and very rarely a *pituitary tumour* (p.518) causes the problem.

Certain disorders of the ovary may also produce symptoms of hormone upset. These include *cancer of the ovary* (p.593), *ovarian cysts* (p.592), and a rare disorder, the Stein-Leventhal syndrome, which also causes swellings in the ovary.

What are the symptoms?
The main symptom of any abnormality in sex-hormone production is irregular or absent periods (see *Amenorrhoea,* p.583). If the pituitary gland is causing the problem, there may also be symptoms of disturbance of the other hormones it produces (see the articles on the *Pituitary gland,* p.515).

In some disorders of the ovary (such as ovarian cysts) the production of the male sex hormone, testosterone, also rises; this may result in increased hairiness (*hirsutism*), the development of skin spots, deepening of the voice, and weight increase.

How common is the problem?
Disturbances of sex-hormone production are common, but most cases, though perhaps worrying, are not harmful to general health.

What should be done?
If your periods become irregular or cease altogether, consult your doctor, who will examine you to make sure no serious disorder is present. If the doctor suspects an underlying disorder, you will probably be referred to a gynaecologist for more examinations, blood tests, and perhaps an *X-ray* of the pituitary gland. If tests reveal an underlying disorder, it will be treated accordingly. Otherwise, treatment is not usually given unless you wish to become pregnant (see *Infertility,* p.607).

Hypothalamus and pituitary gland
The hypothalamus – an area at the base of the brain – and the pituitary gland just below it act together to control the production of sex hormones by the ovaries and other glands.

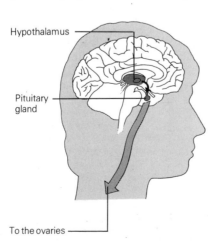

Hypothalamus

Pituitary gland

To the ovaries

The breast

Each breast consists of about 15 to 20 groups of milk-producing glands embedded in fatty tissue which gives the breast its characteristic shape. From each group of glands a milk duct runs to the nipple. Around the nipple is a dark area, the areola, which contains small sebaceous (lubricating) glands that keep the nipple supple.

During pregnancy, the release of certain hormones causes the breasts to enlarge and eventually produce milk (see *Pregnancy and childbirth*, p.616). The breasts may also become a little larger, and sometimes tender, before a period, as a result of the change in hormone levels.

The most serious disorder of the breast is breast cancer. Yet this disease can be successfully treated provided it is diagnosed in its

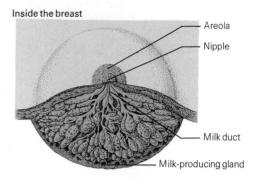

Inside the breast

- Areola
- Nipple
- Milk duct
- Milk-producing gland

early stages. It is therefore very important that you become familiar with the shape and consistency of your breasts (see the box opposite). Report any changes (especially new lumps) to your doctor right away.

Lumps in the breast

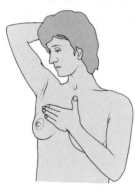

Detection of lumps
Lumps in the breast rarely cause symptoms, and may only be noticeable during regular self-examination.

Some women have naturally lumpy breasts. These are due to the make-up of their breast tissue, and are usually no reason for concern. If a new lump appears in a breast, there are five possible causes of this. The first is a *cyst*, which is a fluid-filled sac of tissue. The second is an infection, though in such cases there are usually other symptoms (see *Breast abscess*, p.590, for more information on symptoms and treatment). The third cause of a breast lump is fibro-adenosis, which is a thickening of the milk-producing glandular tissue. The fourth is a *benign* tumour. None of these is harmful to health. A fifth possible cause is a *malignant* (cancerous) tumour.

What are the symptoms?
A new lump in the breast may cause no discomfort at all and you may not notice it until you carry out an examination of your breasts (see "What should be done?" below). Occasionally, however, a lump is slightly tender (or even painful), often especially so just before a period.

What should be done?
Make a regular examination of your breasts each month, so that you will detect a new lump early. The box opposite shows how to do the examination. To help you remember, arrange a fixed time for the examination – whenever you start on a new pack of contraceptive pills, for example. If you detect any lump in the breast, whether painful or not,

see your doctor within a day or two. You should also see your doctor if a lump you have always had changes in some way – becomes painful, or harder, or bigger. Your doctor will examine you and may well refer you to a specialist. The specialist will also carry out an examination and, depending on the results, may arrange for one or more diagnostic test to find out whether there is a problem, and, if so, what the cause is. Tests include *mammography*, *thermography*, and a *biopsy*.

What is the treatment?
The treatment depends on the nature of the lump. If it is a cyst, the fluid will be drained through a needle into a syringe. This is a simple procedure (it may not even require a local anaesthetic) which usually clears up the problem. However, you will need to have regular check-ups for about two years to make sure the lump does not return.

When the cause of the lump is thickening of the glandular tissue in the breasts (fibro-adenosis), treatment is not essential. However, if such a lump feels tender or painful, your doctor may prescribe tablets to clear up the problem. The tablets contain either sex hormones (for example, the contraceptive pill) or drugs that affect your hormone balance. In addition, your doctor will probably advise you to wear a brassiere that will provide you with firm support.

If diagnostic tests show that the lump is a tumour, you will need to go into hospital to

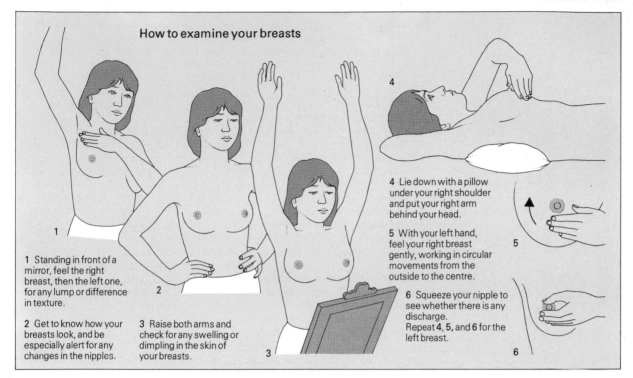

How to examine your breasts

1 Standing in front of a mirror, feel the right breast, then the left one, for any lump or difference in texture.

2 Get to know how your breasts look, and be especially alert for any changes in the nipples.

3 Raise both arms and check for any swelling or dimpling in the skin of your breasts.

4 Lie down with a pillow under your right shoulder and put your right arm behind your head.

5 With your left hand, feel your right breast gently, working in circular movements from the outside to the centre.

6 Squeeze your nipple to see whether there is any discharge.
Repeat **4, 5,** and **6** for the left breast.

have it removed. The type of operation depends on the nature of the tumour. If it is benign, it is usually necessary to remove only the tumour itself, involving a hospital stay of only a few days. After the operation, you will need to have regular check-ups for about two years. For the treatment of a malignant tumour see *Breast cancer*, below.

Breast cancer

Why a *malignant* tumour should develop in the breast is not known. At first the tumour remains localized in the breast. When it has grown to about 25mm (1in) across, it usually starts to spread (*metastasize*) via the bloodstream and the lymphatic system to other parts of the body. In about 10 per cent of cases, the disease affects both breasts.

What are the symptoms?
A lump, which may or may not be painful, develops in the breast, most commonly in the upper, outer part. The lump is usually detected by handling the breast; it is most unusual for it to be seen as a noticeable bulge. Sometimes the skin over the lump becomes creased. There may also be a dark-coloured discharge from the nipple, or the nipple may become indented (retracted – see *Nipple problems*, p.591).

How common is the problem?
Cancer of the breast is one of the most common cancers in women: about 1 woman in 20 develops the disease. It is most common in women in their 40s and 50s and is slightly more prevalent among childless women, women with a family history of the disease, and women who have a late *menopause*.

What are the risks?
When breast cancer is diagnosed early, the prospects for a cure are good. If untreated, or treated too late, the disease will prove fatal.

What should be done?
Monthly examination of the breasts will enable any new lump, or change in a long-standing lump, to be detected early (see *How to examine your breasts*, above, for instructions on how to do this). For women over 50 and women who have a pronounced family history of breast cancer, some areas of Britain have an *X-ray* screening programme to detect the disease in its early stages. Ask your doctor for further information about this and about the possibility of *thermography*.

Any lump that develops in the breast must, even if it is painless, be reported to your doctor right away. If the doctor confirms the presence of the lump, you will be referred to a specialist, who will decide whether the lump is due to breast cancer or to one of certain other disorders. *Mammography* or a *biopsy* (taking a sample of the lump for examination) will probably be carried out.

What is the treatment?

The most usual treatment is to remove the whole breast (see *Breast removal,* opposite), sometimes together with the lymph glands from the armpit next to the breast. Occasionally only part of the breast is removed and some surgeons insert a silicone prosthesis to replace the tissue removed and so preserve the shape of the breast. In addition to the operation, *radiotherapy* or *cytotoxic* drugs may be used. The length of time spent in hospital during treatment varies considerably from case to case.

For a woman to lose a breast is naturally distressing. However, she will receive much sympathy from friends and hospital staff. Indeed, she may be surprised to learn how many other women have also had the same operation – surprised, since she will not have suspected it; this is because a breast prosthesis (a "falsie") worn in the brassiere can be matched to the other breast and is quite undetectable to sight or touch. Most women who have had a breast removed quickly come to terms with the change and find any problems smaller than they had anticipated.

What is the long-term outlook?

If the tumour has been removed at an early stage, either a complete cure or many years of good health can be expected. After treatment, yearly or half-yearly check-ups will be carried out, but in some cases these can be discontinued after a few years. If the cancer does recur, it can be held in check for many years by drugs, radiotherapy, and perhaps further surgery.

As with many other cancers, mental attitude plays a vital part in the treatment of breast cancer. For reasons that are little understood, a woman who has a positive attitude to her illness and is determined to fight it is more likely to be cured.

Breast abscess

An *abscess* is an infected area of tissue. A breast abscess (sometimes called mastitis) forms when microbes enter the breast tissue through the nipple and infect the milk ducts and glands. As the microbes multiply, they cause a red, tender swelling or lump in your breast. The glands in the armpit next to the affected breast may also be tender, and you may have a raised temperature.

How common is the problem?

Breast abscesses are uncommon. Each year only 1 woman in 700 receives treatment for the complaint. Two-thirds of cases occur in women who have recently had a baby (see *Breast problems,* p.641). This is because cracked nipples, which often occur after childbirth, make it easier for microbes to gain entry to the breast tissue. For some reason the problem is more common in women who are not breast-feeding. New mothers can reduce the risk of an abscess developing by taking good care of their nipples, so that they do not become cracked. Whether you are breast-feeding or not, you should see your doctor if an abscess develops.

What is the treatment?

The treatment is the same whatever the cause. You may be given *antibiotic* tablets to control the infection, and perhaps aspirin to reduce any pain and fever.

It is quite safe to continue breast-feeding with the affected breast unless your doctor advises otherwise. Sometimes it may be necessary to massage your breast gently during feeding, to expel all the milk.

Occasionally the antibiotic alone will not clear up the problem, and you will need to go into hospital for a day or two to have the abscess drained. A small cut is made at the edge of the areola, the brownish skin surrounding the nipple, to allow the pus to drain out. The scar left by the cut is undetectable. The drainage allows the antibiotics to clear up the infection quickly.

Galactorrhoea

The breasts normally produce milk only after a woman has given birth to a baby and, in some cases, for a few days before. If milk production occurs at any other time in a woman, or at any time in a man, it constitutes a condition known as galactorrhoea. The milk is usually produced in small quantities by both breasts and is whitish or greenish.

How common is the problem?

Galactorrhoea is rare in women and even rarer in men. It is usually due to excessive production of the hormone prolactin. Prolactin is made by the pituitary gland and stimulates milk production. Galactorrhoea can be due to *hypothyroidism* (p.516), a disorder of the pituitary gland such as a *pituitary tumour* (p.518), or to certain types of oral contraceptive or tranquillizer, but may occur for no apparent reason. In women, galactorrhoea is often coupled with an absence of periods (see *Amenorrhoea*, p.583).

What should be done?
If you think you have galactorrhoea, consult your doctor. Make an exact note of the nature of the discharge. This will help your doctor to make a diagnosis. If a pituitary tumour is suspected to be the cause of the problem, the doctor may arrange for you to see a specialist for appropriate diagnostic tests.

What is the treatment?
If tests fail to reveal any cause for your galactorrhoea, you will probably not need any treatment. You can help control the condition by not handling your breasts and therefore not stimulating the release of milk. If the discharge is caused by a pituitary problem, however, your doctor may prescribe drugs to correct the hormonal imbalance and so stop the abnormal milk production.

Nipple problems

Most nipple problems are a minor irritation rather than a danger to health. But in rare cases a nipple disorder may be an early sign of a serious disease. In such cases do not delay in consulting your doctor. (For information on cracked nipples after childbirth see *Breast problems*, p.641).

Nipple discharge
A small amount of whitish or greenish discharge from the nipple is likely to be breast milk, especially if it comes from both nipples. If this occurs at any time in a man, or in a woman at any time other than just before or following the birth of a baby, it is called *galactorrhoea* (see opposite).

Any discharge which is dark in colour (usually dark red due to blood) should always be reported to your doctor. A likely cause is a tiny *benign* tumour called a duct papilloma, which can be removed during a short operation; but the cause may be *breast cancer* (p.589). Note which nipple the discharge comes from, and whether it emerges from one nipple duct or many, to help your doctor's diagnosis. The doctor will examine your breasts and if possible collect a sample of the discharge for analysis. You may also have to visit a specialist for further tests, such as *mammography*, to be carried out.

Nipple retraction
Long-standing nipple retraction (indentation) often first appears at puberty and usually affects both nipples. Such retraction is harmless, though it may make breast-feeding a little difficult. However, recent retraction may be a sign of breast cancer and must be reported to your doctor straight away.

Cysts or boils in the areola
The areola is the brown area around the nipple. It contains sebaceous glands which exude a waxy substance to lubricate the nipple. If the duct of one of these glands becomes blocked, a *cyst* (a fluid-filled sac) forms in the duct. If the gland itself then becomes infected, a boil will result.

You should consult your doctor if you have such a cyst or boil. In general, treatment is much the same as for a cyst or boil elsewhere on the skin – see *Sebaceous cysts* (p.261) and *Boils* (p.251).

OPERATION: **Breast removal** *(mastectomy)*

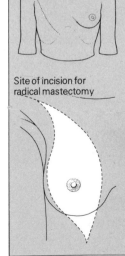

Site of incision for radical mastectomy

If a lump in the breast is found to be malignant it may be removed (a "lumpectomy") or, if there is a danger of the cancer spreading, a mastectomy may be advisable.

During the operation You may be given a simple mastectomy, to remove the breast; a radical mastectomy, to remove the breast, the lymph glands from the armpit, and both pectoral (chest) muscles; or a modified radical mastectomy, in which the pectoral muscles are left in place. It is also possible to have a subcutaneous mastectomy, leaving in place the skin and superficial tissues, beneath which a silicone replacement breast is inserted. You are under general anaesthetic throughout the operation, which takes between 1 and 2 hours.

After the operation You will have a drainage tube removing fluid from the site of the incision, and will probably stay in hospital for a week to 10 days.

Convalescence You may be given radiotherapy or cytotoxic drugs and will have check-ups every 6 or 12 months after postoperative treatment has ended.

Ovaries, uterus, and cervix

The two ovaries and the uterus (womb), which lie in the lower part of the abdomen, are the main female organs of reproduction.

The ovaries lie one on each side of the uterus, to which each is connected by a tube known as the fallopian tube. Each ovary contains thousands of eggs. Each month during your fertile years, one egg ripens and is released into its fallopian tube. As the egg travels slowly down the tube towards the uterus, it may be fertilized by a sperm. If this happens, when the fertilized egg reaches the uterus it burrows into its soft, thick lining, and you are pregnant (see *Pregnancy and childbirth*, p.616). If the egg is not fertilized, it is expelled from the uterus along with the thick, blood-filled uterine lining (called the endometrium) as menstruation (the period).

The uterus is a pear-shaped organ whose walls are composed of powerful muscles. At the lower front end of the uterus is its narrow, thick-walled neck, the cervix, which leads into the top of the vagina.

The disorders included in the following pages are mainly structural abnormalities, growths, or infections in the ovaries, uterus, or cervix. Disorders of the menstrual cycle are dealt with under *Menstruation and the menopause*, p.583.

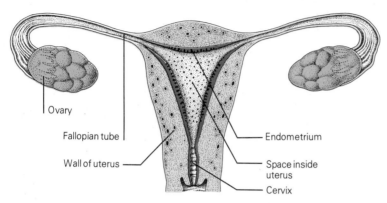

Ovary

Fallopian tube

Wall of uterus

Endometrium

Space inside uterus

Cervix

Ovarian cysts

An ovarian *cyst* is a sac full of fluid which grows on or near an ovary. The cyst, which occurs for no known reason, can grow to a considerable size and in very rare cases may interfere with the production of sex hormones in the ovary.

In some cases, an egg develops abnormally within the ovary and forms a small cyst called an egg cyst. Egg cysts usually cause few if any symptoms and tend to disappear completely within a few months.

What are the symptoms?
An ovarian cyst often produces no symptoms, but you may notice a firm, painless swelling in the lower abdomen, or pain during intercourse. A large cyst can press on the area near the bladder, causing difficulty in emptying it. When hormone production is affected, you may have various symptoms such as irregular vaginal bleeding and an increase in body hair (see *Hypothalamic-pituitary abnormalities*, p.587). If a cyst becomes twisted, it causes severe abdominal pain, nausea, and fever.

How common is the problem?
Ovarian cysts are not common; each year only 1 woman in 2,000 is treated for the condition. Quite often a cyst which has caused no problems is discovered at a routine medical check-up or during a regular examination at a family planning clinic.

What are the risks?
The most immediate risk from an ovarian cyst is that it may become badly twisted or burst, causing *peritonitis* (p.470). In the long term there is a slight risk that an untreated cyst may turn into a *malignant* tumour (see *Cancer of the ovary*, opposite).

What should be done?
Consult your doctor if you have the symptoms described above. If the doctor's examination reveals an abnormal growth, you will be referred to a gynaecologist for further examinations, perhaps including *laparoscopy*.

What is the treatment?
The usual treatment for a cyst is surgical removal. Often this can be done without damaging the ovary, but occasionally the entire ovary and possibly the fallopian tube have to be removed.

If you have completed having your family or are past the menopause, your gynaecologist may advise surgery to remove both ovaries and perhaps your uterus as well (see *Removal of the uterus*, p.594) to avoid the slight risk of malignancy.

Cancer of the ovary

Cancer occurs in an ovary when abnormal tissue develops there and forms a *malignant* tumour. It is not known what causes the cancer, but sometimes it arises in a long-standing *ovarian cyst* (opposite).

Cancer of the ovary is very difficult to detect in its early stages. Because the ovaries are deep within the lower abdomen, any swelling is often not noticed until the disease is well advanced. At this stage there may also be lower-abdominal pain, loss of weight, and general ill-health. Sometimes the tumour produces fluid which causes the whole abdomen to swell (a condition known as *ascites*). If not diagnosed and treated promptly, the cancer spreads (*metastasizes*) and can prove fatal within a few months.

How common is the problem?

Cancer of the ovary is a rare disorder, especially in women who are under 40. Only 1 in every 6,000 deaths among women is caused by the disease.

What should be done?

A woman who notices any of the symptoms described should see her doctor right away. If cancer is suspected, a short hospital stay will be arranged, during which a gynaecologist will carry out an internal examination, perhaps including *laparoscopy*. If cancer is present, an operation will be necessary to remove the affected ovary and, if the disease has spread, as much of the cancerous tissue as possible. In many cases the other ovary and the uterus will be removed at the same time to prevent development of further tumours.

Radiotherapy treatment or *cytotoxic* (anti-cancer) drugs are usually given to prevent a recurrence of the disease, or to slow down its progress if it has already spread. If the tumour produces fluid, this can be drawn off periodically with a needle and syringe – a swift, painless procedure known as *paracentesis*. If the disease cannot be completely cured, treatment permits at least several years of fairly normal life.

Fibroids

A fibroid is a *benign* tumour of the uterus (womb). The tumours (there are usually more than one) develop either within the muscular wall of the uterus or on the outside or inside of the wall, attached to it by a stalk of tissue. Fibroids vary considerably in the extent and rate of their growth. Some take many years to grow to the size of a pea; others may reach 75mm (3in) or more across within the course of only a few years.

What are the symptoms?

Many women with fibroids have no symptoms, especially if the fibroids are small. Those who do have symptoms usually experience heavy, prolonged, and sometimes painful periods. A large fibroid can sometimes be felt as a hard, painless lump in the lower abdomen. If it presses on the area near your bladder, it can prevent you from emptying the bladder easily. It may also make sexual intercourse painful.

How common is the problem?

Roughly 20 per cent of women over 30 have fibroids. They are most common in women between the ages of 35 and 45.

What are the risks?

Occasionally, a fibroid attached to the uterus by a stalk becomes twisted and loses its blood supply, or it may start to wither away. Either of these developments may produce sudden sharp pain low in the abdomen. If this happens, an emergency operation may be required to remove the fibroid. A fibroid may become big enough to prevent conception; and in some cases it enlarges rapidly during pregnancy, when it may cause pain, a miscarriage, or obstruction during delivery. If you have any of the symptoms described, see your doctor, who will examine you. Occasionally,

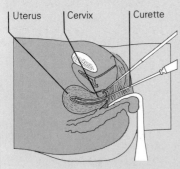

OPERATION: D and C (*dilatation and curettage*)

In this operation, the neck of the uterus (cervix) is dilated (dilatation) so that the uterine lining can be scraped (curettage). It is done to discover the cause of heavy periods (see *Menorrhagia*, p.585), to terminate a pregnancy (see *Unwanted pregnancy*, p.625), or to treat an incomplete miscarriage.

During the operation You will probably be under a general anaesthetic. Your cervix is widened with a dilator, the lining of the uterus is scraped with a curette, and the scrapings are taken away for analysis in a laboratory. The operation takes between 30 minutes and an hour.

After the operation You will have bleeding from the uterus for a few days and may have some pelvic and back pain. You will probably be able to leave hospital in 1 or 2 days.

Convalescence Sexual intercourse and tampons should be avoided for several weeks, but most normal activities can be resumed after a few days.

Uterus | Cervix | Curette

symptomless fibroids are discovered at a routine check-up at a family planning or some other clinic.

What is the treatment?

Small, symptomless fibroids do not require treatment. You will simply have to visit your doctor every six or 12 months for an examination to check that the fibroids are not growing too large. In women over 45, they tend to get smaller or disappear altogether.

If your fibroids are causing long, heavy periods, or they are big enough to present problems in conceiving, your doctor will refer you to a gynaecologist. The gynaecologist may decide to admit you to hospital for an examination and a *D and C* (p.593) to confirm the presence of fibroids and exclude other diseases of the lining of the uterus.

Troublesome fibroids are removed surgically. If you do not intend to have children in the future, you will probably be advised to have the entire uterus taken away (see *Removal of the uterus*, below). If you want to have children, fibroids can often be surgically removed without damaging the uterus.

Cancer of the uterus

Cancer of the uterus starts in the lining (endometrium) of the uterus. After growing in the lining, the cancer invades the wall of the uterus and, if untreated, spreads to the fallopian tubes, ovaries, and other organs.

What are the symptoms?

In women who are past the menopause there is slight bleeding from the vagina, and in women who are still having periods spots of blood may appear between periods. There may also be a vaginal discharge, which can range from a watery, pink fluid to a thick, brown, foul-smelling one. The disease may cause intermittent pains, like period pains.

How common is the problem?

Cancer of the uterus is the fifth most common form of cancer in women. It occurs mainly between the ages of 50 and 60 in women who have not had children.

What should be done?

It is essential that a woman who has any irregular vaginal bleeding, or bleeding six months after her last period, or an abnormal discharge consults her doctor as soon as possible. The cancer grows and spreads very slowly. Therefore the risk that it will prove fatal is much lower than in many other cancers. If symptoms are reported early, there is a high chance of complete cure. If cancer is suspected, a *D and C* (p.593) and a cervical smear (see *Vaginal examination and cervical smear test*, p.599) will be necessary.

What is the treatment?

If cancer of the utcrus is confirmed, the uterus is removed (hysterectomy – see *Removal of the uterus*, below), together with the ovaries and fallopian tubes in case the disease has spread. *Radiotherapy* is sometimes given also, to prevent any further spread of the

---

OPERATION: ## Removal of the uterus
(hysterectomy)

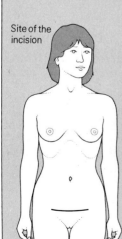

Site of the incision

The uterus, and sometimes also the ovaries and fallopian tubes, may be removed to cure any of a number of gynaecological complaints, especially in women past the menopause.
During the operation There are 2 basic methods for performing a hysterectomy. The most common method is to remove the uterus through an incision in the lower abdomen. With the other (much rarer) method an incision is made at the top of the vagina through which the uterus can be removed. The top of the vagina is then stitched together. Each operation takes between 1 and 2 hours and is done under general anaesthetic.
After the operation You will probably have a drainage tube at the site of any abdominal incision, and may have some vaginal bleeding

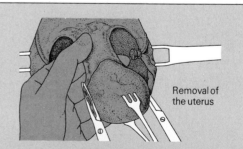

Removal of the uterus

and discharge for a few days. You will be encouraged to get out of bed and walk about the day after the operation, and you will be able to go home 7 to 10 days afterwards.
Convalescence Convalescence may take anything from 2 weeks to 2 months, depending on the general state of your health. In a woman who has not yet reached the menopause, removal of the ovaries will bring about an early menopause.

cancer. A week before the operation a *radium implant* may be left in the uterus for about 36 hours, or external radiotherapy may be given after the operation. Sometimes, as an alternative, a radium implant is inserted into the top of the vagina after the operation.

In some cases hormone treatment may be successful in restricting the tumour's growth. If the cancer is detected at a fairly early stage, the prospects are excellent: 80 per cent of women operated on in these circumstances are completely cured.

Tropho-blastic tumours

(including hydatidiform mole)

A trophoblastic tumour is a rare type of growth that occurs during pregnancy. It grows in the placenta, and usually appears during early pregnancy, when it prevents the fertilized egg from developing into a baby. The tumour can also grow in placental tissue left behind in the uterus after childbirth or a miscarriage; it can appear at any time up to five years after the pregnancy.

A trophoblastic tumour is either *benign* (when it is often called a hydatidiform mole) or *malignant*. It is a rare disorder. The benign type occurs in about 1 in 2,000 pregnancies; the malignant type in 1 in 40,000. A benign growth remains confined to the uterus, but a malignant growth, if untreated, rapidly invades the wall of the uterus and passes via the bloodstream to other parts of the body.

What are the symptoms?
The main symptoms of a trophoblastic tumour are irregular vaginal bleeding and excessive morning sickness.

What should be done?
If a woman has a combination of the symptoms described, she should consult her doctor without delay. An *ultrasound scan* and a urine test will be carried out. A trophoblastic tumour causes excessive production of the hormone HCG, normally made by the placenta. This hormone passes into the urine and can be easily detected by chemical analysis. If a trophoblastic tumour is present, the growth is removed in much the same way as an unwanted pregnancy is (see *Unwanted pregnancy*, p.625). No further treatment is necessary for a benign tumour apart from regular check-ups over the next two years to make sure it does not recur.

If the tumour is found to be malignant, it may be necessary to undergo *removal of the uterus* (opposite). *Cytotoxic* drugs will be given for several months to prevent any spread, and regular check-ups, as for benign tumours, will be necessary. The prospects for a complete cure are good.

Endo-metriosis

The tissue lining your uterus is called the endometrium. Each month part of it grows and becomes engorged with blood, and then is shed as a period. Endometriosis is a condition in which fragments of endometrium somehow escape and develop in other places – within the wall of your uterus, or in your ovaries, or (less commonly) in the fallopian tubes, the vagina, the intestine, or even in scars that form in the abdominal wall after surgery. Each month the fragments of endometrium bleed like the lining of the uterus, but because they are embedded in tissue the blood cannot escape. Instead blood blisters form that irritate and scar the surrounding tissue, which in turn forms a fibrous cyst (sac) around each blister.

What are the symptoms?
In the majority of cases symptoms are absent, or so mild that they pass unnoticed, and require no treatment. If you have symptoms, these include a dragging abdominal or back pain during periods; the pain often becomes worse towards the end of the period. In some cases periods are unusually heavy (see *Menorrhagia*, p.585) and sexual intercourse may be painful.

How common is the problem?
Because endometriosis is linked to menstruation, it can occur only during the fertile years. It appears most often between the ages of 30 and 40, and is more common in women who have not had children. Endometriosis in its mild form is common; but cases severe enough to require treatment are rare.

What should be done?
If you are suffering from painful periods of the kind described, see your doctor. You may be referred to a gynaecologist, who will probably perform a *D & C* (p.593) and a *laparoscopy* before making a firm diagnosis.

What is the treatment?
Your doctor may decide to prescribe the combined oestrogen-progestogen contraceptive pill, which will relieve your symptoms. If the condition is severe, drugs, or

large doses of hormones, will be given to stop your periods for several months; this allows your body to disperse the abnormal tissue.

If endometriosis has affected the ovaries, treatment will be surgical removal of the blisters or cysts as for an *ovarian cyst* (p.592). In severe cases that fail to respond to treatment, you may be advised to undergo *removal of the uterus* (p.594) – especially if you have completed your family.

Pelvic infections

(pelvic inflammatory disease, salpingitis)

This disorder occurs when microbes invade the uterus and spread to the fallopian tubes, ovaries, and surrounding tissues, causing infection and inflammation. The infection may not have any obvious cause but it is often introduced via the vagina, during sexual intercourse (see *Gonorrhoea*, p.611). Very occasionally it occurs after the fitting of an intra-uterine contraceptive device (IUD) or after a miscarriage or abortion.

A pelvic infection can be either acute, causing sudden severe symptoms, or chronic, producing milder symptoms gradually.

What are the symptoms?
If you have an acute pelvic infection, it causes pain or tenderness in your lower abdomen, and you will probably have a fever. Chronic pelvic infection results in recurrent mild, dragging pain in the lower abdomen, and sometimes backache. In both acute and chronic infections you may have pain during intercourse, your periods may be upset (for example, they may be early or heavy), and you are likely to have an abnormally heavy and smelly vaginal discharge.

How common is the problem?
The disease is not common; each year only 1 woman in 1,000 is treated for it. It is most common in young, sexually active women.

What are the risks?
If the infection is neglected, an *abscess* may form on a fallopian tube or ovary, causing damage and scarring and possibly resulting in *infertility* (p.607). Very rarely, the infection spreads swiftly, causing *peritonitis* (p.470) or even *blood poisoning* (p.421).

What should be done?
See your doctor as soon as symptoms occur, so that treatment can be started early. The doctor will take a *swab* from the inside of your vagina, to identify the microbes that are causing the infection.

What is the treatment?
An *antibiotic* is prescribed to clear up the infection. Paracetamol or something stronger is given to help relieve abdominal pain. Your doctor will recommend rest in bed until the symptoms have disappeared, and no sexual intercourse for three or four weeks. This treatment usually leads to a complete recovery. If there is no improvement after about five days, you may be admitted to hospital, where an internal examination and perhaps *laparoscopy* will be carried out to check on the diagnosis. Further treatment with a carefully chosen antibiotic will usually clear up the problem. But if the examination reveals an abscess, surgery may be advisable.

Prolapse of the uterus or vagina

Your uterus, vagina, and other lower abdominal organs are held in place by strong muscles and ligaments at the base of your abdomen. These muscles are known as the pelvic-floor muscles. Prolapse of the uterus or vagina occurs when the muscles and ligaments become weak. Stretching or slackening of the muscles often occurs as a result of childbirth, and it takes place naturally as you get older. The muscles and ligaments no longer hold the uterus firmly in place, so it falls and causes the vagina to sag downwards. This gives rise to the *prolapse* – a bulge of the front or back wall of the vagina. More rarely the uterus may descend so far that it bulges out of the vagina, forming a complete prolapse. (The same weakness can also lead to *stress incontinence*, p.601.)

What are the symptoms?
A lump or bulge appears in the vagina and may project outside. This causes a feeling of heaviness and discomfort, and also backache, especially at the end of the day or after lifting or straining. In some cases the symptoms of stress incontinence appear, but in others the prolapse has the opposite effect and makes it harder to empty your bladder. If the back wall of the vagina has descended you may find defecation difficult, and pushing too hard makes matters worse.

How common is the problem?
Minor degrees of prolapse are common, especially for a few months after childbirth and in later life. Each year 1 woman in 250 consults a doctor because of the problem.

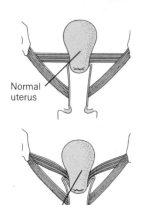

Normal uterus

Prolapsed uterus

What are the risks?

Prolapse can be uncomfortable and inconvenient, but there are no risks to general health unless it is allowed to worsen. Protrusion of a large part of the vagina or uterus can lead to soreness, ulceration, and infection.

What should be done?

Exercises to tone up the pelvic-floor muscles after childbirth may well avert prolapse (see below). If you think you have a prolapse, consult your doctor so that he or she can confirm the diagnosis and exclude any other more serious cause of your symptoms.

What is the treatment?

Your doctor will probably recommend self-help measures to relieve the problem; surgery is required in only a few cases.

Begin self-help measures by going on a diet if you are overweight. Eat plenty of high-fibre foods, so that you can defecate without straining. You can strengthen the muscles of your pelvic floor by exercising them regularly; your pelvic-floor muscles are the muscles you would use to interrupt a flow of urine in mid-stream. Exercise them for several minutes every day (these exercises are also advised following childbirth).

Retroversion of the uterus

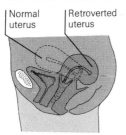

Normal uterus   Retroverted uterus

Normally the uterus is tilted upwards and forwards and lies immediately behind the bladder. In about 20 per cent of women, however, it inclines downwards and backwards and lies close to the rectum; it is then said to be retroverted. This is not a disease but a natural condition.

In nearly all cases, retroversion is completely symptomless and does not require treatment. Occasionally it causes backache, especially during a period.

In some cases, pain is felt during sexual intercourse, when the penis strikes an ovary during deep penetration. See your doctor if this happens to you. The doctor may advise different positions for intercourse, but if the pain is particularly troublesome, you may be referred to a gynaecologist. After ensuring that the pain is not caused by some other pelvic disease, the gynaecologist may decide to move the uterus temporarily into the normal position by inserting a special pessary into the vagina. If this gets rid of the pain, he or she may advise an operation, called a ventrosuspension, to move your uterus permanently into the new position.

Cervical erosion

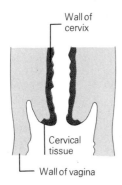

Wall of cervix

Cervical tissue

Wall of vagina

Cervical erosion
Cervical erosion occurs when some of the cells forming the vulnerable lining of the inner part of the cervix (between the uterus and vagina) have spread to cover the tip of the cervix.

The lining of the canal of your cervix consists of a delicate, mucus-secreting, red tissue called columnar epithelium. The lining normally gives way at the mouth of the cervix to a stronger, pink tissue called squamous epithelium, which covers the outside of the cervix and lines the vagina. A cervical erosion is an extension of columnar epithelium to some of the outer part of your cervix, where it normally discharges a small amount of mucus and may bleed following intercourse. The condition is not a disease and carries no serious risks. It is not even a true erosion, since the area has not been made raw by friction. However, because the epithelium is so delicate, once it has extended beyond the mouth of the cervix it is susceptible to infection, and more pronounced cases – which produce more discharge – may require treatment.

How common is the problem?

Some women are naturally prone to developing a cervical erosion. In others it occurs during or after pregnancy, or while taking the oestrogen-progestogen contraceptive pill. The extent of the condition fluctuates considerably in anyone who is affected.

What should be done?

Provided you have a *vaginal examination and cervical smear test* (p.599) regularly to detect any more serious problem, you need do nothing. If, however, the discharge is such that you have to change your pants more than twice a day, see your doctor. Do the same if you have bleeding after intercourse.

After examining you to confirm the presence of a cervical erosion, the doctor will take a cervical smear to discover whether you have *cervical dysplasia* (p.598) as well. He or she may also take a *swab* from the upper vagina, to find out if any infection is present.

What is the treatment?

The extended columnar epithelium can be destroyed by *cauterization*; this allows squamous epithelium to grow over the area. The cauterization, which is painless, is often done as out-patient treatment or during a 24-hour hospital stay. For about two or three weeks afterwards, you will probably have a heavy watery discharge as the cauterized tissues heal. When this stops, you should have no more trouble and will be able safely to resume sexual intercourse.

Cervical dysplasia

In some women who have the condition known as *cervical erosion* (p.597), the delicate red skin on part of the outside of the cervix reacts to the acidic mucus produced in the vagina by changing as best it can into the thicker, pink skin that lines the vagina. This change from one type of skin to another is called metaplasia. Usually this change causes no trouble, but in 1 woman in 250, for no known reason, an abnormal development of cells takes place in an area of metaplasia. This abnormality, which is also symptomless, is known as cervical dysplasia.

What are the risks?

Most cases are symptomless and carry no risk to health, but there is a risk that certain types of dysplasia – if left untreated – may develop into *cancer of the cervix* (below) within about 10 or 15 years.

What should be done?

All women should have a regular *vaginal examination and cervical smear test* (opposite). If a smear suggests dysplasia, you will be advised to see a gynaecologist, who will examine your cervix with a special microscope called a *colposcope* and carry out a *biopsy*.

Depending on the type of dysplasia present, you may or may not need treatment.

What is the treatment?

The area of dysplasia is removed by an operation called a *cone biopsy* or destroyed by *cauterization* or a *laser beam*. A general anaesthetic is given for a cone biopsy, which involves a hospital stay of one or two days, and two weeks' rest at home afterwards. A cone biopsy has the advantage of allowing a more detailed examination of the area. The other procedures are painless and can be done during an out-patient visit to hospital. In very rare cases, a cone biopsy can lead to a tendency to miscarry, and any woman who has had the treatment should tell her doctor about it if she becomes pregnant.

A woman with dysplasia who has completed her family, especially if she is suffering from heavy or painful periods as well, may be advised to undergo *removal of the uterus* (p.594) to prevent any future risks of cancer of the uterus developing.

After treatment for dysplasia, it is essential that you have a cervical smear once a year for a period of five years, then once every three years, so that any recurrence can be detected.

Cancer of the cervix

This form of cancer most often develops in women who have had a certain type of *cervical dysplasia* (above) for several years and who have not received treatment for the condition. There are two main symptoms. The first is a watery, bloody discharge, which may be copious and offensive-smelling. The second is vaginal bleeding between periods, or following the menopause, or after intercourse. In advanced cases there is also dull backache and general ill-health.

How common is the problem?

Cancer of the cervix, although one of the most common cancers in women, is an uncommon disease. Only about 1 woman in every 80 is treated for it. It is most prevalent among women over 40.

What are the risks?

Left untreated, cancer of the cervix will spread to nearby organs, and may eventually prove fatal. However, if detected early and given appropriate treatment, this cancer can, more than most, be completely cured.

What should be done?

See your doctor regularly for a *vaginal examination and cervical smear test* (opposite).

This allows early detection of those types of cervical dysplasia that carry a risk of future cancer of the cervix. The dysplasia can then be treated to reduce the risk.

If a woman has any of the symptoms described, she must see her doctor. The cause of the symptoms is likely to be a relatively minor disorder such as *cervical polyps* (opposite) but it is unwise to take any chances. If the doctor suspects cancer, the woman will be referred to a gynaecologist for an examination, a cervical smear, and a *biopsy* of the cervix to show whether cancer is present.

What is the treatment?

Cancer of the cervix is treated by removing the cervix along with the rest of the uterus, ovaries, and fallopian tubes (see *Removal of the uterus*, p.594), and/or by *radiotherapy*. Radiotherapy is usually carried out by *radium pellets* placed against the growth for two or three sessions of between 18 and 36 hours each, usually before the operation. It may be followed by further external radiotherapy of the lower abdomen. The choice of treatment will be made after a full discussion with the patient.

The chances of treatment providing a complete cure when cancer has not spread

Vaginal examination and cervical smear test

A vaginal examination is carried out routinely in family planning clinics as part of your regular check-up. It is usually done by your family doctor only if he or she suspects that you have a gynaecological problem or are pregnant. The doctor inserts two fingers of one hand into your vagina and presses against your lower abdomen with the other hand, feeling for any abnormalities. The procedure is quite painless as long as you do not tense up.

At family planning clinics you will also have a cervical smear test (also called a "Pap" test) done at least every 5 years (but usually more often), to detect conditions that may cause *cancer of the cervix* (opposite). The vagina is held open by a *speculum* while a few cells are scraped from the cervix with a spatula. The cells are then sent for laboratory examination.

The test is said to be negative if the cells are normal, and positive if they are abnormal. If the results are inconclusive, the test is repeated several months later until the results are definite. Your doctor will arrange for the necessary treatment if the results are found to be positive.
If you are not attending a family planning clinic, it is a good idea to arrange regular cervical smear tests through your family doctor.

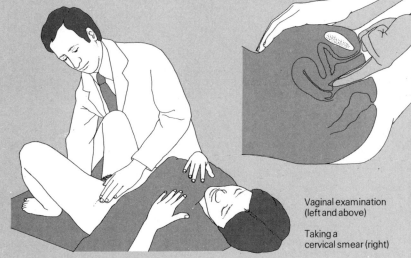

Vaginal examination (left and above)

Taking a cervical smear (right)

beyond the uterus are extremely high – much higher than in most cancers. The treatment will, however, prevent a woman from having children. Even if the reproductive organs are not removed, the ovaries will cease working as the result of radiotherapy. In younger women, the treatment may produce some symptoms of the menopause which may need to be treated (see *Menopause*, p.586).

Following treatment of the cancer, regular check-ups and tests are carried out over the next five years or so.

Cervical polyps

A cervical polyp is a grape-like growth of the delicate mucus-producing tissue that lines the canal of the cervix. Polyps usually occur singly, but may be multiple, and can grow up to 20mm (almost 1in) across. They usually produce a heavy, watery, bloody discharge from the vagina, and sometimes bleeding after sexual intercourse, or between periods, or after the *menopause* (p.586).

What should be done?
Cervical polyps are common and harmless. Even so, if you have the symptoms described, report them to your doctor straight away, since *cancer of the cervix* (opposite) produces similar symptoms. Do *not* take any risks. You will probably be referred to a gynaecologist, who will perform a *vaginal examination and cervical smear test* (above).

What is the treatment?
If a polyp is present, it is removed – a quick, painless procedure that requires no anaesthetic – and is then examined for signs of cancer. Once removed, the polyp is not likely to recur, and you should have no further problems. When a polyp has also been causing irregular bleeding, you may need a *D and C* (p.593) to ensure that some more serious disorder is not causing the bleeding.

Bladder and urethra

The bladder is a muscular-walled sac in which urine collects. It is situated in the lower abdomen. Urine trickles slowly into the bladder from the two kidneys via two narrow tubes called the ureters. The stored urine is passed when the bladder muscles contract and release the urine past the relaxed *sphincter* into the urethra, a short passage whose opening lies in front of that of the vagina.

Disorders of the urinary tract that affect both sexes are dealt with elsewhere (see *Disorders of the urinary tract*, p.500). The problems included here are either those which affect women only or those, like cystitis, which affect women and men but do so in different ways.

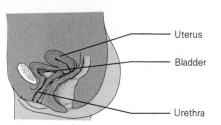

Uterus

Bladder

Urethra

Cystitis in women

Cystitis is inflammation of the bladder. This is nearly always caused by bacteria travelling up the short passage of the urethra and infecting the bladder. The infecting organism is most commonly a microbe that is normally found in the bowels. There are several other urinary-tract problems that produce symptoms similar to cystitis. These include *chronic urethritis* and *irritable bladder* (opposite).

What are the symptoms?
You feel a frequent urge to urinate, but when you try to do so only a small amount of urine is passed. This smells strongly, may have blood in it (*haematuria*), and burns or stings as you pass it (*dysuria*). The urge to urinate is sometimes so strong that you cannot control it before you reach a lavatory (this is called "urge incontinence"). You may also have a raised temperature and perhaps a dull pain in your lower abdomen.

How common is the problem?
Cystitis is a very common complaint. Most women suffer from it at some time. It is particularly common in pregnancy – especially the first few months.

What are the risks?
Cystitis is annoying and inconvenient, but presents little risk to general health. Very occasionally, an untreated infection of the bladder spreads to the kidneys (see *Acute pyelonephritis*, p.502).

What should be done?
See your doctor if you have the symptoms of cystitis. The doctor will probably supply a small container in which you provide a "mid-stream" specimen of urine. You should first wash your vulva thoroughly with clean cotton wool and water. Then, in the middle of passing urine, catch a small amount in the sterile container. The sample is then analysed for the presence of microbes.

What is the treatment?
Self-help: Drink plenty of fluids. Try to empty your bladder completely each time you urinate, and follow the self-help measures described for chronic urethritis (opposite). Always wipe yourself from front to back after you have used the lavatory.

Professional help: Your doctor may give you a course of *antibiotics* right away, especially if your symptoms are severe. If these fail to cure the condition, the doctor will prescribe a different antibiotic on the basis of the laboratory analysis of your urine sample. This should clear up the trouble.

If you have more than two or three attacks of cystitis, your doctor will arrange for you to see a specialist – a gynaecologist or *urologist* – to discover whether you have any urinary-tract abnormality that is encouraging the infection. The specialist will examine you, and may ask for further mid-stream specimens of urine. Sometimes an *intravenous pyelogram* (a special *X-ray* of the kidneys and bladder) and a visual examination of the inside of the bladder (*cystoscopy*) are also necessary. If these examinations and tests reveal an abnormality of the urinary tract, this will be treated accordingly. If not, the specialist may put you on a long course of antibiotics, for a month or more. This should clear up the problem – but you should bear in mind that cystitis is a complaint that may well recur.

Stress incontinence

At the base of your abdomen you have a sheet of muscles known as the pelvic floor. These muscles support the base of the bladder and close off the top of the urethra (the short channel through which you pass urine). In stress incontinence, the pelvic-floor muscles are weak. When you exert pressure on them – by coughing, for example, or laughing, or lifting something – you cannot help losing a little urine. This happens only when the muscles are under stress; you have no trouble when you are resting or sleeping.

Some degree of stress incontinence is extremely common. The pelvic-floor muscles are weakened by childbirth and by being overweight, and also become naturally weaker during middle age although the problem becomes less common in the elderly. Weak pelvic-floor muscles can also lead to *prolapse of the uterus or vagina* (p.596), which will require its own treatment.

What should be done?

If you have troublesome stress incontinence, see your doctor, who will probably refer you to a specialist.

You may be asked to provide a "midstream" specimen of urine, which will show whether a urinary-tract infection could be aggravating the condition. You may also be asked to undergo a special *X-ray* of your bladder called a *micturating cystogram*.

Treatment for stress incontinence is based on exercises to strengthen your pelvic-floor muscles. If you are overweight, go on a diet (see *Obesity*, p.492). If these measures fail to cure the condition, there are two other possible methods of treatment. You can have an operation to tighten up your pelvic-floor muscles or, alternatively, the specialist may advise you to keep a specially designed pessary, or a large tampon or sponge, in your vagina during the day.

Irritable bladder

An irritable bladder is one that contracts uncontrollably. You have a sudden urge to pass urine, and often pass a small amount before you can reach a lavatory (a problem called "urge incontinence"). You may have to get up quickly at night to urinate.

Why certain people have an irritable bladder is not known, but it sometimes occurs in conjunction with stress incontinence, prolapse of the uterus or vagina, or an infection of the urinary tract. It is a common, inconvenient, and occasionally distressing complaint but is not harmful to general health.

What should be done?

See your doctor, who will examine you and arrange for you to provide a "mid-stream" specimen of urine (for details see *Cystitis in women*, opposite). This will be analysed for

indications of any urinary-tract infection. The doctor may also arrange for a special *X-ray* of your bladder to be taken while you are passing urine (a *micturating cystogram*) and for a visual examination of the inside of your bladder (*cystoscopy*).

If you have an irritable bladder, your doctor will advise you to try to hold on to your urine for as long as possible in order to strengthen your bladder muscles. You may also be given a drug to relax your bladder muscles or dampen down the nerves that control contraction.

If none of these treatments improves the condition, the doctor may recommend that you enter hospital for a short operation to stretch your urethra. This procedure may need to be repeated if there is no significant improvement the first time.

Chronic urethritis

This common disorder is a recurrent inflammation of the urethra. It is often caused by bruising during sexual intercourse, especially if you are not relaxed. Less commonly, an infection is responsible.

The symptoms of chronic urethritis are similar to those of *cystitis in women* (opposite), except that they last for only one or two days after intercourse. Because the symptoms of chronic urethritis and cystitis are so similar, and because the disorder is common in women who have just started having intercourse, chronic urethritis is sometimes called "honeymoon cystitis".

What should be done?

Adopt the following self-help measures each time you have intercourse: Drink a glass of water beforehand; use a vaginal lubricant; relax as much as possible; and empty your bladder completely soon afterwards.

What is the treatment?

You should see your doctor so that a sample of urine can be analysed for any infection. If there is an infection, it can be treated by *antibiotics.* If chronic urethritis still persists, your doctor may advise an operation to stretch your urethra or vagina.

Vagina and vulva

The vulva is the area around the opening to the female urinary and reproductive systems. It consists of two folds of tissue (the "lips") which lead to the vagina, the passage between the vulva and the uterus (the womb).

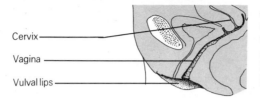

Cervix

Vagina

Vulval lips

Projecting into the top of the vagina is the cervix (the neck of the uterus), and just in front of the opening to the vagina is the opening to the urethra, the narrow tube down which urine is passed from the bladder.

The tissues of the vulva, and to a lesser extent the vagina, are basically similar to skin tissue, and are liable to skin problems such as warts or severe itching (called pruritis). The area is also prone to infections of various kinds, perhaps because some microbes thrive in its generally rather moist conditions.

Vaginal thrush

Vaginal thrush occurs when the fungus candida albicans grows in the vagina (the same fungus causes *oral thrush* – see p.451). Many women harbour small amounts of the fungus, but normally these are prevented from growing and causing symptoms by small amounts of acid produced by harmless bacteria in the vagina. The fungus develops only if the bacteria are destroyed. Vaginal deodorants, *douches*, or *antibiotics* may kill off the acid-producing bacteria and allow the fungus to increase. Similarly, hormonal changes that occur if you are pregnant or on the contraceptive pill can change conditions in the vagina and allow thrush to develop.

Vaginal thrush is very common and presents no risk to general health.

What are the symptoms?
The main symptom is irritation of the vagina and the rest of the genital area. You may notice an unusual thick, white discharge and you may have some pain or soreness during sexual intercourse. There is a tendency to urinate more often than usual and the urine may sting or burn.

What should be done?
To prevent thrush occurring, avoid wearing nylon underclothes (unlike cotton, nylon cannot "breathe" and therefore offers a warm, moist breeding area for the infection), do not use vaginal deodorants or powders, and do not douche your vagina.

If you have developed the symptoms of thrush, consult your doctor, who will probably examine you and take a *swab* from your vagina for laboratory examination.

What is the treatment?
The usual treatment for vaginal thrush is an antifungal drug given in the form of a pessary (vaginal suppository) or cream. This normally clears up the problem. However, if you suffer from repeated attacks, your doctor may prescribe a cream for your sexual partner to apply to his penis. This is because it is possible for a man, while unaffected by the disorder himself, to carry and reinfect you with the fungus. If your vaginal thrush recurs, and you are taking the contraceptive pill, the doctor may recommend some other form of contraception.

Trichomonal vaginitis
(*trichomonas*)

Trichomonal vaginitis is a vaginal infection caused by trichomonas, a tiny one-celled organism. The symptoms of the infection are very similar to those of *vaginal thrush* (above), except that the discharge is noticeably different: it is usually heavy, unpleasant-smelling, and greenish-yellow in colour.

The infection is common and presents no serious risk but can be irritating and painful. And because it is *contagious*, it is likely that your sexual partner will also be affected;

although infection causes no symptoms in a man, he can reinfect you at any time during sexual intercourse.

What should be done?
If you have symptoms of the disorder, consult your doctor, who will probably take a swab from the inside of your vagina for laboratory analysis. Treatment is by a short course of drugs, in tablet form, which your doctor will prescribe for you and your partner.

Pruritis vulvae

Usually, vulval itching is caused by an identifiable disorder such as an infection, an allergy, or a generalized skin condition. When no such cause can be found, the itching is called pruritis vulvae. In young women the condition seems to be associated with anxiety or some emotional problem, such as trouble with a sexual relationship. It also occurs in older women, when it is thought to be due to an upset in the production of sex hormones, particularly a fall in the level of oestrogen. This happens most commonly after the *menopause* (p.586).

What are the symptoms?
If you have pruritis vulvae, your genital area is very sensitive, easily irritated, and intensely itchy. It may be sore and dry, especially during intercourse, and you may also have a thin white discharge. Older women may find bladder control difficult.

How common is the problem?
This problem is common, particularly in the over-45s. There are no dangers directly associated with the condition, but there is a risk that white patches of abnormal skin called leukoplakia will form in the irritated area. If this happens, there is a slightly increased risk of *cancer of the vulva* (below).

What is the treatment?
Self-help: It is important to try not to scratch the itchy area, since this will only make the irritation and any soreness worse. Wash the area with water and unscented soap once a day only and apply a soothing cream. Do not use talcum powder, vaginal deodorants, or *douches*, which are likely to increase the irritation. During intercourse, use a jelly specially made for lubricating the vagina. Wear cotton underwear and avoid nylon tights. If the condition does not improve within two weeks, see your doctor.

Professional help: Your doctor will examine you and probably prescribe a cream containing *steroids* or hormones to relieve the irritation. If there are also patches of leukoplakia, you will be advised to go into hospital and have them removed.

Vulval warts
(condyloma acuminatum)

Warts are small, occasionally itchy areas of viral infection on the skin. Warts on the vulva are fairly common, and are much the same as those on other parts of the body (see *Warts*, p.252). Because they are mildly *contagious*, warts on your vulva may have spread from those you have on your fingers, or perhaps from your sexual partner if he has *penile warts* (p.577). They spread more easily in moist conditions, and are more common in disorders which produce an increased vaginal discharge, such as *vaginal thrush* (opposite). They may also develop during pregnancy, when there is a natural increase in the moistness of the vagina.

In rare cases, vaginal warts that are neglected for many years become *malignant*. So if you think you have vulval warts, see your doctor. He or she will examine you to confirm the presence of warts and discover whether you have any other vaginal infection that may be encouraging their spread. If you have, then the warts may disappear when this other infection is treated.

What is the treatment?
Your doctor may treat any small warts by applying an anti-wart paint to them. The paint often makes the area sore and, as the doctor will tell you, must be washed off thoroughly eight hours later. The treatment may have to be repeated a few weeks later. If it fails, or if the warts are large or inaccessible, they can be removed in hospital. You will be given a general anaesthetic and the warts will be burned away by *diathermy*. If your partner has penile warts, these must be treated as well to prevent you becoming reinfected.

Cancer of the vulva

Cancer of the vulva is extremely rare, especially in women under 60. It starts as a small hard lump, which grows into an ulcer with thick, raised edges and a moist, red centre. Cancer of the vulva tends to grow very slowly, and early detection and treatment usually lead to a complete cure. What causes the cancer is not known, but it is believed that long-standing infections or irritations of the vulva may play a part in its onset.

Always report any lump or ulcer on the vulva to your doctor. If the doctor suspects cancer, you will be referred to a specialist, who will carry out a *biopsy* of the area. The usual treatment is surgery; either the growth and surrounding skin are removed (simple vulvectomy), or the growth, the lymph glands in the groin, and the skin between the two areas are removed (radical vulvectomy). Sometimes *radiotherapy* is given as well.

Sexual problems of women

Sex hormones secreted by the developing female embryo determine the formation and growth of the genitals. Because of the appearance of these genitals at birth, the baby is recognized and reared as a girl. Her awareness of being a girl is usually so firmly fixed during childhood that no reversal after the age of five is possible. At puberty, further female body characteristics appear, such as breast enlargement and pubic hair. These changes, combined with the attitudes of those around her, confirm the individual's sense of being female. In some women the normal pattern of female development is somehow changed or interrupted, with resultant sexual variations. The following articles include two such sexual variations: female homosexuality (also known as lesbianism) and female transsexualism (a sense of being a man imprisoned in a woman's body).

Also discussed is loss of sexual desire. The common term "frigidity" is not used because of its imprecision; as well as loss of sexual desire, it can mean lack of arousal – which is discussed as a special problem of couples (see *Lack of orgasm*, p.615).

Female homo- sexuality
(lesbianism)

Female homosexuals (lesbians) are erotically attracted to other females. In the past, female homosexuality used to be either ignored or deplored. Even today, when the rights of homosexuals are gradually being established, social prejudice can still create problems for a woman who otherwise fully accepts her homosexuality.

There is no known cause of lesbianism. It is not related to physical appearance and seems to be due largely to psychological rather than physical or hormonal factors.

Homosexual behaviour appears to be much less common in women than men; most studies indicate that between 2 and 4 per cent of adult women are exclusively lesbian. Many more, however, have had occasional homosexual experiences. These usually occur during adolescence, and are especially common in single-sex institutions such as girls' boarding schools.

What should be done?
If you are attracted to other girls in a situation where you are deprived of male company, do not assume that you will always be unresponsive to men. You are unlikely to become exclusively lesbian unless your sexual desires and fantasies are concerned only with females and remain that way even when you have plenty of chances to establish heterosexual relationships.

If you are homosexual, it may take a long time for you to realize and accept the fact. A young woman under social pressure to conform to accepted sexual patterns will sometimes do so in spite of her true orientation.

Once you realize that you are lesbian, you are likely to seek a stable sexual partnership which provides emotional security as well as physical satisfaction. If you find such a relationship, you will probably feel that you have no problem. You may, however, be less fortunate, and become anxious or depressed because you seem unable to find the right partner or because you feel uncomfortable in work or social life. In this event you will do well to seek guidance from a counselling agency such as the *Albany Trust* (p.768), or ask your doctor to refer you to a psychiatrist. An effort to "cure" your homosexuality is unlikely; most psychiatrists believe that the best course for an unhappy lesbian is to learn to accept her sexual orientation.

Female trans- sexualism

If you are a female transsexual, you are probably convinced that you belong to the male sex even though you have a female body. Most transsexuals have been dissatisfied with their sex since childhood and become obsessed with the desire to gain social acceptance as a male. Though you may have homosexual affairs, you think of yourself not as a woman making love to another woman but as the male partner in a heterosexual relationship. Female transsexualism appears to be very much rarer than the male equivalent (see *Male transsexualism*, p.581).

What should be done?
If you are severely troubled by your conviction that you are really male, your doctor can arrange a consultation with a psychiatrist,

who will assess your problem and help you to understand it. After your doctor and psychiatrist have discussed your condition with you, it may be agreed that the most beneficial course is for you to accept fully the fact of your male character and that, to further this, you should take regular doses of the male sex hormone testosterone to promote hair growth on your face and chest, to decrease feminine fat, and gradually to deepen your voice.

The most that a female transsexual can generally hope for is to acquire the external appearance of a man. Although it is relatively easy for a surgeon to amputate the breasts and remove the uterus and ovaries so that menstruation ceases, surgery to create male genitals is so difficult and the results so unsatisfactory that it is rarely advised. Most psychiatrists feel that before undergoing any surgery a woman should have a probationary period of living as a male for several years.

Loss of sexual desire in women

The clitoris, inner vulval lips, and vaginal lining of a woman who is sexually aroused become engorged with blood, in the same way that a man's penis becomes erect. However, because the body changes in a woman are less obvious than those in a man, they are often unrecognized, or seen, wrongly, as unimportant to a woman's enjoyment of sex.

The male sex hormone testosterone probably plays a part in maintaining sexual desire (sometimes called *libido*) in both sexes. In a woman testosterone is produced in small amounts in the adrenal glands and ovaries. A drop in the level of testosterone in proportion to the levels of the female sex hormones oestrogen and progesterone may be a factor in the reduction of sexual interest. If you lose your desire for sex to what seems an abnormal degree, however, the long-term reason is more likely to be psychological than physical. (Do not confuse loss of desire with difficulty in becoming aroused, which is a different matter – see *Sexual problems*, p.614)

Loss of desire sometimes begins as a physical problem. Many women find that their interest and enjoyment in sex is greater when they are in their late 30s and early 40s, and that it declines gradually after this age. Many women experience a certain loss of sexual interest after some significant event such as painful loss of virginity, childbirth, or gynaecological surgery. A woman whose ovaries and adrenal glands have been surgically removed (as treatment for cancer, say) may lose her desire because all sources of testosterone have also been removed. Certain drugs can reduce sexual desire, particularly those, such as alcohol and sleeping pills, that depress the central nervous system. *Steroids* may also reduce sexual interest, since they counteract the stimulating action of testosterone. Such counteraction is also caused by oestrogen-containing drugs' such as the contraceptive pill or hormone-replacement therapy for the *menopause* (p.586). Even when loss of desire has begun as a physical

problem, it may be perpetuated and aggravated by psychological problems. It is common for a woman to experience some loss of desire after stress. Problems in the relationship between a woman and her sexual partner can often cause loss of desire but this may be accompanied by a corresponding increase in sexual interest in other people, which can lead to further conflicts within the relationship. Finally, any chronic or painful illness can cause you to become generally depressed and lose interest in sex.

What should be done?

If loss of sexual interest worries you or creates difficulties with your partner, consider the advice given under "Self-help" below. If this does not resolve the problem, consult your doctor, who, after examining you, may advise you to see a specialist, probably a psychiatrist.

If you have never had much interest in sex, and you and your partner are satisfied with things as they are, you have no problems. There is no evidence to suggest that a relatively sexless life is in any way unhealthy.

What is the treatment?

Self-help: If you suspect a reason for your loss of libido, try to solve the problem for yourself. For example, try reducing your intake of alcohol or sleeping pills. It may also help to have a frank talk with your partner. Even if you fail to get to the root of the trouble, this may be the first step towards professional counselling for you both.

Professional help: Your doctor may feel that you need treatment for an underlying physical condition.

A woman whose hormonal balance has changed because she is past the menopause or has had certain reproductive organs removed (because of cancer, for example) may be helped by being given testosterone treatment, either as tablets or in the form of a pellet implanted in the thigh.

Special problems of couples

Introduction

The outlook for couples – that is, sexual partners – with problems has changed markedly during the recent past. Advances in surgical methods and the discovery of new drugs have transformed the prospects for many couples who would otherwise be infertile or suffer from chronic infection of the genital tract. But it is not only medical and surgical procedures that have changed. Attitudes too have changed, and sexual problems which would never have been considered as candidates for treatment or counselling can now be resolved.

The problems in this section of the book are divided into three groups. The first group deals with infertility and contraception. The choice of a contraceptive should be made by both you *and* your partner. There are several reliable techniques available, each with its advantages and disadvantages; you would be well advised to consult one of the helpful leaflets provided by the *Family Planning Association* (p.768) and also talk to your family doctor before you settle on one particular method. Contraceptives can be supplied without charge, either by the Family Planning Association or on prescription from your doctor;

and certain types are available over the counter. (If you have unprotected intercourse and do not want pregnancy to result, see your doctor within 24 hours. He or she may be able to arrange for *post-coital* contraception.)

The second group of problems in this section is concerned with sexually transmitted diseases. The term *venereal* diseases used to be applied to these disorders. The three main venereal diseases were syphilis, gonorrhoea, and non-specific urethritis. During recent years, though, it has been discovered that certain other diseases – among them glandular fever and acute hepatitis B – can also be transmitted if not by sexual intercourse itself, then by intimate sexual contact. The diseases covered in the following pages are those spread primarily (if not exclusively) by sexual contact.

The third group of problems included here are sexual problems. As emphasized above, these should be looked upon as difficulties for both partners to tackle. A frank exchange of views with your partner is of the utmost importance in these circumstances, and in some cases can solve the problem there and then.

Sexual intercourse

Sexual intercourse between a man and a woman can take place when the man's penis becomes erect enough to penetrate the woman's vagina. If the woman is also sexually aroused, the opening to her vagina widens slightly and glands in the vaginal lining secrete a lubricant fluid, making penetration by the penis easier.

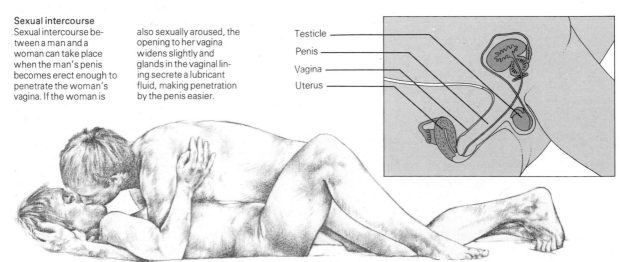

Testicle

Penis

Vagina

Uterus

Infertility and contraception

One of the greatest social changes this century has been the achievement of control over our fertility. However, health considerations, religious views, reliability, and sheer convenience may modify a couple's choice of contraceptive method.

Paradoxically, some couples are unable to achieve what many other couples spend most of their lives seeking to avoid – conception. However, modern diagnostic techniques coupled with sophisticated surgery and new drugs are able to offer otherwise infertile couples an eventual pregnancy.

For free information on contraceptives contact your doctor or a *Family Planning Clinic* at a local medical centre or hospital (see p.768 for address of the head office). The table (below) shows how many pregnancies, on average, can be expected if 100 healthy young couples use a given contraceptive technique (or none at all) for one year.

The contraceptive pill	less than 1
The IUD	2
Condom plus spermicide	3
Diaphragm plus spermicide	3
Condom	15
Diaphragm	15
Natural (rhythm)	20
Spermicide	25
No contraception	90

Infertility

After one year of regular, unprotected intercourse, 10 couples out of 100 will have failed to conceive (see the table above). There are very many causes of infertility or low fertility; only the more common ones are dealt with here. Among them are faulty egg or sperm production, structural abnormalities of the reproductive tract, and psychological factors such as stress and anxiety.

If you plan to have a baby, make sure you know the basics of sexual intercourse. Identify your most fertile days – see *Natural (rhythm) methods,* p.610 – and ensure your life style is not contributing significantly to low sperm production.

What is the treatment?

If you have not conceived in 12 months, you should *both* visit your doctor. Initially your doctor will establish whether intercourse is frequent enough and suitably timed, and also whether you might have a psychological or sexual difficulty such as partial or occasional *impotence* (p.614) which requires its own treatment. Should a correctable condition come to light, you will be advised on treatment and told to try again for several months. If you are still unable to conceive, you will probably be referred to a special fertility clinic for further tests.

The first test for the male partner is a microscopic examination of semen to check that it contains sufficient numbers of healthy sperm. (For information about how sperm are produced, see *Special problems of men,* p.570.) Many factors can contribute to a low sperm count – among them emotional stress, overwork and tiredness, an excess of alcohol, and a raised temperature within the scrotum (caused by a *varicocele,* p.573, for example).

A few days' abstinence from sex before ovulation takes place allows a build-up of sperm numbers. In some cases drug or hormone treatment can boost sperm production, and occasionally it is possible to concentrate sperm using a *centrifuge,* and then by *artificial insemination* introduce them into the partner's uterus. If there are no sperm in the semen, a *biopsy* of testicular tissue will confirm whether sperm are being manufactured. Surgery may be done to open up any blockage in the sperm ducts, but little can be done if there are very few or abnormal sperm.

The first tests for the female partner are to check that ovulation is occurring normally (if you have irregular or infrequent periods, ovulation may be faulty). If it is not, about half of all non-ovulating women can be helped by being given hormone injections or one of the "fertility drugs". You must take these drugs exactly as prescribed to minimize the risk of multiple pregnancy.

A blockage in the fallopian tubes, perhaps due to a previous *pelvic infection* (p.596), may be detected by several techniques – among them *laparoscopy* and *insufflation.* In some cases surgery can repair abnormal tubes. In others, the recently developed technique of removing a ripe egg from the ovary, fertilizing it with the partner's sperm, and then placing it in the uterus to continue development, offers hope for the future.

Contraception

The contraceptive pill

There are 3 main types of contraceptive pill – the combined oestrogen/progestogen pill, the triphasic pill, and the progestogen-only pill – all of which are available only on prescription. All three work by releasing synthetic hormones into your system to reduce in several ways your chances of becoming pregnant.

The combined pill: The combined oestrogen-progestogen pill is the most widely used and the most effective. It works by preventing ovulation (the monthly release of the egg), by making the mucus in the cervix hostile to sperm, and by affecting the endometrium (the lining of the uterus) so as to

Taking the pill
Oral contraceptives are reliable so long as they are taken regularly according to the instructions on the pack. However, vomiting or diarrhoea that lasts for more than 24 hours may expose you to the risk of pregnancy. At such times, continue taking the pills, but use some other method of contraception in addition until you are halfway through your next pack of pills.

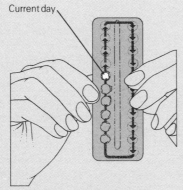

Current day

make implantation of a fertilized egg there highly unlikely. You can expect the combined pill to be 100 per cent effective if you take it according to the instructions on the packet. Very occasionally other drugs (especially certain *antibiotics* or anti-epileptic drugs) taken simultaneously or a severe gastrointestinal upset can cause the pill not to work, but most "failures" of the combined pill are due to the woman not taking it as prescribed.

You should use an additional contraceptive method for 2 weeks when you start taking your first packet of pills. The pill is usually taken for 21 or 22 consecutive days, followed by 6 or 7 pill-free days. You are likely to have less blood loss than during a normal period and you may also find that pain during periods and symptoms of *premenstrual tension* (p.585) are lessened.

Some women find that being on the pill makes them feel better generally, and their skin and hair condition improves. A few women experience side-effects such as nausea, breast discomfort, or spotting of blood between periods ("breakthrough" bleeding). There are a number of different types of combined pill and if you are not happy with one type, your doctor may decide to prescribe another.

It is important to have regular blood-pressure and other check-ups when taking the pill, because it can cause *high blood pressure* (p.382). If this happens, you will probably be advised to change to another method of contraception. Serious risks are very small unless you have suffered from or have a family history of *deep-vein thrombosis*

(p.405), *coronary thrombosis* (p.379), or *stroke* (p.268). If there is a history of any such disorder in your family, your doctor will certainly keep a closer check on your health and will probably advise you against taking the pill at all. Your doctor may also advise you against the pill if you have *sickle-cell anaemia* (p.422) or *diabetes mellitus* (p.519), which can predispose you to circulatory troubles. Another method of contraception may be recommended for a woman who has had *jaundice* (p.485).

The longer you take the pill and the older you are, the more you are at risk from a circulatory disorder. If you are over 35, and especially if you smoke, you should seriously consider changing to another form of contraception. Do not be too worried about giving up the pill if you are over 35. Other methods of contraception are generally a little less effective; but then your fertility is also decreasing, and a less effective method should be adequate. Signs that the pill is not the right contraceptive for you are pain in the legs or chest, swollen legs or ankles, severe or unusual headaches, *migraine* (p.285), and disturbed vision. You should report any of these symptoms to your doctor without delay.

The combined pill is not recommended immediately after childbirth, especially if you are breast-feeding, as it may reduce your milk supply.

Apart from those women mentioned as being especially at risk, most women on the pill are at very little risk. In fact the risks of a normal pregnancy and labour are higher than those associated with the pill.

The triphasic pill: Like the combined pill, the triphasic pill contains both oestrogen and progestogen and is taken for 21 days in every 28-day cycle. Unlike the combined pill, there are three different strengths of hormone in the triphasic pill, so the pills must be taken in the correct sequence for them to work. An advantage of taking the triphasic pill is that the total intake of artificial hormones is slightly reduced. The side-effects and risks are similar to those of the combined pill.

Progestogen-only pill: This is taken every day without a break, even through your period. Unlike the other types of pill, it does not prevent ovulation and you are slightly more at risk of becoming pregnant when taking it, especially if you do not remember to take it at about the same time every day.

The progestogen-only pill seems to be suitable for women of all ages. Side-effects are virtually unknown, and it can be taken by women who are breast-feeding. A disadvantage with this type of pill is that some women fail to have regular periods and may worry that they have become pregnant.

Progestogen injection: An injection of progestogen into the woman's arm or buttocks can provide at least 2 months' contraception. But because the injection can be effective for up to 2 years, and it is "irreversible" during this time, you should probably not consider this form of contraception if you wish to become pregnant in the next year or so. These injectable contraceptive hormones are licensed for only limited use in Britain, and their long-term effects are as yet unknown.

The IUD (coil)

An intra-uterine device (IUD) is a moulded piece of plastic, sometimes with copper added, inserted into the uterus through the cervix. Exactly how the IUD works is not known, but it is a highly reliable form of contraception (see the table on p.607), and the reliability increases with length of use. Fitting an IUD must be done by a doctor or other trained person. It takes about 5 minutes and usually requires no anaesthetic (it is particularly easy for the device to be fitted about 6 weeks after childbirth). Fitting may cause mild discomfort, and it is a good idea for you to take things easily for the rest of the day. Devices may need to be replaced every few years.

If you cannot tolerate the side-effects of an IUD (see below) or if you wish to have children – or if, by some misfortune, you become pregnant with the IUD in place – your doctor will remove it by pulling on the threads projecting from the cervix. (You should *never* try to do this yourself.) Because you have been ovulating regularly while using the IUD, you should be fertile as soon as it is removed.

Advantages: If you have an IUD, you have to make no preparations at all before intercourse and you do not have to remember anything other than to have check-ups by your doctor when advised.

Drawbacks: About 10 per cent of IUDs are expelled accidentally – hence the importance of a periodical check that the device is in place. If your IUD has been expelled, it may be worth trying again as the device will probably then be retained. The IUD also has several side-effects. Your periods may become longer, heavier, and more painful, especially for the first few months after the device is fitted. Between periods you may have some slight bleeding and intermittent pain. Also, some women have an increased mucus discharge but this is nothing to worry about. In addition, the presence of

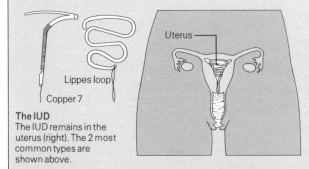

The IUD
The IUD remains in the uterus (right). The 2 most common types are shown above.

Lippes loop

Copper 7

Uterus

the device may interfere with the reproductive system's natural defences against infection. For this reason many doctors advise women who have more than one sexual partner not to use an IUD, since they appear to be at greater risk of catching a *sexually transmitted disease* (p.611). For the same reason, women who have not yet had any children but plan to do so in the future are sometimes advised against the IUD because a severe *pelvic infection* (p.596) can cause *infertility* (p.607). Finally, any pregnancy that does occur with an IUD still in the uterus is more likely than average to be an *ectopic pregnancy* (p.629).

The sheath (condom)

The sheath is basically a tube-shaped piece of thin latex rubber, closed at one end, which is rolled on to the erect penis before intercourse. When you ejaculate, sperm are trapped in the closed end of the sheath; during withdrawal of the penis following intercourse, the sheath should be held at the base to prevent it slipping off, and consequent spillage of sperm. For maximum reliability you should use the sheath in conjunction with some form of spermicide; some sheaths are already pre-lubricated with spermicide.

Advantages: The sheath is easily and widely available and there is a variety of designs. Wearing a sheath gives some protection against catching a sexually transmitted disease.

Drawbacks: Putting the sheath on to the erect penis tends to interrupt love-making, and the man may have reduced sensation in his penis.

The cap (diaphragm)

A cap is a rubber or plastic device that fits snugly over the cervix (the neck of the womb) where it presents a physical barrier to sperm. There are several designs of cap; the commonest is the diaphragm. Initially, a doctor will select a suitable design and size of cap for you, and show you how to fit it. Thereafter you fit the device yourself before intercourse

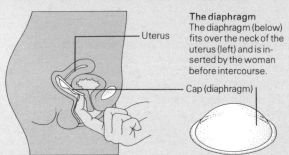

Uterus

The diaphragm
The diaphragm (below) fits over the neck of the uterus (left) and is inserted by the woman before intercourse.

Cap (diaphragm)

(not necessarily immediately before), remove it no less than 6 hours after intercourse, and clean it carefully ready for next time. *Always* use the cap in conjunction with a spermicide.

Advantages: The cap has very few (if any) side-effects on health, and is largely unobtrusive to either partner.

Drawbacks: You are advised to see your doctor every 6 or 12 months to check that all is well. A few women (and men) are allergic to the material caps are made of, and some couples feel that having to insert cap and spermicide reduces spontaneity in love-making.

Spermicides

These are chemicals that kill sperm. They are widely available and come in the form of cream, jelly, foam, *pessary*, or a spermicide-impregnated film, and are inserted into the vagina shortly before each session of intercourse. A spermicide should be used along with a sheath or cap (see the table on p.607). Very rarely, a spermicide may provoke an allergic reaction and cause itching and redness in the genital area.

(Continued overleaf)

Natural (rhythm) methods

The natural or rhythm methods of contraception do not employ any artificial aids, but are based on identifying the day in your menstrual cycle when you ovulate (release an egg). Intercourse on the few days before or after ovulation may result in conception, so these are the "unsafe" days when you should avoid sex. There are three common methods for determining your unsafe days:

The calendar method: Before you start this method, keep an accurate record of the lengths of your cycles for at least 12 months (in all calculations day 1 is the first day of your period). Then, to calculate your unsafe days, subtract 18 from the number of days in your shortest cycle, and 11 from your longest cycle. This gives you two numbers which are the days between which sex is unsafe. For example, if your shortest cycle is 25 days and your longest 30, days 7 to 19 inclusive are your unsafe days.

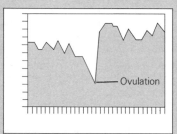

Temperature method
Before using the temperature method of contraception, you should record your temperature every morning for several months until you have established whether your temperature consistently falls and then rises at the same point in every cycle.

Ovulation

The temperature method: In most women, body temperature rises slightly (about 0.5°C – roughly 1°F) just after ovulation and does not fall again until the next period starts. To record this temperature change take your temperature each day as soon as you wake up, with a thermometer specially designed to detect a slight temperature change, and record it on a chart. In each cycle your unsafe days last from the last day of your period until temperature has been raised for three consecutive days.

The mucus-inspection method: At the time of ovulation the mucus in the cervix changes from being thick and sparse to being a thin, clear, profuse discharge which can be pulled out into long threads. You can learn to recognize these changes by examining your own mucus and recording its appearance. When the mucus reverts to the scanty, thicker state the fertile days are over.

How reliable are natural methods? In general, natural methods are not as reliable as artificially aided techniques (see the table on p.607). The calendar method used alone is the least reliable as it is always working retrospectively, and women with very irregular cycles may find, if they adhere strictly to this method, that they have no safe days at all. A combination of the temperature and mucus-inspection methods (called the sympto-thermal method) offers greatest reliability of all the natural methods if it is carried out under the guidance of your doctor or a member of the *Family Planning Association* (p.768). But in the end what really counts is your motivation as a couple and consequent willingness to abstain from sex on the unsafe days.

Sterilization

If you are sure that, whatever the circumstances, you never want another child, sterilization offers a virtually 100 per cent safe form of birth control. You must, however, be *absolutely certain* about your decision, because sterilization must be regarded as an irreversible procedure.

Because sterilization is simply a sealing off of the tubes that carry sperm or eggs, it has no effect on the production of sex hormones. If you are a man, you will produce sperm-free semen; women will produce eggs but these cannot reach the uterus, and simply die and disintegrate. Sterilization does not affect masculinity or femininity in any way.

Sterilization is available free on the National Health Service and it is definitely advisable to discuss the matter with your family doctor or a family planning counsellor before deciding on further action. Whichever partner is intending to be sterilized, the surgeon will usually ask for the written consent of both of you before performing the operation.

Male sterilization (vasectomy): Vasectomy is usually performed as an out-patient procedure, using a local anaesthetic, and takes only about 20 minutes (see diagram). Your doctor will probably ask you to wear a pair of close-fitting underpants or a jock-strap, to ease any dragging feeling you may have in the testicles for a few days after the operation. There may be some bruising of the scrotum, but this will usually disappear within a few weeks.

After the operation you will remain fertile until sperm already present in the vas deferens have been ejaculated or die. So for the first 16 weeks or so after the operation you will be advised to use some other means of contraception.

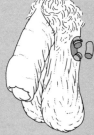

Vasectomy
A vasectomy is usually done under a local anaesthetic. The surgeon makes 2 small incisions in the scrotum, then cuts each of the 2 vas deferens and ties the ends. Additional contraception should be used until 2 samples of ejaculate are found to be sperm-free.

During that time you will have to return to the hospital with a specimen of semen at least twice. When two consecutive specimens have been found to be sperm-free you are sterile. How soon you have sexual intercourse after the operation depends entirely on how you feel.

Female sterilization: Female sterilization usually requires a general anaesthetic but is an operation that causes very little discomfort, takes only about 15 minutes to perform, and requires merely a 24-hour stay in hospital or attendance at an out-patients' clinic. In the most commonly performed operation, a tiny cut – which leaves virtually no scar – is made just below the navel. Through this a *laparoscope* is inserted, and an attachment to this instrument is used to seal off the tubes by *electrocautery* or tiny metal or plastic clips. Alternatively, the tubes may be cut and tied through a small abdominal incision (a *mini-laparotomy*).

Sexually transmitted diseases

A sexually transmitted disease (otherwise known as a *venereal* disease) is an infection transferred from person to person during sexual contact. The most common way to catch such a disease is by sexual intercourse; other ways are by various forms of sexual contact, such as oral or anal sex.

If you suspect you have caught a sexually transmitted disease, *consult a doctor without delay.* This can be your own doctor, or a doctor at a clinic specializing in such diseases (you need not go to your family doctor first). Only about half the patients who attend such clinics are diagnosed as suffering from a sexually transmitted disease; the other half are reassured that there is nothing wrong, or diagnosed as having some other minor complaint. All visits to clinics are treated in the strictest confidence.

There are two excellent reasons for seeking prompt medical help. The first is that, though sexually transmitted diseases are curable with modern treatment, they may be less easy to cure if there is a delay. The second reason is that you can unknowingly pass on the infection during its *incubation period*, before symptoms appear. Once the condition is identified, you should abstain from sexual relationships until you are cured, and also ensure that your sexual contacts visit a doctor as soon as possible.

In addition to the diseases in this section, there are other conditions that may be transmitted sexually. These include *trichomonal vaginitis* (p.602), *penile warts* (p.577), and *vulval warts* (p.603), as well as some forms of hepatitis (see *Acute hepatitis B*, p.486) and various tropical diseases.

Gonorrhoea

Gonorrhoea (popularly known as the "clap") is an infection caused by neisseria gonorrhoeae, a bacterium transmitted by sexual intercourse and other forms of sexual contact. In men, the infection usually starts in the urethra (the passage through which urine is passed) or, in those who indulge in anal sex, the rectum. In women the cervix may be infected as well as the urethra, and in some cases the rectum is also affected whether anal sex has taken place or not. Gonorrhoea can affect the throat after oral sex.

What are the symptoms?
In the man, symptoms appear within a week or two of the infection being contracted. The first thing you notice is a little discomfort on passing urine. At the same time there may be a slight discharge of pus from the tip of your penis. If the condition is not treated, the discharge becomes thicker and more profuse.

If you are female, gonorrhoea may cause no symptoms at all. In other cases there may be an alteration and increase in your vaginal discharge, or, if the infection is in the rectum, there may be a feeling of dampness there or some pus on the faeces. Urinary symptoms are not common. Gonorrhoea of the throat occasionally makes it sore.

How common is the problem?
Each year, about 1 person in 1,000 visits a hospital clinic because of gonorrhoea. It is more common in people with several sexual partners. Two-thirds of sufferers are male.

What are the risks?
In a very few cases (more often in women than in men), the infection spreads from the genital region and causes a form of arthritis and spots on the skin; in women, it can spread to nearby organs such as the uterus and fallopian tubes. Rarely it can go on to cause *urethral stricture* (p.578) in the man.

What should be done?
As soon as you suspect you have gonorrhoea, see your doctor or go to a clinic which specializes in sexually transmitted diseases. It is important not to have any sexual relations until your problem has been treated.

The diagnosis of gonorrhoea is made from laboratory examinations of samples of secretions taken from the infected area. The sample is obtained from an infected urethra by means of a small wire loop; the procedure causes only minor discomfort. In women with suspected gonorrhoea, samples are usually taken from the cervix, urethra, and rectum.

What is the treatment?
Gonorrhoea is cleared up by a course of *antibiotics* given as tablets or capsules, or, less commonly, by injection. Your doctor may advise you not to drink alcohol during the course of the treatment.

Non-specific urethritis (NSU)

NSU is an infection of the urethra, the passage through which urine flows from the bladder to the outside. The disease is transmitted from person to person during sexual intercourse, but for many years the exact nature of the microbes causing the infection remained unknown because of technical difficulties in isolating and identifying them (hence the name "non-specific" urethritis). Modern laboratory techniques have shown about 45 per cent of NSU cases are caused by a bacterium called chlamydia trachomatis; there are probably other microbes that cause NSU which have not yet been identified.

What are the symptoms?

In a man, the symptoms of NSU take anywhere between one and five weeks (the *incubation period*) to appear after the infection has been contracted. The first noticeable symptom is a slight tingling at the tip of the penis – sometimes felt only when you urinate first thing in the morning. The tingling may be accompanied by a scanty, clear discharge – again sometimes only early in the day. If the infection is untreated, the discomfort may become worse and the discharge slightly heavier and thicker. Eventually the symptoms fade away, but the infection may remain dormant and, unless treated, can still be transmitted to another person during sexual intercourse. In a woman, NSU usually causes no symptoms at all, or it may produce a slight increase in vaginal discharge.

How common is the problem?

Statistics from hospital clinics specializing in sexually transmitted diseases show that each year 1 person in 500 catches NSU and that 80 per cent of these sufferers are male. This makes NSU the most common of the sexually transmitted diseases.

What should be done?

If you have the symptoms described, see your doctor or visit a clinic specializing in sexually transmitted diseases. Do not have intercourse until the problem is diagnosed and treatment is completed. The doctor will examine you and take a sample of urethral discharge for laboratory examination. If the diagnosis is NSU, the treatment is relatively simple. You will be given a course of *antibiotics*, which will clear up the condition provided you complete the course as prescribed and do not resume sex until the course is finished. Women who are sexual partners of men with NSU also need to be examined, and even when they are symptom-free will usually also be given treatment.

Syphilis

This potentially serious but rare disease is caused by the bacterium treponema pallidum which is transmitted during sexual intercourse or some other form of sexual contact. The bacteria enter through a small cut or abrasion or through the moist mucous membranes that line the urethra (the passage through which urine flows), the rectum, the vagina, and the mouth.

The disease goes through several stages. In the first (primary) stage, a sore called a *chancre* develops where the infection entered the body. In men this is usually on the penis (or the anus in homosexuals). In women it is usually on the vulva (the external genitals). The sore is painless, feels hard underneath, and is highly infectious. It may be accompanied by the painless enlargement of nearby lymph glands. Unfortunately, not only can the sore take anywhere from nine to 90 days to develop (which may make it difficult to identify which person you caught it from) but it can easily pass unnoticed. After a few weeks, it disappears of its own accord.

The second stage starts several weeks after the development of the sore. In about 75 per cent of cases a rash, which does not itch, appears all over the body, including the palms and soles. You may also notice painless swellings of lymph glands, and moist wart-like lumps around the anus (even when this is not the original site of infection) and sometimes in the armpits. Like the primary sore, these are extremely infectious. After several weeks the rash disappears spontaneously, and the disease enters the so-called latent phase which is symptomless.

Antibiotic treatment has made it exceedingly rare for the latent stage of syphilis to progress to the late stage, when serious complications, such as *aortic incompetence* (p.399), or an *aneurysm* (p.407) in the aorta, or neurological problems can occur. It is only

Diagnosing syphilis
A diagnosis of syphilis can be made by using an instrument called a loop to remove some of the substance inside the sore, then examining it under a microscope.

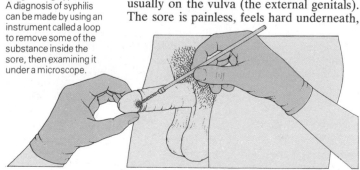

in people who have not had their syphilis treated (and then only in a third of these cases) that serious complications develop.

How common is the problem?
In an average year, 1 person in 12,000 visits a hospital clinic because of syphilis. Almost 90 per cent are men; most are homosexual.

What should be done?
If you notice any symptoms that suggest syphilis, go as soon as possible to a doctor –

either at a clinic specializing in sexually transmitted diseases or to your own doctor. The diagnosis is made from analysis of blood samples and scrapings from the sore or rash. You should avoid all sexual relations until you are either cleared of having the disease or are completely cured of it.

Treatment is simple – a two-week course of antibiotic injections will clear up the infection. To make certain that there is no relapse, however, regular blood tests will be arranged for two years after treatment.

Herpes genitalis

The herpes virus, which is responsible for the infection that produces *cold sores* (p.451) on the face and mouth, is the most common cause of ulcers on the genitals. Herpes genitalis affects both sexes and particularly people who have not had cold sores on the face. It is caught either during sexual intercourse with a person whose genitals are infected or after oral sex with someone who has cold sores. Herpes genitalis may recur after the original infection (sometimes over a period of many years), and so the disorder can crop up during a faithful sexual relationship of long standing.

It is not known exactly what precipitates attacks of herpes. They seem to occur when you feel run-down. Many people find that intercourse reactivates the infection.

What are the symptoms?
After an *incubation period* of usually less than 10 days there is an itchy feeling on the shaft of the penis or on the vulva (the female exterior genitals), followed by the appearance there of a crop of small blisters. In some cases these also occur on the thighs and buttocks. After

about 24 hours the blisters burst to leave small, red, moist, painful ulcers, which sometimes go on to form a hard crust. The glands in the groin may become enlarged and painful, and you may also feel generally unwell and have a raised temperature.

The attack generally lasts about two weeks. Half of those affected have no further problems, but the other half have, over the following months or even years, recurrent attacks. These tend to be progressively milder and become less and less frequent.

What should be done?
If you think you are having a first attack of herpes genitalis, see your doctor or attend a clinic specializing in sexually transmitted diseases. Although there is no cure for the disorder, you will be given one of several antiviral ointments and liquids that make the ulcers less painful and cause them to heal more quickly. Recurrent attacks often clear up fairly quickly whether treatment is given or not.

During an attack, avoid intercourse to lessen the possibility of transmitting the infection to your partner.

Pubic lice

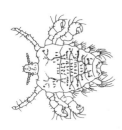

Pubic louse, magnified about 20 times.

Pubic lice, also known as crab lice (or, popularly, as "crabs"), are blood-sucking lice that usually appear only in the pubic hair and the hair around the anus. Occasionally, however, in very hairy people, they occur in other body hair and sometimes on the eyebrows and eyelashes. The louse, which can be seen clearly if you look closely, is from 1 to 2mm (about $\frac{1}{10}$ in) across and resembles a minute, flat crab. The female's pale, shiny eggs ("nits"), which can just be made out with the naked eye, are attached so firmly to hairs that normal washing will not remove them. Pubic lice are almost always caught after sexual contact with someone who already has the infestation.

What are the symptoms?
It will usually be several weeks before you know you have caught pubic lice. This is the time it takes for the lice to breed and appear in noticeable numbers. Many people have no symptoms; others experience itching in the pubic region, particularly at night.

What should be done?
If you have pubic lice, go to a clinic that specializes in sexually transmitted diseases or to your doctor. You will be given a lotion or cream which kills the lice and their eggs. At the same time the doctor may advise a checkup to make sure that you do not have any other sexually transmitted diseases.

Sexual problems

Sometimes a couple are deprived of the full enjoyment of sexual intercourse – or even prevented from engaging in it at all – by physical or psychological problems. These problems are discussed separately in the following articles, but many couples suffer from a combination of problems often stemming one from another. For example, premature ejaculation by a man may result in lack of orgasm for his partner. Advice and treatment are far more successful if such problems are tackled by both partners.

For problems that primarily affect the individual – transsexualism, for instance – see *Sexual problems of women*, p.604, and *Sexual problems of men*, p.580.

Impotence

A sexually impotent man is one who fails to get or maintain an erection. Most males have probably experienced temporary impotence at some time, generally due to a psychological rather than a physical problem. Even if impotence initially has a physical cause, it is often exaggerated by anxiety about inadequate sexual performance.

Among the physical factors that can cause impotence are stress, fatigue, chronic illness, and excess alcohol. Other causes are surgery or disease affecting the spinal cord or genitals, and the side-effects of certain drugs.

What should be done?
Discuss your impotence with your partner. Impotence can be caused merely because your partner is not aware of the particular type of stimulation you need. Always choose a place and time for love-making free from anxiety and conducive to sexual arousal. If impotence persists, consult your doctor, who will first look for and treat any specific physical cause for your problem. In some cases the doctor may prescribe regular doses of testosterone or an anti-anxiety drug; in other cases sex therapy may be advisable at a specialist clinic. Here impotence is likely to be treated as a problem for both you and your partner. You will probably attend about 10 therapy sessions and be given sexual exercises, designed for your particular problem, to perform at home. Such treatment has a good chance of restoring full potency.

Premature ejaculation

Premature ejaculation is male orgasm immediately after, or even before, the penis penetrates the vagina. Habitual premature ejaculation is frustrating for both partners and may produce impotence in the man and loss of sexual interest in the woman. A man who has not previously suffered from the problem may begin having trouble if he has an infection such as *prostatitis* (p.576) or urethritis (see *Urethritis in men*, p.578), or has one of certain diseases of the nervous system. The cause is usually psychological, however. Control over the timing of orgasms is basically something you learn, much as you learn bladder and bowel control. If your initial sexual experiences are rushed or anxious, your learning process may be retarded; and worry can make it worse.

At the beginning of a relationship, rapid ejaculation is so common that it can be regarded as normal. As the relationship continues, most men develop control. However, habitual premature ejaculation is probably the most common male sexual problem.

What should be done?
At the start of a relationship do not worry; you should soon develop more control. If you remain incapable of control, talk about the problem with your partner. Relaxation before sex may help by reducing your anxiety. If you are unable to solve the problem yourself, see your doctor, who may want to examine you to rule out a physical cause of the condition before advising treatment. If there is no physical cause, you may be referred to a sex therapist who will give you advice to follow when you are making love. The therapist may recommend that you and your partner temporarily abandon sexual intercourse and try substituting other forms of body contact; and when you are on the verge of having an orgasm, you or your partner can delay it by squeezing the penis firmly just beneath the glans. When this exercise is repeated at regular intervals, control increases dramatically, and intercourse can then be resumed. The results of such therapy, which can be repeated if necessary, are usually excellent.

Lack of orgasm

Lack of orgasm is nearly always caused by underlying psychological problems. However, it may follow on from loss of sexual arousal or impotence due to a physical complaint – for example, damage to the nervous system by accident or disease, or a side-effect of a drug. Lack of orgasm is extremely rare among men, but only about 1 in 3 women regularly reaches orgasm through intercourse alone – without additional stimulation of the clitoris – and about 10 per cent of women never reach orgasm under any circumstances (including masturbation).

If you are dissatisfied with the frequency or ease with which you or your partner reaches orgasm, have a frank discussion about the matter. You may find that you need to change your sexual techniques. For example, it may help to spend more time stimulating each other's genitals with fingers or mouth before intercourse. A vibrator may also be helpful.

If the problem persists, see your doctor, who may refer you to a specialist clinic. The doctor is unlikely to prescribe drugs unless they are needed for associated problems. Your therapist at the clinic will provide both sessions at the clinic and exercises to be carried out at home – for example, stimulating orgasm by picturing erotic fantasies at the peak of sexual activity.

Painful intercourse
(*dyspareunia*)

Painful intercourse affects most women at some time in their life; in men it is rare. Often the cause is physical in a man, but there is frequently a psychological reason in women. Whatever the sex of the sufferer, both partners are affected.

Painful intercourse in women

There are two types of female dyspareunia, superficial and deep. The superficial type of pain – irritation or a burning sensation – is experienced in the vulva or vagina. Usually it is caused by lack of sexual arousal: the vagina remains dry, and penetration by the penis is consequently painful (see *Loss of sexual desire in women*, p.605). Another cause of superficial dyspareunia is an uncommon condition known as *vaginismus*. This is an involuntary *spasm* of the muscles surrounding the vaginal entrance, which becomes virtually closed, while at the same time the thighs may be drawn together and the back arched. Women with vaginismus try to avoid penetration during intercourse, vaginal examinations, and the use of tampons.

Physical conditions that can cause superficial dyspareunia include *pruritis vulvae* (p.603), cystitis (see *Cystitis in women*, p.600), *haemorrhoids* (p.483), surgical scars, and allergy to douching solutions, deodorants, or spermicides.

If you have deep dyspareunia, which is less common than the superficial type, it generally feels as if the penis has hit a tender spot inside your abdomen. There may also be some pain after intercourse, backache, and *dysmenorrhoea* (p.584). Deep dyspareunia is most commonly caused by a *pelvic infection* (p.596), *endometriosis* (p.595), or some abnormality of an ovary.

If you cannot identify and deal with the cause of painful intercourse yourself, see your doctor. If the trouble seems to be physical, you may be referred to a gynaecologist. Otherwise you (and possibly your partner) may be advised to consult a sex therapist.

Self-help: Try using an artificial lubricant if part of the problem seems to be a dry vagina. Avoid any positions that you find particularly uncomfortable.

Professional help: Gynaecological treatment will be related to the underlying cause – for instance, *antibiotics* for an infection, or sex therapy for lack of sexual arousal.

Painful intercourse in men

Male dyspareunia is commonly experienced in the penis. It may be due to an infection of some kind in the genital area (see *Sexually transmitted diseases*, p.611). Chemical contraceptive and douching agents used by the woman can also inflame the skin of the penis, and some men are allergic to rubber condoms. Your penis may suffer discomfort if your partner has a dry vagina, or if she has an *IUD* (p.609) and the threads attached to it are protruding into the vagina. In this last case, ask a doctor to trim the threads. Male dyspareunia can also be caused by a tight foreskin (see *Phimosis*, p.711).

Pain may also be experienced in the penis (or more deeply) during ejaculation. This can be due to urethritis (see *Urethritis in men*, p.578), *urethral stricture* (p.578), or a problem of the *prostate gland* (p.574).

If you cannot remedy the problem yourself, see a doctor. For a sexually transmitted infection, the doctor will provide appropriate treatment for the disorder. Circumcision may be advised for a tight foreskin. In other cases the doctor may refer you to a *urologist* for specialist diagnosis and treatment or, if no physical cause is suspected, to a sex therapist.

Pregnancy and childbirth

Introduction

A healthy young woman having sexual intercourse two or more times a week without using any method of contraception has a 90 per cent probability of conceiving a child within 12 months. Conception occurs shortly after a mature egg (*ovum*) has been released from one of your two ovaries, approximately halfway through your menstrual cycle (for more information on ovulation see *Menstruation and the menopause*, p.583). The egg travels along the fallopian tube towards the uterus (womb). If you have sexual intercourse during this time, the millions of sperm that your partner has ejaculated may travel from your vagina through the uterus, and up to the fallopian tube. Here one sperm and the egg come together, and fertilization takes place. The fertilized egg reaches the uterus a few days later and embeds itself in the lining of the uterus. This happens at about the time your next period would have been due. So, by the time you are beginning to suspect that you might be pregnant, the embryo is already developing rapidly in your uterus.

A full-term pregnancy lasts about 38 weeks from conception. Conception usually occurs midway through a woman's menstrual cycle but, because the exact day is rarely known, doctors calculate a pregnancy from the first day of a woman's last period. This means that a woman who has conceived midway through a regular 28-day cycle will be said to be four weeks pregnant two weeks after conception, and this method of dating her pregnancy two weeks ahead will continue until delivery. So the entire pregnancy will be said to have lasted on average 40 weeks.

The articles in this section are divided into general problems of pregnancy – ranging from the almost universal problem of heartburn to the comparatively rare disorder of Rhesus incompatibility – and disorders that tend to occur in either early, mid-, or late pregnancy. The events that you can expect in a normal delivery and most common problems of childbirth are described, as well as the modern techniques available to help you during pregnancy and childbirth. Any problems that might affect the mother shortly after childbirth are also discussed. Problems particularly affecting the newborn baby are described in the section *Special problems of infants and children* (p.644).

German measles (rubella) and pregnancy

If you contract *German measles* (p.699) during pregnancy, there is a risk that your baby will be born with a defect, such as heart disease or deafness. The risk is highest if you catch the illness in early pregnancy. When infection occurs during the first 4 weeks, more than 50 per cent of babies are born with a major defect. By the 13th week that figure has dropped to 8 per cent, and it steadily decreases from then on. The type of defect also depends on at what stage during pregnancy the mother is in contact with German measles.

If you have had (or been immunized against) German measles, you are unlikely to catch it again. However, do not rely on your own or a relative's memory that you have had the illness but make absolutely sure by asking your doctor to give you a blood test. If the test shows you have not had the disease, your doctor will immunize you against it with an injection of vaccine that gives you a mild form of the disorder. You must avoid conception for 3 months after the injection, since during that time the disease, though mild, could still harm a developing baby.

If you fail to take the precautions described and do develop German measles in early pregnancy, you will be given the opportunity to have the pregnancy terminated – and thus to avoid the considerable risk of giving birth to a severely handicapped child. Remember that any tests you may be offered can only show whether your child has certain congenital deformities (see *Screening for congenital defects*, p.630); for example, mental deficiency and deafness are only detected months after the child has been born.

Conception

Egg production

A woman has 2 ovaries, 1 on each side of the uterus, which contain many thousands of immature eggs. After puberty, 1 egg normally ripens each month in 1 of the ovaries. The maturing egg and about 100 other cells that cluster around it and nourish it together form what is called a follicle. This follicle is filled with fluid and protrudes from the ovary. About halfway through the menstrual cycle, the follicle bursts and the ripe egg is expelled (ovulation) and drawn into the entrance of the fallopian tube nearby. The diagram on the right shows the successive stages in development and bursting of the follicle, as indicated by the arrow.

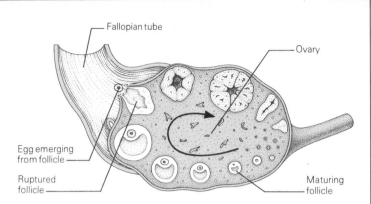

Sperm production

Sperm are minute, tadpole-shaped cells made in the many coiled tubes, called seminiferous tubules, in the 2 testes. The sperm pass from the testes into the epididymis, then into the vas deferens and seminal vesicles where they are stored until ejaculation.

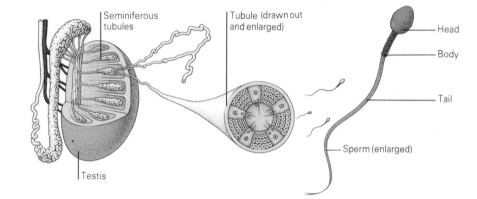

The path of the fertilized egg

As the egg is fertilized by a sperm and begins to divide, it passes along the fallopian tube to the uterus.

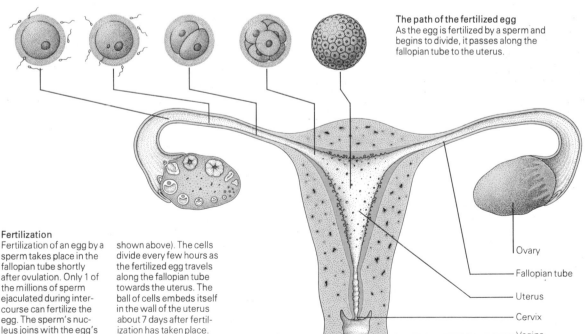

Fertilization

Fertilization of an egg by a sperm takes place in the fallopian tube shortly after ovulation. Only 1 of the millions of sperm ejaculated during intercourse can fertilize the egg. The sperm's nucleus joins with the egg's nucleus and the process of cell division begins (as shown above). The cells divide every few hours as the fertilized egg travels along the fallopian tube towards the uterus. The ball of cells embeds itself in the wall of the uterus about 7 days after fertilization has taken place.

The growing embryo

Until about the 12th week of pregnancy, the developing baby is known as an embryo. From 12 weeks until delivery, it is called a fetus. The embryo develops extremely rapidly. At 5 weeks it is about the size of a grain of rice, but by 12 weeks it is about 60mm (2½in) long.

At 28 days the largest, most developed organ is the heart. The limbs first develop as buds; the nervous system, eyes, and ears are all present by 6 weeks. The proportions of a developing embryo are very different from those of an adult human being. The illustrations below show the embryo at different stages of development and (in outline above each illustration) at life size.

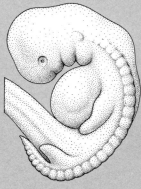
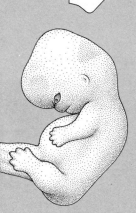
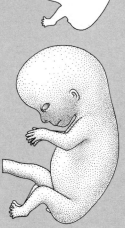
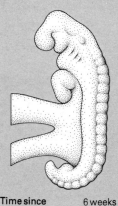

Time since last period

6 weeks

7 weeks

9 weeks

10 weeks

Your changing shape

During the first weeks of pregnancy, there is little visible change in your body, although your breasts may seem a little larger and feel tender and heavy. By about the 12th week, the expanding uterus is too large to stay hidden in the pelvis and can be felt through the abdominal wall. By the time you are 20 weeks pregnant, your abdomen may be swollen and, instead of being indented, your navel may be protruding. Towards the end of pregnancy the baby's head may move down slightly to settle in the pelvic cavity. This makes your breathing easier, but means that you may need to pass urine more often.

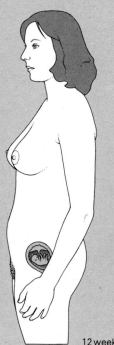

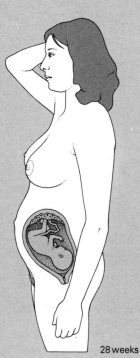
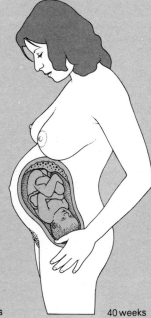

12 weeks

28 weeks

40 weeks

The placenta

At first the baby developing in the uterus is nourished by the mother's bloodstream via "roots" or trophoblasts growing into the lining of the uterus. By about 20 days these are recognizable as the placenta. The fetus is attached to the placenta by the umbilical cord extending from what will be the baby's navel. Fetal blood flows to the placenta and there absorbs substances from – and expels waste products into – the mother's blood in much the same way that your blood takes up oxygen from – and expels carbon dioxide into – your lungs. Maximum exchange of substances is facilitated by the villi, which provide a large surface area within the placenta.

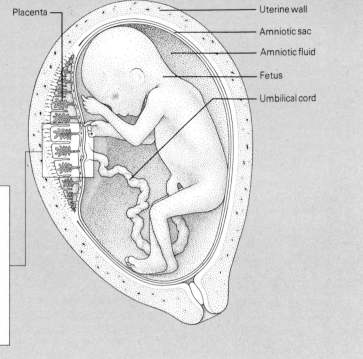

Placenta
Uterine wall
Amniotic sac
Amniotic fluid
Fetus
Umbilical cord

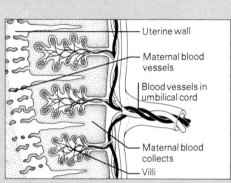

Uterine wall
Maternal blood vessels
Blood vessels in umbilical cord
Maternal blood collects
Villi

Genetic counselling

As medical understanding of inherited diseases has improved, genetic counselling services have been provided by specialists or specialist units in hospitals. These are to help couples who come from families with a history of some inherited disease and who are worried that they might give birth to a child with the disease.

Children born with cystic fibrosis, sickle-cell anaemia, thalassaemia, or certain other inherited diseases acquire them from parents who, though healthy, are both *carriers* of the disease (see *Genetics*, p.704). Tests are now becoming available to show whether couples are carriers of such diseases or not. If both parents are carriers, the risks of their having a child with the disease can be calculated, and they will also be told about the severity of the disease, whether treatment is available, and whether the diagnosis can be made before the baby is born. As an example, if both prospective parents are found to be carriers of thalassaemia, they will be told that there is a 1 in 4 chance that a child will be affected; that, if they decide to have a child, the mother should have tests carried out early in pregnancy because the disease is of crippling severity; and that, if the fetus is found to have thalassaemia, the pregnancy can be terminated. When parents have religious or other objections to termination of pregnancy, the tests will not be carried out, since

they involve a slight risk for the fetus (see the box on *Special procedures in pregnancy*, p.639).

In some cases, matters are less clear-cut than in the example above: the detection of carriers may not be completely reliable, and diagnosis before birth may not be possible. In these circumstances, the counsellor will probably study the pattern of the disease over several generations before assessing the risks. There is also a high risk of certain inherited diseases – for example, *haemophilia* (p.424) – being passed on when only one parent is a carrier.

If you and your partner have any worries that you might give birth to a child with an inherited disease, you should ask your doctor for genetic counselling. And you should make sure the doctor refers you only to a specialist or specialist clinic: calculation of the risks of inherited disorders is too critical to be made by anyone other than an expert.

Apart from possibly having to undergo tests to determine whether you are carriers, you will also be asked for details of the health of your parents and other relatives – so have this information with you, in written form, when you go for counselling. In every case, the genetic counsellor can only give advice; he or she cannot guarantee that a baby will be normal, and eventually the decision whether to go ahead and have a child has to be taken by the couple themselves.

General problems of pregnancy

The problems dealt with on the following pages may occur at any time throughout the nine months of pregnancy. In some cases, even the diagnosis of pregnancy itself may not be very straightforward. On the other hand, many women claim that they just "know", at a very early stage, when they are pregnant. Others can only tell if they have some of the recognized early symptoms of pregnancy. These symptoms include: missing a period when previously regular; having a short, scanty period and tender, swollen breasts with darkening of the nipples; nausea; more frequent urination; an increased vaginal discharge; feeling more tired than usual; suddenly going off some foods, or having a peculiar taste in the mouth.

Diagnosis of pregnancy

If you have been having unprotected sexual intercourse and you miss two periods after having previously been regular, then you may well be pregnant and should see your doctor for confirmation. At this stage, the doctor can usually diagnose pregnancy by a vaginal examination. However, if you have had trouble with previous pregnancies or you do not wish to have a child, you will want to know whether you are pregnant at an earlier stage. In this case, as soon as you suspect you are pregnant, you should have a pregnancy test. This can be arranged through your doctor, your local family planning clinic, or a reputable commercial pregnancy-testing service; alternatively, you can carry out your own test, with a kit obtained from a chemist's (see *Do-it-yourself pregnancy testing*, below).

Once your pregnancy has been confirmed, and if you wish it to continue, your doctor will arrange for you to attend an ante-natal clinic run either by the doctor or by the hospital in which you are planning to have your baby. You will probably attend your first ante-natal clinic when you are twelve weeks pregnant and should continue to attend regularly throughout your pregnancy.

Diet during pregnancy

When you are pregnant, much of what you eat goes to your baby to enable him or her to develop healthily. It is therefore essential that you eat regular, well-balanced meals. Meat, fish, cheese, beans, lentils, and eggs are excellent sources of protein; dairy products are rich in calcium; eggs, liver, kidneys, wholemeal bread, dried fruit, and green vegetables will supply you with the iron you need to avoid *anaemia during pregnancy* (p.623); and fresh fruit and vegetables provide vitamins. (For further information see *Eating and drinking sensibly*, p.24.) If you gorge yourself you will of course put on weight.

And while excessive weight gain may not necessarily be harmful, it will nevertheless make it much harder for you to regain your figure after your baby is born. An occasional alcoholic drink does not seem to harm the fetus but if you usually drink alcohol daily you should cut your intake (see *The effects of alcohol*, p.33). Smoking during pregnancy can definitely cause your baby to be underweight at birth and also increases the risk of premature delivery. If you find it impossible to give up smoking, you must at least try to cut down on the number of cigarettes you smoke (see *The dangers of smoking*, p.38).

Do-it-yourself pregnancy testing

Kits for do-it-yourself pregnancy testing are available from any chemist's. They work by reacting with a hormone called *HCG*, which is present in the urine of pregnant women about 2 weeks after the first missed period. The most widely used type of kit contains a chemical solution which, when mixed with a few drops of urine in the test tube provided, will, if you are pregnant, almost always form a dark ring in the tube. If no ring forms, this means that you are probably not pregnant. The negative result is less reliable than the positive; it may well be false if you are taking anti-depressant drugs, nearing the menopause, or having irregular or infrequent periods. Always follow the manufacturer's instructions carefully. For testing purposes, the urine should be passed first thing in the morning, before you drink anything. The concentration of HCG is then at its highest.

Physical activity during pregnancy
(including sex)

Pregnancy is not an illness, and most women are advised to carry on with their everyday activities very much as they usually would.

Exercise: Contrary to popular belief, there is no reason why you should avoid physical activity while you are pregnant, unless otherwise advised by your doctor. Regular exercise, especially walking or swimming, will probably help you to feel well and stay fit, although there is no evidence that it will aid the development of your baby. It is wise to avoid strenuous sports, especially those that carry a danger of injury – for example, horse riding. But as a general rule, after discussion with your doctor, you can feel safe to continue the forms of exercise you enjoy as long as you are careful not to strain yourself.

Travel: Travelling may make you tire more easily than usual, and you should allow for this in planning any journeys. Most airlines will not carry women who are in the last weeks of pregnancy because of the risk of an unexpected delivery. If you are planning to fly, you should check with the airline before you start your journey. Try to avoid travelling if you suffer either from travel sickness or morning sickness. If you have to make a long journey in these circumstances, discuss with your doctor the choice of an *anti-emetic* (anti-sickness) drug; under no circumstances should you yourself choose and take such drugs while pregnant.

If your doctor has given you any records concerning your pregnancy, you should always carry these with you so that in an emergency the doctors treating you can be fully acquainted with your condition. Avoid travelling far from home if you have recently had a threatened *miscarriage* (p.628), if you are within about two weeks of the expected time of delivery, or if your pregnancy has some complications that would require the specialist knowledge of your local hospital in the event of an emergency.

Work: Most women stop working at about the 28th week of pregnancy, which is when they become eligible for the state maternity benefit and grant. If your doctor thinks your work is too strenuous, or if you have had problems with any previous pregnancies, he or she may advise you to give it up before that time. However, if you feel well, there is no medical reason not to continue working until much nearer the time of the birth.

Sex: If your pregnancy is normal, you can safely have sexual intercourse throughout its entire term. Pregnancy makes some women feel more like having intercourse, but others lose the desire altogether; in such cases, sexual desire almost always returns to normal after pregnancy.

If you have had repeated miscarriages during past pregnancies, or if you have recently had a threatened miscarriage, it is probably better to avoid intercourse until about the 16th week of your pregnancy.

In the last four weeks of pregnancy it is advisable to have intercourse while lying on your side since you will probably find this position more comfortable. In this position, penetration by your partner is not so deep and there is therefore less risk of a premature labour being precipitated.

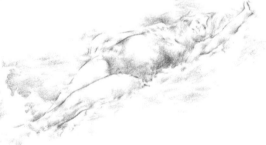

Swimming
This is an excellent form of exercise for anyone, but especially for pregnant women as the baby's weight is supported by the water.

Nausea and vomiting during pregnancy
(morning sickness)

Many women are affected by nausea and vomiting during early pregnancy. This happens most frequently in the morning, often immediately after waking, but it can happen at any time if you allow yourself to become over-tired or wait too long between meals. Vomiting usually begins during the first month and continues until the 14th to 16th week. It is usually minor and harmless, though unpleasant. Only in a small percentage of cases does it develop into severe vomiting, known as hyperemesis; this drains the body of fluids and chemicals and harms general health.

How common is the problem?
About 1 in 15 pregnant women sees a doctor because of the condition, and it is estimated that 0.5 per cent of all pregnant women who vomit develop hyperemesis. Vomiting is most common in first pregnancies.

What should be done?
If you have begun vomiting during your pregnancy, avoid greasy foods and do not go too long without eating; take frequent small meals instead of a few large meals. If you experience nausea on waking, try eating some dry toast or a cream cracker before you

get up. Never take any drugs for your nausea or vomiting without consulting your doctor.

If your vomiting is making you very miserable, see your doctor. He or she will examine you, both to assess whether the vomiting is affecting your physical health and to check on the unlikely chance that some disorder such as a urinary infection is the cause of the vomiting. A reassuring examination alone may well be enough to enable you to put up with your symptoms until they eventually disappear. If not, your doctor may prescribe an antivomiting drug for you.

Hyperemesis requires hospital treatment. Antivomiting drugs are given, and fluids and chemicals are replaced by *intravenous drip*.

Heartburn during pregnancy

Heartburn is a burning pain in the centre of the chest and upper abdomen, sometimes accompanied by an unpleasant taste in the mouth or belching. Despite its name, it has nothing to do with the heart. For further information see *Hiatus hernia* (p. 456).

The complaint affects almost half of all pregnant women. This is because during pregnancy the muscle that helps to close off the upper part of the stomach from the oesophagus (gullet) becomes lax (as do many other muscles during pregnancy) and allows digestive acid from the stomach to enter the oesophagus and irritate its sensitive lining. In late pregnancy the enlarging uterus presses on the stomach and aggravates the condition. Heartburn is harmless and nearly always disappears after delivery.

What should be done?

You can minimize heartburn by eating small meals frequently. This means that there is always food in the stomach to soak up much of the acid. If this does not solve the problem, go to your doctor, who will probably prescribe an antacid to be taken regularly.

Where to have your baby (home or hospital)

Most babies in Britain today are born in hospital. A few women are delivered at home; some who would prefer home birth are advised against it by their doctors. What *are* the relative merits of hospital and home deliveries?

Hospital facilities and specialist staff make the maternity department of your local hospital the safest place for delivery. During labour you will probably be attended by a midwife (a nurse with training in the procedures of childbirth and post-natal care). If your delivery is expected to progress smoothly, you may be in the care of a "pupil" (trainee) midwife, with only occasional checks from senior staff. If anything threatens to go amiss, however, expertise and experience are immediately available; an *obstetrician* is always on call in virtually every maternity department. In addition, there are such aids as monitoring equipment, fetal *tocographs* (p.640), and newborn-baby revival units for use in case of unexpected complications.

At a home confinement, with only a midwife and/or doctor (usually a GP) in attendance, there may be risks. But advocates of home delivery maintain that unforeseen complications are rare and that home delivery is a calmer, more peaceful, and more private affair. The bright lights, noise, and general hospital hubbub are absent, and the baby is welcomed into the family circle without delay.

To some extent, of course, your decision must be governed by where you live. In an inner-city area you may find that no local GP is prepared to deliver babies at home. In a rural area where the choice is between a small hospital and your comfortable house, home delivery may be preferable. If there is even a slight possibility of trouble, a hospital maternity unit with specialist techniques is the only practical choice. For a first baby, it is always wise to go into hospital, but if you have had one or more problem-free births and your pregnancy is proceeding normally, you need not fear home delivery. If your doctors resist your request for home delivery even though no complications seem likely, and if you are determined to have your baby at home, consult your local branch of the *National Childbirth Trust* (p.768). Although, for obvious reasons, doctors prefer pregnant women not to change from one type of care to another after making an initial decision, you will have to change to more specialized care if complications develop at any stage of your pregnancy.

If you decide to have the baby in hospital, you can often choose one of several types of hospital care. You can have the baby in a consultant unit, under the care of a particular obstetrician's team (though your obstetrician may not actually deliver the baby). Or you can give birth in a general-practitioner unit, where it may be possible for your family doctor to attend you. Or if you want to have your baby in hospital and go home as soon as possible, you may be able to do this under what is known as the "domino" scheme, which provides care by a particular midwife, who will accompany you into hospital for the birth, go home with you for a day or two afterwards, and then visit you regularly.

To find out the various options open to you, talk to your family doctor as soon as pregnancy is confirmed. Ask, too, about "shared care" – an arrangement that permits a woman who wants to have her baby in hospital to remain under the care of her family doctor throughout pregnancy while seeing the consultant obstetrician at occasional intervals.

Anaemia during pregnancy

Haemoglobin is the red blood pigment that carries oxygen to the body's tissues. If the haemoglobin in your blood falls below an adequate level, you become anaemic. The most common cause of a low level of haemoglobin is a deficiency of iron in the body (see *Iron-deficiency anaemia*, p.419); another cause is often an inadequate amount of folic acid (see *Pernicious anaemia and folic-acid deficiency*, p.420).

Even if you take in a normal amount of iron and folic acid in your diet, you may become anaemic when you are expecting a baby; during pregnancy the blood becomes more dilute as its volume is increased; and later in pregnancy the baby will need an increasingly large proportion of iron and folic acid.

What are the symptoms?

You may not notice a slight degree of anaemia, but if it is pronounced, the symptoms include paleness, weakness, tiredness, breathlessness, fainting, and palpitations.

What are the risks?

Anaemia in pregnancy makes you less able to cope with a sudden large loss of blood, as in a *post-partum haemorrhage* (p.638). It also makes you more vulnerable to infection after having the baby. If you become severely anaemic, there is a risk that the baby will suffer from a lack of oxygen in the uterus and will not have enough iron reserves to combat possible jaundice in the first few weeks of life.

What should be done?

You can help prevent anaemia during pregnancy by eating foods especially rich in iron – liver, beef, wholemeal bread, eggs, and dried fruit. Eat citrus fruits and fresh vegetables; the vitamin C in these helps iron to be absorbed more efficiently. Make sure you eat plenty of green vegetables, since these are the best source of folic acid.

What is the treatment?

Early in your pregnancy, your doctor will check whether you are anaemic by performing a simple blood test. Even if this shows that you are not anaemic, the doctor will probably prescribe tablets of iron and folic acid to supplement your natural intake. These tablets used to make many people nauseated or constipated but have now been improved to minimize their side-effects. If, despite this improvement, you find the side-effects troublesome, tell your doctor, who will probably be able to prescribe another type of tablet that may be more suitable for you.

In the unlikely event that you develop severe anaemia, the treatment given will be that described for iron-deficiency anaemia.

Constipation during pregnancy

Constipation is common in pregnancy, and is probably caused mainly by increased laxity of the digestive-tract muscles. In late pregnancy it is aggravated by the pressure of the enlarging uterus (womb) on the bowel. Constipation is rarely a dangerous condition and is nothing to worry about.

You can help to avoid constipation by eating plenty of fresh fruit and vegetables and other foods with a high fibre content (see *The components of a healthy diet*, p.25), by drinking plenty of fluids, and by not delaying going to the lavatory when you feel the need to.

What is the treatment?

Do not take laxatives without consulting your doctor, since some can irritate the intestine. If your constipation is very bad, see your doctor, who will probably prescribe a medicine to soften the faeces.

Varicose veins during pregnancy

Many women suffer from *varicose veins* (p.409) during pregnancy, especially in the later stages. As the uterus enlarges, the flow of blood from the leg veins up to the abdomen is slowed. This sometimes produces pressure which causes the veins in your calves and thighs to become swollen and painful. The veins around the entrance to the vagina may also be affected.

What should be done?

Rest with your feet up as often as possible. If you are working and you spend a lot of time on your feet, tell your employer about your condition so that some periodic relief from standing can be arranged.

Support stockings and tights relieve the discomfort of varicose veins considerably and can stop the veins from becoming more swollen. You can either ask your doctor to prescribe them or buy them over the counter. Always put them on first thing in the morning *before* you get out of bed and keep them on until last thing at night.

The veins usually become considerably less swollen after you have had your baby.

Sleeping problems during pregnancy

Many women find it difficult to get to sleep when they are pregnant. This may be due to worrying about the baby or to physical problems: the need to pass urine more often, *heartburn during pregnancy* (p.622), the baby kicking, or the sheer difficulty of getting comfortable. Anxiety about the loss of sleep (which actually has no harmful effects) makes it even harder to fall asleep, and so a vicious circle tends to develop.

What should be done?

First read the article on *How to get a good night's sleep* (p.20). It may also help if before going to bed you do some of the relaxation exercises you have learnt at your ante-natal classes. During the later stages of pregnancy, when the developing baby may be pressing on a nerve, it can sometimes help if you lie on your side with a pillow placed under your knees or your hips. If none of this works, it is best to accept that you are going to have a wakeful night and not worry about it. Take a varied amount of reading matter to bed with you or do household chores during these wakeful hours. Then try to catch up on your lost sleep at some other time, when you do start to feel tired.

If, despite following this advice, you are distressed that you are missing your normal sleep, do *not* take any drugs but see your doctor. He or she *may* be able to prescribe a sedative, but would much rather that you coped without. The doctor will be even less keen to prescribe a sedative if you are in the first 14 weeks of pregnancy – when there is the risk that the drug could harm the baby – or if you are nearing delivery – when the drug could make the baby very sleepy after birth, causing breathing difficulties.

Backache during pregnancy

When you are pregnant, the ligaments and fibrous tissue that normally lock your joints firmly together become slightly more elastic. This is to allow your pelvis to expand at the moment of birth and so facilitate straightforward delivery. However, this loosening of the joints also has an adverse effect: it makes them more susceptible to strain. This applies particularly to the joints of your spine, because during pregnancy these come under additional strain, anyway: the growth of your uterus shifts your centre of balance and your stance becomes abnormal. So even standing for any length of time can give you what is known as either non-specific backache or sciatica (see *Backaches*, p.546).

What should be done?

Follow the advice given in the box on *How to protect your back* (p.547). In particular always bend at the knees rather than from the waist when picking things up. And you can reduce the strain on your back during pregnancy to a minimum by keeping your weight within reasonable proportions. Your ante-natal clinic will give you advice and teach you exercises. For *treatments for backache*, see p.548. Like many other problems of pregnancy, backache usually disappears after your baby is born.

Relieving backache
A gentle exercise for relieving backache is to kneel on all fours and arch your lower back a few times. When you relax, never allow your back to hollow, as this can cause more backache.

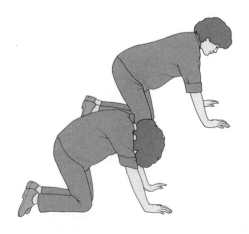

High blood pressure and pregnancy

At routine check-ups in early pregnancy some women are found to have *high blood pressure* (p.382). This may have been present for some time before pregnancy, or it may be due to the anxiety of expecting a baby. In cases of anxiety, the pressure will gradually subside to normal, and stay there, as the mother gains in confidence. But in cases of pre-existing high blood pressure, although the pressure usually falls slightly during the middle weeks of pregnancy, it rises again at the end. There are generally no symptoms.

Pre-existing high blood pressure is not as serious a problem in pregnancy as is blood pressure that develops in late pregnancy; the latter can be a sign of *pre-eclampsia and eclampsia* (p.631). However, if not controlled it can lead to haemorrhage, intra-uterine death or retarded fetal growth.

What should be done?

The earlier pre-existing high blood pressure is discovered, the greater your chances of having a safe pregnancy. That is why it is important to see your doctor as soon as you suspect you are pregnant. If you are found to have high blood pressure, you will be given frequent examinations. Not only will the pressure be monitored but blood and urine tests will also be performed to check on the function of your kidneys and the well-being of your baby. *Ultrasound* (p.639) may also be used to ensure that your baby is developing at a normal rate.

You will be advised to rest, and if your blood pressure is above a certain level, you may well be prescribed an antihypertensive drug to lower it. Most women with the condition can have a normal delivery, but if your blood pressure is very high, you may be advised to have a *Caesarean section* (p.640) a week or so before the baby is due.

Heart disorders and pregnancy

Pregnancy always involves the heart in extra work, and if your heart already has some serious underlying defect, such as may be caused by a *congenital heart disorder* (p.656), there is a risk of *heart failure* (p.381).

What should be done?

If you have a severe heart disorder, you should consult your doctor before deciding to have a baby; if you become pregnant, with or without the doctor's go-ahead, you will probably come under the care of a specialist.

Although a doctor usually knows if a woman has a heart disorder, sometimes a disorder is revealed only under the stress of pregnancy. Any such disorder may produce a heart murmur, which will be detected by the doctor during a routine examination, but a murmur does not necessarily denote a disorder, and in fact the vast majority of heart murmurs discovered in early pregnancy are completely insignificant. If the doctor does suspect a heart disorder, an *electrocardiogram* and other tests may be carried out.   (*Continued overleaf*)

Unwanted pregnancy

The news that you are pregnant is not always welcome. If, after careful consideration, you decide that in no circumstances can you take care of the child you are expecting, there are two courses of action open to you. You can complete the pregnancy and have the child adopted or, if you act early enough in your pregnancy, you may be able to have the pregnancy terminated (popularly called an "abortion"). Termination is legal in Britain only if two doctors agree that the operation is necessary on the grounds of your physical or mental health, if there is a substantial risk that the child will be abnormal, or if the health of your other children may be adversely affected.

In some parts of Britain you may find difficulty in having your pregnancy terminated on the National Health Service. Of the variety of private services that offer a termination for a fee, some are run purely for commercial reasons and should be avoided. Your doctor should be able to tell you of a reputable clinic or one that is supported by abortion charities and so charges lower fees.

The following organizations give advice to those who have an unplanned pregnancy: the *Brook Advisory Centres* (free clinics that will also give advice to those under 16); the *British Pregnancy Advisory Service* (a private charitable organization); the *National Council for One-Parent Families* (free advice on all aspects of pregnancy); the *Family Planning Association* (a charitable organization). Addresses are given on p.768.

The two methods most commonly used for terminating pregnancy during the first 12 weeks are *D and C* (p.593) and removal of the contents of the uterus by suction apparatus inserted through the vagina. After the 13th week, the pregnancy is usually terminated by *induction of labour* or, rarely, by a very early *Caesarean section* (p.640); at this stage the risks of termination become substantial, and usually an abortion will be delayed as late as this only if there has been a need to wait until this stage before a suspected abnormality of the fetus can be diagnosed as certain. Termination is illegal after 28 weeks.

What is the treatment?

The main treatment is rest, so that extra strain is not placed on a heart already under stress. You may be given *antibiotics* to take throughout your pregnancy since at this time your heart is more susceptible to bacterial infections. Any heart failure will be treated as necessary. If you smoke, you will be told to make every effort to stop.

When you go into labour, the doctor's main aim will be to secure an easy delivery for you, one with the minimum of pushing, since this puts a strain on the heart. *Episiotomy* and *forceps* (p.640) may be used for this reason.

Drugs and pregnancy

A pregnant woman should take no drugs during pregnancy – except those prescribed by her doctor as part of her care. This applies not only to prescribed medicines you may have left over from a previous illness, but also to over-the-counter medicines. Abstinence from smoking and a strict limit on alcohol intake are also important.

Most drugs, and many foods, can pass from the mother's bloodstream through the placenta into the developing baby. A few drugs may cause the baby to develop abnormally, especially if taken during the first 2 to 3 months when the baby's major organs and parts of the body are developing, so a woman should avoid drugs if there is the slightest possibility that she might be in the early stages of a pregnancy that has not yet been confirmed.

The most important exceptions to this general ban on drugs during pregnancy are the iron and vitamin supplement tablets that expectant mothers are given at the ante-natal clinic. These will not harm the baby – indeed, they are important for the baby's normal, healthy development.

If you have a long-term medical condition such as diabetes or epilepsy, always inform your doctors about your intention to become pregnant. And it is vital that, when you become pregnant, you take your drugs and plan your diet precisely as advised by the doctor, in order to safeguard your health and the health of your baby.

A third exception to the ban may be drugs that your doctor prescribes if you are ill during pregnancy. Since the thalidomide tragedy of the early 1960s, doctors are reluctant to provide what may be "non-essential" preparations such as sleeping pills, tranquillizers, or anti-emetics (antinausea drugs). However, a few pregnant women do need such drugs, and also drugs such as *antibiotics* to combat infection. In these essential cases the doctor will select a well-established drug that has been carefully scrutinized for use during pregnancy (a process called *teratological* screening).

Finally, if you ever have doubts about whether any drug – no matter how mild – is safe to take while pregnant, check with your doctor beforehand.

Diabetes and pregnancy

Diabetes mellitus (p.519) increases the risks of complications in pregnancy. About 15 per cent of all babies carried by women with severe diabetes die before or shortly after birth, despite every precaution; and the risk to the mother's life during pregnancy is about twice as high as average.

For every woman known to have diabetes before pregnancy there are several who are found to be mildly diabetic during pregnancy; these are mainly women with a family history of the disease. Women who have previously had a baby weighing more than 4.3kg (9½lb) may also prove to have mild diabetes in subsequent pregnancies.

What should be done?

You will be given a glucose-tolerance test (see *Diabetes mellitus*, p.519) if diabetes in pregnancy is suspected, especially if sugar is found in your urine on routine laboratory analysis of two or more specimens. You should not worry about this – glucose is commonly found in the urine of non-diabetic pregnant women, and the test is simply a precautionary measure.

What is the treatment?

If you are found to have diabetes, you will receive the appropriate treatment. And you may well be admitted to hospital for the last 10 weeks or so of the pregnancy, so that the diabetes can be controlled precisely and the baby's condition monitored.

After the 36th week of pregnancy, the risk to the baby's life begins to rise steeply, and delivery will usually be by *induction of labour* or *Caesarean section* (p.640).

Rhesus incompatibility

Rhesus incompatibility is an incompatibility between the Rhesus blood group of the mother and that of the fetus. It occurs only if the mother is Rhesus negative and the fetus is Rhesus positive (through having inherited Rhesus positive *genes* from the father). See the boxes entitled *Genetics* (p.704) and *What are blood groups?* (p.428).

When any baby is born – and also sometimes after a *miscarriage* (p.628), an abortion (see *Unwanted pregnancy*, p.625), or an accidental haemorrhage (see *Ante-partum haemorrhage*, p.631) – some of the baby's blood enters the mother's circulation. Most Rhesus negative women have their first baby without any problems, but the mother may, after the birth, become "sensitized" to any Rhesus positive blood that has entered her circulation, and in any later pregnancy *antibodies* may pass from her bloodstream into that of the developing baby and start destroying the baby's red blood cells. The situation does not occur if the father's ABO blood group is incompatible with the mother's.

How common is the problem?

About 85 per cent of the population are Rhesus positive. This means that a Rhesus negative woman having a child has an 85 per cent chance of having the child by a Rhesus positive man. However, only one Rhesus negative woman in 20 seems to develop antibodies after her first pregnancy, and, in women who do, modern diagnosis and treatment have made problems very rare.

What are the risks?

Rhesus incompatibility produces no symptoms in the mother. In the cases when it occurs, the baby is at risk of developing *haemolytic anaemia* (p.423) and *neonatal jaundice* (p.647) at birth or, in extreme cases, of being stillborn. These risks are substantially increased with each successive Rhesus-incompatible pregnancy.

What should be done?

At the beginning of pregnancy you will automatically be given a blood test to determine (among other things) whether you are Rhesus negative or positive. If you are Rhesus negative, then your partner's blood will also be tested and, if the results show that there is a chance that the baby will be Rhesus positive, you will have regular blood tests throughout your pregnancy.

If it is your first pregnancy, the tests are aimed at making sure that yours is not a rare case where antibodies develop before the baby is born. If it is a subsequent pregnancy, the tests are carried out to make absolutely sure that the treatment given after your previous pregnancies was effective (see "What is the treatment?" below). If you had your first pregnancy before modern treatment was available, then antibodies may well have formed already and the blood tests will show their concentration in your body.

What is the treatment?

The development of a *serum* called Anti-D has largely made the danger of Rhesus incompatibility a thing of the past. The serum is given by injection to the mother soon after every delivery (and after a miscarriage or accidental haemorrhage) and destroys any of the baby's red blood cells in the mother's circulation before the mother's body has had time to develop antibodies. In the rare cases when antibodies develop, the baby may be given an intra-uterine transfusion.

Rhesus disease in pregnancy

When a Rhesus negative mother gives birth to a Rhesus positive baby, some of the baby's blood can escape into the mother's bloodstream during labour (1). If the mother is not given an injection of anti-D serum within 48 hours of labour, she will develop antibodies to Rhesus positive blood (2). If she becomes pregnant with another Rhesus positive baby, her antibodies may cross the placenta and destroy this baby's red blood cells (3).

Key
- ⊟ Rhesus negative blood
- ⊞ Rhesus positive blood
- ▲ Antibodies

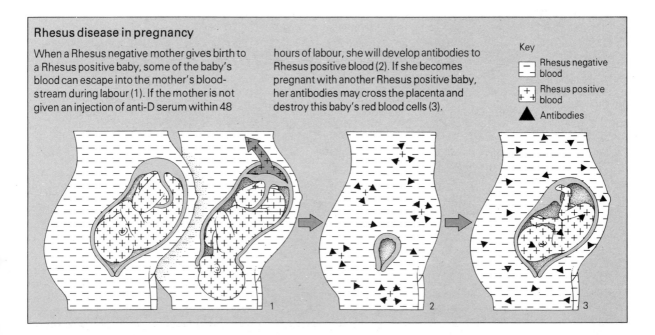

Complications of early pregnancy

During the first three months after conception, the fetus is developing rapidly. It is during this period that it is most vulnerable, since all of its major organs are forming. Almost inevitably, most pregnant women experience at least one of the minor complaints, such as nausea or constipation, mentioned in the previous pages. More serious complications include threatened or completed miscarriage, and ectopic pregnancy.

Miscarriage

A miscarriage (known medically as an abortion) occurs when a pregnancy ends spontaneously before the beginning of the 28th week of the pregnancy, counted from the first day of the last period. After that time, the spontaneous premature ending of a pregnancy is termed a stillbirth if the baby is born dead or a premature delivery if the baby is born early but alive. When a pregnancy is ended artificially, this is known popularly as an abortion, medically as a termination of pregnancy (for further information see *Unwanted pregnancy*, p.625).

A miscarriage may occur because the fetus has some abnormality; because the uterus has some structural defect; or because of some hormonal imbalance in the mother. Miscarriages from falls or other minor accidents to the mother are rare, because the fetus is well protected inside the uterus.

Miscarriages can be grouped into different categories. It is not unusual for some women to experience what is termed a "threatened" miscarriage in early pregnancy. This is usually indicated by a small amount of bleeding from the vagina. In many such cases the pregnancy then proceeds normally.

An "inevitable" miscarriage, however, is one in which the fetus has died and in which, no matter how much care is taken once the symptoms of the miscarriage have appeared, the pregnancy will be aborted.

The term "incomplete" miscarriage is used for a miscarriage in which parts of the fetus and placenta have remained in the uterus after most of its contents have been expelled.

A "missed" miscarriage means that the baby has died in the uterus but that there are no noticeable symptoms.

"Recurrent" miscarriages seem to occur mainly in women who have an imbalance in their sex hormones. Such miscarriages normally happen early in pregnancy, but some occur after the third month, when they may be due to an incompetent cervix.

What are the symptoms?
The first symptom you are likely to notice at the start of an abortion is bleeding from your vagina. This can range from a few drops of blood to a heavy flow. The bleeding either starts with no warning or is preceded by a brownish discharge.

A threatened miscarriage is often painfree. But if the fetus is dislodged and the miscarriage is "inevitable", the uterus begins to contract and pain will be felt in the lower abdomen or back. The pain may be either dull and constant or sharp and intermittent. At some stage during a miscarriage you may pass some solid matter out of the vagina. Try to keep this material in case your doctor wants to examine it.

In an incomplete miscarriage, bleeding and pain may go on for several days, either constantly or intermittently. With a missed miscarriage, you may well have no bleeding or pain, but the symptoms of early pregnancy will disappear and your breasts will probably feel less full. Often the only symptom is that your doctor discovers that your uterus has not increased in size since your previous antenatal examination.

How common is the problem?
Each year about 1 in every 10 pregnant women sees a doctor about a miscarriage.

Vaginal bleeding in pregnancy

If you have bleeding from your vagina at any stage during pregnancy, you should tell a doctor straight away, or, if the bleeding is heavy, call for an ambulance and lie down while you are waiting. Bleeding in early pregnancy may be due to *cervical erosion* (p.597), but it can be the sign of an impending miscarriage. Bleeding in late pregnancy may be an *ante-partum haemorrhage* (p.631), although a slight blood-stained discharge may be the "show" indicating that labour is about to begin (see *Childbirth*, p.634).

What are the risks?

Miscarriages generally present no risks to a woman's health. If you fail to see your doctor about an incomplete miscarriage and allow it to drag on, you will eventually become anaemic and the tissue in your uterus may become infected.

What should be done?

If you are pregnant and have bleeding from the vagina, with or without pain, tell your doctor and rest at home. If the bleeding stops or is fairly light, the doctor may simply tell you to continue resting. If the bleeding is heavy or you have severe pain, the doctor will probably send you to hospital.

If, after you have had bleeding, it seems that the pregnancy is continuing, your doctor may arrange for you to have another pregnancy test, and perhaps *ultrasound* (p.639), to confirm the pregnancy. It is best not to have sexual intercourse for a few weeks after you have had bleeding.

Recurrent abortions due to hormone imbalance can be diagnosed by blood tests and by a microscopic study of samples of mucus that have been taken from the neck of the uterus. In the case of a threatened miscarriage, there is nothing that can be done medically, and you will probably be told simply to rest in bed as much as possible.

What is the treatment?

If your miscarriage is inevitable, incomplete, or missed, you will usually have the remains of the fetus and placenta removed from your uterus under general anaesthetic. If you have had recurrent miscarriages, you will be referred to a gynaecologist. If the cause is discovered to be a ·sex-hormone deficiency, you will be given the appropriate hormone to correct the imbalance. If the cause is a fault in your cervix, you may need a minor operation (see *Incompetent cervix*, p.630).

After a miscarriage you are likely to be depressed by your loss. However, you can safely start trying to conceive again as soon as you like afterwards – though ideally you should wait until you have had at least one normal period, since your doctor can then estimate more accurately the likely delivery time of the baby.

Ectopic pregnancy

In ectopic (or tubal) pregnancy your egg is fertilized by a sperm in the normal way but develops outside the uterus, usually in one of the fallopian tubes. The placenta burrows into the surrounding tissue, which usually tears and causes internal bleeding. This tissue is unfitted to sustain a placenta and fetus, and it is impossible for the pregnancy to continue. You will experience constant, severe abdominal pain, which will probably be followed by bleeding from the vagina.

Each year about 1 woman in 20,000 is treated for ectopic pregnancy. Such a pregnancy usually occurs for no apparent reason – but it is known that you are more at risk of having one if you have had some abnormality of your fallopian tubes from birth or if they have been previously operated on or infected, or if you are using an *IUD* (p.609).

What should be done?

If during pregnancy you develop abdominal pain that lasts for more than a few hours, see your doctor right away. If you delay, you run the risk of suffering severe internal bleeding and consequent *shock* (p.386).

Your doctor will examine you carefully, since the abdominal pain of ectopic pregnancy can be confused with that of several other conditions, including a miscarriage, appendicitis, and infection of the fallopian tubes. You may be referred to a hospital. There *ultrasound* (p.639) can often enable an accurate diagnosis to be made, but sometimes it can be confirmed only by *laparoscopy*.

Once an ectopic pregnancy is confirmed, any loss of blood you have suffered is treated with a blood transfusion and an operation is performed immediately. The fertilized egg, placenta, and surrounding tissue are removed and the torn blood vessels are sealed.

Even if one of your fallopian tubes has been damaged by an ectopic pregnancy, any subsequent pregnancy should proceed normally, although your future chances of conception are slightly reduced.

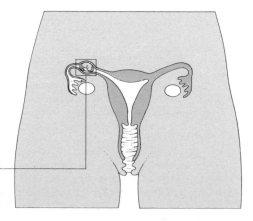

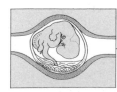

The position of an ectopic pregnancy
Except in rare cases, an ectopic pregnancy occurs in a fallopian tube when, for some reason, the fertilized egg has not travelled into the uterus.

Complications of mid-pregnancy

During the middle three months of pregnancy, many women say their health has never been better. Their sense of well-being may be caused by the fact that the baby's development is now proceeding at a less hectic rate. Most women start attending ante-natal clinic when they are about 12 weeks pregnant. At the clinic, their general health is assessed and they are given iron and folic-acid tablets.

Blood and urine samples are examined and blood pressure is checked at every visit.

The main complications that can occur at this stage are an incompetent cervix and hydramnios. Hydramnios is rarely serious, provided it is recognized early; and although an incompetent cervix may cause a miscarriage, such a disorder can easily be treated during any subsequent pregnancy.

Incompetent cervix

In this condition the cervix opens up during pregnancy, usually at some time after the 14th week, causing an inevitable *miscarriage* (p.628). Often the cervix is weak because of damage during a previous delivery or a gynaecological operation, but sometimes the cause of the weakness is unknown.

If it is known or suspected that you have an incompetent cervix, a miscarriage can be prevented by an operation in early pregnancy.

While you are under a general anaesthetic, a piece of stout thread is sewn through the cervix (in the manner of an old-fashioned purse string) and tightened, holding the cervix firm. After the operation you may be given a drug to lessen the chances of the operation stimulating *premature labour* (p.636). The thread is cut when labour starts or at about the 38th week of pregnancy if labour has not begun by then.

Hydramnios

Hydramnios is usually a harmless condition which can occur in the later stages of pregnancy and in which there is an excessive amount of amniotic fluid around the baby. In most cases, the swelling of the uterus is only slightly greater than normal and the condition produces either no symptoms or gradual onset of increasing breathlessness, indigestion, and a tense ache in the abdomen. In rare cases, the swelling is greatly pronounced, the onset of the symptoms described is sudden and accompanied by nausea, and there is a risk of premature labour.

Hydramnios is found to be more common than average in diabetic mothers, in women suffering from *pre-eclampsia* (p.631), and in those with a multiple pregnancy (see the box on *Twin pregnancy*, p.633).

What should be done?
For a minor case of hydramnios, your obstetrician will probably advise you simply to take a little more rest. For hydramnios of sudden onset, you will be told to rest completely and may be given drugs to relax your uterus and reduce the risk of premature labour.

Screening for congenital defects

Women who have had previous children with *spina bifida* (p.654) or *Down's syndrome* (p.653) or who are over 36 are usually offered a screening test so that they can choose whether or not to terminate the pregnancy if their baby is found to be affected by either disorder. (See the box on *Genetic counselling*, p.619.)

The amniotic fluid (the fluid surrounding the baby in the uterus) around a fetus with spina bifida usually contains a raised level of the protein AFP. (However, you may also have a raised level of AFP if you are expecting twins or are beyond the 18th week of pregnancy.) If your blood, tested between the 16th and 18th weeks of pregnancy, shows a raised level of AFP, you will probably then have *ultrasound* (p.639) to discover whether you are expecting twins or if you are in fact beyond the 18th week of pregnancy. If it is found that neither of these is the cause, *amniocentesis* (p.639), the withdrawal of a sample of amniotic fluid from the uterus, will show whether your baby has spina bifida.

Amniocentesis is also used for screening for Down's syndrome. The *chromosomes* in the sample of amniotic fluid are examined under a microscope, and from this it can be determined whether the baby has the disorder.

Complications of late pregnancy

Any complications that occur in the last few months of pregnancy will probably be dealt with in hospital. Because most babies stand a better chance of survival the nearer full term they are born, some maternity treatments are designed to prevent the expectant mother from going into labour too early – chiefly by making her rest, and by giving drugs to relax the uterine muscles so that they do not begin the contractions of childbirth. However, if the obstetrician suspects that the baby is having difficulties inside the uterus, hospital treatment may then be designed to bring forward labour so that the baby is born as quickly and as safely as possible.

It is imperative that you continue to attend the ante-natal clinic during these last weeks, so that any possible complication can be diagnosed and treatment started before you and your baby have been seriously affected.

Pre-eclampsia and eclampsia

(toxaemia of pregnancy)

Pre-eclampsia is a disease of late pregnancy in which the mother's blood pressure rises and there is an excessive amount of fluid in the body. Why this happens is not known. If, in addition, the mother's urine contains protein, she is in danger of developing the more dangerous condition of eclampsia, in which the blood pressure increases drastically.

What are the symptoms?
In mild pre-eclampsia you may feel perfectly well. You should therefore attend all your ante-natal check-ups, so that the condition can be detected and treated at an early stage. Severe pre-eclampsia, which can develop during the last few weeks of pregnancy, is signified by headaches, blurred vision, intolerance of bright lights, nausea and vomiting, and swelling of the ankles. You may then be on the verge of developing eclampsia, the symptoms of which are convulsive fits and sometimes unconsciousness.

Pre-eclampsia is a common condition, particularly in first pregnancies, whereas eclampsia is now rare.

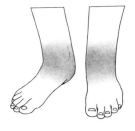
Swollen ankles may indicate pre-eclampsia

What are the risks?
Mild pre-eclampsia presents practically no risk to you or your baby. Only the rare conditions of severe pre-eclampsia and eclampsia are dangerous. If you have either, your placenta, which provides your baby with oxygen and food, functions less efficiently. In eclampsia, there is also a definite risk to the life of the mother.

What is the treatment?
Your doctor may prescribe a drug to control your blood pressure. You can help lower it yourself by plenty of rest and reducing the amount of salt in your food.

In the rare event that you do develop the symptoms of impending eclampsia, you will probably be admitted to hospital, where you will be given drugs to lower your blood pressure, remove excess fluid from your body, and inhibit your fits.

Your obstetrician may decide that your labour should be induced (see *Induction of labour*, p.640), since once your baby is born all the symptoms of pre-eclampsia clear up.

Ante-partum haemorrhage

Ante-partum haemorrhage is any bleeding from the vagina at any time after the end of the 28th week of your pregnancy. Bleeding before this time is known as a threatened miscarriage (see *Miscarriage*, p.628).

Ante-partum haemorrhage may be the result of *placenta praevia* (p.632); a burst vaginal varicose vein; damage to the cervix; or separation of the placenta from the uterine wall (accidental haemorrhage).

In most cases – that is, mainly those that do not involve the placenta – ante-partum haemorrhage is mild and harmless. An accidental haemorrhage can cause *retarded fetal growth* (p.632), however, and if placental bleeding is heavy it can endanger the life of both baby and mother.

If you have bleeding during pregnancy, ask your doctor to visit you at home right away. In all cases, you will probably be admitted to hospital. There you will have blood tests and a close watch will be kept on the general condition of you and your baby. If a considerable amount of blood has been lost, this will be replaced by blood transfusions and the baby will need to be delivered as soon as possible, either by *induction of labour* or *Caesarean section* (p.640).

Placenta praevia

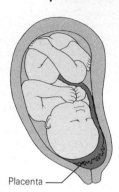

Placenta

In placenta praevia, the placenta develops low in the uterus – near, or sometimes over, the exit. Any part of the placenta that is near the exit is poorly supported and vulnerable to damage. The condition occurs in about 1 pregnancy in 200.

In some cases, the placenta appears to be low in the uterus early in pregnancy but, as pregnancy develops, the upwardly expanding uterus carries the placenta up with it.

What are the symptoms?

There may be no symptoms, but if the placenta becomes partly detached from the uterus, you will have sporadic, painless bleeding from the vagina usually late in the pregnancy. If you have bleeding from the vagina during pregnancy, with or without pain, call your doctor at once and go to bed.

What is the treatment?

In the case of a slight degree of placenta praevia fairly early in pregnancy, your doctor will probably have your baby's condition constantly monitored and normal labour may eventually be possible.

If placenta praevia is severe, there will be heavy bleeding. You will require a blood transfusion – perhaps in your home – and you may be given sedation. The baby will be delivered by *Caesarean section* (p.640), to prevent the possibility of the placenta being damaged by the emerging baby and thus depriving the baby of oxygen.

Premature rupture of membranes

When labour starts, the membranes surrounding the baby in the uterus rupture, releasing amniotic fluid – your "waters break". But occasionally the membranes rupture prematurely, before labour begins.

The main risks of premature rupture are that it will encourage you to go into *premature labour* (p.636) or allow an infection to enter the uterus and affect the baby.

What should be done?

If you think your membranes have ruptured prematurely, contact your doctor, who will probably arrange for you to go into hospital, where you may be given *antibiotics* to prevent any infection. If your expected delivery date is in two or three weeks' time, labour will probably be induced (see *Induction of labour*, p.640), but if the expected date is further ahead, you will be kept in hospital under observation and may well be given a drug to relax the muscles of the uterus and so lessen the chances of premature labour.

Sometimes a small tear in the membranes will heal naturally and allow the pregnancy to continue normally without the use of drugs.

Intra-uterine death

This is the death of a baby in the uterus after the 28th week of pregnancy. Intra-uterine death may be caused by severe *pre-eclampsia* or *eclampsia* (p.631), accidental haemorrhage (see *Ante-partum haemorrhage*, p.631), *post-maturity* (p.633), a severe abnormality of the baby, or *diabetes mellitus* (p.519) in the mother; in some cases the cause is not known.

What are the symptoms?

If the mother no longer feels any movement from the baby, her doctor will suspect intra-uterine death. If the doctor cannot hear any heartbeat, special tests will be carried out. If these show an absence of heartbeat, intra-uterine death is confirmed. The aim then is to carry out a delivery as soon as it is considered safe to do so.

If the mother does not go into labour spontaneously, labour is brought on artificially (see *Induction of labour*, p.640), taking measures to avoid infection.

Clearly the chances of a woman who has had one intra-uterine death having another depend on the cause: in such cases, the obstetrician will discuss in detail the possibilities with the mother.

Retarded fetal growth

In some pregnancies, the placenta fails to supply enough nourishment. The result is that the baby's development in the uterus is stunted. The deficiencies of the placenta may be caused by, among other conditions, severe pre-eclampsia or eclampsia, high blood pressure, accidental haemorrhage, placenta praevia, heart disease, diabetes mellitus, or they may occur for no apparent reason.

What are the symptoms?

There are no very obvious signs that a baby's growth is retarded. However, the doctor's suspicions may well be aroused if you do not continue to gain weight, or if you actually lose weight, in late pregnancy, or if your uterus has not grown at the expected rate for your stage of pregnancy. Sometimes the doctor is alerted because the baby's movements in the uterus become less frequent.

What are the risks?

After birth, the baby has less body fat and therefore less resistance to cold than normal, and is prone to *hypoglycaemia* (p.522).

What should be done?

Pregnant women should attend all their antenatal check-ups. If you are beyond the 30th week of your pregnancy, and you think your baby is not moving as much as before, count the movements accurately. Choose two days of the week on which you are not going to leave the house, and on each day make a note of each group of movements you feel after 9am. If they reach 10 by 5pm on both occasions, then you probably have nothing to worry about. If the number does not reach 10 on one or both days, contact your doctor or midwife. Your baby is, as likely as not, perfectly well (there is a complete absence of movement in some normal pregnancies), but it is wise not to take chances.

Investigative tests may include blood or urine tests, to measure the level of one of your hormones, and *ultrasound* and *fetal tocography* (p.639), to examine the baby.

If it is discovered that your baby's growth is retarded, your doctor will decide when is the best time for the baby to be delivered. You may have to have the baby in a hospital that can provide him or her with specialized treatment and care. Labour may have to be brought on artificially (see *Induction of labour*, p.640) or the baby may have to be delivered by *Caesarean section* (p.640).

Post-maturity

Ideally, labour starts when your baby is fully mature. When labour is delayed so long after this stage that harm can come to the baby, the condition is known as post-maturity. An ageing placenta can fail to provide a large baby with enough oxygen and this can result in brain damage or even death – the stillbirth rate in post-mature babies is almost double that in babies born at the right time. If your obstetrician suspects post-maturity, labour will probably be brought on artificially (see *Induction of labour*, p.640). A close watch will be kept on your baby, and if he or she appears to be in difficulty, delivery will be hastened by the use of *forceps* or *Caesarean section* (p.640).

Twin pregnancy

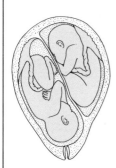

Twins occur as the result of either the splitting of a single egg or the parallel development of 2 eggs. They account for 1 in 80 of all pregnancies in this country (triplets, by comparison, are very rare: they occur in only 1 in 6,400 pregnancies), and are more common among black women than white. Out of every 10 pairs of twins 7 are binovular (that is, 2 eggs have been fertilized by 2 sperm). These are known as fraternal twins. Identical (monovular) twins have developed from 1 egg that has split shortly after fertilization. In the case of fraternal twins, there are 2 placentas; with identical twins there is only 1 placenta; so it is by carefully examining the placenta after delivery that the doctor is able to discover whether twins are fraternal or identical.

The outlook for both the expectant mother and the twins is good, particularly if the mother has the necessary amount of rest. But, of course, there are risks attached to every pregnancy, and in a twin pregnancy the risks of premature labour, anaemia, pre-eclampsia, placenta praevia, and post-partum haemorrhage are slightly greater.

A multiple pregnancy is usually diagnosed by your doctor during a routine ante-natal examination, and confirmed by *ultrasound* (p.639). As soon as the doctor suspects a multiple pregnancy, he or she will advise you to rest in bed as much as possible to reduce the risk of premature labour, especially in the latter part of your pregnancy. To combat the increased risk of your becoming anaemic, the doctor may prescribe more than the usual amount of iron and folic-acid tablets.

If you experience contractions in late pregnancy or have a watery discharge from your vagina, contact your doctor; you may be going into premature labour – in which case you will be admitted to hospital and possibly given a drug to relax the muscles of the uterus.

Childbirth

There are several signs that tell you when your baby is about to be born. The first sign in a normal labour comes when you feel contractions of the muscles of the uterus. At first these may seem like irregular bursts of indigestion-like pain or twinges of backache. As the birth approaches, the contractions come at more regular intervals, with increasingly less time between each contraction. Even then, they may vary in severity.

Contractions on their own are not always a reliable sign that labour has started. Throughout pregnancy, the uterus has been contracting in preparation for labour (although these contractions are rarely noticeable until the last few weeks of pregnancy), and if contractions are unaccompanied by any other signs and do not increase in frequency, then you are probably not in labour.

As labour starts, the mucous plug that, during pregnancy, has formed a barrier between your uterus and vagina will be expelled as a blood-stained discharge – the "show".

Another sign of labour may be the bursting of the membranes surrounding the amniotic fluid in which the baby floats. You may either have a slow trickle of fluid from your vagina, or there may be a sudden gush. In either case, rupture of the membranes is usually a sign that delivery is not far off.

If you are having your baby in hospital, you go through the "prepping" procedure. You are given a vaginal examination to see how far your labour has progressed and in what position the baby is lying. You will probably also be given an enema to empty your bowels. In some hospitals, it is also the custom to shave off all or part of the pubic hair as a precaution against infection.

Labour can be divided into three stages. The first stage starts with the first contractions. With each contraction, the cervix – the baby's exit from the uterus – is gradually pulled open and up, until it merges with the walls of the uterus and is fully opened, or *dilated*. Full dilation occurs when the opening of the cervix is 10cm (100mm) in diameter. At this point the uterus, cervix, and vagina have merged to form the birth canal.

The average duration of the first stage of labour is 12 hours for a first baby and six to eight hours for a subsequent birth. However, for some women having their first baby, the first stage can last for more than 24 hours (though every effort is made to prevent this);

and for some women who have had several children it may last only a few minutes.

When the cervix is fully dilated, there is a transition period between the first and second stages of labour. For some women, labour seems to come to a temporary halt at this point, while others feel hot, then cold, and may even vomit. As the second stage begins, contractions become much more powerful and are usually accompanied by an urge to push the baby out and down the birth canal. The baby's negotiation of the birth canal causes pressure on the rectum and may make you feel that you want to defecate.

You will be advised to push only when you are having a contraction, so that the two forces combine to expel the baby and you conserve energy between contractions. However, when delivery is imminent, you may be told to stop pushing, as a too forceful push could result in the baby's head tearing the tissues of your vagina. Ideally the baby's head should be eased out.

The second stage of labour ends when the baby emerges completely from your birth canal. The second stage lasts on average anything up to an hour for a first baby, and up to 30 minutes for a subsequent baby.

After the baby is delivered, the umbilical cord connecting the baby to the placenta inside the uterus is tied and clipped in two places – about 100mm (4in) and 150mm (6in) from the baby's abdomen. The cord is then cut between these two points.

The third stage of labour is delivery of the placenta (the afterbirth). Your uterus continues to contract in an effort to separate the placenta from the wall of the uterus and to expel it. This is marked by some extra bleeding and by the umbilical cord moving a little further out of the vagina. To speed up the expulsion of the placenta in order to prevent the possibility of *post-partum haemorrhage* (p.638), the midwife may pull gently on the cord while pressing upwards on your abdomen with the other hand. The third stage of labour usually lasts about 15 minutes.

After the placenta has been delivered, you may be given an injection to reinforce your body's efforts to make the uterus contract firmly, and so prevent excessive bleeding. Any tears or incisions that have been made in the vagina are cleaned and stitched and you may be able to hold your baby in your arms while this is being done.

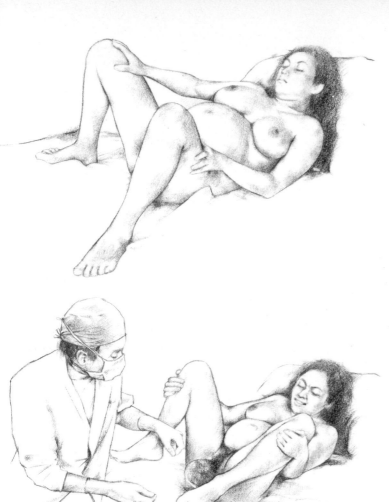

The 3 stages of labour

During the first stage of labour the mother experiences regular contractions that increase in strength and frequency.

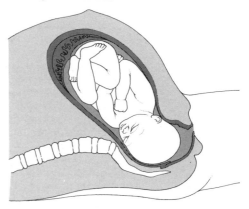

When the cervix is fully dilated, the baby moves down the birth canal. The head rotates and appears at the opening. As it emerges it rotates again to help the shoulders out.

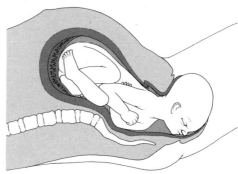

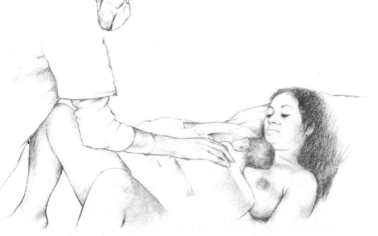

After the baby has been born, the mother's uterus continues to contract to expel the placenta and prevent excessive bleeding from the wall of the uterus as the placenta is peeled away. This completes the third stage of the labour.

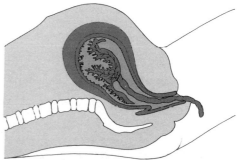

Premature labour

A premature labour is one that takes place well before the expected date of delivery and results in the birth of a pre-term baby (one that is less than 37 weeks old). If a baby is abnormally light, but born at full term, this is not considered premature labour but is the result of *retarded fetal growth* (p.632).

Severe *pre-eclampsia and eclampsia* (p.631) cause about a third of all premature labours. *High blood pressure* (p.624), *placenta praevia* (p.632), accidental haemorrhage (see *Ante-partum haemorrhage*, p.631) and several other causes probably account for a further proportion.

How common is the problem?
About 5 per cent of pregnancies end in premature labour, and in about half of these the cause is unknown.

What are the risks?
The earlier in a pregnancy that a baby is born, the less are the baby's chances of survival. Premature babies who survive are at risk from *respiratory distress syndrome* and *neonatal jaundice* (p.647); this risk is greater the more premature the birth.

What should be done?
If you think you are starting labour prematurely (see *Childbirth*, p.634, for the symptoms of labour), contact your doctor at once. If the doctor is not immediately available, arrange for transport – or call an ambulance – to take you to your maternity hospital as soon as possible. Warn the hospital that you are coming. (If the hospital is at some distance, telephone the hospital for advice.) In hospital you will be examined to see whether your labour actually has started, because there are many false alarms.

What is the treatment?
If the obstetrician decides that you are in the very early stages of labour, you may be prescribed a drug to relax the muscles of the uterus and so prevent labour. If it is decided to let the labour go ahead, you are likely to have an *episiotomy* (p.640) to allow a free passage for the baby's head. *Forceps* (p.640) may also be used to protect the head. Afterwards the baby will be put into an incubator to be given oxygen, kept warm, and, if necessary, fed by a tube inserted down the throat and into the stomach.

Pain relief in labour

The intensity of pain in labour varies considerably from woman to woman. It is partly governed by your mental attitude: if you are frightened or tense, you will feel pain more acutely. That is why you should attend relaxation exercises and information sessions at an ante-natal clinic.

You may not need pain relief during labour, but if you do, there are various methods available.

If you are suffering pain during the first stage of labour, and the doctor or midwife is fairly sure that delivery is not imminent, you

Epidural anaesthesia
The injection for an epidural anaesthetic is given between contractions, with the mother lying on her side and curled up as much as possible to allow the anaesthetist to insert the needle between the vertebrae (backbones).

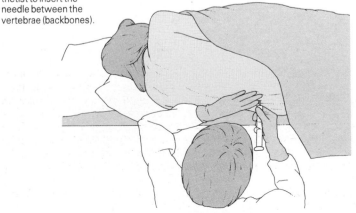

may well be given an injection – usually in your thigh – of a general painkilling drug. The drug is not given late in labour, because it might well affect the baby's breathing.

A common, more short-term method of relieving pain at the end of the first stage of labour and during the second stage is to allow you to inhale a combination of nitrous oxide and oxygen (gas-and-air) from a cylinder attached to a mask that you hold to your face whenever you need relief. It takes 20 to 30 seconds to be effective, so you should inhale at the start of a contraction rather than waiting until the pain begins to peak. You cannot inhale too much because the mixture makes you too drowsy to hold the mask in your hand for very long.

Vaginal pain can be relieved by a local anaesthetic injected into the tissues of the vagina. The anaesthetic is often used before a delivery by *forceps* or an *episiotomy* (p.640).

Many hospitals offer a painkilling method called epidural anaesthesia. This consists of an anaesthetic injected into the base of your spine to numb temporarily the nerves running to the lower half of your body, so that you feel nothing. However, if the anaesthetic is given quite late during the first stage of labour, you may be unable to push the baby out and may then require a forceps delivery.

Prolonged labour

Prolonged labour is usually due to one of two things. One is a "lazy" uterus, whose muscles fail to produce sufficiently strong or regular contractions. The other is an obstruction to normal delivery, as occurs in *disproportion* (below), when the baby's head is too large for the mother's pelvic canal, or in *malpresentation* (below), when the baby's position in the uterus makes delivery difficult.

A "lazy" uterus can be stimulated to contract more by the *intravenous* infusion of a certain hormone into your bloodstream (see *Induction of labour*, p.640). In some cases of prolonged labour, delivery will need to be by *Caesarean section* or by *forceps* (p.640), depending on the stage of labour that has been reached and the position of the baby in relation to the mother's pelvis.

Mal-presentation

The position of the baby in the mother's pelvic cavity immediately before birth is called the presentation. The most common presentation is for the baby to be head down, with the crown (occiput) settled into the outlet of the pelvic cavity and the baby facing the mother's back. This presentation positions the baby for the easiest passage through the birth canal. The baby may be in one of several other positions – malpresentation – which in some cases can cause *prolonged labour* (above) or even the need for delivery by *forceps* or *Caesarean section* (p.640).

Two of the more common types of malpresentation are occipito-posterior and breech presentation. An occipito-posterior baby is head down but facing the mother's front. In this case, the mother will probably have severe backache and labour is likely to be extremely prolonged; delivery by Caesarean section or forceps may be necessary. In

a breech presentation – common in *premature labour* (opposite) – the baby is buttocks down. In this case, the baby's head is more vulnerable to pressure as it passes along the birth canal, which is not sufficiently enlarged by the buttocks.

In some cases of breech presentation, the obstetrician will have been able to manipulate the baby externally – feeling the baby through your abdomen – into the normal presentation during the last few weeks of pregnancy. If breech presentation persists, but the mother is young and healthy, the obstetrician may decide to allow labour to start naturally, while being prepared to carry out a Caesarean section if the labour proves to be difficult or prolonged.

Other forms of malpresentation are very rare. When they occur, delivery is usually by Caesarean section, less commonly by forceps, with the mother under a general anaesthetic.

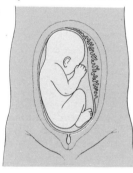

Breech presentation
In a breech presentation (above) the baby's buttocks will be first to pass down the birth canal. The canal may not be dilated enough for the baby's head to follow easily.

Occipito presentations
In an occipito-posterior presentation (right), the baby's chin is pushed down on to the chest, so that he or she cannot flex the neck to negotiate the curve of the birth canal as in the more common occipito-anterior presentation (far right).

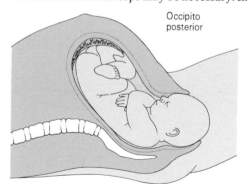

Occipito posterior

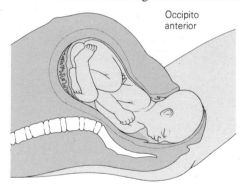

Occipito anterior

Disproportion

The term disproportion describes any case in which the mother's pelvic cavity is too narrow for the passage of her baby's head. This can happen in some small-boned women and in some women under 1.5m (5ft) tall; in certain cases when a woman's pelvis is disproportionately small because of a serious injury; and if the baby's head is abnormally large, as in *hydrocephalus* (p.655).

If your doctor suspects disproportion, you will be given an internal examination and

later an *X-ray*, in the 37th week of pregnancy. If these reveal severe disproportion, the baby may be delivered by *Caesarean section* (p.640). An X-ray can show some cases to be borderline, however; in these cases, normal labour will be allowed to proceed, but the baby's condition will be monitored closely throughout, and if there is any sign of risk to the baby, an emergency Caesarean section or a *forceps* delivery (p.640) will be performed.

Post-partum haemorrhage

Post-partum haemorrhage is excessive loss of blood from the uterus or vagina after delivery. A common cause is failure of the uterine muscles to contract firmly enough to control the bleeding produced by separation of the placenta from the uterus. Such deficient contractions can result from exhaustion if you had a very long labour; or from a previous weakening of the muscles of the uterus, as occurs when the uterus has been stretched excessively by a *twin pregnancy* (p.633) or by a large number of pregnancies. Bleeding may occur if parts of the placenta remain inside the uterus and prevent it from tightening up as much as possible. A haemorrhage can also occur when the vagina has been torn during the delivery.

Bleeding from the uterus is controlled by drugs that encourage the uterus to contract. If fragments of placenta remain in the uterus, they are removed manually. If bleeding is from a torn vagina, the tear will be stitched up layer by layer after the area has been numbed by a local anaesthetic.

Retained placenta

Normally, after delivery the placenta separates from the wall of the uterus and – with the help of the midwife, who may pull gently on the umbilical cord – is expelled from the vagina. But occasionally the placenta becomes trapped in the uterus – in some cases because it has not separated completely from the wall of the uterus. If it has not been expelled 30 minutes after delivery, it is called a retained placenta.

A retained placenta is removed manually by an obstetrician while you are under a general anaesthetic. When it has been taken out, you are given a drug to encourage your uterus to contract further and thus prevent excessive bleeding.

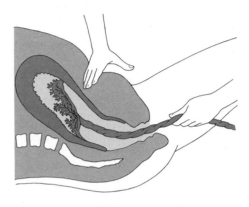

Aided expulsion of the placenta

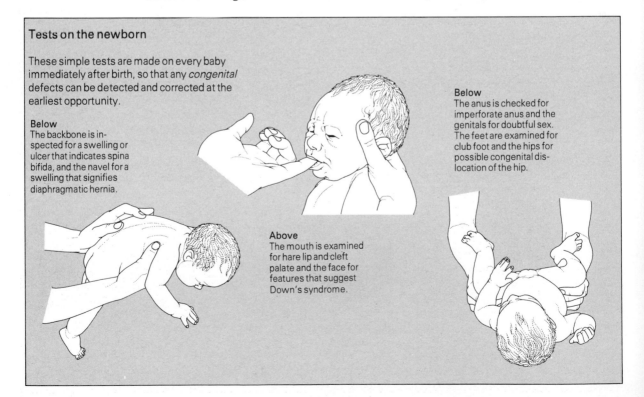

Tests on the newborn

These simple tests are made on every baby immediately after birth, so that any *congenital* defects can be detected and corrected at the earliest opportunity.

Below
The backbone is inspected for a swelling or ulcer that indicates spina bifida, and the navel for a swelling that signifies diaphragmatic hernia.

Above
The mouth is examined for hare lip and cleft palate and the face for features that suggest Down's syndrome.

Below
The anus is checked for imperforate anus and the genitals for doubtful sex. The feet are examined for club foot and the hips for possible congenital dislocation of the hip.

Special procedures in pregnancy

Amniocentesis

This is the withdrawal, through a hollow needle, of a sample of amniotic fluid (the fluid that surrounds the baby in the uterus and which contains cells that have been shed by the baby). The needle is inserted through the abdomen and the wall of the uterus, after the abdomen has been numbed with a local anaesthetic.

Amniocentesis is carried out if there is a possibility that the baby has *spina bifida* (p.654), *Down's syndrome* (p.653), or some other serious abnormality. This possibility exists if you have already had an abnormal child, if there is a family history of some abnormality, or if you are 36 or over. The procedure is usually carried out between the 16th and 18th weeks of pregnancy. *Ultrasound* (below) is used first, to locate the exact position of your baby and placenta.

Tests of amniotic fluid identify a great proportion of abnormal babies. In these cases the mother is offered the opportunity of having the pregnancy terminated. If you do not approve of termination in any circumstances, there is rarely any point in running the slight risk of your pregnancy that amniocentesis entails.

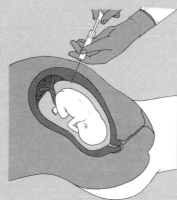

Amniocentesis
Amniocentesis – the withdrawal of a sample of amniotic fluid from the uterus – is usually done only if the obstetrician suspects some abnormality that can be diagnosed only by examination of cells shed by the baby into the fluid. The sample of fluid is spun in a centrifuge to remove the cells for examination.

Ultrasound

In ultrasound, a device transmits sound waves through the body tissues, records the echoes as the sounds encounter objects within the body, and transforms the recordings into a picture. When used on a pregnant woman, the transmitter/recorder is moved over the surface of the abdomen which will first have been covered with a film of oil. The picture is improved if the woman drinks plenty of water beforehand and does not urinate.

Ultrasound is used to measure the size and shape of the fetus to help establish the stage of a pregnancy; to detect some abnormalities; to confirm the presence of twins; to show a baby's rate of development if *retarded fetal growth* (p.632) is suspected; to ascertain the position of the baby in the uterus during late pregnancy (see *Malpresentation*, p.637); and to locate the position of the placenta if *placenta praevia* (p.632) is suspected. Ultrasound is a painless procedure and cannot harm you or your baby.

Tocography

This is a method used in certain pregnancies to record the unborn baby's heart rate and movements and the contractions of the uterus. These can be detected from about the 30th week of pregnancy onwards. Two flat metal recording devices, linked to a monitor, are strapped to the mother's abdomen. If the membranes have ruptured, an electrode may also be attached to the baby's scalp to allow more precise monitoring. Tocography is used in cases when the

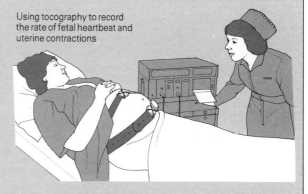

Using tocography to record the rate of fetal heartbeat and uterine contractions

fetus is especially at risk – for example, if you have *pre-eclampsia* or *eclampsia* (p.631); when *ultrasound* (left) or other tests indicate that the pregnancy may not be normal; and when *induction of labour* (p.640) is carried out and tocography allows the doctor to measure the response of you and your baby to the drugs administered. Tocography is also being used more frequently in what are expected to be normal labours, in case an unexpected risk to the baby should suddenly develop.

Fetoscopy

In fetoscopy a hollow needle that holds a telescopic probe and light is inserted through the mother's abdomen into the uterus, allowing the doctor to observe the baby. The baby's position has first been ascertained with the help of *ultrasound* (left). The probe can be manoeuvred to take blood samples for analysis – usually from the umbilical cord.

Fetoscopy may be used when the doctor has reason to believe that the baby may be abnormal in such a way that only tests on the baby's blood can confirm. For example, both parents may have a mild form of *thalassaemia* (p.422), in which case there is a strong possibility that the baby will have a more severe form of the disease. If the parents are totally opposed to termination of pregnancy whatever the circumstances, there is rarely any point in the mother running the slight risk to the pregnancy entailed by fetoscopy.

Special procedures in childbirth

Induction of labour

This is a deliberate initiation of labour by a doctor. It is usually carried out when it is considered that the risks of allowing the pregnancy to continue outweigh the risks of induction – as is often the case in *retarded fetal growth* (p.632) or *post-maturity* (p.633). The doctor first examines you internally to assess the state of your cervix. If the cervix is not ready for labour to begin, the doctor will insert into your vagina a pessary containing a substance that causes the uterus to contract and the cervix to dilate (open). The doctor then locates the membranes around the amniotic fluid in which the baby floats, and makes a small, painless cut in the membranes to drain the fluid away.

Sometimes these procedures alone are enough to initiate labour. If labour is slow in starting, however, a synthetic form of the hormone oxytocin is slowly passed into your blood-stream by *intravenous drip*. The hormone encourages the uterus to contract as in natural labour. However, in about 1 in 50 inductions of labour, the uterus fails to respond and a *Caesarean section* (right) or emergency delivery using *forceps* (right) is then required.

The progress of induced labour is monitored throughout by *tocography* (p.639), or, less commonly, by frequent physical examination. Usually labour will proceed safely to a normal delivery. But because, even with the most modern methods, it is difficult to be sure about the exact stage of a pregnancy, there is always a slight risk of premature delivery. If labour does not progress successfully after induction procedures, Caesarean section may be necessary.

Episiotomy

This is a cut sometimes made during labour to widen the opening of the vagina. Episiotomy is commonly done at premature births, especially when a *forceps* delivery (right) is necessary, because the premature baby's head is less resistant to pressure. Or it may be done to avoid the baby's head tearing the vagina and the muscles around the vagina as it emerges from the birth canal. The cut is made after the injection of a local anaesthetic. In an emergency, however, there may be no time for an injection; but in such cases, the

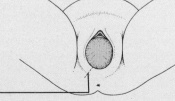

The most common incision for an episiotomy is medio-lateral – from the vagina out to the side.

Medio-lateral incision

skin of the vagina will be so stretched that it will be numb and you will feel no pain from the cut. Blood on the baby's head is usually from the episiotomy. After delivery, the cut is carefully sewn up, usually with catgut that gradually dissolves away. The cut heals rapidly, although the scar may cause a little discomfort for a few weeks.

Forceps

Obstetrical forceps consist of two wide, blunt blades made to fit around a baby's head. The blades are shaped so that they cannot press too far in on the baby's head. They are used to assist delivery when, for example, your uterus is not contracting efficiently or the baby shows signs of *asphyxia* (p.646) and so needs to breathe oxygen as soon as possible;

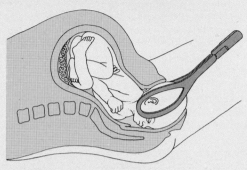

Cross-section of birth canal, showing baby being helped out by forceps

to protect the baby's head in a breech presentation (see *Malpresentation*, p.637) or in *premature labour* (p.636); or to turn the baby's head to a more favourable position for delivery. In nearly all cases when forceps are used you are first given an *episiotomy* (left).

Ventouse

The ventouse (also known as vacuum extraction) is a device that is sometimes used instead of *forceps* (above) when the mother is having difficulty in labour or when the baby is in danger of being asphyxiated. It consists of a cup connected to an air pump. The cup is placed on the baby's head and the air pump creates a vacuum that sucks the baby down the birth canal. The swelling (caused by the suction) on the head of a baby born with the aid of a ventouse disappears within a week and has no ill-effects.

Caesarean section

When it is impossible or unsafe for a baby to be delivered through the birth canal, a horizontal or vertical incision known as a Caesarean section is made in the lower part of the mother's abdomen and uterus, and the baby is delivered through this. Caesarean section is necessary if there is marked disproportion, severe placenta praevia, unsuccessful induction of labour, signs of asphyxia in the baby, and in many cases of malpresentation. Like any operation, Caesarean section carries with it some risks, and if a normal vaginal birth is possible, it is preferable. Usually the mother is given a general anaesthetic for the operation, but some doctors use an epidural anaesthetic. The most common incision for a planned Caesarean section is the unobtrusive "bikini-line" cut made just below the top of the pubic hairline.

Post-natal problems for the mother

Some women see pregnancy only as a preparation for childbirth and do not look beyond the baby's birth. However, changes that have been taking place gradually in your body over a period of nine months are reversed more quickly after the delivery. Adjusting to this and learning how to cope with the demands of the baby (especially if it is the first one) can cause many women to feel depressed for the first week or two after delivery.

Before your baby was born, you probably gave some thought to whether to breast-feed or bottle-feed, and may have been given conflicting advice on the advantages and disadvantages of each method. Medical research has shown that breast-feeding has several advantages over bottle-feeding. Artificial milk is similar in composition to breast milk, and if it is given in the correct quantities babies thrive on it; even so, it lacks certain constituents of breast milk that are beneficial to your baby. For example, breast milk can help protect your baby against any infections to which you yourself are immune. The composition of breast milk also seems to vary with the baby's needs, whereas the composition of artificial milk stays constant. This means that you can put your baby to the breast as often as he or she seems to want it without the baby gaining weight too quickly, whereas your baby may become overweight with too many bottle feeds. Breast-feeding may also strengthen the bond between you and your child. On a day-to-day basis there are advantages and disadvantages with both methods. In most women, breast milk is always available and requires no preparation. However, there may be times when you are tired or ill and would like your partner to attend to the baby. Unless you have been able to express a feed into a bottle beforehand, then bottle-feeding is more practical.

Some women decide to breast-feed, try for a few days, then give up, convinced that the baby is not getting any nourishment. It can be difficult to develop a satisfactory routine, especially if you have never breast-fed before. A few women soon find that they cannot produce enough milk for their babies and have to change to bottle-feeding. If this happens to you, remember that those first few feeds will have already given your baby a good start towards a certain amount of immunity to infections.

About six weeks after the baby is born, you will have a post-natal check-up. The doctor examines you to make sure that your uterus and bladder are in the correct position and that any scar tissue is healing satisfactorily. This is the time to mention any problems that you may be having, either with your body or in adjusting to the new baby.

Breast problems

If you decided during pregnancy to breast-feed your baby, your doctor will probably

Using a breast pump
Some breast pumps can be converted to bottles for immediate use.

have advised you on the care and preparation of your breasts. For example, an inverted nipple may have needed to be drawn out (see *Nipple problems*, p.591) and you should have massaged your nipples regularly to make them supple. Even so, problems can arise during the first few weeks of breast-feeding, and these should be dealt with quickly if breast-feeding is to be as convenient and enjoyable as possible.

Engorgement
In most women, a few days after delivery, their milk supply arrives so quickly and forcibly that the breasts become tightly swollen and sore; they are said to be engorged. (This can also happen when a woman decides to stop breast-feeding and milk accumulates in her breasts.) A baby is unable to suckle from a swollen nipple, so some excess milk has to be removed before you can breast-feed – by

expressing the milk either by hand or by a breast pump. The breasts should also be softened by being bathed in hot water. If your breasts are engorged because you have stopped breast-feeding, you should support them with a firm bra and take *analgesics* if necessary. After a few days the build-up of milk will prevent more milk from being produced and your breasts will gradually become less tense and painful.

Cracked nipples

You may feel a sharp pain in your nipple when your baby is suckling, which probably means that there is a thin crack in the nipple. This can happen if the baby is dragging on the nipple end rather than sucking the whole nipple, or if you do not dry your nipples thoroughly after each feed. Tell your doctor, who will probably recommend a soothing cream to apply to the nipple. The crack should take only a few days to heal, but in the meantime it is important that you do not give the baby the affected breast.

Blocked milk duct and abscess

If you feel a small, hard lump in your breast, you may have a blocked milk duct. Try massaging the breast and bathing it in hot water. If the lump does not disappear straight away, see your doctor immediately, since the lump may be a *breast abscess* (p.590) caused by infection. Your doctor will examine the breast and may well give you *antibiotics* to treat the infection. You can go on feeding your baby from the affected breast while undergoing the treatment. If the abscess is not treated early enough, you may have to have a small operation to drain it.

Milk production
Milk is produced within sinuses in the breast. The baby's sucking stimulates milk to flow along ducts leading from the sinuses to the areola. A blocked milk duct may become infected, causing an abscess.

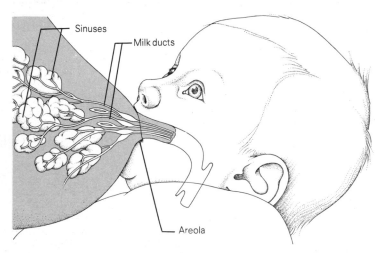

Sinuses

Milk ducts

Areola

Puerperal fever

Puerperal fever is fever caused by infection of the genital tract within two weeks after childbirth. Since the development of *antibiotics* and the use of antiseptics, puerperal fever has become extremely rare. If you have a marked fever shortly after childbirth, your doctor may suspect puerperal fever.

There is a slight risk that the infection, if not recognized and treated early enough, can spread to the bloodstream, causing blood poisoning, or to the uterus and fallopian tubes, causing infertility.

Once the possibility of any other infection causing the fever has been excluded, cotton-wool swabs from your birth canal and samples of your urine will be sent for laboratory analysis. You will then be given an antibiotic to stop the infection spreading.

Depression after childbirth

Many women feel low or miserable a few days after childbirth – the so-called post-natal "blues". This is so common as to be almost a normal part of pregnancy and probably has several causes. The sudden change in your body hormones caused by the birth can affect your mood, and there may be a sense of anti-climax after an event that you have anticipated for several months. You are very tired and even a little afraid and lacking in confidence. The "blues" go away quite quickly with the support and understanding of your friends and family.

It is normal, too, to feel mildly depressed occasionally during the first few weeks of motherhood. The tiredness that is inevitable when you are looking after a new baby, the sudden change in your life style, the feeling, especially if you have been working, that your horizons and your circle of friends have shrunk, all contribute to this.

A few women do become more seriously depressed after childbirth, to the extent that they are unable to look after themselves and the baby. Such a depressive illness (see *Depression*, p.297) usually starts within about a month of the baby's birth. The symptoms are tiredness, a feeling of failure and inability to cope as a mother, and quite often aggressive feelings towards the baby, possibly provoked by *excessive crying* (p.651) – which may induce a sense of guilt. You may experience a loss of pride in your appearance and home, a withdrawal into yourself and away from others, and a fading appetite or, conversely, you may start eating compulsively.

What should be done?

Your main aim must be to avoid becoming over-tired. It is not only by crying for a feed that a baby in the same bedroom can disturb you, but also by restless sleep and making noises while awake – so, as you need all the sleep you can get, you should move the baby to a nearby room at an early stage. This will not prevent the baby from being heard if hungry. You should also arrange a shift system with your partner, whereby you take turns to see to the baby if he or she is very unsettled or distressed. Try to obtain help during the day from family or friends who are willing to do shopping for you or to look after the baby while you get some rest. If you feel depressed, try to share the problems with your partner or anyone else close to you who is a good listener; another mother with a baby can be especially understanding.

If, after these measures, you find that you still cannot shake off your depression, that you are unable to care for your baby properly, and that you seem to have lost interest in everything, you should consult your doctor. He or she will probably prescribe an *antidepressant* drug. If your depression is very severe, the doctor may suggest that you go into hospital for treatment. If this is necessary, you or your partner should ask the doctor to arrange for you to be admitted to a hospital that has a mother and baby unit, however far away. Although you may feel that the baby is the cause of your illness, a separation at this stage may make it even more difficult for you to develop a close relationship with him or her.

Sex after childbirth

After a straightforward delivery, there is no medical reason why you should not resume sexual intercourse as soon as you feel ready for it. Some people start intercourse a few days after the birth of their child; others prefer to wait until the routine post-natal examination, about six weeks after the birth, has given them the all-clear.

If you wish to avoid becoming pregnant again, you will need to consider methods of contraception: do not depend on breast-feeding to prevent ovulation. Even if you have not yet had a normal period, you may be fertile. (Some women re-establish their former monthly cycle within six weeks of the birth, others may take months, and others never return to what they once regarded as normal. If at all worried, consult your doctor.) Certain methods of birth control may not be suitable immediately after childbirth, so it is wise to discuss the problem with your partner and doctor before leaving hospital. Your vagina may be extremely tender for the first 10 days or so after the birth, or possibly for several weeks if you had an *episiotomy* (p.640) or your vagina was torn during labour. If intercourse is painful, leave it for a while. If it is still uncomfortable or painful after your six-week post-natal check-up, see your doctor. Vaginal pain may be caused by an area of raw skin persisting in the vagina or a stitch not dissolving – both of which can be treated by your doctor.

You may find that your vagina has lost some elasticity, resulting in less satisfying intercourse for both you and your partner. You can gradually tone up the muscles around your vagina by practising interrupting a flow of urine in mid-stream.

Looking after a new baby can be extremely tiring and emotionally exhausting, leaving you no energy for sex. Adopt the measures for avoiding over-tiredness suggested in *Depression after childbirth* (opposite).

Your partner may feel left out of the developing relationship between you and your baby, and may need the reassurance of your continuing affection and attention. Just as he needs to realize that you are going through a difficult period of adjustment, you should make an effort to understand that he too may be feeling confused and vulnerable now that he no longer has your undivided attention. Involve him in the care of the baby and he will feel that the baby belongs to both of you; this will have the added bonus of giving you more time to rest, so that you are then not too tired to enjoy sex.

Avoiding discomfort
Intercourse after childbirth may be more comfortable if you adopt a position whereby your partner's weight is not pressing on your breasts and there is no undue friction on your vagina.

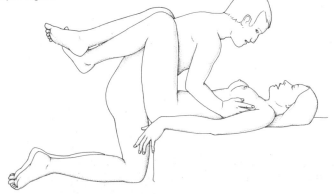

Special problems of infants and children

Introduction

This section of the book deals with problems that affect infants and children from birth until they enter puberty (at about 11 to 13 years of age). Some of the problems are confined to infants and children; others can affect anybody, but a baby or child who is affected may require special diagnostic tests or different treatment from that given to an adult. Furthermore, the outlook for certain diseases is very different in childhood and middle age.

The first group of articles in this section concerns special problems of the newborn and infants up to one year old. Telling whether a newborn baby is ill can be difficult, especially if he or she is your first. Sometimes, obvious symptoms show that the baby is unwell: for example, a rash, a fever, or diarrhoea. At other times you will realize from changes in your baby's behaviour that something is wrong, but the cause may be by no means obvious. If your baby cries loudly and persistently and does not quieten when picked up, or if he or she is listless or refuses feeds, see your doctor. (In many cases, there is an appropriate self-diagnosis symptom chart in Part II of this book to help you decide what to do.)

The next few groups of articles are concerned with *congenital* disabilities – defects which are present at birth, and which usually result from faulty development in the uterus. Sometimes the defect is chemical, and symptoms may be delayed for weeks or months. Modern surgical and drug treatments have greatly improved the outlook for many affected children.

Most of the remaining disorders in this section are grouped according to the part or parts of the body they affect. In childhood, especially, physical disorders may affect general well-being. Disorders of the nervous system and psychological problems, eye and ear defects, asthma, and any chronic illness can have a profound effect on a child's ability to learn and therefore on the prospects for his or her adult life.

Respiratory disorders are very common in childhood, accounting for almost half of all illness. Fortunately – like the digestive disorders – they are usually easily diagnosed and treated. In contrast, many blood and urinary disorders may go undetected because they give rise to mild,

varied, and sometimes apparently unrelated symptoms. Abnormal-looking urine, for example, can escape even an attentive parent's notice, but once detected, should always receive prompt medical attention because of the possibility of serious disease developing later in life.

Finally, there is a series of articles that deals with the most common infectious diseases in infants and children. If you suspect that your child has one of these infections, check the appropriate self-diagnosis symptom chart in Part II, or see *Symptom comparison of infectious diseases* (p.702). If in doubt, it is always wise to consult your doctor. And every child should be protected against major infections by a full course of recommended immunizations (see *Immunization*, p.701).

Should I have my son circumcised?

Parents often feel that their baby boy needs to be circumcised because they cannot pull his foreskin back over the head of the penis. An unretractable foreskin is, however, quite normal in a very young baby, because at birth the foreskin is still joined to the tissues of the end of the penis, and it is only gradually that the two separate – at some time after the baby is six months old. By the time the boy is three, the foreskin should be fully retractable; but it should not be forced back to speed up the process (see *Phimosis*, p.711, for further information).

In some cases, however, the foreskin remains fixed, and then circumcision will be necessary. The operation is straightforward, and requires only one or two days in hospital. Occasionally a too-tight foreskin can be freed simply by a small incision known as a dorsal slit being made in it, under anaesthetic.

It is sometimes thought that circumcision reduces the risk of disease, but provided you teach your son to keep his uncircumcised penis clean, the presence of the foreskin is unlikely to be a risk to health.

Milestones

All children acquire mental and physical skills in much the same order (a child will probably not stand before he or she has learned to sit, for example). However, the rate at which these skills are acquired varies enormously. The age given below for each milestone in a child's development is only a rough average.

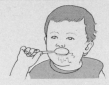

Your child will probably be able to:

- Smile at 6 weeks

- Raise head and shoulders from a face-down position at 3 months

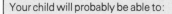

- Roll over from a face-down position on to the back at 6 months

- Remain in a temporary sitting position (when placed there) at 7 months

- Babble without meaning at 7 months

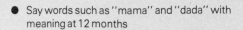

- Try to feed himself or herself with a spoon at 8 months

- Sit up unsupported at 8 months

- Say words such as "mama" and "dada" with meaning at 12 months

- Stand unsupported for a second or two at 12 months

- Walk unaided at 15 months

- Understand simple commands at 18 months

- Achieve bowel control at 20 months

- Stay dry during the day at 2 years

- Talk in simple sentences at 2 years

- Stay dry through the night at 3½ years

- Get dressed and undressed (with a little help) at 4 years

- Hop, skip, and draw a figure with separate body and limbs at 5 years

Growth charts

These charts show the normal height and weight for boys (right) and girls (far right) from the ages of 1 to 12. Because children's growth rates vary, the charts show an acceptable range of height and weight for each year of growth. You can assume that your child's growth is normal if his or her weight and height fall within the shaded areas above his or her age.

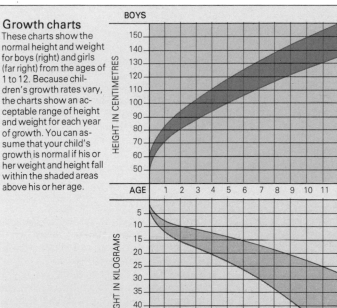

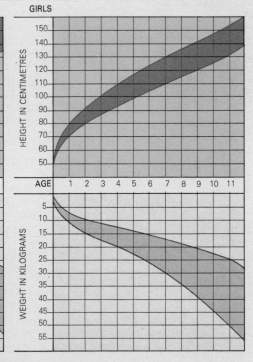

Height and weight conversions
1 inch = 2.5 centimetres
1 pound = 0.45 kilograms

Newborn and early infants

The disorders described in the following articles most commonly affect children during the first year of life. Some disorders, such as asphyxia and respiratory-distress syndrome, occur mainly in infants who are premature or who go through a difficult delivery. Many such infants are unable to cope unaided with the stresses of life outside the uterus and must be treated in hospital during the critical period following birth. Other problems are extremely common in early infancy and can often be treated at home. But infections which are usually mild in adults can be serious in infants; gastroenteritis, for example, usually requires special treatment and is discussed here. Finally, there are rare disorders such as Down's syndrome, caused by an error in the child's *chromosomes*.

Asphyxia

Some newborn babies have asphyxia – that is, they fail to breathe. The brain controls breathing, and what causes the asphyxia is failure of the baby's brain to function normally. Sometimes this happens because the placenta, which supplies oxygen to the baby in the uterus, fails to maintain an adequate supply of oxygen to the brain during the stresses of labour. This often happens when the baby is undersized in relation to the term of the pregnancy or is considerably overdue. Sometimes the baby's brain is damaged during delivery. In very rare cases its functioning is also impaired when the mother is given a painkilling drug, such as pethidine, shortly before delivery. Occasionally, the brain is malformed because of some fault which has occurred during development in the uterus.

What are the symptoms?
The baby fails to breathe or cry when born. In milder cases, the skin is blue and the limbs feel quite stiff (though there may be movement in them). In very severe cases, the baby is ashen, immobile, and limp.

How common is the problem?
About 10 per cent of newborn babies need some help with their breathing; but with improvements in obstetrics the number of infants affected should decline. A mother who smokes during pregnancy is more likely to give birth to a baby who is undersized and who may therefore have asphyxia at delivery (see *The dangers of smoking*, p.38).

What are the risks?
The risk of permanent brain damage (after four or five minutes' lack of oxygen) or even death (after 10 minutes' lack) is low, since all obstetricians and midwives are fully prepared for resuscitating an asphyxiated baby within seconds of delivery. The risk is slightly higher at a home birth, because specialized equipment is not usually immediately available.

What should be done?
In the unlikely event of your having to revive an asphyxiated newborn baby – or any baby who has stopped breathing – quickly wipe the secretions out of the baby's throat with a handkerchief or any clean piece of material, then use mouth-to-mouth resuscitation (see *Accidents and emergencies*, p.802).

What is the treatment?
Deficiency in the oxygen supplied by the placenta is usually detected during labour, in which case the asphyxia can be prevented or minimized by an emergency delivery (see *Special procedures in childbirth*, p.640).

If the baby is born asphyxiated, secretions of fluid from the uterus, together with mucus, are quickly sucked out of the baby's mouth, nose, and throat through a special tube. In mild cases of asphyxia, the baby is then made to gasp, inhaling oxygen, which causes the brain to initiate breathing.

If this technique is not successful, a special oxygen mask may be placed over the baby's face and oxygen pumped under pressure into the respiratory tract, or the inside of the baby's nose can be tickled with a tube through which oxygen is flowing.

If the baby's breathing has been depressed by drugs given to the mother shortly before delivery, their effect can be reversed by injecting the baby with another drug.

In severe cases of asphyxia, oxygen is passed into the lungs through a tube inserted into the trachea (windpipe), and artificial respiration is started. Breathing usually begins within a few minutes. Occasionally, when the brain has been damaged during delivery or is underdeveloped, artificial respiration may need to be continued for up to several weeks.

Respiratory-distress syndrome

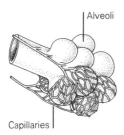

Inside the lung
When a baby is born and takes his or her first breath, alveoli (air sacs in the lungs) fill with air, and oxygen from the air passes into the baby's blood flowing through capillaries surrounding the alveoli.

The baby in intensive care
A baby with respiratory-distress syndrome may need artificial respiration using a mechanical ventilator. This will be provided in a neonatal intensive-care unit, where newborn babies with any serious or life-threatening illnesses are cared for.

After a baby's first breath has expanded the lungs, the alveoli (small air sacs) in the lungs are kept open by a chemical called surfactant. However, in some very small premature babies and in very large babies born of diabetic mothers, the lungs are deficient in surfactant, and the alveoli start to close up again within a few hours of birth. The baby then develops what is called the respiratory-distress syndrome – that is, has increasing difficulty in breathing.

What are the symptoms?
A few hours after birth, the baby's breathing becomes progressively more laboured and rapid. As the baby breathes in, the chest sinks instead of expanding; on breathing out, the baby makes a grunting noise.

How common is the problem?
The more premature the baby, the more likely the problem; it is very common in babies weighing less than 1.5kg (about 3lb) at birth. It is also fairly common in the abnormally

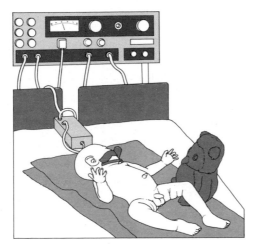

large babies often born to diabetic mothers (see *Diabetes and pregnancy*, p.626).

What are the risks?
In the past, the baby's severely reduced intake of oxygen often resulted in permanent brain or lung damage, or death. These risks have been reduced because nowadays the disorder is anticipated during pregnancy in many cases, and intensive care is available immediately after birth.

What is the treatment?
When it is suspected that a birth may well be premature, the adequacy of surfactant in the fetus's lungs is determined by taking a sample of the mother's amniotic fluid (the fluid surrounding the baby in the uterus). If the surfactant is inadequate, it may be increased by giving the mother an injection of a drug. (This would not be done if the birth was imminent, as the drug takes about 24 hours to work.) A recent form of treatment is to give the baby artificial surfactant after delivery.

A baby who has developed, or is in danger of developing, a severe degree of the respiratory-distress syndrome must be cared for in a neonatal intensive-care unit. There the baby is given artificial respiration with a ventilator and the levels of oxygen, carbon dioxide, and chemicals in the blood are carefully monitored. Eventually the baby responds by producing adequate surfactant, and the treatments can be discontinued. Ideally, every mother considered likely to have a baby who may develop the respiratory-distress syndrome should be delivered at one of the hospitals with an intensive-care baby unit. But in practice, the baby is often born elsewhere and then transferred (in a specially equipped ambulance) to such a hospital. Provided the baby has suffered no serious lack of oxygen, the chances of normal physical and mental development are excellent.

Neonatal jaundice

Many babies show a slight yellowing of the skin (jaundice) soon after birth. This condition is normally no cause for concern, and usually clears up within a few days.

Jaundice is caused by an excess in the bloodstream of the yellowish-brown chemical bilirubin, a natural waste product of the continuous breakdown of red cells in the blood. Normally, bilirubin is removed from the bloodstream by the liver, which uses it to help form bile. Some bile is stored in the gallbladder, from where it passes through the main bile duct to the digestive tract, where it

helps digestion of fats. The rest of the bile passes directly from the liver through tiny bile ducts to the main bile duct, and then into the digestive tract. When any part of this process fails to work, bilirubin accumulates in the blood, turning the skin yellow. In newborn babies, this most often results when the immature liver, not yet functioning normally, does not process bilirubin fast enough. The jaundice that results is known as physiological or normal jaundice (see *Jaundice*, p.485).

In a few babies, jaundice results when excessive breakdown of red blood cells (haemolytic disease) releases too much bilirubin into the bloodstream. The most common cause of haemolytic disease in newborn babies is that the blood of the fetus is Rhesus positive and *antibodies* enter it from the Rhesus negative blood of the mother (see *Rhesus incompatibility*, p.626).

Malformation or total absence of the baby's bile ducts causes what is known as obstructive jaundice. Bile, and with it bilirubin, cannot pass from the liver, causing the bilirubin to build up in the bloodstream.

What are the symptoms?

In all types of jaundice, the baby's skin and the whites of the eyes turn slightly yellow. In haemolytic disease this happens within the first day of birth, in physiological jaundice after about two days, and in obstructive jaundice after about a week. In physiological jaundice and mild haemolytic disease, the yellowness is slight and normally disappears after a few days. But in severe haemolytic disease and obstructive jaundice the discoloration grows more pronounced and remains until treatment is carried out. A baby with physiological jaundice or haemolytic disease is sometimes lethargic and reluctant to feed. In obstructive jaundice the baby may have diarrhoea and fails to gain weight.

How common is the problem?

Physiological jaundice is very common; it occurs in well over half of all babies. Haemolytic disease is uncommon, and obstructive jaundice is extremely rare.

What are the risks?

Haemolytic disease carries the remote risk that a very high level of bilirubin in the blood will cause brain damage. But this almost never occurs, because once a doctor has diagnosed the disease treatment is carried out straight away, and a constant check is kept on the level of bilirubin in the blood. In obstructive jaundice the blockage will cause fatal liver damage unless it can be corrected.

What is the treatment?

In most cases of physiological jaundice, the baby is simply given plenty of water to drink. When the level of bilirubin is high, the baby may be exposed to ultra-violet light (*phototherapy*), which helps the liver form the chemicals necessary to process bilirubin.

Mild cases of haemolytic disease disappear without treatment. Severe cases are treated by exchange blood transfusion. The treatment for obstructive jaundice is surgery. If the main bile duct is malformed, the chances of repairing it are good; if the many, tiny bile ducts are malformed, the outlook is poor.

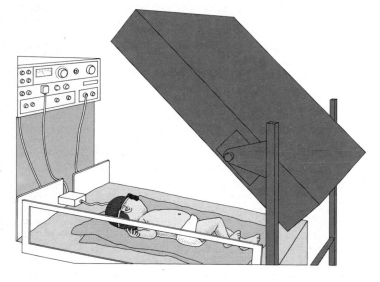

Treatment for jaundice Rays from an ultra-violet lamp (phototherapy) help to lower the amount of bilirubin in the blood. The baby's eyes will be covered so that they are not harmed by the rays from the lamp.

Cot death

Cot death – also known as crib death, or SIDS (Sudden Infant Death Syndrome) – has long been a mystery. An apparently healthy baby is laid down to sleep, and some time later is found dead. About 1 baby in 5,000 dies in this way, most commonly between three and 18 weeks of age. It is known that the baby dies suddenly and peacefully, usually while asleep, but in nearly all cases no explanation for the death is discovered. Suffocation, which might seem an obvious cause of death, is in fact extremely rare. Research has shown that the risk of cot death is higher in the winter and in bottle-fed babies, and that it may be linked to the baby becoming overheated from too many bedclothes.

What should be done?

Losing a baby in this way can be emotionally shattering for the parents, and they generally need the comfort of relatives and friends, together with the reassurance of their doctor that there was nothing they could have done to prevent the tragedy. Help and information can also be obtained from the *Foundation for the Study of Infant Deaths* (p.768). Some couples find that starting another pregnancy soon after helps to alleviate their grief.

In the event of a cot death, it is unfortunately essential for an *autopsy* to be done. This occasionally reveals a cause of death, which helps further research on the prevention of cot death.

Feeding problems

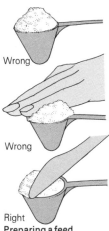

Wrong

Wrong

Right

Preparing a feed
When preparing your baby's feed, do not over-fill the measuring spoon or compress the powder (top two diagrams). Fill the cup loosely and level off the powder with a knife (bottom diagram).

There are a number of problems that may affect your baby during or just after feeds. This article covers the more common and less serious of them. However, if your baby persistently fails to take adequate milk and does not gain weight at the normal rate, there may be some serious problem; in that case, consult your doctor or health visitor without delay. (For problems affecting the breast-feeding mother see *Breast problems*, p.641.)

Crying during or after feeds
Although many mothers believe that a baby who cries after feeding is suffering from wind and babies must always be "burped", few paediatricians would subscribe to this view.

A bottle-fed baby may cry because the feed has not been mixed to the correct consistency. If it is too dilute, the baby cries because he or she is undernourished (an additional sign of undernourishment is that the baby passes small, firm, dark green motions). If the feed is too concentrated the baby, apart from becoming fat, will take in too much salt and will cry because he or she is thirsty. To remedy the problem, always make up an artificial feed according to the manufacturer's instructions (see diagrams, left). If your baby seems to want more feed, then continue feeding; most babies stop when they have had enough.

Another reason for crying, especially in hot weather, may be thirst. Try giving some sterilized water in a bottle or on a spoon. Finally, your baby may cry after a feed simply because he or she wants attention.

Poor feeding
During their first few weeks, some babies start to feed actively but soon fall asleep. If your baby does this, wake him or her and try to stimulate further feeding. The phase soon passes in a healthy baby; but if it continues, or if your baby has been feeding slowly or uninterestedly for a few days, see your doctor.

Regurgitating after feeds
Most babies bring back a little milk, particularly when they burp – this is called *posseting*, and is quite normal. Some babies – usually very active ones – regurgitate quite a lot but this usually ceases after solids are introduced into the diet, and generally clears up completely by nine months. If this does not happen, or if there is true vomiting, which may be due to a disorder such as *congenital pyloric stenosis* (p.660), consult your doctor.

Gastro-enteritis in infants

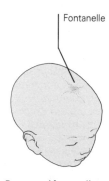

Fontanelle

Depressed fontanelle
If the soft spot on the top of your baby's head seems abnormally sunken, suspect dehydration – perhaps due to gastroenteritis – and call your doctor without delay.

In gastroenteritis, the stomach and small intestine become inflamed. The disorder may be no more than a mild tummy upset, but at the other extreme can cause continuing loss of fluid and vital body chemicals in the faeces which leads to *dehydration* (for general information on *gastroenteritis* see p.459).

Bottle-fed babies are more prone to the disorder than breast-fed babies, mainly because breast milk contains *antibodies* which shield the digestive tract against infection.

What are the symptoms?
Loose, green, watery stools are passed frequently. In mild cases, the baby remains happy and feeds well, but in more severe attacks the baby is miserable and irritable, feeds poorly, may vomit, and has a slightly raised temperature. Signs of dehydration are a dry mouth, sunken eyes and *fontanelle* (the soft spot on the top of the head), lethargy, and irritability. In severe dehydration, the skin loses elasticity, all feeds are refused, and the baby's temperature may be high or low.

How common is the problem?
With the increasing prevalence of breast-feeding, infantile gastroenteritis is much less common than it used to be. Most cases are mild or are treated before severe dehydration can occur. If dehydration is allowed to reach an advanced stage, it can cause brain damage or even death.

What should be done?
You can treat mild gastroenteritis yourself by adopting the measures described under "Self-help" below. But see your doctor at once if your baby has symptoms of dehydration, or vomits all feeds in a six-hour period.

If you are bottle-feeding your baby, check that you are sterilizing bottles and teats thoroughly. Never put the teat of a bottle or a dummy in your own mouth and avoid handling it before giving it to the baby.

What is the treatment?
Self-help: If you are bottle-feeding your baby, cut out the baby's feed of milk for 24 hours and substitute cooled boiled water containing a level teaspoonful of glucose and half a teaspoonful of salt to each half-litre. On the second day, replace this liquid with an artificial-milk feed of a quarter of the usual amount of baby-milk powder to the usual amount of water; on the third day use half the normal amount of powder; and on the fourth day three-quarters the amount. During this

four-day course give the normal daily volume of fluid, but in small amounts every hour or so. From the fifth day, it should be safe to return to normal bottle-feeding.

If you are breast-feeding your baby, consult your doctor or health visitor for advice. **Professional help:** Call your doctor if you are at all worried about your baby. In mild cases, he or she will simply give advice on feeding and fluids and may prescribe an antidiarrhoeal drug. A baby suffering from a serious attack will be admitted to hospital and given fluids and vital chemicals, perhaps by *intravenous drip*. After a time, artificial-milk feeds will be given in a similar way to that described above.

Nappy rash

Certain irritants can inflame the skin on a baby's buttocks, thighs, and genitals and cause nappy rash. The irritants are chiefly chemicals in the faeces, ammonia produced by a reaction between bacteria in the faeces and urine (when the rash is called ammonia dermatitis), and soap or detergent left in nappies by inadequate rinsing. Most babies have nappy rash at some time.

See p.234, **Visual aids to diagnosis, 4.**

What are the symptoms?
The baby's skin over the area covered by the nappy becomes red, spotty, sore, and moist. The rash varies in severity. Ammonia dermatitis is characterized by a smell of ammonia often strong enough to make your eyes water when you change the nappy.

What are the risks?
There are no serious risks associated with nappy rash. However, in boys, ammonia often inflames and swells the foreskin of the penis, causing the baby pain and occasionally difficulty in passing urine. Sometimes the area of the nappy rash can become affected by a fungal infection.

What should be done?
Nappy rash is generally a problem the parents can deal with themselves. But if the treatment described fails to clear up the rash within a few days, see a doctor.

What is the treatment?
Part of the treatment, and the way to ensure that the problem does not recur, is to sterilize and rinse the baby's nappies thoroughly, and to change them promptly. Ordinary washing of nappies is often not enough to rid them of microbes from the baby's faeces, so you must sterilize the nappies. Boil them for some time, or soak them in a solution of one of the antiseptics manufactured specially for the purpose (re-use the solution you used for sterilizing the baby's bottle). After washing the nappies, rinse them several times to remove all traces of soap or detergent.

A more expensive way of achieving the same objective is to use disposable nappies.

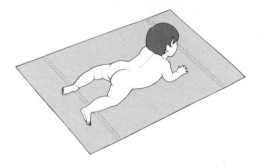

How to ease nappy rash
Help to clear nappy rash by allowing your baby to spend as much time as possible with his or her nappy area exposed in a warm, dry atmosphere.

Any baby who suffers from nappy rash must have his or her nappies changed often – very often if the baby passes faeces at frequent intervals, as many babies do.

Plastic pants normally have no bearing on whether the baby gets nappy rash. If nappies are not changed often enough, however, the waterproof pants, by keeping the nappy area moist, can aggravate the rash.

There are several treatments for the actual rash. One is to expose the baby's buttocks to a warm, dry atmosphere. Take the baby's nappy off and lay him or her chest down, with face turned to one side, on soft towelling underlaid by a waterproof sheet. Any faeces or urine produced should be cleared up immediately and the rash bathed with warm water but not soap. The towelling should then be changed if necessary. Afterwards, pat the affected area dry with a soft towel, and lightly sprinkle the rash with talcum powder.

You can obtain various creams from a chemist to relieve nappy rash. Ammonia dermatitis can be relieved – and prevented from the start – by the use of a silicone barrier cream containing zinc oxide and calamine. This cream acts as a barrier against both microbes and moisture. It should be applied liberally to a boy's foreskin that has been inflamed by ammonia.

If the rash persists, see your doctor, who may be able to give further advice and prescribe a special cream to speed up healing.

Seborrhoeic eczema

(including cradle cap)

See p.234,
Visual aids to diagnosis, 5.

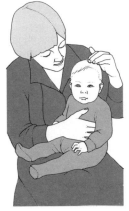

Avoiding infection
Seborrhoeic eczema and cradle cap often clear up of their own accord. However, it is important that the rash is not allowed to become infected. Wash and pat dry your baby regularly, making sure that no trace of moisture is left on the skin. Rub the baby's head with baby oil if the scales are unsightly.

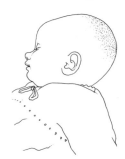

This common skin disorder occurs during the first two years of life, usually during the first three months. It occurs most commonly on the head (when it is also known as cradle cap), but can also appear on the face, the neck, the armpits, and the groin. (For general information see *Eczema*, p.253.)

In cradle cap, scurf appears on the scalp, followed by yellow, greasy, scaly patches that sometimes extend over the eyebrows and behind the ears. Seborrhoeic eczema on the face takes the form of small red blotches and pimples, which become redder when the baby cries or gets hot. Elsewhere, the eczema occurs as red patches with areas of scaling.

The eczema does not irritate and has no effect on general health. In the rare cases when it becomes infected the patches become soggy, and ooze yellowish fluid.

The cause of eczema is unknown, but sometimes it can be triggered off by *nappy rash* (opposite) which starts in the groin and works its way up the body.

Each year about 1 baby in 100 is taken to a doctor because of seborrhoeic eczema.

What is the treatment?

The disorder usually heals of its own accord, and there is normally no need to see a doctor. Keep the affected areas clean and dry by bathing them in the normal way and dusting them with talcum powder. If cradle cap is unsightly, rub the scales gently with baby oil or petroleum jelly; this loosens them and they can be washed away.

Alternatively, your doctor may prescribe a special cream to loosen the scales.

If the eczema becomes infected, see your doctor who may prescribe an *antibiotic* cream to clear up the infection. For seborrhoeic eczema that results from nappy rash, the doctor may prescribe a mild *steroid* cream.

Excessive crying

During the first few weeks of life the average baby sleeps a great deal but, when awake, cries lustily and often. A baby who cries feebly and infrequently may be seriously ill.

It is only from about six weeks of age onwards, when the baby is becoming aware of his or her surroundings, that there are some wakeful periods without crying. The number of these periods increases as the baby grows, until by the age of six months the baby may spend, on average, a total of three or four hours a day without crying, but, instead, gurgling and playing.

Some newborn babies cry for much of the time they should be sleeping, and when they are about six months old cry for much of the time they should be playing. Crying of this degree can be termed excessive.

Much of a placid baby's contentment stems from the mother's contentment. In the same way, the anxious mother transmits her anxiety to her baby, who may then sleep badly and cry excessively. A vicious circle can evolve: the more the baby cries, the more anxious the mother becomes. She may also get cross with the baby for crying so much, causing the baby to cry even more.

Excessive crying is much more common in a first than a subsequent baby. This is because the first-time, inexperienced mother is often anxious about her competence to look after a new young life. The mother rarely realizes that her own emotional state may often be the major cause of a baby's excessive crying. She puts the crying down to teething, or tummy ache, or pain in passing urine. Here are some details about the potential causes of crying:

Teething: Babies cut their first teeth between the ages of six months and two years (see *Teething problems*, p.685). Where the tooth emerges, the gum is often slightly swollen and inflamed, and the discomfort makes the baby cry. But the inflammation rapidly subsides, and, even if several teeth are coming through, teething should not cause crying on and off for more than a few days.

It is inevitable that the occasional illness will coincide with the eruption of a tooth, but it is wrong to attribute such conditions as diarrhoea or convulsions to teething.

Tummy ache: There is no reason why the simple milk diet (whether natural or otherwise) of the normal baby should cause tummy ache (see *Feeding problems*, p.649). If the baby cries uncontrollably for several hours each evening, it is more likely that the cause is so-called 3-month or 10-week *colic* (sharp tummy ache). But, although some doctors consider that the baby has a genuine physical pain, others believe that this is an example of the baby reacting to the tension of the mother at the end of a hard day; and they believe that the crying stops after 10 to 12 weeks because by then the mother has become more competent and confident in her handling of the baby, and has communicated this new calmness to the baby.

Passing urine: Sometimes a baby cries at the same time that he or she passes urine. This leads some mothers to believe that passing urine is painful for the baby and that this is the cause of the excessive crying. In most cases, however, the crying precedes urination and, in fact, aids it. Crying increases pressure in the tummy, which causes the bladder to empty more thoroughly.

In a minority of babies who cry excessively, there is something actually wrong. The baby may have an infection – indicated by a raised temperature, a runny nose, cough, vomiting, diarrhoea, poor feeding, or general failure to thrive. Do not forget that the baby may be lonely and needing comfort; this is the probable cause if the crying stops when the baby is picked up. Occasionally, crying is due to

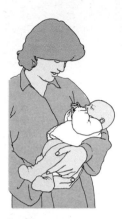

One cause of crying
If your baby stops crying when picked up, he or she may simply need comfort and attention.

unsuitable, or not enough, food. If you have made certain that your baby is not ill, lonely, or inadequately fed, then you must face the fact that he or she is simply sensing and reacting to your own emotional state.

What should be done?
If you are tired from night sessions with the baby, try to snatch a few hours' sleep during the day, at the same time as your baby. Let housework take second place; the well-being of you and your child is much more important. Accept any offers of help, particularly from a willing partner. If you are breast-feeding a particularly demanding baby, and if feeding is well established, treat yourself to the occasional evening out while a competent relative or friend bottle-feeds the baby with artificial or expressed breast milk.

If you still find yourself under considerable strain, to the extent that you feel yourself getting really angry with your baby, see your health visitor or doctor at once. They will find practical ways of helping you to cope and so relieve your anxiety.

Birthmarks

See p.233,
Visual aids to diagnosis, 1–3.

A birthmark is any area of discoloured skin that appears at birth or shortly afterwards and persists for at least several months. (Discolorations that disappear a few days after birth are usually bruises, brought about during labour or during delivery with forceps.) A birthmark may be either a conglomeration of tiny blood vessels in the skin (known as a *naevus*) or a discoloration on the surface of the skin (called a pigmented spot).

There are three main types of naevus. A capillary naevus is a flat, pink or pinkish-brown area. Many babies have capillary naevi at birth, most of which gradually fade and disappear before the baby is 18 months old. A strawberry naevus is a bright-red, raised area usually no bigger than a 50p piece. It can occur on any part of the body. At birth it is so small that it is not noticed for a few days. It grows rapidly for a few weeks, then increases in size proportionately with the baby. Occasionally, when there is fatty tissue under the naevus, the red area lies on top of a soft lump, about 10mm (roughly ⅓in) above the skin level. When the baby is about six months old, small, scattered white areas can be seen in the naevus. They spread, gradually replacing the red tissue, while at the same time the area becomes flatter. The naevus has usually disappeared by the time the child is about three years of age, leaving a slightly pale area of skin. The third type of naevus is the port wine

stain – a purplish-red, often extensive and sometimes partly raised area that generally occurs singly, on the face or limbs. Generally a port wine stain persists into adult life, though sometimes it may fade slightly.

The other type of birthmark, a pigmented spot, is most commonly a flat, irregularly-shaped, coffee-coloured spot (often called a "café au lait" spot). Usually there are only one or two small spots, but in some cases the spots are multiple or large, or both. Some babies are born with pigmented moles that have hair growing on them. Pigmented spots are generally permanent.

Why birthmarks occur is unclear. They have little medical significance, and the only real problem that they may cause is disfigurement. Large, unsightly birthmarks that persist can be treated by *plastic surgery* (p.260) or other measures when the child has reached the age of three or four. A surgeon will sometimes hasten the spontaneous disappearance of a strawberry naevus by injecting hot salt water into it while the baby is under an anaesthetic. A simple, makeshift way of dealing with an unsightly birthmark is to cover it with a special skin-coloured cream that can be bought from a chemist. A large strawberry naevus occasionally bleeds, either spontaneously or after a blow, but pressing on the wound with a finger for several minutes usually stops the bleeding.

Down's syndrome

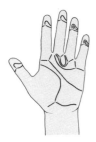

Normal hand

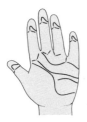

Hand of child with Down's syndrome

Visual signs of Down's Syndrome Before techniques for analysing chromosomes were developed, Down's syndrome was often suspected from the distinctive crease patterns on the typically short, broad hands of an affected child.

In the normal human body all cells except egg cells and sperm cells each have 46 *chromosomes*. Egg cells and sperm cells each have 23 chromosomes. When an egg cell is fertilized by a sperm cell, the two cells come together to provide the developing baby with the normal 46 chromosomes in each cell.

Sometimes, however, an egg cell (or occasionally a sperm cell) has a certain chromosome (number 21) in duplicate – so that the fertilized egg has 47 instead of 46 chromosomes, and the child has 47 chromosomes in each cell. Such a child has Down's syndrome.

What are the symptoms?
Babies with Down's syndrome are recognizable at birth by their facial appearance. The eyes slope upwards at the outer corners (which is why such children were formerly called mongols), the facial features are small, and the tongue is large and tends to stick out. Other characteristics include a flat back to the head, and sometimes the little finger curves towards the third finger.

Children with Down's syndrome are invariably mentally handicapped and need to be educated in a special school. But they can be active participants in family life because they are responsive, loving, and even-tempered, and many can enjoy music.

How common is the problem?
Down's syndrome affects 1 in every 1,000 babies born. A mother is at greater than average risk of having a baby with this abnormality if she is over 40; or if she or the father has some rare chromosomal abnormality. For women at risk the test of *amniocentesis* (p.639) is carried out and a termination is offered if the test is positive.

For a young woman with normal chromosomes who has had an affected child, there is only a remote risk of any further children being affected by Down's syndrome.

What are the risks?
About a quarter of children with Down's syndrome also have some form of *congenital*

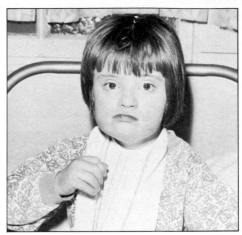

Typical facial features Most children with Down's syndrome have small facial features, with upward-slanting eyes.

heart disorder (p.656). There is a slightly higher than normal incidence among them of *intestinal atresia* (p.662) and *leukaemia* (p.426). And they are particularly prone to respiratory and ear infections.

What should be done?
Unless parents find it a continual strain, it is much better to bring up a child with Down's syndrome in a family and not in a special children's home. Support is available from the health visitor and local social services. There is also a national organization, *Down's Children's Association* (p.768), which can help.

Children with Down's syndrome attend special schools staffed by teachers who are trained to deal with mentally handicapped children and to help them attain their full potential. The staff, in cooperation with the parents, try to teach the child not only speech but self-help such as feeding, dressing, and using the lavatory.

People with Down's syndrome can be trained to do simple but useful jobs. They will always, however, need a protective environment, and have to be cared for by their family or in a home for the mentally handicapped.

Doubtful sex

During the first three months of pregnancy, the embryo secretes hormones that regulate the development of sex organs. If this development is abnormal, then at birth the baby's sex organs will be malformed.

Minor defects in the sex organs can nearly always be corrected by surgery. But in rare cases – fewer than 1 in 1,000 babies – the defect is considerably more pronounced,

sometimes to such an extent that doctors are in doubt about the baby's true sex. In such cases, cells scraped from the inside of the baby's mouth are tested shortly after birth to reveal the true genetic sex of the child. Surgery is then carried out – sometimes over a period of years – to correct the appearance of the sex organs. In most cases, the child will grow up to lead a normal sex life.

Congenital disorders of the central nervous system

The central nervous system (described in detail elsewhere – see *Disorders of the brain and nervous system*, p.266) consists of the brain and spinal cord. It develops within the first two months of pregnancy, from a strip of cells running along the back of the embryo. The edges of the strip gradually curl inwards to form a tube of cells. The front part of this tube expands and forms the brain; the back part becomes the spinal cord. Surrounding and within the brain and spinal cord – cushioning these delicate organs – is a liquid, cerebrospinal fluid, produced by the brain. As the skull bones and spinal column develop, they provide further protection for the brain and spinal cord.

A *congenital* disorder of the central nervous system is a fault, present at birth, in the brain and/or spinal cord. In spina bifida some part of the spinal column, and usually the spinal cord inside it, are defective. In hydrocephalus, there is an excess of cerebrospinal fluid in and around the brain.

Congenital disorders of the central nervous system tend to run in families. If a couple has one affected child, or have any relatives who have had such a child, they should request a consultation with a genetic counsellor, (see *Genetic counselling*, p.619) to discuss the risks involved in any subsequent pregnancy.

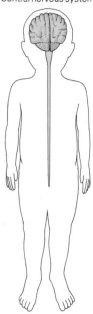

Central nervous system

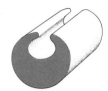

Development of the spinal cord
The spinal cord begins to develop when the embryo is about 20 days old. A groove appears in the centre of what will be the baby's back.

Over the course of a few days the groove deepens and the edges curve towards each other.

Within 3 days of the groove appearing the edges have fused to form the tube that develops into the spinal cord.

Spina bifida

In a child born with spina bifida, part of the bony spine that helps protect the spinal cord fails to develop properly. The nerves of the spinal cord in that area are exposed and unprotected and may also be defective. Usually the affected region is the lower spine. The spinal nerves in that region control the muscles of the legs, bladder, and bowels, and a child born with the disorder will usually have some paralysis of the legs and incontinence. In some children the defect in the spine is so mild as to cause hardly any physical handicap; the only visible defect may be a small dimple in the skin somewhere on the baby's back. But in others the loss of function in the lower part of the body is complete; and there is a large, purplish-red membrane covering a gap in the spine. Between the two extremes is a whole spectrum of disability ranging from minimal to severe.

How common is the problem?
About 1 in every 700 babies born in Britain has spina bifida; a proportion of these babies also have *hydrocephalus* (opposite).

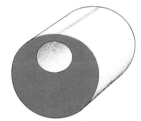

Cross-section of normal spine
Skin on back
Spinal fluid
Spinal cord
Vertebra

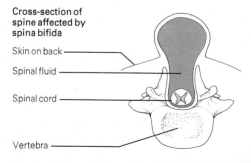

Cross-section of spine affected by spina bifida
Skin on back
Spinal fluid
Spinal cord
Vertebra

What are the risks?

The fragile membrane on the baby's back may be damaged before it can be treated. If infection enters the cerebro-spinal fluid through the damaged area, meningitis (see *Meningitis in babies and children*, p.668) develops. Infections of the bladder are common in more severe cases, and with hydrocephalus there are additional risks.

What is the treatment?

There is no cure for spina bifida: defects in the formation of the spinal cord cannot be rectified, and any paralysis will be permanent. In most cases, an operation to repair the membrane on the child's back is carried out shortly after birth, but little can be done to repair the defective spinal nerves.

Parents are encouraged to join a local branch of the *Association for Spina Bifida and Hydrocephalus* (p.768) for help and support.

What are the long-term prospects?

Prospects for the child with spina bifida vary considerably, according to the severity and extent of the disorder.

From time to time, operations may be necessary to correct deformities of the legs or to enable the child to achieve bladder control (although many sufferers manage to achieve this naturally when young).

Mentally normal sufferers can attend school – an ordinary school for the rare children with only minimal paralysis of the legs, or a special day school for those who are physically handicapped.

Hydro-cephalus

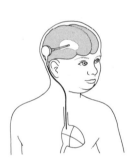

Treatment for hydrocephalus
When hydrocephalus does not clear up spontaneously, the surgeon may insert a tube (shunt) behind the child's ear to drain off the fluid from the brain into a main blood vessel.

The brain is bathed by fluid called cerebrospinal fluid. The fluid is secreted in the cavities (*ventricles*) inside the brain and passes into the space around the brain, where it is absorbed into a membrane surrounding the space. If, in the developing fetus, the membrane is defective, or the flow of the fluid is blocked, the fluid builds up within the cavities of the brain. The result is that the increasing pressure causes the brain to swell. This is called hydrocephalus ("water on the brain"). To accommodate the swelling, the loosely connected bones of the skull spread apart, and the head grows larger than normal. In severe cases of the disorder the brain may be permanently damaged.

Hydrocephalus may also occur late in infancy as a result of damage to the brain from an infection or a tumour.

What are the symptoms?

The early stages of the disorder may be suspected at birth if the baby's head circumference is significantly larger than the average of 350mm or 13½in. If it is, the head is measured frequently during the early weeks, and if its rate of growth is excessive, investigations, including *X-rays*, are carried out.

How common is the problem?

Abour 1 in every 10,000 babies born has hydrocephalus alone; the disorder occurs more often in association with spina bifida.

What are the risks?

When hydrocephalus is well advanced at birth, serious brain damage and underdevelopment are inevitable, and early death of the child from infection is likely.

What is the treatment?

It is possible to detect the disorder in the uterus by X-rays and *ultrasound*. When the disorder has become well advanced during pregnancy, it may be necessary – for the mother's own safety – to have the baby delivered by *Caesarean section* (p.640).

If the hydrocephalus is not too advanced, it can be relieved after birth by an operation. The baby is given a general anaesthetic and a small hole is drilled in the skull. A fine tube with a one-way valve is inserted in the hole

Normal baby   Hydrocephalic baby

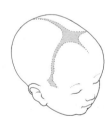 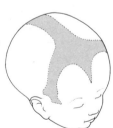

and installed between the brain at one end and, at the other, a major blood vessel leading into the heart. By this means, fluid drains from the brain into the bloodstream.

After the operation the size of the baby's head gradually becomes normal. During the first year the baby will need regular checkups, about once a month. As the child grows, the tube may become blocked, and the child will become irritable and may start to vomit. If this happens, see your doctor immediately. If a blockage of the tube is suspected, the child will be taken into hospital to have the blockage removed or the tube replaced.

Congenital heart disorders

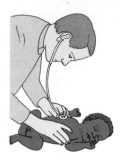

Many congenital heart disorders are detected by examination with a stethoscope.

About 8 babies in every 1,000 are born with a heart abnormality of some kind. This *congenital* abnormality (congenital means "present at birth") may be so minor that it needs no treatment and does not affect the life of the person. At the other extreme, it may be so severe that, despite treatment, the baby is likely to die. (For the various kinds of congenital heart disorders see pp.658–9.)

The development of abnormalities
The heart of a fetus starts to develop early in pregnancy and is complete by the third month. Any abnormality of development during this vital period will cause a congenital heart disorder, or, possibly, more than one. An abnormality may result if the mother has German measles or one of certain other infections during early pregnancy (see *German measles and pregnancy*, p.616), or if the child has defective chromosomes (see, for example, *Down's syndrome*, p.653).

Some drugs taken early in pregnancy can also cause heart abnormalities in the developing fetus. For this reason, a woman who is or thinks she may be pregnant should never take drugs unless they have been approved by a doctor who is aware of her condition.

There is a slight tendency for congenital heart disease to run in families. If either

---

How the circulation alters after birth

The heart before birth
Inside the uterus, the baby is submerged in fluid and so cannot obtain oxygen by breathing. Instead, the baby obtains oxygen from the mother's blood via the placenta. Before birth, therefore, the baby's lungs need only the same amount of blood as other body tissues whereas the placenta needs a copious supply for oxygenation. To achieve this there are 2 bypasses in the fetal heart (shown as black arrows in the diagram). One is the ductus arteriosus, which channels deoxygenated "used" blood (grey) – which, after birth, would be bound for the lungs – into the aorta and thence along the umbilical artery to the placenta for oxygenation. The other bypass is the foramen ovale, which takes the oxygenated "fresh" blood (brown) returning from the placenta along the umbilical vein, and diverts it through the right atrium into the left atrium, and then via the left ventricle along the aorta to the body tissues.

From body tissues

Blood flow through ductus arteriosus

Aorta

Blood flow through foramen ovale

To body tissues

Umbilical vein from placenta

From body tissues

Umbilical artery to placenta

The heart after birth
Within seconds of birth, the baby starts to breathe and becomes dependent on the lungs rather than the placenta for oxygen. The ductus arteriosus, which carried deoxygenated blood to the placenta, and the foramen ovale, through which oxygenated blood from the placenta passed through the heart, are no longer needed. Both close completely over a period of several weeks. Oxygenated blood now comes from the lungs and enters the left atrium, not the right, while deoxygenated blood passes along the pulmonary artery to the lungs. The umbilical blood vessels tighten, become sealed off, and eventually shrivel away. The umbilical cord, which connected the baby to the placenta, is cut and it too shrivels up and drops off after a few days.

Note: For general information about the structure of the heart and blood vessels see p.371.

From body tissues

Pulmonary artery to lungs

Aorta

From body tissues

To body tissues

Pulmonary vein from lungs

parent has or has had congenital heart disease, there is a 4 per cent chance of a child having the same or a similar condition. In such cases, it may be wise to consult a genetic counsellor before having a baby (see *Genetic counselling*, p.619). However, because the affected parent has survived to adulthood, the chances of the child being severely affected by the disease are slim.

In most cases of congenital heart disease it is not known what causes the abnormality.

Symptoms

In many cases of congenital heart disease there are no symptoms and the abnormality is discovered during a routine examination of the heart. In others, symptoms are marked. Sometimes they appear at birth; sometimes they do not develop until childhood or much later. Symptoms are not directly related to the need for any treatment; many symptomless cases require surgery to prevent trouble occurring later in life.

A common feature is blueness of the skin (*cyanosis*). This occurs when the abnormality has caused an excess of deoxygenated blood to circulate through the system. Mild *heart failure* (p.381) in a baby shows itself as difficulty in feeding (because the baby finds it an effort to suck), being underweight as a result, and crying for shorter than normal periods. In a baby with severe heart failure, these signs are more pronounced: the breathing is rapid and distressed, and the baby will almost certainly have cyanosis or heart failure.

Children with congenital heart disease may become breathless on exertion and their physical development tends to be poor; if they have heart failure, they may be breathless and cyanotic even while resting.

Heart murmurs

Diagnosis of a congenital heart disorder is most commonly made by examination with a *stethoscope*. In a perfectly healthy heart, the stethoscope picks up sounds of the ventricles contracting and the closing of the heart valves. Most other sounds are known as heart murmurs, but the presence of a murmur does not necessarily mean there is an abnormality in the heart, or that the heart is seriously unhealthy. For example, a heart murmur can be detected if the baby's blood flow is greatly increased because he or she has developed *anaemia* (p.419). The doctor can usually detect which murmurs are a sign of some abnormality and which are not. Each abnormality generally produces a particular type of murmur – as when, in *congenital pulmonary stenosis* (p.658), for example, the blood has

to pass through a narrower channel than normal; and in most cases the doctor can diagnose the abnormality present.

Some children with perfectly normal hearts are found to have heart murmurs; such children should be treated in exactly the same way as any other healthy individual.

Special diagnostic tests

Once the doctor has detected an abnormality, further investigations are carried out in hospital. An *X-ray* of the chest shows up certain abnormalities in the shape and size of the heart chambers. An *electrocardiograph* (*ECG*) records the electrical impulses produced by the heartbeat, and in so doing it reveals any enlargement of the chambers of the heart. In addition, an *ultrasound* investigation may be carried out to reveal the relative thickness of the heart chamber walls and the condition of the valves. These procedures cause no discomfort, and no anaesthetic is needed. In certain cases, an investigation called *cardiac catheterization* is required. The baby or child is anaesthetized or sedated, and a tube called a *catheter* is passed along a blood vessel, usually in the leg, until it reaches the heart. It is then watched on an X-ray screen as it is manipulated into the chambers of the heart through the various openings. The catheter also enables measurements to be made of the pressure of, and amount of oxygen in, the blood in each chamber of the heart. Finally, an X-ray cinefilm is taken of a liquid opaque to X-rays passing through the catheter into the blood vessels of the heart and lungs; this shows the shape and size of the chambers and valves. Armed with information from these procedures, heart specialists and surgeons can diagnose the problem and decide on the best possible treatment.

Treatment

Most cases of congenital heart disease require an operation to correct the abnormality. Unless the disorder is so severe that it requires immediate surgery, the operation is delayed until early childhood, when the rate of success is considerably higher than in infancy because of the greater capacity of the child's system to withstand open-heart surgery. With modern surgical techniques, the success rate for most heart operations on children is now very high, and children who have had successful operations can, in most cases, expect to live a normal life.

Heart failure in infants is treated with drugs, which may need to be given for several years, until surgery is possible.

Congenital aortic stenosis

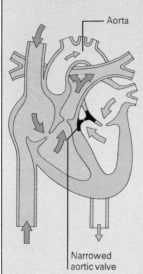

Aorta

Narrowed aortic valve

This is a narrowing of the aortic valve, and sometimes of the aorta itself, restricting the flow of blood to the body. It accounts for 6.5 per cent of all congenital heart disorders; the disease is almost totally confined to boys.

Effects Usually none; in rare cases, babies develop severe heart failure and cyanosis. Children may suffer from shortness of breath, chest pains, and blackouts. Rarely, sudden death without preceding symptoms can occur.

Treatment In all cases, an operation is performed to relieve or remove the constriction, occasionally when the child is between 8 and 10, but more often when the child has grown up and is rather better able to withstand heart-valve surgery.

Ventricular septal defect (hole in the heart)

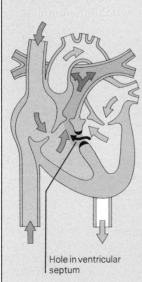

Hole in ventricular septum

This is a hole in the ventricular septum, usually the upper part. Blood flows from the left ventricle into the right, sometimes in large quantities so that excess blood passes through the lungs. In 25 per cent of cases the hole gradually closes by itself. It accounts for 31 per cent of all congenital heart disorders.

Effects Most babies and children have none, or they may tire easily and have shortness of breath on exertion; occasionally there is severe heart failure or pulmonary hypertension.

Treatment A small hole usually does not require treatment. For a larger hole, open-heart surgery is needed and is usually delayed until the child is between 5 and 10. If there is an earlier danger of pulmonary hypertension, a simple preliminary operation is carried out.

Congenital pulmonary stenosis

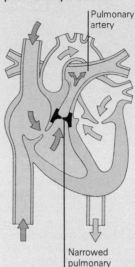

Pulmonary artery

Narrowed pulmonary valve

A narrowing of the pulmonary valve, or, more rarely, of the pulmonary artery or the upper right ventricle, reducing the flow of blood to the lungs. It accounts for 9 per cent of all congenital heart disorders.

Effects Usually none. Some babies and children have cyanosis, shortness of breath on exertion, and tire easily; in others, there may be severe heart failure, which can lead to sudden death.

Treatment If the stenosis is mild, no treatment is necessary. If it is moderate or severe, surgery has to be carried out to relieve or remove the constriction.

Atrial septal defect

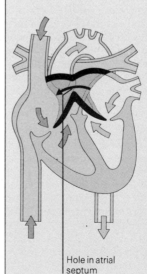

Hole in atrial septum

This is a hole in the atrial septum. Blood passes from the left atrium into the right, sometimes in large amounts so that excess blood circulates through the lungs. Spontaneous closure of the hole is rare. Atrial septal defect accounts for 11 per cent of all congenital heart disorders. Girls are more commonly affected than boys.

Effects Most babies and children have none or they may tire easily and have shortness of breath on exertion. If the disorder is not detected and treated in childhood, pulmonary hypertension may develop in late adolescence.

Treatment Except when the hole is very small and there is therefore no danger of pulmonary hypertension developing later, an operation is necessary to repair the defect. The operation is usually performed when the child is between 5 and 10.

Coarctation of the aorta

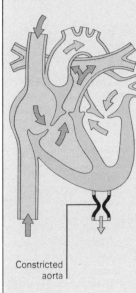

Constricted aorta

A constriction of the aorta, which reduces the supply of blood to the lower parts of the body. It accounts for 9 per cent of all congenital heart disorders.

Effects In some cases there are no symptoms. In others, symptoms appear in early childhood: headaches, weakness after exercise, weak or absent pulse in the groin, and sometimes coldness in the legs. In a few cases, when the aorta is extremely constricted, severe heart failure occurs in infancy.

Treatment Surgery is necessary in all cases, even when there are no symptoms. The operation, by which the constriction is removed and the two parts of the aorta joined together, is usually carried out when the child is between 4 and 8.

Fallot's tetralogy

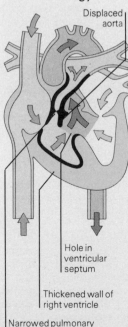

Displaced aorta

Hole in ventricular septum

Thickened wall of right ventricle

Narrowed pulmonary valve

In this disorder, 4 abnormalities occur together – a hole in the upper ventricular septum; a displacement of the aorta to the right, so that blood from both ventricles enters it; a narrowed pulmonary valve; and a thickening of the wall of the right ventricle. Fallot's tetralogy accounts for 6 per cent of all congenital heart disorders.

Effects From birth, cyanosis, clubbing of the fingers and toes, and underdevelopment. After exercise the child is short of breath and squats to relieve the discomfort.

Treatment In all cases an operation to correct all the abnormalities is carried out before the child is 5.

Patent ductus arteriosus

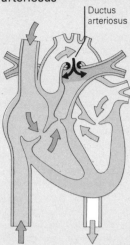

Ductus arteriosus

The ductus arteriosus fails to close after birth. Blood from the aorta flows through it into the pulmonary artery, so that excess blood passes through the lungs. The disorder accounts for 8 per cent of all congenital heart disorders.

Effects Usually none; in a few cases, during the first year of life, shortness of breath on exertion, frequent respiratory infections, and cyanosis. Pulmonary hypertension may develop.

Treatment In some cases, if the diagnosis is made early, the defect can be closed with drug treatment. In all other cases, a simple operation to close the duct is carried out before the child is 5.

Transposition of the great vessels

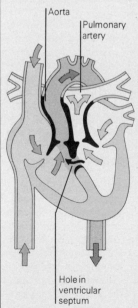

Aorta

Pulmonary artery

Hole in ventricular septum

In this disorder, the aorta and pulmonary arteries are transposed, so that oxygenated blood from the lungs passes through the pulmonary artery and back to the lungs, instead of through the aorta and to the tissues. There is usually a hole in the septum that allows some oxygenated blood to pass into the right side of the heart and the aorta. It accounts for 4.6 per cent of all congenital heart disorders.

Effects From birth, cyanosis, clubbing of the fingers and toes, and underdevelopment.

Treatment In all cases an emergency procedure to create a larger hole in the septum is performed before the baby is 3 months old; this is done by inserting a tube into the heart via a vein. A second operation, performed before the child is 5, creates two artificial blood vessels in the upper heart and restores the circulation to normal.

Congenital disorders of the digestive system

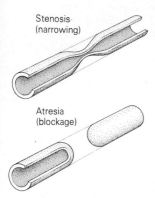

Stenosis
(narrowing)

Atresia
(blockage)

Stenosis and atresia
The two main types of
congenital digestive-tract
abnormality are stenosis
(a narrowing, or some-
times thickening of the
wall) and atresia (a com-
plete blockage creating
two dead-ends).

The digestive tract (described fully on p.435) is a continuous tube that digests food, absorbs nutrients from it, and eliminates what remains as waste matter. The glands connected to the tract include the pancreas, which passes digestive juices into the small intestine, and the liver, which empties bile into the small intestine (see *Liver, gallbladder, and pancreas*, p.485).

While still in the uterus, the baby receives all its nourishment from the mother via the placenta. It is only after birth, when the baby must start feeding, that any malformations of the system that occurred during development in the uterus reveal themselves.

The system is affected mainly by two kinds of malformation. The first is *stenosis* – a narrowing of a tube or duct, sometimes almost to the point of closure. The second is *atresia* – a gap in a tube or duct that separates it into two distinct, sealed-off sections. Why these malformations occur is not known.

Clearly, any serious abnormality in the digestive tract will affect the baby's capacity to digest and absorb food, but there are more immediate dangers, too. In particular, with disorders that cause vomiting, there are two serious risks. One is that the baby may inhale the vomit, which can cause suffocation or lead to death from pneumonia. The other risk is that the baby's failure to retain body fluids due to prolonged vomiting can eventually lead to death from *dehydration*.

The most common disorders of the digestive system are described in this section. They can all be treated by operations which, except in the case of bile-duct atresia, have a high success rate. The baby is prepared for an operation by having the stomach washed out and by being fed with *intravenous fluids* to keep the digestive tract empty and to maintain the correct balance of water and chemicals in the body. With most operations, the baby is under a general anaesthetic. He or she generally recovers from a successful operation within 48 hours; and usually by a week later the stitches have been removed and the baby is back at home.

Congenital pyloric stenosis

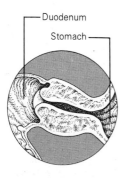

Duodenum

Stomach

Pyloric stenosis
The walls of the baby's
pylorus are thickened and
so obstruct the passage
of milk from the stomach
to the intestine.

The pylorus is a short muscular tube about 20mm (just under 1in) long with a normal internal diameter of approximately 5mm ($\frac{1}{5}$ in). It connects the stomach to the duodenum, the first section of the intestine. In pyloric stenosis (the cause of which is unknown), the wall of the tube thickens, and the passageway inside narrows. As a result, little or no milk can pass from the stomach into the intestine and the baby cannot absorb nourishment from the milk.

What are the symptoms?
Between two and eight weeks after birth the baby begins vomiting violently after feeds. The fierce stomach contractions made by the baby to force the feed through the narrowed pylorus are unsuccessful and instead force it up the oesophagus (gullet) and out of the mouth – sometimes as much as several feet away. This is called "projectile vomiting". Usually, the vomit contains a lot of milk curds and mucus and smells unpleasant. Initially, the vomiting does not interfere with the baby's well-being or desire to feed. But the baby soon begins to lose weight, becomes anxious and restless, and passes smaller stools less and less frequently. If the baby is not treated, he or she tends to feed reluctantly and becomes listless – partly because the constant vomiting upsets the delicate balance of body chemicals.

How common is the problem?
About 1 in every 150 boys born, and 1 in every 775 girls, suffer from the complaint. It is more common in first-born boys than in other boys, and it tends to run in families. The condition has also been known to occur in identical twins.

What are the risks?
If the disorder is untreated, severe cases can lead to death from *dehydration* and chemical imbalances in the body fluids.

What should be done?
If your baby is vomiting in the way described, contact your doctor immediately. If the doctor suspects pyloric stenosis, he or she will examine the abdomen and watch the baby feeding, looking for the violent abdominal contractions (visible gastric *peristalsis*) that are symptomatic of pyloric stenosis. The contractions resemble a golf ball travelling from left to right beneath the surface of the skin.

Several examinations – or on rare occasions, a *barium meal* – may be necessary before the diagnosis can be confirmed.

You may hear the doctor refer to the enlarged pylorus as a pyloric tumour. But there is no cause for alarm; the word "tumour" as used in this context is a common medical term for any *benign* swelling.

What is the treatment?
Self-help: Until medical help is obtained, feed the baby more often than usual, but reduce the normal amount of each feed.

Professional help: In all cases, simple surgery known as Rammstedt's operation clears up the trouble.

Surgery consists of making an incision in the abdomen and then making a deep cut along the outside of the tightly swollen pylorus; this immediately allows the passageway inside the pylorus to expand enough to allow food to pass through.

After the operation, the baby is given gradually increasing feeds, until within 48 hours feeding is back to normal. The success rate of the operation is almost 100 per cent.

Oesophageal atresia

In this disorder, there is a complete absence of part of the oesophagus (gullet). The top part, leading from the mouth, is a dead-end, and so there is no passageway into the baby's stomach. As a result, at birth the baby cannot swallow secretions from the mouth and nose, and instead they may enter the trachea (windpipe) and partially block it.

The blockage hinders the baby's breathing. There are continual bubbling noises in the throat, and sometimes the baby's skin turns blue. When the doctor removes the secretions with a suction tube, the symptoms vanish; but they return as soon as the secretions build up again. Any attempt to feed the baby results in the feed filling up the oesophagus and then spilling over from the sealed-off top section of the gullet into the windpipe, making the baby cough and splutter.

When these symptoms occur, the doctor will suspect oesophageal atresia, and will test for it by passing a tube down the baby's oesophagus. If the tube will not enter the stomach the diagnosis is confirmed. About 1 in every 3,500 babies has the disorder.

What is the treatment?
Once oesophageal atresia is diagnosed, urgent treatment is essential. An operation is

performed to open up and join the two separate sections of the oesophagus. Surgery generally clears up the trouble completely, and there are usually no long-term problems.

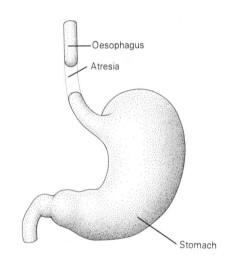

Oesophageal atresia
The only cure for this disorder is an operation to join the 2 separated parts.

Bile-duct atresia

Bile, a fluid produced in the liver, is responsible for many essential processes in the body, among them carrying a chemical called bilirubin away from the liver and out of the system (see *Neonatal jaundice*, p.647). The bile travels through a series of tiny ducts in the liver and some of it is stored in the gallbladder. As bile leaves the gallbladder it is joined by bile flowing through larger ducts outside the liver. All the ducts eventually join to form the main bile duct leading to the duodenum (part of the small intestine).

Very rarely, a baby is born with parts of the bile ducts missing, with the result that bile is trapped in the liver. Bilirubin cannot be removed in the bile, and so builds up in the bloodstream. This causes a prolonged *jaundice* (yellowing of the skin – see p.485), usually starting in the second week. The baby may also pass pale faeces and dark urine.

What should be done?
Any baby who has the symptoms described above should be examined by a doctor. If

atresia seems likely, the surgeon will carry out an operation called a *laparotomy*, which is performed when the baby is about two months old. The inside of the abdomen is examined and if there is atresia of the ducts outside the liver, it is possible in some cases to join the gallbladder to the duodenum, thus enabling bile to flow directly from the liver to the intestine. If the operation is unsuccessful, *cirrhosis of the liver* (p.487) will gradually develop and almost certainly lead to death in early childhood.

If the bile ducts outside the liver appear normal, a small piece of liver is removed for examination (*biopsy*). Examination of the fragment under a microscope will show whether the baby has atresia of the small bile ducts in the liver. Unfortunately there is no successful treatment for this condition at present, and the child usually succumbs to cirrhosis of the liver within a year or two. Liver transplantation is a possible hope for the future in some of these cases.

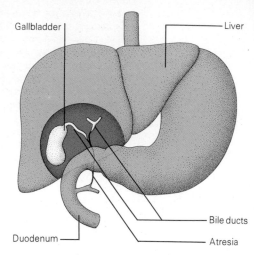

Atresia in the bile duct below the gallbladder (above) can be cured by joining the gallbladder to the duodenum and so bypassing the lower part of the main bile duct. Atresia higher up in the many smaller bile ducts is less easily treated.

Intestinal atresia and stenosis

In intestinal *atresia*, the baby is born with part or parts of the small intestine missing. In intestinal *stenosis*, part of the upper intestine is narrowed almost to the point of closure.

Within a few hours of birth a baby with intestinal stenosis or atresia starts to bring up green vomit, so-coloured because it contains bile, a liquid produced in the liver and passed into the intestine. The vomiting continues at intervals, and if the condition is not treated, the vomit may eventually contain blood as well as bile. The baby's abdomen swells as wind accumulates in the intestine.

About 1 baby in every 2,000 has one of the disorders; diagnosis is confirmed by *X-ray*.

What is the treatment?

Because the baby may die if severely affected, it is essential that an operation is carried out right away – in atresia, to open up and join together the separate parts of the intestine; in stenosis, to widen the constricted intestine. The results of early surgery are excellent, and the baby is normally left without any long-term problems.

Intestinal stenosis
The upper intestine (in this case, the duodenum) can be narrowed to such an extent that the baby's only chance of survival is an early operation to widen the intestine.

Duodenal stenosis

Intestinal atresia
When a newborn baby is suffering from intestinal atresia, it is possible that more than one part of the intestine may be defective (as shown right).

Duodenal atresia

Small-intestine atresia

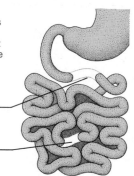

Hirschprung's disease

Bowel movements consist of the intestine contracting and pushing its contents down towards the rectum. In about 1 baby in 5,000 the lower parts of the large intestine, including the rectum, have no nerve cells to control the necessary contractions, and through not functioning normally they are narrow and rigid, and allow through little faecal matter.

What are the symptoms?

The baby has severe constipation. Apart from noticing that the baby's motions are infrequent and hard, the mother or medical staff will probably also see that the baby's abdomen is swollen and tight.

In some cases, vomiting begins a few hours after birth. The vomit is green and may eventually contain blood (see *Intestinal atresia and stenosis*, opposite).

Diagnosis of the disease is confirmed by an *X-ray*, for which a *barium enema* is given, and by a *biopsy* of the rectum.

What should be done?
If your baby is passing fewer motions than usual, and especially if he or she begins to vomit, consult your doctor without delay.

What is the treatment?
An operation is carried out to remove the affected part of the intestine and sew together the normal sections. Surgery has a high success rate, and the long-term outlook is good.

Imperforate anus

The anal canal forms the final section of the digestive tract and ends with the anus. (For general information on this part of the body see *The anus*, p.483). Some babies are born with the canal imperforate (closed). There is either a membrane stretching across the canal; or the canal fails to develop (*atresia*) and the digestive tract ends at the rectum, with no connection between the rectum and the anus. In a few cases, there is an additional problem: the muscles in the wall of the anus that control the opening of the bowels are insufficiently developed.

What should be done?
Examination of the baby after birth will reveal the presence of an anal membrane but not an atresia. An atresia should be suspected if, within 12 hours after birth, the baby has not passed a green-black substance, called *meconium*, which has accumulated in the intestine. The diagnosis is confirmed when a

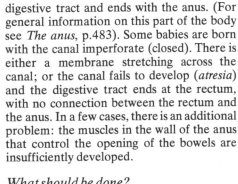
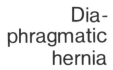

Large intestine

Rectum

Anal membrane

finger or thermometer inserted into the anus meets a blockage – the end of the rectum.

How common is the problem?
Imperforate anus is rare. In Britain about 1 baby in every 1,000 is born with the disorder.

What is the treatment?
Surgery is necessary to remove the membrane or to open up the end of the rectum and join it to the anus. The operation is usually successful, and the long-term outlook is entirely satisfactory except in those cases when the muscles of the anus are weak. In such cases the child will suffer from either severe constipation, when the stools are normal, or poor bowel control, when the stools are soft. The child may then need an operation called a colostomy (see *Colostomy and ileostomy*, p.482); this creates a kind of artificial anus in the abdomen and allows the contents of the intestine to be collected in a bag.

Dia-phragmatic hernia

The diaphragm is a large sheet of muscle that separates the chest from the abdomen. Some babies are born with an opening in the diaphragm, through which part of the intestine may protrude into the chest (see also *Hiatus hernia*, p.456, and general information on *hernias*, p.537). When this happens, the intestine can compress the lungs and make the baby breathless.

The disorder is usually detected during the examination given just after birth, and the diagnosis is confirmed by a chest *X-ray*.

What is the treatment?
Surgery is performed as soon as possible. The baby's chest is opened up, the intestine pushed back into place, and the opening in the diaphragm sewn up. The operation is usually completely successful, and as long as the lungs have developed properly while the baby was in the uterus, there should be no long-term effects.

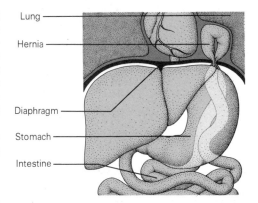

Lung

Hernia

Diaphragm

Stomach

Intestine

Risks of diaphragmatic hernia
In congenital hernia of the diaphragm, part of the intestine protrudes through the diaphragm to press on a lung (usually the left lung). This causes the baby to have breathing difficulties. In severe cases, the baby may also have cyanosis (a bluish tinge to the skin). The usual treatment is surgery to reposition the intestine and repair the diaphragm.

Congenital disorders of the skeleton

The four disorders discussed below – dislocation of the hip, club foot, and hare lip and cleft palate – can all be inherited, but more often they result from an uninherited error in development before birth. Hare lip is included in the following pages because, although it does not affect the skeleton, it often occurs in conjunction with cleft palate. The exact nature of these developmental problems is not clear.

If the defect is slight, the baby's general health will not be affected. If it is more severe and left untreated, the child will have difficulty in learning to walk or, in the case of hare lip and cleft palate, in learning to speak. Feeding problems can also result from hare lip and cleft palate. For these reasons – in addition to the psychological strain on the child who must cope with the defect – these disorders are best treated within the first few years.

Congenital dislocation of the hip

Some babies are born with the ball-shaped head of the thigh bone lying outside the cup-like socket in the pelvis; the socket is shallow and poorly formed. One or both hips may be affected. The cause of the condition is not known; most babies who have it are born by *breech* birth but this may be a consequence of the dislocation rather than a cause. About 1 baby in 60 is born with a suspected dislocation; six times more girls than boys are affected. The disorder runs in families.

What are the symptoms?
When the doctor manipulates the baby's hip joints during the routine test just after birth, a clicking is usually heard or felt if the baby has the disorder. However, clicking can also be made by movements of the ligaments, and in a few cases it is not possible to diagnose the condition with certainty, even after several tests. *X-rays* are usually not taken; doctors are reluctant to use them on the hips of very young babies, because of the slight possibility of damage to the genital area.

What is the treatment?
In most cases, tests will confirm a diagnosis of dislocated hip and the doctor will apply light splints to the baby's thighs to correct their position. These are usually worn for about nine months. If the doctor suspects a dislocated hip but cannot confirm the diagnosis, he or she will advise the mother to use double nappies folded into rectangles instead of triangles. These keep the baby's thighs spread apart, and over a period of months will usually correct any dislocation by keeping the ball of the thigh bone constantly in the socket. In a few cases, the hip will remain dislocated after this treatment. If this happens, the hips will usually be X-rayed to confirm the diagnosis. If a definite dislocation is revealed,

then the treatment is to put light splints on the baby's thighs to keep them more firmly apart.

In cases when the disorder is not detected until childhood, the child may need one or more operations to correct the dislocation. The child is given a general anaesthetic and stays in hospital for several weeks. After the operation, plaster casts are applied to the legs for several months.

If corrected early, the defect is often completely cured and the child is able to walk

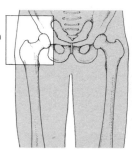

Normal hip joint
In a normal hip joint the ball at the top of the thigh bone fits neatly into the socket in the pelvis.

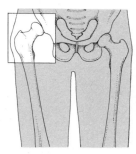

Dislocated hip joint
In a dislocated hip joint the thigh bone is displaced and does not fit into the socket in the pelvis.

normally and suffers no adverse effects in later life. A child whose dislocation is corrected surgically may have problems in walking throughout life.

Club foot

(talipes)

A baby with club foot is born with one or both feet bent either downwards and inwards, or upwards and outwards. Many babies with normally formed feet persistently turn them inwards, but you can push them back to the proper position; in club foot you cannot.

The problem, which sometimes runs in families, affects about 1 in 500 babies. With modern medical care, nearly all cases are detected at birth and eventually cured.

What is the treatment?

If the defect is only slight, the doctor will show the baby's mother how to manipulate the foot regularly each day until it settles into normal position. In more pronounced cases, as much correction as possible is done by manipulation, then splints (or plasters) are put on the foot to prevent it growing back to its former position. Periodically, the splints are removed, the foot is manipulated further back to the normal position, and new splints are put on. This is repeated over a year or more, until the foot is normal.

In severe cases of club foot, an operation (or, rarely, more than one) is necessary to correct the deformity. The results of such surgery are very good.

Hare lip and cleft palate

Hare lip is a vertical split in the upper lip. It may be partial, or extend right up to the base of the nose (which sometimes appears flattened), and it affects either one side of the lip or, less commonly, both sides. Sometimes the gap is continued in the upper gum. This gap, called a cleft palate, runs along the midline of the palate, extending from behind the teeth to the cavity of the nose. Cleft palate usually occurs as an extension of hare lip, but in some cases may occur as an isolated disorder. A cleft palate sometimes makes feeding and swallowing difficult, and may make any regurgitated milk come through the nose instead of the mouth.

How common is the problem?

About 1 baby in 1,000 is born with one or both of these defects. The problem sometimes runs in families, occasionally affecting several children in the same family.

In most cases of hare lip and cleft palate, the reason for the defect is unknown. However, in rare cases, the condition may occur as one of a group of disorders caused by a *chromosome* abnormality.

What are the risks?

Unless treated, hare lip causes psychological distress because of its appearance; cleft palate may cause serious speech difficulties.

What is the treatment?

An operation to repair the defect is carried out when the baby is older. Until then, treatment varies according to the degree of the defect. Many babies need no interim treatment; they feed and swallow quite well. Some bottle-fed babies may need a larger than normal hole in the teat, or may have to be switched to spoon feeding. Regurgitation of milk through the nose usually clears up by itself after a few weeks.

In severe cases of cleft palate, a special plate may need to be fitted on the roof of the mouth each time the baby is due to be fed. A special brace may also be fitted on the upper gum if the parts of the gum in the region of the clefts are out of line.

Surgery is carried out on a hare lip when the baby has attained a weight of about 4.5kg or 10lb (about 12 weeks old). If the nose is flattened, this will require further surgery later on. Cleft palate is repaired by an operation when the baby is about a year old, before he or she learns to speak. For each operation,

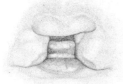

Hare lip
A hare lip can vary in severity from a small notch in the upper lip to a split extending to the nose (as shown right).

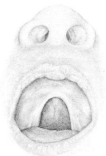

Cleft palate
A cleft palate can be an extension of a hare lip or it can occur without any corresponding damage to the lip (as shown right).

the baby is given a general anaesthetic and is usually in hospital for a week or so.

The results of the operations are usually excellent, improving appearance and allowing the development of normal speech. When a speech defect does develop, *speech therapy* can often help.

Skin

Many skin problems that affect adults can also affect children (see *Skin, hair, and nail disorders*, p.250, for a general description of these problems). The two disorders discussed here occur mainly in children. Infantile eczema is an allergic reaction (see *Allergies*, p.705) and, while it is not a serious condition, it may signal that the child will develop other allergies such as *asthma* (p.355) or *allergic rhinitis* (p.345) in later life. Infantile eczema, however, is not *contagious* (catching), unlike ringworm, which is extremely contagious.

Infantile eczema

See p.234,
Visual aids to diagnosis, 6.

Infantile eczema (also called infantile atopic dermatitis) is a red, scaly, itchy, sometimes weeping skin condition. It starts during the first years of life and may persist (see *Eczema*, p.253). Each year, about 1 baby in 10 is taken to the doctor because of eczema.

What are the symptoms?
In mild cases, the skin is only slightly dry, red, and scaly, and is affected in only small areas. In severe cases, the rash covers large areas of the body. Little red pimples appear, and as the baby scratches them they begin to form large weeping areas which become encrusted.

What are the risks?
If the eczema weeps, infection may occur, particularly in the nappy area. Certain immunizations may produce blistering on the skin affected by eczema, and should be postponed until treatment has reduced the rash.

What should be done?
Mild forms of the disorder require no treatment other than soothing applications of petroleum jelly or olive oil. For more severe cases, you should consult your doctor.

What is the treatment?
Self-help: Make sure that clothes in direct contact with your baby's skin are made of cotton. Do not use any ointments or creams without first consulting your doctor, but use emulsifying ointment dissolved in the bath water instead of soap to wash the skin and help remove crusts.

Professional help: If the baby is troubled badly by itching, the doctor will probably prescribe an *antihistamine* drug. Severe phases of the disorder are treated with *steroid* ointments or creams. If the eczema is infected, an *antibiotic* can be prescribed.

In some children infantile eczema disappears after a few months. In others, the condition fluctuates for several years, particularly on the hands and feet and on the inner creases of the elbows and knees. Most children have outgrown the disorder by the time of puberty, but in about 10 per cent of all cases the problem remains throughout life.

Ringworm

See p.237,
Visual aids to diagnosis 20 and 21.

Ringworm is a fungus called tinea which infects the skin and causes scaly, itchy patches to develop. In children it usually affects the scalp, the trunk, or the feet. Ringworm of the feet is known as *athlete's foot* (p.256).

When ringworm affects the scalp, the skin flakes and itches, and bald patches develop. Ringworm on the trunk starts as a small, round, red patch which is scaly and itchy. The patch gradually grows bigger until it is about 25mm (1in) across: as it gets bigger, the central area heals, leaving a red ring on the skin (hence the name). After a week or two, other patches may appear nearby.

Ringworm is *contagious* and can even be caught from a pet dog or cat. It is far more common in children than in adults; about 1 child in 100 has the condition.

What should be done?
There is no self-help for an infection of ringworm, so do not delay in taking your child to the doctor as soon as symptoms appear. The doctor will generally prescribe an ointment or a cream, which should be applied at least twice daily to the affected areas. If the scalp is affected (or the trunk very severely) a syrup containing an antifungal agent will be prescribed.

Any child with ringworm should stay away from school until the condition clears. Dispose of any combs, hairbrushes, or hats the child has used, and if a pet is also suffering from ringworm, you should take it to a vet for treatment. If the child follows the full course of treatment, ringworm of the scalp and trunk is usually cured and is unlikely to recur.

Nervous-system and psychological disorders

The first three disorders discussed below are caused by an abnormality or disturbance in the nervous system. The second, meningitis, can usually be cured completely, with no long-term effects. Convulsions, on the other hand, may recur (see *Epilepsy*, p.287). The third disorder, cerebral palsy, is more severe and often requires special schooling and, rarely, full-time institutional care.

The three psychological disorders included here range in severity from sleeping problems, which are usually no cause for concern, to autism, which is a serious disorder and may need special treatment and education.

Convulsions in children

A convulsion is a fit or seizure caused by unusual nervous activity in the brain. They occur more often in children than in adults, because a child's brain is still developing and therefore is more sensitive to disturbances than is the brain of an adult.

The causes of convulsions in children vary. In most cases the cause is either unknown (this is called *idiopathic* epilepsy; see *Epilepsy*, p.287) or a raised temperature from some minor infection (a *febrile* convulsion). However, convulsions may also occur in children with *cerebral palsy* (p.669), a *brain tumour* (p.281), or meningitis (see *Meningitis in babies and children*, p.668). Alterations to body chemistry, as when a diabetic child receives too much insulin (see *Diabetes mellitus*, p.519), can cause convulsions.

What are the symptoms?
Grand mal convulsion (also called a major seizure): This is the most common type of convulsion. The child suddenly falls to the ground unconscious, with arms and legs held stiff. After a few seconds, the arms and legs, and sometimes the face, start to twitch or jerk rhythmically, often violently. The fit usually lasts about two minutes, and during this time the child may pass urine or faeces.

During the next few minutes, the child slowly regains consciousness, and is then irritable and may complain of a headache. Soon after this, the child falls deeply asleep for several hours. On waking, he or she is completely back to normal.

Most febrile convulsions, when the child has a high temperature, take the form of grand mal convulsions. Other grand mal convulsions may be the result of epilepsy, especially if they recur without the child having an obviously high temperature. One or two short-lived grand mal convulsions are extremely unlikely to be harmful, but several prolonged attacks can damage a temporal lobe of the brain and give rise to psychomotor convulsions (which are discussed below).

Petit mal convulsion: This minor convulsion, which can occur many times in one day, is often mistaken for "daydreaming". The child suddenly becomes motionless, and stares vacantly for a few seconds; occasionally, he or she may totter or fall. After the convulsion the child is usually unaware of what has happened. Nearly all children who suffer from petit mal convulsions grow out of them.

Psychomotor convulsion: For no apparent reason the child suddenly stops and stares, then acts in a frightened or aggressive manner. This behaviour may cease, or it may progress to a full-scale major convulsion that lasts for a few minutes. Afterwards the child is unaware of what he or she has been doing.

Infantile spasm: With a sudden jerk, the baby or child doubles up at the waist for a second or two. This convulsion, which occurs several times each day, first appears at about the age of three months and occasionally continues for several years.

How common is the problem?
About 1 child in 25 has one or more convulsions at some time. They tend to run in families, and are more common among mentally handicapped or *spastic* children.

What are the risks?
There are very few risks attached to the actual convulsions themselves. The most serious of these risks is that a prolonged grand mal convulsion may result in permanent brain damage, which will show itself as a mental handicap or cerebral palsy.

What should be done?
Convulsions are often a cause of great concern to parents, but most convulsions do not harm the health of the child in any way. Even so, a child who has a convulsion for the first time should be seen by a doctor within 24 hours; however, if *any* convulsion lasts for

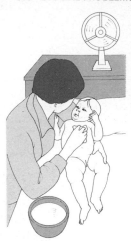

Avoiding febrile convulsions
A child who has had previous convulsions caused by a fever is at risk from further convulsions if he or she becomes feverish again. Try to keep the child cool – for example, use a sponge soaked in tepid water and have a fan going nearby.

more than five minutes, summon an ambulance immediately. If a child has a grand mal convulsion, follow the advice described in *Dealing with an epileptic fit* on p.289. Do not attempt to restrain movements or to force anything between the teeth to prevent tongue-biting. For other types of convulsion, simply move aside any possibly harmful objects. Try to make a note of the details of any convulsion and describe it to the doctor to help with the diagnosis.

All first convulsions (except a first febrile convulsion whose cause is known to be a fever) are followed by investigative medical tests. The more severe the convulsion, the more likely will be hospital admission for more extensive tests.

A complete physical examination and an *electroencephalogram* (*EEG*) recording are carried out in most cases; these may be followed by a skull *X-ray*, a *CAT scan*, and *cerebral angiography*.

What is the treatment?

Self-help: If your child has an infection, and has had a previous febrile convulsion, take steps to reduce the child's temperature and so avoid a possible recurrence of the convulsion. Give junior aspirin, and inform your doctor of the infection. Take the child's temperature every two hours; if it is above 38°C (about 100°F), remove some of the child's clothes, sponge the face and upper body with tepid water, and set an electric fan going nearby to keep the child cool.

Professional help: If convulsions are found to be due to an underlying disorder such as a brain tumour or meningitis, treatment will be given for that disorder. Any recurrent convulsions, whether associated with mental handicap, cerebral palsy, or any other cause, will be treated by long-term drug medication. Such treatment will probably need to be taken for several years, and in some cases it will have to be lifelong.

Psychomotor convulsions are usually difficult to treat. Combinations of various drugs are effective in some cases. In a few children who are severely affected, surgery may be carried out to remove all or part of the temporal lobe in the brain.

It is always wise to inform your child's teachers if he or she is having convulsions, particularly if a dose of drugs is necessary during the school day. And once the frequency of convulsions has been lessened by drugs, the child should be encouraged to take part in all normal activities unless advised otherwise by the doctor.

If a child under drug treatment has been completely free of convulsions for at least two years, the drugs may then be stopped for a trial period of observation, in the hope that the condition has been cured.

Meningitis in babies and children

Meningitis is an inflammation of one or more of the three thin layers, the meninges, covering the brain. The inflammation is nearly always the result of an infection. Often it is not related to another infection, although it is occasionally caused by bacteria or viruses that are already causing a more general infection, such as *mumps* (p.700) or *acute infection of the middle ear* (p.333). Such an infection may spread to the meninges by means of the cerebro-spinal fluid that bathes them. Meningitis can also result, in rare cases, from a penetrating head injury (see also *Meningitis*, p.273).

What are the symptoms?

The baby or child has a high temperature (up to 39°C, about 102°F), and, if he or she is old enough to talk, will be miserable and irritable and complain of a severe headache. The neck is held stiffly, or even arched backwards, and if you attempt to bend the head forwards, this will be resisted. The child may become unusually quiet and withdrawn, and turn away or shield the eyes from any bright lights (*photophobia*). There may be vomiting and convulsions (see *Convulsions in children*, p.667). In severe cases, there is occasionally a rash of small purplish spots on the body.

In very young babies, the *fontanelle* (the soft spot on top of the head), instead of being slightly sunken as normal, is bulging and taut, due to the inflammation causing increased pressure of the cerebro-spinal fluid within.

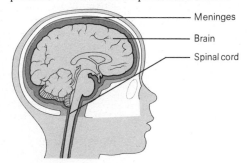

— Meninges
— Brain
— Spinal cord

The meninges
The brain and spinal cord are covered by 3 layers – the meninges – which become inflamed when infection causes meningitis to develop.

How common is the problem?

Meningitis in children under 14 is very rare; each year only 1 child in 2,500 contracts the disease. Because it is occasionally a *contagious* illness, meningitis can occur as a minor epidemic in an enclosed community such as a boarding school.

What are the risks?

The risks for babies and young children are greater than those for older children and adults, because an inability to communicate may prevent the disorder from becoming detected early – and if the infection is bacterial the meningitis may, without treatment, then progress to a dangerous stage. In that case, the younger the sufferer, the more chance there is of brain damage resulting in some form of mental handicap or *cerebral palsy* (below), or even death. However, most cases are detected early enough for successful treatment, and recovery is complete.

What should be done?

If your baby or child has the symptoms described, telephone the doctor without delay. If the doctor suspects meningitis, the baby or child will be admitted to hospital, where a *lumbar puncture* test will confirm the diagnosis. For a bacterial infection, *antibiotics* will be given; if viruses are responsible, the disease will usually clear up by itself. Fluids that have been lost by vomiting are replaced via an *intravenous drip*.

Cerebral palsy

Cerebral palsy is a paralysis of the muscles (primarily those of the limbs) caused by a brain abnormality. The affected part of the brain is unable to control certain muscles, making them stiff and difficult to use. The degree of the child's handicap varies. Either certain limbs are completely immobile or the child's movements are weak and poorly controlled. Simple movements such as reaching for a cup may be jerky and only accomplished after several fruitless attempts.

Defectiveness of this kind is called spasticity, and children with cerebral palsy are commonly called *spastics*. Many of these children have a degree of mental handicap, though some are highly intelligent. Spastic children may also have some degree of deafness; visual defects, most often squint (see *Squint in children*, p.674); and convulsions (see *Convulsions in children*, p.667).

For most children, the exact cause of cerebral palsy cannot be determined. What is known is that it is definitely not inherited, so having one spastic child does not increase the likelihood of having another. Cerebral palsy may result from faulty development or from brain damage occurring before, during, or shortly after birth. Later on, brain damage can be caused by a *brain injury* (p.276), meningitis (see *Meningitis in babies and children*, opposite), or severe convulsions.

What are the symptoms?

In many cases, cerebral palsy is unrecognized until well into the baby's first year. Floppy muscles can be an early indication of the disorder, but many spastic babies do not have this symptom. The main symptom, stiffening of the limbs, does not usually occur until the baby is at least six months old. When this happens, normal muscle balance is disrupted and the limbs settle in typical abnormal positions. For example, affected arms are usually tucked in to the side, with elbows and wrists bent; legs may be crossed like scissors; and the foot may point downwards from the ankle. The baby may move very little, and what movement there is will be clumsy. In addition, the baby may find it difficult to suck and swallow. The normal *milestones* (p.645) of infant development, such as walking and speech, may be delayed. Children who walk very late or fail to walk will be unable to explore their environment and learn from their experience at a vital stage of their development, a condition made worse if there is also defective vision or hearing.

When speech is considerably delayed – as is often the case when the child is deaf – it may be distorted and extremely difficult to understand. Spastic children of average or high intelligence can become extremely frustrated by being deprived of normal development and ability to communicate, and may have emotional problems as a result.

How common is the problem?

Cerebral palsy is the most common crippling disorder of childhood. Throughout the world, about 1 child in 300 is affected. It is slightly more common in babies who are premature or very small (under 2.5kg or 5½lb) at birth.

What are the risks?

Stiff muscles can very quickly become fixed, further restricting the child's movements. The child may fail to walk and need to be confined to a wheelchair.

There is a serious risk that an intelligent child will fail to be recognized as such,

Types of cerebral palsy
Cerebral palsy does not always affect the whole body. Sometimes only the legs are affected, and this condition is known as paraplegia. About a third of all children with the disorder are affected down one side of the body, and this is known as hemiplegia. Those children most severely affected – with paralysis of all four limbs – are said to have quadriplegia.

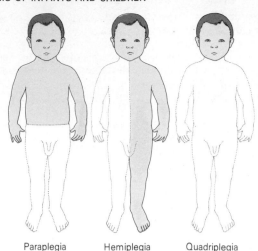

Paraplegia   Hemiplegia   Quadriplegia

especially if movement and communication are very difficult. For this reason, it is essential that the child's mental ability and development are assessed regularly, and that vision and hearing are tested so as not to further handicap the child's ability to learn (see *Learning problems*, p.673).

What should be done?
See your doctor if you are concerned about your baby's progress. Most health districts organize routine checks of all babies, so there is little chance of a case of cerebral palsy passing undetected. Parents of spastic children are encouraged to contact *The Spastic Society* or the *National Society for Mentally Handicapped Children* (p.768).

What is the treatment?
Abnormalities of the brain, such as those causing cerebral palsy – while they do not get any worse – cannot be made any better. But this certainly does not mean that nothing can be done for your child. The aim of treatment is to detect the extent of any handicaps – physical, mental, visual, or auditory – and, as far as possible, to reduce these to a minimum.

Such treatment cannot be provided by the child's parents alone. Caring for a child with cerebral palsy involves teamwork on the part of parents, doctors, *physiotherapists*, *speech therapists*, teachers, and, in some cases, *occupational therapists*.

Physiotherapy is provided at special schools, clinics, and in the child's own home and is aimed at preventing, as much as possible, the development of fixed deformities by relaxing stiffened muscles and finding beneficial positions for the affected limbs. With physiotherapy, some children who have never been able to walk learn to do so with

the aid of appliances such as a walking frame and callipers. Speech therapy may not only improve the child's speech but also help with feeding and swallowing difficulties.

Operations by an *orthopaedic surgeon* can correct the fixed stiffness in deformed limbs and make movement easier. Surgery enables some children who would otherwise be confined to a wheelchair to walk with the aid of appliances. Deafness in many spastic children can be lessened by a hearing aid. A squint can be corrected by surgery, and spectacles are prescribed for other visual defects. Muscle-relaxant drugs are sometimes prescribed to lessen stiffness in the limbs, and drugs are used to treat any convulsions.

The spastic child is regularly examined by a *paediatrician* or community medical officer, sometimes with the help of an educational psychologist, to assess his or her general progress and intelligence. They will discuss with parents what educational arrangements would be best suited to the child.

Many children who have mild cerebral palsy have normal or near normal intelligence and can attend an ordinary school. Spastic children who are moderately to severely handicapped and have normal intelligence will need to attend a school for the physically handicapped. For spastic children who have subnormal intelligence, there are day schools for the mentally handicapped. Finally, those children who are profoundly handicapped and mentally subnormal need to attend a day school for the physically and mentally handicapped.

To you as a parent, your child's progress may be slow, and improvement may seem a long way off. But never let impatience lead you to try an unorthodox type of treatment without first discussing the matter fully with the team of professionals who have been treating your child.

What are the long-term prospects?
The prospects for children with cerebral palsy depend on the degree and type of handicap(s). For children able to attend a normal school, there should be few problems; most grow up to lead a relatively normal life in society. For the majority of spastics, who attend schools for the physically handicapped, there are greater problems; but the sophisticated devices available today at these schools help spastic children to communicate with others and enable some of them to play an active role in society when they grow up. In many cases, though, they will always require an environment tailored to meet their specific needs.

Sleeping problems in children

Normal sleep patterns

Most babies, in the early weeks of life, wake once or twice during the night, but by the age of nine months are sleeping through the night. At one year, babies will sleep on average for about 16 hours in every 24; two or three hours of this will be during the day.

By the time they have reached the toddler stage (18 months), children begin to vary enormously in the amount of sleep they need. Some toddlers will require relatively little sleep and will wake up early each morning. Leave plenty of safe toys in the child's cot overnight, to enable you to get your normal sleep in the morning. Such a child is usually very active during the day, needs no day-time nap, and is not tired until bedtime.

By the age of three, many children will have reached the same stage and given up their daily nap. And by the age of five, nearly all children will be awake throughout the day.

Lessening the chance of sleeplessness

Do not make yourself too readily available to a child during the night, otherwise he or she may become dependent on your attention and become sleepless if deprived of it. For example, at the stage when a baby has given up night feeds, you should not immediately go and pick up the baby if he or she starts crying. Listen outside the door of the baby's room. In most cases, the crying will stop after a few minutes, and the baby will go back to sleep. If the crying continues, however, you should go in because the baby may be unwell or uncomfortable. Try not to take a child into your own bed if he or she wakes during the night; this can create a habit which is extremely difficult to break.

Some children have trouble falling asleep, though they may sleep well during the night. In this case, try to ensure that the child is not disturbed – by an older brother or sister repeatedly entering the bedroom, for instance. You should also never send a child to bed as a punishment. Over a period of time, the child may come to associate going to bed with punishment, may eventually fear going to bed and, once in bed, sleep badly.

What to do about sleeplessness

If, despite your precautions, your child finds it very difficult to get to sleep, or wakes a lot in the night, you may be tempted to ask your doctor for a sedative for the child. (*Never* give a child your own sleeping tablets.) But it is wiser not to treat the problem with drugs: the child may come to rely on them and acquire a habit that is hard to break. The fact is that most children grow out of the problem naturally, within one or two months of its onset. If, however, sleeplessness does become a persistent problem, consult your doctor, who may refer you to a child psychiatrist.

Nightmares and sleepwalking

Nightmares usually only become a problem after the age of four. In most cases, they are caused by a disturbing incident, or a frightening story or television programme. Occasionally, they are an indication that the child is under stress as a result of problems at home or school. They are hardly ever the result of physical illness – except a fever. Some children have night terrors; they usually scream, may talk or babble, and appear terrified, but are difficult to wake and cannot say what has frightened them. Sleepwalking in itself is not serious, but may be another nocturnal sign of emotional disturbance.

The immediate remedy for nightmares and night terrors that have woken a child is comfort and reassurance from the parent. Try to reach your child as soon as possible, and turn

Hyperactive children

There are many more hyperactive children in the US than in Britain, even taking into account the greater population in the US. This probably reflects the doctors' attitudes, rather than the state of child health. A formal medical diagnosis of hyperactivity in Britain is rare, whereas such a diagnosis is more common in America.

The hyperactive child is physically and mentally restless. He or she has a short attention span, is prone to temper tantrums, and has boundless energy and little need of sleep. American doctors believe that such aberrant behaviour is due to "minimal brain dysfunction" that cannot be detected or demonstrated by any diagnostic tests. It is believed the dysfunction can be a result of birth trauma, an unspecified food allergy, or marginal vitamin deficiency, and drugs may be used to treat it.

British doctors view hyperactivity as primarily a behavioural phenomenon and suggest that it is mainly caused by an imbalance of activity levels between various family members. Because there is no formal diagnosis, there is no set treatment; instead, the doctor is likely to encourage greater awareness and tolerance among family members as regards activity and individualistic behaviour.

the lights on to reassure the child that it was "only a dream". Never ask questions about the fear on the spot; this may only make the child feel worse. Instead, take his or her mind off the disturbance, and talk soothingly about something pleasant.

A child who has a nightmare or night terror and does not wake up will probably drift back into a peaceful sleep. Unless the problem persists, it is better not to wake the child. It is also best not to wake a sleepwalking child, but gently guide him or her back to bed. Once you have discovered a child sleepwalks, fix a gate across the top of the stairs to prevent a serious fall during any further episodes.

If the child is old enough, it may be a good idea to discuss the nightmares or sleepwalking the next morning. Try to find out what the underlying trouble is, so that you can deal with it. If you are unsuccessful in this and if the nightmares or sleepwalking become a serious problem, see your doctor, who may arrange a consultation for both the child and you with a child psychiatrist.

Autism

Autism is an inability from birth – or a loss of the ability within the first 30 months of life – to develop normal human relationships, even with close relatives such as parents. In many of its symptoms it is similar to *schizophrenia* (p.295). What causes the disorder is not known, though in some cases it has been suggested that there may be links between the child's problem and emotional disturbances in the family as a whole.

What are the symptoms?
The symptoms, if not present from birth, develop quite suddenly, perhaps over as little as a few days. Symptoms vary greatly, but follow a general pattern. As a baby the autistic child will have difficulty with feeding and toilet training. He or she will not give, or will cease to give, smiling recognition to the parent's face, and noticeably avoids looking into other people's eyes. It will become increasingly apparent that such children live in a world of their own. Speech, facial expressions, and other forms of communication are absent or unintelligible. In some cases a few words are spoken, but are repeated interminably for no sensible reason. An autistic child makes no distinction between people, other living things, and inanimate objects, treating them all in the same manner. He or she cannot evaluate situations, and so reacts inappropriately to them – for example, becoming fiercely agitated if taken into new but harmless surroundings, but running across a dangerously busy road without fear.

By not communicating, the autistic child remains isolated from other family members. He or she may be unpredictably violent at one moment, and then sit completely still, in some strange position, for hours on end. An autistic child may adopt strange postures and mannerisms. And although an autistic child may have normal intelligence, he or she may give the impression of being subnormal – or in some cases deaf.

How common is the problem?
About 1 child in 3,000 is autistic – and the disorder seems to affect five times as many boys as girls. The illness is not inherited, and there are no known predisposing factors.

What are the risks?
There is always a risk that unsupervised autistic children may be injured because of their inability to recognize dangerous situations.

What should be done?
If you feel that your child has always been, or has suddenly become over the past few days, unreasonably withdrawn or uncommunicative, take him or her to your doctor. If the doctor suspects that the child is autistic or mentally subnormal, you and your child will be referred to a child psychiatrist.

What is the treatment?
Once autism has been diagnosed, a full discussion will usually be arranged between you, your doctor, and any specialists involved. Unless the autistic child causes unbearable stress and tension in the family, you will probably be encouraged to look after the child at home. The more care, attention, and stimulation you can give, the better the chances of an improvement in the condition. You will have support from your child psychiatrist, and you may wish to contact the *National Society for Autistic Children* (p. 768). There are also in existence a few specialized units where an autistic child will be encouraged to establish contact with the rest of society. Later the child will probably have to attend a special school for the educationally subnormal.

What are the long-term prospects?
Some autistic children recover sufficiently over several years to grow up as relatively normal members of society. Unfortunately, others need lifelong specialized care.

Learning problems

Learning starts at birth. It depends upon the baby's ability to see and hear clearly (see *Can my baby see and hear properly?*, p.675) and the normal development of physical and mental abilities and personality (see *Milestones*, p.645). These aspects of the baby's progress are checked at a clinic, usually when the baby is 6 weeks, 9 months, and 18 months old.

But learning problems may well develop between the last check-up at 18 months and school age, and during this period it is up to parents to alert their doctors if they feel their child is not learning as quickly as his or her playmates. In many cases, there will prove to be nothing wrong with the child's basic learning abilities, and he or she will go on to catch up with other children. Once a child reaches school age, any undisclosed learning problems will soon be detected in the classroom.

Whenever any child is suspected of having learning difficulties, at whatever stage of development, he or she will be referred to a *paediatrician* for a thorough physical examination. This will reveal any hearing or sight problems, or any other physical problems such as, for example, deafness produced by *glue ear* (p.675), or poor vision caused by a squint (see *Squint in children*, p.674).

If a detected physical problem cannot be cured, or if the learning problem cannot be identified as physical, the child will be given an IQ test by an educational psychologist, to uncover any mental subnormality (see below). The test is invaluable in separating out the physically but not mentally handicapped child from the majority of handicapped children, who are both physically and mentally handicapped. The test is also designed to identify children with much more subtle problems, such as dyslexia (see below) or *autism* (opposite).

Mental subnormality

One child in 50 is sufficiently mentally subnormal to be unable to keep up with other children of the same age. These children are called educationally subnormal (ESN) – either to a moderate (M) or severe (S) degree – and must be educated in special schools. If a series of tests and continuous assessments indicate that your child is mentally subnormal, a team of professionals will discuss alternatives with you, and how best to cope with your child.

Dyslexia

Some children who have great difficulty in learning – particularly, learning how to read –

have no physical problems and have a normal IQ. The problem these children face is faulty interpretation and use of the knowledge they have acquired. The most well-known example is dyslexia. This is when a child has difficulty in reading and spelling because he or she confuses certain letters whose shape is the same but whose positioning is different – for example, b, d, q, and p. Dyslexic children usually overcome their difficulty through tuition given at their ordinary school. Parents are encouraged to contact the *British Dyslexia Association* or the *Dyslexia Institute* (p.768) for valuable advice and information on special tuition courses.

The education of handicapped children

Many slightly mentally and/or physically handicapped children attend ordinary schools. If they are unable to cope with the work there, a place will be sought for them in a special school. But the number of such schools is very limited. Current policy in Britain encourages the education of handicapped children in normal schools whenever possible.

Severely mentally and/or physically handicapped children need specialized tuition and care in a special school. These are run either by the State or by societies who cater for a specific handicap – for example, The *Spastic Society* (p.768). They are either day, boarding, or long-stay schools. Unfortunately, there is always a shortage of places for children who need them.

The outlook for handicapped children

Physically handicapped children of normal intelligence have every hope of doing well in life. Within reasonable limitations, they should be encouraged to become independent and to train for an occupation.

Children who are slightly mentally handicapped are much more at the mercy of society. They need realistic support and encouragement from their family to enable them to grow up with some confidence and independence. Armed with this, they should be able to do some sort of work. Sheltered workshops and even sheltered hostels exist for adults at the lower end of this category who need a protected environment.

Both children who are severely mentally subnormal and those who are mentally and physically handicapped may be quite incapable of launching out into an adult world. Such children may have to spend their whole life in some form of institution – either a mental hospital or a home for the chronically sick.

Eyes and ears

A child learns about the world largely by watching and listening. Even a minor problem with either the eyes or ears, if untreated, may interfere with the child's development (see *Learning problems*, p.673). Therefore it is vital to check the development of your baby's vision and hearing. Be certain to take your baby to the clinic for the routine eye and ear tests carried out at six to nine months.

Until then, check the baby's progress by doing the tests described opposite (see *Can my baby see and hear properly?*).

If your child has sticky eyes, a squint, a discharge from or crusting around the ear, or seems inattentive, see your doctor. Many childhood eye and ear problems – particularly squint and glue ear – can be cured completely with early diagnosis and treatment.

Squint in children

In someone who squints (or is "cross-eyed"), the two eyes do not look at the same object: one eye focuses on what the person wants to observe; the other, unaligned, eye looks elsewhere, usually inwards, but occasionally outwards or even upwards or downwards.

Visual symptom
A squint is rarely obvious in the first weeks of life. It usually becomes apparent as the baby learns to use the eyes.

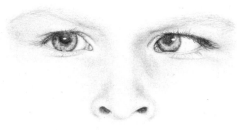

A squint may be constant or may come and go, and may affect one eye or both eyes alternately. It usually first appears in infancy or early childhood, when the eyesight is developing. It is most commonly associated with another kind of defect in the eye – for example, pronounced short sight or long sight. Most children who squint do not see double, because their brain ignores what is seen by the squinting eye. This eye will become "lazy" (*amblyopic*): that is, as a result of having its vision suppressed, it will become defective, discerning less and less detail.

How common is the problem?
Squint is fairly common. Each year about 1 child in 300 is taken to see a doctor because of a suspected squint.

What should be done?
If a baby under three months old has a squint that comes and goes, there is no need to worry; the baby is simply still learning to use his or her eyes. In cases of intermittent squint past this age, and in all cases of constant squint, you should take the baby or child to

your doctor. The doctor may be able to tell you that the squint is only apparent; many young children have a fold of skin over the inner corner of each eye that often gives the illusion of a squint.

If the doctor suspects a true squint, then you and your baby will be referred to an *ophthalmologist*, who will carry out tests to discover the cause of the squint and devise the best course of treatment.

What is the treatment?
If the eye is lazy, then a patch is worn over the good eye for as long as possible – at least several hours – each day. This forces the child to use the lazy eye. The treatment is usually effective only before the age of seven or so; after this age the laziness becomes ingrained and is very difficult to cure. Spectacles may also need to be worn if the child is short- or long-sighted. In some children, the combination of patch and spectacles clears up the problem within a few months.

If a child has a severe squint, surgery may be carried out, both to help the child use the lazy eye and to improve the child's appearance for psychological reasons by straightening the eyes. The operation strengthens or weakens some of the muscles that move the eyeball, and usually requires only a few days' stay in hospital. Whatever the treatment, it may be carried out at a local hospital or clinic. Patching is usually done under the supervision of an *orthoptist*.

What are the long-term prospects?
The prospect of a squint and "lazy" eye being cured is very good if treated early. After the age of seven, remedying the squint itself is still possible but there is an increased risk that the lazy eye will gradually become so disused that patching will not be successful and the eye effectively goes blind.

Medical myth

A child with a squint soon grows out of it.

Wrong. You should never assume a squint will disappear naturally. It is never too early to show a possible squint to your doctor; the sooner treatment is started, the better the prospects of a total cure.

Glue ear

(also called secretory otitis media)

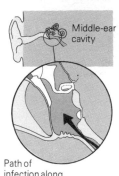

Path of infection along eustachian tube

Some children have repeated attacks of *acute infection of the middle ear* (p.333), which is usually caused by an infection of the nose and throat, such as a *cold* (p.342), passing along the eustachian tube from the back of the nose to the middle-ear cavity. Attacks are more frequent in children because their short eustachian tubes make it easy for microbes to reach the middle ear. Repeated infections cause the eustachian tube to become swollen and blocked, allowing a sticky fluid produced by the infections to collect in the middle ear, causing the condition known as glue ear.

What are the symptoms?
The main symptom is deafness in the affected ear. This is rarely total; in most cases sounds are muffled or faint. The deafness is caused by the sticky fluid preventing the eardrum and middle-ear bones from vibrating freely. The child may also have earache or a sensation of fullness in the ear.

If your child seems unusually inattentive or is having trouble at school, it is possible that the cause is partial deafness from glue ear (see *Learning problems*, p.673).

How common is the problem?
Glue ear is a fairly common disorder; about 1 child in 100 suffers from it. The condition is very rare indeed in adults.

What are the risks?
If the condition is not detected or treated after several months, there is a danger that the bones of the middle ear may become cemented together, causing permanent deafness in the affected ear.

If the child is at a stage when speech is developing, the deafness may retard this development and, later on, affect the child's performance at school.

What should be done?
If you suspect deafness after any ear infection, see your doctor, who will examine the affected ear with an *otoscope*. This instrument gives a clear view of the eardrum and often allows the doctor to gauge the severity of any glue ear present.

What is the treatment?
In mild cases, when there is not much fluid in the ear and hearing loss is minimal, the doctor will probably prescribe decongestant tablets or an antihistamine in the form of tablets or medicine. These reduce the swelling of the eustachian tube and so allow the fluid to trickle out of the middle ear down the tube and into the nose and throat.

In more severe cases, the child has to go into hospital to have the fluid removed. Under general anaesthetic, a very fine needle is passed through the eardrum and the fluid sucked out with a syringe, or a small cut is made in the eardrum (*myringotomy*). Usually, a tiny plastic tube (called a grommet or stopple) is inserted into the hole in the eardrum to allow air to enter and dry out the middle ear. It is generally left in place for several months, after which it drops out or is removed, and the hole in the eardrum heals naturally.

If the *adenoids* (p.677) are swollen as a result of repeated infections, and so are blocking the entrance to the eustachian tube (or, rarely, are acting as a reservoir of infection), your doctor may advise their removal.

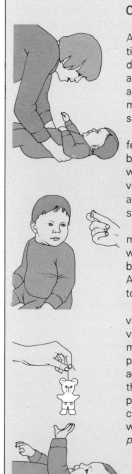

Can my baby see and hear properly?

All babies undergo a thorough general examination just after birth but this may be too early to detect defects of vision and hearing. Between 4 and 6 weeks of age the baby's vision is tested again at a baby clinic. During your baby's first few months, you can check his or her progress yourself by trying the simple tests described below.

All babies are short-sighted during the first few weeks of life, but at about 6 weeks, your baby should smile or stare if you bring your face within about 500mm (20in). Test your baby's vision at 3 months by dangling a familiar toy about 200mm (8in) away; the baby's eyes should follow its movement.

You can check on your baby's hearing at 3 months by making a loud noise near the baby, when he or she is crying. The baby should react by ceasing to cry and becoming temporarily still. At 4 months, the baby should turn his or her head to look for the source of the sound.

If you have any worries about your baby's vision or hearing, mention them to your health visitor or doctor. Make sure you keep all appointments at the baby clinic, especially for the full physical examination carried out on all babies aged 6 to 9 months. This examination includes thorough tests of vision and hearing, and any problems that have arisen can be detected and cured before they have a chance to interfere with the baby's development (see *Learning problems*, p.673).

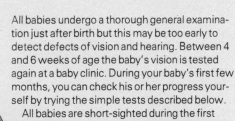

Respiratory system

The most common cause of respiratory-system disorders in children is infection. Because the respiratory tract in a child is short, infectious microbes can pass easily from one infected part to another. This is why recurrent coughs and colds in babies and children often lead to infections elsewhere in the respiratory tract. (For a discussion of the respiratory system in general see *Disorders of the respiratory system*, p.340.)

Before the widespread use of *antibiotics*, many respiratory infections which are now considered minor – for example, tonsillitis – often led to serious complications. Today even pneumonia, once a "killer disease", is often treated at home.

One major risk of respiratory infections is that your child may have difficulty in breathing (see *Stridor and croup*, p.678). Even if there are no other symptoms, if your child is short of breath and starts to turn bluish about the lips (*cyanosis*), get the child to hospital (see also the advice in *Accidents and emergencies*, p.801).

Tonsillitis in children

The two tonsils at the back of the throat are part of the ring of *lymph glands* that guard the entrance to the respiratory and digestive systems. Very small at birth, they enlarge gradually, reaching maximum size at age six or seven. Thereafter they shrink but do not disappear, as *adenoids* (opposite) do. The tonsils are relatively large at early school age, when the respiratory tract begins to be attacked by a variety of new microbes; they are thought to act to keep the microbes away from the lower respiratory tract.

Tonsillitis is an acute viral or bacterial infection of the tonsils, sometimes causing them to become abnormally swollen as well as inflamed. It occurs mainly in school-age children, occasionally in adolescents and adults (see *Tonsillitis*, p.351).

Medical myth

Surgical removal of tonsils is a safe minor operation, which would benefit most children.

Wrong. Like any operation, tonsillectomy carries a small risk which increases with age. Except in severe cases of recurrent tonsillitis – or if swollen tonsils interfere with swallowing or breathing – the operation is usually unnecessary.

What are the symptoms?
The illness starts suddenly with sore throat and difficulty in swallowing; within a few hours the child becomes feverish and may seem quite ill. The painful irritation in the throat makes some children vomit or cough. In a very few cases, the child has a febrile convulsion (see *Convulsions in children*, p.667). Young children often complain of stomach pain. Glands on either side of the neck and in the angle of the jaw may swell and become tender. They can be felt as small, knob-like protuberances. Sometimes the swellings persist for several weeks after the main symptoms have subsided.

How common is the problem?
Virtually every child has one or more attacks of tonsillitis, which is very *contagious*. Frequent attacks usually lessen after the age of seven as resistance develops.

What are the risks?
Before the advent of *antibiotics*, tonsillitis could lead to *rheumatic fever* (p.393) or some form of *glomerulonephritis* (p.504), but such complications are rare today.

What should be done?
Try the self-help measures recommended under "What is the treatment?" below. If, despite these, fever and reluctance to eat because of pain last for more than 24 hours, consult your doctor, who will examine the child's tonsils and determine whether the condition is present.

What is the treatment?
Self-help: The child should be kept indoors (but not in bed, unless he or she requests otherwise) in a warm – not overheated – room. Symptoms can usually be relieved by "junior" aspirins or paracetamols and plenty of fluids, which should be sipped regularly. Do not force the child to eat or drink. If he or she asks for cold desserts to cool the throat, there is no harm in giving these. A cooling fan, or frequent sponging of the face with tepid water, also helps to reduce the child's temperature. In most cases, children with tonsillitis respond swiftly to these measures.
Professional help: The doctor will probably prescribe an antibiotic drug; ensure your child takes the full course as instructed. The tonsillitis should clear up in a few days.

If attacks of tonsillitis are so severe and frequent that they affect general health, then surgical removal of the tonsils (tonsillectomy – see opposite) may be the only answer. This operation was performed frequently in the past, but most doctors nowadays recommend it only as a last resort.

OPERATION: **Tonsils removal**
tonsillectomy

Removal of the tonsils is carried out for recurrent attacks of tonsillitis that are interfering with general health or education. The operation is usually done when the child is 6 or 7; it becomes more difficult as the patient gets older.

During the operation Under a general anaesthetic, the child's mouth is held open and the tongue is pulled forward to reveal the inflamed tonsils. The tonsils are then carefully cut away and the raw area is left to heal naturally.

After the operation There may be some bleeding of the raw areas, but this is not usually serious. The child should be out of hospital in 2 or 3 days, and most children are back to normal in 2 weeks.

Plenty of ice cream serves to both soothe the sore throat and cheer up the child.
See also information on operations, p.738.

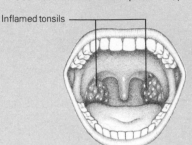
Inflamed tonsils

Adenoids

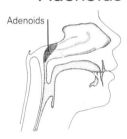
Adenoids

Position of adenoids
The adenoids are sited at the back of the nasal passage.

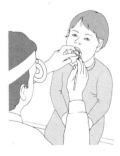

Examining adenoids
Because the adenoids are awkwardly situated, the doctor needs to use a special long-handled mirror to examine them.

Adenoids, which are two glandular swellings at the back of the nose, above the tonsils, are found almost exclusively in pre-adolescent children. Exactly what they do is not clear, but it is thought that they assist the body's defences against respiratory-tract infections. They are never troublesome unless they grow too big. Normally, adenoids begin to enlarge at about the age of three; from about five, they begin to get smaller, and they disappear at puberty. In a minority of children, however, they grow even larger from the age of five and eventually obstruct the airway from the nose to the throat, or block the opening of the eustachian tube from the middle ear into the nose. A child to whom this happens is commonly said to have "adenoids".

What are the symptoms?
If the airway from the nose is blocked the child breathes mainly through the mouth, snores when asleep, and is likely to speak with a nasal twang. The flow of secretions at the back of the nose is obstructed, bacteria multiply in the stagnant fluid, and the adenoids become infected. Infected secretions drip from the child's nose during the day, and accumulate in the throat at night, causing an irritating cough. The infection may also spread along the tube to the middle ear. This can cause *glue ear* (p.675).

How common is the problem?
Troublesome adenoids are much less common now that *antibiotics* usually prevent infections from becoming chronic. Few children today have the typical "adenoidal face" – open mouth, runny nose, and nasal speech.

What are the risks?
There are no serious risks if infection is kept under control. If infections are neglected and followed by chronic ear trouble, partial deafness may result.

What should be done?
If your child has a repeatedly blocked nose, frequent earaches, or an irritating cough in the night, consult your doctor. After examining the child, the doctor may refer him or her to a specialist. The specialist will probably examine the adenoids by reflecting a light onto them from a mirror held at the back of the throat – a procedure that is rather uncomfortable. In some cases, the specialist may find that the adenoids are not enlarged but that the opening at the back of the nose is unusually small. In such an event, surgical removal of the adenoids is necessary.

What is the treatment?
Infections caused by abnormally enlarged adenoids are treated with antibiotics when necessary. Surgical removal of the adenoids (adenoidectomy) is carried out less often today, because the adenoids shrink of their own accord as the child reaches puberty. However, when repeated earaches interfere with a child's education or persist despite antibiotic treatment, adenoidectomy may be the only answer (see *Tonsils removal*, above, which is a similar operation occasionally carried out at the same time). The child is generally in hospital for about three days or so, and there are no long-term effects from the operation except to remove the problems caused by the troublesome adenoids.

Stridor and croup

Stridor is a wheezing or grunting noise made when a child breathes through a larynx or trachea that is narrower than normal. The narrowing can be due to one of several problems – an *inhaled foreign body*, for example (see the box below) – but is usually due to swelling of the lining of the air passages following a respiratory infection, often a cold (see *Recurrent coughs and colds*, p.680). A sudden attack of stridor in association with a respiratory infection is called croup.

What are the symptoms?
In addition to the characteristic sound of stridor, a child with croup will have symptoms of the respiratory infection, plus a hollow-sounding cough, and hoarseness. Older children may complain of discomfort in the area of the larynx or the front of the chest.

Usually attacks of croup occur at night. The child wakes with a sudden loud crowing noise, which becomes louder when he or she inhales. The child is likely to be alarmed and bewildered. In most cases, the attack subsides in a few hours, though some children get recurrent attacks.

What should be done?
If your child has difficulty in breathing and turns bluish, especially around the lips, see *Accidents and emergencies*, p.801, for first-aid treatment and get the child to a doctor or hospital as quickly as possible. If your child has stridor and is not already being treated for a respiratory infection, consult your doctor about the cause of the problem.

What is the treatment?
Self-help: During an attack of croup, be calm and reassure the child, who may be frightened. Panic – whether your own or the child's – will only make the situation worse. If your child has had previous episodes, the doctor may have provided you with drugs to ease the attack.

Professional help: If the child has an underlying respiratory infection which is caused by bacteria, *antibiotics* will be prescribed.

A child who is having extreme difficulty in breathing will be admitted to hospital, where the staff will give oxygen, and perhaps *steroids* (as an injection or throat spray) to reduce inflammation in the air passages. If the throat is seriously obstructed, it will be necessary either to pass a tube through the mouth into the trachea or – in the most severe cases – to make an incision in the trachea and insert a tube to enable the child to breathe. The tube is usually removed within 24 hours. Rarely, breathing has to be maintained artificially with a *respirator*. Most children admitted to hospital with stridor make a complete recovery within a few days.

Inhaled foreign body

If a child inhales a foreign body – for instance a bead or a peanut – it can partially or completely block the air passage. If your child has sudden difficulty in breathing or turns bluish about the lips (*cyanosis*), see *Accidents and emergencies*, p.803, for first-aid treatment and get the child to a doctor or hospital as quickly as possible.

If an inhaled foreign body causes only a partial blockage, the child will have sudden *stridor* (see the article on this page) and possibly a cough. In this case, take the child to hospital, where a doctor will look for the inhaled object through a *bronchoscope* and, if possible, remove it there and then.

Occasionally an inhaled foreign body passes further down into the lung, causing a small area of inflammation and infection (see *Pneumonia in children*, opposite). Such an object can be removed with a bronchoscope, and *antibiotics* are given for the infection.

Bronchiolitis

The greater part of the lungs consists of millions of tiny tubes called bronchioles, which convey air between the larger airways, the trachea (windpipe) and the bronchi, and the tiny air sacs called alveoli where oxygen is exchanged for carbon dioxide.

In bronchiolitis, the lining of the bronchioles is infected by a virus. The virus usually starts by causing a *cold* (p.342) and then spreads to the lungs. The infected lining swells, almost completely blocking the passage of air in and out of the alveoli and so preventing the baby from getting sufficient oxygen. Bronchiolitis occurs almost exclusively in babies.

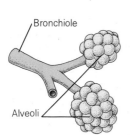

Bronchiole

Alveoli

What are the symptoms?
The baby has a cold that suddenly becomes worse after a day or two. He or she then starts to breathe quickly and with difficulty; in some cases, the chest fails to expand when breath is drawn in. The baby is limp, unable to feed, and may turn blue (*cyanosis*).

Bronchiolitis is not common and most cases are swiftly diagnosed. In rare cases *heart failure* (p.381) or pneumonia (see *Pneumonia in children*, opposite) can result.

What should be done?
If your baby shows any of the symptoms described, consult your doctor immediately.

You should be especially watchful if your baby has a cold which, instead of getting better after two or three days, suddenly gets worse. If cyanosis has developed, the baby will be admitted to hospital and put into an oxygen tent immediately. In some cases, *antibiotic* drugs may be given. In very severe cases, an anti-inflammatory *steroid* drug may be given to reduce the swelling in the bronchioles and allow the baby to breathe more easily. With prompt treatment, most babies recover completely from the condition.

Pneumonia in children

Pneumonia is an inflammation of the lungs, usually caused by an infection. For general information on this disease see *Pneumonia* (p.359). In children, pneumonia is most commonly caused by a viral infection that has started in the upper respiratory tract. It develops to produce patchy inflammation – sometimes called "bronchopneumonia" – usually in the lower parts of both lungs.

Bronchopneumonia can also develop as a complication of *measles* (p.699) or *whooping cough* (p.701). Children suffering from *cystic fibrosis* (p.685) are also susceptible to bouts of serious bronchopneumonia, and it can also be caused by an *inhaled foreign body* (opposite) which has travelled down into the lung.

Some older children get what is sometimes referred to as "lobar" pneumonia – inflammation of one or more lobes of the lung by the pneumococcus bacterium.

What are the symptoms?
A child who contracts bronchopneumonia starts by having a cold for two or three days. The child's temperature then rises to about 38.5°C (101°F) and he or she develops a dry cough, starts breathing more quickly than normal, and in some cases may wheeze. In very serious cases, breathing difficulties cause the child to turn blue (*cyanosis*).

The onset of lobar pneumonia is quite different. There is no cold. The child becomes ill suddenly, and his or her temperature rises to about 40°C (104°F). Breathing is rapid, and the child has a dry cough. *Pleurisy* (p.361) may develop, causing pain in the chest.

How common is the problem?
Each year about 1 child in 300 suffers from pneumonia. Bronchopneumonia is much more common than lobar pneumonia, but is still quite rare; it develops in only a few upper respiratory-tract infections.

What are the risks?
The high temperature that is brought on by pneumonia can in some rare cases cause a *febrile* convulsion (see *Convulsions in children*, p.667). On rare occasions, the inflamed areas of the lungs are gradually replaced by fibrous tissue, which, if extensive, may

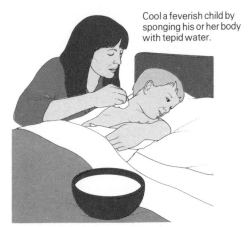

Cool a feverish child by sponging his or her body with tepid water.

give rise to *bronchiectasis* (p.363). Fatal pneumonia in children is rare.

What should be done?
If your child develops a temperature and starts having difficulty breathing, call the doctor; this is a matter of urgency if the child is less than six months old.

Most cases of pneumonia in children can be treated at home; hospital admission is only necessary in very severe cases.

What is the treatment?
Self-help: If the doctor decides that the child can be treated at home, there are several things you can do to relieve symptoms and hasten recovery. The high temperature can be lowered by giving "junior" aspirin and cooling the body by sponging with tepid water. Give plenty of fluids, and persuade the child to rest quietly as much as possible.

Professional help: It is mainly the child's own resistance to the infection that brings about a recovery. *Antibiotics* act against bacteria but have no effect on viruses, which cause most cases of bronchopneumonia. Antibiotics are used against lobar pneumonia, and when there is some doubt about whether a virus or bacterium is responsible for the infection. Antibiotics are usually given by mouth, unless the infection is very severe.

A normally healthy child will nearly always recover completely from pneumonia – usually after about a week.

Recurrent coughs and colds

It is quite normal for a young child to have a number of coughs and colds in winter, and it is nothing for you to worry about. Most children keep catching colds during the start of school life (some actually spend more time at home than at school), because at school the child is exposed to all kinds of new viruses. Gradually, however, the child acquires increasing immunity to them and has far fewer colds.

A child's cold is often accompanied by a cough – chiefly because, instead of blowing mucus into a handkerchief, he or she tends to sniff it down into the throat. The mucus irritates the throat, so in an attempt to get rid of it, the child coughs. Quite often a child with a cold has some abdominal pain and he or she may vomit.

When to consult your doctor
In rare cases, recurrent coughs and colds are a symptom of a serious underlying disorder. In such illnesses, the child appears generally unwell for most of the time, and when this happens, consult your doctor.

In some children, cold symptoms are caused not by a cold but by an allergy (see *Allergic rhinitis*, p.345). If your child sneezes and has a runny nose and watering eyes during the summer months, he or she probably has hay fever – an allergy to pollen. If the symptoms occur throughout the year, the child may be allergic to dust or pet hair.

If a recurrent cough is not accompanied by a cold, or if it is accompanied by wheezy breathing – which may indicate *asthma* (p.355), or in rare cases, *cystic fibrosis* (p.685) – you should consult your doctor.

Certain symptoms indicate that complications may have set in. See your doctor if a baby with a cold cries continually, refuses to feed, is restless, and has a hot skin. Consult the doctor also if your child has a cold and then develops earache or pain in the face or forehead, or runs a high fever (above 39°C or 102°F), or is persistently hoarse, along with a nagging, dry, painful cough.

What you can do for recurrent coughs and colds
In some cases, a child with recurrent colds will cough a lot at night. This may be because the room is too cold and the air is irritating the throat, or because it is too warm and the air is making the throat dry. Adjusting the temperature of the room may solve the problem.

Babies with colds sometimes have trouble feeding. This is no cause for concern if the feeding difficulty lasts only a day or two. You can help by keeping the baby's nose clear of obstructing mucus, to allow easy breathing.

Try giving an older child a hot drink before bed, to help clear the back of the nasal passages. Your doctor may prescribe a cough mixture.

Examination by the doctor

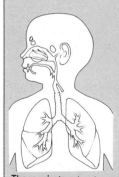
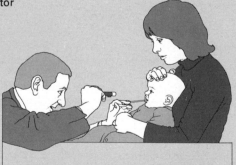
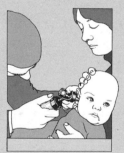

Ear examination
Respiratory infections often travel along the eustachian tube, causing infection of the middle ear. It is important that such an infection is treated with antibiotics, as it could lead to persistent ear trouble in later life.

The respiratory tract
Infections of the respiratory tract – the nose, throat, trachea (windpipe), and lungs – tend to be more common during childhood than at any other time.

Throat examination
The doctor will examine a child's throat to see whether the tonsils or adenoids are inflamed. Although tonsillitis and enlarged adenoids are not usually dangerous, they may lead to breathing difficulties. If your child has been wheezing or grunting, the doctor will suspect stridor and may want to check how far the inflammation has spread before making a diagnosis.

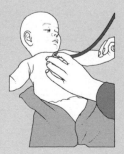

Chest examination
A chest examination will ensure that your baby's cold is not developing into a more serious disorder such as bronchopneumonia or bronchiolitis.

Blood

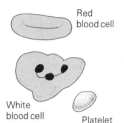

Red blood cell

White blood cell

Platelet

The blood disorders discussed here vary greatly in their effect on the child. These disorders, because their symptoms are varied and usually mild, may go undetected. For a child with iron-deficiency anaemia or anaphylactoid purpura, a delayed diagnosis is not likely to have any permanent ill-effects, and the disorder is treated in the usual way. But a child who has leukaemia, a cancer affecting white blood cells, has the best chances of recovery if the disease is caught early. Recent research in the treatment of leukaemia has much improved the prospects for children with the disease. Even so, leukaemia requires intensive treatment, and may prove a great strain on both the child and the family. For further information, read *Malignant diseases in childhood*, p.695.

Anaphyl-actoid purpura

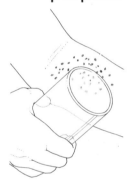

The glass test
Press a glass tumbler against the rash. If the rash is purpuric, it will still be visible under pressure (see p.239, **Visual aids to diagnosis**, 29).

In anaphylactoid purpura, a rash appears just beneath the surface of the skin, due to an abnormal reaction between *antibodies* – which the body has produced to act against some substance taken into the system – and blood vessels. The vessels become inflamed and porous, producing the rash. In most cases, the antibodies are made to combat an infection by streptococcus bacteria; but they can be produced in reaction to a food or drug.

The disorder most commonly affects children aged between two and 10.

What are the symptoms?
Usually the child will have had a sore throat two weeks before the onset of the rash. The rash, which does not irritate, consists of purplish-red, irregularly shaped spots, ranging from the size of a pinhead to 25mm (1in) across and occurring on the ankles, shins, buttocks, and elbows. When the spots appear, some children feel generally unwell and have a slight temperature. The rash is not present all the time but tends to come and go. Some children may also have swollen joints, or a tummy ache that is often severe and persistent. Occasionally, blood is passed in the faeces, indicating bleeding in the bowel, or in the urine, signifying kidney damage (see *Glomerulonephritis*, p.504).

Anaphylactoid purpura is very rare; it is more common in boys than in girls.

The main risk faced by a child with this disorder is permanent kidney damage. Other, less likely dangers are *intussusception* (p.683) or massive bleeding in the bowel or other internal organs.

What should be done?
If your child has any of the symptoms described, consult your doctor. Treatment will not be required in most cases, which will clear up spontaneously after a month or two – though in some children the problem recurs for up to two years before finally disappearing. If there are signs of kidney damage, certain special tests such as a kidney *biopsy* may be advised. To relieve very painful tummy ache, the doctor may prescribe anti-inflammatory *steroid* tablets.

Iron-deficiency anaemia in children

Anaemia is an insufficiency of haemoglobin, the red, iron-containing pigment in the blood that carries oxygen to the tissues of the body. Of the various types of anaemia, the most common in children is iron-deficiency anaemia (see *Iron-deficiency anaemia*, p.419, for general information on this disease). The most likely cause of this disorder is inadequate iron in the diet. Unfortunately, the disorder tends to diminish appetite, which makes the problem worse. In most babies, it does not matter that the natural or artificial milk on which they are fed contains little iron, because they can draw on stores of iron built up before birth; premature babies, however, have low stores and may therefore tend to suffer from iron-deficiency anaemia.

A less common cause of iron-deficiency anaemia in children is failure to absorb iron in the diet, as in *coeliac disease* (p.684).

What are the symptoms?
Mild anaemia may produce no obvious symptoms. Signs of more pronounced anaemia (of any type) include several or all of the following: paleness, especially at the fingertips and on the lining of the lower eyelids; tiredness; weakness, and, less commonly, fainting; breathlessness; palpitations, especially on exertion; inactivity; and loss of appetite.

What should be done?

If your child is less active than his or her playmates, and especially if breathlessness follows minimal activity, take him or her to the doctor. Do *not* try to treat anaemia yourself by giving iron pills or tonics.

The doctor will take blood samples for analysis. Further tests may then be required at hospital. If the diagnosis is iron-deficiency anaemia caused by lack of iron in the diet, the doctor will prescribe iron for three months or longer, usually in liquid form. The doctor will also make recommendations about diet. For a baby going on to semi-solids, tinned baby foods provide plenty of iron, as do meat, eggs, and green vegetables.

Leukaemia in children

Leukaemia is a cancer affecting white blood cells, which protect the body against infection. Acute lymphatic leukaemia is the type that accounts for most cases of leukaemia in children. (For a full definition of leukaemia and a description of the disease in adults see *Leukaemia*, p.426.)

Acute lymphatic leukaemia affects the lymphocytes and the cells that form them, the lymphoblasts. These abnormal lymphoblasts cause swelling of the lymph glands and infiltrate the bone marrow. They circulate in the bloodstream to affect various parts of the body, including the liver, spleen, and surface of the brain and spinal cord. In the bone marrow, the leukaemic cells interfere with the marrow's production of red blood cells, platelets, and other white blood cells.

What are the symptoms?

The main symptoms of acute lymphatic leukaemia are: anaemia, marked by progressive paleness, tiredness, and general sickliness; thrombocytopenic purpura (see *Thrombocytopenia*, p.425), characterized by a purplish-red rash; pains in the limbs; severe headaches; swollen glands in the neck, behind the angle of the jaw; an enlarged spleen, which the doctor will be able to feel in the upper left abdomen; susceptibility to infections, especially *pneumonia* (p.359); and sores and ulcers in the mouth and throat.

How common is the problem?

Any form of leukaemia in children is extremely rare; each year, only 1 child in 10,000 suffers from the disease.

What are the risks?

Because of recent advances in treatment, children with leukaemia have a much better outlook than ever before. But the treatment itself involves a risk that the child may contract a serious infection which, because his or her resistance is low, may be fatal.

What should be done?

If you are worried that your child might have leukaemia, take him or her to the doctor, who will carry out an examination and probably be able to relieve your worry on the spot. If the possibility of leukaemia cannot be ruled out immediately, the doctor will arrange for your child to go to hospital, where a blood sample and a *biopsy* of bone marrow will be taken. Laboratory analysis of these will show whether or not the disease is present.

What is the treatment?

Treatment is carried out in hospital where the child is usually first given a blood transfusion. The basic treatment is one or more courses of *cytotoxic* (anti-cancer) and *steroid* drugs, given in varying combinations. Some are given as tablets, others by *intravenous drip*.

In most cases, a course of *radiotherapy* is also given, and any infection is treated by large doses of *antibiotics*.

To protect your child against the risk of serious infection, he or she will be isolated from other patients, and when you visit, you will have to wear a mask and gown. A young child in particular may be bewildered and upset, and you must try to overcome your own distress in order to offer all the reassurance you can. An older child will probably realize the seriousness of the illness. (For advice on how best to cope, see *Malignant diseases in childhood*, p.695.)

In nearly all cases, treatment causes symptoms to abate after several weeks. The disease is then said to be in remission, and you will probably be allowed to take the child home. Over the next year or so, he or she will be expected to attend regular hospital checkups and will be given doses of drugs to ensure, with your essential help, that he or she is able to lead as normal a life as possible.

If symptoms recur or worsen, your child may need to be re-admitted to hospital.

What are the long-term prospects?

A complete cure for the disease now seems possible. About 50 per cent of children who have received modern intensive treatment for acute lymphatic leukaemia have survived at least five years; and some of them are still alive and healthy after much longer periods.

Digestive system and nutrition

A healthy digestive system and a sound diet are essential for a growing child. Several of the disorders described below are the result of the digestive system's inability to handle certain foods (for a full description of *Disorders of digestion and nutrition* see p.434). Most of these disorders (phenylketonuria, for example) are detected soon enough after birth to prevent the child ever eating the foods which can be harmful. If your child has such a disorder, your doctor will advise you of a suitable diet. A child who keeps strictly to the special diet need never suffer the symptoms of the disorder.

Intussusception

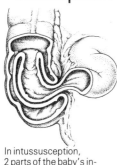

In intussusception, 2 parts of the baby's intestine are telescoped together.

In this rare disorder a part of the intestine, usually the small intestine, telescopes into the intestine ahead of it. What causes the telescoping is not known. It can happen at any age, but occurs most often in babies about six months old and is more common in boys.

What are the symptoms?
A previously healthy baby may suddenly scream violently as a wave of muscular contraction passes along the telescoped intestine. The screaming may carry on for several minutes. The baby then becomes pale and limp, and may vomit. He or she may pass a motion of blood-stained mucus, like red jelly. In some cases the uncontrollable screaming recurs every few minutes.

What should be done?
See your doctor as soon as possible if the above symptoms occur. By feeling the child's abdomen, the doctor may be able to make a firm diagnosis of intussusception. If not, the baby will be admitted to hospital for a *barium enema* examination. This will confirm a tentative diagnosis of intussusception – and may also, as the barium is forced along the intestine, push the telescoped intestine back into place (which will show up on the *X-ray*). If the barium does not do this, the baby will have an operation in which the abdomen is opened and the gut is pushed back into its normal position. The results of the operation are usually excellent, and the baby has no further problems.

Encopresis

Encopresis is an uncommon condition in which a child regularly soils his or her underclothes, despite having been toilet-trained. In most cases, large amounts of hard faeces accumulate in the rectum and lower bowel (where you can sometimes feel them as a lump in the abdomen), and the soiling material is a liquid which may contain mucus and which has trickled past the blockage. Because of this, parents often think that the child has diarrhoea and do not realize that he or she is actually constipated. They also do not realize that often the child cannot control the passing of these liquid motions. Whatever the reason for your child soiling his or her pants, you should try to adopt an understanding attitude rather than punishing the child for "dirty habits", since such punishment can do nothing to cure the problem. The constipation may be the result of some problem with the toilet-training of the child – this may have been either too strict or inadequately supervised, so that the child does not clear his or her bowels properly (see also *Constipation in children*, p.688).

In a few cases, encopresis takes the form of soiling underclothes with solid faeces. This is nearly always due to an emotional disturbance, usually within the family, although sometimes at school.

What is the treatment?
A child with the first type of encopresis must be taken to the doctor. The treatment is to give several *enemas* or *suppositories* to clear the rectum and lower bowel. Your doctor may be able to do this at the surgery, but usually the procedure is carried out in hospital. At home, you should encourage your child to go to the lavatory twice each day, at regular times. In some cases, your doctor may prescribe laxatives to be taken daily, sometimes over a long period.

If your child soils his or her pants with solid faeces, try instituting the toilet routine described above. But if the problem persists, you should see your doctor, who may recommend a consultation with a child psychiatrist. This is likely to involve not just the child but the whole family.

Coeliac disease

(also called gluten enteropathy or non-tropical sprue)

Coeliac disease is an allergy of the small intestine. When it comes into contact with gluten (a protein present in most grains), the membrane lining the intestine loses its fluffy texture and becomes smooth. As a result, the intestine is less able to absorb nutrients (see *Malabsorption*, p.475). The disease is nearly always discovered and diagnosed in infancy or early childhood.

What are the symptoms?
Symptoms usually start within a few weeks of cereals being introduced into the baby's diet (at about four or five months). The baby starts to put on less weight (or even loses weight) and may have a poor appetite, which slows down progress even more. Several times each day he or she passes loose, pale, bulky, offensive-smelling faeces, together with a lot of wind. The wind may make the baby's stomach swell, and this will contrast with his or her undernourished appearance. In some cases, ulcers develop in the mouth.

How common is the problem?
The disease is rare. A child with a relative who has the disorder has a slightly higher risk than average of being born with it.

What are the risks?
In the very rare cases when a mild form of the illness is not detected in infancy, the child's growth may be permanently stunted. An affected child will also be susceptible to dangerously severe infections.

What should be done?
If your child has the symptoms described, see your doctor. If the doctor suspects coeliac disease, he or she will arrange for the child to enter hospital for tests on the blood and the faeces. If these disclose the likelihood of the disease, a *biopsy* of the lining of the small intestine is carried out. This will confirm whether the child has coeliac disease or not.

What is the treatment?
The principle of treatment is to exclude wheat, rye, and other grain gluten from the baby's diet. Your doctor will arrange for you to discuss this special diet with a dietician. Rice and maize can be eaten, but the child will have to eat special bread and biscuits, and you must make any cakes or pastry with a special gluten-free flour; all of these can be prescribed by your doctor. Within a few weeks of starting on the diet, the child's symptoms clear up, and he or she starts to gain weight and thrive in the normal way.

Although the diet is restrictive (gravies, many processed foods, and confectionery all contain gluten), it need not be dull.

What are the long-term prospects?
If you have coeliac disease you can look forward to a normal life, apart from the diet. As you reach adulthood you may find that you can eat limited quantities of gluten-containing foods with no apparent ill-effects. However, most doctors believe that such foods are best avoided.

Recurrent tummy aches and headaches

Some children who are otherwise healthy suffer from sudden tummy aches or headaches every few days, weeks, or months. They may look pale and want to lie down. Generally the pain lasts a few hours, but it can last all day. When asked to locate the tummy ache, the child usually points to the navel. Sometimes tummy aches are accompanied by vomiting, diarrhoea, or a slight fever, or by all three; when this happens regularly, the condition is often referred to as "the periodic syndrome" or "abdominal migraine".

Many children are rid of such tummy aches and headaches by puberty; a few continue to have them in adult life, or may develop *migraine* (p.285).

Only a small proportion of children with recurrent tummy aches have an underlying physical problem. This can be kidney trouble, or, more rarely, a peptic ulcer (a disorder almost entirely confined to boys). Food allergies may cause the pains in some children. But in the great majority of cases, the root cause is probably psychological. Headaches, too, are seldom a symptom of a serious underlying disorder. It is estimated that 90 per cent of recurrent headaches in children are the result of emotional stress at home or in school – for example, the birth of a new baby causing a shift in the parents' attention away from the child, or the approach of important examinations.

In many cases, the trouble seems to "run in the family": one or both parents have frequent headaches or migraine and have had the same sort of tummy aches in their own childhood. It is not known whether the tendency is inherited in the genes (see *Genetics*, p.704) or the result of parental influence.

What should be done?
If your child has recurrent tummy aches or headaches, take him or her to the doctor, to check that there is no physical trouble producing the pains. If there is no physical cause for tummy aches, the doctor may suggest that you try noting whether the pains occur consistently after the child has eaten a particular food (this may lead you to identify a food allergy). For a severe headache, give aspirin or paracetamol.

In many such cases the underlying disorder may be psychological. If symptoms persist, your doctor may arrange for you and your child to see a child psychiatrist.

Cystic fibrosis

Cystic fibrosis is a rare *congenital* disease in which several glands in the body do not function properly. Another name for this disorder is fibrocystic disease of the pancreas, so-called because abnormalities of the pancreas cause some of the main problems. For example, the pancreas fails to produce *enzymes*. These enzymes are normally concerned with the digestion, in the small intestine, of proteins, carbohydrates, and fats, breaking them down into simpler substances that can then be absorbed in the bloodstream. (For a fuller description of the function of the pancreas see *Liver, gallbladder, and pancreas,* p.485.) The result is that the child's food is only minimally broken down (by a small number of enzymes produced in the intestinal wall), and it passes out of the body with its fats and most other nutrients unabsorbed (see *Malabsorption,* p.475).

Cystic fibrosis is also marked by a malfunctioning of the glands in the lining of the bronchial tubes. Instead of producing the normal thin mucus that traps germs and is then coughed up, the bronchial glands produce a thick, sticky mucus that tends to stagnate in the tubes. Microbes are able to multiply readily in mucus-clogged airways, causing serious respiratory infections such as *pneumonia* (p.359). (*Continued overleaf*)

Teething problems

A baby's first milk teeth, the incisors, usually appear during the first year and seldom give much trouble. The gum may be a little inflamed, there may be more dribbling than usual, and the baby will probably chew a lot on the fingers or a teething ring, but there is unlikely to be any real pain.

The first and second molars, which are usually cut between the ages of one and three, are much more likely to cause problems. The gum may be tender and make eating painful, the cheek on the affected side of the mouth may be hot and flushed, and the child will probably be miserable for a few days. Unfortunately, there is little that can be done. Rubbing the gum gently and giving a cool drink now and again may ease the pain a little.

It is very easy to overlook real illness in a child by attributing symptoms to teething. If a child of teething age shows signs of distress, see your doctor. Clutching one side of the face, for example, may be a sign not of teething but of earache.

There are considerable variations in the ages at which teeth appear, and the ages given should be considered only as averages. Some children have one tooth or more at birth; others have none at a year. Early or late teething is of no importance and should not be a cause of worry.

Permanent teeth may appear immediately after the milk teeth fall out; or, if they appear before the milk teeth fall out, the dentist may have to extract milk teeth early (see *Crowded and badly occluded teeth,* p.440).

Permanent (adult) teeth and when they appear

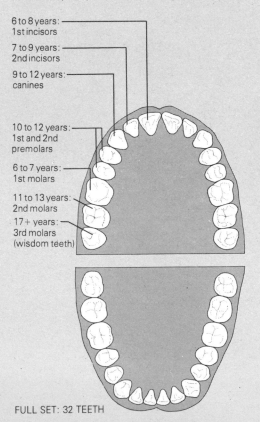

6 to 8 years:
1st incisors

7 to 9 years:
2nd incisors

9 to 12 years:
canines

10 to 12 years:
1st and 2nd premolars

6 to 7 years:
1st molars

11 to 13 years:
2nd molars

17+ years:
3rd molars
(wisdom teeth)

FULL SET: 32 TEETH

Milk (baby) teeth and when they appear

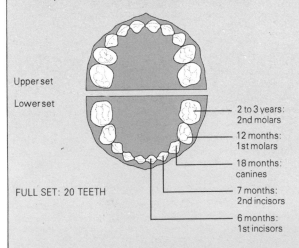

Upper set

Lower set

2 to 3 years:
2nd molars

12 months:
1st molars

18 months:
canines

7 months:
2nd incisors

6 months:
1st incisors

FULL SET: 20 TEETH

Other glands are also affected (their type and number varying from case to case), but usually without serious consequences.

What are the symptoms?
Symptoms sometimes occur immediately after birth: mucus secretions in the baby's intestines make the first bowel motions too thick and sticky for the baby to pass.

In all cases, the child gains little weight right from birth because hardly any nutrients are absorbed from the child's feeds. Intestinal contents pass out of the body as large, pale, greasy-looking faeces that float in water and have a foul smell. The child has recurrent respiratory infections, accompanied by a cough and fever, and these tend to be more severe and persistent than normal.

How common is the problem?
About 1 in every 1,500 babies is born with the disease, which tends to run in families (see *Genetics*, p.704).

What are the risks?
Repeated bouts of pneumonia are common and usually lead to bronchiectasis, which in turn makes the lungs even more susceptible to pneumonia; eventually, this may prove fatal. However, although modern treatment has improved the prospects for many children, a large number do not reach adulthood.

What should be done?
If cystic fibrosis is known to run in your family, your baby's first bowel movements will be tested to discover whether he or she has the disease. If the disorder is diagnosed this early, immediate treatment can lessen respiratory infections and lung damage, and lengthen the child's life expectancy.

In cases when abnormal faeces and failure to put on weight are obvious soon after birth, the doctor will follow up the symptoms. But in some cases, when respiratory infections are the predominant feature and do not develop until some weeks after birth, you may be the first person to discover that something is wrong; in that case, consult your doctor as soon as possible. Hospital tests will then be carried out to confirm the diagnosis.

Although the child will grow up underdeveloped and tend to miss school a lot, parents are advised not to over-protect the child and should encourage him or her to be as active as possible.

If cystic fibrosis runs in your family and you are considering having a child, or if you want another child after having had one who has the disease, you should seek *genetic counselling* (p.619) through your doctor.

What is the treatment?
Extracts of animal pancreas, in powder or granule form, are given to replace the missing enzymes from the pancreas, and the amount of fat in the child's diet is reduced. With this treatment, the child puts on weight and the stools become much more normal.

To keep the lungs as free of mucus as possible, the child needs to have daily *physiotherapy*, which includes postural drainage (see *Bronchiectasis*, p.363). This can be carried out at home; the physiotherapist will show you what to do. Respiratory infections are treated with large doses of *antibiotics* which, in severe cases, may be given by aerosol inhalation, so that they can act directly on the lungs.

The *Cystic Fibrosis Research Trust* (p.768) provides valuable advice and support for the parents of afflicted children.

Lactose intolerance

The lining of the small intestine normally produces an *enzyme* called lactase, which breaks down lactose (the sugar in human and powdered cow's milk), enabling it to be absorbed into the bloodstream. A severe attack of gastroenteritis (see *Gastroenteritis in infants*, p.649) can sometimes temporarily damage the intestinal lining, which then produces little or no lactase. The result of this is not apparent at first, because, until the diarrhoea and vomiting caused by the gastroenteritis stop, the baby is taken off milk and given boiled water. It is only when cow's milk is gradually reintroduced that a reaction to the deficiency of lactase occurs: the lactose in the milk is not absorbed into the bloodstream but ferments in the gut, causing vomiting and frothy, explosive diarrhoea.

What is the treatment?
If the doctor treating the gastroenteritis suspects that the return of the diarrhoea is not a symptom of recurring gastroenteritis but of lactase deficiency, he or she will put the baby on to a synthetic milk containing little or no lactose. If this improves the condition, the diagnosis is confirmed, and the baby continues with the synthetic feed. The intestine will eventually return to normal. Determining when this has happened is done by periodically trying the baby with cow's milk until it no longer causes diarrhoea.

Hepatitis in children

Hepatitis is inflammation of the liver. It is caused by a virus that enters the body through the mouth and is carried to the liver in the bloodstream. Of the various forms of hepatitis, the only one likely to affect children is *acute hepatitis A* (p.486) – so-called because the virus concerned is called the type A virus. The disease, which develops between two and six weeks after the initial infection, is milder in children than in adults.

What should be done?
A child who develops *jaundice* (p.485) and other, flu-like, symptoms should see a doctor, who will usually advise bed rest. One symptom of the disease is severe loss of appetite. Give the child frequent glucose or sugary drinks, and keep encouraging him or her to eat. After about two weeks in bed the child usually feels well enough to get up, and after a further two weeks he or she should be able to return to school.

Hepatitis is a *contagious* (catching) disease, and while the child is ill he or she, together with other members of the family, should avoid contact with other children. The family should be even more careful than usual about washing hands after using the lavatory and before meals. And the lavatory pan and any potties should be cleaned several times a day with an antiseptic lavatory-cleaner.

The outlook is excellent. There are no after-effects of the disease except the beneficial one of immunity from further attacks.

Growth disorders

If you consult the *Growth charts* on p.645, you will see that there are wide ranges of heights and weights in normal, healthy children – differences due mainly to hereditary factors. Usually, it is only if your child's size falls outside the normal range for his or her age that one of the following growth disorders may be responsible.

Nutritional disorders
The most common nutritional problem among children (and adults) in the Western world is *obesity* (p.492). Obesity needs to be treated not only because it is harmful to the child's health but because it often persists into adult life, when it increases the risks accompanying many diseases. At the other extreme is malnutrition, which may be due to social factors or to illness such as *coeliac disease* (p.684) and *cystic fibrosis* (p.685).

Delayed puberty
Puberty normally starts in girls at about $11\frac{1}{2}$ and in boys at about $13\frac{1}{2}$. Delay in its onset is often hereditary (see the section entitled *Special problems of adolescents*, p.706).

Hormonal disorders
These illnesses – mainly caused by inadequate hormone production by the pituitary gland or thyroid gland – are the least common of the growth disorders. They include *gigantism* (p.516), *dwarfism* (p.516), and *hypothyroidism* (p.526).

Permanent impairment of growth may also be caused as a side-effect of certain severe chronic diseases – for example, *congenital heart disorders* (p.656), *sickle-cell anaemia* (p.422), *thalassaemia* (p.422), *rheumatoid arthritis* (p.552), and chronic kidney trouble.

What should be done?
If you are concerned about your child's size, take him or her to the doctor. After an examination, your doctor will probably be able to reassure you that there is nothing wrong. If an underlying disorder is suspected, your doctor will arrange for appropriate diagnostic tests.

Rickets

A child with rickets usually has misshapen (bowed) legs

If a child has inadequate calcium in the blood, the bones are not as strong as they should be. The leg bones bend (usually outwards) under the weight of the child, causing bowleggedness. This is rickets, which usually first shows itself between the ages of one and two.

The main cause of calcium deficiency is not enough vitamin D – or, less commonly, not enough calcium – in the diet (see *Vitamins*, p.494). Occasionally, lack of sunshine, from which the body manufactures some vitamin D, contributes to the deficiency. (The equivalent in adults is *osteomalacia*, p.543.)

In the past, rickets was a fairly common disease in Britain because of the large number of poorly-nourished children living in built-up, smog-bound city areas. Today it is extremely rare. Vitamins are given routinely to infants, and nearly all modern children have an adequate mixed diet, which provides them with sufficient quantities of vitamin D and calcium. They also get enough sunshine. The only children at risk are a small percentage who are on a poor diet; these are additionally at risk if they are dark-skinned and can therefore absorb little sunshine.

What is the treatment?

You will be advised to give your child a balanced diet, supplemented daily by vitamin D (in tablet or liquid form) and large quantities of calcium, usually in milk. Do not give excessive doses of vitamin D, as these can be harmful. This treatment hardens the bones, and unless the child is already markedly deformed, he or she develops normally. In the rare cases when the legs are noticeably affected, operations may be needed to correct this; the results are usually excellent.

Phenyl-ketonuria

To develop and function the body needs protein, which is made up of chemicals called amino-acids. Normally, excess amounts of any amino-acid taken into the body are broken down into harmless constituent chemicals. In phenylketonuria (known for short as PKU), the body, through an inherited defect, lacks the *enzyme* necessary to break down one of these amino-acids, phenylalanine. The main danger is that if excess phenylalanine accumulates in the still-developing body of a fetus or infant, it damages the nervous system.

In the rare cases when a baby with PKU develops in the womb of a mother who herself suffers from the disorder, the baby is affected by the high level of phenylalanine in the mother's body and he or she is likely to be born with a small, deformed brain and, in some cases, also a deformed heart. If, as is usually the case, the mother is only a "carrier" of the disorder, or has the disorder but is on a low-phenylalanine diet, the baby with PKU is normal at birth. A blood test for PKU, called the Guthrie test, is given to all babies at six days old. If the test reveals PKU, treatment starts immediately.

The disorder is extremely rare in Britain, affecting only 1 in 12,000 babies born. But it is becoming slightly more common as modern treatment allows more sufferers to reach adulthood and have children.

What is the treatment?

The baby is immediately given special bottle feeds low in phenylalanine (a certain amount of which is essential to the body). No breast-feeding is allowed. When the baby progresses to specially selected solids, the milk feed is continued as the protein source. The child with PKU has to keep to a diet based on vegetables and salads. To provide the necessary protein, vitamins, and minerals, the diet is supplemented with a number of special proprietary foods. (For further information contact the *National Society for Phenylketonuria*, p.768.)

The low-phenylalanine diet is quite expensive and requires a lot of imagination and careful preparation if the child is not to find it monotonous. For this reason, doctors are anxious to establish whether at a certain age the child's organs are sufficiently well-developed to resist damage caused by high levels of phenylalanine, so that he or she can then safely progress to a normal diet. Trials indicate that a normal diet might be possible at about the age of 10 or 12.

A woman with treated phenylketonuria who is eating normal food should revert to the special low-phenylalanine diet before becoming pregnant. This is to ensure that her own body level of phenylalanine falls to a point where it will not damage the baby developing in her uterus.

Constipation in children

Like adults (see *Constipation and diarrhoea*, p.474) the bowel habits of children vary. A child should be regarded as constipated only if he or she does not pass any faeces for a period of at least four or five days.

A diet deficient in *fibre* is responsible for many cases of constipation. Ensure your child has enough fibre by including fruit, vegetables, and bran in his or her diet (see *The components of a healthy diet*, p.25). Babies of six months or more can be given bran in the form of wholemeal cereals, but check with your doctor first.

A child may also become constipated during an acute infection, through drinking less or sweating more than usual. Rather than giving the child a laxative, encourage him or her to take as much fluid as possible.

Another cause of constipation is an *anal fissure* (p.484), a small tear in the anus which makes the passing of faeces painful. Severe constipation, lasting for two weeks or more, may be a symptom of *Hirschprung's disease* (p.662) or of *hypothyroidism* (p.526).

If your child is constipated, take him or her to the doctor. Do not try to cure the condition yourself by giving a laxative.

Medical myth

Sugar or fruit juice should be added to the bottle feed of a constipated baby.

Wrong. This treatment will probably cause diarrhoea.

Urinary tract and sex organs

The urinary tract consists of the two kidneys; the two tubes called ureters leading from the kidneys to the bladder; the bladder itself; and the tube leading from the bladder to the outside, the urethra. (See *Disorders of the urinary tract*, p.500, for details).

Urinary problems in children should always receive medical attention. In particular, urine that looks abnormal must be reported to your doctor. This is because if there is some abnormality in your child's urinary tract, then early diagnosis and treatment will virtually remove the risk of *chronic kidney failure* (p.512) developing in later life.

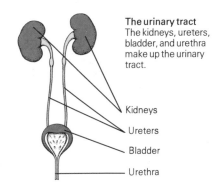

The urinary tract
The kidneys, ureters, bladder, and urethra make up the urinary tract.

Kidneys

Ureters

Bladder

Urethra

Bed-wetting
(enuresis)

Medical myths

Children who wet the bed sleep more deeply, and generally pass more urine, than other children.

Wrong. Children who wet the bed sleep as deeply and pass as much urine as other children.

Cutting down on drinks before bed-time prevents bed-wetting.

Wrong. This measure is unlikely to have a marked effect on the problem.

By the age of about three and a half, approximately 75 per cent of all children are dry at night; but the other quarter continue to wet the bed, and in a few cases also wet their clothes during the day. The medical term for this incontinence is enuresis. If the child becomes enuretic after a long period of dryness following successful toilet-training, this is known as secondary enuresis.

The cause of enuresis, especially secondary enuresis, can be psychological. For example, it may be stress resulting from the arrival of a new baby or separation from the mother. In a small minority of cases, there may be an underlying physical cause, such as an infection (see *Urinary infections in children*, below), *spina bifida* (p.654), of which continuous dribbling is one symptom, or *diabetes mellitus* (p.519), which is also marked by constant thirst. But in most cases, the cause of bed-wetting is unknown.

Enuresis often runs in families, and can continue for a number of years. The problem is slightly more common in boys.

What should be done?
At some time during the late evening, wake the child to give him or her the opportunity to use the lavatory. If, after a few weeks, this fails to have any effect and the bed-wetting continues, consult your doctor to make sure there is nothing physically wrong. The doctor will take a sample of urine for analysis, and – in rare cases – the child may be referred to a *paediatrician* for further tests.

The same principles that apply to toilet-training should also be followed to deal with bed-wetting. Praise the child for any dry nights, and encourage him or her to keep a record of them; but never scold or punish the child for wet nights or record them. This can deeply hurt the child, who, after all, has no control over the problem.

What is the treatment?
If the child is seven or over, the doctor or paediatrician may suggest the use of an alarm machine, which rings loudly and wakes the child as soon as the first drop of urine is passed into the bed. This has the eventual effect on many children of making them wake up whenever they feel the need to urinate, before they have passed any urine.

Whatever the underlying cause and the measures used, the problem will nearly always clear up before adolescence.

Urinary infections in children

In a urinary-tract infection, microbes – usually bacteria – gain access to and multiply in the urinary tract. The process of infection is much the same in children as in adults – see *Infections, inflammation, and injury*, p.502, for further information. However, the site of the infection and the symptoms it causes rarely are as clear-cut in children as they are in adults. For example, a baby with a urinary-tract infection may simply have an unexplained fever and feed poorly. An older child suffering from an infection is likely to have a fever, feel generally unwell, and appear to forget previous bladder training.

How common is the problem?

Infections of the urinary tract are quite common during childhood. In an average year in Britain, 1 child in 100 is diagnosed as having the problem. During the school years, 25 times more girls than boys are affected.

What are the risks?

There are few risks from one or two isolated bouts of infection. But if the problem recurs, it may be that the child has some underlying abnormality of the urinary tract (see *Chronic pyelonephritis*, p.503, for further details). It is essential that any such abnormality is detected and treated as soon as possible in order to prevent chronic pyelonephritis.

What should be done?

Take your child to the doctor if you suspect that he or she has a urinary infection. The doctor will carry out an examination and will probably take a sample of urine for laboratory analysis. If the result indicates a problem, your child will be referred to a hospital specialist for diagnostic tests, including an *intravenous pyelogram (IVP)* and a *micturating cystogram*.

What is the treatment?

Self-help: Ensure that your child follows all the doctor's instructions as regards drinking extra fluids or eating specific foods. Encourage the child to empty his or her bladder completely when using the lavatory; going again a few minutes later will help this. And although symptoms of the condition may subside a few days after starting a course of drugs (see "Professional help" below), the course must be completed as prescribed.

Professional help: The infection itself is usually treated by a course of *antibiotics*, in tablet or liquid form. If tests have revealed any underlying abnormality of the tract, a long course of antibiotics will be given to prevent the infection recurring, and corrective surgery may need to be carried out.

Nephritis

There are several forms of the disease called *glomerulonephritis* (see p.504 for a general description, and see also *Nephrotic syndrome*, opposite). One form that affects children in particular is usually called nephritis. It develops in a child who has had a streptococcal (bacterial) infection, usually a sore throat, two or three weeks previously. The body makes certain chemicals called *antibodies* to fight the invading bacteria, which they do successfully. But through some fault in the body's immune system the antibodies persist and begin to harm the kidneys. The kidneys become inflamed, unable to produce normal amounts of urine, and they allow blood to leak into the urine.

What are the symptoms?

The symptoms appear over a few days. One main symptom is a reduced amount of urine which looks smoky or reddish-brown because of the blood in it. The other main symptom is accumulation of fluid in the body due to reduced urine output. The fluid (*oedema*) appears as swellings around the eyes and face, or even over the whole body. In addition, some children suffer from a headache and raised temperature.

How common is the problem?

Nephritis is rare; it complicates only a small fraction of streptococcal infections. In an average year, 1 child in 3,000 of school age receives medical attention for the problem.

What are the risks?

There are few risks associated with nephritis. Occasionally the build-up of fluid in the body causes the child's blood pressure to rise dramatically; this results in a severe headache, vomiting, and perhaps convulsions. Consult your doctor without delay should this happen.

A child who suffers from repeated attacks of any urinary problem, including nephritis, runs the risk of long-term damage to the kidneys. The result after many years could be *chronic kidney failure* (p.512). If this applies to your child, discuss the situation with your doctor, who may arrange for a specialist examination.

What should be done?

Nephritis is a problem that requires medical attention. Abnormal-looking urine in particular should always be reported to the doctor. If after a physical examination the doctor suspects nephritis, blood and urine samples will be collected. Laboratory analysis of the urine sample will confirm the diagnosis while analysis of the blood sample should reveal which antibodies are causing the nephritis.

What is the treatment?

The doctor will usually advise that the child rests quietly, in bed if he or she is very ill. In addition, the child will be put on a restricted diet that aims to reduce amounts of salt, fluids, and protein (meat, fish, eggs). The diet continues until urine amounts are back to normal and is designed to ease strain on the kidneys and to counteract accumulation of fluid in the body.

Drugs that aid recovery include a course of *antibiotics* to eradicate any remaining bacteria, and a *diuretic* to increase the amount of water lost in the urine.

Certain children who are considered at risk will be admitted to hospital so that any complications can be dealt with straight away. If blood pressure rises to a dangerously high level, further drugs are given to control it (see *High blood pressure*, p.382). But even with complications, prospects for a full recovery within a week or so are excellent.

Nephrotic syndrome

Like *nephritis* (opposite), nephrotic syndrome is a form of *glomerulonephritis* (see p.504 for a general description of this disease). For most children with nephrotic syndrome, the cause is unknown. In nephrotic syndrome the tiny filtering units in the kidneys, the glomeruli, are damaged. One result is that proteins leak from the blood through the glomeruli into the urine. Also, the volume of urine is much reduced, so that fluid which should be passed out of the body starts to accumulate in the tissues just under the skin.

Oedema in children
A child with a kidney disorder may develop oedema. This is characterized by a puffy face and swollen abdomen and ankles.

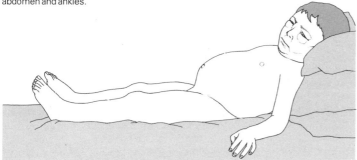

What are the symptoms?
There are two main symptoms of nephrotic syndrome. The first is the gradual appearance, over several weeks, of generalized swelling throughout the child's body, due to accumulation of fluid (*oedema*). The swelling is especially noticeable around the eyes and face, and the abdomen may be distended.

The second main symptom is a much reduced output of urine – perhaps as little as one fifth of the normal output. The urine usually looks normal.

How common is the problem?
Nephrotic syndrome is uncommon. It affects a slightly higher number of children than nephritis. The condition usually starts

between the ages of two and four, and it is slightly more common in boys.

What are the risks?
A child with the syndrome is vulnerable to a variety of infections – for example, *peritonitis* (p.470). But the main risk is that in about 10 per cent of cases the condition cannot be completely cured, despite intensive treatment. As these children grow up, most of them develop *chronic pyelonephritis* (p.503).

What should be done?
Consult your doctor if your child appears to be developing oedema. The doctor will examine the child and take a sample of urine for laboratory analysis. If results of the analysis suggest nephrotic syndrome, you will be referred to a hospital specialist for further tests on samples of blood and urine (and, if necessary, a *biopsy* of the kidney).

What is the treatment?
Self-help: Although the condition often requires hospital treatment, you can help your child by ensuring that he or she keeps to a special diet and takes any drugs exactly as advised by the doctor. Food should be cooked and served without salt, and the food itself should contain plenty of protein – fish, meat, eggs, and cheese. The doctor may also advise a restricted fluid intake.

Professional help: Usually the child is admitted to hospital, where treatment by diet and drugs is more easily supervised. The drugs used are *steroids*. They are given in high doses at first but the amount is gradually reduced and stopped after about eight weeks. The symptoms clear up by the end of the second week, and the child is allowed home.

In about half of cases there is complete recovery with no after-effects. The remainder will have another attack of the condition after several weeks or months; treatment as described will again relieve the symptoms. In a small proportion of sufferers attacks continue to recur, and often a prolonged course of drugs over six months or a year will eventually cure the condition.

Wilm's tumour

In this disorder, which almost exclusively affects children under five, a *malignant* tumour forms on one of the kidneys. The main symptom of the tumour is a hard lump on one side of the abdomen; there may also be blood in the urine and abdominal pain.

How common is the problem?
Wilm's tumour is very rare; it accounts for 5 per cent of cancer deaths in children between two and 12 years of age.

What are the risks?
The risks are those of all cancers: that the malignant cells will spread to other parts of the body. However, the recent advances in treatment have greatly improved the outlook for children affected by the disease.

What should be done?
If you notice the symptoms described, consult your doctor. If he or she suspects a tumour, the child will be given a special *X-ray* test, known as an *intravenous pyelogram* (*IVP*).

What is the treatment?
If Wilm's tumour is diagnosed, the affected kidney is removed surgically. The child will also be given *cytotoxic* (anti-cancer) drugs, to destroy any remaining cancer cells; and *radiotherapy* may also be used for this purpose. Over 80 per cent of children are cured.

Undescended testes
(*cryptorchidism*)

In boys, the testes (the male sex glands) develop inside the abdomen from the same tissue that forms the ovaries in girls. Normally, by a month before birth, they have descended through the abdominal wall into the sac called the scrotum.

In a very small proportion of boys, one or both testes fail to descend by birth, for reasons that are not known. The condition does not cause the baby any pain or problems with urinating.

Usually, undescended testes do eventually descend during the boy's first few years, and regular medical check-ups are carried out by your doctor until this happens.

What should be done?
Undescended testes may eventually cause infertility if not corrected. If either or both testes have not descended by the time the boy is five or thereabouts, an operation known as an orchidopexy is carried out to lower the testis or testes into the normal position. This involves a stay of two or three days in hospital. Once the testes are descended, there should be no further problems.

Vulvovaginitis

Vulvovaginitis is redness, itching, and soreness of the vulva, the opening to the vagina (see *Vagina and vulva*, p.602, for a description of this part of the body). It affects only a small proportion of girls, those who have a particularly sensitive vulva (see also *Pruritis vulvae*, p.603). In many cases, no cause can be found for the condition. In other cases, it is brought about by infection from faecal microbes; by a skin allergy to wool or nylon; by bed-wetting; by *threadworms* (p.703); or, very rarely, by the child having inserted a foreign body into the vagina.

What are the symptoms?
The soreness can produce a frequent desire to urinate, and this urination is sometimes painful; some parents may mistakenly believe that their daughter has a bladder disorder. If a foreign body has been inserted in the vagina, there may be a foul-smelling discharge.

What should be done?
In all cases, you should take your daughter to visit a doctor. If he or she suspects that a foreign body in the vagina is causing the trouble, an anaesthetic will be given and the vagina will be examined and any object removed. This should cure the trouble.

What is the treatment?
In most cases, self-help by careful hygiene is the answer. After opening her bowels, the girl should wipe herself in a backward direction only. She should take a bath daily, and the vulva should also be washed after defecation. After all bathing, the area should be dried thoroughly but gently, and dusted with medicated talc, and then a silicone ointment ("barrier cream") applied. The silicone ointment, obtainable from a chemist's, forms a protective barrier against faecal viruses. Knickers should be changed daily. They should be made of cotton – or, if of some other material, have a cotton gusset – and be loose-fitting.

If you follow the above measures carefully, and keep to any advice your doctor gives you, the condition should eventually clear up and leave no after-effects.

To keep infection from the urinary tract, always wipe from front to back.

Muscles, bones, and joints

The most common cause of muscle, bone, or joint problems in children is injury (see *Injuries*, p.532). Most childhood injuries heal quickly and well. In addition to injuries, there are a few disorders which are especially troublesome in children. One of these is rheumatic fever. It is very rare, but severe or recurrent bouts can lead to valvular heart disease (see *Heart valves*, p.392). A bone infection, called osteomyelitis, can also have serious complications, but is usually treated successfully. Still's disease, a rare *autoimmune* disorder, will normally have run its course when the child reaches puberty. Muscular dystrophy, however, is an inherited disease that causes progressive wasting of the muscles; intensive research is being carried out to find a cure for this disease.

Rheumatic fever in children

Rheumatic fever is a disease which most commonly attacks children of school age, particularly those in the six-to-eight age group. It is usually, but not always, characterized by a painful swelling of certain joints (for a general description of the disease as it affects adults, see *Rheumatic fever*, p.393). The disease originates in a throat infection caused by a particular strain of streptococcus bacterium. The body produces specific *antibodies* to destroy the bacteria, but in some children the antibodies also attack the tissues of the joints; less commonly, they attack the tissues of the heart, or the tissues of both heart and joints. Inflammation of the joints has no long-lasting effect, but recurrent inflammation of the heart can occasionally cause permanent damage to the heart valves.

Few children infected by the streptococcus bacterium contract rheumatic fever. Their susceptibility is at least partly hereditary, and is intensified if they are undernourished and live in cold, damp, overcrowded homes.

What are the symptoms?
The symptoms of rheumatic fever appear between one and four weeks after the initial sore throat. If the joints have been affected, one or two become red, swollen, and painful to move (this condition is known as acute rheumatic arthritis); the child also has a fever, loss of appetite, feels generally unwell, and is often pale and sweaty. The inflammation of the joints usually disappears after about 24 hours, but if by this stage the disease has not been treated, other joints may in turn become temporarily inflamed. The disease is characteristically described as "flitting from joint to joint". The wrists, elbows, knees, and ankles are most commonly affected. The hips and shoulders occasionally become inflamed; the fingers and toes scarcely ever. If the heart alone has been affected (this is called acute rheumatic carditis), there are often, in mild cases, no obvious symptoms. The only symptoms are vague ones such as tiredness, paleness, and general sickliness. There is a danger in these mild cases that it is not thought necessary to consult the doctor, and the condition remains undiagnosed.

Severe cases of heart trouble are marked by definite symptoms, chiefly breathlessness, especially during exertion or when the child is lying down, and the accumulation of fluid (*oedema*) under the skin of the legs and back.

In some cases of rheumatic fever a rash appears, usually on the chest, back, and abdomen. The rash consists of reddish circles with pale centres; they are usually 20 or 30mm (about 1in) across and keep changing in shape. The rash does not itch.

Nodules, or little swellings, sometimes appear – particularly when the heart is affected. They develop just below the skin, over bony prominences such as the elbows, knees, knuckles, and the back of the head. They are usually round, about 5 or 10mm across, and firm and painless.

How common is the problem?
Rheumatic fever is no longer the widespread problem that it used to be. Even within the last 20 years the number of cases has decreased by seven or eight times. This is the result partly of *antibiotic* treatment of the initial infections. It is also the result of general improvements in living conditions, diet, and hygiene, which have made the bacterium responsible for the disease less common and have increased people's resistance to it.

What are the risks?
Unless it is severe, a single attack of rheumatic fever is unlikely to lead to valvular heart disease (see, for example, *Mitral stenosis*, p.395, and *Aortic incompetence*, p.399). The

risk of heart disease lies in one or more further attacks. At one time, a child who had had rheumatic fever was more likely than other children to have an attack in the future, but today the long-term prescription of *antibiotics* for a child who has had one attack should protect the child from further streptococcal throat infections. The child who still runs a risk of developing heart disease is the one whose attack of rheumatic fever has passed unnoticed (see "What are the symptoms?" above) and for this reason it is wise to consult your doctor whenever your child has a sore throat.

In very severe cases of rheumatic fever affecting the heart, there is a slight risk of *heart failure* (p.381).

What should be done?
If your child has any of the symptoms described, put him or her to bed and consult your doctor. If the doctor suspects rheumatic fever, a *throat swab* will be taken, together with a sample of the child's blood for hospital laboratory tests. The doctor will also examine the child carefully, listening to the chest with a *stethoscope*, to discover whether the heart has been affected.

What is the treatment?
If the attack is mild, the child can rest in bed at home until tests show the attack is over.

In more severe cases, the child is admitted to hospital. There the pain and swelling of inflamed joints is quickly eased by fairly high doses of soluble aspirin. When the heart has also been affected, the drug may be continued (in smaller doses) after the inflammation has disappeared.

In particularly severe cases, especially when the heart is seriously affected, a course of more powerful anti-inflammatory drugs, perhaps *steroids*, may be prescribed. In the rare event of actual heart failure, further drugs (such as anti-arrhythmics and diuretics) may be given. Whenever the heart is affected, the child must be propped up in bed with pillows to ease any breathlessness that might occur. In all cases, an *antibiotic* drug is prescribed to get rid of any bacteria that remain from the original throat infection, and to prevent further attacks.

What are the long-term prospects?
Today the long-term prospects are good. After any attack of rheumatic fever, mild or severe, doctors now prescribe *antibiotics* to be taken daily over a period of years to prevent a further attack. For those children whose hearts have been damaged by rheumatic fever, the antibiotics may have to be taken for the rest of their lives. In rare cases, valvular heart disease does develop – usually through undiagnosed attacks of rheumatic fever, or further attacks through failure to take the antibiotics regularly. But with modern treatment, most sufferers can lead a normal or near-normal life.

Muscular dystrophy

Muscular dystrophy is a progressive wasting and weakening of the muscles. There are several forms of the disease. Some of them are very rare, and affect both boys and girls. The most common and well-known form, with which this article deals, is Duchenne muscular dystrophy, which affects only boys. This disease starts during childhood (usually before the age of five) and initially affects the muscles of the shoulders, hips, thighs, and calves. In time, it spreads to all muscles, causing progressive crippling and immobility.

Like *haemophilia* (p.424), some cases of Duchenne muscular dystrophy are inherited through female "carriers" of the disease. But spontaneous cases, arising in families with no history of the disease, also occur.

What are the symptoms?
The boy develops a waddling gait, with the feet wide apart. He has trouble climbing stairs, falls easily, and finds it difficult to get up. He can also scarcely raise his arms above his head. The affected muscles sometimes look larger than normal; this is due to fatty tissue replacing wasted muscle tissue. In most cases, the limbs and spine become deformed, until by the time of adolescence the boy is confined to a wheelchair.

What are the risks?
Because the sufferer cannot exercise his chest properly, he becomes more susceptible to serious chest infections.

What should be done?
If your son shows a combination of the signs that suggest muscular dystrophy, consult your doctor. Hospital tests will show whether the boy has the disease or not.

Any woman from a family with a history of the disease should consult a doctor before deciding to have a child (see *Genetic counselling*, p.619). If a carrier gives birth to a boy, there is a 50 per cent chance that he will have muscular dystrophy. If the woman decides to

Visual sign
A distinctive sign of muscular dystrophy is when a child starts having problems in getting into an upright position.

go ahead and have a child, the sex of the fetus can be tested during early pregnancy (see *Amniocentesis*, p.639). If the fetus is male, the mother will be given the opportunity to have the pregnancy terminated.

What is the treatment?
No cure has yet been found for the disease. *Physiotherapy* treatment is given to help minimize deformities; but even so it is likely that the boy will need to attend a school for the physically handicapped. Eventually, by about the age of 20, the sufferer will probably succumb to a fatal chest infection.

For the parents of boys afflicted with this disease, the *Muscular Dystrophy Group of Great Britain* (p.768) provides valuable help and guidance.

Osteo-myelitis

Osteomyelitis is an infection in an area of bone. The condition can be either acute or chronic. Despite its apparent inertness, bone is an active, living tissue and is honeycombed by blood vessels (see *Bone diseases*, p.543, for further details). In osteomyelitis, bacteria from, for example, a contaminated skin wound get into the blood and set up an infection in the bone. Or, in some cases, the infection may affect an area of bone after a minor injury to the bone two or three weeks previously. The area becomes inflamed and pus forms just as in a skin infection such as a *boil* (p.251). Usually only a single area in one of the limb bones near a joint is affected, but rarely (and especially in younger sufferers) more than one bone becomes infected. Sometimes the infection does not spread but is walled off in a cavity of bone. There it remains dormant, perhaps for years, until for some reason the sufferer's natural resistance is lowered, and the condition flares up.

What are the symptoms?
Symptoms usually develop over two or three days. The main symptom is pain and excruciating tenderness in the affected area, particularly when the joint near it is flexed. An infant or younger child will be reluctant to move an arm or a leg, and will probably scream with pain if the limb is touched or moved. If a leg bone is infected, then the child

---

Malignant diseases in childhood

Malignant diseases (cancer) in childhood are extremely rare. Only 0.8 per cent of all hospital admissions of children under 14 are for cases of cancer (and this figure includes repeated admissions of the same children).

If your child develops cancer, the doctors in charge of the case will discuss with you the nature of the disease, the necessary treatment, and the outlook for the child. Treatment will probably be given at a special hospital *oncology* unit. It may involve surgery, *radiotherapy*, and *cytotoxic* (anti-cancer) drugs. You must be prepared for the distressing side-effects that often occur with the last two treatments: for example, vomiting, loss of hair, and weakness. The child may need repeated *X-rays*, *biopsies*, and other tests, and in some cases may need to spend days or weeks in a limited-access, germ-free isolation unit.

The cure rate in childhood cancer is on average greater than 50 per cent, but varies considerably according to the disease concerned. For example, cases of recovery in some forms of leukaemia are as low as 10 per cent, but in *Hodgkin's disease* (p.433) the cure rate is as high as 80 per cent.

You are probably the best judge of how much to tell your child about the illness. If you are unsure about this, ask the advice of the doctors involved. Whichever course you adopt, talk to your child at the earliest opportunity, before there is any chance of his or her being wrongly, and perhaps alarmingly, informed about the illness by another child in the hospital.

After some time, your child may be allowed to leave hospital, depending on the nature of the disease and the stage it has reached. Once the child is home, it is important not to treat him or her in an over-protective or any other special way. Try to make your child's home life, and your expectations of him or her at school, as normal as possible. In the case of a child with one of the less curable cancers, it may be difficult to encourage success at school when you know he or she may never live to benefit; but, for your child's sake, you must try to preserve the appearance of normality. To help you cope with this difficult time, ask your doctor to put you in touch with local self-help groups formed by other parents of children with cancer. Their experiences may be of help to all your family in learning how to come to terms with the disease.

is reluctant to walk and, if forced to do so, he or she has a pronounced limp.

A generally ill appearance and a high temperature accompany the pain, and if the condition is not treated within another day or two the skin over the infection will have become red and swollen.

How common is the problem?
Osteomyelitis is a rare condition in the Western world. It occurs most frequently between the ages of five and 14, and is more common in boys than in girls.

What are the risks?
In the extremely unlikely event of the condition being completely neglected, the bacteria can spread and multiply in the blood, causing *blood poisoning* (p.421). A more likely, though still rare, risk is that the infection will eat away a considerable area of bone and may even spread into the neighbouring joint. If this happens, the result is likely to be permanent stiffness or deformity of the joint.

Another risk is that the infection will spread upwards and break through to the skin surface. This appears as an *abscess* which discharges pus and which refuses to heal until the underlying bone infection is treated.

What should be done?
If your infant or child has symptoms of osteomyelitis, then consult your doctor without delay. If the doctor's physical examination confirms your suspicions, hospital admission will be necessary right away. To confirm the diagnosis, blood tests and *X-rays* of the area will be carried out.

What is the treatment?
The main treatment is a course of *antibiotic* drugs, given in tablet or liquid form (or perhaps at first in an *intravenous drip*). If necessary, a short operation is carried out to drain and clean out the abscess. In some cases, the doctor will decide to immobilize the affected limb in splints or a plaster cast. Once the infection is on the wane the child will be allowed home, but your doctor's instructions as to taking antibiotics and exercising the affected area must be followed until the condition is cured.

Still's disease

Still's disease is believed to be an intermittent malfunctioning of the body's defence mechanism. Chemicals called *antibodies* produced to combat any invading microbes, attack the body's own tissues. Why this *auto-immune* condition should develop is not known. The antibodies cause inflammation of joints, various organs, and other parts of the body.

The disease starts most commonly between the ages of two and five and comes and goes over a number of years, usually clearing up by puberty. The attacks each last on average for a few weeks, and tend to lessen in severity. Medical opinion is divided as to whether or not the illness is a juvenile form of *rheumatoid arthritis* (p.552).

What are the symptoms?
The child usually has, for at least part of the time, a raised temperature. The temperature often swings from normal in the morning to about 39.5°C (103°F) in the evening. Appetite is poor, resulting in loss of weight. Sometimes a rash of red pimples breaks out over the trunk and limbs. *Anaemia* (p.419) develops in many cases.

Sites of inflammation vary considerably from child to child. The front of one or both eyes may become red and painful; the lymph glands in the neck and armpits may swell; the outer membrane of the heart may be inflamed, giving rise to chest pain; and the lungs may be damaged – signified by a bad cough. In a large proportion of cases the joints become swollen, stiff, and painful. Most commonly the knees, ankles, elbows, and joints of the neck are affected, usually gradually, but sometimes abruptly. Over the years, the joints may become deformed in a few sufferers, and the muscles of the affected limbs become weaker.

How common is the problem?
Still's disease is rare: each year only 1 new case occurs in every 2,500 children under 14. Girls are affected about twice as often as boys. Occasionally more than one member of a family is affected by the disorder.

What are the risks?
Although the child may be extremely ill, especially at the onset of Still's disease, it is rare for the disorder to be fatal. In a small proportion of cases, inflammation of the joints leads to partial or crippling deformity. Very rarely, inflammation of the eyes can lead to partial or complete blindness.

What should be done?
If your child has a combination of the symptoms described, see your doctor, who will

usually refer you both to a *paediatrician*. A physical examination and laboratory analysis of blood samples are usually sufficient for a firm diagnosis to be made. If it is only the joints that are swollen and there are doubts about the cause, a *biopsy* of the membrane called the *synovium* (which encloses the joint) will be carried out.

What is the treatment?

Self-help: The child should have plenty of rest but should be allowed to get up when he or she feels like it. Give the child an *analgesic*, such as junior aspirin, to ease the pain. This can also have the effect of relieving inflammation of the tissues. Provide a nutritious, balanced diet containing plenty of protein, and encourage the child to eat. For children who have inflammation of the joints in the fingers and hand, special cutlery (available through the NHS) is a great help. If the child cannot get to school, contact your local education authority, who may be able to provide a home tutor.

Professional help: Your doctor will treat the disease in much the same way as he or she would treat rheumatoid arthritis. *Corticosteroid* drugs may be necessary during the early stages, but they are rarely used as a long-term treatment. They are extremely valuable in bringing relief to inflamed joints and will also be given in the form of eye drops if the eyes have been affected.

Severe anaemia may be treated by a blood transfusion. In addition, *physiotherapy* exercises are advised when the joints are affected. These are exercises both for the parent to perform on the joints and for the child to do alone. It is important that the child does the exercises as well as he or she is able; do your utmost to give encouragement and praise.

What are the long-term prospects?

Once the disease has run its course, the child will usually enjoy normal health. In only a few cases will there be a legacy of deformed joints or damaged sight, and of these cases only a small proportion will be serious.

Flat feet, bow legs, and knock knees

From the time most children begin to learn to walk until the onset of puberty, their legs and feet gradually change shape. Flat feet, bow legs, and knock knees are stages through which all children pass to some degree, and are usually no cause for concern.

At birth, a normal baby has flat feet. Arches develop slowly over the first 6 years. Until the age of 2, the child tends to have bow legs – that is, when the ankles are touching, the knees are not. As the child learns to walk, this tendency is increasingly reversed until, at the age of 3 or 4, he or she tends to be knock-kneed – when the child stands knees together, the ankles do not touch. Over the next few years, the knees and ankles become more aligned until by the teens the legs and feet appear normal.

In the vast majority of children with flat feet, bow legs, or knock knees, no treatment is necessary. Be sure that your child has well-fitting shoes and plenty of opportunity to exercise his or her growing feet and legs. In some children one or more of these variations in posture may persist into adolescence and even adulthood. Only rarely are they caused by a disease such as *rickets* (p.687). If your child's feet or legs seem to be developing abnormally, or your child's walking seems slow to progress, consult your doctor.

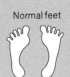

Normal feet

Flat feet

Flat feet
A child with flat feet has no arches and therefore makes a different foot imprint from a child whose arches have developed.

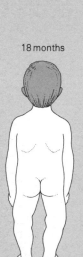

18 months

4 years

Bow legs and knock knees
A child will usually have bow legs until the age of 2 (far left). From this age until the child is about 4 the knees gradually come together and the child will probably be knock-kneed (left) for a few years.

Childhood infectious diseases

An infectious disease is a disease caused by microbes that enter and multiply within the body. Certain infectious diseases are usually caught during childhood and, once you have had the infection, you are very unlikely to catch the same one again (why this is so is explained below). The more common childhood infections are described in the following articles. (For other infectious diseases see *General infections and infestations*, p.558.)

The childhood infectious diseases described here are *contagious* – that is, they spread from one person to another. The causative microbes, which can live outside the body for only a few hours, are usually spread in tiny droplets coughed or sneezed into the air ("droplet infection") and by direct (for example, hand-to-hand) contact. Such diseases often spread through a school as a minor epidemic.

Microbes usually enter the body through the thin lining of the respiratory or digestive tract. Once inside, there is an *incubation period* during which they are not sufficiently numerous to cause any symptoms, and the child is usually unable to infect other people. As the microbes increase in numbers and spread via the bloodstream and the *lymphatic system* (p.432), symptoms begin to appear and the child becomes able to infect others.

Meanwhile the body is fighting the infection in various ways. One way is to manufacture special molecules, called *antibodies*, that disarm or destroy the microbial invaders. (Each disease initiates manufacture of its own particular kind of antibody.)

Once the body has suffered a particular disease it can recognize any reinfection straight away, and antibodies destroy the microbes before they get a foothold. So once you have had the disease, you become immune – that is, you cannot have the same disease again. This is called natural immunity. Sometimes microbes infect a child but the body is able to destroy them even before they cause symptoms. Such children are immune afterwards, although they have not apparently suffered from the disease. Also, the body can be stimulated to produce antibodies against a certain disease by injection of an artificially prepared, harmless version of the microbe concerned. The process of becoming immune – whether by natural or artificial means – is called *immunization* (p.701).

Caring for a feverish child

The various aspects of health care that apply to all the childhood infectious diseases discussed in the following pages are summarized here. More specific information for each disease is included in the separate articles.

General risks of childhood infectious diseases
One rare, though possible, risk of an infectious disease is *encephalitis* (p.274). It is heralded by drowsiness or sleepiness, when it is difficult to wake the child fully; headache; fear of bright lights; and, perhaps, unconsciousness. Encephalitis is serious; it usually comes on a week or so after the infectious disease has cleared up. If you suspect it, contact your doctor at once.

Other risks include febrile convulsions (see *Convulsions in children*, p.667), ear infections such as *acute infection of the middle ear* (p.333) and respiratory-tract infections such as pneumonia (see *Pneumonia in children*, p.679). Refer to the pages indicated and become familiar with the symptoms of these complications; if they occur in your child, consult the doctor without delay.

Any child who develops an infectious disease runs a risk (though only a very slight one) of the complications described above. However, certain children are at special risk and should receive special attention. They include infants under 1 year old; children taking a course of *steroid* drugs; and children who already have a long-term disease – diabetes mellitus, asthma, or cystic fibrosis, for example. If you feel your child is at risk, inform your doctor as soon as symptoms of an infectious disease appear. Contact the doctor also if you know that such a child has been exposed to other children who have since developed an infectious disease. For some diseases (such as measles and chickenpox) the doctor is able to provide temporary protection by giving an injection of ready-made *antibodies* (called "gamma-globulins") which either prevent the child from developing symptoms or make the symptoms much less severe. This form of protection lasts from 4 to 6 months (see *Immunization*, p.701).

How to look after the child
To avoid spreading the infection, keep the child at home, but you do not need to isolate him or her from your other children as they almost certainly have already been exposed to the causative microbes. Junior aspirin or paracetamol, given according to the instructions on the bottle, will lower a raised temperature and ease headaches and muscular aches. (For more details, see *Nursing sick children*, p.764.)

Measles

See p.239,
Visual aids to diagnosis, 26.

Measles is a highly *contagious* disease caused by a virus that spreads throughout the body but affects chiefly the skin and respiratory tract. The *incubation period* of the disease is 10 to 14 days. (See *Childhood infectious diseases*, opposite, for further information.)

What are the symptoms?
The following account of symptoms describes a typical case of measles.

During the first day or two the child becomes miserable, with a raised temperature, runny nose, red watering eyes, dry cough, and perhaps diarrhoea. By the third day the temperature falls and tiny white spots, like grains of salt, appear inside the mouth. On the fourth and fifth days the temperature rises again and the characteristic measles skin rash appears. The rash starts on the forehead and behind the ears as small (2 or 3mm, about $\frac{1}{10}$ in), dull-red, slightly raised spots. The spots gradually spread to the rest of the head and body (but not usually the limbs). As they spread the spots get bigger and join together. By the sixth day the rash is fading, and after a week all symptoms have gone.

Some children with measles complain of headaches and are lethargic. In rare cases, sufferers say that light hurts their eyes. Usually this is no cause for concern, but it is best to mention it to your doctor.

How common is the problem?
In Britain, measles is much less common than it once was; this is due to an immunization programme introduced in the late 1960s. Each year the disease affects 1 child in 50.

What should be done?
You must notify your doctor if you suspect a case of measles; all cases are recorded by the health authorities. If it is an isolated case, the doctor will probably visit you; but if there is a local epidemic, then a telephone description of the symptoms may be enough for a diagnosis. But at the first sign of any complications – such as ear problems, or the symptoms of *encephalitis* (p.274) – consult your doctor without delay.

What is the treatment?
Self-help: There are several ways in which you can make the child more comfortable and guard against possible risks – see *Caring for a feverish child*, opposite. Because measles is so contagious, it is not practicable to try and prevent other members of the family who have not already had the disease from developing it.

Professional help: Because measles is a viral infection, your doctor is unlikely to prescribe *antibiotic* drugs, which are not effective against viruses. (They do, however, work against bacteria, and are used in the event of complications such as ear problems or pneumonia – see *Pneumonia in children*, p.679.)

In the vast majority of children who catch measles, the disease disappears within 10 days and the only after-effect is lifelong immunity to another attack.

German measles
(rubella)

See p.239,
Visual aids to diagnosis, 27.

German measles is a *contagious* disease caused by a virus called the rubella virus. It is a very mild infectious disease – in the majority of children who catch it, it causes no more inconvenience than a common cold. Once inside the body, the virus has an *incubation period* of between 14 and 21 days before it starts to cause any symptoms. (See *Childhood infectious diseases*, opposite, for further information.)

What are the symptoms?
For the first two days the child has a slightly raised temperature, and perhaps swollen glands behind the ears, down the side of the neck, and on the nape of the neck. The rash appears on the first or second day. It consists of flat, reddish-pink spots about 2 or 3mm ($\frac{1}{10}$ in) across, which appear first on the face, then spread rapidly to the body. The rash lasts for only a day or two. By the fourth or fifth day all symptoms have faded away.

How common is the problem?
German measles is slightly less common than *measles* (above), though it is not as highly contagious and so does not occur in epidemics – spreading through a school, for example – in quite the same way.

What are the risks?
Like other childhood infectious diseases, German measles carries the risk of *encephalitis* (p.274), though this occurs in only 1 case in 6,000. A more common complication, particularly in adults, is stiff, swollen joints (see *Infectious arthritis*, p.553).

Because German measles is such a mild disease, little specific treatment is required – see *Caring for a feverish child* (opposite) for further information. But the disease is known to cause damage to babies developing in the uterus. It is therefore essential to contact any pregnant woman who has been exposed to someone suffering from German measles –

either during the disease itself, or within one week before the rash appears. In addition, telephone your doctor before you take a child who may be infected to the surgery, to avoid infecting any pregnant women there.

All girls aged 13 or 14 are offered immunization against the disease to prevent them catching it at a later time, when they might be pregnant (see *Immunization*, opposite, and *German measles and pregnancy*, p.616).

Chickenpox
(*varicella*)

See p.239,
Visual aids to diagnosis, 28.

This mild infectious disease is caused by the herpes zoster virus (sometimes called varicella zoster) which is the same virus that, after years of dormancy, may cause *shingles* (p.562). The virus affects chiefly the skin and lining of the mouth and throat. There is an *incubation period* of between one and three weeks before symptoms appear (see *Childhood infectious diseases*, p.698).

What are the symptoms?
The main (and often first) symptom of chickenpox is a rash in which groups of small, red, sometimes painful, fluid-filled spots appear on many parts of the body. After a few days the spots burst or dry out, and then crust over. They are very itchy.

In addition to the rash, a child may also have a slightly raised temperature, but in general does not appear ill. However, adults who catch the disease often have flu-like symptoms (see *Influenza*, p.559) for a few days before the rash appears. Children recover very quickly – usually within 10 days – but adults take longer.

How common is the problem?
Chickenpox is a fairly common childhood disease, though not quite as common as *measles* (p.699). It is rare in adults.

What are the risks?
There are very few risks associated with chickenpox. A rare possible complication is *encephalitis* (p.274). If the spots are scratched excessively, they may become infected and start to produce yellow pus.

What is the treatment?
Calamine cream or lotion applied to the spots will help relieve itching. If spots in the mouth or around the eyes are painful, your doctor will prescribe a soothing mouthwash or eyewash. Adults who suffer flu-like symptoms should take soluble aspirin or paracetamol according to the instructions on the container. (See *Caring for a feverish child*, p.698, for general treatment.)

Chickenpox is invariably a mild disease, and a complete recovery with consequent lifelong immunity can be expected.

Mumps

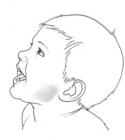

Visual symptom
A child who is developing mumps will probably feel generally unwell before noticing a tender swelling just in front of the ear.

Mumps is a common infectious disease caused by a virus. After an *incubation period* of two to four weeks, the salivary glands (see *Mouth and tongue*, p.450) swell. The parotid gland, just in front of the ear, is particularly affected. (See *Childhood infectious diseases*, p.698, for further information.)

What are the symptoms?
One parotid gland, at the side of the face, under the ear, begins to swell. A day later, the parotid gland on the other side may also swell. The swellings are usually accompanied by a raised temperature and a general feeling of being ill. Occasionally, the salivary glands under the jaw add to the swelling, and it may be painful to open your mouth or to swallow.

How common is the problem?
Mumps is probably the most common childhood infectious disease. It is not as *contagious* as, for example, *measles* (p.699), so it is uncommon for mumps to spread swiftly through a school.

What are the risks?
A fairly common risk of mumps is swelling and inflammation of the testes in a boy, or of the ovaries in a girl. This occurs about three or four days after the neck glands swell, and is more common when the disease occurs in an adult. A boy or man will notice the swelling and it can be very painful for a day or two. Invariably, the swelling goes down after a few days, leaving no after-effects. It is excessively rare for the swelling to cause sterility.

Another risk of mumps is *acute pancreatitis* (p.490), felt as a stomach ache which usually passes within a few days. Other risks of mumps, and general treatment for the disease, are described in the box entitled *Caring for a feverish child*, p.698.

Mumps is generally a mild disease. You should contact your doctor if the salivary glands (or the testes) are very painful. The doctor may prescribe an anti-inflammatory *steroid* drug to reduce the pain and swelling if it is severe. The usual outcome of mumps is complete recovery within about 10 days.

Immunization

Immunization is the process by which people become immune (resistant) to specific diseases. There are 2 ways in which people become immune to disease. If you catch an infectious disease, such as measles, your body produces *antibodies* which attack and destroy the measles-causing microbes. Your symptoms disappear, and you recover from the disease. If, later on, you are exposed again to the same microbes, the antibodies you have already produced will destroy the microbes before they can cause any symptoms. This type of immunity is called natural immunity. (See *Childhood infectious diseases*, p.698, for further details.)

You can also be made immune to a disease artificially, without ever suffering from it. Artificial immunity can be temporary (also called passive) or permanent (also called active). The best-known example of passive immunity is the protection given to newborn babies by antibodies that have entered their blood from the mother before birth. Later in life, if you need temporary immunity the doctor will inject (*inoculate*) you with ready-made antibodies. This temporary (passive) immunity lasts up to 6 months. To ensure permanent (active) immunity, the doctor will inject you with a vaccine containing dead or harmless versions of the particular microbe. Your body will produce antibodies to fend off the microbes and, while you do not suffer the symptoms of the disease (except, in some cases, a slightly raised temperature), you do become immune to it. The term *vaccination* originally applied only to immunization against smallpox, but it is now generally used to refer to the process of injecting a person to give immunity. Sometimes a disease is caused by *toxins* (poisons) formed by bacteria; in such cases the vaccine is made from the toxin and not from the bacteria.

The chart above shows how a child's immunizations are usually scheduled to offer maximum protection against serious infectious disease. If your child has ever had convulsions, if there is a history of convulsions in your family, or if the child is ill, be sure to tell your doctor before the child's immunizations begin.

People who plan to travel abroad may need special immunizations before leaving – see *Going abroad*, p.566.

AGE	VACCINE	METHOD
First few weeks	BCG (see *Tuberculosis*, p.563)	Injection
3 to 6 months	DTP Poliomyelitis	Injection/1 By mouth
6 to 8 months	DTP Poliomyelitis	Injection/2 By mouth
10 to 14 months	DTP Poliomyelitis	Injection/3 By mouth
16 to 24 months	Measles	Injection
5 years	DT Poliomyelitis	Injection By mouth
10 to 13 years	BCG	Injection
13 to 14 years (girls)	German measles	Injection
16 to 18 years	Tetanus Poliomyelitis	Injection By mouth

Key to vaccines
BCG = Tuberculosis vaccine
DTP = Diphtheria, tetanus, and pertussis (whooping cough) vaccine
DT = Diphtheria and tetanus vaccine

Whooping cough

(pertussis)

Whooping cough is a *contagious* disease that affects chiefly the respiratory system. Bacteria called bordetella pertussis infect the lungs, causing the airways (bronchi) to become clogged with thick mucus. The extremely severe bouts of coughing characteristic of the disease may persist for several weeks. Symptoms develop after an *incubation period* of between one and two weeks. (See *Childhood infectious diseases*, p.698.)

What are the symptoms?
The early symptoms are like those of an ordinary *cold* (p.342) – runny nose, dry cough, and slightly raised temperature. But unlike an ordinary cold, the symptoms do not improve after a few days, but worsen. The nasal discharge thickens, and the coughing becomes more severe until it occurs continuously in bouts up to a minute long. Because the child cannot breathe in during a bout of coughing, his or her face goes deep red, or even blue (*cyanosis*), from lack of oxygen. At the end of each bout of coughing, as the child gasps for breath, he or she makes a "whooping" noise that gives the disease its name. (Babies tend to whoop less loudly.)

Quite often, vomiting occurs after a bout of coughing. The severe coughing phase of the disease can last from two to 10 weeks. Gradually the coughing and vomiting become less severe and less frequent, though a cough may persist for several months.

How common is the problem?
Whooping cough was rare in countries like Britain during the 1960s, due to a thorough immunization programme. But as the numbers of children protected against the disease falls, so the disease becomes more common.

Symptom comparison of infectious diseases

	Incubation period	Raised temperature	Skin rash	Swollen glands	Cough
Measles	10 to 14 days	Day 1	Day 4, dull-red blotches	Very slight	Day 1
German measles	14 to 21 days	Day 1, slight	Days 1 or 2, flat, light-red spots	Day 1, side and back of the neck	None
Chickenpox	7 to 21 days	Day 1	Day 1, crops of red spots becoming blisters	None	None
Mumps	14 to 28 days	Day 1, slight	None	One or both sides of the face	None
Whooping cough	7 to 14 days	Week 1	None	None	Week 1, becoming worse; week 2, severe and "whoop" develops

In England and Wales in 1976 there were 4,300 recorded cases; whereas in 1978, there were almost 70,000.

What are the risks?
There are several dangerous risks associated with whooping cough; the younger the child, the greater the risks. Bursting of blood vessels in the brain during a bout of coughing, *encephalitis* (p.274), or cyanosis can cause death, but fatalities are extremely rare in children aged over six months.

Although these complications may not be lethal, they can produce permanent brain damage. Another risk, *pneumonia* (p.359), produces permanent lung damage in 1 child in 100 who has the disease.

What should be done?
A child who has been immunized against whooping cough (see *Immunization*, p.701) –

while he or she may get a mild case at some time – is unlikely to be seriously ill with the disease. The process of immunization does itself carry a very slight risk of encephalitis, so it is not advised for children who have had one or more convulsions in the past, or whose near relatives have had convulsions. Otherwise, immunization should be carried out because risks associated with it are minimal compared with the risks of the disease itself.

If your child is not protected by immunization, and he or she develops a cough that does not clear up within a week but seems to get worse, inform your doctor. The doctor may be able to diagnose whooping cough after a physical examination.

What is the treatment?
Self-help: Most children can be nursed at home – see *Caring for a feverish child* (p.698) for general advice. The doctor will probably make regular visits during the severe coughing phase. Get medical help without delay if you notice that the baby or child turns blue during a bout of coughing.

Do not give cough-suppressant medicines as the cough, though distressing, does help to prevent mucus from clogging the lungs. You can counteract the tendency to vomit after coughing by feeding the child small, frequent meals just after the bouts of coughing.

During a bout of coughing a baby is best lying face down with the foot of the cot raised; children usually prefer to sit up and lean forward. There is little else to do except comfort and reassure the child.

Professional help: If started in time, a course of *antibiotics* may reduce the severity of the cough. If the cough is very severe, a baby or young child may be admitted to hospital where oxygen can be given in a tent or by a face mask or a *ventilator*.

Scarlet fever

In this infection, streptococcus bacteria enter the body via the tonsils. Once inside, the bacteria multiply and produce a poison – *toxin* – that circulates in the blood. After an *incubation period* of between one day and one week, the amounts of toxin are sufficient to cause symptoms. Some of the symptoms are the same as those of tonsillitis – see *Tonsillitis in children*, p.676. (See also *Childhood infectious diseases*, p.698.)

What are the symptoms?
On the first day the child develops a high temperature (as high as 40°C, about 104°F); a red, sore throat; and a furred tongue. In

some children the tonsils have a whitish coating and occasionally the sufferer may vomit.

On the second day a bright-red (scarlet) rash appears on the child's face, leaving a clear area around the mouth; by the third day this rash – which may itch – has spread to cover the rest of the body and the arms and legs. Meanwhile the temperature starts to fall and the tongue takes on a bright-red strawberry-like appearance. By the sixth day the rash has faded. Both skin and tongue begin to peel leaving a red, raw surface underneath. Peeling can last another 14 days.

Scarlet fever has become a rare disease. It is at least 10 times less common than, say, measles (p.699) or *mumps* (p.700). It hardly ever affects adults. Besides being less common than it once was, scarlet fever is also less dangerous. The main risks, both very rare and occurring about two or three weeks after the rash, are rheumatic fever (see *Rheumatic fever in children,* p.693) and a form of kidney trouble in which the kidney tissue becomes inflamed (see *Glomerulonephritis*, p.504).

What should be done?
Contact your doctor if you suspect your child has scarlet fever. Follow the advice given in *Caring for a feverish child* (p.698); in addition, the doctor will prescribe an *antibiotic* drug to act against the streptococcus bacteria. If you make sure that the child takes the complete course of antibiotics, a full recovery is virtually certain.

Diphtheria

Diphtheria is a dangerous disease that still occurs in less developed parts of the world. But, thanks to an extensive immunization programme in Britain, the disease has almost been eradicated from this country; in 1978 there were only two recorded cases. To ensure the programme's continuing success, it is essential that your children receive the appropriate injections for lifelong protection (see *Immunization*, p.701).

The symptoms of diphtheria include raised temperature, rapid pulse, enlarged neck glands, and, occasionally, a thick, yellow nasal discharge. But the characteristic symptom is a greyish membrane that grows on the tonsils. Swelling of the throat may become severe enough to prevent breathing. Inform your doctor at once should these symptoms appear in a member of your family. If diphtheria is diagnosed, all personal contacts will be traced and their immunity confirmed. Hospital treatment involves injections of powerful *antibiotics* and *antitoxins*, and – if breathing is blocked – a *tracheotomy*.

Tuberculosis in children

Tuberculosis (TB) is an infectious disease caused by the tubercle bacteria. It occurs in two stages. The first stage used to affect mainly children, but nowadays, besides being much rarer than it was, because of extensive immunization, it develops chiefly in young adults. The second stage invariably occurs in adults. Because the two stages are interlinked, they are both described in full in one article – see *Tuberculosis*, p.563.

Threadworms
(also called pinworms)

Threadworms are tiny white worms, about 10mm (⅜in) long, that are much more common in children, especially schoolchildren, than in adults. They originally enter the system as eggs in contaminated food. The eggs hatch in the intestine, and about two weeks later the female worm lays eggs around the anus. This may cause irritation, and if the child scratches the anus, he or she picks up some eggs on the fingers. Sucking the finger or eating food with unwashed hands will then cause reinfection. By contaminating food, sheets, and towels, the child may pass on threadworms to other members of the family.

The condition does not affect general health but can be irritating unless treated; scratching the anus may make it slightly inflamed. The worms, which are most active at night, can sometimes be seen in the faeces or around the child's anus; they look like small white threads. In some cases, however, the child does not have any symptoms.

If you see threadworms, or your child's anus constantly itches, the entire family should visit the doctor.

What is the treatment?
Self-help: The whole family should exercise scrupulous hygiene. Hands should be washed after going to the toilet, after handling a pet (which may also be infected), and before touching any food. Fingernails should be clipped short to lessen the chance of eggs being trapped under them. Children should wear pyjamas, rather than a nightgown, so that, when itching, their fingers are less likely to come into direct contact with the anus. Sheets, pillowcases, nightwear, and underwear should be frequently changed, boiled, and ironed to kill any worms or eggs on them. If you have any pets, consult a vet.
Professional help: The entire family will be treated, even those who have no symptoms. They will be given a short course or one large dose of a drug that kills and flushes out the worms; the treatment is usually repeated after two weeks. Anal inflammation is relieved by a cream or ointment, which may also contain chemicals to kill the eggs. These measures, combined with good hygiene, invariably clear up the problem.

Genetics

Children are commonly said to "take after" their fathers or mothers in some mannerism or habit, and especially in physical features such as the shape of the nose or the colour of hair. Genetics is the scientific study of the process of biological inheritance and tells us how and why certain traits run in families.

Every baby develops from a single cell, the fertilized egg, which contains the information necessary for the development of inborn mental and physical characteristics. This information is carried in 23 pairs of rod-shaped *chromosomes*. Every pair of chromosomes is composed of one contributed by the mother and one by the father, and each chromosome contains thousands of *genes* – the factors that determine specific features of the child such as blood group and the colour of eyes and hair. What those features will be depends on how the chromosomes from each parent were shuffled in the process of maturation of the sperm and eggs, and how the genes in one chromosome of a pair link up with their opposite numbers in the other chromosome. There are two types of gene: dominant and recessive.

When we say that a gene is dominant, we mean that the feature it determines will appear in the next generation regardless of the character of its opposite number in the other chromosome of the pair. Features determined by recessive genes will not show up in a child unless both parents contribute chromosomes containing that recessive gene. For example, blue eyes are recessive, brown eyes are dominant. So a child will inherit blue eyes only if both parents contribute a gene for blue; if one parent contributes blue and the other brown, the child will have brown eyes. If both you and your partner have blue eyes, there are *no* genes for brown in either of you since a gene for brown, being dominant, would have given you brown eyes; and so your children must be blue-eyed. On the other hand, even if both of you are brown-eyed, there may be genes for blue eyes lurking in the chromosomes of each of you; and so, perhaps to your surprise, you may have one or more blue-eyed children.

Single-gene disorders

Most serious genetic disorders are caused by a single defective gene, which is usually recessive. In other words, the condition will not occur in a child unless both parents contribute the disease-determining gene to the fertilized egg. An example of this kind of disorder is *cystic fibrosis* (p.685). About 1 in every 20 persons carries a gene for cystic fibrosis, usually without being aware of it. Only if two carriers have a child (a chance of 1 in 400) can the disease occur in the next generation – but the next generation *can* include carriers.

The pattern is complicated when – as in *haemophilia* (p.424) – the defective gene is carried in one of the chromosomes that determine the sex of a child. Females have two identical sex chromosomes (known as X chromosomes); males have one X chromosome and one that is differently structured (known as Y). If the sperm that fertilizes an egg carries an X chromosome, the baby will be a girl; if the sperm carries the Y chromosome, it will be a boy. Haemophilia is a sex-linked disease in that the gene that governs the clotting ability of blood is carried in an X chromosome, never in a Y. If

An example of an inherited disease

Cystic fibrosis is known to be caused by an inherited genetic abnormality involving a single defective gene. The defective gene is recessive, which means that only someone who inherits it from both parents will have cystic fibrosis. Thus, whereas most people have two normal genes (NN), one on each of the chromosomes, a cystic-fibrosis sufferer always has two cystic-fibrosis genes (CC). In people with only one C gene – the other being N – the dominant N defeats the recessive C. But such people, though free of the disease themselves, are carriers. That is, they can transmit it to future generations.

If two carriers have a child, it may be neither diseased nor a carrier (NN); it may be a carrier (NC); or it may be the unfortunate inheritor of defective genes from both parents (CC), in which case it will have cystic fibrosis. The diagram on the right shows the various possibilities.

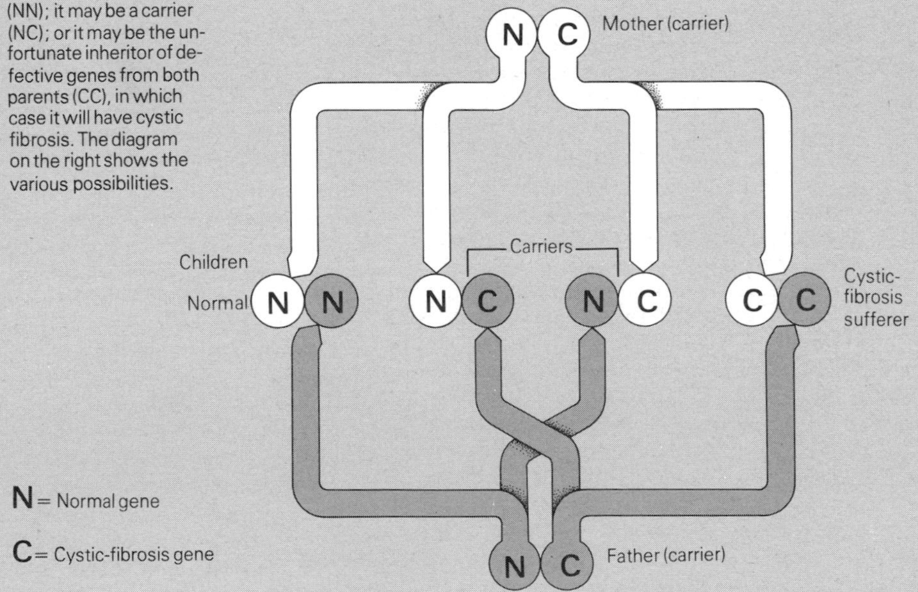

N = Normal gene

C = Cystic-fibrosis gene

Mother (carrier)

Children

Normal

Carriers

Cystic-fibrosis sufferer

Father (carrier)

Telfast ® **120mg Film Coated Tablets**

Fexofenadine 112mg
(as fexofenadine hydrochloride 120mg)

Aventis

Please read this leaflet carefully before you start to take your medicine. If you are not sure about anything or have any questions ask your pharmacist or doctor.

What is in your medicine?

The name of your medicine is Telfast 120mg Film Coated Tablets. Each tablet contains 112mg of the active ingredient fexofenadine (as 120mg of fexofenadine hydrochloride). The tablets also contain microcrystalline cellulose, pregelatinised maize starch, croscarmellose sodium, magnesium stearate, hypromellose, povidone, titanium dioxide (E171), colloidal anhydrous silica, macrogol 400 and iron oxide (E172).

Each pack contains 30 tablets which are peach in colour and capsule-shaped.

What you should know about Telfast 120mg Film Coated Tablets

Fexofenadine hydrochloride, the active ingredient of Telfast 120mg Film Coated Tablets, is one of a group of medicines called antihistamines.

The company responsible (also known as the Marketing Authorisation Holder) for this product in the UK is Aventis Pharma Ltd., 50 Kings Hill Avenue, Kings Hill, West Malling, Kent, ME19 4AH, UK and in the Republic of Ireland is Aventis Pharma Ltd., Citywest Business Campus, Dublin 24, Republic of Ireland.

The product is made by
Sanofi Winthrop Industrie,
30-36 avenue Gustave Eiffel,
37100 Tours, France.

What are Telfast 120mg Film Coated Tablets for?

Telfast 120mg Film Coated Tablets contains fexofenadine hydrochloride, which is an antihistamine.
Antihistamines relieve the symptoms such as sneezing, itchy, runny nose and itchy, red and watery eyes, that occur with hayfever (seasonal allergic rhinitis).

When should you not take Telfast 120mg Film Coated Tablets?

DO NOT take Telfast 120mg Film Coated Tablets if you have ever had a reaction to any of its ingredients (See 'What is in your medicine?' for list of ingredients).

Before taking your medicine

Before taking your medicine always tell

your doctor or pharmacist if you:

- are pregnant
- could be pregnant
- are breast feeding
- have ever had heart problems

Driving and Telfast 120mg Film Coated Tablets

Tests show that Telfast 120mg Film Coated Tablets does not cause drowsiness so that you can usually drive while you are on treatment with Telfast 120mg Film Coated Tablets. However, there may be rare exceptions so make sure that you are not affected in this way before driving or carrying out tasks requiring concentration.

Taking your medicine

Take your tablets with water before meals.

If you use an indigestion remedy containing aluminium and magnesium, it is recommended that you leave about 2 hours between the time that you take Telfast 120mg Film Coated Tablets and your indigestion remedy. This is because it may affect the action of Telfast 120mg Film Coated Tablets by lowering the amount of drug absorbed.

Adults and children aged 12 years and over:

Take one tablet once daily.

If you accidentally take too many tablets, ask your doctor for advice or go to the nearest hospital.

After taking your medicine

In tests, the most common side effects of Telfast 120mg Film Coated Tablets were headache, dizziness, tiredness/sleepiness, sickness, diarrhoea, sleeping disorders, bad dreams, nervousness, faster heart beat and palpitations, but these occurred to the same extent when dummy (placebo) tablets were used instead.

Other side effects experienced have included allergic skin reactions like rash and itching. Very rarely, chest tightness or wheezing, unexpected swelling and flushing may occur. If this occurs, you should stop taking the tablets and seek medical advice.

If you notice anything unusual or have any unexpected effects tell your pharmacist or doctor.

Storing your medicine

Do not use your medicine after the expiry date on the box. Return unwanted tablets to the pharmacist.

Keep your medicine in a safe place where children cannot reach or see it.

This leaflet was last revised in 09/2006

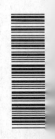

TE238A - *173889*

both parents contribute a defective X chromosome to the fertilized egg, the pairing of the abnormal blood-clotting genes means that the resultant female baby will have haemophilia. This happens very rarely, however. If, as happens much more often, the mother contributes a defective X chromosome and the father contributes a Y chromosome, there are two inevitable results of the union:

1 The offspring will be a boy (because he has one X and one Y chromosome).

2 Although the abnormal gene is recessive, it cannot be overcome by a dominant gene since there is no gene for blood clotting on the differently-structured Y chromosome; and so the boy child will be haemophiliac.

It also follows that:

1 All daughters of a haemophiliac man will be carriers.

2 Only some of the daughters of a carrier may be carriers (since they can inherit the normal X chromosome rather than the one with the defective gene).

3 A man with haemophilia cannot pass the defective gene on to his sons because they will inherit his Y chromosome, on which there is no gene for blood clotting.

In a few single-gene diseases the defective gene is not recessive but dominant. This means that anybody who inherits the faulty gene from either parent is bound to have the condition. For an example, see *Huntington's chorea* (p.293) which is particularly tragic in that symptoms do not appear until middle age. As a consequence, many sufferers from the disease do not know they have it until after they have had children and possibly passed the abnormal gene to them; or, alternatively, knowing that Huntington's chorea runs in one branch of their family, they refrain from having children and then discover, too late, that they themselves have not inherited the disease and would not, therefore, have passed it on.

Multiple-gene disorders

Single-gene diseases, as shown above, clearly illustrate the way in which inheritance works. Many disorders, however, are inherited not through single genes but through more than one; and here the picture becomes much more complex. Many disorders are characterized as tending to "run in families" (see, for instance, *Coronary artery disease*, p.374 and *Asthma*, p.355). What that rather vague phrase means is that there is a genetic element present in susceptibility to the disorder but that it cannot be readily isolated and defined. Also, the interaction between genes may be influenced by environmental factors such as upbringing and diet.

If you suspect or know that you and/or your partner might pass a genetic disease along to your children, you should seek advice from an experienced *genetic counsellor* (p.619).

Allergies

Allergies are a range of physical disorders caused by hypersensitivity to substances eaten, inhaled, or brought into contact with the skin. This hypersensitivity results from a misdirected response by the body's natural immune system. Your natural immune system exists in order to protect you from infection by invading microbes such as bacteria or viruses (see *General infections and infestations*, p.558). It does this by manufacturing *antibodies* that kill or neutralize the invaders. What seems to happen in allergic people is that the antibodies fight the wrong battles: they go to work against normally harmless substances (termed *allergens*).

The form that an allergy takes depends on both the type of antibody and the part of the body in which the battle between antibody and allergen takes place. In food allergies, for example, the offending substance may cause symptoms affecting the intestines (as in coeliac disease), or it may be absorbed into the bloodstream, travel around the body, and so come into conflict with antibodies in the blood vessels (causing, say, a headache) or in the skin (causing a rash). In the type of allergic rhinitis commonly known as hay fever, airborne pollens are inhaled, and the reaction occurs in the lining of the nose. In asthma, inhaled dust or pollen causes a reaction in the lungs.

In an allergic reaction, immune-system cells release irritant chemicals such as *histamine*. These substances cause the various symptoms characteristic of allergic attacks – headaches, excessive production of mucus, and skin conditions such as redness, spottiness, and itching.

Who is susceptible?

Some people develop one or more allergies in infancy and suffer all their lives – though most children "grow out" of their asthma or eczema. Other people develop an allergy at some time and either do or do not react consistently to the offending allergen. Susceptibility seems to run in families (see *Genetics*, opposite) but there is no way to predict whether a given member of a family will be affected. Sufferers commonly have several allergic diseases – asthma and eczema, for instance, often occur together.

What is the treatment?

Theoretically the best "treatment" is total avoidance of exposure to the allergen; but this is feasible only in certain cases – if you know you are allergic to, say, shellfish or penicillin. More often the allergen is either difficult to identify or virtually impossible to avoid – pollen, for example, or animal fur. Where an allergen has been identified, it is occasionally possible to *desensitize* the sufferer by a course of injections that acclimatize the body to increasing doses of the offending substance.

The mainstays of modern treatment for allergies are drugs that reduce or counteract allergic reactions – for instance, cromoglycate (which, by blocking the action of immune-system cells, can prevent an allergic reaction from developing) or antihistamines. For details consult the individual articles dealing with allergy-based disorders.

Special problems of adolescents

Introduction

Adolescence – the period of transition from childhood to adulthood – is generally considered to last approximately from puberty, when secondary sexual characteristics start to develop and (in girls) when menstruation begins, to age 18. The changes normally start to occur soon after the age of 10 or 11 in girls, and soon after the age of 12 or 13 in boys. The physical climb towards maturity tends to reach a plateau soon after the age of 17 or 18 in both sexes. In the intervening years there are physical, mental, and emotional pressures that can make adolescence a peculiarly difficult time. Thus, though individual variations are great, it makes practical sense to use the words "adolescent" and "teenager" as synonyms.

Some of the problems discussed in the following pages are primarily physical, others are psychological, but it is seldom possible to make sharp distinctions between the two categories. For example, young people suffering from acne often react in a highly emotional way and the disorder can colour their whole adolescent life. And some degree of psychological trouble is always at the root of the development of anorexia nervosa, a serious and possibly fatal medical condition.

It is frequently hard to say whether the teenagers themselves or their parents are most affected by such teenage concerns as the temptations of sexual experimentation, drugs, and alcohol. You will, therefore, find intermingled advice to both adolescents and the older people concerned with them in the following pages. The key to a healthy transition to adulthood is very often a healthy relationship between the generations.

Early or late development

Although the hormonal changes that indicate the onset of puberty usually begin at about the age of 10 or 11 in girls and about 12 or 13 in boys (see the tables opposite), there are wide variations in adolescent growth patterns, and most of these can be considered normal.

An adolescent's development is affected by a number of factors. Girls' development tends to start earlier than boys', and development patterns are also influenced by heredity; a girl whose mother started her periods comparatively late is likely to develop late herself. Similarly, a boy's development is likely to follow the pattern of his father's.

Whether an adolescent develops early or late is also affected by his or her general health. Undernourishment or illness during childhood may delay the onset of puberty. In addition, a child who is smaller or thinner than average is likely to be a late developer.

Whatever her age, a girl will not normally have her first period until she weighs at least 45kg (7 stone). In addition, a girl who very quickly loses a lot of weight after she has started having periods may stop having them – this may be an early sign of *anorexia nervosa* (p.709).

The body in late adolescence
By the age of 17 or 18, most boys are sexually mature – the genitals have grown; facial and body hair has appeared; the voice has deepened; and there have been changes in the bones and muscular development resulting in the typical male body shape of broad shoulders and narrow hips. Many girls reach sexual maturity by the time they are 16, by which time the breasts have developed and the pelvis has broadened; underarm and pubic hair has grown; and fatty deposits have been laid down to give a typically female shape.

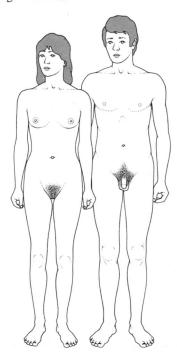

Normal adolescent development

Physical development in adolescent girls

	Average age when change begins	Average age when change ceases to be conspicuous	Remarks
Increase in rate of growth	10 to 11	15 to 16	Conspicuous growth that begins before 9 or failure to grow by 15 warrants consultation with your doctor. Final average height is between 1.52 and 1.76m (5ft and 5ft 10in).
Breast development	10 to 11	13 to 14	Noticeable development of breasts (one of which may begin to "bud" before the other) is usually the first sign of puberty. If change does not occur by 15, there may be cause for concern.
Emergence of body hair	Pubic hair: 10 to 11 Underarm hair: 12 to 13	13 to 14 15 to 16	Ages of first appearance of body hair are extremely variable.
Development of apocrine sweat glands	12 to 13	15 to 16	The apocrine sweat glands are responsible for increased underarm sweating, and a type of body odour not present in children.
Menstruation	11 to 14	15 to 16	Menstruation often begins with extremely irregular periods, but by 16 a regular period (3 to 7 days every 28 days) becomes evident. Menstruation beginning before 10 or failing to begin by 16 warrants consultation with your doctor.

Physical development in adolescent boys

	Average age when change begins	Average age when change ceases to be conspicuous	Remarks
Increase in rate of growth	12 to 13	17 to 18	If conspicuous growth fails to begin by 15, consult your doctor. Final average height is between 1.63 and 1.86m (5ft 4in and 6ft 1in).
Enlargement of genitals	Testicles and scrotum: 11 to 12 Penis: 12 to 13	16 to 17 15 to 16	As testicles grow, the skin of the scrotum darkens. The penis usually increases in length before broadening. Ability to ejaculate seminal fluid usually begins about a year after the penis starts to lengthen.
Emergence of body hair	Pubic hair: 11 to 12 Underarm and other body hair: 13 to 15 Beard: 13 to 15	15 to 16 17 to 18 17 to 19	Development of hair is extremely variable and largely dependent on genetic inheritance. The spread of hair up the abdomen onto the chest usually continues into adulthood.
Development of apocrine sweat glands	13 to 15	17 to 18	See remarks in the table for girls (above).
Voice change	Enlargement of the larynx (voice-box) begins at 13 to 14, and the voice deepens at 14 to 15	16 to 17	Growth of the larynx may cause the appearance of a prominent Adam's apple.

Medical disorders

Adolescent males and females are more or less susceptible to any of the general illnesses in this book. The four complaints – acne, anorexia nervosa, scoliosis, and phimosis – discussed below, however, are almost exclusively adolescent. Complaints that can affect people of all ages but to which teenagers seem especially prone are discussed in sections dealing generally with such problems. See, for instance, *Glandular fever*, p.562, and *Hodgkin's disease*, p.433.

Teenagers and/or parents who are worried about whether or not physical development is proceeding normally should study the tables on the previous page. Note the broad range of ages within which such changes as the growth of body hair, the beginning of menstruation (*menarche*), and maturation of bodily structure occur. Many boys and girls begin to develop characteristic signs of adolescence earlier or later than the average ages indicated in the tables, but such variations are rarely a sign of a medical disorder. If changes begin to occur very early (before the age of 10) or no signs of puberty have appeared by the age of 16, consult a doctor.

Acne

(acne vulgaris, or common acne)

See p.240,
Visual aids to diagnosis 30.

Almost every part of your body is covered with hairs, most of them virtually invisible. Each hair grows from a follicle (a tiny pit in the skin), and within each follicle is a sebaceous gland that produces an oily substance to keep the skin lubricated. If there is an over-production of oil and some of it becomes trapped because excess skin has blocked the follicle, the blocked pit may become inflamed. The result is a spot, which may be just a red lump or may become a pus-filled pimple. Most teenagers have a few pimples or spots – mild acne.

Acne can be caused by taking certain drugs such as *steroids* or anti-epilepsy medicines, but it is usually a problem of adolescence; it begins at puberty and clears up in the late teens or in the early twenties. Sometimes acne persists into adulthood, for some reason particularly in men.

The reason why so many adolescents suffer from acne is that the level of hormones in the body rises at puberty. This leads to increased production of oily substance (called *sebum*) by the sebaceous glands, and to excess production of the top layer of skin cells that can block the ducts of the glands.

What are the symptoms?

Spots are usually concentrated on the face, but there are often additional spots on the nape of the neck, the back, the chest, and upper arms. Squeezing or picking at pimples may further damage the skin and worsen the spots. As individual acne spots heal, others appear. Each healed spot leaves behind a purplish mark, which normally fades away; but some *cystic* spots take weeks to clear up and may occasionally leave visible scars.

How common is the problem?

Over half of all young men aged 14 to 18 have acne to some degree. It is slightly less common in adolescent girls, many of whom tend to develop spots mainly around the time of their periods. Severe acne leading to permanent scars is rare, however. Some types of acne seem to run in families, especially if there is a tendency to greasy skin.

What are the risks?

Acne poses no direct risks to general health, but many adolescents feel self-conscious and embarrassed about their spots. It is risky to pick at spots on your face because if you do this the chances of infection and eventual permanent scarring are increased.

What should be done?

If you have mild acne, the self-help measures suggested below should keep it under control. If it becomes severe, consult your doctor. But remember that you are probably more aware of your spots and they look more unsightly to you than they do to other people.

What is the treatment?

Self-help: There are a number of common myths about the causes of acne, but there is no good evidence that what you eat affects your spots; nor are they affected by masturbation. You should wash your skin twice a day (not more often unless it becomes abnormally dirty or oily) – but spots are not caused by dirty skin. Sunshine, though, often helps to clear up acne. Do not squeeze or pick at your spots, as you may only make matters worse. You can buy acne lotions containing specific anti-acne chemicals without a prescription,

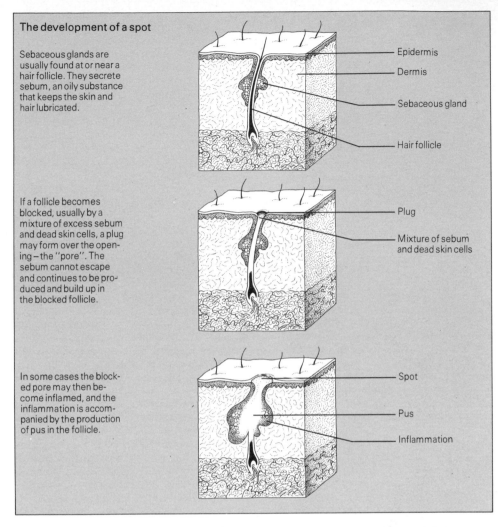

The development of a spot

Sebaceous glands are usually found at or near a hair follicle. They secrete sebum, an oily substance that keeps the skin and hair lubricated.

- Epidermis
- Dermis
- Sebaceous gland
- Hair follicle

If a follicle becomes blocked, usually by a mixture of excess sebum and dead skin cells, a plug may form over the opening – the "pore". The sebum cannot escape and continues to be produced and build up in the blocked follicle.

- Plug
- Mixture of sebum and dead skin cells

In some cases the blocked pore may then become inflamed, and the inflammation is accompanied by the production of pus in the follicle.

- Spot
- Pus
- Inflammation

and these sometimes help. Beware of vigorously over-treating your spots, as this may further damage your skin.

Professional help: If your acne is severe enough to warrant professional help, your doctor will probably prescribe a special preparation that makes the skin peel and has an antiseptic action to prevent new spots from forming. If this treatment does not work, the doctor may prescribe small, regular doses of *antibiotics* for up to six months. Even more prolonged treatment with special drugs may be needed for persistent, severe acne. Both treatments produce a gradual improvement; but there is no simple, instant cure.

What are the long-term prospects?

If you are left with bad scarring after your acne has cleared up, you may be advised to have the top layer of the affected skin shaved off by a plastic surgeon (see *Plastic surgery*, p.260). This should leave the skin smooth.

Anorexia nervosa

Anorexia nervosa – a refusal to eat that can lead to extreme loss of weight, hormonal disturbances, and even death – is primarily an illness of adolescent girls. Though generally treated as a disease in itself, it is often a symptom of a psychological problem closely associated with family background. Anorexic girls may use their refusal to eat as a tool for manipulating their parents, whose increasing concern about the problem gradually turns each mealtime into a battle.

Although the cause of the illness is not yet understood, one explanation is that it arises from a subconscious desire to retreat from oncoming maturity. The teenage girl diets in order to make her body retain its pre-adolescent shape. This rejection of normal sexuality may be triggered off by an early sexual experience that has led to feelings of fear or guilt. Or, sometimes, an emotionally insecure girl, overhearing a casual comment that she is too fat, may decide she must lose weight to gain friends.

What are the symptoms?

The illness usually starts with dieting in a normal way, but the girl eats less and less every day. She gives false reasons for doing so, insisting, for example, that her legs or arms are still too fat. The less she eats, the less she wants. Even if she becomes skeletally thin, she still sees herself as plump and does not eat sensibly. Sometimes, however, she may go on "binges", gobbling up quantities of a particular food – and then vomiting. To counter family pressure, she may hide food and throw it away, claiming she has eaten it. When her weight drops to about 12kg (almost 2 stone) below normal (see *Weight chart* on p.28, for approximate normal weights), she stops having periods (see *Amenorrhoea*, p.583) and her body may become more hairy.

At the beginning of the illness, a sufferer from anorexia nervosa is often abnormally energetic. She may cook large meals for others while starving herself, and she will insist that she feels fine. But her skin begins to look sallow and papery, and she eventually becomes obviously ill. Constipation is likely to develop, but whether or not she is constipated, she may take large doses of a laxative

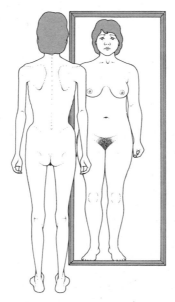

Advanced anorexia nervosa
Even after having dieted to such an extent that she looks painfully thin to observers, a girl with anorexia nervosa sees herself as still being overweight.

in the belief that by hurrying food through her system she will keep from growing fat. In later stages of the illness she may lapse into full-scale *depression* (p.297).

How common is the problem?

Anorexia nervosa is fairly common; in this country about 1 teenage girl in 100 is probably afflicted. Only 1 in 2,000 male adolescents has the condition, but the incidence is increasing. It is, however, primarily a disorder of Western society.

What are the risks?

A teenager who tries to keep her weight down by taking large numbers of laxatives and vomiting frequently may undergo dangerous changes in blood chemistry because of the abnormal loss of body fluids. Many teenagers go through a temporary phase of excessive dieting, but only a minority develop anorexia nervosa. Of those who do, about 5 per cent die, mainly by committing suicide as a result of depression. A small number die as the result of secondary infections (stemming from undernourishment) or *dehydration* (caused by excessive use of laxatives). Some adolescent girls literally starve themselves to death.

What should be done?

If your teenage daughter has an unrealistic image of herself as being too fat and seems to be dieting excessively, see your doctor without delay. Treatment of anorexia nervosa becomes increasingly difficult as the condition progresses. The disorder can be reversed fairly easily before about 12kg (about 2 stone) have been lost, but after this, treatment is likely to be more prolonged. After examining the girl, your doctor may decide that she is not actually ill and may simply give you and her some advice on how to avoid trouble. If her condition is diagnosed as anorexia nervosa, the doctor will probably arrange for immediate referral to hospital.

What is the treatment?

Even in its early stages anorexia nervosa is best treated in hospital. Treatment varies considerably, but the hospital doctor will discuss the illness with the sufferer and help her to decide on a suitable weight. They will then agree on the type of diet she should have in order to gain weight at a healthy rate. If possible, the girl will be given a room to herself, where she can be closely supervised. While in hospital she may also be given *psychotherapy*, and at least some of this treatment will take place in the presence of the girl's parents. The more she brings personal and family problems into the open – problems of which her parents may be unaware – the better the chance of solving them.

When the girl reaches a suitable weight and no longer seems reluctant to accept physical and emotional maturity, she is permitted to go home. Before she leaves the hospital, the family will be given advice on how to treat her and how to recognize the onset of another attack if one occurs.

What are the long-term prospects?

For a year or two after an apparent cure the girl will be asked to visit the hospital periodically as an out-patient. This is because up to 60 per cent of girls who seem to have recovered from anorexia nervosa have further attacks. Although many parents assume that this disorder represents merely a transient phase of adolescence, some anorexia sufferers have difficulty with their diets for many years, alternating starvation with gorging.

Scoliosis
(curvature of the spine)

Scoliosis is a sideways curvature of the spine that causes the ribcage to lose its symmetry. Sometimes spinal curvature is a *congenital* abnormality present at birth, and sometimes it may be caused by developmental problems such as paralysis or weakness of the spinal muscles. In adolescence, however, scoliosis may appear for no apparent reason in a previously normal individual. It is nearly 10 times more common in girls than in boys.

What should be done?

Even a minor degree of spinal curvature should be shown to the doctor. Early diagnosis is important because the deformity may rapidly get worse if untreated; and, as a consequence, the lungs may be affected to a point where there are recurrent chest infections and shortness of breath. The doctor will probably ask the child to stand up straight

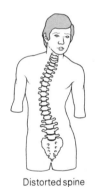

Distorted spine

with the heels together, then bend forward. If the curvature is caused by scoliosis, the back will remain curved as the child bends. The doctor will probably refer the child to a specialist, who will carry out periodic physical examinations in order to monitor the progress of the curvature.

What is the treatment?

If scoliosis is caused by a spinal abnormality, the underlying problem must be diagnosed and treated accordingly. The scoliosis of adolescence is, however, difficult to treat. *Physiotherapy* will be used to improve posture and tone up spinal muscles. If this fails to correct the curvature, the sufferer may have to wear a spinal brace. Such braces are fitted by orthopaedic surgeons, and, kept in place permanently for a year or so, they nearly always help to straighten the curvature.

Phimosis
(tight foreskin)

"Phimosis" is the technical term for a tightness of the foreskin that prevents it from being comfortably drawn back over the glans (or tip) of the penis. The difficulty cannot generally be detected before a boy reaches the age of about five because foreskins are normally small and tight in the very young. Most commonly, phimosis is discovered in adolescence, when although there may be

little or no pain on passing urine, the condition causes extreme pain in the penis when it becomes erect.

What should be done?

Never use force to pull back a foreskin; it can damage the tissues. Consult your doctor, who may recommend *circumcision* – a relatively minor operation.

Circumcision
A tight foreskin is normal until a boy is about 3 or 4. If it causes any trouble after that age, the doctor will probably recommend circumcision. A general anaesthetic is usually given and the foreskin is cut away around the glans penis.

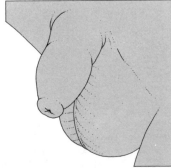

Phimosis

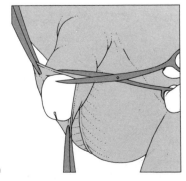

Circumcision

Psychological and behavioural problems

In adolescence, the emotional ferment that accompanies the natural physical changes is often exacerbated by conflicting pressures – those presented by the individual's own age group as well as by his or her family and society in general. The articles in this section summarize the most common problems and suggest ways of trying to cope with them.

Rebelliousness

The hallmarks of adolescence are self-consciousness, self-awareness, and self-centredness. Coupled with these is an inner conflict that seems to be a prerequisite for growing up – a stubborn determination to assert independence, along with a continuing need to rely on adult support (emotional as well as financial). So typical adolescents demand the right to question and criticize the behaviour and standards of their parents, but resent parental efforts to shape and control their own behaviour.

Parental pressures on them to conform or to take jobs they do not want, uncertainty about the future, and the almost universal adolescent worries about boy/girl relationships all play a part in the development of difficult or moody behaviour.

Your adolescent children are unlikely to reject your values totally, but neither will they completely accept them. Quiet, cooperative teenagers may be as much cause for concern as their extremely rebellious brothers or sisters. Some clashes between parents and normal teenage children are inevitable. This problem usually becomes troublesome in the turbulent middle years of adolescence, between 13 and 16.

What are the symptoms?

Teenagers are often moody and sullen. They tend to strike know-it-all postures, to reject advice from their elders, and to view all situations from only one standpoint – their own. Yet – and this is one reason for the sullenness – they are inwardly much less confident than they seem. For instance, they tend to attach extreme importance to outward appearance. Their adoption of outrageous fashions or freakish hair styles may seem to their elders like an unpleasant flouting of convention. But it probably simply reflects the need of teenagers to be like their friends, and to adopt fashions and a life style obviously different from those of their parents. Lacking self-confidence, most teenagers need the protective colouring that comes from dressing and behaving like the rest of their group.

With intense self-consciousness they are also acutely aware of their physical defects, which they magnify out of all proportion to the reality. Parents whose teenagers are convinced that life is in ruins because of spots or curly hair may find it hard to persuade their children that a clear skin or straight hair is not the only passport to happiness.

Since they have a continuing need for adult support, some adolescents form a close relationship with grown-ups who do not belong to the school and family circle. The confidant may be a respectable neighbour or youth leader, but it may also be someone of whom the parents would disapprove (if they knew of the relationship). This yearning to have someone to lean on – someone unlike the finger-wagging parent – rarely leads to harmful results; and the relationship generally lasts for only a short time.

Towards the end of adolescence, between the years of 16 and 18, when most young people have left school (and especially if they have begun to earn money), rebelliousness fades. The teenager will still be critical, but criticism gradually becomes more constructive and is aimed at matters other than those of direct personal concern. Some intolerance of older people's ways may well linger on, but the unpredictable turbulence, uncertainty, and moodiness of the mid-adolescent phase almost always passes. The young person approaching 20 is likely to show an increasingly mature willingness to compromise and is readier to accept advice.

What should parents do?

Successful relationships between parents and adolescents depend on communication, and this is not always easy. Adolescents cannot be expected to be patient and tolerant and to treat their parents like equals; it is the parents who must bear these burdens – and so the advice in the following paragraphs is directed to older people.

(If you are an adolescent, however, do not ignore what follows. You can help your parents through these difficult years just by knowing that they want to help, not hinder, in your voyage towards maturity. Remember, too, that they may be facing their own difficulties at this time. Your mother may be thinking of looking for a job now that you do not need her quite so much. Your father may have growing business concerns. Their own parents, now becoming old, may be an increasing cause for concern. All such "mid-life crises" may affect their tolerance of and sympathy towards your special problems.)

The basic question for many parents is this: Should you continue to enforce your old standards, with disciplinary measures to back them up if necessary, or should you relax the rules, after discussing them reasonably with your adolescent son or daughter? Too much parental concern is an obvious irritant; too little may be interpreted by the teenager as lack of concern. You must base your decisions on standards for behaviour and discipline in your own family, but mothers and fathers should always try to present a united front to their teenage children. Begin by agreeing on issues that both parents feel are vital for the teenager's health and safety. You may, for example, insist on your right to know where adolescents are at a given time, to make it an unbreakable rule that they should never drive a car after drinking alcohol, etc. And you may feel strongly about other issues – for example, the level of rudeness you are prepared to tolerate. Then, having agreed on the important ground rules, try to be flexible in other areas such as dress or speech habits, which, though they may irritate you, do not matter in quite the same way.

Teenagers' anxieties about appearance tend to focus mostly on hair, skin, or weight. Give what practical help you can. If your daughter is really overweight, for example, help her to modify her diet. Whatever the problem and however trivial it may seem,

never laugh it off. It is only in very late adolescence that the confidence comes to accept oneself as one really is, and to believe that others can do the same.

What is abnormal behaviour?

Very seldom does adolescent rebelliousness reach a point so critical that professional help should be sought. But there are some circumstances in which such help becomes essential. Refusal to go to school (which may stem from unreasonably high parental expectations or from bullying) is an example. Once a pattern of truancy is established, it can be virtually impossible to reverse, and so you should consult a teacher at the school (and preferably a child guidance counsellor also) if the problem arises in your family. Similarly, if your child rejects your guidance so totally as to seem to be menacing his or her position in a law-abiding society, do not hesitate to ask your doctor to refer you to a counsellor or social worker before it is too late.

Occasionally the stresses of adolescence precipitate mental illness. Short periods of gloom are common, but if a teenager's mood remains sombre for more than a few days, and if symptoms of depressive illness – insomnia, loss of appetite, or withdrawal from friends as well as family – begin to appear, see your doctor without delay. Occasionally, too, the swings of mood that are a common feature of adolescence may become so extreme that medical help should be sought. (For the symptoms of *manic depression* see p.298.) Finally, a very few adolescents, unable to cope with what they see as a disaster (often the break-up of a love affair), take drastic action to escape harsh reality. Boys tend to resort to alcohol or physical violence in these circumstances, while girls more commonly resort to drug overdose. In such cases emergency medical help is essential.

The dangers of addiction

Anyone who drinks, smokes, or takes drugs may become addicted (see *Alcoholism*, p.304; *Drug addiction*, p.305; and *The dangers of smoking*, p.38); but the danger is most serious among teenagers, who tend to be attracted to assertive "sophisticated" gestures and to have a fairly short-term outlook. Fortunately, few adolescents are likely to experiment with hard drugs, if only because they are difficult to come by. The use of soft drugs, though, is quite common. In many circles cannabis is easily obtained and casually used. Cigarettes and alcohol are also available at nearly all teenage gatherings. Parents

do, therefore, have some cause for worry. Adolescence is characterized by a desire to experiment, a sense of almost limitless powers and possibilities, and a need to test oneself to the utmost. Adolescents, too, are particularly susceptible to the pressures of their peers. They need to feel part of a group. If the group pattern involves the use of drugs, alcohol, or cigarettes, it is often difficult for a teenage boy or girl to resist the temptation to conform. And as one experiment frequently leads to a second, experimentation can easily become habitual use, if not addiction. Most smokers, for example, started to smoke in adolescence. Statistics suggest that whereas young people who do not smoke before the age of 20 are unlikely to start, 85 per cent of those who smoke while teenagers become permanently "hooked".

What should parents do?
Where drugs are concerned, the best thing you can do is to make sure that the adolescent knows the risks he or she is running. The fact that drug addiction presents a more immediate danger than smoking or drinking may make your appeal to the good sense of your children more convincing. Assume that all adolescents are exposed to temptation at some time, and discuss with them the best way to refuse any offer of drugs. Your advice will carry most weight if it is supported with facts. To make clear the hazards of flirting with drug addiction, recommend a reading of that article, with special attention to the facts on the chart accompanying the article.

There is no medical evidence that cannabis is as risky as drugs such as heroin. Because most teenagers know this, you would probably weaken your argument by over-stating the case against cannabis. Do point out, however, that there is a danger of becoming psychologically dependent on smoking cannabis. Any such dependence is bound to be

harmful, even if the drug itself may not endanger an adolescent's physical health.

Efforts to discourage young people from smoking cigarettes have not been very successful. It is hard to combat the constant battle for the minds of the young by tobacco-industry promoters, who portray smokers as successful, suave, and in happy control of life's events. Whether or not adolescents start to smoke depends largely on their social surroundings and on the availability of cigarettes. Friends who smoke are the main influence, but family environment is also important. Teenagers are quick to resent double standards. You are in no position to point out the evils of tobacco with a cigarette dangling from your lips. The best way to encourage your children not to smoke is not to smoke yourself. Refusing to permit children to smoke at home, even though they may smoke elsewhere, has the advantage that it cuts down their consumption of cigarettes.

Drinking is in a slightly different category since, while "No smoking" is the only sensible rule, it should be possible to learn to drink sensibly. Drinking in young people can be a serious problem – not simply because of the possible risks of alcoholism later on, but because of the disastrous consequences here and now of having had too much to drink. People in the late teens are the group most at risk from road accidents, and driving under the influence of alcohol is one of the most common causes of accidents. But adolescents need to learn most things for themselves, by doing rather than just being told the facts.

Most youngsters soon discover how alcohol affects them, and only an occasional teenager fails to learn how to cope with both the pleasant and unpleasant effects. The best place in which to acquire social skills – which include the ability to recognize when one has had enough alcohol and to say no to any more – is in the home. Restrained parental drinking almost always leads to restraint in the drinking habits of the younger generation.

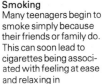

Smoking
Many teenagers begin to smoke simply because their friends or family do. This can soon lead to cigarettes being associated with feeling at ease and relaxing in virtually any situation.

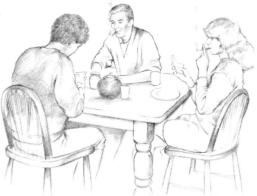

Exploring sex

In the early years of adolescence (ages about 12 to 15) the closest friendships are generally made with people of the same sex. Often these friendships are so intense that some parents begin to worry about possible homosexuality. Remember, however, that even though homosexual feelings are common and quite normal during this period, the homosexual phase of adolescence is nearly always transient (see *Male homosexuality*, p.580, and *Female homosexuality*, p.604). In

time the teenager becomes increasingly aware of himself or herself as either male or female and begins to seek relationships with people of the opposite sex. In spite of modern permissiveness, however, sexual intercourse before late adolescence (around the age of 17 or 18) is probably the exception rather than the rule. Instead, virtually all teenagers masturbate, a practice that is harmless.

Parents and children tend to have unrealistic views of one another's sexuality. Many

Developing relationships
Social development is part of adolescence, and the extent to which sexual exploration is involved depends on both peer-group behaviour and the example set by parents.

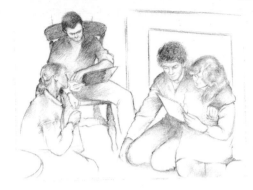

adolescents find it difficult to believe that their parents are still interested (or, indeed, were ever interested) in sex. Parents often feel strongly that, even though their teenage children may be able and eager to have sexual relationships, they are not emotionally ready for sex. Adolescence is a time for experimenting, though, and most adolescents are going to experiment to some extent in this area as in any other. Research indicates that few teenagers are promiscuous. If your children seem sensible in other ways, you have no reason to suppose they will suddenly go off the rails sexually.

What should parents do?

The period of sexual transition is less difficult if you can come to terms with your child's sexuality. Unless you can acknowledge openly the fact that your teenagers are growing up sexually as well as in other ways, they will remain unconvinced that you trust them and are ready to give them any help or advice they may need. To begin with, do not worry about masturbation or in any way emphasize its "risks". There are none; and nothing you do or say should arouse guilt feelings in your youngsters. Masturbation is a universal practice and a harmless one. On the other hand, do not hesitate to speak out about the real risks of irresponsible sexual intercourse – unwanted pregnancies, *sexually transmitted diseases* (p.611), and frustrating and unsatisfactory emotional involvements.

You have a responsibility to make sure that your adolescent children know the facts of life, including the unpleasant ones. If you find it impossible to talk to them yourself, make sure they have received adequate sex education at school, or provide a book on the subject. They should also know about contraception (see *Infertility and contraception*, p.607) and how to get contraceptive advice.

At best, your attitude should encourage confidence in your sons and daughters. Confidence, along with an understanding of the complexities of sexual relationships, almost always leads to a sense of responsibility. And a responsible adolescent is well on the way towards knowing how to withstand pressure to become involved in relationships that he or she does not want.

Adolescent pregnancy

Details about various methods of contraception appear elsewhere in this book (see *Infertility and contraception*, p.607). If you think that you and another person may start a full sexual relationship, however, it is vitally important to get some personal advice. Do not hesitate to consult your family doctor. Most doctors will not disclose the facts of any such interview to parents without permission. If you prefer to talk about contraception with someone who might view your situation more objectively than would your doctor, try one of the family planning clinics run by local authorities. Or go to one of the *Brook Advisory Centres* (p.768), which give advice to the young, whether married or unmarried.

If you are a girl, remember that pregnancy is a possibility even if your periods have not yet started; the first ovulation may (though rarely) take place before the first period. Remember, too, that the consequences of a pregnancy may be unpleasant not only for you but for your baby.

Unplanned birth to an unmarried teenage girl is a poor start to life. Moreover, there are higher risks, for both mother and baby, attached to having a baby when you are under 16. So always use a contraceptive.

If you become pregnant (see *Pregnancy and childbirth*, p.616) – or if you are responsible for a pregnancy – it is important to tell your parents at once. Although many girls are terrified of breaking the news to their parents, they often find that, once the initial shock is over, parents can be extremely helpful and supportive. Remember that your parents are as likely to feel upset and guilty about the pregnancy as you are, and it may take them a little while to adjust to it.

You should see your family doctor without delay. The earlier help is sought, the more options are open to a pregnant youngster. If you decide to have an abortion, for example, it is safer and easier if done in the first few weeks, preferably within the first 3 months.

Special problems of the elderly

Introduction

Like all ageing machines, a human body that has been around for a number of years tends to work less efficiently than it did when "new". But this does not mean that illness is an inevitable part of old age. Certainly your lungs, kidneys, heart, and other organs will be less efficient at 60 than they were at 20, but ageing should not be equated with unavoidable breakdown. You need neither expect nor accept illness as an integral part of growing old.

Because of the natural process of ageing, some of the disorders covered in other sections of this book – arteriosclerosis and osteoarthritis, for example – tend to occur with greater frequency in older people; but they are not exclusively diseases of old age. The problems discussed in this section, however, are those that affect only or primarily the elderly.

How old is an "old" person? There is a good deal of truth in the saying that "you're as old as you feel". Many people of 75 or 80 and beyond are as alert and active as they were at 60, whereas a few 60-year-olds appear to have already crossed the threshold of "senility". The advances being made in medical and health care, coupled with increasingly positive attitudes to the problems of ageing and improved methods of social support, may well push old age further and further into the future for most of us who are alive today. Our prospects for a happier and healthier, as well as a longer, life are excellent.

The physical and mental disorders that affect today's elderly people sometimes pose as great a problem for their families as for the sufferers themselves. For this reason most of the following articles contain advice for concerned relatives intermingled with direct advice to the elderly. If you have family members who are over 65, you should be aware of the several organizations in this country that specialize in providing assistance and advice for old people. In virtually every area, for instance, there are local representatives of such groups as *Age Concern, Council and Care for the Elderly*, and *Help the Aged* (see p.768 for addresses). Ask your doctor or local health visitor to put you in touch with any of these groups; they provide a varied range of supportive facilities, including, in some cases, advice on financial matters.

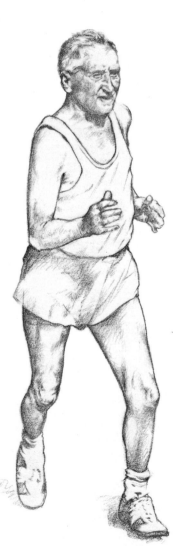

The ageing process

On average, a 75-year-old man will be 75mm (3in) shorter than he was when he was in his prime.

Over the years, a gradual loss of elastic tissues causes the skin to wrinkle and sag.

Between the ages of 30 and 75, the heart's efficiency decreases by about 30 per cent and the lungs' by 40 per cent.

The liver's efficiency decreases by 10 per cent, while the kidneys may be 40 per cent less efficient.

Thinning of the bones causes them to become lighter and more brittle.

The effect of age on different organs varies, but all become more susceptible to fatigue and disease. However, not everyone reaches the same stage at the same chronological age.

Planning for retirement

Now that so many people retire earlier and live longer, it seems likely that the majority will spend a quarter of their adult life in retirement while remaining physically and mentally active for much of this time. Yet some people approach this major period of their lives with no idea of how they are going to manage financially and no plans for activities to fill their new abundance of free time.

Financial planning for your retirement is essential. If possible, work out at least 5 years in advance how much you will have to live on and, if this amount seems only just adequate, before you retire try to renew, one by one, any expensive household items that show signs of wearing out. If necessary, seek professional advice – perhaps from your solicitor or bank manager – about how best to manage any investments as well as your pension.

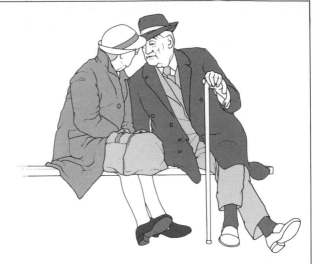

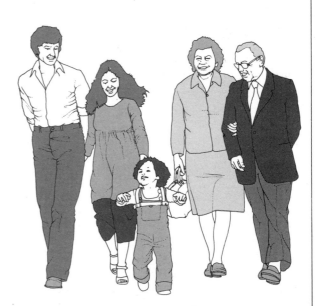

Activities

If you have always had interests and hobbies outside the sphere of your job, retirement will give you the opportunity to devote more time to them. It will also give you the chance to take up new interests – your local library will have information on any afternoon and evening classes run by your local authority. If your job was your main interest in life and you find the idea of giving it up depressing, some kind of voluntary work may be the ideal way for you to keep in touch without jeopardizing your pension rights.

Relationships

Good friends and neighbours are one of the best insurance policies for a happy old age. Think carefully before moving to another area when you retire, because it can be difficult to make new friends and fit into a new community as you become less active.

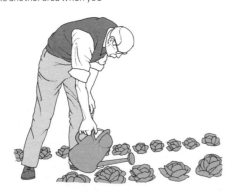

Incontinence

Incontinence is the uncontrollable, involuntary discharge of urine or faeces. Incontinence in the elderly – like incontinence in the young – is usually brought on by an underlying condition such as a urinary-tract disorder, constipation, immobility, or medication for some other problem. Incontinence is not an unavoidable part of "growing old", and it should not be accepted as such. It is, however, much more common in old people than in the young. This is because the efficiency of the muscular *sphincters* and the tone of various ligaments connected with the urinary and digestive tracts gradually diminish with age.

In general, the problem of incontinence disappears if the underlying condition is treated successfully. That condition might be, for example, a urinary-tract infection (see *Infections, inflammation, and injury*, p.502) or trouble with the *prostate gland* (p.574). Similarly, certain gastrointestinal diseases or too little *fibre* in the diet can often lead to a loss of bowel control. In all such cases treatment of the causative condition usually cures the incontinence.

One specific type of faecal incontinence that tends to occur chiefly in the elderly is brought on by faecal *impaction* – the accumulation of a hard mass of faecal matter somewhere in the bowel. The partial blockage upsets the mechanism by which faeces are regularly expelled, but the blockage is not complete enough to prevent the more liquid portion of bowel contents from seeping past and leaking out. If the blockage becomes big enough, it can press on the bladder and give rise to urinary incontinence as well.

A few people become incontinent as the result of a severe disorder such as *stroke* (p.268), *spinal-cord injury* (p.278), or *senile dementia* (p.724). In at least some of these cases it is unlikely that the basic disorder will respond to treatment. The accompanying incontinence must then be dealt with as a problem in its own right.

How common is the problem?

About 1 person in 5 over the age of 65 suffers from incontinence to at least a small degree. The great majority of these are incontinent of urine only. Some can no longer go several hours without passing urine; if their bladders are full, they may dribble urine when they cough or sneeze. Others may have a powerful urge to urinate even though there may be hardly any urine to pass.

Only a small proportion of sufferers are faecally incontinent; faecal incontinence on its own can sometimes be a sign of *depression* (p.297). Incontinence of both the bladder and bowel is extremely rare except among some very old, bedridden people.

What should be done?

Regardless of age, you should consult your doctor if you have episodes of involuntary urination or defecation. After examining you, the doctor may want specific diagnostic tests to find out whether the incontinence is due to an underlying condition such as urinary infection. If it is and the condition is reversible, you will be treated for it. If, however, the cause turns out to be irreversible, much can be done to moderate the more unpleasant effects.

What is the treatment?

Self-help: You may be able to re-establish some control over your bladder and bowels by using the toilet at frequent, regular intervals. Make sure your living and sleeping quarters are close to the toilet, and keep a chamber-pot or commode within reach of your bed. Wear garments that are easy to manage without fiddling with small buttons or catches. All lavatory facilities should be made as easy as possible to use; it sometimes helps, for example, to have handrails installed alongside the toilet. If you are becoming somewhat forgetful, use memory aids or even an alarm clock to remind you to follow a routine of, say, two-hourly visits to the lavatory. For urinary incontinence, drink sparingly, especially at bedtime; for faecal incontinence, eat plenty of high-fibre foods and remember that uncontrollable bowels tend to open about an hour after every meal. (For further suggestions see *Caring for the sick at home*, p.754.)

Professional help: Your doctor may be able to prescribe a drug that stabilizes activity of the bladder so that urges to pass urine are fewer and further apart. Unfortunately, effective bowel-stabilizing drugs have not yet been developed, but a course of laxatives or other drugs may improve matters. Enemas will clear any faecal impaction, and this should allow your bowels to resume their regular habits.

There are a number of bodily incontinence aids for people who need them. Your doctor, district nurse, or local centre for the elderly can tell you about them and can help you procure any that may be appropriate. A typical example is specially designed underwear, which soaks urine up into a porous outer layer and neutralizes the odour, leaving the inner layer (next to the skin) relatively dry. As well as avoiding embarrassment and reducing damage to outer clothing, such underwear minimizes skin problems around the genitals caused by incontinence.

In some cases of urinary incontinence a feasible treatment is *catheterization*: the insertion into the bladder of a plastic tube that drains urine into a bag. The bag is emptied at intervals. For persistent faecal incontinence, surgery to tighten or reinforce the anal sphincter is occasionally advisable. A recent development that aids certain sufferers is a tiny electrical device that is surgically implanted near the outlet from the bladder or rectum. A steady stream of minute electrical impulses stimulates muscles of the sphincter, allowing it to stay closed for longer periods but still to open when you want it to.

Accidental falls

Everyone has an occasional fall, but falls among adults are most common and most serious in people over 65. Many old people neglect the precautions listed in *How to guard against falls* (p.720) and live in houses packed with objects that are potential booby traps. Many neglect their vision and general health. And some slowing of the reflexes is inevitable with age. Unfortunately, too, your bones become more brittle as you age. Finally, you become increasingly susceptible to disorders (such as Parkinson's disease and various circulatory and arthritic conditions) that may affect your ability to retain your balance; and the drugs taken to control these disorders sometimes cause dizziness as an unpredictable side-effect.

How common is the problem?

Falls are by far the commonest type of accident in people over 65. Deaths from falls, or due to complications directly stemming from falls, account for more than half of all accidental deaths of old people in Britain. One recent estimate suggests that in the elderly population about 3 million falls need medical attention each year – an average of nearly 1 fairly bad fall for every 3 old people. In a typical orthopaedic ward for women, about half the patients are likely to be elderly women with broken bones. The corresponding proportion of elderly men is lower, probably because women's bones tend to become more brittle than men's.

What are the risks?

Many falls, even in people over 65, cause nothing worse than a bruise. Fragility of skin and small blood vessels, however, makes bruising more serious and extensive in the elderly after even a minor fall. There is always a risk, too, of falling against or upon something that is itself dangerous. Half of all deaths from burns in this country, for instance, occur among the aged, who may accidentally stumble into heating appliances or knock pans of boiling liquid over themselves. And an apparently gentle blow on the head can cause delayed bleeding within the skull (see *Subdural haemorrhage*, p.272). Broken bones, especially so-called broken hips, which are in fact thigh bones (femurs) broken near the top, are peculiarly common in the elderly; chances of a hip fracture resulting from a fall apparently increase twofold for each five years you attain past the age of 50.

Apart from the injuries of the fall itself, there may be several indirect consequences of the accident. If, as sometimes happens, a solitary victim lies immobilized and undiscovered for long hours or days, the result may be *hypothermia* (p.723), *pneumonia* (p.359), psychological problems, or even death. Moreover, if broken bones necessitate a stay in hospital, a long period of enforced immobility may further weaken ageing bones and muscles. And some old people who have had serious falls lose confidence in their ability to get about. They become less and less active, and therefore less and less confident – a vicious circle that can prematurely lead to bedridden inactivity.

What should be done?

Guard against falls by following the recommendations in the box on p.720. If you live alone, work out some way of alerting others swiftly in case you have an accident. Some elderly people always carry a noise-making device such as a whistle. Some have understandings with neighbours; they agree on a daily sign that will let the neighbours know they are well. If the sign is omitted on any day, then the neighbours are alerted to the possibility that they may have had an accident. (A word of warning, though: be careful not to develop a routine or set of signals that can prove useful as a guide for possible housebreakers.) It is also wise to agree on a schedule of telephone calls or visits to and from friends and relations, who will be alerted if the schedule is disrupted without any prior warning.

Remember that even a few days off your feet may cause weakness and stiffness of muscles and joints, making balance more unsteady. So keep as active as you can. If you begin to feel that you are less steady on your

How to guard against falls

Because anyone can have a bad fall, the following suggestions are worth considering regardless of age. Apart from toddlers, though, the people most likely to fall are the elderly. If you are over 65 (or if you are in any way responsible for the well-being of an old person), try to follow as many of these recommendations as are applicable in your situation. Since you probably need to spend money in order to put some of them into effect, you may want to find out whether you qualify for financial aid. Consult your local post office, social security office, or centre for the elderly.

1 If you need glasses, wear them. But never walk around with glasses on your nose that are meant only for reading; take them off before moving about.

2 If you are even slightly unsteady on your feet, use a walking stick. Do not hesitate to use a frame outdoors as well as in the house if you feel safer with one.

3 Wear well-fitting shoes or slippers with non-slip soles. Avoid long shoelaces, which can easily come undone and trip you up.

4 Store frequently used clothes and other items in places where you can reach them without standing on a stool or chair. If you must climb up to get something, use a stable stepladder or sturdy chair; better still, get someone to do the reaching for you.

5 Make sure carpets and other floor coverings are secured around the edges, and tack down worn spots. Never use loose mats and rugs on shiny, polished floors.

6 See to it that potential hazard spots such as steps and stairs are brightly lit. White paint on either side of a flight of stairs will help to lighten any dark corners.

7 Have a bedside lamp or low-wattage night light in your bedroom so that you never have to grope about in the dark when getting out of bed.

8 A strong banister running along all indoor and outdoor steps is advisable. Try to install one wherever such a support is lacking.

9 Fit secure handrails in convenient places near the bath and toilet, and use non-slip mats both inside and alongside the bath or shower.

10 Do everything possible to minimize clutter in rooms frequented by the elderly. Children's toys, especially those on wheels, are a particularly dangerous hazard.

11 Do not permit wires from electrical appliances to run loosely along the floor; wherever possible, wires should be secured to walls or skirting boards.

Safety in the house
There are a number of easy adjustments that can be made in the home to reduce hazards for an elderly person.

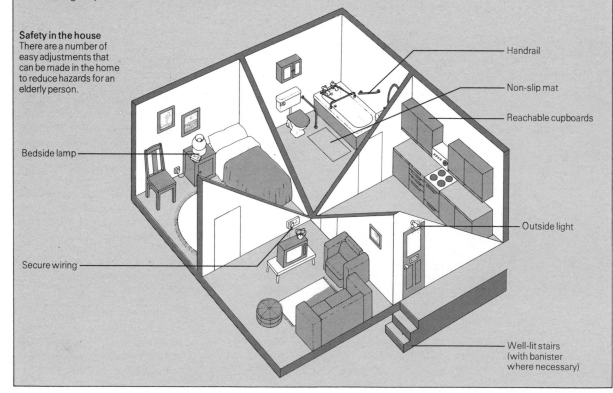

Handrail

Non-slip mat

Reachable cupboards

Bedside lamp

Outside light

Secure wiring

Well-lit stairs (with banister where necessary)

feet than you ought to be, consult your doctor. Since there are several possible causes of unsteadiness, the doctor may order a series of tests, including blood tests and *X-rays*, to determine whether your problem is a treatable underlying disorder. Always see your doctor, too, if you have had a bad fall, even though you have suffered no apparent ill-effects; it always pays to be cautious.

What is the treatment?

If you are present when someone falls, or if you find someone apparently immobilized by a fall, carry out appropriate first-aid measures (see *Accidents and emergencies*, p.801). An elderly person who is in pain should be seen by a doctor without delay. If you find anyone unconscious, you should summon medical help at once; if your doctor is not available, call an ambulance.

The pain and discomfort of a fall, even if no bones have been broken, may be considerable. It is important to relieve the pain as quickly as possible so that the person can keep moving. Bed may seem to be the most comfortable place, but it is all too easy for someone who is already stiff and sore after a fall to become quite bedbound and immobile. Painkillers may be needed, and cold compresses will reduce the pain and swelling of bruises. Application of heat can relieve any muscle stiffness.

Elderly people who have had treatment in hospital for broken bones (or any other type of disorder) are normally provided with home-help services during a recovery period following release from hospital. Ask your doctor to put you in touch with the proper agency for providing nursing and housekeeping assistance.

The failing senses

It is an inescapable fact that our sense organs – most notably the mechanisms of sight and hearing – are likely to deteriorate as we advance into old age. Often, though, declining sensitivity turns out to be at least partly caused by factors other than ageing.

Such cases can be treated and the senses either restored or improved. Even when the fault cannot be reversed, modern technical aids can significantly improve your ability to see and hear. So take advantage of them. The world need not recede into silent darkness as you pass through the so-called "twilight years".

The eyes: Only about 1 person in 20 over 50 years of age is likely to have keen enough eyesight to read, walk, and drive

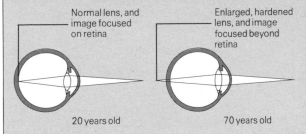

Normal lens, and image focused on retina

Enlarged, hardened lens, and image focused beyond retina

20 years old   70 years old

without glasses. Nine out of 10 people over 65 suffer from *presbyopia* (p.311), a condition in which the lens of the eye becomes stiff and so focuses less easily on nearby objects. There is no cure for ageing eyes themselves, but you should visit an optician regularly (see *Going to the optician*, p.312) for a check-up. A new pair of glasses may compensate for your failing eyesight; or – even more important – an examination may reveal an underlying and treatable disorder such as *cataract* (p.319) or *glaucoma* (p.320).

The ears: In Britain about 150,000 people over 65 are known to be sufficiently hard of hearing to have consulted their doctors about the problem. Probably 10 times as many have trouble hearing but have not sought medical help. This is unfortunate because increasing deafness may be due to an easily treated underlying cause such as an accumulation of wax in the ear. Wax accumulates faster as you get older (see *Wax blockage*, p.330). So it is wise to ask your doctor about the possibility of syringeing your ears whenever you notice that your sense of hearing seems impaired.

There is no magic cure, of course, for the gradual deterioration of the mechanism in the ear. Do not hesitate, however, to ask your doctor to prescribe a hearing aid, and make a point of persevering in its use until you have learned how to make the most of it. (For information on types of aid and their usage see *Hearing loss and hearing aids*, p.335.)

Other senses: Among other senses that often become less keen as you grow old are taste, smell, and balance. Do not worry if food tastes and smells less appetizing than it used to. This will not affect your well-being as long as you continue to eat a sensible and varied diet. Balance is a more serious matter since unsteadiness can lead to *accidental falls* (see p.719 for further advice). And there is one kind of sense perception – sensitivity to changes in temperature – that can be life-threatening if it deteriorates greatly.

The skin of healthy young adults can detect a temperature drop of only $\frac{1}{2}$°C (about 1°F) in the surroundings. In old age this sensitivity can diminish so much that you may fail to notice a drop of up to 5°C (about 9°F). That is one reason why elderly people tend to suffer more than the young from *hypothermia* (p.723). If you do not have thermostatically controlled central heating, you will do well to keep a thermometer in your living room so that you will be warned if the temperature falls below a safe level.

Skin problems of the elderly

(including senile purpura)

One reason why ageing skin becomes increasingly thinner, more wrinkled, and less flexible is that there is a gradual change in the nature of the fibrous and elastic elements in the skin that account for its suppleness and smoothness. This and other physical changes are irreversible; and as the ageing process continues, the skin may also become more susceptible to some of the disorders that can affect younger skin (see *Skin, hair, and nail disorders*, p.250). In addition, blotches and oddly pigmented patches of skin tend to appear in old age with increasing frequency and for no apparent reason. These may come and go, and in general they are not a cause for concern. One such development that is particularly common is known as senile purpura (which is an indication of nothing more serious than ageing skin).

Senile purpura

Reddish-brown or purplish areas, sometimes as big as 50mm (about 2in) in width or length, may appear anywhere on the body but are usually most noticeable on legs, forearms, or the backs of the hands. These markings are caused by bleeding under the skin; blood seeps slowly from tiny vessels that have become damaged by loss of elasticity in the skin. Although the blood is gradually reabsorbed, the underlying defect is irreversible and so the spots are likely to recur. They are harmless, and you need not see a doctor about them unless you want reassurance that the markings are really senile purpura, and not a treatable disorder.

Itching

Another irritating by-product of old age may be the development of extremely dry, itchy skin. If you are troubled by constant itching, see your doctor, who will examine you for signs of a possible underlying condition such as *jaundice* (p.485). If, as is likely, there is no cause other than age, the doctor will probably recommend an over-the-counter "moisturizing" ointment or lotion – one containing lanolin, for example – to relieve the itching.

Trigeminal neuralgia

(tic douleureux)

This kind of neuralgia ("neuralgia" means "pain from a damaged nerve") almost never affects anybody under 50 and is most common among people over 70. The trigeminal nerve is a major nerve in the face. If it is damaged the result is severe pain, which is usually felt in only one side of the face. We do not know what causes the nerve damage or why the condition is much more likely to occur in older people. Although not a life-threatening disorder, it can be extremely distressing and even disabling.

The pain of trigeminal neuralgia shoots through the affected side of the face along the track of the nerve. It may last for a few seconds or as much as a minute or more, and while it lasts it can be agonizing. It may be triggered off just by touching a sensitive place somewhere on the face or even after having been sitting in a draught.

Sometimes attacks occur for no apparent reason every few minutes over several days or weeks. They may then fade away, but stabbing pains usually return at decreasing intervals, and attacks may eventually become almost continuous. In some cases occasional muscular *spasms* accompany the pain and cause a facial tic (twitching).

What should be done?

If you have what seems to be trigeminal neuralgia, consult your doctor, who may want a careful examination of your sinuses and ears and may also suggest that you see your dentist before a firm diagnosis can be made. The reason for this is that infections of the sinuses, ears, or teeth often cause facial pain that may be mistaken for neuralgia. If you are suffering from trigeminal neuralgia, the doctor will probably prescribe a drug that prevents attacks in most cases. It must be taken exactly as prescribed; your doctor will supply regularly increasing doses until all pain has stopped, after which the dose is gradually reduced. If the drug does not work in your case, your doctor may recommend an operation to destroy the trigeminal nerve by either cutting through it or injecting alcohol around it. Any such procedure is done under general anaesthetic by a *neurosurgeon*. Until recently this left part of the face permanently numb. However, newly developed techniques have substantially improved the results of operative treatment, and most patients can now confidently expect a cure without this unpleasant development.

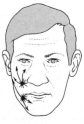

Sites of the pain

Functions of the trigeminal nerve
The trigeminal nerve supplies sensation to the face, teeth, mouth, and nasal cavity, and produces movement in the muscles of the jaw.

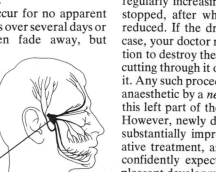

Trigeminal nerve

Hypothermia

Hypothermia is a state in which body temperature falls more than 2°C (about 4°F) below the healthy norm of 37°C (98.6°F). Death is a possibility if hypothermia persists for more than a few hours; and a person whose body temperature drops below about 25°C (77°F) has only a 30 per cent chance of recovery. Anyone can become hypothermic and freeze to death if exposed to extreme cold for some time without adequate protection. And hypothermia is always a risk for people who swim in the sea around Britain at any time of year, but particularly in summer when conditions on land can be deceptively warm. Most of its victims in Britain, however, are elderly (chiefly people over 75). There are two main reasons for this. First, the ageing body becomes progressively less capable of maintaining an even temperature when subjected to external cold. Secondly, the body mechanism that detects a drop in its own temperature gradually loses its sensitivity; some old people do not realize they are dangerously cold (see *The failing senses*, p.721).

What are the symptoms?
If you find an old person sitting or lying listlessly in cold conditions, always suspect hypothermia even if he or she is covered by several blankets or layers of clothing. Early symptoms of hypothermia are likely to include drowsiness, mental confusion, and pallor. Loss of consciousness follows. The hypothermic individual's hands and feet will obviously feel cold to the touch, but a much more telling indication of hypothermia is a cold abdomen. The best way to determine whether body temperature is dangerously low, of course, is to use a thermometer (see *Taking a temperature*, p.755).

How common is the problem?
In an average winter in this country more than 9,000 elderly people are admitted to hospital because of hypothermia, and at least 500 die of it. However, it is likely that many more people whose deaths have been attributed to other causes, such as *heart failure* (p.381), have in fact died of hypothermia. The vast majority of sufferers are old men and women living alone in poor home conditions. But even the relatively well-off may suffer physically from the social isolation that can come with old age.

What should be done?
To begin with, take preventive measures if you have elderly relatives or neighbours. Visit them as often as you can in cold weather, and do everything possible to ensure that they have plenty of warm clothes and blankets, that they eat well, and that their living quarters are kept at a temperature of at least 20°C (68°F). Make certain, too, that they are taking advantage of any government services or benefits such as fuel-bill subsidies that they may require. All post offices and social security offices can provide information and advisory leaflets for people over 65. In addition, there are many special organizations – Meals on Wheels, for instance – that are prepared to assist the elderly in a variety of ways (see p.768 for some names and addresses).

If you find an old person in what appears to be an early stage of hypothermia, take him or her to a nearby doctor or call for medical help. If the sufferer is already unconscious and you cannot get your own doctor, ask for an ambulance. (The unconsciousness may be due to a condition other than hypothermia – a stroke or heart attack, for example – and emergency treatment is obviously necessary in any case.) While waiting for professional help to arrive, do what you can to warm the cold body gradually. Additional coverings and a warm drink – *not* an alcoholic drink – may help if the hypothermic person is still conscious. Be gentle. Do not pile very heavy coverings on sufferers; do not try to force them to eat or drink; do not chafe their hands or feet roughly in order to restore warmth (see *Accidents and emergencies*, p.809).

What is the treatment?
The key to treatment of hypothermia is gentle, gradual re-warming of the chilled body, and this is precisely what is done by doctors in or out of hospital. The treatment *must* be gradual because over-swift application of heat can cause sudden enlargement of blood vessels at the surface of the body. If this happens, a rush of blood into the swollen vessels may rob vital inner organs of the blood that they need.

Preventing hypothermia
Elderly people may become dangerously cold without realizing it, so they should be encouraged to keep their living quarters at a minimum temperature of 20°C (68°F) even if they do not feel cold.

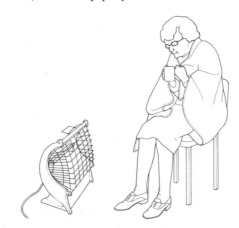

Senile dementia

Dementia is a disorder in which a formerly normal brain ceases to function normally and the sufferer becomes forgetful, confused, and out of touch with the real world. The condition is very rare among people under 65 (see *Pre-senile dementia*, p.293). Senile dementia (dementia affecting the elderly), on the other hand, is common. The deterioration of the mind is due sometimes to the progressive wasting of irreplaceable brain cells; sometimes – and when this happens, there is a greater possibility of any treatment being successful – to gradual narrowing and hardening of the arteries that carry blood to the brain (see *Arteriosclerosis*, p.404).

Senile dementia, which may develop over several years, is by definition progressive and incurable. Do not assume, however, that signs of confusion or impaired intellectual capacity in someone over 65 are always due to senility. There may be an underlying – and treatable – cause. For example, chest or urinary-tract infections, strokes, heart attacks, and hypothermia can result in mental confusion; and so can a low blood-sugar level, hypoglycaemia, or the use of certain types of drug. The confusion, agitation, and drowsiness resulting from any such underlying condition are different from the symptoms of senile dementia in two respects: they tend to develop rapidly over the course of a day or two, and they are likely to clear up with appropriate treatment of the basic trouble. In some cases, when senile dementia is developing, the condition may seem worse than it is because of problems with eyesight and hearing that already exist.

Moreover, actual dementia is sometimes caused by long-standing abuse of alcohol or drugs or by vitamin deficiency, hypothyroidism, syphilis, or brain trouble such as a tumour or subdural haemorrhage. And very often the mental signs of "senility" lessen when any such condition is treated. An additional common problem in the elderly is depressive illness (see *Depression*, p.297), which sometimes mimics the symptoms of dementia. These symptoms are unfortunately often attributed to dementia when they may be caused by treatable depression.

The following paragraphs deal exclusively with true senile dementia, which has a slow, insidious onset and which is not caused by an underlying, treatable disorder. Many elderly people in an early stage of the condition realize that they are beginning to lose their mental grip, but they can do little to arrest its progress. The advice in this article is therefore directed to close relatives and friends rather than to the sufferers themselves.

What are the symptoms?

The first symptom is a gradual loss of memory, particularly of recent events. You will begin to notice that the elderly person cannot remember what has happened a few hours (or even moments) earlier, although he or she can recall happenings of many years ago. This is a classic symptom of an old memory and does not necessarily mean that dementia will progress, though it can do. As weeks and months pass, powers of reasoning and understanding may dwindle, and there may also be a loss of interest in all familiar pursuits, even in such simple activities as watching television or seeking news of friends. Eventually there may be a deterioration of personality.

Senile dementia often culminates in emotional and physical instability. Some sufferers tend to swing between moods of apathetic withdrawal and overactive aggressiveness, and they may behave in uninhibited and antisocial ways. Table manners deteriorate; personal cleanliness is neglected; and usual politeness disappears. Sometimes sufferers may even become violent if impulsive behaviour is frustrated. A few old people lose their sexual inhibitions, too, and this can lead to embarrassing physical approaches to young persons of either sex. Any or all such symptoms lead slowly but progressively towards decay of intellect and emotion.

How common is the problem?

The older the age group, the greater the likelihood of senile dementia. In Britain about 1 person in 10 over the age of 65 has the condition, but the figures rise to 1 in 5 over the age of 80. This means that, in the population at large, about 1 family in every 10 includes at least one elderly member suffering from senile dementia.

What are the risks?

You are taking risks whenever you leave demented old people alone or permit them to continue living alone after they have progressed beyond an early stage of senility. Because of forgetfulness and inability to concentrate, there is a constant danger of accidental misuse of fire, gas, and kitchen tools. Combined with possible physical disabilities such as deafness or impaired vision, mental confusion makes it difficult for sufferers to take medicines as prescribed, to cross streets in safety, or even to use the bathroom. Without supervision they are apt to eat badly and to neglect personal hygiene. The results can be distressing, especially if – as often happens – they begin to suffer from *incontinence* (p.718), malnutrition, or a disease caused by

Drugs and the elderly

Even minor disorders of old age often need treatment, at least in part, with pills, capsules, or liquid medicines. As a result, you may well be taking several different drugs – probably in different forms and on different schedules – at one time. In such an event it is only too easy to become confused about which medicines to take at which intervals, or to forget whether the correct dose of a given drug is 1, 2, or 3 pills. Research studies indicate that about 4 in every 10 elderly people who are under doctors' care do not take their medicine precisely (or, in many cases, even approximately) as prescribed by the doctor.

The following list of Dos and Don'ts should help you to avoid making serious mistakes. (The list has been compiled primarily for people over 65. But it contains good advice for anyone who uses drugs for medical reasons – and this means practically everybody.)

Dos

Do use whatever memory aids you find useful to help you re-member to take your medicines, tablets, etc. regularly as prescribed. For ex-ample, a drug that is meant to be taken at the same time once a day might always be taken at bedtime, and it might be a good idea to take a three-times-a-day drug after each meal. Write down a check-list of all the drugs you are taking, and up-date the list as soon as there are changes. It will also help if

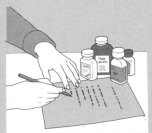

you prepare your list in the form of a calendar upon which you can tick off each dose of every drug as you take it (above).

Do make sure that all contain-ers are clearly labelled with the contents and times of dosing; if you have trouble reading a pharmacist's writing, ask for the label to be rewritten in larger, clearer characters. If you are taking different drugs for different disorders, you could write the name of the disorder on the relevant container to avoid confusion when you need to take a particular drug.

Do ask your doctor to give you a drug in the easiest possible form to take. For instance, if you find it difficult to pour a liquid medicine into a measur-ing spoon without spilling some, it may be possible to get the same drug in tablet form. Similarly, if your fingers cannot easily cope with the lids of child-proof containers, your pharmacist may agree to put your pills in simple screw-top bottles (below).

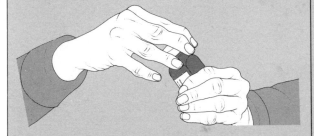

Do inform *all* the doctors you deal with – for example, your general practitioner and any hospital doctors or specialists – of *all* the drugs you are taking, even those you have bought over the counter (show them your check-list if you can). This will help prevent double treat-ment or dangerous interactions of various drugs.

Don'ts

Don't be a drugs magpie, per-mitting unused residues to ac-cumulate in your medicine cabinet. Keep drugs that you are currently using (including those, such as antihistamines or paracetamol, that you need to take only occasionally), and discard partially used supplies of all other drugs (right).

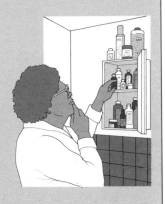

Don't start taking a drug again after a long interval without consulting your doctor. Today's symptoms may be due to a dis-order entirely different from the one for which last year's drug was prescribed. Moreover, some drug that you may now be taking might interact dangerously with the old one. And many drugs have a limited "shelf life", after which they become less effective and some can even be harmful.

Don't keep containers of pills on your bedside table unless absolutely necessary; there is too much risk of sleepily taking either the wrong medicine or an overdose of the right one. This can happen especially if, in-stead of switching on the light, you trust to your sense of touch to find the pills (right).

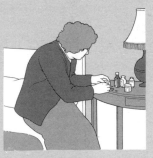

Don't leave similar-looking drug containers grouped together. To avoid confusion, ask your pharmacist, if necessary, to change the packaging of a drug. But you yourself should not transfer the contents of one container to another without making absolutely sure that the new container is correctly and clearly labelled.

lack of vitamins (see *Vitamins*, p.494). If a relative of yours in the early stages of senility is still going about without companionship, be sure that he or she always carries some mark of identification – for example, a bracelet inscribed with name and address or, at the very least, a piece of paper carrying your own address and telephone number.

What should be done?

If you suspect that an elderly relative or close friend is beginning to suffer from dementia, you should gently persuade (or take) him or her to see a doctor, preferably the family doctor, who will be familiar with the person's history and may already have suspected signs of the condition. The doctor may refer you to a *geriatrician*, if necessary. After making a physical examination and carrying out tests of memory and reasoning power, the doctor will probably search for the symptoms of a possible underlying disease – the pallor of vitamin B_{12} deficiency, for example – that might be causing mental deterioration. If loss of memory or confusion has developed with extreme rapidity, the doctor will be unwilling to make a firm diagnosis of senile dementia without further tests. If, however, you have noticed a slow deterioration, and if the sufferer is well past 65, and there seems to be no good reason for him or her to be suffering from depression, your suspicion is likely to be confirmed.

What is the treatment?

Although no medical cure is possible, your doctor will undoubtedly help you decide what to do next. Some practical help can be given to both the old person and those who care for him or her. In the early stages of senility, when many old people are still able to live alone, their friends can help by organizing memory aids such as lists and routines, and by making sure that adequate food and warmth are provided. There are risks to this procedure (see "What are the risks?" above); but unless they have become very confused, most of the elderly do better in familiar – even if muddled – surroundings than in homes for the aged. Visits by an efficient, sympathetic health visitor or district nurse, along with regular attention from a service such as Home Help or Meals on Wheels, will help many people to maintain some degree of independence in spite of increasing senility.

If you feel responsible for the well-being of a senile relative, you should take as much advantage of community services as you can. In many places, for instance, there are day-care centres where old people are looked after for several hours, provided with lunch, and given some kind of *occupational therapy* (see *Community health care*, p.743). Your doctor may also be able to arrange for your relative to be admitted to hospital or a home for the elderly (see the box below) for brief periods so that you can have an occasional holiday. And the doctor can advise you how to cope with such specific problems as incontinence. For information on home-nursing techniques see the section entitled *Caring for the sick at home* on p.754.

What are the long-term prospects?

Eventually your aged relative may well require the skilled and constant care that are available only in long-stay hospitals or homes. If the doctor strongly recommends this form of care, you will be doing the old person the best possible service by accepting the recommendation.

Special care for the elderly

One of the effects of age on a person is often increasing inability to cope – either mentally or physically – with everyday chores. Many old people are fiercely independent and may try to hide any disability because they are afraid of being "put into a home" and thereby losing all autonomy. However, in Britain only 6 per cent of old people are in residential care – either state-run or private. The other 94 per cent are either largely independent, or dependent on friends or relatives, or living – and to a large extent coping – at home while being supported in some way by various community services.

Most congenial for many old people is a system whereby they are cared for by relatives who live with or near them. However, this can be a tremendous burden on the families involved. For this reason, the family doctor may make arrangements for day care or short holiday care, when the elderly person goes to a special centre or residential home for a week every few months, or for 1 or 2 days every week, so relieving the strain on relatives.

Full-time residential care, run either privately or by the social services department of the local authority, is usually recommended only for old people for whom any of the alternatives is impractical. Many old people adapt well to institutional life after the initial upheaval, but in some cases it has been found that loss of independence leads to loss of initiative, intellect, and personality. The warden-supervised sheltered homes that are now being provided by some local authorities may be the answer for the many old people who need a certain amount of daily care but want to retain a measure of independence.

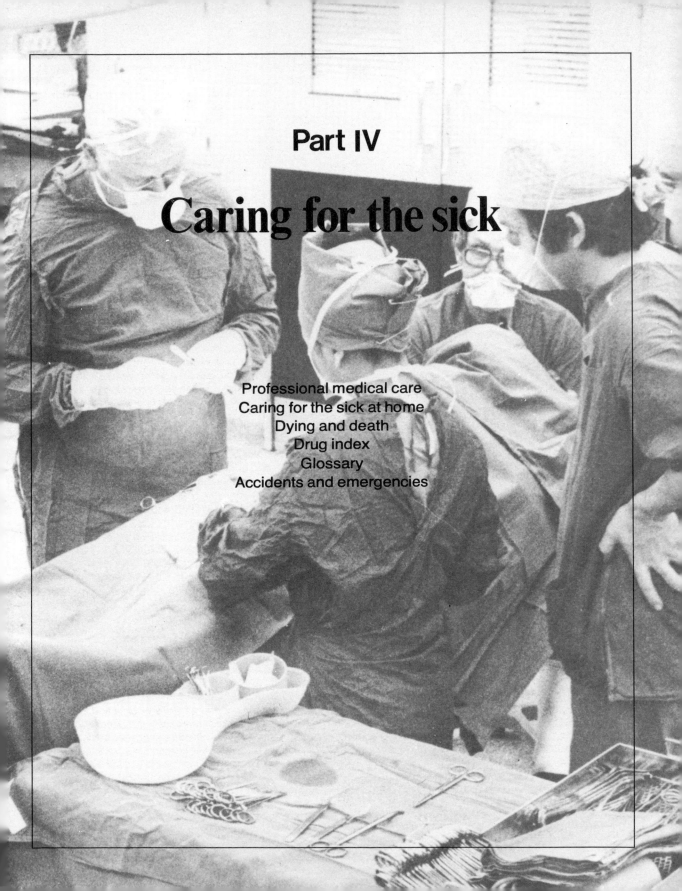

Part IV

Caring for the sick

Professional medical care
Caring for the sick at home
Dying and death
Drug index
Glossary
Accidents and emergencies

Professional medical care

Introduction

The world of professional medicine is divided into three parts – primary care, secondary care, and community medicine. The key member of the primary care team, to whom you as a member of the public have direct access, is the family doctor (general practitioner). He or she is the person most of us consult when we have a medical or health problem. As a practitioner of general medicine, your family doctor is likely to be able to treat most minor illnesses and also cope with some major ones – many GPs have a special interest in, say, *paediatrics* (the care of infants and children), or *obstetrics* (the care of pregnant women and women in childbirth), or some other speciality. For detailed diagnosis and expert treatment of major illnesses, however, your family doctor will sometimes hand you over ("refer you") to the key member of the secondary team – the specialist hospital doctor. Each local health authority has a community physician who organizes preventive services such as immunization and also watches for and controls outbreaks of infectious diseases.

The information in the following section is organized largely according to the primary/secondary care distinction. The first pages deal chiefly with the family doctor – how to find one and sign on, and the services he or she provides, along with details concerning the allied professionals such as the pharmacist (chemist). The next group of articles deals with the secondary care team of hospital doctors, nurses, and associated specialists, together with descriptions of the different types of hospital and how they are organized.

All Western countries spend between 5 and 10 per cent of their Gross National Product on the medical care of their populations; but the systems of health-care finance vary from one country to another. Britain pays for almost all of its medical services out of taxation – that is, all earning members of the population contribute payments in the form of direct taxation. As a patient of the British National Health Service, you pay no fees to your general practitioner, and hospital care is also free. Most people pay only small amounts towards the cost of drugs, dental treatment, and spectacles, since the cost of these items is heavily subsidized by the NHS. A few individuals are outside the system; they arrange for all treatment as private patients and pay in full for the treatment they need. Many others have limited health insurance for some types of treatment.

In most industrialized countries other than Britain, the only medical care funded by general taxation is for the mentally handicapped, the chronically mentally ill, and those elderly persons who have no means to pay for their treatment. In such countries, all other treatments – both in and out of hospital – are paid for by the patient. The patient is then reimbursed for all or most of the fees he or she has paid, by an insurance scheme. In some countries the insurance policy is arranged directly by the state; in others, several independent insurance companies provide alternative policies.

Halfway between the British system and the insurance-based scheme lies the concept of "health-maintenance programmes". Participants – usually whole families – pay a fixed sum per year to the organization that runs the programme, and in return they receive as much or as little medical care as they need. In contrast to insurance-based schemes, and in line with the British system, doctors and hospitals have no direct financial relationship with their patients. The three approaches outlined above can be combined in several ways; and within any one country different systems may be operating at any one time.

Each system of health-care funding has its advantages and disadvantages. Insurance-based systems are said to provide doctors and patients with the most "realistic" setting for medical care, but they rarely provide adequate financial cover for the expensive, long-term treatment needed for chronic illness such as regular *dialysis* for the kidney-failure patient. In these circumstances prolonged illness may still cause families serious financial hardship. Nor do insurance-based systems provide for the poor and needy, alcoholics, and vagrants. On the other hand, taxation-based schemes are usually under-financed, with too little investment spending on new buildings and new equipment. In almost every country the potential cost of developing medicine is outstripping the financial resources available.

General practice

The bulk of general medical care in Britain is provided by the general practitioner – often called the GP or family doctor. The GP treats a wide variety of symptoms and illnesses in patients of all kinds, but does not specialize exclusively in any particular group of patients or part of the body. About 90 per cent of patients are dealt with personally by the GP; the remaining cases are referred by the GP to a hospital specialist.

British general practice is based on the idea of a GP as a personal doctor who knows his or her patients and their background and can use this knowledge in helping them when they are ill. GPs have a continuing responsibility for the care of their patients and have to be available to them – or arrange for a deputy to be available during holidays, for example – 24 hours a day, seven days a week.

Registering with a GP

Your first step in obtaining general medical care under the National Health Service is to register with a GP who is under contract to the NHS. Even though any NHS GP is legally bound to provide you with any emergency treatment you may need, whether you are registered or not, you should register with a GP before you actually need one. Then, if you become ill, you will not have to waste time finding a doctor, and your doctor will have immediate access to your records.

Anyone over 16 has the right to choose his or her GP; parents choose for children under 16. If there are several GPs in your area, you may choose which one to register with. To discover the GPs in your area, you should consult the medical list in your local main post office or public library or the office of your local Family Practitioner Committee – the body responsible for organizing the services of local GPs, dentists, pharmacists, and opticians. You can find the address of the committee on your medical card or in the telephone directory.

The medical list gives the name and address of each local GP within the NHS. It states whether he or she works alone or with other doctors, what the surgery hours are, and whether the surgery runs an appointments system. A "C" after the doctor's name indicates that the doctor provides a contraceptive service, giving patients advice on methods of contraception and prescribing oral contraceptives. An "M" indicates that the doctor is a qualified *obstetrician* and will provide any woman with all or part of the care she needs when having a baby. Even if a doctor is not an obstetrician, he or she may still provide some maternity care.

The Family Practitioner Committee will not recommend a doctor. Its list merely enables you to discover a doctor near you who might provide you with a suitable service. The list will not tell you whether the doctor provides his or her own out-of-hours service or uses a *deputizing service* (p.731), whether the doctor works with nurses, midwives, and health visitors, or if the doctor has a special interest – for example, in children (*paediatrics*), or in the elderly (*geriatrics*). To find out the answers to any of these questions, you will have to go along to the surgery and ask either the doctor or the receptionist. You are also entitled to ask the doctor's attitudes on abortions, vasectomies, home deliveries, and other contentious matters that concern you and your family. It is a good idea to ask your friends, relatives, or neighbours who are patients of the doctor for their opinions.

Once you have chosen your doctor, you should go to the surgery and tell the doctor's receptionist that you would like to register as a patient. Take your medical card with you (if you have not got one, contact the Family Practitioner Committee). The doctor does not need to see you before accepting you as a patient. If the doctor accepts you, he or she will sign the card and will send it to the local Family Practitioner Committee. The committee will register you on the doctor's list of patients, arrange for your medical records to be transferred from your previous doctor, and send you a new medical card.

What to do if you cannot find a doctor

Just as you have a right to choose your family doctor, so the doctor has a right to choose his or her patients, and you may find that the doctor of your choice will not take you on to the list of patients. This may be because you live out of the doctor's area or the list is full (although the doctor does not have to give you a reason). You may also be removed from a doctor's list at any time – again without any need for a reason to be given. If this happens, the doctor is, however, obliged to give you any necessary treatment until you have found another doctor.

If you have difficulty in finding another doctor – because you have just moved to a new area, or if you have been removed from a doctor's list – contact your local Family Practitioner Committee. It will assign you to a doctor of its own choice.

If your doctor moves away or retires, the Family Practitioner Committee will arrange for you to be transferred to another doctor. If your former doctor is replaced, you will probably be placed on the list of the new doctor. If you do not accept the committee's transfer, you must find a new doctor yourself.

Temporary patients

If you move away from home for less than three months, you may apply to a doctor in the new area for treatment as a temporary resident. You must tell the doctor how long you are likely to be in the area. You will also need to show the doctor your medical card, or quote your NHS number (which is on the card), or give the name of your family doctor.

Changing your doctor

You have the right to change your doctor at any time. If you need to do this as a result of moving house, you simply follow the procedure already described above. If you want to change your doctor for any other reason, you must first make sure the new doctor you have chosen is willing to accept you, and then do one of two things. The first alternative is to take your medical card to your present doctor, say that you want to change to a new doctor, and ask him or her to sign part B of the card, which shows consent to the change; you then fill in the card and take it to the new doctor. The second alternative is to write to your local Family Practitioner Committee, supplying details of the change you want to be made and enclosing your card; the committee will then arrange the transfer (which will not take effect until 14 days after the committee received your letter) and they will send you a new card. (These methods of changing your doctor and the relevant addresses are also given on your medical card.)

How a general practice works

Most GPs work in group practices and in conjunction with a variety of other health-care staff – receptionists, health visitors, nurses, midwives, and sometimes social workers and remedial therapists – to make up what is known as a "primary care team". The strength of such a team lies in its being able to practise more preventive medicine than could a single GP, and also in providing long-term help for the chronically ill. Often each doctor in the group will have a particular specialist interest – in child health, or sexual counselling, for example – and patients can arrange to see the appropriate group doctor, even if they are not on his or her list.

The basic service that a GP provides is regular surgeries, usually held twice a day, in the morning and evening. More and more GPs are running their surgeries on an appointments system, both to regulate their work and to prevent their patients having to wait in the surgery too long. Some GPs, however, still run a traditional open-access surgery at which the patient just turns up and waits his or her turn to see the doctor. At some surgeries, the two systems are combined, with booked-appointment periods and some open-access periods. Whatever the system, if your case is urgent you will be given priority. If you have difficulty in convincing a receptionist that you need to see a doctor right away, or if you do not want to discuss the details of your condition with the receptionist, ask to speak to the doctor personally.

Seeing other doctors: Some general practices enable you to see any doctor in the group. There are advantages in this. For example, if you want an immediate appointment and your doctor is booked up, you may be able to see one of the others. Or you may find that one of the other doctors is more sympathetic than the one you are registered with or has a special interest in a condition you suffer from – in which case you can always make appointments to see that doctor or make sure of attending at the times he or she is taking surgery.

The primary care team: There are several important members of the primary care team besides the GP. One of these is the practice nurse, who is usually employed by the doctor and works within the surgery. She may hold her own separate clinics (for procedures such as dressings, injections, and immunizations), which do not coincide with the time of the doctor's surgeries; and you may have to make appointments to attend these.

The district nurse is employed by the local health authority. She provides nursing care in the patient's own home – for patients just discharged from hospital, patients with a chronic (long-term) condition, and patients who are terminally ill.

The district midwife – who is, again, a local health authority employee – works with GPs in providing ante- and post-natal care and attends the confinements of women who have their babies at home.

The health visitor also works for the local authority. She is a nurse (and may also be a midwife) trained in the preventive and social aspects of health care. Unlike the district nurse, who looks after people who are already ill, the health visitor educates families in staying healthy. Health visitors are responsible for visiting newborn babies once they have returned home from hospital or, if they have been born at home, once they have passed from the care of the midwife. They give advice to parents on looking after the baby and check on the baby's development by carrying out simple tests of hearing, vision, and coordination. Health visitors also visit the handicapped, the elderly, and people with infectious diseases, who cannot leave their homes; they advise such people on home management and hygiene. Their work partly overlaps with that of social workers, to whom they may refer any difficult social problems they come across.

In a few areas, GPs can also call on the help of community *physiotherapists* and dieticians, who may be based at a hospital, health centre, or community clinic. These specialists may visit patients in their homes.

Health centres: A health centre is a purpose-built unit from which one or more group practices may operate. Since it is owned by the local health authority, the health centre may also provide premises for dentists, chiropodists, and other health service staff.

Emergencies: If you are too ill to visit the surgery, you can ask the doctor to come to your home. In such a case, you must try to let the doctor know as early as possible in the day, preferably before mid-morning, so that the doctor can plan his or her rounds for the day. If your condition is serious and you cannot get hold of your doctor (for instance, because he or she is out visiting other patients) or any of the other doctors in the practice, then ring 999 and ask for an ambulance to take you to hospital.

If you fall ill outside surgery hours, you should telephone your family doctor if he or she runs an out-of-hours service. Explain your symptoms as exactly and clearly as possible, so that the doctor can judge whether your condition warrants a visit. If your condition is not serious enough for this, the doctor will give you advice on self-treatment over the telephone and ask you to ring again should your condition get worse. In serious cases, the doctor may arrange for an ambulance to take you to hospital – either to the accident and emergency department or to a ward to which your direct admission has been arranged by the doctor.

A GP cannot be on call every night and every weekend, and the doctor you speak to may well not be your own. Doctors in group or partnership practices often have a rota to take over one another's out-of-hours work. Any doctor you contact at your own practice will have access to your medical records should they be needed.

Deputizing services: Some doctors arrange for their out-of-hours work to be done by a deputizing service. This is usually a commercial organization and not run by a Family Practitioner Committee. Nevertheless, the medical aspects of the service are monitored by a committee of local doctors, and the local Family Practitioner Committee also limits the amount of medical service that a general practice can pass on to a deputizing service.

If your doctor is using a deputizing service, you will be referred, on telephoning your doctor, to the service's telephone number. Some services employ nurses to answer the calls, and they may be able to give you advice over the telephone. But if you particularly ask for a doctor to visit you, the service will send one. The deputy doctor will probably give you a letter to take to your own doctor in the morning, explaining what treatment has been given so that your own doctor can arrange any necessary follow-up care.

Examination and diagnosis
Often the most useful aid in helping your doctor to decide what is wrong with you is your description of your symptoms. For that reason, the doctor will ask you detailed questions about them – how much distress they are causing you, when they first appeared, whether you have had them before, and so on. To help the doctor in a diagnosis, and to save time, you should anticipate the most obvious questions before you go along to the surgery and prepare accurate answers to them: for example, try to remember *exactly* when your symptoms started. After questioning you, the doctor may then examine you, possibly with the aid of an instrument. Some GPs routinely measure the blood pressure of their older patients, whether or not their complaint warrants it. In this way they use the opportunity of the patient's visit to discover whether he or she is suffering from *high blood pressure* (p.382) – a potentially risky condition that does not always produce symptoms.

Tests: Nearly all GPs have access to the *X-ray* and *pathology* departments of the nearest general hospital, which can provide them with more specialized forms of investigation than their own examination; and, if necessary, your doctor may send you to the hospital for an X-ray or a blood, urine, or faeces test. (There are some simple blood and urine tests that your doctor can perform in the surgery, and some group practices have their own *electrocardiograph* – a machine that measures the functioning of the heart; in both cases, this will save patients a trip to the local hospital.)

The hospital sends the results of any tests to your doctor. On the basis of the results, the doctor then decides whether you need further tests, whether he or she can treat you, or whether you need to see a specialist.

Drugs

Your doctor will prescribe for you any drugs that you need. In most cases you will need to take the prescription to a chemist's, but sometimes the doctor can provide you with the drug personally, as is often the case at a rural practice.

In towns and cities, chemists usually take it in turns to stay open in the evening so that medicines prescribed at evening surgery can be dispensed that evening. You can discover the rota of evening openings by consulting your local newspaper or asking your doctor or the doctor's receptionist.

If you are on long-term drug treatment, you will not usually have to see the doctor each time you need a new prescription. Instead, you simply telephone the receptionist at the surgery and request a repeat prescription, which you can pick up later in the day. But if you are on long-term treatment, your doctor will want to see you regularly in order to keep a check on your condition.

Prescription charges: Under the NHS you pay a flat-rate charge (the "prescription charge") for the drugs you receive on each prescription, irrespective of their real cost. There is an exception to this: some contraceptives are prescribed free. The following groups of people are exempt from having to pay prescription charges:

- Children up to and including the age of 16
- Women aged 60 and over
- Men aged 65 and over
- Pregnant women (who must get a certificate from their midwife or doctor)
- Women with children under 1 year old
- People on supplementary benefit or family income supplement
- People suffering from certain specified long-term illnesses

If you consult a doctor privately, he or she cannot give you an NHS prescription for drugs. You will be given a private prescription and will have to pay the full cost of the prescribed drugs.

Charges

If you are registered with a GP as an NHS patient you pay nothing for the doctor's medical services. The doctor also provides certain medical certificates free of charge; these include the certificates you need to claim sickness benefit. Your doctor may, however, charge you if you need a private certificate of sickness to show your employer or a certificate of fitness to drive certain vehicles. You will also have to pay for any vaccinations needed to visit certain countries and for an International Certificate of Vaccination.

If you are consulting a doctor for treatment as a temporary resident, the doctor is entitled to ask you to produce your medical card and, if you cannot, to charge you for his or her services. The doctor will then give you a receipt, so that you can reclaim the fee from your local Family Practitioner Committee when you return home.

For private consultations see *Private medicine*, p.746.

Pharmacists (chemists)

General pharmacists who work in chemists' shops are contracted to dispense drugs to NHS patients and also supply them to private patients. If you are unsure about any aspect of the drugs your doctor has prescribed – for example, whether you can drink alcohol or drive after taking the drug – then ask the pharmacist (or telephone your doctor).

Pharmacists can also advise you about minor disorders and about various medicines and dressings they sell without prescription. Always make sure your doctor has signed the prescription before you leave the surgery, otherwise the pharmacist will not make it up. And never attempt to obtain prescribed drugs from a pharmacist without a prescription; under no circumstances will he or she provide you with them.

Referral to hospital

If your doctor refers you to a specialist (also known as a consultant), the doctor will make an appointment for you to attend the specialist's out-patient clinic. This is usually held in a large hospital, where the specialist has easy access to X-ray and pathology departments. But in some cases, specialists hold clinics in a small cottage hospital or a health centre.

If you want to see a private specialist, your GP can arrange this for you.

If you are too ill to attend the out-patient clinic, your doctor will probably arrange for the specialist to visit you at home. If your condition is severe, you may be admitted to hospital there and then, as an in-patient. Once your doctor has referred you to a specialist, the specialist is responsible for your care until he or she discharges you and refers you back to your own doctor.

Some GPs are in charge of beds in a cottage (community) hospital. If your family doctor is such a GP and if your condition is one which the GP can treat but which needs nursing care that is not available at home, the GP may admit you to one of these beds and look after you while you are in hospital.

Hospitals

A large part of the hospital service is provided by the district general hospital. This usually contains beds for major medical and surgical cases. Often there are beds for maternity and children's cases, and sometimes for acute psychiatric and geriatric cases. The district general hospital also has operating theatres, *X-ray* departments, various laboratories, and out-patient clinics.

In addition to the general hospitals, there are many single-speciality hospitals. These include maternity, eye, and children's hospitals – but by far the largest in number are hospitals for the mentally ill and the mentally handicapped. Between them, these last two specialist hospitals account for about half the hospital beds in Britain.

Many single-speciality hospitals, especially in large cities, are centres for post-graduate training and research and they build up a considerable expertise in their speciality. If you have an especially rare condition, you may be sent some distance to such a specialist centre for sophisticated treatment.

A teaching hospital is one attached to a medical school, from which students go to the hospital for practical training. However, most teaching hospitals have the much wider function of also being district general hospitals. They have a wide range of specialities that often include some of the most sophisticated and least common, such as neurosurgical units for brain surgery and renal units that carry out kidney transplants. Teaching hospitals often have particularly difficult cases referred to them.

As expensive, high-technology medical equipment has increasingly been concentrated in large hospitals, so small general hospitals have been closed down. However, others have been transformed into community (cottage) hospitals. These are generally run by a group of GPs, who admit certain of their own patients to the beds. The patients include those who need more nursing care than is available at home, those whose families normally care for them but are away on holiday, and those who no longer need the expensive facilities of a large hospital but still require nursing.

Nearly all community hospitals are in rural areas. But a few are being developed in cities, to cater for large numbers of elderly and other sick people who cannot be properly cared for at home.

Accident and emergency admissions

Planned admissions to hospital are outnumbered by sudden admissions following major accidents and medical emergencies, such as a heart attack, stroke, or diabetic coma. Anyone who suffers such an accident or emergency in the home should, in most cases, call his or her general practitioner who will, on the evidence given over the phone, be able to decide what is the best course of action. If the doctor is not available, it is best to dial 999 and ask to be taken by ambulance to the nearest major accident and emergency department of a hospital or, if possible, make your way (in a friend's car, for instance) to such a department. Some small general hospitals and community hospitals run a casualty service – and occasionally this is available only between certain hours – but such a service is usually only able to deal with minor accidents and emergencies.

Sometimes the accident and emergency department of a city hospital is full and has to divert an ambulance to another hospital, which in a city will not be far away. However, a full department will usually accept people who have made their own way to the hospital.

Some people who are not seriously injured or ill go to an accident and emergency department as though it were a general practitioner's surgery. This is usually in city areas, where many people are temporary residents and are not registered with a GP. The duty doctor in the hospital will treat such patients only if he or she thinks it absolutely necessary. They will not be treated until all the major cases have been dealt with, and in a busy department this may mean a wait of several hours.

When you get to see the doctor on duty, he or she will assess what is wrong with you and start any necessary immediate treatment. You may then be sent to the X-ray department to discover whether you have any broken bones or other injuries, and you may also have to supply blood and urine specimens for analysis. If the doctor needs advice or a second opinion, he or she will call upon a more senior colleague – a registrar from the medical or surgical team on duty, or the specialist (consultant) in charge of the accident and emergency department.

Once you have been given any necessary treatment and it has been determined exactly what damage you have sustained or how serious your disorder is, you may be admitted to the hospital as an in-patient. As alternatives, you may be transferred to another hospital as an in-patient, be referred back to your GP for further treatment or follow-up care (such as removing stitches), or be asked to return to the accident and emergency department – or a specialist out-patient clinic at the hospital – for follow-up care.

Hospital staff

Until the advent of the National Health Service the staff of most hospitals consisted almost entirely of doctors and nurses. However, hospitals have changed and expanded greatly over the last 30 years or so, and most of the growth has been, not in the numbers of doctors and nurses employed but in the numbers of employees in fields allied to the medical profession. For example, as medical techniques and procedures such as post-operative therapy and diagnostic processes have become more technical and specialized, people are being trained and employed purely as physiotherapists, radiographers, and laboratory technicians, and to do some jobs that used to be done by doctors. There is also a large body of domestic staff in every hospital doing much of the work that used to be part of the nurses' duties, and so allowing the nurses to concentrate on actually nursing their patients.

Despite the fact that so many jobs that were formerly done by doctors and nurses have now been delegated, there are more doctors and nurses attached to each hospital, allowing for shorter working days yet still providing full 24-hour cover.

The National Health Service has become an enormous concern. It is the largest single employer of labour in Britain, requiring a large and efficient administrative department whose members are rarely seen by the average patient but who ensure the smooth running of the system.

The staffing structure of a typical general hospital

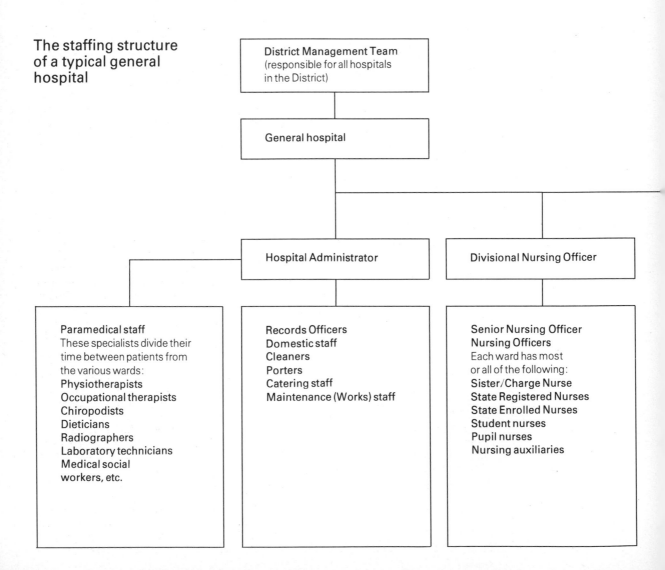

District Management Team (responsible for all hospitals in the District)

General hospital

Hospital Administrator

Divisional Nursing Officer

Paramedical staff
These specialists divide their time between patients from the various wards:
Physiotherapists
Occupational therapists
Chiropodists
Dieticians
Radiographers
Laboratory technicians
Medical social
workers, etc.

Records Officers
Domestic staff
Cleaners
Porters
Catering staff
Maintenance (Works) staff

Senior Nursing Officer
Nursing Officers
Each ward has most
or all of the following:
Sister/Charge Nurse
State Registered Nurses
State Enrolled Nurses
Student nurses
Pupil nurses
Nursing auxiliaries

Out-patients

Far more people attend hospital as out-patients than are admitted to hospital beds. Hospital out-patients fall into two main categories. Some are sent to hospital by their GP for X-rays or tests, as a necessary preliminary to treatment by the GP. Others are referred by their GP to a specialist's out-patient clinic. (A few specialists, particularly those who do not rely heavily on X-rays, blood tests, and other hospital diagnostic help, hold some of their out-patient clinics in health centres – see the information on the different types of general practice in *How a general practice works*, p.730.)

The GP writes to the hospital or specialist asking for an urgent or routine appointment for you. You then receive directly from the hospital a letter notifying you of the date of your appointment. Waiting lists for specialist out-patient appointments vary considerably from speciality to speciality and from area to area. If you have to wait more than a few weeks for a routine appointment, it is worth asking your GP if he can refer you to a specialist a little farther afield, who might give you an earlier appointment.

Seeing a specialist: When you arrive for your appointment, you may have to wait a long time to see a doctor: the medical staff may be busy elsewhere with more serious, emergency cases. Each specialist has a team of assistant doctors. On your first visit to the clinic, you will, if you have been referred to a particular specialist, usually see that specialist personally (or, if not, his or her senior registrar, the most senior assistant in the team).

The specialist will probably ask you to provide a full history of your complaint, will question you about your symptoms, and will perhaps carry out an extensive examination and send you to other parts of the hospital for X-rays, certain blood tests, or other tests. (Simple blood tests and urine test may be done on the spot, by the staff within the clinic.) On the evidence gathered, the specialist will decide either to treat you at the clinic or to refer you back to your GP, with the test results and advice to the GP on how to manage your condition.

If you are treated at the clinic, this will probably be by one of the specialist's junior assistants, and if the treatment goes according to plan and there are no complications, you may well not see the specialist again.

Many specialists run regular clinics for all their patients with a particular disorder – diabetes, for example. This arrangement makes it easier for specialist staff such as dieticians to attend and give advice and treatment when needed.

The specialist may think you should see another specialist – perhaps one with a particular knowledge of the condition you have. He or she will usually do this through your GP, but, if the second specialist works in the same hospital, you will probably be referred to that specialist directly.

Admissions by a specialist

If a specialist decides to admit you to hospital after seeing you as an out-patient, you will be admitted immediately if your case is an urgent one. If it is not, you will be put on the specialist's waiting list or, less usually, booked in for a definite date some weeks, or even months, ahead. Being given a definite date rather than being put on a waiting list has the advantage of giving you plenty of notice to make such arrangements as taking time off work or getting someone to look after your children while you are in hospital.

Waiting lists: As with out-patient appointments, waiting lists for admission vary greatly in length. Notice of admission is often only a few days. Patients are usually chosen earlier or later from the waiting list according to how severe their condition is, how long they have been waiting, and how soon a bed in an appropriate ward becomes available. However, some empty beds are not taken up – perhaps because a patient has moved, been treated elsewhere, or recovered. Anyone who lets the specialist know that he or she can come into hospital at a few hours' notice may well be telephoned and given the opportunity of taking up an empty place right away.

Chairman, Medical
Advisory Committee

Consultant
Each consultant heads a team or
"firm" of doctors. A full team would
be as follows:
Senior Registrar
Registrar
Junior Registrar
Senior House Officer   often called
House Officer   "Housemen"

In hospital

Many hospitals issue in-patients with a booklet explaining hospital routine, services available, who to discuss problems with, and other information. If the booklet is sent to you in advance of your admission, it may include a list of what you should take with you into hospital. You are usually advised to take essential items such as nightwear (including a bedjacket or cardigan, dressing gown, and slippers), flannel, soap, towel, toothbrush, toothpaste, hairbrush, comb, nail scissors or nail file, and something to read.

You will also need some money to buy items from the hospital shop or the travelling shops that are taken through the wards. If you take in a large amount of money, you can give it to the hospital administration for safe keeping. Many of the larger hospitals now include a bank.

Admission procedure

Hospitals usually admit patients through a central admissions office. A clerk takes down your name, address, next of kin, and other details. You may be given a means of identification, often a bracelet, which has your name and hospital number on it and which you should wear throughout your stay. If you are on a special diet or you need a certificate to claim sickness insurance, you must let the clerk know. When these formalities are over, you are taken to the ward. (In some hospitals your details are taken down in the ward, to which you are admitted straight away.)

Older hospitals generally have large, dormitory-style single-sex wards, but in more modern hospitals the wards consist of several rooms, with men in some and women in others. Whatever the age of the hospital, it will usually have some single rooms for those whose condition requires isolation.

Things to take to hospital
Soft holdall or case
Towel
Nightclothes
Slippers
Flannel or sponge
Soap
Talcum powder
Deodorant
Toothpaste
Toothbrush
Brush
Comb
Shaving equipment
Cosmetics
Sanitary towels (for women)
Money

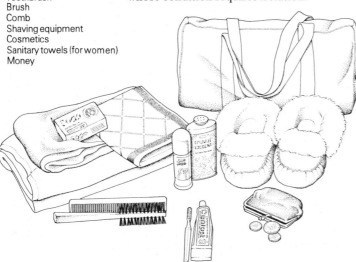

Hospital doctors

A specialist (consultant) will be in charge of your case, but you will probably see less of the consultant than of his or her junior staff (see *Hospital staff*, p.734). The most junior of these, a junior house officer (HO), does the more basic medical tasks on the ward – among them, arranging tests and investigations, performing some of the simpler of these, and writing up patients' notes – under the supervision of one or more senior house officers (SHOs) or registrars. Registrars are doctors training to be consultant specialists. They generally look after the medical administration of the ward on behalf of the consultant. Senior registrars are those in the final stages of their training. They may deputize for the consultant in supervising operations and conducting ward rounds, when the team of doctors review the progress of each patient and decide on future treatment.

The junior house officer is usually the first doctor to visit you after you have settled into your bed. He or she takes down a detailed history from you, asking you to describe your symptoms, your current treatment, and any illnesses in other members of the family (a routine question and nothing to worry about). You may be asked the same questions several times during your stay; other doctors need the information, and they prefer to obtain it from you rather than your case notes.

If you enter a teaching hospital, you will probably see less of your consultant than in a general hospital, and more of the junior doctors. You will also see medical students who are part of the consultant's team. They may help the junior house officer with tasks such as taking a medical history and will accompany the consultant and registrars on their ward rounds. As a patient, you are helping medical students, together with nursing, radiography, and other students, gain valuable experience if you allow your case to be used for teaching purposes; but you do have the right to refuse this.

If you have any questions about your treatment, talk to the junior house officer first. If you are not satisfied, ask to see your registrar or consultant (see *Patients' rights*, p.748). If relatives of a patient want to talk to a particular doctor, they should ask the ward sister to make an appointment.

Nurses and other staff

Every ward is staffed by nurses 24 hours a day, on a shift system (see *Hospital staff*, p.734). The nursing team consists of a ward sister (or charge nurse, the male equivalent of a sister), who is in charge; state-registered nurses (SRNs), who have had three years' training; state-enrolled nurses (SENs), who have had two years' training; student nurses, who are training to be SRNs; and pupil nurses, who are training to be SENs. In addition, auxiliary nurses – who have received no formal training – will probably help with some nursing tasks. Other permanent ward staff include ward clerks (who do administrative work), cooks, and cleaners.

A wide range of other people visit hospital wards. They include hospital administrators, laboratory technicians, physiotherapists, pharmacists, chaplains, social workers, hairdressers, volunteers who run the trolley shops, and porters.

Wards

In a general hospital, wards are divided basically into three types: general medical wards, general surgical wards, and specialist wards.

The occupants of a general medical ward are people who need non-surgical treatment of an unspecialized kind. Some are admitted as emergency cases – for example, after a heart attack or a diabetic coma. Others are admitted for such investigations as blood or urine tests, *X-rays*, *intravenous pyelograms*, *ultrasound*, *biopsies*, or *endoscopies*. Treatment is mainly by drugs but may also include physiotherapy, diet, and exercise.

General surgical wards contain mainly patients who need an operation for a specific disorder but who are otherwise healthy. Other patients will be those who need surgical treatment for serious injuries.

If you are entering hospital for an operation to treat a disorder, you will usually be admitted a day or two before the operation. This enables X-rays and other preliminary investigations to be carried out, doctors to assess your condition accurately, and preparations for the operation to be made.

All other wards come under the broad heading of specialist wards. They include wards for children, the elderly, and people who need specialized treatment – for example, for mental illnesses or diseases of the joints. Other examples of specialist wards are maternity wards and intensive-care units; the latter are for seriously ill patients who may well be on life-support systems. Each specialist ward will usually include some patients who need medical treatment with drugs and others who need surgery.

Ward routine: If you are feeling fairly well, you will not be expected to stay in bed all day. Indeed, after an operation you may be encouraged to get up quite promptly. Wards usually have day rooms, where more mobile patients can watch television and eat. You are expected to get up early (in some hospitals, at 6am) and to have an early breakfast, lunch, and supper. The hospital's booklet will state the times of meals. It will also tell you what the visiting hours are. In some hospitals, these are now much more generous than they used to be and exclude only a few hours in the day. In other hospitals, however, visiting hours are confined to short periods in the afternoon or evening, and children may be barred – even from visiting their parents. Even so, if you are in such a hospital and your visitors can come only at a certain time or have to travel a long way, you will probably be able to arrange with the ward sister to see them outside the normal visiting hours.

The children's ward is very different from all other wards. Mothers are encouraged to be with their children throughout the day; and many wards have accommodation to allow mothers to stay the night. There are playleaders for the younger children and sometimes teachers for the older ones.

The psychiatric ward is also rather different from the others in its routine. Since the patients are not physically ill, they spend their time up and dressed, talking to their therapists or undergoing other treatment.

Social services in hospital

Your admission to hospital may create financial or practical problems for your family. If this is the case, ask to see the medical social worker, who can provide assistance (for example, by helping your family with financial matters or providing a home help). The assistance may also be available after you have been discharged.

The medical social worker can also be particularly helpful if you are receiving social security benefits. These benefits are reduced or withdrawn when you are admitted to hospital (on the grounds that the NHS is providing you with free food and accommodation) and the rules concerning them are complicated; you may need the social worker to explain them to you. The rules are given in full in a pamphlet, obtainable from your local post office or doctor's surgery.

The social worker can also get free fares to and from the hospital for the following patients (and, in some cases, their visiting relatives): war pensioners receiving treatment for their pensioned injury; people living in the Highlands and Islands who have to travel over a certain distance and pay more than a certain amount; those on supplementary benefit or family income supplement; and other people with low incomes.

Having an operation

At some stage you will be asked by a doctor to sign a consent form for your operation. If there is anything you do not understand in the form, ask the doctor about it before you sign. You will be visited by doctors from the surgical team, and you will probably also see the anaesthetist, whose job is to give you a general anaesthetic and keep a check on your basic body functions (such as heartbeat and breathing) during the operation.

On the morning of the operation you do not have anything to eat or drink. The reason for this is that if your stomach is not empty, the anaesthetic may cause you to vomit while you are unconscious – which could be dangerous. Any necessary shaving, to remove hair from the area to be operated on, is carried out. You are then dressed in a clean theatre gown to minimize the risk of infection. An hour or so before the operation is due, you are given an injection that makes you sleepy and your mouth dry. The anaesthetic itself is given – usually by injection – in the operating theatre.

Except when blood vessels are being stitched, internal and membranous areas that have been cut or injured will be closed with dissolving stitches. Small skin incisions will usually be closed with nylon thread or clips, and larger incisions may be held together by large supporting stitches. Non-dissolving stitches are usually removed 7 to 10 days later.

After some types of surgery, particularly abdominal surgery, you may have to be fed or given fluids through a tube inserted into a vein for a day or two. Other tubes (drainage tubes) may also be used to drain off fluids and pus.

Anaesthetist
The anaesthetist administers anaesthetics and is an expert in treatment of surgical shock, maintenance of body fluids, and relief of post-operative pain.

Surgeon (house officer)
The house officer, the registrar's junior, obtains experience in theatre before deciding in which particular branch of medicine to specialize.

Surgeon (consultant)
The consultant heads a team or "firm" of doctors and decides which operation is necessary.

Nurse
All nurses spend some time in the operating theatre, assisting the theatre sister and surgeons and learning basic skills.

Theatre sister
The theatre sister is responsible for supplying the surgeons with the necessary instruments and for all aspects of the smooth running of the theatre.

Instrument trolley

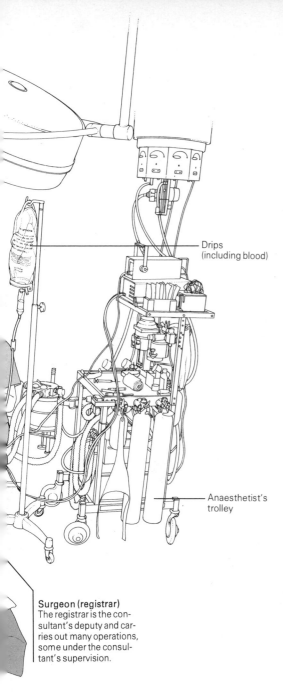

Drips
(including blood)

Anaesthetist's
trolley

Surgeon (registrar)
The registrar is the con-
sultant's deputy and car-
ries out many operations,
some under the consul-
tant's supervision.

Intensive care

After having a major operation, a patient may need to be maintained on an artificial *ventilator* or breathe with the help of an oxygen mask for some hours, and may also need continuous electronic monitoring of blood pressure, heart rate, and other vital body functions. The equipment necessary to provide post-operative intensive care is usually concentrated in a unit where the patients are cared for by specialist medical and nursing staff. Most patients remain in the intensive-care unit, under constant supervision, for only a few days and are then transferred to a normal ward to continue their recovery.

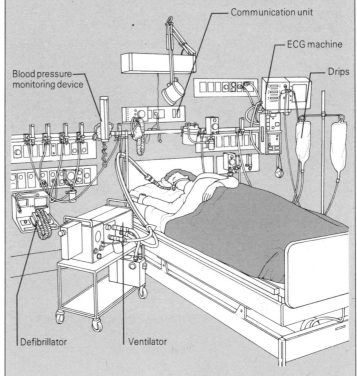

Communication unit

ECG machine

Drips

Blood pressure
monitoring device

Defibrillator

Ventilator

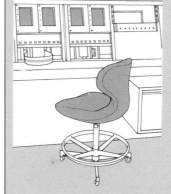

Central control station
Intensive-care units typically house between 4 and 12 patients and usually have a central console, which allows a single member of the nursing staff to keep a check on all the patients. The recordings made of each patient's vital functions are shown on the console, and all the instruments are fitted with automatic alarms.

Diagnostic tests

Some diagnostic tests, such as blood and urine tests, are given routinely to most patients, whereas others, such as X-rays or bronchoscopy, will only be given to confirm or rule out a particular disorder suspected by the doctor.

Recently, some tests that carried a risk to the patient or caused discomfort – for example, X-rays in pregnancy or cerebral angiography – have been replaced by new "non-invasive" tests that are risk-free and painless – for example, ultrasound and the CAT scan.

The introduction of fibre-optics has also been a major advance in diagnostic tests, since they allow doctors safely to examine a variety of body cavities, from the stomach to the interior of the knee joint, without the need for a major operation.

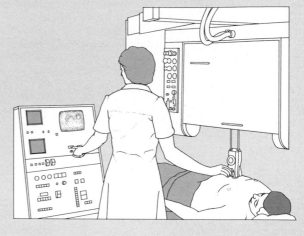

Ultrasound (above)
Ultrasound, a method of converting sound waves into a visual pattern, is used to obtain information about soft body tissues. It is particularly useful in examining pregnant women, as it does not expose the developing fetus to potentially harmful X-rays. The procedure is harmless and painless.

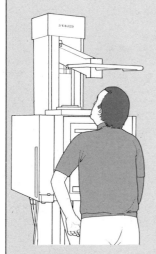

Having an X-ray (above)
A chest X-ray is completely painless. You stand with your chest and arms pushed against the plate, then breathe in deeply and hold your breath while the picture is being taken.

CAT scan (below)
This CAT (computerized axial tomography) scan shows a horizontal 2D slice of the body across the shoulders. In a CAT scan, as in a conventional X-ray, the denser areas of the body show as lighter areas on the image, and vice versa.

The large black areas in the centre of this picture are the lungs, and a vertebra (one of the many that go to make up the backbone) can be seen clearly as a white circle around the grey area of the spinal cord. A shoulder blade projects from each side of the spine, and the shaded area opposite the spine represents the muscle and fat tissues of the patient's chest.

What the X-ray shows (right)
X-rays reveal dense areas of the body such as bone, and are usually taken to show up any damaged or distorted bones. Because softer tissues also show up if they are filled with air or fluid, X-rays are especially useful in revealing disorders of the lung. This lung abscess, filled with air and fluid (right), shows up as a white area against the darker area of the lung around it.

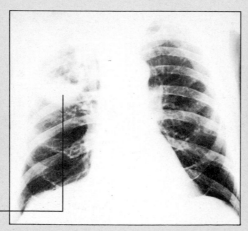

Abscess

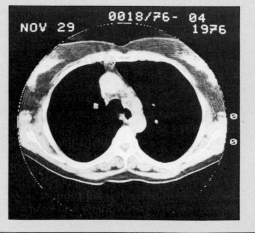

Endoscopy

Endoscopy is a procedure by which a special tube, equipped with a lighting and lens system, is used to examine a body cavity. Different types of endoscope are used for different parts of the body. For example, a broncho-scope is used to examine the lungs, a cystoscope to examine the bladder, and a laparoscope to examine the abdominal (including female reproductive) organs.

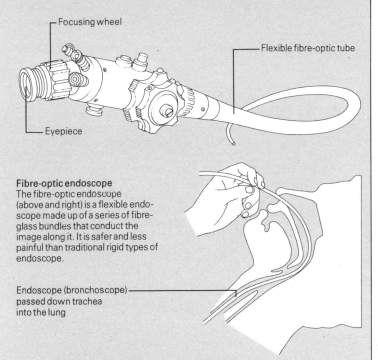

— Focusing wheel

— Flexible fibre-optic tube

— Eyepiece

Fibre-optic endoscope

The fibre-optic endoscope (above and right) is a flexible endoscope made up of a series of fibreglass bundles that conduct the image along it. It is safer and less painful than traditional rigid types of endoscope.

Endoscope (bronchoscope) passed down trachea into the lung

Biopsy

A biopsy is the removal of a small sample of body tissue that can aid diagnosis after it has been carefully analysed during examination under a microscope.

Blood test

Analysis of a blood sample can provide information on, among other things, the quantities and health of red and white blood cells and platelets. It can also show the pathologist the proportions of vital chemicals contained in the blood, such as glucose, sodium, urea, and cholesterol, which can be important in indicating the presence of certain diseases.

Urine test

A urine sample provides a guide to the health of the urinary tract. It is examined for bacteria, pus cells, evidence of bleeding, and the presence of protein. The proportion of certain chemicals in the urine is also important; for example, the treatment of diabetes depends on the amount of glucose in the sufferer's urine.

Discharge from hospital

You are usually given a day or two's notice of when you are to be discharged from hospital. If you are still feeling weak, this gives you plenty of time to arrange for a friend or member of the family to collect you by car or, if this is not possible, to book hospital transport to take you home. Occasionally, however, when your bed is urgently required, you may be discharged at very short notice. If you discharge yourself before your doctor considers you well enough to leave hospital, you may be asked to sign a form stating that you left against medical advice.

Before you leave, you may be prescribed a special diet to be followed at home or told about exercises or restrictions on your activities, and you may be given a supply of drugs. If you need more drugs when the supply runs out, you usually obtain them from your GP.

When you are discharged, you should give the hospital staff the address at which you can be contacted in the near future. If you will be unable to work and will need to claim sickness benefit for some time after your discharge, ask for a medical certificate.

If you are going to need home nursing or a home help, the provision of these by your local social services department will normally be arranged, shortly before you leave hospital, by the medical social worker. However, if you are discharged at short notice, these services may be difficult to arrange quickly, especially at the weekend; in such a case, the medical social worker or ward sister will probably be able to provide help from some other source, often a voluntary body. In some cases, a GP will arrange visits from a district nurse or health visitor (see *Community health care*, p.743).

Usually, after discharge from hospital, you will be asked to attend an out-patient clinic at least once. There, one of your specialist's junior staff will check on your progress. (But if you are at all worried about your condition at any time before or after attending the clinic, get in touch with your GP.) In some cases, a discharged person is not given an out-patient appointment, but is returned straight to the care of his or her GP.

If you need further physiotherapy treatment or follow-up advice on diet after you leave hospital, you will normally need to return to the hospital for these. If you need occupational therapy, this may be provided at an out-patient clinic of the hospital, at a local community health clinic. For those who are unable to attend clinics, the therapist may treat you in your own home.

Dental care

Dental treatment under the National Health Service is provided by the general dental service (self-employed dentists under contract to the NHS), and can be obtained from local health clinics, the school health service, the hospital service, and dental surgeries.

General dental practice differs in several ways from general medical practice:

1. General dental treatment under the NHS is not free – you have to pay something towards its cost.

2. You do not have to register with a dentist, as you do with a general practitioner, in order to obtain treatment. A dentist who accepts you for a course of treatment under the NHS simply has to make you dentally fit at the time and has no obligation to treat you subsequently – though in practice most dentists have regular patients.

3. Dentists tend to do much more private work than GPs do, and some place limits on their NHS work. So if you want NHS treatment from a dentist, you must make this clear at the outset. You should also ask if there is any kind of treatment the dentist will not do on the NHS; otherwise you could find yourself unwittingly liable to private fees for some parts of your treatment. It is also wise to find out whether the dentist has a long waiting list for NHS appointments.

4. A dentist is allowed to provide you with NHS treatment on some occasions and private treatment on others if you wish; whereas a GP cannot do this.

5. You have no absolute entitlement to NHS dental treatment as you have to NHS medical treatment. If you cannot find a dentist who will treat you under the NHS, your local Family Practitioner Committee is not obliged to find you one. This means that if, for example, you live in an inner city area, you may find it difficult to discover a dentist who will give you NHS treatment. You may have to either pay for private treatment or, if the city has a dental hospital, get treatment (in most cases, free) at the hospital.

Dental charges

All NHS dental check-ups are free (see *Going to the dentist*, p.447). Adults are entitled to two check-ups a year, children to three, and expectant and nursing mothers to four. If the dentist examines you before deciding whether to accept you as an NHS patient and then declines to accept you, the check-up still costs you nothing. In such a case, the dentist may refer you either to another dentist or to a hospital. If a dentist accepts you for treatment, he or she will ask you to sign a form which states that you consent to treatment, agree to any examination by a regional dental officer (as a check on the work of the dentist), and undertake to pay any necessary charges.

NHS treatment and dentures are free for the following groups of people: children under 16; full-time students between 16 and 21; expectant mothers; women who have had a child within the previous 12 months; anyone on supplementary benefit or family income supplement; anyone who has free prescriptions and free milk because of low income; and dependants of people in the last two categories. Ask at any main post office or social security office for a leaflet that gives full details about free dental treatment. Anyone not on supplementary benefit but unable to pay for NHS treatment may be able to obtain reduced charges by filling in the appropriate form, which is available from the dentist. And people over 16 but under 21 who have left school receive free treatment but pay for dentures and alterations to them.

For everyone else, only examinations, repairs to dentures, and the emergency stopping of bleeding are free on the NHS. Otherwise, there is a standard charge for each form of dental treatment (including any *X-rays* taken) and for each type of denture. Details of charges are given in a leaflet obtainable from your social security office.

There is no fixed scale of charges for private treatment, and the dentist can, within reason, charge what he or she likes.

Housebound patients: If you are genuinely housebound – for example, if you are obviously bedridden – you can ask the dentist to visit you. If you live up to eight kilometres (five miles) from the surgery, there is no charge for the visit under the NHS; for longer distances you pay a fee. The cost of treatment is then the same as normal.

Community health services and hospitals

Schoolchildren can obtain treatment either from a general dental practitioner or through the school dental service. The main function of the school service is to ensure that all children have their teeth examined, to see if treatment is needed, and to give advice on dental hygiene. If the parents wish, the service can also carry out necessary treatment.

Some health clinics provide dental examinations for pregnant women and free dental care for handicapped people, as well as advising on dental hygiene. This preventive aspect of dentistry tends to be neglected in the general service because dentists do not get paid for it under the NHS contract.

Hospitals: If you live in a city with a dental hospital, you can attend its out-patient department to obtain any ordinary treatment. In most cases, this is free. You will be treated by a dental student under the supervision of a consultant dentist. Dentists and GPs sometimes refer patients to a dental hospital for specialist dental treatment or oral surgery. This is always free.

Dental emergencies

If you break a tooth or have severe toothache while you are on a course of NHS treatment from a dentist, he or she is legally bound to treat the emergency on the NHS. This is part of the dentist's obligation to make you dentally fit during the course. However, most emergencies occur between courses of treatment, when the dentist is under no legal obligation to treat you; and, in practice, many dentists will accept you for emergency treatment only as a private patient. If you need urgent dental treatment outside practice hours, or you cannot obtain it from a dentist for any other reason, either contact your GP or go to the accident and emergency department of a general hospital or the out-patient department of a dental hospital.

Care of the sight

Care of the sight under the National Health Service is provided by the general ophthalmic service. This is made up of ophthalmic medical practitioners and ophthalmic opticians (see *Going to the optician*, p.312).

Everyone who qualifies for National Health Service treatment can have a free sight test at an eye centre or ophthalmic optician's once every 12 months. For tests more frequent than this, there is a charge for each extra test. However, in exceptional cases – such as a child with rapidly progressing short sight – the extra tests are free.

Anyone who wishes may have a private sight test, for which a fee is charged. In this case the person must also obtain any spectacles privately and pay for their full cost.

Those entitled to free NHS spectacles are children under 16, full-time students between 16 and 21, people already obtaining free milk and prescriptions, hospital patients, and those whose income is below a certain level. (Ask for the relevant leaflet, obtainable from any main post office or social security office, which gives full details.) Everyone else must pay a fixed proportion of the cost of the spectacles . The lenses are usually available at an NHS-subsidized price, but the charges for private frames as opposed to NHS frames are usually much higher. And luxury items, such as lenses that darken in sunlight, must usually be obtained and paid for privately.

If you are housebound, you can either pay for an optician to visit you or alternatively ask your doctor if he or she can arrange for a hospital eye consultant to visit you and treat you under the NHS.

Any optician must give you a sight test under the NHS, but he or she has the right to refuse to fit you with NHS spectacles. If every optician in your area were to do so, you would have to write to your local Family Practitioner Committee, which would order one of the opticians to treat you.

Community health care

Community health care is provided by various medical and other trained staff, who are usually based at health clinics. Community health workers include health visitors, community nurses, and midwives, all of whom visit people in their homes; there are also local authority social workers, who help the ill, handicapped, and elderly. Certain public health duties are carried out by local health authorities and by occupational or industrial health services at places of work.

Ante-natal care

A pregnant woman who receives ante-natal care has her condition and that of her unborn baby constantly monitored. She is advised about her diet, the bad effects of smoking, and other matters. A woman should start obtaining ante-natal care as soon as she discovers she is pregnant, so that if there is anything wrong with her or her baby there is a chance of it being detected early.

You can obtain ante-natal care from the ante-natal clinic, from a GP on the *obstetric* list (see *General practice*, p.729), or from both clinic and GP ("shared care"). If you are having your baby at home, the ante-natal clinic available to you will be at your local health clinic; if the baby is to be delivered in hospital, the hospital will provide care at its own ante-natal clinic or at sessions held at the health clinic – which is often easier for a mother with young children to attend. Many health clinics also hold relaxation and exercise classes to help you through labour, and evening "parentcraft" classes to teach parents how to look after the new baby.

Post-natal care

Some days after the birth of a baby, the hospital or home midwife hands over the home care of the mother and child to the health visitor. The health visitor carries out simple examinations of the baby to make sure he or she is developing normally, and gives advice on feeding and generally looking after the baby. She may, in some cases, take a blood sample from the baby, to be tested at a laboratory for signs of the rare disease *phenylketonuria* (p.688), which if detected early can be treated by diet. (In other cases, this blood test is performed in hospital.)

The health visitor will also advise you to take your child regularly to the child care clinic at your local health centre until the child starts school. At the clinic a medical officer will perform various screening tests on the child's hearing, vision, and movements, carry out immunizations, and, with the health visitor, will answer any questions you have about feeding, sleeping, crying, or other aspects of the baby's behaviour. Most child care clinics also welcome casual visits from mothers with any problems. Some GPs run their own children's clinic for the young children in their practice, again usually in conjunction with a health visitor. You are free to attend whichever clinic you prefer.

If the health visitor, medical officer, or your GP thinks that your child's condition requires more specialized investigation, he or she will refer you and the child to a specialist in that field – such as an audiologist for hearing or an ophthalmologist for vision – at the health clinic.

Health clinics also sell low-cost powdered milk and baby foods on the National Health Service, and many run mother-and-baby groups and clubs for mothers and toddlers.

Other health-clinic services

Your local health clinic may provide services other than those mentioned above. The most common of these is the family planning clinic, where both men and women can go for advice and practical guidance on contraception, and where some contraceptives can be prescribed and obtained free of charge. Another service that may be provided is the "Well woman" clinic, which women can attend for screening tests such as breast examination or a cervical smear, to make sure that any potentially serious conditions such as cancer of the breast or cervix are detected in the early stages. At these clinics women can also talk generally to the staff and receive advice on any specifically female health problems.

Many health clinics have a noticeboard giving information on local groups and clubs such as Stroke clubs, Handicapped children groups, and so on.

Dental care is provided at some clinics for children, pregnant women, mothers with children aged under one year, and, in many districts, the handicapped.

In theory, chiropody (care of the feet) is available under the NHS not only to the elderly but to the same groups that qualify for dental care. In practice, however, nearly all chiropody sessions are devoted to the elderly; because elderly feet are so prone to problems, old people may need professional care of their feet simply in order to get about; they may be so immobilized that the chiropodist has to visit them in their own home. Even so, because of the shortage of chiropodists in the NHS, elderly people may still have to wait a considerable time before they can get either a clinic appointment or a home visit from the chiropodist. (If you have decided on private treatment, look up Chiropodists in the yellow pages of the telephone directory. State-registered chiropodists have the letters SRCh after their names.)

To find out about the services provided by health clinics in your area, telephone one of the clinics (listed in the telephone directory under your Area Health Authority), or you can contact your local Community Health Council (also listed in the directory).

The school health service

The school health service aims at ensuring that no child is prevented from receiving the full benefits of his or her education by health problems such as long periods of illness, or defects of vision, hearing, or speech. The service also continues the programme of immunizations started in infancy. Another part of the service's work is concerned with the teaching of mentally and physically handicapped children.

The way that the school health service is run varies slightly from one education authority to another, but you can expect your child to have at least two medical examinations during school life. The first is usually performed around the time of school entry, either at the school itself or in a local health clinic. You will be told when your child is to be examined and invited to attend. Obviously it is better if you can be there because you will then be able to discuss any problems with the doctor or nurse.

School medical examinations are an extension of the pre-school check-ups carried out at your local health clinic. Normally the service does not provide treatment but refers a child with a disorder to his or her GP. School doctors not only carry out routine examinations, but examine children specially referred to them by school nurses, teachers, or parents. In addition, school doctors treat children with visual defects or minor ailments, provide immunizations, follow up the condition of children with physical deformities, and deal with special problems. School doctors and nurses usually also give talks and show films on various aspects of health, as part of the school curriculum.

School dental clinics: Mobile dental clinics under the school health service provide several routine examinations for children during their school years. The clinics provide mainly a screening and preventive service and dispense advice on dental hygiene. However, the school dentist may also give a child treatment if the parents wish.

Care at home

Medical care of people in their own homes is provided when necessary by health visitors, district nurses, and midwives.

The main role of health visitors is to call on families with very young children and the elderly. They give advice on diet and hygiene and generally help prevent and detect illness. They also advise on when children need to see their GP and when handicapped elderly people would benefit from an aid that can be provided by the local authority. Health visitors are an important link with other parts of the health service in general.

The district nurse, too, visits people at home, and often provides a valuable link with GPs and hospitals. Her or his duties include providing more nursing care for sick people than their families can give them, caring for people who have been discharged early from hospital but still need nursing, and nursing chronically sick or terminally ill patients in their own homes.

Midwives deliver, or help doctors to deliver, babies born at home. They also visit the mother regularly during the first 10 days or so after the birth to make sure that everything is going well with her and her child, until the health visitor takes over and begins to make routine calls.

Social workers and home helps: The functions of social workers include helping people with long-term illnesses or handicaps to maintain their independence and helping rehabilitate the disabled and the mentally ill.

Among the practical aids and services the social worker can offer are arranging sheltered accommodation for the handicapped; hostels for the mentally ill; *occupational therapy*; braille teaching for the blind; aids in the home, such as handrails to assist walking; and financial help with the installation of telephones and extensions.

Home helps visit those who are unable to carry out, or need assistance with, everyday activities such as house cleaning, shopping, and the preparation of meals. They do this work mainly for the elderly, but they also stand in for parents who fall ill, become unable to look after their children, and cannot find home help elsewhere.

Meals on Wheels: The Meals on Wheels service provides regular hot meals to anyone who is handicapped or housebound and cannot manage to buy or cook food. The service is run by the local authority, often with voluntary help from the Women's Royal Voluntary Service or other organizations. The cost of the meals is subsidized, and they are free for anyone who cannot afford them.

Public health

One of the few occasions when your doctor is authorized to breach the confidentiality of your medical records is if you are found to be suffering from a notifiable disease. Such diseases include certain types of food poisoning, infectious diseases such as measles, and infestations such as lice. The doctor has to notify the local medical officer for environmental health, whose job is to keep an eye on the number of reported cases of any notifiable disease, and to take action to minimize the risk of an epidemic or to curb it if it develops. If you have a notifiable disease, you may be asked to list all the people you have had contact with, the places you have been, and the food you have eaten, so that the medical officer and his or her staff can trace the source of the infection and contact any other people who may be at risk.

The local health authority and the medical officer have certain statutory powers in connection with notifiable diseases, to protect the public's health. These include the power to remove a person with such a disease to an isolation hospital or to restrict the person to home, and to examine and take specimens of blood and urine from anyone with whom the affected person has had contact.

Another responsibility of the medical officer is to remove to hospital elderly and infirm people who have a chronic illness, people who are living in insanitary conditions, and those who are unable to look after themselves – even with the assistance of a home help – and who have no-one else to look after them.

Occupational health
All workplaces are legally obliged to have first-aid kits, and all factories with over a certain number of employees should have people qualified in first aid on their staff. Some employers go much further than this and run an occupational health service for their workers. The services vary in size. Small businesses may employ only a trained nurse. Many larger organizations, however, have doctors, nurses, and occupational hygienists, to ensure that workers are physically fit for their jobs and that those jobs are not presenting unnecessary health risks to the workers

(for more information on this aspect see *Safety and environmental health*, p.42). The medical staff examine workers periodically during employment. They also check the fitness of workers who have had an accident or been ill and help to rehabilitate those who are unable to continue with their job. They do not usually, however, provide any major treatment but refer a sick or injured worker to his or her family doctor.

The code of ethics for occupational doctors demands that they must have a person's permission to disclose that person's medical record to management or a trade union official. Occupational doctors may, however, recommend to management or union (without disclosing why) that a worker should change jobs in the interests of health.

Private medicine

Apart from health care provided free or for a small charge by the National Health Service, private treatment is also available for which you pay the full amount.

In the case of certain private practitioners – including a fairly small number of general practitioners, some specialists, and most practitioners of *alternative medicine* (p.752) – treatment is exclusively private and unavailable under the NHS. In other cases, private treatment is offered as an alternative to NHS treatment by practitioners who provide both, with specialists providing the bulk of this alternative private medical care.

The proportion of specialists who do a considerable amount of private practice varies greatly among different specialities (it is highest in the surgical specialities) and in different parts of Britain (it is much higher in England than elsewhere).

Private specialist treatment
There are few advantages in electing to have a private rather than an NHS general practitioner; but private as opposed to NHS specialist treatment can, under certain circumstances, offer considerable benefits. The circumstances and the benefits are these. First, you may be suffering from a distressing and uncomfortable, but not life-threatening, condition – a hernia, for instance, or varicose veins, or a cataract. Treatment for these cases under the NHS tends to get delayed as priority is always given to people with more urgent conditions; whereas private specialist treatment offers early admission. Secondly, you will, as a private patient, have the opportunity of choosing your own hospital admission date – which is rare under the NHS. Thirdly,

the private patient is usually treated by the senior specialist in person and not, as tends to be the case with NHS treatment, by a junior doctor. Fourthly, if you wish, you can have a private room.

If, however, your condition is one that requires urgent hospital admission – for example, a burst ulcer or acute appendicitis – there may well be no advantage to you in choosing private medicine rather than the treatment provided by the NHS. Indeed, often in such urgent cases the specialist admits a would-be private patient to an NHS bed, either because a private bed cannot be made available soon enough or because the specialist considers that in the circumstances NHS medical facilities are better than those in a small private clinic. In such a case you do not pay privately for your treatment and are considered to be an NHS patient.

If your GP advises specialist treatment and you wish this to be private, the GP will refer you to a suitable specialist. By consulting a private specialist or receiving treatment from one, you do not, of course, forfeit your entitlement to future NHS treatment.

In recent years many private beds in NHS hospitals have been phased out and there has been increased building of private hospitals. If you are admitted to a private bed in an NHS hospital, you will probably find that your private room is in a wing separate from the main wards; the visiting hours may be more flexible than in the rest of the hospital, and you may have a greater choice of menu.

Health insurance
Many people cover themselves against the cost of private medicine by taking out health

insurance with a provident association, a body that uses members' subscriptions to pay members' fees for treatment and to support private hospitals. The largest association in Britain, BUPA (British United Provident Association), runs its own private hospitals throughout England and also supports the Nuffield Nursing Homes Trust, the largest group of private hospitals in England.

Both BUPA and the other major provident association, PPP (Private Patients Plan), have three levels of benefit, based largely on different standards of hospital. A subscriber who might request admission to an expensive private London clinic would pay higher subscriptions than someone who would want a private bed in a provincial NHS hospital.

Generally speaking, a provident association will accept as members only people who are reasonably healthy at the time of joining. The association will not accept people over 65 as new subscribers; neither will it cover payments to a private GP, dentist, or practitioner of alternative medicine. It may, however, cover payments for private health screening (see *Health-screening clinics*, below).

As a private patient, you have to pay the full cost of your treatment – the specialist's fees, the charge for any hospital stay, and the surgeon's and anaesthetist's fees if you have had an operation. If you are insured, you will be paid benefits to a pre-established amount, which may or may not cover the full cost of treatment. Any difference you pay yourself.

Health-screening clinics

In several British cities there are now private health-screening clinics, where you pay to have a medical examination. There is a standard range of tests available – including *X-rays*, *mammography*, blood tests, and *electrocardiography* – plus any other tests indicated as necessary by the questionnaire you originally fill in. At some clinics the charge is reduced for members of provident associations. You do not need to be referred to the clinic by your GP, but if the clinic decides you need treatment, it will send the GP a copy of its report.

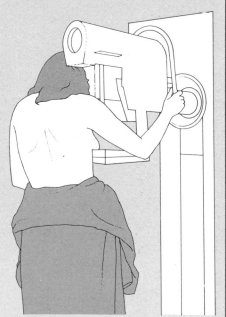

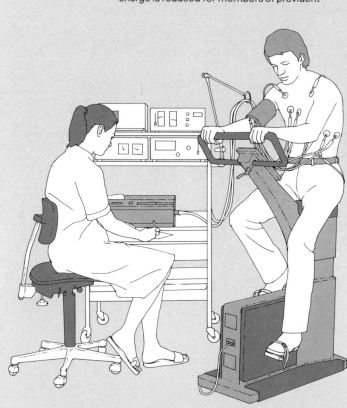

Exercise ECG (left)
Most health-screening clinics carry out an exercise ECG, which may show up any heart abnormalities not evident while the patient is resting.

Mammography (above)
Regular 6-monthly screening by mammography has been shown to detect breast cancers before they are noticeable during self-examination or even physical examination by a doctor.

Patients' rights

In most cases, to obtain treatment under the National Health Service you must first be registered with a general practitioner; but if you are injured in an accident or taken ill suddenly, any GP or accident and emergency department of a hospital will provide you with treatment.

In theory, you have the right to choose your GP and to change him or her when you like (and the GP has the right to refuse to accept you on his or her list or to remove you from it). In reality, your choice may well be limited to the doctors in practices close to your home, since most GPs will not accept patients living a long distance away from their surgery. If you cannot find a GP who will accept you, you must ask your local Family Practitioner Committee to allocate you one. The doctor chosen by the committee cannot refuse to accept you (for further information see *General practice*, p.729).

You have no absolute entitlement to the services of a dentist or optician under the NHS, as you do with a GP. In fact, in some parts of the country it is difficult to find a dentist who will provide NHS treatment. You should have no trouble in finding an optician who will give you an NHS eye test, but if you need spectacles the optician may be unwilling to provide you with NHS frames and may try to persuade you to select from the much wider and generally more expensive range of frames available privately.

You cannot demand hospital treatment. You obtain it only if a doctor considers it necessary. If your GP thinks you need specialist treatment, he or she will refer you to a specialist; if you have any preference for an individual specialist, you will be referred to him or her, as far as possible. In some cases, though, it may not be feasible for you to see the specialist of your choice. Some types of specialist hospital, such as hospitals for the elderly and for mentally ill patients, have a catchment area, and if you live in the catchment area of a hospital that specializes in your problem, you will automatically be referred to a specialist at that hospital.

In most illnesses, your doctor will tell you what is wrong with you if you ask. A problem sometimes arises if you have a serious or potentially fatal illness, in which case the doctor may decide not to tell you (though almost always your relatives will be told), because he or she regards this approach as being in your best interests. If you do want to know what is wrong with you, and the likely outcome, you should make this clear to the doctors treating you. If you keep asking questions you will be told what you want to know.

You should also tell your relatives that you wish to know the truth; then, once your doctor learns this from them, he or she will probably agree to tell you.

Once the specialist has explained your condition to you and before treatment has begun, you may wish to ask either the specialist or your GP about the range of possible treatments and their relative advantages. You can also ask your GP to refer you to another specialist for a second opinion. If you refuse the treatment suggested by the specialist, he or she may well be unwilling to treat you in any other way – in which case you will have to ask your GP to recommend a specialist who will treat you in the way you want.

Compulsory admission to hospital

There are only three sets of circumstances in which you have to enter hospital and be compulsorily detained there. The circumstances are as follows: if you are suffering from a form of mental illness that threatens the health and safety of yourself or others; if you are suffering from a notifiable disease that has to be reported to the local health authority; or if you are living in insanitary conditions and can either no longer look after yourself or find anyone else to look after you.

The most usual mechanism by which a mentally ill person can be made to enter a mental hospital against his or her will is the use of one of the 72-hour detention orders under the Mental Health Act (1959). A relative or social worker may apply for the order, supported by the patient's GP; or the police may detain the sick person. Less often the initial order is for 28 days' detention.

After a 72-hour detention has elapsed, a decision has to be made by all concerned whether the person should be released or there should be an application for a 28-day order. This application must be initiated by a relative or social worker, but this time it needs the support of two doctors, one of whom must be a psychiatrist.

At the end of 28 days, detention can be extended for another year by a further order, obtained in the same way. This order can be renewed for another year, but on this and all subsequent occasions the application must be made by the hospital. Subsequent renewals (and there is no limit to the eventual number of renewals) will be for two years each.

Relatives can appeal against the detention of an individual in a mental hospital. Since the procedure is rather complex, it is sensible to ask the help of *MIND*, the charity that looks after the interests of the mentally ill. For the address, see p.768.

Consent to treatment

In general, your consent to the medical treatment you are given in hospital or by your GP is taken as implied – implied by your having asked for help and not refused the treatment offered you. The principal exceptions are when you are specifically asked to consent in writing to having an operation, or you are taking part in medical research.

A surgeon will not perform an operation on you without your written consent, unless it is an extreme emergency or you are unconscious and alone. A parent's consent is generally sought before an operation on a child; but this matter is not defined in law. The consent of the husband is usually required before a surgeon will sterilize the wife; and similarly the wife's consent is required before a vasectomy to sterilize the husband.

In some cases – for example, in some types of cancer – you may be asked to consent not to one specific operation but to whatever procedure the surgeon finds necessary during the preliminary exploratory surgery. If you are asked to give such general consent, before you sign you may wish to find out from the surgeon what the possible procedures are, and if you are unhappy discuss the matter with the surgeon.

Another case in which you may be asked for your written consent is if, while you are in hospital, you are asked to allow investigations of your condition in order that information can be gained that could well help other patients. This is consent for medical research. Before obtaining your written consent, the doctors in charge will explain to you what they want to do, why they want to do it, and what the likely effects on you will be. If you find the project alarming or upsetting, you may refuse to take part.

Confidentiality

All doctors keep to themselves anything you tell them (except in certain exceptional circumstances, some of which are given below). The case notes that contain this confidential information are always kept in secure conditions, but in some specialities – such as psychiatric illness and sexually transmitted diseases – extra precautions are taken to maintain the patient's confidentiality. In clinics for sexually transmitted diseases, for example, the notes are filed under numbers rather than names. You have a legal right to expect that any doctor who treats you will not disclose without your consent any medical information about you to anyone other than the doctors and medical staff involved in your case. These other doctors and medical staff

will be bound in the same way. The exceptions are laid down by law. For example, if you have a highly infectious condition, the local medical officer for environmental health must be informed; those addicted to heroin and certain other drugs have to be notified to the chief medical officer; a doctor may have to give information to the police under the Road Traffic Acts; courts can order the disclosure of records; and all deaths, births, and stillbirths must be notified to the local authority.

Complaints

There are some circumstances in which you may feel you have grounds to make a complaint. You may be unhappy about the medical treatment you receive (whether from a GP or in hospital), or you may be faced with a long wait for treatment. If you are in hospital, an aspect of your care – such as the nursing or the food – may seem to raise problems. In such situations, discuss the matter straight away with the person concerned.

If you are making a serious complaint, remember that you are much more likely to gain the cooperation of the person concerned if you adopt a calm and reasonable attitude.

In many cases your dissatisfaction will have been the result of a misunderstanding. In such a case the matter will probably be resolved quickly after a short discussion, with no ill-feeling on either side.

If it is not easy to contact the person concerned, make an appointment to see him or her at the earliest opportunity. Before you attend the appointment, it might help you both if you write a letter setting out your complaint as clearly as possible.

Occasionally you may not know whom to approach with a complaint. In that case, use the chart on the next two pages, which also indicates the procedure you should follow if your problem remains unsolved. The chart deals with those complaints that are most likely to arise. For the addresses of the various bodies mentioned in the chart, consult a telephone directory (in some cases the organization will appear under the general heading of National Health Service). Alternatively, contact the *General Medical Council* (see p.768 for central address) or ask at a post office, a Citizen's Advice Bureau, or your doctor's surgery.

If you are ever in any doubt about your best course of action concerning a complaint, the first person to see is your own family doctor. If he or she is unsympathetic, you should then contact the *Patients' Association* (p.768) or your local Community Health Council.

How to make a complaint (before using this chart read *Patients' rights*, p.748)

Medical negligence

This occurs if you suffer because the standard of your treatment falls below the standard expected of your doctor, dentist, optician, or pharmacist.

Ethical misconduct

This occurs if a doctor, dentist, optician, or pharmacist behaves in a dishonest or improper way or abuses his or her professional knowledge or privileges – for example, if he or she discloses details of your case to non-medical people without your consent, or makes improper advances to you.

Administrative negligence

This occurs if your treatment is unreasonably slow or delayed or is unsatisfactory due to rudeness, indifference, or unreasonable behaviour on the part of the staff; or if your physical surroundings are not up to reasonable standards of warmth and comfort.

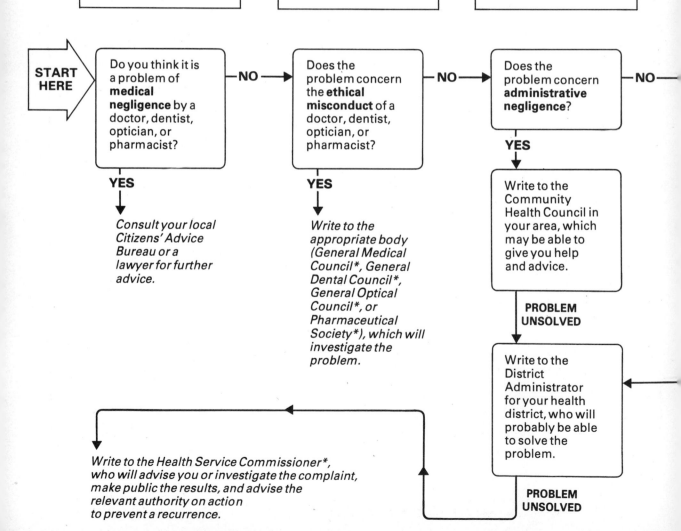

START HERE

Do you think it is a problem of **medical negligence** by a doctor, dentist, optician, or pharmacist? —**NO**→

YES

Consult your local Citizens' Advice Bureau or a lawyer for further advice.

Does the problem concern the **ethical misconduct** of a doctor, dentist, optician, or pharmacist? —**NO**→

YES

Write to the appropriate body (General Medical Council*, General Dental Council*, General Optical Council*, or Pharmaceutical Society*), which will investigate the problem.

Does the problem concern **administrative negligence**? —**NO**—

YES

Write to the Community Health Council in your area, which may be able to give you help and advice.

PROBLEM UNSOLVED

Write to the District Administrator for your health district, who will probably be able to solve the problem.

PROBLEM UNSOLVED

Write to the Health Service Commissioner*, who will advise you or investigate the complaint, make public the results, and advise the relevant authority on action to prevent a recurrence.

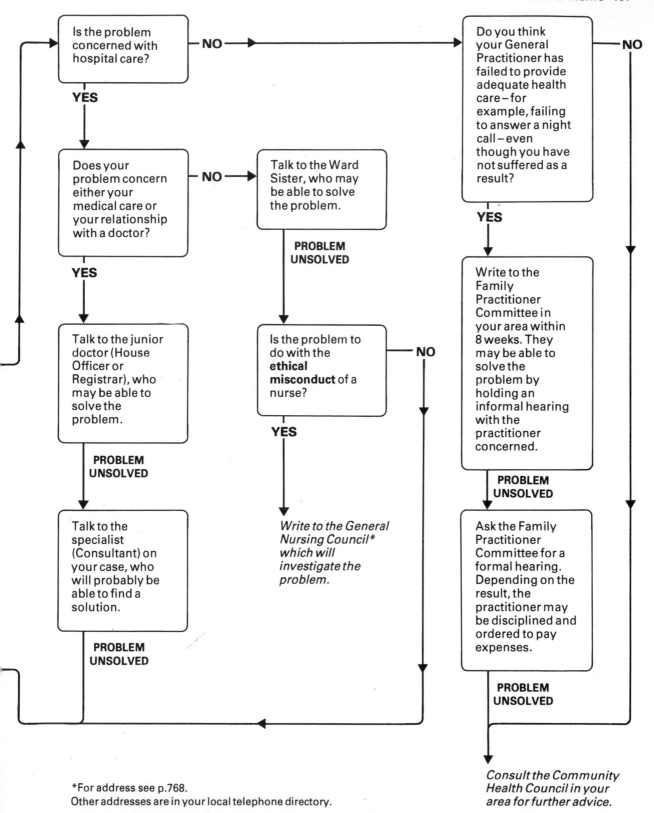

Is the problem concerned with hospital care?

NO →

YES ↓

Do you think your General Practitioner has failed to provide adequate health care – for example, failing to answer a night call – even though you have not suffered as a result?

NO →

YES ↓

Does your problem concern either your medical care or your relationship with a doctor?

NO →

Talk to the Ward Sister, who may be able to solve the problem.

PROBLEM UNSOLVED

YES ↓

Write to the Family Practitioner Committee in your area within 8 weeks. They may be able to solve the problem by holding an informal hearing with the practitioner concerned.

PROBLEM UNSOLVED

Talk to the junior doctor (House Officer or Registrar), who may be able to solve the problem.

PROBLEM UNSOLVED

Is the problem to do with the **ethical misconduct** of a nurse?

NO

YES ↓

Write to the General Nursing Council* which will investigate the problem.

Talk to the specialist (Consultant) on your case, who will probably be able to find a solution.

PROBLEM UNSOLVED

Ask the Family Practitioner Committee for a formal hearing. Depending on the result, the practitioner may be disciplined and ordered to pay expenses.

PROBLEM UNSOLVED

Consult the Community Health Council in your area for further advice.

*For address see p.768.
Other addresses are in your local telephone directory.

Alternative medicine

Alternative (or fringe) medicine is any form of medicine other than that conventionally practised throughout the Western world. The main types of alternative medicine practised in this country are acupuncture, osteopathy, homoeopathy, herbalism, naturopathy, and chiropractic (for descriptions see these two pages). Each therapy has its conception – which differs from that of conventional medicine – of how an illness develops and how the body overcomes it.

Any form of alternative medicine can be used to treat any illness. However, each type of medicine is considered especially suited to certain disorders or problems. Thus osteopathy is used predominantly for joint and back troubles, and acupuncture for pain relief anywhere. Many practitioners of alternative medicine practise more than one type of medicine and can therefore choose whichever they consider to be the most suitable for any given case.

If you are ill, you should consult your general practitioner about your problem. But if he or she can offer no treatment for your condition or has provided treatment that you are not happy with, there is no reason for you not to turn to alternative medicine for help. However, if the reason for taking this step is that you are unhappy with the treatment your GP is giving you, or if you have a serious condition, you should first discuss with the GP your intention of trying alternative medicine. He or she can then warn you about the possible pitfalls of alternative medicine, and, in the case of serious disorders, actual risks to your health.

Some GPs and specialists practise forms of alternative medicine themselves, but most who do so charge for the treatment. In rare cases a GP or a specialist will provide treatments such as acupuncture or homoeopathy on the National Health Service.

Most information about alternative medical treatment can be gained from books on the subject. But if you are considering treating yourself, it is not wise to rely on self-taught knowledge alone – an actual practitioner of alternative medicine should also be consulted for the knowledge and practical experience he or she can offer.

Finding a good practitioner of alternative medicine (that is, one whose treatment is successful) is not easy. It is true that most branches of alternative medicine are governed by a society that awards qualifications to those who have passed its courses (such practitioners have letters after their name), but the quality of training given on such courses is highly variable. The only way that you may be able to gain some idea of the standard of training and qualifications given is by writing to or telephoning the appropriate society and asking for information. Even so, most alternative medical practice is of a rather intuitive nature, and a successful practitioner will not necessarily have qualifications or even belong to a society. Perhaps the best way of choosing a practitioner is – as in so many other spheres – on the personal recommendation of someone whose judgement you trust. And a further word of warning:

You should bear in mind that there is no guarantee the alternative therapy you have chosen will work. And you should also realize that your rights as a patient are far less than those you have with conventional medicine (see *Patients' rights*, p.748) – cases of malpractice in alternative medicine are extremely difficult to prove.

Acupuncture

Acupuncture is a form of medicine that has been developed in the East over thousands of years. Several hundred critical points have been mapped on the body, and it is believed that each illness is characterized by the "disturbance" of a particular combination of several of these points. To relieve the disturbance and thus cure the illness, fine needles are inserted into the skin at each of the appropriate points. Acupuncture is used particularly to treat disorders marked by pain.

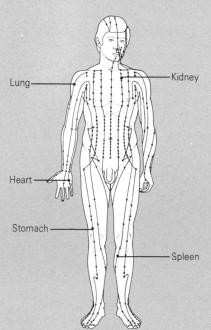

Lung

Kidney

Heart

Stomach

Spleen

Meridian lines
These lines provide a guide for acupuncturists, showing at which points the needles should be inserted to influence the flow of energy to various areas of the body. There are 14 main lines covering the body, each line representing an internal organ. If the organ is diseased, according to practitioners of acupuncture its particular energy flow will be disturbed, and the needles are used to correct the flow. Needles inserted at the correct points can also sometimes have the same effect as giving an anaesthetic.

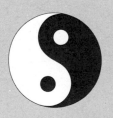

Yin and yang
Shown left is the symbol for yin and yang, the Chinese concept of the balance in everything of yin (passivity or water) and yang (activity or fire). Disease results from their imbalance; many forms of alternative medicine make use of this concept.

Osteopathy

Osteopathy was devised late in the last century. The system is based on the idea that faulty alignment of bone structure causes many disorders, often indirectly – for example, an unbalanced pelvis can upset the functioning of the entire body and lead to an apparently unconnected problem such as headache or asthma. The osteopath first probes the sick person's body with the fingertips to discover the whereabouts of the faulty alignment. Treatment ranges from massage to powerful manipulation of the areas concerned.

Chiropractic

Chiropractic was founded soon after osteopathy, in the late 1800s, and is similar in its treatment. But whereas osteopathy is concerned with faulty bone structure, the underlying idea of chiropractic is that disorders result from faulty working of the nervous system. In addition, chiropractics concentrate upon one part of the body rather than looking on the body as an integrated whole, as osteopaths do. They chiefly treat specific joint, muscle, or bone disorders, and they rely mainly on the study of *X-rays* to show them the problem areas. Treatment consists mainly of a more forceful manipulation of the joints than is used in osteopathy, and is carried out on a special adjustable couch.

Homoeopathy

This is a system of treatment devised in the late 1700s at about the same time that orthodox medicine began to develop. A disorder is treated by giving to the sick person a small dose of one of various substances that, if given in a large dose to a healthy person, would produce the symptoms of that disorder. Whichever substance is chosen depends on the physical and mental nature of the person, as revealed by a preliminary examination.

Naturopathy

This is a medical system that was devised in the 1800s to treat disease without resorting to drugs. It is based on the idea that any disorder is brought about by a faulty diet and way of life. Treatment consists of correcting these and is sometimes accompanied by exercise, massage, special baths, and sunbathing. In addition, vitamin preparations and herb teas may be recommended. Naturopathy is used mainly to treat chronic diseases and inexplicable ill-health and as a preventive regimen to keep illness at bay.

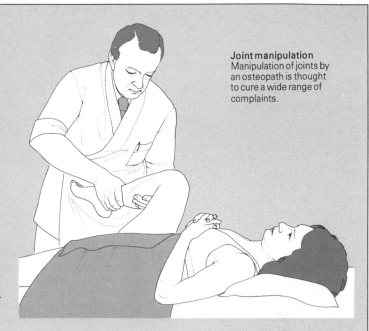

Joint manipulation
Manipulation of joints by an osteopath is thought to cure a wide range of complaints.

Herbalism

Herbalism is an ancient system of treatment from which orthodox medicine ultimately developed. It uses many of the drugs that are used in orthodox medicine but in the natural, unrefined, unconcentrated forms in which they occur in herbs instead of in the artificial, purified forms in which they are prescribed in conventional medicine. In their natural state, as plant extracts, the drugs limit side-effects and are considered by herbalists to provide a much more wholesome treatment. They are administered in teas, liquid medicines, tablets, or creams. Herbalists believe that there is a natural remedy for every ailment.

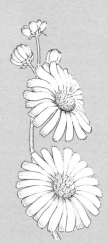

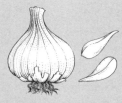

Garlic
Garlic has traditionally had many uses in herbalist medicine and is now proving of interest to orthodox physicians because of its ability to lower concentrations of fat in the blood.

Caring for the sick at home

Introduction

Nowadays, it is recognized that the sick and injured should be cared for, whenever possible, in their own homes. Besides relieving the pressure on hospital services, home care is usually more reassuring and more pleasant for the patient – and probably, therefore, more conducive to a speedy recovery.

At one end of the scale there are the long-term sick or disabled invalid and the elderly, bed-ridden patient who both need virtually full-time care and attention. More often, though, the problem will be the simpler and more temporary one at the other end of the scale – the bouts of flu and childhood infectious diseases, for instance, that are a recurrent and inevitable part of family life.

You should not feel intimidated at the prospect of having to take on the role of a home nurse, even if you have had no previous experience of the sick-room. Home nursing calls for a mixture of common sense and a caring approach that virtually anyone – man or woman – is able to provide. Difficult nursing procedures and sophisticated, expensive equipment in the home are very seldom called for. The basic nursing skills – taking a temperature, making a bed, preventing bedsores, and a knowledge of the best way to move an immobile patient are all simple procedures that are easily learned and are usually all that is needed. Many such routine nursing procedures are described and illustrated in this section. Your principal aim is to keep the patient comfortable, clean, and fresh. When horizons are limited to bed and bedroom, small things tend to be magnified. However ill the patient feels, he or she can be made to feel better on fresh, cool, unwrinkled sheets. If you are caring for someone who is likely to be bed-bound for some time, one or two pairs of non-iron (but *not* nylon) sheets will make your task of laundering bed-linen much easier.

You need never feel, if you are caring for a sick member of your family, that the responsibility is entirely your own. If more complex care is needed than you are able to give, your doctor will arrange for the district nurse or health visitor either to carry out special procedures (injections or changing dressings, for example) or simply to dispense guidance and advice.

Long-term sickness or disability is a great strain on the whole family, particularly on the person who has to cope with the bulk of the nursing care. But it is important that the nurse's responsibility does not become overwhelming. An exhausted nurse is unlikely to be efficient. Hence, the whole burden of care should not fall on one person. Every member of the family can fetch and carry, help with bed-making, and provide company in the sickroom. Outside agencies, too, should be called upon if their help is needed: articles in the previous section (see *Community health care*, p.743) describe the various services available – home helps, for example, and Meals on Wheels. Financial assistance is provided, too, which those who are nursing the sick or disabled may be entitled to. And equipment can often be hired or borrowed to make nursing easier. Commodes, bedpans, urinals, and other nursing aids, for example, may be borrowed from the Social Services Department, or hired from the local medical loans department of the *British Red Cross Society* (see p.768 for the head-office address).

Children and the elderly pose special nursing problems, the former because they make by far the most demanding patients, both emotionally and physically; the latter because of the special risks (such as stiffness in the joints and loss of muscle tone) attached to enforced physical inactivity in the elderly. The advice given in this section and elsewhere in the book will help you to deal with the difficulties involved in caring for both the young and the old (see also *Special problems of infants and children*, p.644, and *Special problems of the elderly*, p.716).

Convalescence can be an even more difficult time than illness for both patient and nurse. The better the patient feels, the more irritable and impatient for recovery he or she is likely to become. On occasion, though, the reverse may be true, and a patient who has been well nursed may be reluctant to abandon the "security" of his or her disorder. So it is vital in the middle of the illness that you try to encourage your patient to do whatever he or she can manage. This will make it easier for the patient to recover former independence and self-sufficiency as health returns to normal.

Home nursing in general

In the following pages are included many practical hints and pieces of advice on how to care for a sick person in the home. Give some thought to the day's routine, and the arrangement of furniture and items of equipment, so that problems are minimized for both you and your patient. Your doctor or visiting nurse should be able to provide valuable help and guidance (see *Care at home*, p.745, for further details).

Planning the sick-room

If you are nursing someone who is likely to be ill for some time, plan the sick-room carefully. In a house, it may be better for the sick-room to be a converted ground-floor room rather than an upstairs bedroom, since, in this way, the sick person will not feel so isolated and you will not have to make so many trips up and down the stairs.

Your main aim in arranging the room must be to make things comfortable for the sick person and convenient for yourself. A single bed makes bed-making easier, and, if possible, the bed should be accessible on both sides; if this is not possible, make sure that the accessible side is on the sick person's right (especially if he or she is right-handed, as this should give you room to position a bedside table conveniently on the patient's right), because this is the position in which a doctor prefers to stand when making an examination. If you can, place the bed so that the sick person can see out of the window. Provide a bedside table to hold medicines, a water jug and glass, tissues, a bell (so that you can be summoned if you are needed), and any other necessary items. If the patient is allowed out of bed but cannot easily get to a lavatory, a commode chair (a chair whose seat incorporates a chamber-pot) is essential. You can borrow one (and also a bedpan and, if necessary, a bed urinal for a male) from the National Health Service, through your local health visitor, or from the medical loans depot of your local branch of the *British Red Cross Society* (p.768).

A sick person does not "need" fresh air, but he or she may feel more fresh and comfortable if a window is left slightly open. This is a matter of individual preference and should not be forced on the patient. Whether the room is ventilated or not, it must be kept free from draughts and reasonably warm – at about 21°C (70°F) during the day, 18°C (65°F) at night.

Giving medicines

It is essential for medicines to be taken for the full course, and the specified number of times a day, as ordered by the doctor. You must not go against your doctor's advice and stop giving a sick person medicines just because he or she appears to be getting better.

If a medicine is prescribed, say, four times a day, ask the doctor whether all the doses can be given during the daytime. Always measure the dose of a liquid medicine in the special spoon provided, to ensure accuracy, as teaspoons can vary in size significantly. When you pour the medicine, hold the bottle with the label upwards so that any overflow does not make it illegible. If a sick person finds it difficult to swallow gelatin-coated capsules, wet the capsules first to make them slip down the throat more easily.

Drugs can have predictable side-effects, about which the doctor will warn you (see *Drug index*, p.778). But very occasionally, a sick person has an unexpected allergic response to a drug. Penicillin and related *antibiotics* are among the most common drugs to cause allergy, and the most usual allergic reactions are a rash (see *Urticaria*, p.255), itching, or wheezing. If, after taking a medicine, a sick person develops symptoms that seem unrelated to his or her illness, tell the doctor straight away and ask if you should stop giving the drug until an alternative medicine can be prescribed.

See also *Drugs and the elderly*, p.725, and *Giving medicines to children*, p.764.

Taking a temperature

Normal body temperature is about 37°C (98.6°F) but may vary by about 0.5 to 1°C (1 to 2°F) throughout the day; it is at its lowest in the early hours of the morning. A rise in temperature (a fever) is not in itself dangerous unless it exceeds 40°C (104°F), the level at which the body's own temperature-control system begins to become ineffective. A rise in temperature is usually caused by an infection. While the temperature is rising, the sick person feels cold and shivery.

You can measure a person's temperature by using either a clinical thermometer or a temperature indicator strip.

The clinical thermometer: The clinical thermometer is a small glass tube marked with a scale and with a mercury-filled bulb at one end. As the mercury is heated by your body, it expands and rises up the tube to a point on the scale (which has an arrow indicating normal body temperature). A small kink in the tube prevents the mercury sinking back into the bulb when the thermometer is removed from the warmth of the body. Before you buy a clinical thermometer examine it carefully, warming the bulb in your hand, to ensure that

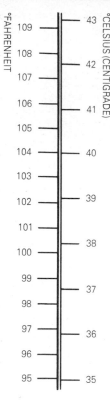

Temperature
conversion scale

the mercury column and the markings are clear enough for you to see them easily.

A thermometer in the mouth gives a fairly accurate reading of body temperature. But it is easier to take the temperature of a young child by putting the thermometer in the arm-pit. In this case, the reading will be about 0.5°C (1°F) lower than that given when the thermometer is in the mouth. Note: You should never leave a baby or young child alone with a thermometer.

The temperature indicator strip: This is a reusable plastic strip that is placed on the forehead. The strip is divided into chemically impregnated panels, each with a temperature printed on it. The different chemicals on each panel cause the panel to glow when they reach a certain temperature. You can read your own temperature by watching the strip in a mirror. You can obtain a strip at any chemist's. It does not give the precise reading of a thermometer, but it indicates temperature as accurately as is needed for home nursing purposes. (It is all too easy for you and the person you are nursing to become obsessed with the use of a thermometer and to monitor faithfully every small rise and fall of temperature even though they have no real clinical significance.) A strip has the addi-tional advantage of being easier to use, espe-cially in the case of a young child.

Whether you use a thermometer or strip, never take a temperature immediately after

the person has had a bath, a meal, a hot drink, or a cigarette (which a sick person should not be smoking anyway), since you may then get a false reading.

If a sick person has a fever, do not try to "sweat it out" by keeping the room too warm or by putting extra blankets on the bed – this may make the person's temperature rise even further. Instead, to help bring the tempera-ture down, give some soluble aspirin or

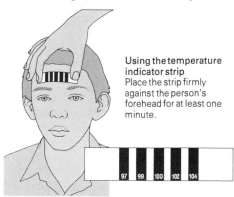

Using the temperature
indicator strip
Place the strip firmly
against the person's
forehead for at least one
minute.

paracetamol according to the directions on the bottle and not more than once every four hours. While the person's temperature is fall-ing, he or she will sweat profusely. To replace the body fluids and salt lost in this way, give plenty of water, fruit drinks, and soup or nourishing drinks such as those that are made with beef extract.

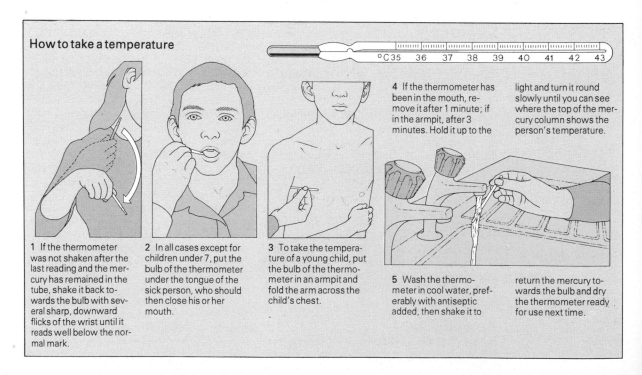

How to take a temperature

1 If the thermometer was not shaken after the last reading and the mercury has remained in the tube, shake it back to-wards the bulb with sev-eral sharp, downward flicks of the wrist until it reads well below the nor-mal mark.

2 In all cases except for children under 7, put the bulb of the thermometer under the tongue of the sick person, who should then close his or her mouth.

3 To take the tempera-ture of a young child, put the bulb of the thermo-meter in an armpit and fold the arm across the child's chest.

4 If the thermometer has been in the mouth, re-move it after 1 minute; if in the armpit, after 3 minutes. Hold it up to the light and turn it round slowly until you can see where the top of the mer-cury column shows the person's temperature.

5 Wash the thermo-meter in cool water, pref-erably with antiseptic added, then shake it to return the mercury to-wards the bulb and dry the thermometer ready for use next time.

Bed-making

Sheets for the sick person's bed should be made chiefly of cotton – which is sweat-absorbent – and not of nylon. Non-iron cotton/polyester sheets will save you a lot of work when you change the bed.

A bed-bound person needs his or her bed to be made twice a day – morning and evening – and to be tidied more often. Change the sheets every four or five days – more often if the sick person is sweating a lot or if you just want to make him or her more comfortable. Always draw the bottom sheet tightly over the bed so that there are no wrinkles (which make the sheet uncomfortable for the sick person) and tuck it in well. Arrange the pillows so that they support the shoulders as well as the head. The most comfortable arrangement for someone who is forced to lie on his or her back is two pillows placed at an

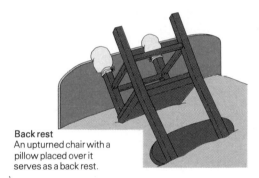

Back rest
An upturned chair with a pillow placed over it serves as a back rest.

angle to each other with a third lying across them If the sick person prefers only one pillow, pull it well down so that the neck and shoulders as well as the head are supported.

Once the sick person can sit up, he or she will need either a back rest (which can be bought, or improvised from an upturned kitchen chair), or at least extra support with more pillows. Also provide something, such as a bolster, to support the feet and prevent the person sliding down the bed.

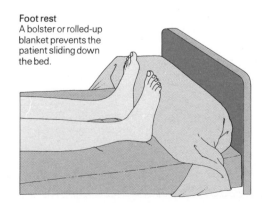

Foot rest
A bolster or rolled-up blanket prevents the patient sliding down the bed.

Changing the sheets

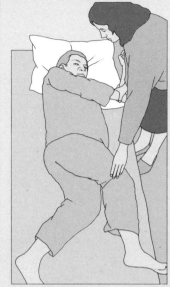

1 If the sick person cannot get out of bed at all, there is still an easy way of changing the bottom sheet. First, turn the person on one side.

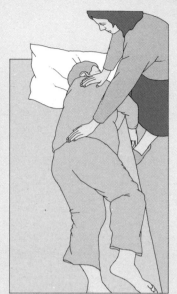

2 Move the person to the edge of the bed, making sure that he or she is lying in a stable position.

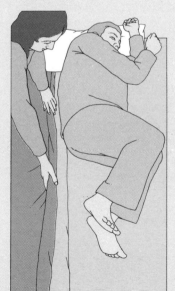

3 Roll one half of the old sheet lengthwise up against the person, then roll one half of the clean sheet lengthwise and put it on the bed with the rolled up half in the centre of the bed.

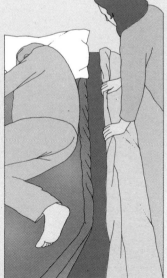

4 Roll the person on to this clean half, and take off the old sheet. Finally, unroll the rest of the clean sheet, stretch it tight, and tuck it in.

Drawsheets

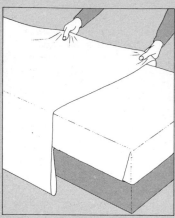

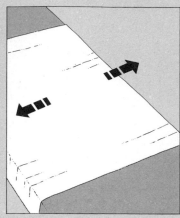

1 A drawsheet is an ordinary sheet folded in such a way as to provide the sick person with a clean, unwrinkled sheet to lie on without your having to remake the bed.

First, move the patient out of the bed (see p.761 for instructions on how to move an immobile patient). Then take and fold the sheet in half lengthwise and put it over the bed crosswise so that it extends from the sick person's head to his or her knees and so that it overlaps the bed more on one side than the other.

2 Tuck one side in, pull the sheet tight, and tuck in the other side. When you want to provide a fresh area beneath the patient, untuck both ends of the sheet, pull it along to a new position, and tuck in both sides tightly again. For the comfort of the patient, make sure the drawsheet is kept very taut.

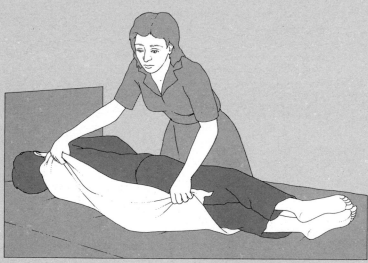

3 A drawsheet can also be used as an aid to moving an immobile or very weak person. If you want to move the person sideways, first untuck the end of the drawsheet opposite to that side of the bed to which you want the person to move. Then cross to that side of the bed and, leaning across the bed and holding the free far end of the drawsheet, use it to roll the person towards you. To move the person up the bed, you need someone's help. Both ends of the drawsheet are untucked, each of you holds one end, and the person is lifted on the drawsheet to the desired position.

Hospital corners

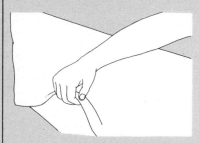

1 Hospital ("mitred") corners make a neat and comfortable finish to the sick-room bed. Place the bottom sheet in position and tuck in at the ends. With one hand, lift the side of the sheet about 400mm (16in) from the head of the bed.

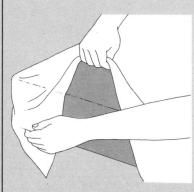

2 Tuck the flap of sheet which hangs between the side of the bed and your hand under the mattress with your other hand. Then let the side of the sheet fall to form a fold at the side of the bed.

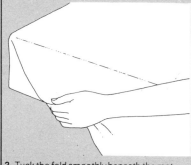

3 Tuck the fold smoothly beneath the mattress. Repeat at the other 3 corners of the bed. Place the top sheet and blankets over the bed, tucking in each one across the bottom of the bed. Lifting and tucking the top sheet and blankets together, make hospital corners at the bottom of the bed only.

Giving food, drink, and special diets

Remember that meals may be the highlights of a monotonous day for the bed-bound patient, so make them as tempting and attractive as you can. Bear in mind, too, that, unless the doctor advises a particular kind of diet, you can safely give the sick person whatever he or she wants to eat – the invalid is nearly always the best judge of what is suitable. The chances are that small helpings of simple food will be all that is wanted until the appetite returns to normal. Do not worry too much if your patient seems to have little appetite. Someone who is in bed all day needs fewer calories than does someone going about his or her regular daily activities. The important thing is to make sure that the little he or she does eat is providing a balanced diet (see *What is a balanced diet?*, p.26). As long as a low-protein diet (below) is not necessary, you should give frequent, small meals, containing plenty of protein and vitamins. Give plenty of fluids – again, whatever non-alcoholic drinks the sick person prefers. However, an occasional glass of sherry or stout will probably do no harm and may even be beneficial in some illnesses if that is what your patient would like. (Spirits are best avoided.)

If the doctor has ordered a special diet and one which you will have to provide for quite a long time, you should get a special cookery book on the subject. This may well be available in a health food store, where you can often obtain dietary instant-food preparations, such as cholesterol-free cake mixes.

Low-salt diet: The doctor may recommend a low-salt diet for someone who is suffering from liver disease (see *Liver, gallbladder, and pancreas*, p.485), kidney disease (see *Disorders of the urinary tract*, p.500), or *high blood pressure* (p.382). The average daily intake of salt is normally about 10g (⅓oz). This can be cut to about 5g simply by adding no extra salt at table, and to about 3g if no salt is added during cooking. If the doctor considers it necessary to restrict the salt intake even further, he or she will advise you on providing a special diet which does not contain, for example, any cured meat or fish, cheese, tinned food other than fruit, food made with bicarbonate of soda or baking powder, or salted butter or margarine. The flavour that a salt-free diet lacks can be provided by the use of a salt-substitute. If the sick person has kidney disease, check with the doctor whether any salt-substitute you buy has to be free of potassium, which is unsuitable for some kidney-disease patients.

Low-protein diets: A low-protein diet may be recommended by the doctor for some kidney disorders. Such a diet will involve a reduced intake of meat, fish, eggs, dairy products, and other protein-rich foods. Because protein provides part of the body's energy needs, extra sugar or glucose should be given to make up for this loss of protein.

Feeding a sick person: A sick person who is elderly or very ill may need to be spoon-fed. If so, feed the person with minced or pureed foods, since these are the easiest both to give and to swallow. Make sure the person is in a comfortable position before you start, and tuck a napkin beneath his or her chin. Taste the food to check that it is at the right temperature. Old people eat slowly, and spoon-fed meals tend to be lengthy; you may find that the food stays hot for a longer period if you use a special child's dish with a hollow base that you fill with hot water. When giving fluids, provide an angled straw (available from most chemists'), which allows the person more control over intake than would sips from a cup, especially if the person is lying flat on his or her back.

Someone who is seriously ill may be able to take only liquid foods. To provide enough nutrition, a liquid diet should include milk, egg in milk, sugar, and fruit juices or fruit purees. To add extra nourishment to soups, broths, and milky drinks, thicken them with a

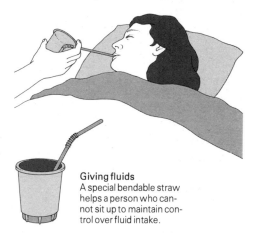

Giving fluids
A special bendable straw helps a person who cannot sit up to maintain control over fluid intake.

meal-replacement substance, which you can buy at a chemist's. These meal substitutes are made in a number of flavours so try to choose one which will tempt your patient's appetite. Check regularly with the doctor that the diet you are providing is nutritious enough.

If a stroke has paralysed one side of a person's body, food may tend to collect in the paralysed cheek. If the person cannot remove the food with a finger, wipe it away with a cotton-wool bud, holding the cheek gently away from the teeth.

Giving a bedpan

A commode (a chair which incorporates a chamber-pot in its seat) is the most comfortable aid for bladder and bowel relief of a sick person. But if someone is too ill or disabled to get out of bed, a bedpan – and, for a male, a bed urinal – will have to be used. Most people who are not used to a bedpan find it inhibiting, especially if someone else is present – so make sure the sick person has complete privacy while he or she is using the pan (but stay within calling distance).

Before you give a bedpan, warm it in hot water, dry it well, and sprinkle the rim with talcum powder to make it easier for the pan to be slipped under the buttocks. If the person cannot lever himself or herself up, let him or her use the pan lying down: lift the hips while you manoeuvre the pan beneath the buttocks, open end towards the feet. The easiest way to give a bedpan to a totally helpless person is to turn him or her on one side, put the pan against the buttocks – pressing it down into the bed as much as possible – and roll the person back on top of it. When the pan has been used, hold it firmly and roll the person on to the side away from you as you pull the bedpan away. Then wipe the person clean before gently moving him or her back into a more comfortable position.

After use, bedpans and urinals must be washed thoroughly in water containing washing soda. Always put them back in the same place so that they can be found in a hurry. A urinal should be left within easy reach of the bed so that the sick person has no need to call or ring for it. Keep it in an empty plastic bowl or bucket to lessen the possibility of spills, especially at night.

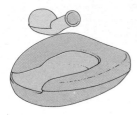

Bedpan and urinal
One or both of these items are essential for an immobilized patient. Your doctor or nurse may be able to arrange for them to be lent to you by a local organization.

Preventing bedsores

Anyone who is confined to bed for a long time is liable to develop bedsores, especially if he or she is paralysed or can manage only restricted movement. The sores occur on those parts of the body – most commonly, the elbows, knees, heels, shoulder blades, and hips and buttocks – that bear the weight of the body or rub constantly against the bedclothes. The elderly and people with certain blood disorders are more likely than others to

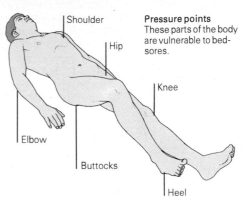

Pressure points
These parts of the body are vulnerable to bedsores.

Shoulder

Hip

Knee

Elbow

Buttocks

Heel

develop bedsores if confined to bed. Bedsores can also develop if areas of skin in contact with moisture, such as sweat or urine, are not cleaned regularly.

A bedsore starts off as a patch of tender, reddened, inflamed skin. Later, the skin becomes purple; then it breaks down and an ulcer develops. As soon as ulcers appear, you should consult the doctor for expert treatment. The ulcers generally take a long time to heal completely.

Bedsores can be prevented. Someone confined to bed can, unless he or she is paralysed or otherwise immobile, still "exercise" and move to support the weight by different parts of the body. Every hour or so, a period of wriggling the toes, rotating the ankles, flexing the arms and legs, tautening and relaxing muscles, stretching the whole body, and then moving into a new position will both stimulate circulation and prevent joints stiffening. If the sick person cannot move, you must change his or her position as often as you can – at least every two hours, but ideally more often than this – so that the pressure of the body on any particular area is relieved. This is most easily done, especially if the sick person is a good deal heavier than you, by using a *drawsheet* (p.758). Otherwise, *lift* the person into a new position (enlisting someone else's help if necessary); dragging the person may damage the skin and increase the chances of bedsores developing.

Giving a bedpan
It is easier if someone helps you lift the patient while you place the pan in position.

Use a bed-cradle to keep the weight of the bedclothes off the sick person's legs and feet. You may be able to borrow one through your health visitor or from the medical loan depot of the local *British Red Cross Society* (p.768). If not, you can improvise using a stool or a clean wooden box with the sides cut out. If the person is lying permanently on his or her side, support the upper part of the arms and legs on soft pillows to cushion the elbows and knees. A pillow placed between the ankles

Relieving pressure
Use plenty of soft pillows or cushions to relieve the pressure that can lead to bedsores.

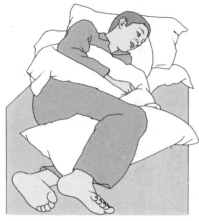

should be enough to stop them rubbing against each other.

Make sure that the sheets are always clean, dry, crumb-free, and pulled as tight as possible to prevent wrinkling (see *Bed-making*, p.757). If the sick person is likely to be bed-ridden for a long time, it is worth buying a sheepskin (preferably a synthetic, washable one) for the person to lie on, to cushion the whole body. Sheepskin boots can be bought to protect the heels and ankles.

Whenever you wash the sick person, keep the skin on places vulnerable to bedsores particularly clean and dry. If you notice any reddening, sponge the area with surgical spirit, cover it with a soft dressing, and try to keep body weight off it for the next day or two until the redness disappears.

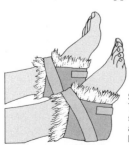

Sheepskin boots
These help to protect the skin of the heels and the ankles from developing bedsores.

Moving an immobile patient

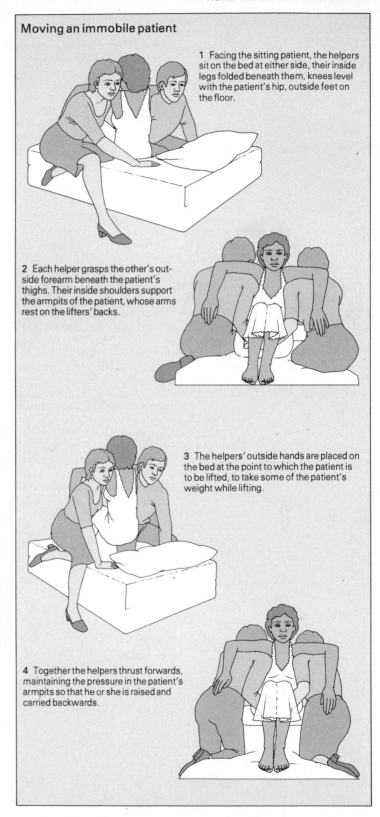

1 Facing the sitting patient, the helpers sit on the bed at either side, their inside legs folded beneath them, knees level with the patient's hip, outside feet on the floor.

2 Each helper grasps the other's outside forearm beneath the patient's thighs. Their inside shoulders support the armpits of the patient, whose arms rest on the lifters' backs.

3 The helpers' outside hands are placed on the bed at the point to which the patient is to be lifted, to take some of the patient's weight while lifting.

4 Together the helpers thrust forwards, maintaining the pressure in the patient's armpits so that he or she is raised and carried backwards.

Dealing with vomiting

Most people prefer to be left alone while they are vomiting, but others find it comforting to have their forehead supported by someone's hand. If a sick person has required your presence in this way, you can help further by offering him or her water afterwards to rinse out the mouth and sponge the face. Always make sure that a person with nausea is in the recovery position if there is any possibility of him or her falling asleep or becoming unconscious (see *The recovery position*, p.805). Vomiting is rarely a dangerous condition unless the vomit is inhaled, when it can result in suffocation.

After a vomiting attack, do not give the person solid food for several hours, but do give water or fruit drinks to replace lost body fluids. There are no medicines that you can buy over the counter to cure vomiting. If the person is vomiting repeatedly, call in the doctor, who, provided he or she does not discover any underlying cause of the vomiting, might prescribe anti-emetics (anti-vomiting drugs). Later, when the vomiting attacks are over, the doctor will probably advise you to give soup, beef tea, a fruit drink, or tea if the sick person will take any of these. Let the sick person's own inclinations about food guide you as his or her appetite returns.

Coping with incontinence

Some loss of bladder control is common in elderly people or in those who have some degree of paralysis below the waist. For a full description of the problem and how to cope with it, see *Incontinence*, p.718.

Relieving a stuffy nose

A stuffy nose can be relieved by giving an inhalant. The best method is to use gelatin-coated capsules of liquid inhalant. Cut the tip off a capsule and squeeze the contents on to a

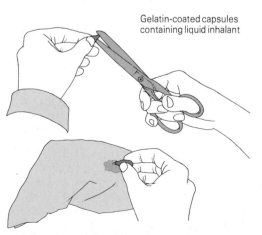

Gelatin-coated capsules containing liquid inhalant

clean handkerchief, from which the sick person can then inhale the vapour. This kind of inhalant is especially useful for giving to children who cannot sleep because of a stuffy nose. Sprinkle the inhalant, very lightly, directly on to the pillow.

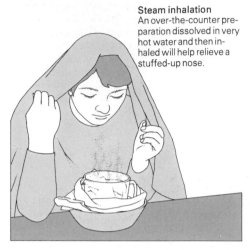

Steam inhalation
An over-the-counter preparation dissolved in very hot water and then inhaled will help relieve a stuffed-up nose.

You may prefer to use the traditional method of steam inhalation. Pour boiling water into a jug, and add the correct dose of inhalant. If your patient is bed-bound and cannot sit at a table to inhale from the jug, put the jug into a flat-bottomed washing-up bowl to catch any of the hot liquid that may be spilt on the bed. A towel draped over both the sick person's head and the jug will allow as much vapour as possible to be inhaled. The inhalation should last for about 10 minutes. (See *Self-help for a blocked or runny nose*, p.344.)

Keeping a sick person clean

A sick person will almost certainly feel better if he or she is able to wash at least twice a day. If the person is bed-bound, you can protect the bed by placing a large towel over the bottom sheet before providing a basin of water and toiletries. If you are going to give your patient a bed bath (an all-over wash in bed), make sure the room is warm, and provide a second large towel to be draped over those parts of the body not being washed, so that the person does not become chilled. It is a good idea to offer the sick person a bedpan before bathing him or her (cleanliness reduces the possibility of bedsores developing around the genital area).

Washing hair

Having clean hair will also boost a sick person's morale. If the person cannot get up, it is possible to give him or her a shampoo in bed.

There are several techniques for washing the hair of a person confined to bed. Whichever technique you use, make sure that the bed is protected by a piece of waterproof sheeting. It is probably easiest if you can place a bowl of water on a table slightly lower than the bed. Move the sick person up the bed, so that his or her hair dangles over the edge into the bowl. At the same time, support the neck and shoulders with a pillow. Do not attempt to wet your patient's head by dipping it into the bowl. It will be more comfortable for him or her if you pour jugs of water carefully over the hair, letting the water drain back into the bowl as you wash and rinse.

After washing the person's hair, part-dry it with a warm towel and finish with an electric hair dryer.

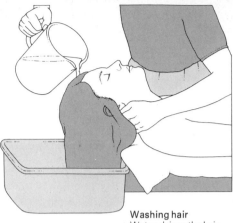

Washing hair
Wet and rinse the hair over a bowl near the bed.

Giving a bed bath

If a sick person is unable to give himself or herself a bed bath, you can give one. Ensure that the room is warm before removing any bedclothes. Cover the patient's body with a large towel and place another one underneath the body to protect the bedclothes (if the person is immobile or too heavy to lift, you can get the second towel into position in the same way that you can a clean bottom sheet – see *Changing the sheets*, p.757).

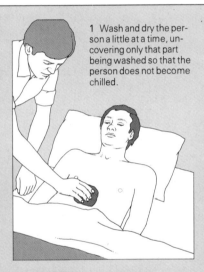

1 Wash and dry the person a little at a time, uncovering only that part being washed so that the person does not become chilled.

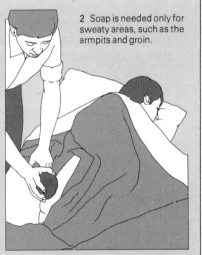

2 Soap is needed only for sweaty areas, such as the armpits and groin.

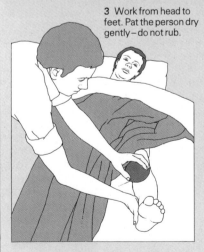

3 Work from head to feet. Pat the person dry gently – do not rub.

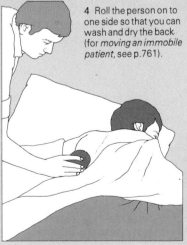

4 Roll the person on to one side so that you can wash and dry the back (for *moving an immobile patient*, see p.761).

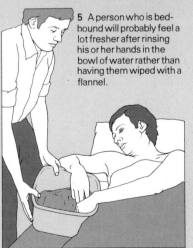

5 A person who is bedbound will probably feel a lot fresher after rinsing his or her hands in the bowl of water rather than having them wiped with a flannel.

Nursing sick children

In general, children are not affected by illness as badly as older people are, but when they are, they take up far more time than virtually any other patient. You should be prepared for this; the sick child needs at least one "nurse", preferably one of his or her parents, on hand almost constantly in order to raise morale and promote a speedy recovery. (For specific information on the various childhood illnesses see *Special problems of infants and children*, p.644.)

Should you keep the sick child in bed?
Unless the doctor has told you the child needs to stay in bed, you can let the child decide whether he or she feels well enough to be up.

It is the child who is neither very ill nor yet well enough to be permanently up who will make most demands on your time and company. In this case, it is wise to make up a bed downstairs (commandeer a sofa, camp bed, or air bed), so that you do not have to keep climbing the stairs and the child has the television and your household activities as distractions. Children learn a great deal through play and, if your child feels well enough, you can make up for his or her lost schooling to some extent by providing much-needed stimulation, as well as entertainment, through the games you play together.

Giving medicines to children
It is important that a sick child takes the full course of medicine prescribed by the doctor. Because small children cannot swallow pills easily, their medicines are usually prescribed in liquid form. To prevent spillage, it is best, after pouring the dose into the measure spoon provided with the medicine, to transfer it to a slightly larger spoon. It can be difficult to get a child to take an unpalatable medicine – in which case, you should sit the child on your knee, give him or her a pleasant drink to hold, ready to be swallowed after the medicine, and (because most taste buds lie at the front of the tongue) tip the medicine into the child's mouth as far back as you can. Show by your manner that you automatically assume the child will take the medicine – if the child senses that you expect trouble, he or she will provide it. Sometimes bribery helps, in the form of a favourite sweet or biscuit put in view nearby and promised as soon as the child has taken the medicine.

If the child refuses to take the medicine, try mixing it with a spoonful of something he or she likes – jam or chocolate spread, perhaps. Do not mix the medicine with a drink, since it will probably stick to the sides or bottom of the drinking vessel and be left behind. If you still have no success, ask the doctor if the medicine can be given in tablet or capsule form. A child of three or older may be able to swallow a tablet or capsule whole with the aid of a drink (a capsule should be wetted first to make it slippery). If the child cannot do this, you may be able to get him or her to take a tablet by crushing it (this should not be done with a capsule) and mixing it with a spoonful of jam or whatever else the child likes. With luck, the spoonful will slip down without the child even tasting the medicine.

Dealing with a raised temperature
A raised temperature is not dangerous provided it does not exceed 40°C (104°F). Only very rarely does a fever have any harmful effects – for example, in a few susceptible children a high temperature may cause *febrile convulsions* (for more information see *Convulsions in children*, p.667).

Unless a child's temperature is 39°C (102°F) or higher all you need to do is make sure that he or she drinks plenty of fluids and is kept lightly clothed or covered.

At about a level of 38°C, you can, if the child seems miserable or uncomfortable, give junior aspirin or paracetamol, according to the dosage on the bottle and no more than once every four hours. When it is time for a second or subsequent dose, first take the child's temperature again; if it has started to fall, do not give the medicine. If the child is asleep, do not wake him or her up; the sleep will very probably do as much good as the aspirin or paracetamol.

If the child's temperature continues to rise in spite of the medicine and reaches 39°C (102°F) or higher, call the doctor and in the meantime relieve the discomfort of the fever by fanning the child or by sponging his or her face, neck, arms, and legs with warm water and leaving them to dry naturally – the evaporation of the water cools the skin.

If your child has had a febrile convulsion in the past, make sure the doctor knows about

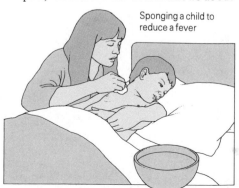

Sponging a child to reduce a fever

this. The doctor will probably recommend that you try to lower the child's temperature at an early stage by giving aspirin or paracetamol at the first sign of a raised temperature and sponging the child as soon as he or she feels at all hot.

Feeding the sick child

Unless the doctor has recommended a special diet, let the child eat what he or she feels like rather than what you think is suitable. Provide smaller helpings than usual, and do not worry if the child does not eat much; a child who is ill in bed needs less energy than usual. In cases of raised temperature, vomiting, or diarrhoea, it is important to give the child plenty to drink. Again, let the child choose. If he or she wants fizzy lemonade or cola, this does not matter. It is not what is drunk that counts, but the quantity drunk.

Dealing with a vomiting child

Children vomit easily, and often without warning, at the beginning of an illness. However, sudden vomiting does not necessarily indicate the onset of an illness – a child may vomit from excitement or for no apparent reason. A vomiting child will need your comfort and help. Support the child's head with one hand pressed against the forehead, or place your hand firmly on his or her tummy during the vomiting. Afterwards, give the child a glass of water to rinse out the mouth and wash his or her face. Provide plenty of fluids to avoid dehydration. (See also *Dealing with vomiting*, p.762.)

Keeping the sick child occupied

Whereas sick adults usually like to be left alone, sick children, unless they are very ill, usually want company or entertainment. The younger the child, the greater will be the demands on your time, because the child will be more dependent on you for his or her distractions, entertainments, and amusement.

Generally, a sick child will neither feel like concentrating on one thing for very long nor want to do anything intellectually demanding. And he or she will probably want to play with familiar toys and games rather than learn to cope with something new. All children tend to "regress" a little in developmental terms when they are ill, and should be given toys and activities meant for a slightly younger age group. A child who is confined to bed will need a flat surface – a bed-table or, failing that, a large tray – for toys and games, and to serve as a drawing board.

The activities suggested here for a sick child are absorbing, undemanding, and suitable for doing in or out of bed.

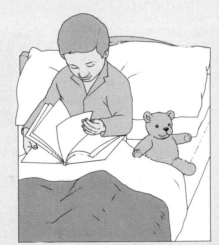

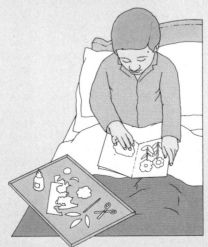

1 Sticking pictures in a scrapbook. Instead of buying a scrapbook, you may be able to make one yourself from rolls of old wallpaper. Give the child the book, a stack of old magazines, round-ended scissors, and a stick of solid glue.

2 Making felt pictures. Glue a piece of felt about 200mm (8in) square on to a sheet of stiff cardboard. From differently coloured pieces of felt, cut out the shapes of figures, animals, houses, trees, and other objects – or draw the outlines on the pieces of felt for the child to cut out. The felt cutouts stick naturally to the felt base, and the child can arrange them to create pictures, and perhaps make up an accompanying story.

3 Cardboard modelling. Provide old cardboard cartons, tubes, and other containers, round-ended scissors, and a stick of solid glue.

4 Dough modelling. Mix equal parts of flour and salt with enough water – and food colouring if you like – to make a stiffish dough. Give the child a rolling pin and pastry cutters, and, if he or she is in bed, put a plastic tablecloth over the bedclothes.

Nursing old people

The increasing likelihood of illness in old age means that elderly people tend to spend more and more time at home, perhaps in bed. Many families with ageing relatives can obtain practical advice and assistance from the local community health services (see *Community health care*, p.743) and organizations such as *Age Concern* (p.768).

Old people are especially vulnerable to chilling, and more so if their resistance is lowered by illness. Make sure that the temperature in the sick-room never goes below 18°C (65°F) and keep it higher if possible (see *Hypothermia* p.723). For further details of the individual complaints that affect old people see *Special problems of the elderly*, p.716.

Food

The appetite of an old person who is sick will probably be small. It is therefore important that the food that is taken is nutritious. Each day give at least one protein meal (one containing meat, cheese, fish, or eggs), about half a litre (three-quarters of a pint) of milk, and some high-*fibre* foods, such as fruit, vegetables, or bran cereal.

Coping with senility

Many old people remain mentally alert and independent to the end of their life. Some, however, become senile – mentally and physically feeble. If you are looking after a sick person who is senile, make the fullest possible use of your local health visitor and district nurse. Through them it may be possible for you to make use of the Meals on Wheels service and the laundry service, and get help once or twice a week with giving the sick person a bath. Many local authorities provide day centres for old people which give whoever is looking after them some relief from nursing. (See also *Senile dementia*, p.724.)

Caring for the convalescent

After a long illness, it takes a certain amount of time for a person who may be up and about again, to get back to former routine and activity. This transitional time – when the patient is neither ill nor fully recovered – is termed convalescence. During this period, all strenuous activities – physical and mental, and sports and leisure pastimes as well as work – must be resumed *gradually*. The importance of this slow return to everyday life cannot be over-emphasized.

General care

People convalescing from an illness often become bored and frustrated by their enforced inactivity, especially if they were very active before their illness. Radio, television, recorded music, newspapers, books, amusements, and company will help to occupy them and lessen the frustration. Best of all, if the person's work is such that it can be done at home, is for him or her gradually to ease back into a working routine.

However, there is another side to all this. The convalescent may well believe himself or herself to be more fully recovered than is actually the case, may consequently tackle too much too soon, and as a result overtax his or her strength. Loss of strength may cause the person to become depressed by an unaccustomed loss of concentration, and suffer a setback in convalescence. It is your job to try to prevent this. Ask the doctor what it is reasonable for the convalescent to do, and if the person shows signs of going beyond this limit, gently but firmly persuade him or her to stop. The doctor will also tell you if the convalescent needs a special diet and, if necessary, can also organize professional help for you in caring for the person.

If it is difficult to provide regular care for a convalescent person who no longer needs close medical supervision in hospital, your doctor might be able to arrange for him or her to stay in one of the convalescent homes that are run by the NHS.

The dangers of inactivity in the old

It is all too easy for an old person who is supposed to be convalescing and recovering to become unnecessarily bed-bound. With such inactivity comes a rapid physical deterioration: unused muscles become weak and flabby, joints stiffen, and constipation, bed-sores, and weak bladder and bowel control may develop. The bed-bound patient is also more prone to *thrombosis* or *embolism* and more likely to suffer from severe respiratory infections such as pneumonia. You must therefore encourage the convalescent to get up and about as soon as possible and to stay active (see *Accidental falls*, p.719, for more advice).

Getting out of bed

Anyone who has been ill and bed-bound for some time will feel weak and probably dizzy when getting out of bed for the first time. So persuade the person to sit still on the edge of the bed for a few minutes before attempting to stand. Put a chair covered with a blanket beside the bed. When the person feels steady, stand in front of him or her so that the person can use your hips or shoulders as a support while standing up, and provide extra support by holding the person under the armpits. Then help to lower the person on to the chair and wrap the blanket around him or her. Once the convalescent person feels stronger, a few steps can be tried, leaning on your arm or nearby furniture for support.

Physiotherapy

Someone who has been weakened or temporarily disabled by illness or injury may need a course of *physiotherapy* during convalescence, to regain muscle strength or the flexibility of the limbs. Physiotherapy usually includes exercises and massage, and sometimes heat or electrical treatment. Usually it is arranged through, and given in, a hospital out-patient department or local clinic. In a very few areas, National Health Service physiotherapy is carried out in the sick person's home, but otherwise any home physiotherapy must be paid for privately; if private physiotherapy is chosen, make sure the practitioner has the letters MCSP, MCsP, or SRP after his or her name.

"Active" exercises are those that sick people can carry out for themselves after having been taught by the physiotherapist. "Passive" exercises are those given if the person cannot move his or her own limbs; the physiotherapist will manipulate them instead, to prevent joint and muscle stiffness. If you are caring for someone in this condition, ask the physiotherapist to show you how to give these "passive" exercises.

Occupational therapy

Anyone who has had a long illness or a lengthy stay in hospital may be helped at home by *occupational therapy* to recover any lost skills and to adjust to living in the outside world again. The doctor will ask for the therapist to visit the sick person. If necessary, the therapist will arrange for the sick person to be provided with, and taught to use, aids for such everyday activities as bathing and dressing. If the person is in a wheelchair and the home needs to be modified, the therapist can also give advice on how to do this – for example, by widening doors and converting steps to a ramp – and on how to apply for a grant for such alterations.

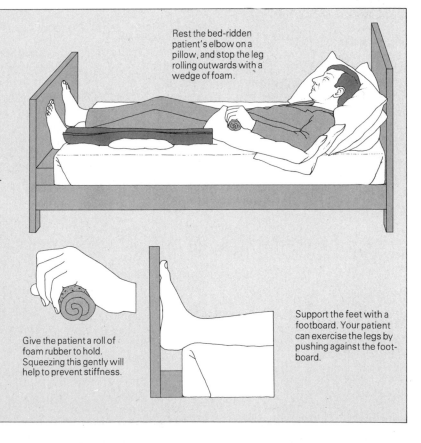

Preventing limbs from stiffening

A period of bed rest is often necessary after a major illness or operation. Although sick people tend to prefer to stay in a position they find comfortable, they should be encouraged to move around in bed as much as possible, to prevent the joint stiffness and loss of muscle tone which may follow prolonged inactivity. You can help to prevent joint stiffness, first of all by carefully placing and supporting the patient's limbs in the most comfortable, natural, and strain-free positions, and resting them on pillows, cushions, or foam-rubber rolls. Encourage the patient to exercise each joint through its whole range of movement several times each day. If he or she is quite immobile, you should do this for him. Gently bend and straighten each elbow and wrist, and the fingers and thumb of each hand. Raise each leg in turn, bending and straightening the knee and ankle.

Rest the bed-ridden patient's elbow on a pillow, and stop the leg rolling outwards with a wedge of foam.

Give the patient a roll of foam rubber to hold. Squeezing this gently will help to prevent stiffness.

Support the feet with a footboard. Your patient can exercise the legs by pushing against the footboard.

Helpful organizations

The organizations in the following list provide special services involving the health and welfare of the British public. Addresses and telephone numbers are those of the central or head office. Many organizations, especially those linked with the National Health Service, have branches throughout the country; for addresses that you cannot find here or in the telephone directory, consult your doctor or ask at your local health clinic.

Action on Smoking and Health (ASH)
27 Mortimer Street
London W1

01-637 9843

Age Concern
Bernard Sunley House
60 Pitcairn Road
Mitcham, Surrey

01-640 5431

Al-Anon (*for the families of alcoholics*)
61 Great Dover Street
London SE1

01-403 0888

Alcoholics Anonymous
11 Redcliffe Gardens
London SW10

01-834 3202

Albany Trust (*for counselling on sexual problems*)
Beauchamp Lodge
2 Warwick Crescent
London W2

01-286 8235

Association for Spina Bifida and Hydrocephalus
Tavistock House North
Tavistock Square
London WC1

01-388 1382

Asthma Society and Friends of the Asthma Research Council
12–14 Pembridge Square
London W2

01-229 1149

Back Pain Association
Grundy House
31–33 Park Road
Teddington, Middx

01-221 2347

British Diabetic Association
10 Queen Anne Street
London W1

01-323 1531

British Dyslexia Association
4 Hobart Place
London SW1

01-235 8111

British Epilepsy Association
Crowthorne House
New Wokingham Road
Wokingham, Berks

Crowthorne 31822

British Humanist Association
13 Prince of Wales Terrace
London W8

01-937 2341

British Kidney Patient Association
Bordon, Hants

Bordon 2021

British Medical Association
BMA House
Tavistock Square
London WC1

01-387 4499

British Migraine Association
178A High Road
Byfleet
Weybridge, Surrey

Weybridge 52468

British Pregnancy Advisory Service
58 Petty France
London SW1

01-222 0985

British Red Cross Society
9 Grosvenor Crescent
London SW1

01-235 5454

British Rheumatism and Arthritis Association
6 Grosvenor Crescent
London SW1

01-235 0902

Brook Advisory Centres
(*for advice on contraception*)
153A East Street
London SE17

01-708 1234

Chest, Heart and Stroke Association
Tavistock House North
Tavistock Square
London WC1

01-387 3012

Cheyne Centre for Spastic Children
61 Cheyne Walk
London SW3

01-352 8434

Colostomy Welfare Group
2nd Floor
38–39 Eccleston Square
London SW1

01-828 5175

Council and Care for the Elderly
13 Middlesex Street
London E1

01-621 1624

Cystic Fibrosis Research Trust
5 Blyth Road
Bromley, Kent

01-464 7211

Disabled Living Foundation
346 Kensington High Street
London W1

01-602 2491

Down's Children's Association
Quinborne Community Centre
Ridgeacre Road
Quinton, Birmingham

021-427 1274

Dyslexia Institute
133 Gresham Road
Staines, Middx

Staines 59498

Family Planning Association
27–35 Mortimer Street
London W1

01-636 7866

Foundation for the Study of Infant Deaths
5th Floor
4 Grosvenor Place
London SW1

01-235 1721

Friedreich's Ataxia Group
12C Worpleston Road
Guildford, Surrey

Guildford 503133

Gam-Anon (*for the families of gamblers*)
Address and telephone number as for Gamblers Anonymous (below)

Gamblers Anonymous
17–23 Blantyre Street
London SW10

01-352 3060

General Dental Council
37 Wimpole Street
London W1

01-486 2171

General Medical Council
44 Hallam Street
London W1

01-580 7642

General Nursing Council
23 Portland Place
London W1

01-580 8334

General Optical Council
41 Harley Street
London W1

01-580 3898

Health and Safety Executive
1 Chepstow Place
London W2

01-229 3456

Health Service Commissioners
Church House
Great Smith Street
London SW1

01-212 7676

Help the Aged
Help the Aged International Centre
Langley Road
Slough, Bucks

Ileostomy Association of Great Britain and Ireland
Amblehurst House
Chobham
Woking, Surrey

Chobham 8277

Inspector of Anatomy
(*for advice on the donation of organs for transplant or research*)
Alexander Fleming House
Elephant and Castle
London SE1

01-703 6380

Migraine Trust
45 Great Ormond Street
London WC1

01-278 2676

MIND (National Association for Mental Health)
22 Harley Street
London W1

01-637 0741

Multiple Sclerosis Society
286 Munster Road
London SW6

01-381 4022

Muscular Dystrophy Group of Great Britain
Natrass House
35 Macauley Road
London SW4

01-720 8055

National Association of Funeral Directors
57 Doughty Street
London WC1

01-242 9388

National Childbirth Trust
9 Queensborough Terrace
London W2

01-221 3833

National Council for One-Parent Families
255 Kentish Town Road
London NW5

01-267 1361

National Organisation for the Widowed and their Children (CRUSE)
126 Sheen Road
Richmond, Surrey

01-940 4818

National Society for Autistic Children
1A Golders Green Road
London NW11

01-458 4375

National Society for Cancer Relief
30 Dorset Square
London NW1

01-402 8125

National Society for Mentally Handicapped Children and Adults (MENCAP)
123 Golden Lane
London EC1

01-253 9433

National Society for Phenylketonuria
26 Towngate Grove
Mirfield, Yorks

Mirfield 492873

Parkinson's Disease Society of the UK
81 Queen's Road
London SW19

01-946 2500

Patients' Association
(*advisory service to protect the interests of all patients*)
11 Dartmouth Street
London SW1

01-222 4992

Pharmaceutical Society
1 Lambeth High Street
London SE1

01-735 9141

Pre-Retirement Association of Great Britain and Northern Ireland
19 Undine Street
London SW17

01-767 3225

Psoriasis Association
7 Milton Street
Northampton

Northampton 711129

Release (*for advice on problems related to drug taking*)
1 Elgin Avenue
London W9

01-289 1123

Royal National Institute for the Blind
224 Great Portland Street
London W1

01-388 1266

Royal National Institute for the Deaf
105 Gower Street
London WC1

01-387 8033

Royal Society for the Prevention of Accidents
Cannon House
Priory Queensway
Birmingham

021-233 2461

Samaritans (*for advice for anyone in distress*)
17 Uxbridge Road
Slough, Bucks

Slough 32713
For local branches see telephone directory

Standing Conference on Drug Abuse (SCODA)
3 Blackburn Road
London NW6

01-328 6556

Spastic Society
16 Fitzroy Square
London W1

01-387 9571

Stillbirth and Perinatal Death Association
37 Christchurch Hill
London NW3

01-794 4601

Women's National Cancer Control Campaign
1 South Audley Street
London W1

01-499 7532

Dying and death

Introduction

Most of us hope for a long life and a swift death, but only a quarter of the population have this wish fulfilled. Most people die gradually over a period of weeks or months. This gradual period of dying may seem less desirable to the individual, but is often better for his or her relatives, who have more time to adjust to their loss and prepare for the complex practical procedures attendant upon death. The articles that follow deal with these matters fully, and also give advice on helping the bereaved, including those coping with a child's death.

Chief causes of death

Each year in Britain, with a population of around 50 million, about 600,000 people die. The statistics in this table show the chief causes of death for a recent year. The figures fluctuate from year to year, but the general trends remain the same. Apart from accidental deaths (see the table of *Chief causes of accidental death* on p.42), the major causes of fatalities in middle and old age are heart disease, stroke, and cancer.

Age group	Annual number of deaths from all causes per 100,000 people	Chief cause of death (as percentage of total deaths)	Commonest other causes (in order of frequency)
Under 1	140	Birth difficulties such as respiratory distress syndrome, asphyxia, and neonatal jaundice (45%)	Congenital abnormalities; pneumonia and bronchitis; infectious diseases; accidents.
1–4	55	Accidents (28%)	Congenital abnormalities; cancers; pneumonia and bronchitis; infectious diseases.
5–14	27	Accidents (37%)	Cancers; pneumonia; congenital abnormalities; brain and nervous system diseases.
15–24	65	Accidents (55%)	Pneumonia; stroke.
25–44	120	Accidents (17%)	Heart diseases; stroke; breast cancer; lung cancer.
45–64	1,000	Heart diseases (30%)	Lung cancer; stroke; breast cancer; accidents.
Over 64	6,000	Heart diseases (30%)	Stroke; pneumonia and bronchitis; lung cancer.

Terminal illness

Terminally ill people differ in how much they want to know about their condition, and most doctors now believe that their patients have a right to know as much as they want to about their prospects. Sometimes the family find it hard to accept this open approach because of their own psychological responses to death and dying. In reality, many dying people know – or strongly suspect – that they have a fatal illness.

When and what to tell the dying person

You should always let a person with a terminal illness decide the timing and extent of any discussion of death. If the patient does ask questions about the possibility of his or her dying, this indicates that he or she has been thinking about the matter and has, to some extent, already come to terms with it. If no questions are asked, knowledge should not be forced upon the dying patient. This does not mean, however, that you should hold out false hopes of recovery. Someone who is misled in this way will be unable to understand why he or she is growing weaker instead of stronger, and may lose confidence in the doctor's treatment; may be deprived of the chance to put his or her affairs in order; and, worst of all, if he or she suspects the truth, will be denied the opportunity to discuss fears and seek reassurance. You should always bear in mind that an individual's uncertainty about his or her fate often gives rise to greater fear than certainty does.

A dying person will usually make quite clear how much he or she wants to be told about prospects for survival. Someone who is terminally ill usually seeks some reassurance, however, and you should be able to give a comforting answer that is not dishonest.

One almost inevitable question put to the doctor is how much time the dying patient has left to live. Usually only a very approximate answer is possible – for example, "anything from a couple of weeks to several months". A more precise answer than this is likely to be misleading. Someone who is terminally ill may sometimes seem to find it easier to talk about his or her death to someone who is not especially close – for example, a doctor. This may be so even in the case of very close relationships and does not show any lack of affection or trust. In fact, the closer the relationship, the more each partner may want to protect the other, and the longer it may be before they can talk freely together. For the terminally ill patient in hospital, this may make for difficulties. Not only are the hospital staff often too busy to spend time talking with the dying person, but they may find it

difficult to talk about dying anyway, since they see their primary role as being curative. A terminally ill patient may well find that the family doctor is the best person to talk to in the first place. And the doctor can help the person and his or her family to break down any barriers that the prospects of death have erected between them.

Care at home or in hospital

It is never true that "nothing more can be done" for a dying person. When curative treatment is no longer of any use, the dying person still needs relief from troublesome symptoms and pain, and still requires understanding and comfort. Usually such care is best given in the dying man's or woman's own home rather than in hospital. At home, the person can remain more independent, feel more of an individual, and still take a limited part in family life, and so he or she is far less likely to feel isolated. The general hospital is much more geared to carrying out all possible procedures for treating and trying to cure the sick person than to caring for the dying one. So if a choice is offered between home and hospital care, home care is better, provided you can nurse the patient adequately at home. Home care is not usually taxing; pain relief seldom has to be given by injection, and half of all cases of terminal illness do not require difficult nursing care (even in those cases that do, such care will usually be needed only for a few weeks).

If you do plan to look after a terminally ill relative at home, regular visits from the family doctor and district nurse will be essential, together with all possible support from the family and friends.

Hospices

Hospices are small units (often built in the grounds of a general hospital) that are set up especially to care for the dying and to help their families. They are becoming increasingly widespread.

In a hospice a dying person is not troubled with routine hospital measures such as temperature- and pulse-taking. The efforts of the staff are concentrated on relieving pain and any other symptoms, and comforting both the person and his or her family. It might be thought that to see others dying around them would be depressing for terminally ill people, but most patients are reassured rather than distressed, because the deaths occur so peacefully.

Most hospices run a home-care service to support any family that wants to care for a dying relative at home.

Physical and emotional pain

Pain is the most feared symptom of dying. Continuous, long-term pain will usually wear a sick person down regardless of the depth and extent of underlying courage and will permeate his or her whole being, excluding thoughts of anything else.

But such suffering, even in some of the most painful forms of cancer, now seldom, if ever, occurs. *Analgesics* (painkilling drugs) are nearly always given before they are actually needed, so that the pain is not allowed to build up to a level at which the sick person needs to ask for additional quantities of the drug. When analgesics are given regularly in this way, the dose can usually be kept low, so that the person remains not only pain-free but alert and comfortable.

Severe pain is usually controlled by an opiate – in most cases, the drug morphine. The risk that the sick person will become addicted to the drug is more than outweighed by the essential relief from severe pain that the drug provides.

It is not only physical pain that a terminally ill person may have to face, but also the emotional pain that we are all bound to feel at the thought of dying. Anger is a common reaction to the prospect of death; so is depression. Some people may have feelings of guilt or dissatisfaction when they look back on their lives and achievements. But in the end, given loving support from those around them, terminally ill people come to terms with the prospect of death in their own time and their own way.

Often, dying people resent their growing helplessness and fear a loss of dignity. For this reason, and for as long as possible, someone who is dying should be given every opportunity to manage his or her own affairs, should be consulted on family matters, and should be encouraged to help other members of the family to make plans for their future.

Many dying people fear that the moment of death will be unpleasant and violent, and many are afraid of being left to die alone – which may make them seem over-demanding to those caring for them. It is very often possible to dispel these fears quite honestly by telling the person that in nearly all cases someone who is extremely ill feels an overwhelming drowsiness just before the end, lapses without pain into unconsciousness, and dies serenely in his or her sleep.

The approach of death

Towards the very end, the dying person may become restless, or his or her breathing may become noisy, partly because of a constant trickle into the windpipe of saliva that cannot be coughed up, partly because of the lungs becoming waterlogged as the heart fails. If you are caring for the patient at home and these symptoms occur, call your doctor, who will be able to give an injection to make him or her more comfortable. If the patient is still alert, you can make breathing easier either by propping him or her gently up in bed in a sitting position by means of several pillows, or by laying the patient on his or her side, the top arm and leg drawn out a little for support and a single pillow beneath the head.

You should assume that right until the end the dying person can hear what you say, as hearing is one of the last faculties to fail. You may well feel helpless in the presence of a person near to death, because you do not know what it is you have to do apart from providing practical relief of the kind described. But support for someone you love who is approaching death is more a matter of reassurance – of maintaining awareness of a loving presence – than of trying to improve physical comfort. It is the very fact of your being there that is so important; nothing more is necessary than to hold a hand, so that the dying person does not feel alone.

Death

Death occurs when both the heartbeat and breathing have stopped. It is easy for a doctor to ascertain that this has happened, provided that the person is not being given *ventilation* on a life-support system. If the person is, the doctor has to carry out a set series of tests to determine whether the brain is dead. If this is the case, death is established and life support is discontinued.

Delaying death

In order that their lives can be prolonged, people who are suffering from certain serious diseases are only too often obliged to undergo some form of extremely unpleasant treatment. However, as the periods of relative health between each such treatment become shorter and shorter, all the treatment eventually does is to prolong the process of dying unnecessarily and uncomfortably. At this stage, usually by agreement between the sufferer and the doctors, the treatment is stopped and only necessary painkillers and any other comfort-inducing drugs are given. In this way, the sufferer is usually given the chance to die peacefully and gracefully.

Unconscious people who are able to maintain their own breathing and heartbeat but for whom there is no prospect of regaining consciousness may be fed and the functions of their vital organs may be artificially maintained by medical staff in order to keep them alive. But often they are not given life-saving measures, such as *antibiotics* for infections; it is regarded as justifiable to allow a life that is no longer truly a life to draw to an end naturally and with dignity.

Criteria of death

As described above, death occurs when both breathing and heartbeat have stopped. In the case of serious injury (a road traffic accident, say), when life-support equipment is not immediately to hand, it may be possible to maintain breathing and heartbeat for a short time by emergency first-aid procedures (see *Absence of breathing*, p.802, and *Absence of heartbeat*, p.804) until emergency life-support equipment is available. Eventually, though, if the heart and lungs do not begin to function on their own, even the most energetic first-aid measures will prove ineffective.

In a modern hospital, various sophisticated pieces of equipment are available to assist breathing and heartbeat functions and therefore to help maintain life itself. But breathing and heartbeat may cease when the equipment is disconnected. If they do, this shows that the brain stem (the part between the brain and the spinal cord, at the top of the neck) is damaged. The brain stem controls breathing and, to some extent, heartbeat; but once the brain stem is badly injured it will not recover and death is inevitable.

It is not always easy to say for sure if and when the moment of death has arrived. An *electroencephalogram* (*EEG*) of brain activity may not necessarily help, either. The EEG measures chiefly brain waves in the cerebral hemispheres (the parts of the brain dealing with "higher" activities such as speech and memory – see *Disorders of the brain and nervous system*, p.266), so it does not reliably indicate whether the brain stem itself is still active. Under such circumstances "death" is determined by a lengthy series of tests carried out at least twice by different doctors to confirm true brain death.

The practicalities of death

When someone dies, there are several legal formalities to be dealt with before the funeral can be held. They include obtaining a medical certificate of the cause of death (the death certificate), registering the death, engaging an undertaker to organize the funeral, and discovering whether the dead person left a will. There will be further formalities in any of the following cases: if the death has to be reported to the coroner; if the body is to be cremated rather than buried; or if the body is to be donated for medical research or to have organs removed for transplant.

In this article it is assumed throughout that you are either the next of kin of the dead person or his or her executor – that is, someone who has been appointed by the dead person to carry out his or her wishes as set forth in a legally valid will.

The death certificate

Only a registered doctor can certify that someone is dead and state the cause of death. So the first thing to do if someone dies at home is to call the family doctor. In most cases the doctor will have been looking after the person during his or her last illness and will therefore usually have no difficulty in ascertaining the cause of death. If the doctor has seen the person within 14 days before death, he or she is not legally obliged to examine the body before filling in the medical certificate of cause of death. However, in practice, most family doctors do visit the house and see the body before making out the certificate. If the doctor has not seen the person within 14 days before death, he or she is legally bound to examine the body. The doctor also needs to see the body if it is to be cremated – so if a cremation is planned, tell the doctor. You should also tell the doctor if the dead person asked for his or her body to be bequeathed for medical research, or if you and other close relatives wish this (see *Medical use of the body*, p.776).

If the person has died in hospital, one of the doctors who were in attendance will fill in the medical certificate of cause of death. The ward sister will tell the relatives of the death and arrange for them to claim the dead person's possessions. If a person has died in an accident and been brought to hospital, the police will ask the relatives to identify the body. It may be that the dead person has donated certain organs to be used as transplants, or that the surviving relatives wish to donate them. If so, the organs can usually be removed for transplantation only when the person dies in hospital, since removal needs to be carried out promptly after death. If organs are to be donated, you should tell the hospital doctor if he or she has not already asked whether this is what the family want. Once the doctor has filled in the medical certificate, he or she will either send it to the registrar of births, deaths, and marriages for the sub-district in which the person died or give it to you to take to the registrar yourself. The doctor will also give you a notice, known as the notice to informants, which lists those who can register the death (be informants) and which also provides information about how to go about doing so.

Registering a death
A death has to be registered before the body can be disposed of. If the death occurs in a house, the duty to inform the registrar falls – in order of priority – on the following people: any relative who was present at the death or in attendance during the last illness; any relative living in the sub-district where the person died; someone other than a relative who happened to be present at the death; the person arranging the funeral. If the death occurs in some place other than someone's home, it should be registered by any available relative; anyone who finds the body; or the person in charge of funeral arrangements.

A death must be registered by the informant at the office of the registrar for the sub-district in which the death occurred. It must be registered within five days of the death (eight days in Scotland); or, if the registrar is informed of the death in writing and sent the medical certificate of cause of death, both within five days, registration can be carried out within a further period of 14 days – in which case the registrar can issue the necessary form to allow a burial to go ahead, but not a cremation (for the reason why this is so see *Burial and cremation*, opposite). The sub-district in which the death occurred can be discovered by asking at a post office, the town hall, a hospital, or the local citizens' advice bureau. The address of the registrar's office can be found in the telephone directory under Registration of births, deaths, and marriages. Some rural sub-district registrars' offices are closed on certain days of the week, so before going to one the informant should check to make sure that it is open.

A death cannot be legally registered without the medical certificate of cause of death. The informant must either take this certificate with him or her or, if it was posted, make sure it has arrived. The informant also needs to take the dead person's medical card and any war-pension order book. If for any reason the death has been reported to the coroner, the pink form that is issued by the coroner should also be taken along.

The registrar will want to know the date and place of death, the dead person's name (including, in the case of a married woman, the maiden name), the date and place of birth, sex and occupation, whether the person was receiving a state pension or other social-security payment, and the date of birth of any surviving spouse.

After the death has been registered, the registrar will give the informant a death certificate and a certificate of disposal. The death certificate is needed before the death grant and widow's pension can be claimed (two extra copies of the certificate – which must be paid for – should be requested, since a death certificate may be demanded by, for example, an insurance company, as proof of death). The certificate of disposal must be given to the funeral director before the funeral can be arranged. If you are the dead person's executor, or if you are the next of kin and, in the absence of a will, want to take charge of the dead person's affairs, you should ask the registrar for form PR48.

Referral to the coroner
Mention of the coroner usually worries people because the name popularly suggests deaths in which foul play is suspected. In fact, most of the circumstances in which the coroner must be informed of a death are quite innocent. A death is reported to the coroner – generally by a doctor or policeman – in any one of the following situations: if no doctor attended the person during his or her final illness; a doctor did attend but did not see the person within 14 days of death or after death; the cause of death is unknown; if the death was caused by an accident; resulted from abortion, or poisoning; was attended by suspicious circumstances, such as violence or neglect; occurred during an operation or because of failure to recover from an anaesthetic; or appears to have been caused by either industrial disease or industrial poisoning.

In the majority of cases, the coroner will order a post mortem examination to be carried out on the body in order to establish the exact cause of death. If, as is usual, the post mortem clearly establishes the cause of death to the coroner's satisfaction, he issues a pink form, which provides authorization for the registration of the death.

Inquests
If the post mortem fails to reveal the cause of death, and in cases when the death was violent, unnatural, or due to an accident, the coroner holds an inquest, a public court hearing. The coroner may order people to attend

the inquest as witnesses. Anyone with an interest in the death is permitted to attend, and may be represented by a solicitor if he or she wishes, especially if compensation claims are being considered. Sometimes a jury is also present at the inquest.

Once the coroner or jury have given their verdict and the inquest is over, the coroner sends a certificate to the registrar enabling the death to be registered. The coroner may give the next of kin an order allowing burial or cremation before the inquest is over – usually as soon as the body has been identified. If the coroner's enquiries are going to take a long time, the inquest will be formally opened, and then adjourned. Once the inquest has been opened, you may ask the coroner for a letter confirming the fact of death. The letter can serve, instead of the death certificate, as proof of death for social security and insurance claims.

Acting as an executor

If the dead person has left a will, the person appointed as executor – usually the spouse or other close relative – has the duty of arranging the funeral. If there is no will, the duty of serving formally as executor usually falls on one of the dead person's close relatives who is willing to accept the job.

To deal with the dead person's financial and other affairs, the executor must apply to the local probate registry for a grant of probate or letters of administration. The application is made on a special form supplied by the registrar (see *Registering a death*, opposite).

Any instructions left by the dead person referring to the funeral ceremony or stating clearly whether he or she wishes to be cremated or prefers not to be cremated are not usually ignored. However, such instructions are not legally binding on the executor.

The funeral

It is sensible to contact an undertaker or funeral director soon after the doctor has issued a medical certificate of cause of death, and then the funeral director will explain the complexities of registration. Even though you may not feel like shopping around at such a time, it is wise to obtain quotations for the fee from more than one undertaker. Once the death has been registered and you have obtained a certificate of disposal (or the coroner has issued a certificate allowing burial or cremation), you can then make definite arrangements for the funeral.

Undertakers who are members of the *National Association of Funeral Directors* (p.768) offer a basic simple funeral which

provides care of the dead body, a coffin, a hearse, and one car for mourners; you have to see to the burial service or crematorium arrangements, together with any notices in the press (though the undertaker will advise you on what to do). Alternatively, at a greater cost, the undertaker can arrange everything and give you a written estimate of the cost. In either case, you will have to decide on the type of coffin, the type and location of burial service and who is to conduct it, whether the body is to be embalmed, and whether it is to be buried or cremated.

The funeral is usually held somewhere between three and six days after death. Most funeral ceremonies are performed by the church and fall into two parts – the religious ceremony and the committal ceremony at the graveside. Those who want a non-religious ceremony should contact the *British Humanist Association* at the address given on p.768.

Burial and cremation

Under common law, every parishioner has a right to be buried in the parish churchyard unless it is closed to further burials. If this is the case, the dead person will be buried in a cemetery that is maintained by the local authority. Such cemeteries have areas set aside for most main religious denominations.

You will need to find out whether the dead person has already chosen and paid for a plot in a churchyard or cemetery. If he or she has not, you will have to pay for one. You can choose a basic area, which will be part of a common grave filled with other coffins and on which you will not be allowed to erect a headstone. Or, if you prefer to do so, you can pay for the exclusive right to a grave, on which you can have a memorial erected. The undertaker will explain to you the details of how to make all such arrangements.

If a body is to be cremated instead of buried, more formalities are involved. (The reason for the more complex procedure is a need to prevent destruction of the body before the possibility of any crime has been discounted.) The funeral director will explain what forms you need to fill in and where to obtain them. After the cremation, you have the choice of collecting the ashes to keep or bury or scatter yourself or of asking the crematorium to dispose of them for you.

Paying for the funeral

The funeral expenses are the first claim on the dead person's estate. However, the person responsible for the funeral will not be able to obtain the necessary funds from the estate until he or she has applied for and received a grant of probate or letters of administration from the local probate registry (see *Acting as an executor*, p.775). Fortunately, the person who arranges the funeral is allowed to claim the dead person's death grant to help towards the cost of the funeral. In order to claim the grant, you should take the following documents to the local social security office: the death certificate, a marriage certificate if you are claiming for your spouse, the undertaker's estimate or bill, any social security order books, and, if the dead person had one, his or her National Insurance contribution card.

Furthermore, if you are not working full time and have a low income, or if you are on supplementary benefit, you may be able to get state help towards the funeral expenses.

The local authority has a duty to arrange a funeral if no one else will do it. A hospital, too, will arrange the funeral of anyone who dies in the hospital and whose relatives cannot be traced or cannot afford the funeral. The local authority or hospital will claim the death grant in such a case and may also claim a sum from the dead person's estate. Hospitals will also arrange a funeral for a stillborn baby if the parents wish; the baby will then be buried in a common grave or cremated.

Medical use of the body

If a dead person has (either in writing or verbally before two witnesses) expressed a wish that his or her body should not be used for medical research or that the organs should not be removed for transplantation, those instructions cannot be overruled, whatever the wishes of the dead person's surviving relatives. However, if the dead person bequeathed his or her body or organs for use after death, the next of kin is legally allowed to overrule the request. In the absence of instructions by the dead person either way, the next of kin or executor is allowed to donate the body or organs for medical use, provided no close relative forbids it. If for some reason the death has been reported to the coroner, the coroner's permission is needed before organs may be donated.

If the dead person's body is being donated for research, you should, as soon as death has occurred, contact the *Inspector of Anatomy* (p.768), who will make the arrangements. If the organs are to be removed for transplantation, a hospital has to be notified promptly after the person's death; in the case of the eyes, the hospital of your choice must be an eye hospital or a general hospital that has an eye department.

Bereavement

Immediately following the death of someone who has been close to them, many people simply feel desolately numb and empty. For a while they behave almost as if nothing has happened; but eventually they may well be stricken by intense grief. During this period immediately after a loss, delusions of seeing the dead person are common – and this kind of experience, though it may worry you, is quite normal. There is also a tendency to forget quite often that the person is dead and act as though he or she were still alive. Also common after a loss are an idealization of the dead person and feelings of guilt that you did not do more for the person when he or she was alive. Guilt feelings (and intense grief) are much more common in cases of entirely unexpected death than they are when death has occurred after a long-drawn-out illness, when the bereaved person was able to provide loving care (and to anticipate the loss).

A bereaved person should always try to acknowledge his or her loss and not attempt to shut it out of consciousness. Although such activities may be painful, talking about the dead person to relatives and friends and sorting out the person's possessions will help you enormously in coming to terms with the loss.

The intensity of grief normally starts to wane after about six weeks, to be replaced by a more general state of depression and apathy. Grief is usually no longer intense after about six months, although it will probably recur every so often over the following years; and you may, indeed, never become entirely reconciled to your loss. By the end of a year, however, most bereaved people have recovered from the initial blow and have started building a new life for themselves.

Occasionally grief over a loss is so prolonged or intense that it cannot be relieved without professional help by a psychiatrist. Bereaved people most likely to need such help are those whose personality makes them particularly prone to grief, those whose relationship with the dead person has left them with strong feelings of guilt or anger, and those who are socially isolated and unable to communicate their grief.

It is understandable that some people, in the intensity of their grief, may seek comfort through spiritualists. But, by stimulating all over again the desire for the dead person and by denying reality rather than coming to terms with it, spiritualism may, in some people, prolong mourning.

Bereaved husbands, wives, or parents may find most support from others who have suffered a similar loss. *CRUSE* the *National Organization for the widowed and their children* – see p.768 gives practical help and advice to widows and their children.

Helping the bereaved

A bereaved person is likely to need practical help at first, both in continuing a day-to-day existence and in making any necessary decisions. Apart from that, it may seem to you that there is little real comfort you can offer to someone who has suffered a recent loss. But this is not so. In allowing the person to talk to you about his or her loss, you encourage an outlet for the expression of grief that can only be beneficial.

You should *always* take any threat of suicide seriously and discuss the problem immediately with a doctor or social worker.

Do not make the mistake of giving your help only over the first few difficult days and then withdrawing it. The bereaved person will need support throughout the lonely months that follow. The first anniversary of a death, or the first Christmas spent alone, can be a particularly miserable time, when a visit or an offer of hospitality from you would probably be very welcome.

Children and death

Until the age of three, children are extremely unlikely to have any concept of death at all, and not until they are about nine do most youngsters fully understand that death is the absolute end of life and is inevitable.

The bereaved child

Children should be allowed to grieve in their own way and no effort should be made to force them to conform to adult ideas. Young children often appear to recover from a bereavement quite quickly, especially if they can re-attach themselves to someone who may be a substitute for the dead person.

Adults should not try to suppress their own grief in front of a child, since, whether the child wishes to grieve or not, such suppression will make him or her feel excluded. They should give the child every opportunity to ask questions about the death. Some children feel that in some way the death of a loved one may be their fault, and they need the reassurance of a sympathetic and understanding adult that of course this is not so.

If possible, a child should not be asked to cope with any other major changes for at least six months after a bereavement.

The dying child

A child may be better able to face the prospect of his or her own death than the parents can. More than death, the child may fear painful treatment and, if admission to hospital is necessary, separation from his or her parents. The child will be helped to come to terms with death if he or she is told about the nature of the disease and if death is not treated as a taboo subject. The most important thing that loving parents can give their terminally ill child is security, which is evidenced physically by their presence and mentally by their honesty.

It is important for a fatally ill child to lead a normal life for as long as is feasible and not be treated in any special way that will make the child feel different from his or her friends. School work, seeing friends, and normal family activities and discipline should be continued for as long as possible.

If you are given the opportunity to choose between hospital and home care, remember that in most such cases children are much like adults, in that it is much more comforting for a terminally ill child to be looked after at home rather than in hospital (see *Terminal illness*, p.771). However, it is essential for parents who take on home care to have a telephone and a sympathetic family doctor who can be called on in any circumstances and will arrange hospital admission if the parents can no longer cope.

The death of a child

The death of a child inevitably causes more grief than the death of an adult. Added to the normal sorrow of loss are misery and perhaps even rage at the incomprehensible cutting off of a life that had scarcely begun. Sudden death is even more difficult to bear than death that comes at the end of a long illness. For that reason, at the beginning of a child's serious illness, parents should always enquire as to its likely outcome, because if it is a fatal illness they will then have time to try to adjust to the prospect of their child's death.

Two organizations that offer comfort and support to parents of babies who have died are the *Stillbirth and Perinatal Death Association* (which helps after deaths that occur in the uterus or within a week or so of birth) and the *Foundation for the Study of Infant Deaths* (for parents of babies who have died suddenly and unexpectedly). The addresses of these organizations are given on p.768.

Drug index

New drugs are constantly being discovered, and many of the drugs in common use 20 years ago have now been superseded by newer, safer, compounds. At the same time, the sheer numbers of drugs have increased greatly. As a result, this index is highly selective and should not be looked upon as a manual for self-prescription by you and your family.

In general, the fewer drugs you take the better. Except for minor symptoms such as occasional cough or headache, you are well advised to let your doctor prescribe all the medicines you need. What follows is a guide to the more common drugs that your doctor might prescribe.

There are three types of entry in the alphabetical index:

1 General categories, listed according to function – for instance, ANTIBIOTICS or ANTI-ANXIETY DRUGS. These entries describe the major groups of drugs, giving in each case their uses and side-effects and information on ways of administering the drugs (as tablets, in liquid form, etc). Other significant facts applying to the general category (such as the advisability of avoiding alcohol during treatment) are also included.

2 Chemical names of specific drugs – for instance, diazepam. The chemical-name entry relates the drug to its general category and may also give details of its specific effects; whether, for instance, a given drug has an unusual side-effect.

3 Trade names – for instance, Valium (a trade name for diazepam). Entries for trade names are simply identified according to their basic chemical ingredient(s) – given in brackets – and the general category to which they belong. The initial letter of a trade name is capitalized.

Drugs that can be bought without a prescription are marked with an asterisk (*).

acebutolol hydrochloride A BETA-BLOCKER.

acetazolamide A DIURETIC, used for treating glaucoma. Possible side-effects (in addition to those common to the group): loss of appetite, depression.

acetohexamide A HYPO-GLYCAEMIC.

Achromycin (tetracycline) An ANTIBIOTIC.

Actidil* (triprolidine hydrochloride) An ANTIHISTAMINE.

actinomycin D A CYTOTOXIC, given only by injection.

Actrapid MC A short-acting insulin preparation.

Adcortyl (triamcinolone) A CORTICOSTEROID.

adrenaline A BRONCHODILATOR.

Adriamycin (doxorubicin) A CYTOTOXIC.

Afrazine* (oxymetazoline) A DECONGESTANT.

Agarol* A combination of phenolphthalein (a stimulant LAXATIVE) and liquid paraffin (a faeces-softener).

Agiolax* (senna) A stimulant LAXATIVE.

Aldomet (methyldopa) An ANTIHYPERTENSIVE.

Alkeran (melphalan) A CYTOTOXIC.

allopurinol A drug for prevention of gout. Possible side-effects: rashes, fever, nausea, diarrhoea, abdominal pain, drowsiness. It is advisable to drink at least 2 litres (4 pints) of fluid a day during treatment.

Alu-Cap (aluminium hydroxide) An ANTACID.

Aludrox (aluminium hydroxide) An ANTACID.

aluminium hydroxide An ANTACID.

aluminium phosphate An ANTACID.

Alupent (orciprenaline sulphate) A BRONCHODILATOR.

Aluphos (aluminium phosphate) An ANTACID.

alverine An ANTISPASMODIC.

amantadine A drug used for treating Parkinson's disease and as an ANTIVIRAL for treatment of shingles and prevention of influenza. Possible side-effects: nervousness, insomnia, dizziness, swollen ankles.

aminophylline A BRONCHODILATOR. Possible side-effect (in addition to those common to the group): nausea.

amitriptyline hydrochloride A tricyclic ANTIDEPRESSANT, also used for treatment of enuresis.

Amoxil (amoxycillin) An ANTIBIOTIC.

amoxycillin A broad-spectrum ANTIBIOTIC.

amphotericin An ANTIFUNGAL. Possible side-effects: headache, loss of appetite, fever, physical weakness, diarrhoea.

ampicillin A broad-spectrum ANTIBIOTIC.

Ampiclox (ampicillin) An ANTIBIOTIC.

amylobarbitone (sodium) A barbiturate used as a SLEEPING DRUG.

Amytal (amylobarbitone) A SLEEPING DRUG

Anafranil (clomipramine hydrochloride) An ANTIDEPRESSANT.

ANALGESICS Drugs that relieve pain. Two main types: non-narcotic analgesics for mild pain, narcotic analgesics (based on opium) for severe pain. Most non-narcotic analgesics contain aspirin (or aspirin-like substances) or paracetamol, and are also ANTIPYRETICS; some are ANTI-INFLAMMATORIES as well. Many trade-name products are a combination of non-narcotic analgesics, sometimes with codeine, a weak narcotic analgesic; they are no better than single-ingredient preparations. Pain is best relieved by taking regular doses of aspirin every 4 hours, for up to 24 hours. For further information and possible side-effects see specific drugs. Narcotic analgesics may be taken as tablets, suppositories, or by injection. Possible side-effects: nausea, constipation, dizziness, inability to pass urine. All narcotic analgesics cause gradual development of some degree of tolerance and are habit-forming. Risk of addiction from weaker narcotics such as codeine is much lower than from powerful morphine derivatives. Narcotic analgesics are not prescribed for people taking monoamine-oxidase inhibitors or suffering from low blood pressure, asthma, liver damage, or head injury.

Anapolon (oxymetholone) A SEX HORMONE (MALE).

Anovlar 21 A medium-dose oestrogen oral contraceptive.

Antabuse (disulfiram) A drug used to treat alcoholism.

ANTACIDS Drugs that relieve indigestion and heartburn by neutralizing effects of stomach acid. Antacids are taken in tablet or, more effectively, in liquid form or as a powder mixed with water. Possible side-effects: constipation (from aluminium compounds), diarrhoea (from magnesium compounds). In preparations combining different antacids the side-effects may neutralize each other. Antacids may be combined with an ANTISPASMODIC to treat peptic ulcers. It is inadvisable for people with kidney problems to take preparations containing magnesium. Antacids are taken between meals and, because they affect the absorption of many drugs, should not be taken with other medicines.

Anthisan* (mepyramine maleate) An ANTIHISTAMINE.

ANTI-ANXIETY DRUGS Drugs (sometimes called anxiolytics, sedatives, or minor tranquillizers) that suppress anxiety and relax muscles. Some are also used as SLEEPING DRUGS or for relief of premenstrual tension. Possible side-effects: drowsiness, dizziness, confusion, unsteadiness (especially in the elderly). Because they can become habit-forming and users develop tolerance, anti-anxiety drugs are usually prescribed for periods of no more than 4 months of continuous use. To avoid withdrawal symptoms, usage is halted gradually. Effects last for several hours, when it is inadvisable to drive or work with potentially dangerous machinery. Effects of alcohol may be increased.

ANTI-ARRHYTHMICS Drugs for controlling irregularities of heartbeat. The oldest anti-arrhythmics are digitalis and quinidine, both of which are plant extracts. More recently introduced anti-arrhythmics include the BETA-BLOCKERS, verapamil and disopyramide.

ANTIBIOTICS Drugs (strictly naturally occurring substances) that combat bacterial infection. Some are effective only against specific types of bacterium; others – known as broad-spectrum antibiotics – are effective against a wide range. Possible side-effects: nausea, vomiting, diarrhoea, and – especially from use of broad-spectrum antibiotics – secondary infections such as thrush. Allergic reactions, particularly to penicillin and its many derivatives, are common – among them, rashes, fever, painful joints, body swelling, wheezing. In such cases a change of treatment may be advisable.

Once treatment gets under way, the prescribed course should be completed even when cure seems already effected. Failure to finish the course may increase the chances of bacterial resistance to further treatment with the drug.

ANTICANCER DRUGS See CYTOTOXICS.

ANTICOAGULANTS AND THROMBOLYTICS Anticoagulants prevent blood from clotting. Possible side effects: bleeding from nose or gums, bruising, smoky or pink urine, bleeding into the intestinal tract. Because anticoagulants interact adversely with many other drugs, users should carry a warning card and take other medicines only under a doctor's orders.

Thrombolytics help dissolve and disperse blood clots and may be used in patients with recent arterial or venous thrombosis.

ANTICONVULSANTS Drugs that prevent epileptic attacks by depressing the activity of the brain. Once the patient has remained free of fits for 2 or 3 years, the dose will be gradually reduced, and in some cases, may eventually be stopped altogether. Possible side-effects: drowsiness, rashes, dizziness, headache, nausea, indigestion. Abrupt withdrawal can precipitate a convulsion. It is inadvisable to drink alcohol or operate potentially dangerous machinery while taking anticonvulsants.

ANTIDEPRESSANTS There are two main groups of mood-lifting antidepressants: tricyclics and monoamine-oxidase inhibitors (MAOIs). Beneficial effects may take 3 to 4 weeks to develop. Possible side-effects of tricyclics: drowsiness, dry mouth, blurred vision, constipation, difficulty in urinating, faintness on standing, sweating, trembling, rashes, palpitations, impotence (in males). Possible side-effects of MAOIs: dizziness, faintness on standing, headache, trembling, constipation, dry mouth, blurred vision, difficulty in urination, rashes. The MAOIs interact adversely with other drugs and several foods and are usually prescribed only if depression fails to respond to tricyclics. Individuals taking MAOIs are advised to carry a warning card. It is inadvisable to drink alcohol, drive, or use complex machinery after taking any antidepressant.

ANTIDIARRHOEALS Drugs used for relief of diarrhoea. Two main types of antidiarrhoeal are simple absorbent substances (for instance, kaolin, chalk, or charcoal mixture) and drugs that slow down the contractions of the bowel muscle so that the contents are propelled more slowly. Antidiarrhoeals are available in tablet or liquid form. Because effective treatment of diarrhoea can lead to constipation, it is inadvisable to continue using antidiarrhoeals for prolonged periods.

ANTI-EMETICS Drugs for treating nausea and vomiting. ANTI-HISTAMINES and some ANTISPASMODICS are widely used anti-emetics, especially for prevention of motion sickness. Vomiting caused by underlying disease is most often treated with an ANTIPSYCHOTIC. Anti-emetics are usually taken as tablets, but may be taken in liquid or suppository form or given by injection. For possible side-effects see ANTIHISTAMINES, ANTISPASMODICS, and ANTIPSYCHOTICS. It is inadvisable to drive, use potentially dangerous machinery, or drink alcohol after taking an anti-emetic. Anti-emetics are not recommended in cases where the cause of vomiting is not known, and should not be taken for the sickness of pregnancy without a doctor's advice.

ANTIFUNGALS Drugs for treating fungal infections, the most common of which affect the hair, skin, nails, or mucous membranes. Antifungals may be taken in tablet form or applied locally as creams, ointments, or pessaries. Internal fungal infections such as endocarditis are treated by antifungal drugs given by injection. For possible side-effects see specific drugs.

ANTIHISTAMINES Drugs used primarily to counteract the effects of histamine, one of the chemicals involved in allergic reactions. They used to be widely prescribed in allergic conditions such as hay fever, but drugs such as sodium cromoglycate, which have fewer side-effects than the antihistamines, and are as effective in controlling hay fever, are now often used in preference. Many antihistamines are also useful for relief of stuffy or runny nose, nausea, and vertigo; they are therefore common ingredients of cold-cure remedies and are used as motion-sickness preventives. Possible side-effects: drowsiness, blurred vision, dry mouth. It is inadvisable to drive, operate potentially dangerous machinery, or drink alcohol after taking an antihistamine.

ANTIHYPERTENSIVES Drugs that lower blood pressure. The 2 groups of drugs most commonly used are the BETA-BLOCKERS and DIURETICS. People with high blood pressure who do not respond to these are treated with other categories of drugs, referred to in this index simply as ANTIHYPERTENSIVES. These are usually taken as tablets but may be given by injection for rapid effect. For possible side-effects see specific drugs.

ANTI-INFLAMMATORIES Drugs for reducing inflammation – the redness, heat, swelling, and increased blood flow found in infections and in many chronic non-infective diseases such as rheumatoid arthritis or gout. Three main types of drug are used as anti-inflammatories: ANALGESICS, such as aspirin, CORTICOSTEROIDS, and non-steroidal anti-inflammatory drugs such as indomethacin. The analgesics that are especially effective for treating rheumatic conditions also reduce the fever and inflammation of the joints, and minimize changes in the blood found in rheumatic conditions. Drugs such as indomethacin have little effect on pains due to, say, toothache or a bruise, but are very effective in relieving the inflammation – and so the pain – of diseases such as gout. Corticosteroids may be applied locally as cream or eye drops for inflammation of the skin or eyes; they are not generally prescribed for rheumatic conditions unless such disorders have failed to respond to treatment with non-steroid drugs.

ANTIPSYCHOTICS Antipsychotics (sometimes called major tranquillizers) are useful in treating symptoms of severe psychiatric disorders. Some antipsychotics are also used as ANTI-EMETICS, and may also be useful in migraine. They may be taken in tablet, liquid, or suppository form, or given by injection. Possible side-effects: jaundice, tremor, abnormal face and body movements, low temperature.

ANTIPYRETICS Drugs that reduce fever. The most commonly used are aspirin and paracetamol, which are both also ANALGESICS. This double action makes them particularly effective at relieving the symptoms of feverish illnesses such as influenza.

ANTIRHEUMATICS See ANTI-INFLAMMATORIES and ANALGESICS.

ANTISICKNESS DRUGS See ANTI-EMETICS.

ANTISPASMODICS Drugs for reducing spasm of the bowel musculature in order to relieve the pain of conditions such as irritable colon or diverticular disease. Some antispasmodics are used, in combination with ANTACIDS, to treat peptic ulcer.

A few are also used as ANTI-EMETICS. Antispasmodics may be taken in tablet or liquid form or by injection. Possible side-effects: dry mouth, palpitations, difficulty in passing urine, constipation, blurred vision.

ANTIVIRALS Drugs used for treatment of viral infections or provision of temporary protection against infections such as influenza. Few viral disorders apart from herpes simplex (cold sores) and herpes zoster (shingles) respond to drugs, and those that do respond will do so only if treatment is started early. For further information see specific drugs.

Anturan (sulphinpyrazone) A drug used for prevention of gout.

Anusol* A cream or suppository for treatment of haemorrhoids or anal itching.

ANXIOLYTICS See ANTI-ANXIETY DRUGS.

Anxon (ketazolam) An ANTI-ANXIETY DRUG.

APERIENTS See LAXATIVES.

Apresoline (hydralazine hydrochloride) An ANTI-HYPERTENSIVE.

Aprinox (bendrofluazide) A DIURETIC.

Arobon* (ceratonia) An ANTI-DIARRHOEAL.

aspirin* A non-narcotic ANALGESIC, and an ANTIPYRETIC or ANTI-INFLAMMATORY. Aspirin is effective in the treatment of headache and of muscle and joint pains. Although usually taken as tablets, it is less likely to irritate the stomach in soluble form. *Buffered* aspirin and tablets, with a special protective coating which is not broken down until the tablet reaches the intestine, may also reduce gastric irritation. Possible side-effects: stomach pain, vomiting, rashes. High or prolonged doses may cause deafness, noises in the ear, nausea, or headache. Aspirin is available in "junior"-strength tablets, but is not recommended for infants under 1. Aspirin is inadvisable for anyone with abdominal pain, nausea, vomiting, peptic ulcer, a bleeding disorder, or being treated with anticoagulants.

Atarax (hydroxyzine hydrochloride) An ANTI-ANXIETY DRUG.

atenolol A BETA-BLOCKER.

Ativan (lorazepam) An ANTI-ANXIETY DRUG.

Atromid-S (clofibrate) A drug for reducing blood-cholesterol level.

atropine sulphate An ANTI-SPASMODIC and ANTI-EMETIC. Not recommended for people with glaucoma or a tendency to urinary retention.

Atrovent (ipratropium bromide) A BRONCHODILATOR.

Aureomycin (chlortetracycline hydrochloride) An ANTIBIOTIC.
Aventyl (nortriptyline) An ANTIDEPRESSANT.
Avomine* (promethazine theoclate) An ANTIHISTAMINE.
azathioprine A CYTOTOXIC used primarily as an IMMUNO-SUPPRESSIVE. Possible side-effects (in addition to those common to the group): rashes, wasting of muscles.

Bactrim (co-trimoxazole) An ANTIBIOTIC.
barbiturates See SLEEPING DRUGS.
belladonna An ANTI-SPASMODIC containing atropine, extracted from deadly nightshade.
Benadryl* (diphenhydramine hydrochloride) An ANTI-HISTAMINE.
bendrofluazide A DIURETIC.
Benemid (probenecid) A drug used for prevention of gout.
benethamine penicillin An ANTIBIOTIC, given by injection.
Benoral* (benorylate) An ANALGESIC, ANTIPYRETIC and ANTI-INFLAMMATORY.
benorylate* An ANALGESIC, ANTIPYRETIC and ANTI-INFLAMMATORY containing aspirin and paracetamol. (For further information see aspirin and paracetamol.)
benzathine penicillin An ANTIBIOTIC.
benzoctamine hydrochloride An ANTI-ANXIETY DRUG.
Benztrone (oestradiol) A SEX HORMONE (FEMALE).
benzylpenicillin An ANTIBIOTIC.
Berkdopa (levodopa) A drug used for treating Parkinson's disease.
Berkmycen (oxytetracycline) An ANTIBIOTIC.
Berkolol (propanalol hydrochloride) A BETA-BLOCKER.
Berkozide (bendrofluazide) A DIURETIC.
BETA-BLOCKERS Beta-adrenergic blocking agents – beta-blockers for short – reduce oxygen needs of the heart by reducing heartbeat rate. They are used as ANTIHYPERTENSIVES and ANTI-ARRHYTHMICS, for treating angina due to exertion, and for easing symptoms such as palpitations and tremors in patients with anxiety states. Beta-blockers may be taken as tablets or given by injection. Possible side-effects: nausea, insomnia, physical weariness, diarrhoea; overdose can cause dizziness and fainting spells. Discontinuance of treatment should be gradual, not abrupt. Beta-blockers are not prescribed for people with asthma.

Beta-Cardone (sotalol hydrochloride) A BETA-BLOCKER.
betahistine hydrochloride An ANTI-EMETIC, mainly used for treating vertigo or Ménière's disease. Possible side-effects: nausea, headache.
Betaloc (metoprolol tartrate) A BETA-BLOCKER.
betamethasone A CORTICO-STEROID.
bethanechol chloride A stimulant LAXATIVE, also used to treat urinary-tract disorders. Possible side-effects: abdominal cramps, nausea, increased salivation.
bethanidine sulphate An ANTI-HYPERTENSIVE. Possible side-effects: feelings of faintness, swollen ankles, stuffy nose, and failure to ejaculate.
Betnelan (betamethasone) A CORTICOSTEROID.
Betnesol (betamethasone) A CORTICOSTEROID.
Bidrolar* (senna) A stimulant LAXATIVE.
Biogastrone (carbenoxolone) A drug used for healing peptic ulcers.
biphasic insulin injection An intermediate-acting insulin preparation.
bisacodyl* A stimulant LAXATIVE. Possible side-effect: abdominal cramps.
bismuth subgallate A drug given as a suppository for treating haemorrhoids and anal itching.
bleomycin sulphate A CYTO-TOXIC, given only by injection.
Blocadren (timolol maleate) A BETA-BLOCKER.
Bolvidon (mianserin hydrochloride) An ANTIDEPRESSANT.
bran* A bulk LAXATIVE (which is fibrous wheat taken as tablets).
Bricanyl (terbutaline sulphate) A BRONCHODILATOR.
Brocadopa (levodopa) A drug used for treating Parkinson's disease.
bromocriptine A drug for treating Parkinson's disease, also used for suppressing lactation and for treatment of some hormonal disorders. Generally taken in tablet form. Possible side-effects: nausea, constipation, headache, dizziness, drowsiness, confusion, dry mouth, leg cramps, hallucinations.
BRONCHODILATORS Drugs that open up bronchial tubes that have become narrowed by muscle spasm. Bronchodilators, which ease breathing in diseases such as asthma, are most often taken as aerosol sprays, but they are also available in tablet, liquid, or suppository form; in emergencies – for instance, severe attacks of asthma – they may be given by injection. Effects usually last for 3 to 5 hours. Possible side-effects:

rapid heartbeat, palpitations, tremor, headache, dizziness. Because of possible effects on the heart, prescribed doses should never be exceeded; when asthma does not respond to the prescribed doses, emergency medical treatment is needed.
Broxil (phenethicillin potassium) An ANTIBIOTIC.
bumetanide A DIURETIC.
Burinex (bumetamide) A DIURETIC.
busulphan A CYTOTOXIC. Possible side-effect (in addition to those common to the group): skin pigmentation.
Butacote (phenylbutazone) An ANTI-INFLAMMATORY.
Butazolidin (phenylbutazone) An ANTI-INFLAMMATORY.
Butazone (phenylbutazone) An ANTI-INFLAMMATORY.
butobarbitone A barbiturate used as a SLEEPING DRUG.

Cafergot (ergotamine and caffeine) A preparation for treating migraine. Possible side-effect: drowsiness.
calamine A soothing skin preparation in cream or liquid form, used mainly for treating sunburn.
Calpol* Paracetamol in liquid form.
Canesten (clotrimazole) An ANTIFUNGAL.
Cantil (mepenzolate bromide) An ANTISPASMODIC.
carbamazepine An ANTI-CONVULSANT, also used for relief of trigeminal neuralgia. Possible side-effects (in addition to those common to the group): dry mouth, double vision.
carbenoxolone sodium A drug used for healing peptic ulcers.
carbimazole A drug, taken in tablet form, for treating thyrotoxicosis. Possible side-effects: nausea, headache, rashes, aching joints. Carbimazole is not prescribed for nursing mothers.
Cardiacap (pentaerythritol tetranitrate) A VASODILATOR.
Cardophylin (aminophylline) A BRONCHODILATOR.
cascara* A stimulant LAXATIVE. Possible side effects: abdominal cramps, red-tinged urine. It should not be taken by nursing mothers.
Catapres (clonidine hydrochloride) An ANTI-HYPERTENSIVE.
CCNU (lomustine) A CYTOTOXIC.
Cedilanid (deslanoside) An ANTI-ARRHYTHMIC.
Cedocard (isosorbide dinitrate) A VASODILATOR.
CeeNU (lomustine) A CYTOTOXIC.
Celevac* (methylcellulose) A bulk LAXATIVE.

Cellucon* (methylcellulose) A bulk LAXATIVE.
cephalexin A broad-spectrum ANTIBIOTIC.
cephaloridine A broad-spectrum ANTIBIOTIC, given only by injection.
cephradine A broad-spectrum ANTIBIOTIC.
Ceporex (cephalexin) An ANTIBIOTIC.
Ceporin (cephaloridine) An ANTIBIOTIC.
ceratonia* An ANTI-DIARRHOEAL.
Cerubidin (daunorubicin hydrochloride) A CYTOTOXIC.
Chendol (chenodeoxycholic acid) A drug for treating gallstones.
chenodeoxycholic acid A drug taken in tablet form for treating gallstones. Possible side effects: diarrhoea, itching.
Chenofalk (chenodeoxycholic acid) A drug for treating gallstones.
Chloractil (chlorpromazine hydrochloride) An ANTI-PSYCHOTIC also used as an ANTI-EMETIC.
chloral hydrate The oldest sleeping drug, now used mainly for children because it is safe and predictable. Possible side-effects: rashes, stomach irritation. See SLEEPING DRUGS.
chlorambucil A CYTOTOXIC.
chloramphenicol An ANTI-BIOTIC used mainly as an ointment or in drops for ear and eye infections.
chlordiazepoxide An ANTI-ANXIETY DRUG, also used as a SLEEPING DRUG.
chlormethiazole edisylate A SLEEPING DRUG also used in psychosis and to relieve drug/alcohol withdrawal. See SLEEPING DRUGS.
chlormezanone An ANTI-ANXIETY DRUG, also used as a SLEEPING DRUG.
Chloromycetin (chloramphenicol) An ANTIBIOTIC.
chlorothiazide A DIURETIC.
chlorotrianisene A SEX HORMONE (FEMALE).
chlorpheniramine maleate An ANTIHISTAMINE.
chlorpromazine hydrochloride An ANTIPSYCHOTIC also used as an ANTI-EMETIC. Possible side-effects (in addition to those common to the group): tremor, stiffness, nightmares, insomnia, constipation, depression, difficulty in passing urine, menstrual disturbances, rashes, jaundice.
chlorpropamide A HYPO-GLYCAEMIC.
chlortetracycline hydrochloride A broad-spectrum ANTIBIOTIC. See tetracycline to which this preparation is similar.

chlorthalidone A DIURETIC.

Cidomycin (gentamicin) An ANTIBIOTIC.

cimetidine A drug used for healing peptic ulcers. Possible side-effects: diarrhoea, dizziness, rashes. Avoid long-term use.

cinnarizine* An ANTIHISTAMINE primarily for relief of nausea and vertigo.

cisplatin A CYTOTOXIC. Possible side-effects (in addition to those common to the group): deafness, kidney damage.

clindamycin An ANTIBIOTIC, primarily used for bone and joint infections. It is advisable to discontinue use of clindamycin if diarrhoea occurs.

clobazam An ANTI-ANXIETY DRUG.

clofibrate A drug, normally taken in tablet form, for reducing blood-cholesterol level. Possible side-effects: nausea, diarrhoea, aching muscles. Clofibrate is not generally prescribed for people with liver or kidney disease.

Clomid (clomiphene) A drug for treating infertility in women.

clomiphene A drug taken in tablet form for treating infertility in women. Possible side-effects: hot flushes, abdominal discomfort, blurred vision, nausea, vomiting, depression, insomnia, breast tenderness, weight gain.

clomipramine hydrochloride A tricyclic ANTIDEPRESSANT.

clonazepam An ANTICONVULSANT. Possible side-effects (in addition to those common to the group): muscular weakness, clumsiness, mood changes.

clonidine hydrochloride An ANTIHYPERTENSIVE, also used for prevention of migraine attacks. Possible side-effects: dry mouth, drowsiness, depression, swollen ankles. Abrupt withdrawal should be avoided.

clorazepate dipotassium An ANTI-ANXIETY DRUG, also used as a SLEEPING DRUG.

clotrimazole An ANTIFUNGAL. Possible side-effect: local itching.

cloxacillin An ANTIBIOTIC.

codeine linctus A COUGH SUPPRESSANT. Possible side-effect: constipation.

codeine phosphate A mild narcotic ANALGESIC also used as a COUGH SUPPRESSANT and ANTIDIARRHOEAL. Not recommended shortly before, during, or after drinking alcohol, or for infants under 1. Possible side-effects: nausea, dizziness, drowsiness, constipation.

COLD-CURE REMEDIES Although there is no drug that can cure a cold, symptoms can be relieved by aspirin or paracetamol, taken with plenty of fluid.

Cold-cure remedies that contain these drugs are the most effective. Many preparations contain ANTIHISTAMINES and DECONGESTANTS, for drying up nasal secretions and unblocking nasal passages. However, taken by mouth these drugs are unlikely to be effective unless swallowed in doses high enough to produce side-effects outweighing benefits. Possible side-effects: drowsiness, giddiness, headache, nausea, vomiting, sweating, thirst, palpitations, difficulty in passing urine, weakness, trembling, anxiety, insomnia. Cold-cure remedies should be avoided by people suffering from angina, high blood pressure, diabetes, or thyroid disorders, and by anyone taking monoamine-oxidase inhibitors. It is inadvisable to drive or use potentially dangerous machinery after taking a remedy containing an antihistamine. Patent cold-cure remedies are not listed in this index.

Colofac (mebeverine hydrochloride) An ANTISPASMODIC.

Cologel* (methylcellulose) A bulk LAXATIVE.

Conova 30 A low-oestrogen oral contraceptive.

Controvlar (oestrogen and progestogen) A preparation for treating menstrual disorders. See SEX HORMONES (FEMALE).

Cordilox (verapamil hydrochloride) An ANTI-ARRHYTHMIC.

CORTICOSTEROIDS Hormonal preparations used primarily as ANTI-INFLAMMATORIES or IMMUNOSUPPRESSIVES, but also useful for treating malignancies or compensating for a deficiency of natural hormones in disorders such as Addison's disease. Corticosteroids may be taken as tablets, applied locally as cream or eye drops, or given by injection. Possible side-effects of over-use of tablets: swollen ankles, raised blood pressure, fat deposits on face, shoulders, and abdomen, hairiness, flushing, acne, disturbance of menstrual patterns, muscle weakness, mood changes, peptic ulcers, cataract. Corticosteroid tablets also reduce the body's resistance to infection, and they may suppress growth in children. Given as eye drops, they may cause glaucoma; as creams, they may cause rashes, acne, and other skin troubles. In all forms these drugs are used sparingly and for only limited periods. Discontinuance of treatment should be gradual. People taking corticosteriod tablets are advised to carry a warning card, and anyone who has been under such treatment within the

past 2 years should so inform any new doctor, nurse, dentist, or midwife.

Cosmegen Lyovac (actinomycin D) A CYTOTOXIC.

Cosylan* (dextromethorphan hydrobromide) A COUGH SUPPRESSANT.

co-trimoxazole An ANTIBIOTIC.

COUGH SUPPRESSANTS Simple cough medicines, which contain substances such as honey, glycerine, or menthol, soothe throat irritation but do not suppress coughing. They are most soothing when taken as lozenges and dissolved in the mouth; as liquids they are probably swallowed too quickly to be effective. A few drugs – notably codeine and pholcodine – are actually cough suppressants; that is, they can help to control a dry, unproductive cough. For possible side-effects see specific drugs. Ordinary cough medicines are not included in this index.

Crescormon Growth hormone.

Crystapen (benzyl penicillin) An ANTIBIOTIC.

Crystapen V (phenoxymethylpenicillin) An ANTIBIOTIC.

Cyclimorph (morphine) An ANALGESIC.

cyclizine* An ANTIHISTAMINE primarily for relief of nausea and vertigo.

Cyclogest (progesterone) A SEX HORMONE (FEMALE).

cyclophosphamide A CYTOTOXIC.

Cyclo-Progynova (oestrogen and progestogen) A preparation for treating menopausal symptoms. See SEX HORMONES (FEMALE).

cyproheptadine hydrochloride* An ANTIHISTAMINE for treating not only allergic disorders but – occasionally – poor appetite or migraine.

cytarabine A CYTOTOXIC, given only by injection.

Cytosar (cytarabine) A CYTOTOXIC.

CYTOTOXICS Drugs that kill or damage multiplying cells. Cytotoxics are used in treatment of cancer and as IMMUNOSUPPRESSIVES. They are taken as tablets or given by injection, and several cytotoxics, with different types of action, may be used in combination. Possible side-effects: nausea, vomiting, loss of hair. Because cytotoxic action can affect healthy as well as cancerous cells, these drugs may also have dangerous side-effects: for example, they can damage bone marrow and affect the production of blood cells, causing anaemia, increased susceptibility to infection, and

haemorrhage. Frequent blood counts are therefore advisable for anyone having such treatment.

Dactil (piperidolate hydrochloride) An ANTISPASMODIC.

Daktarin (miconazole) An ANTIFUNGAL.

Dalacin (clindamycin) An ANTIBIOTIC.

Dalmane (flurazepam) A SLEEPING DRUG.

danthron* A stimulant LAXATIVE. Possible side-effects: abdominal cramps, red-tinged urine, diarrhoea in infants if taken by nursing mothers.

Daonil (glibenclamide) A HYPOGLYCAEMIC.

Daranide (dichlorphenamide) A DIURETIC.

Daraprim* (pyrimethamine) A drug used for prevention of malaria.

daunorubicin hydrochloride A CYTOTOXIC, given by injection.

DDAVP (desmopressin) A HORMONE used for treating diabetes insipidus.

Debendox (dicyclomine hydrochloride) An ANTISPASMODIC also used as an ANTI-EMETIC.

Decadron (dexamethasone) A CORTICOSTEROID.

Deca-Durabolin (nandrolone) A SEX HORMONE (MALE).

DECONGESTANTS Drugs that reduce swelling of the mucous membranes lining the nose by constricting blood vessels, thus relieving nasal stuffiness. Decongestants are best taken as a nasal spray or drops; overuse, however, can lead to increased stuffiness. They can also be taken by mouth as a constituent of COLD-CURE REMEDIES, but are less effective in this form. Large doses taken by mouth may affect heart rate or the brain.

DEHYDRATING AGENTS See DIURETICS.

Deltacortril Enteric (prednisolone) A CORTICOSTEROID.

Delta Phoricol (prednisolone) A CORTICOSTEROID.

demeclocycline hydrochloride A broad-spectrum ANTIBIOTIC. See tetracycline.

Demulen 50 A medium-oestrogen oral contraceptive.

Depixol (flupenthixol dihydrochloride) An ANTIPSYCHOTIC.

desipramine hydrochloride A tricyclic ANTIDEPRESSANT.

deslanoside A digoxin-like ANTI-ARRHYTHMIC, given only by injection. See digoxin for side-effects.

desmopressin A HORMONE, given either as nasal drops or by injection, used for treating diabetes insipidus.

Deteclo A trade name for tetracycline, an ANTIBIOTIC.

dexamethasone A CORTICO-STEROID.

Dexedrine (dexamphetamine sulphate) An addictive drug seldom used for medical purposes.

dextromethorphan hydro-bromide* A cough medicine. Possible side-effects: constipation. See COUGH SUPPRESSANTS.

DF 118 (dihydrocodeine tartrate) An ANALGESIC.

Diabinese (chlorpropamide) A HYPOGLYCAEMIC.

Diamicron (gliclazide) A HYPOGLYCAEMIC.

diamorphine hydrochloride A powerful narcotic ANALGESIC.

Diamox (acetozolamide) A DIURETIC.

Dianabol (methandienone) A SEX HORMONE (MALE).

Dia-tuss* (pholcodine) A COUGH SUPPRESSANT.

diazepam An ANTI-ANXIETY DRUG, also used as a SLEEPING DRUG.

diazoxide An ANTIHYPERTENSIVE given only by injection. Possible side-effects: palpitations, swollen ankles.

dichloralphenazone A SLEEPING DRUG similar to chloral hydrate.

dichlorphenamide A DIURETIC used in treating glaucoma. Possible side-effects: loss of appetite, depression.

dicyclomine hydrochloride An ANTISPASMODIC and ANTI-EMETIC, often used for treating infantile colic. Not recommended for anyone with glaucoma or with a tendency to urinary retention.

diflunisal An aspirin-like ANALGESIC, ANTIPYRETIC, and ANTI-INFLAMMATORY. For further information see aspirin.

Diganox Nativelle (digoxin) An ANTI-ARRHYTHMIC.

Digitaline Nativelle (digitoxin) An ANTI-ARRHYTHMIC.

digitoxin A digoxin-like ANTI-ARRHYTHMIC. See digoxin.

digoxin An ANTI-ARRHYTHMIC, which also makes the heartbeat stronger and may be used for treatment of heart failure. Side-effects: nausea, palpitations, confusion.

dihydrocodeine tartrate A mild narcotic ANALGESIC. Not recommended for people with respiratory disease or children under 4.

Dimelor (acetohexamide) A HYPOGLYCAEMIC.

Dimenhydrinate* An ANTIHISTAMINE primarily for relief of nausea and vertigo.

dioctyl sodium sulpho-succinate* A faeces-softening LAXATIVE.

Dioctyl-Medo* (dioctyl sodium sulphosuccinate) A faeces-softening LAXATIVE.

diphenhydramine hydro-chloride* An ANTIHISTAMINE.

diphenoxylate hydrochloride An ANTI-DIARRHOEAL.

disopyramide An ANTI-ARRHYTHMIC. Possible side-effects: dry mouth, blurred vision, urinary retention.

Disprin* (soluble aspirin) An ANALGESIC and ANTIPYRETIC.

Distaquaine V-K (phenoxy-methylpenicillin) An ANTIBIOTIC.

distigmine bromide A stimulant LAXATIVE, also used to treat myaesthenia gravis. Possible side-effects: abdominal cramps, nausea, increased salivation.

disulfiram A drug taken in tablet form, for treatment of alcoholism. If taken before, during, or after drinking, disulfiram may cause headache, palpitations, nausea, vomiting, and severe shock.

DIURETICS Drugs that increase the quantity of urine produced by the kidneys, thus ridding the body of excess fluid. Diuretics reduce waterlogging of the tissues caused by fluid retention (dropsy) in disorders of the heart, kidneys, and liver; they are useful in treating mild cases of high blood pressure; they may also decrease fluid pressure within the eye (in glaucoma) or within the lungs (in pulmonary oedema). They are normally taken as tablets. Possible side-effects: rashes, nausea, dizziness, weakness, numbness, tingling in hands and feet.

Dolobid (diflunisal) An ANALGESIC, ANTIPYRETIC, and ANTI-INFLAMMATORY.

Dopamet (methyldopa) An ANTIHYPERTENSIVE.

Dorbanex* (danthron) A stimulant LAXATIVE.

dothiepin hydrochloride A tricyclic ANTIDEPRESSANT.

doxorubicin A CYTOTOXIC, given only by injection.

doxycycline A broad-spectrum ANTIBIOTIC. See tetracycline to which this preparation is similar.

Dramamine* (dimenhydrinate) An ANTIHISTAMINE.

Dryptal (frusemide) A DIURETIC.

Dulcodos (bisacodyl) A stimulant LAXATIVE.

Dulcolax (bisacodyl) A stimulant LAXATIVE.

Duogastrone (carbenoxolone) A drug used for healing peptic ulcers.

Duphaston (dyhydrogesterone) A SEX HORMONE (FEMALE).

Durabolin (nandrolone) A SEX HORMONE (MALE).

Duromorph (morphine) An ANALGESIC.

Duvadilan (isoxsuprine hydrochloride) A VASODILATOR.

Dyazide (triamterene) A DIURETIC.

dydrogesterone A progestogen. See SEX HORMONES (FEMALE).

Dytide (triamterene) A DIURETIC.

Economycin (tetracycline) An ANTIBIOTIC.

Edecrin (ethacrynic acid) A DIURETIC.

Efcortelan (hydrocortisone) A CORTICOSTEROID.

Efudix (fluorouracil) A CYTOTOXIC.

Eltroxin (thyroxine) A drug for treatment of hypothyroidism.

Emeside (ethosuximide) An ANTICONVULSANT.

Enavid (oestrogen and progestogen) A preparation for treating menstrual disorders. See SEX HORMONES (FEMALE).

Endoxana (cyclophosphamide) A CYTOTOXIC.

Epanutin (phenytoin) An ANTICONVULSANT and ANTI-ARRHYTHMIC.

ephedrine hydrochloride* A BRONCHODILATOR and DE-CONGESTANT.

Epilim (sodium valproate) An ANTICONVULSANT.

Equanil (meprobamate) An ANTI-ANXIETY DRUG.

ergotamine A drug taken in tablet or suppository form, for treating acute attacks of migraine.

Erythrocin (erythromycin) An ANTIBIOTIC.

Erythromid (erythromycin) An ANTIBIOTIC.

erythromycin An ANTIBIOTIC.

Erythroped (erythromycin) An ANTIBIOTIC.

Esbatal (bethanidine sulphate) An ANTIHYPERTENSIVE.

Estracyt (estramustine phosphate) A CYTOTOXIC.

estramustine phosphate A CYTOTOXIC.

ethacrynic acid A DIURETIC.

ethinyloestradiol An oestrogen. See SEX HORMONES (FEMALE).

ethisterone A progestogen. See SEX HORMONES (FEMALE).

Ethosuximide An ANTICONVULSANT used primarily for treatment of petit mal epilepsy. Possible side-effects (in addition to those common to the group): clumsiness, mood changes.

ethyloestrenol An anabolic steroid. See SEX HORMONES (MALE).

Eugynon 30 A low-oestrogen oral contraceptive.

Eugynon 50 A medium-oestrogen oral contraceptive.

Fansidar* (pyrimethamine) A drug used to prevent malaria.

Femergin (ergotamine) A drug used for treating migraine.

Femulen A progestogen-only oral contraceptive.

fenoprofen An aspirin-like ANALGESIC, ANTIPYRETIC, and ANTI-INFLAMMATORY used mainly for rheumatic disorders. See also aspirin.

Fenopron (fenoprofen) An ANALGESIC, ANTIPYRETIC, and ANTI-INFLAMMATORY.

Fentazin (perphenazine) An ANTIPSYCHOTIC and ANTI-EMETIC.

figs, syrup of* A stimulant LAXATIVE. Possible side-effect: abdominal cramps.

Flagyl (metronidazole) A drug used for treatment of non-bacterial infections.

floxapen (flucloxacillin) An ANTIBIOTIC.

flucloxacillin An ANTIBIOTIC.

fluorouracil A CYTOTOXIC.

flupenthixol dihydrochloride, an ANTIPSYCHOTIC.

fluphenazine decanoate An ANTIPSYCHOTIC given by injection for treatment of schizophrenia.

fluphenazine hydrochloride An ANTIPSYCHOTIC.

flurazepam An ANTI-ANXIETY DRUG used primarily as a SLEEPING DRUG.

Fortral (pentazocine) An ANALGESIC.

Frisium (clobazam) An ANTI-ANXIETY DRUG.

frusemide A DIURETIC.

Frusetic (frusemide) A DIURETIC.

Frusid (frusemide) A DIURETIC.

Fulcin (griseofulvin) An ANTI-FUNGAL.

FUNGICIDES See ANTI-FUNGALS.

Fungilin (amphotericin) An ANTIFUNGAL.

Fungizone (amphotericin) An ANTIFUNGAL.

Furadantin (nitrofurantoin) An ANTIBIOTIC.

Furan (nitrofurantoin) An ANTI-BIOTIC.

Fybogel* (ispaghula husk) A bulk LAXATIVE.

Fybranta* (bran) A bulk LAXA-TIVE.

gentamicin A broad-spectrum ANTIBIOTIC, normally used as an ointment or given by injection. If taken by mouth, gentamicin can cause physical instability.

Genticin (gentamicin) An ANTIBIOTIC.

Gestone (progesterone) A SEX HORMONE (FEMALE).

Gestone-Oral (ethisterone) A SEX HORMONE (FEMALE).

glibenclamide A HYPOGLYCAEMIC.

glibornuride A HYPOGLYCAEMIC.

gliclazide A HYPOGLYCAEMIC.

globin zinc insulin injection An intermediate-acting insulin preparation.

Glutril (glibornuride) A HYPO-GLYCAEMIC.

glyceryl trinitrate A VASO-DILATOR.

glymidine A HYPO-GLYCAEMIC.

Gondafon (glymidine) A HYPOGLYCAEMIC.

Gravol* (dimenhydrinate) An ANTIHISTAMINE.

griseofulvin An ANTIFUNGAL. Possible side-effects: headache, nausea, rashes, photophobia.

Grisovin (griseofulvin) An ANTIFUNGAL.

growth hormone A HOR-MONE given only by injection for treatment of undersized children.

guanethidine monosulphate An ANTIHYPERTENSIVE. Possible side-effects: feelings of faintness, swollen ankles, stuffy nose, diarrhoea, and failure to ejaculate.

guanoclor sulphate An ANTI-HYPERTENSIVE. Possible side-effects: feelings of faintness, swollen ankles, stuffy nose, diarrhoea, and failure to ejaculate.

Gyno-daktarin (miconazole) An ANTIFUNGAL.

Gynovlar 21 A medium-dose oral contraceptive.

Haldol (haloperidol) An ANTI-PSYCHOTIC.

haloperidol An ANTI-PSYCHOTIC.

hamamelis* A drug given as a suppository for treatment of haemorrhoids or anal itching.

Harmogen (piperazine oestrone sulphate) A SEX HORMONE (FEMALE).

Havapen (penamecillin) An ANTIBIOTIC.

Heminevrin (chlormethiazole edisylate) A SLEEPING DRUG.

heparin An ANTICOAGULANT, given only by injection.

HORMONES Chemicals produced naturally by the endocrine glands. In some disorders – for example, diabetes mellitus – in which too little of a particular hormone is produced, synthetic equivalents or natural-hormone extracts are prescribed for making good the deficiency. Such treatment is known as hormone-replacement therapy. For other uses of hormones – in particular the CORTICOSTEROIDS and SEX HORMONES – and for side-effects, see appropriate entries.

Hormonin (oestriol) A SEX HORMONE (FEMALE).

hydralazine hydrochloride An ANTIHYPERTENSIVE. Possible side-effects: palpitations, swollen ankles, feelings of faintness, nausea, vomiting.

Hydrea (hydroxyurea) A CYTOTOXIC.

hydrocortisone A CORTICO-STEROID.

Hydrocortone (hydrocortisone) A CORTICOSTEROID.

hydroxyurea A CYTOTOXIC.

hydroxyzine hydrochloride An ANTI-ANXIETY DRUG.

Hygroton (chlorthalidone) A DIURETIC.

hyoscine hydrobromide An ANTISPASMODIC also used as an ANTI-EMETIC. Not recommended for people with glaucoma or urinary retention.

HYPNOTICS See SLEEPING DRUGS.

HYPOGLYCAEMICS (ORAL) Drugs that lower the level of glucose in the blood. Oral hypoglycaemic drugs are used in diabetes mellitus that cannot be controlled by diet alone, but does not require treatment with injections of insulin. Possible side-effects: loss of appetite, nausea, indigestion, numbness or tingling in the skin, fever, rashes, jaundice. If the glucose level falls too low, weakness, dizziness, pallor, sweating, increased saliva flow, palpitations, irritability, and trembling may result. Such symptoms should be reported to the doctor.

Hypovase (prazosin hydrochloride) An ANTIHYPERTENSIVE.

Hypurine Isophane (isophane insulin injection) An intermediate-acting insulin preparation.

Hypurin Neutral (insulin injection) A short-acting insulin preparation.

Hypurin Protamine Zinc (protamine zinc insulin injection) A long-acting insulin preparation.

idoxuridine An ANTIVIRAL for herpes infections.

Iliadin-Mini* (oxymetazoline) A DECONGESTANT.

Ilosone (erythromycin) An ANTIBIOTIC.

imipramine hydrochloride A tricyclic ANTIDEPRESSANT, also used for treatment of enuresis.

IMMUNOSUPPRESSIVES Drugs that prevent or reduce the body's normal reaction to invasion by disease or by foreign tissues. Immunosuppressives are used for treating auto-immune diseases (in which the body's defence system, working abnormally, attacks its own tissues) and for helping to prevent rejection of organ transplants. Most drugs used as immunosuppressives are either CYTOTOXICS or CORTICOSTEROIDS.

Imodium (loperamide hydrochloride) An ANTIDIARRHOEAL.

Imperacin (oxytetracycline) An ANTIBIOTIC.

Imuran (azathioprine) A CYTOTOXIC used as an IMMUNOSUPPRESSIVE.

Inderal (propranolol hydrochloride) A BETA-BLOCKER.

Indocid (indomethacin) An ANTI-INFLAMMATORY.

indomethacin An ANTI-INFLAMMATORY, taken in tablet, liquid, or suppository form. Possible side-effects: headache, dizziness, loss of appetite, nausea, indigestion, diarrhoea. It is advisable not to drive or use potentially dangerous machinery after taking indomethacin.

Inolaxine* (sterculia) A bulk LAXATIVE.

insulin A HORMONE, produced by the pancreas, which controls the breakdown of sugar in the body to produce energy. As a drug, insulin is used for treating most young diabetics, and some older diabetics whose diabetes cannot be controlled by diet or by HYPOGLYCAEMICS. Most insulin preparations are extracted from pork or beef pancreases. "Monocomponent" insulins are obtained from a single animal source and are valuable if an allergy develops to one species or another. Many specially purified insulins are also available and these, too, are less likely to cause an allergic reaction. If allergy is a severe problem a "human" insulin may be given synthesized by microbes following *genetic engineering* or by chemical modification of a monocomponent insulin. Insulin is always given by injection, as it is destroyed by the digestive juices. Some preparations act rapidly but have only a short duration, others have a slower onset and a longer duration. The type given depends on an individual's needs, and often a mixture is necessary. Initial treatment is always given in hospital so that the correct dosage regimen can be established. Possible side-effects: hypoglycaemia (which may occur if too high a dose is given, or if the person misses a meal, eats too little carbohydrate, or takes more exercise than usual), with weakness, dizziness, pallor, sweating, increased saliva flow, irritability, trembling, confusion, and coma. Allergic reactions: rashes, itching, swelling of the face and throat, local irritation or lumpiness of the skin.

insulin injection A short-acting insulin preparation.

Intal (sodium cromoglycate) A drug for preventing attacks of asthma and allergic rhinitis.

ipratropium bromide A BRONCHODILATOR. Possible side-effect (in addition to those common to the group): dry mouth.

iproniazid A monoamine-oxidase inhibitor ANTI-DEPRESSANT.

Ismelin (guanethidine monosulphate) An ANTIHYPERTENSIVE.

isocarboxazid A monoamine-oxidase inhibitor ANTI-DEPRESSANT.

Isogel* (ispaghula husk) A bulk LAXATIVE.

isoniazid An ANTIBIOTIC.

Isophane insulin injection An intermediate-acting insulin preparation.

Isordil (isosorbide dinitrate) A VASODILATOR.

isosorbide dinitrate A VASO-DILATOR.

isoxsuprine hydrochloride A VASODILATOR.

ispaghula husk* A bulk LAXA-TIVE.

Juvel A multivitamin preparation.

Kabikinase (streptokinase) A THROMBOLYTIC.

Kaodene* (codeine phosphate and kaolin) An ANTI-DIARRHOEAL.

kaolin* An ANTIDIARRHOEAL.

kaolin and morphine mixture* An ANTIDIARRHOEAL.

Kaopectate* (kaolin) An ANTI-DIARRHOEAL.

Keflex (cephalexin) An ANTI-BIOTIC.

Kenalog (triamcinolone) A CORTICOSTEROID.

Kest* (magnesium sulphate) A fast-acting bulk LAXATIVE.

ketazolam An ANTI-ANXIETY DRUG.

KLN* (kaolin) An ANTI-DIARRHOEAL.

Klyx* (dioctyl sodium sulphosuccinate) A faeces-softening LAXATIVE.

Largactil (chlorpromazine) An ANTIPSYCHOTIC also used as an ANTI-EMETIC.

Larodopa (levodopa) A drug used for treating Parkinson's disease.

Lasix (frusemide) A DIURETIC.

LAXATIVES Drugs that increase the frequency and ease of bowel movements, either by stimulating the bowel wall (stimulant laxative), by increasing the bulk of bowel contents (bulk laxative), or by lubricating them (faeces-softeners). Laxatives may be taken by mouth or directly into the lower bowel as suppositories or in enemas. Bulk laxatives must be taken with plenty of water. If laxatives are taken regularly, the bowels may become unable to work properly without them.

Laxoberal* (sodium picosulphate) A stimulant LAXATIVE.
Ledercort (triamcinolone) A CORTICOSTEROID.
Ledermycin (demeclocycline hydrochloride) An ANTIBIOTIC.
Lentard (insulin zinc suspension) A long-acting insulin preparation.
Lentizol (amitriptyline hydrochloride) An ANTIDEPRESSANT.
Leo Initard (isophane insulin injection) An intermediate-acting insulin preparation.
Leo Mixtard (isophane insulin injection) An intermediate-acting insulin preparation.
Leo Neutral (insulin injection) A short-acting insulin preparation.
Leo Retard (isophane insulin injection) An intermediate-acting insulin preparation.
Leukeran (chlorambucil) A CYTOTOXIC.
Levius* Aspirin, coated for intestinal release.
levodopa A drug, usually taken in tablet form, for treatment of Parkinson's disease. Possible side-effects: loss of appetite, nausea, vomiting, dizziness, faintness on standing, palpitations, involuntary tongue, jaw, or neck movements, abdominal pain, difficulty in passing urine, discoloration of urine, mental disturbances, insomnia. Levodopa is not generally prescribed for anyone with acute glaucoma, and regular use may be inadvisable for people suffering from several other illnesses.
Librium (chlordiazepoxide) An ANTI-ANXIETY DRUG.
liquid paraffin* A faeces-softening LAXATIVE. Prolonged use is inadvisable. Possible side-effect: seepage, which can cause anal irritation.
lithium carbonate A drug used for treatment and prevention of manic and depressive illness, and available only in tablet form. Possible side-effects: nausea, trembling, thirst, passing large amounts of urine, weight gain. Doses must be monitored to prevent toxic effects producing sleepiness, vomiting, diarrhoea, blurred vision, dizziness, unsteadiness, slurred speech.
Loestrin 20 A low-oestrogen oral contraceptive.
Logynon A triphasic oral contraceptive.
Lomotil (diphenoxylate hydrochloride) An ANTI-DIARRHOEAL.
Lomusol (sodium cromoglycate) A drug for preventing asthma and allergic rhinitis.
lomustine A CYTOTOXIC.
loperamide hydrochloride An ANTIDIARRHOEAL.
Lopresor (metoprolol tartrate) A BETA-BLOCKER.

Ludiomil (maprotiline hydrochloride) An ANTIDEPRESSANT.
Luminal (phenobarbitone) An ANTICONVULSANT.
lymecycline A broad-spectrum ANTIBIOTIC. See tetracycline.
Lynoral (ethinyloestradiol) A SEX HORMONE (FEMALE).

Macrodantin (nitrofurantoin) An ANTIBIOTIC.
Magnapen (ampicillin and flucloxacillin) An ANTIBIOTIC.
magnesium carbonate* An ANTACID.
magnesium sulphate* A fast-acting bulk LAXATIVE. Tablets act within 2 hours if taken with plenty of water on an empty stomach.
magnesium trisilicate* An ANTACID.
MAJOR TRANQUILLIZERS See ANTIPSYCHOTICS.
Maloprim* (pyrimethamine) A drug used for prevention of malaria.
maprotiline hydrochloride A tricyclic ANTIDEPRESSANT.
Marevan (warfarin) An ANTICOAGULANT.
Marplan (isocarboxazid) An ANTIDEPRESSANT.
Marsilid (iproniazid) An ANTIDEPRESSANT.
Maxolon (metoclopramide) An ANTISPASMODIC also used as an ANTI-EMETIC.
mebeverine hydrochloride An ANTISPASMODIC.
medazepam An ANTI-ANXIETY DRUG, also used as a SLEEPING DRUG.
Medihaler-Epi (adrenaline) A BRONCHODILATOR.
medroxyprogesterone acetate A progestogen. See SEX HORMONES (FEMALE).
Melleril (thioridazine) An ANTIPSYCHOTIC.
melphalan A CYTOTOXIC.
Menophase (oestrogen and progestogen) A preparation for treating menopausal symptoms. See SEX HORMONES (FEMALE).
mepenzolate bromide An ANTISPASMODIC.
meprobamate An ANTI-ANXIETY DRUG, also used as a SLEEPING DRUG. Possible side-effects (in addition to those common to the group): headache, nausea, diarrhoea, physical weakness, visual disturbances.
mepyramine maleate* An ANTIHISTAMINE.
mesterolone A SEX HORMONE (MALE).
Metamucil* (ispaghula husk) A bulk LAXATIVE.
metformin hydrochloride A HYPOGLYCAEMIC.
methacycline hydrochloride A broad-spectrum ANTIBIOTIC. See tetracycline.

methadone hydrochloride A powerful narcotic ANALGESIC, also used as a COUGH SUPPRESSANT.
methandienone An anabolic steroid. See SEX HORMONES (MALE).
methicillin sodium An ANTIBIOTIC, given only by injection.
methotrexate A CYTOTOXIC.
methyl cellulose* A bulk LAXATIVE.
methyldopa An ANTIHYPERTENSIVE. Possible side-effects: dry mouth, drowsiness, depression, diarrhoea, swollen ankles, and failure to ejaculate.
methyltestosterone A SEX HORMONE (MALE).
metoclopramide An ANTISPASMODIC also used as an ANTI-EMETIC or for treatment of heartburn. Possible side-effects (in addition to those common to the group): drowsiness, constipation, tremor.
Metoprolol tartrate A BETA-BLOCKER.
metronidazole A drug used mainly for treatment of non-bacterial infections such as trichomonas and amoebic dysentery. Possible side-effects: nausea, indigestion, diarrhoea, unpleasant taste in the mouth.
Metrulen (oestrogen and progestogen) A preparation for treating menstrual disorders. See SEX HORMONES (FEMALE).
mexiletine hydrochloride An ANTI-ARRHYTHMIC. Possible side-effects: confusion, nystagmus, palpitations, tremor.
Mexitil (mexiletine hydrochloride) An ANTI-ARRHYTHMIC.
mianserin hydrochloride A tricyclic ANTIDEPRESSANT.
miconazole An ANTIFUNGAL. Possible side-effects: itching, rashes.
Microgynon 30 A low-oestrogen oral contraceptive.
Micronor A progestogen-only oral contraceptive.
Microval A progestogen-only oral contraceptive.
Migraleve* (paracetamol, codeine phosphate, buclizine dihydrochloride, and dioctyl sodium succinate). A preparation for relieving symptoms of migraine.
Migravess (aspirin and metoclopramide) A preparation for relieving symptoms of migraine.
Migril (ergotamine, cyclizine hydrochloride, and caffeine) A preparation for treating migraine.
Miltown (meprobamate) An ANTI-ANXIETY DRUG.
Minihep (heparin) An ANTICOAGULANT.
Minilyn A medium-oestrogen oral contraceptive.
Minocin (minocycline) An ANTIBIOTIC.

minocycline A broad-spectrum ANTIBIOTIC. See tetracycline. Minocycline can be taken only in tablet form. Possible side-effect (in addition to those common to the group): vertigo.
MINOR TRANQUILLIZERS See ANTI-ANXIETY DRUGS.
Minovlar A medium-oestrogen oral contraceptive.
Modecate (fluphenazine decanoate) An ANTIPSYCHOTIC.
Moditen (fluphenazine hydrochloride) An ANTIPSYCHOTIC.
Mogadon (nitrazepam) An ANTI-ANXIETY DRUG used as a SLEEPING DRUG.
Monistat (miconazole) An ANTIFUNGAL.
monoamine-oxidase inhibitors See ANTIDEPRESSANTS.
Monotard (insulin zinc suspension) A long-acting insulin preparation.
morphine A powerful narcotic ANALGESIC, also used as a COUGH SUPPRESSANT and ANTIDIARRHOEAL.
Multilind (nystatin) An ANTIFUNGAL.
Multivite A multivitamin preparation.
MUSCLE RELAXANTS Muscle relaxants relieve muscle spasm in disorders such as backache. Most commonly used are ANTI-ANXIETY DRUGS.
mustine hydrochloride A CYTOTOXIC, given by injection.
Myleran (busulphan) A CYTOTOXIC.
Myotonine Chloride (bethanechol chloride) A stimulant LAXATIVE.

Nacton (poldine methylsulphate) An ANTISPASMODIC.
naftidrofuryl oxalate A VASODILATOR. Possible side-effect (in addition to those common to the group): insomnia.
nalidixic acid An ANTIBIOTIC used primarily for urinary-tract infections. Possible side-effects (in addition to those common to the group): joint and muscle pains, visual disturbances. Sunbathing is inadvisable during treatment.
nandrolone An anabolic steroid. See SEX HORMONES (MALE).
naproxen sodium An aspirin-like ANALGESIC and ANTI-INFLAMMATORY used for treating rheumatic disorders. For further information see aspirin.
Nardil (phenelzine) An ANTIDEPRESSANT.
Natulan (procarbazine hydrochloride) A CYTOTOXIC.
Negram (nalidixic acid) An ANTIBIOTIC.
Nembutal (pentobarbitone sodium) A SLEEPING DRUG.
Neogest A progestogen-only oral contraceptive.

neomycin sulphate An ANTI-BIOTIC used for infections of skin, ears, and eyes. Possible side-effects (in addition to those common to the group): physical instability, rashes, itching.

Neo-NaClex (bendrofluazide) A DIURETIC.

Neoplatin (cisplatin) A CYTOTOXIC.

neostigmine A stimulant LAXATIVE, also used in treatment of myaesthenia gravis. Possible side-effects: abdominal cramps, nausea, increased salivation.

Nepenthe (morphine) An ANALGESIC.

Neulente (insulin zinc suspension) A long-acting insulin preparation.

Neuphane (isophane insulin injection) An intermediate-acting insulin preparation.

Neusulin (insulin injection) A short-acting insulin preparation.

Neutradonna (a combination of ANTACIDS with belladonna) An ANTISPASMODIC.

Nilevar (norethandrolone) A SEX HORMONE (MALE).

nitrazepam An ANTI-ANXIETY DRUG used primarily as a SLEEPING DRUG.

Nitrocontin Continus (glyceryl trinitrate) A VASODILATOR.

nitrofurantoin An ANTIBIOTIC used primarily for urinary-tract infections.

Nivemycin (neomycin sulphate) An ANTIBIOTIC.

Nobrium (medazepam) An ANTI-ANXIETY DRUG.

Noctec (chloral hydrate) A SLEEPING DRUG.

Nolvadex (tamoxifen citrate) A CYTOTOXIC.

norethandrolone An anabolic steroid. See SEX HORMONES (MALE).

norethisterone A progestogen. See SEX HORMONES (FEMALE).

Norgeston A progestogen-only oral contraceptive.

Noriday A progestogen-only oral contraceptive.

Norimin A low-oestrogen oral contraceptive.

Norinyl A medium-oestrogen oral contraceptive, also used for treating menstrual disorders.

Norlestrin A medium-oestrogen oral contraceptive, also used for treating menstrual disorders.

Normacol* (sterculia) A bulk LAXATIVE.

Normacol-X A combination of danthron (a stimulant LAXATIVE) and sterculia (a bulk LAXATIVE).

Normax* A combination of danthron (a stimulant LAXATIVE) and dioctyl sodium sulphosuccinate (a faeces-softener).

Norpace (disopyramide) An ANTI-ARRHYTHMIC.

nortriptyline A tricyclic ANTI-DEPRESSANT.

Norval (mianserin hydrochloride) An ANTIDEPRESSANT.

Nuelin (theophylline) A BRONCHODILATOR.

Nu-Seals Aspirin* (aspirin).

Nuso (insulin injection) A short-acting insulin preparation.

Nystan (nystatin) An ANTI-FUNGAL.

nystatin An ANTIFUNGAL used primarily for thrush infections. Possible side-effects if taken as tablets: nausea, diarrhoea.

Nystavescent (nystatin) An ANTIFUNGAL.

oestradiol An oestrogen. See SEX HORMONES (FEMALE).

oestriol An oestrogen. See SEX HORMONES (FEMALE).

OESTROGENS See SEX HORMONES (FEMALE).

Omnopon (papaveretum) An ANALGESIC.

Oncovin (vincristine sulphate) A CYTOTOXIC.

Orabolin (ethyloestrenol) A SEX HORMONE (MALE).

ORAL CONTRACEPTIVES See SEX HORMONES (FEMALE).

Oratrol (dichlorphenamide) A DIURETIC.

Orbenin (cloxacillin) An ANTI-BIOTIC.

orciprenaline sulphate A BRONCHODILATOR.

Orlest A medium-oestrogen oral contraceptive.

Ortho-Novin 1/50 A medium-oestrogen oral contraceptive.

Otrivine* (xylometazoline hydrochloride) A DECONGESTANT.

Ovestin (oestriol) A SEX HORMONE (FEMALE).

Ovran A medium-oestrogen oral contraceptive.

Ovran 30 A low-oestrogen oral contraceptive.

Ovranette A low-oestrogen oral contraceptive.

Ovulen 50 A medium-oestrogen oral contraceptive.

Ovysmen A low-oestrogen oral contraceptive.

oxazepam An ANTI-ANXIETY DRUG.

oxprenolol hydrochloride A BETA-BLOCKER.

oxycodone A powerful narcotic ANALGESIC, taken only as a suppository.

oxymetazoline* A DECONGESTANT.

oxymetholone An anabolic steroid. See SEX HORMONES (MALE).

Oxymycin (oxytetracycline) An ANTIBIOTIC.

oxytetracycline A broad-spectrum ANTIBIOTIC. See tetracycline, to which this preparation is similar.

PAINKILLERS See ANALGESICS.

Palaprin Forte* (aspirin) An ANALGESIC and ANTIPYRETIC.

Paludrine* (proguanil) A drug used to prevent malaria.

Panadol* (paracetamol) An ANALGESIC and ANTIPYRETIC, in tablet or liquid form.

Panasorb* (paracetamol) An ANALGESIC and ANTIPYRETIC, in tablet form.

papaveretum A powerful narcotic ANALGESIC.

Parabal (phenobarbitone) An ANTICONVULSANT.

paracetamol* A non-narcotic ANALGESIC and ANTIPYRETIC, which can be taken in tablet or liquid form. Less likely than aspirin to cause gastric irritation. Higher-than-normal doses can damage the liver irreversibly. It is unsuitable for sufferers from liver or kidney trouble.

Paramax (paracetamol and metoclopramide hydrochloride) A preparation for relieving symptoms of migraine.

Parlodel (bromocriptine) A drug for treating Parkinson's disease or hormonal disorders, and for suppressing lactation.

Parnate (tranylcypromine) An ANTIDEPRESSANT.

Paynocil* (aspirin) An ANALGESIC and ANTIPYRETIC, to be dissolved on the tongue.

penamecillin An ANTIBIOTIC.

Penbritin (ampicillin) An ANTI-BIOTIC.

Penidural (benzathine penicillin) An ANTIBIOTIC.

pentaerythritol tetranitrate A VASODILATOR.

pentazocine A mild narcotic ANALGESIC. Possible side-effect: visual hallucinations. Not recommended for anyone who has had a heart attack or for children under 6.

penthienate methobromide An ANTISPASMODIC.

pentobarbitone sodium A barbiturate SLEEPING DRUG.

Pentovis (quinestradol) A SEX HORMONE (FEMALE).

Periactin* (cyproheptadine hydrochloride) An ANTI-HISTAMINE.

Peritrate (pentaerythritol tetranitrate) A VASODILATOR.

perphenazine An ANTI-PSYCHOTIC, also used as an ANTI-EMETIC.

Pertofran (desipramine hydrochloride) An ANTI-DEPRESSANT.

Petrolagar No 1* (liquid paraffin) A faeces-softening LAXATIVE.

Petrolagar No 2* A combination of phenolphthalein (a stimulant LAXATIVE) and liquid paraffin (a faeces-softener).

phenelzine A monoamine-oxidase inhibitor ANTI-DEPRESSANT.

Phenergan (promethazine hydrochloride) An ANTI-HISTAMINE.

phenethicillin potassium An ANTIBIOTIC.

phenobarbitone An ANTI-CONVULSANT. Possible side-effects (in addition to those common to the group): restlessness, confusion (particularly in the elderly). Prolonged use may cause dependence.

phenolphthalein* A stimulant LAXATIVE. Effects may continue for several days. Possible side-effects: abdominal cramps, red-tinged urine, rashes.

phenoxymethylpenicillin An ANTIBIOTIC.

phenylbutazone An ANTI-INFLAMMATORY, taken as tablets or suppositories, used especially to treat gout. Possible side-effects: nausea, indigestion, ulceration and bleeding from mouth and digestive tract, swollen ankles, insomnia, dizziness. Prescribed only in limited quantities for short periods of time.

phenytoin An ANTI-CONVULSANT, also used as an ANTI-ARRHYTHMIC. Must be taken only in controlled doses. Signs of overdosage, which should be reported to the doctor: excessive hairiness, nervousness, acne, weight loss, blurred vision, nystagmus, unsteadiness.

pholcodine* A COUGH SUPPRESSANT. Possible side-effects: nausea, drowsiness.

Phyllocontin Continus (aminophylline) A BRONCHODILATOR.

Physeptone (methadone hydrochloride) An ANALGESIC also used as a COUGH SUPPRESSANT.

PILL, THE See SEX HORMONES (FEMALE).

pimozide An ANTIPSYCHOTIC.

pipenzolate bromide An ANTISPASMODIC.

piperazine* A drug used for treating threadworms and roundworms, available in tablet or liquid form. Possible side-effects: nausea, diarrhoea, itching.

piperazine oestrone sulphate An oestrogen. See SEX HORMONES (FEMALE).

piperidolate hydrochloride An ANTISPASMODIC.

Piptal (pipenzolate bromide) An ANTISPASMODIC.

Piriton* (chlorpheniramine maleate) An ANTIHISTAMINE.

pivampicillin A broad-spectrum ANTIBIOTIC.

poldine methylsulphate An ANTISPASMODIC.

Pondocillin (pivampicillin) An ANTIBIOTIC.

Praxilene (naftidrofuryl) A VASODILATOR.

prazosin hydrochloride An ANTIHYPERTENSIVE. Possible side-effects: feelings of faintness, drowsiness, physical weakness. Abrupt withdrawal should be avoided.

Prednesol (prednisolone) A CORTICOSTEROID.

prednisolone A CORTICOSTEROID.

prednisone A CORTICOSTEROID.

Prempak (oestrogen and progestogen) A preparation for treating menopausal symptoms. See SEX HORMONES (FEMALE).

Primolut N (norethisterone) A SEX HORMONE (FEMALE).

Primoteston Depot (testosterone) A SEX HORMONE (MALE).

Primperan (metoclopramide) An ANTISPASMODIC and ANTIEMETIC.

Pro-Actidil* (triprolidine hydrochloride) An ANTIHISTAMINE.

Pro-Banthine (propantheline bromide) An ANTISPASMODIC.

probenecid A drug used to prevent gout. Possible side-effects: nausea, frequent urination, headache, flushes, dizziness, rashes.

procainamide hydrochloride An ANTI-ARRHYTHMIC. Possible side-effects: nausea, diarrhoea, rashes, fever.

procaine penicillin An ANTIBIOTIC, given only by injection.

procarbazine hydrochloride A CYTOTOXIC. It is inadvisable to drink alcohol while under treatment with procarbazine.

prochlorperazine A weak ANTIPSYCHOTIC used primarily as an ANTI-EMETIC.

Proctofibe* (bran) A bulk LAXATIVE.

Progesic (fenoprofen) An ANALGESIC, ANTIPYRETIC, and ANTI-INFLAMMATORY.

progesterone A progestogen. See SEX HORMONES (FEMALE).

proguanil* A drug used for prevention of malaria. Available as tablets, to be taken daily, starting the day before entering a malaria zone and continuing for a month after leaving the area. Possible side-effect: indigestion.

Progynova (oestradiol) A SEX HORMONE (FEMALE).

Proladone (oxycodone) An ANALGESIC.

promazine hydrochloride An ANTIPSYCHOTIC.

promethazine hydrochloride* An ANTIHISTAMINE also used for allergic disorders, nausea, and vertigo.

promethazine theoclate* An ANTIHISTAMINE primarily used for relief of nausea and vertigo.

Pronestyl (procainamide hydrochloride) An ANTI-ARRHYTHMIC.

propantheline bromide An ANTISPASMODIC.

Propranolol hydrochloride A BETA-BLOCKER.

Prostigmin (neostigmine) A stimulant LAXATIVE.

protamine zinc insulin preparation A long-acting insulin preparation.

Prothiaden (dothiepin hydrochloride) An ANTIDEPRESSANT.

Provera (medroxyprogesterone acetate) A SEX HORMONE (FEMALE).

Pro-viron (mesterolone) A SEX HORMONE (MALE).

pseudoephedrine hydrochloride A BRONCHODILATOR and nasal DECONGESTANT.

Pulmadil (rimiterol hydrobromide) A BRONCHODILATOR.

PURGATIVES See LAXATIVES.

pyrazinamide An ANTIBIOTIC used primarily for treatment of tuberculosis. Possible side-effects (in addition to those common to the group): fever, loss of appetite, jaundice.

pyrimethamine* A drug used for prevention of malaria. Available as tablets, to be taken weekly, starting a week before entering a malaria zone and continuing for 4 to 6 weeks after leaving. Possible side-effect: rashes.

Pyrogastrone (carbenoxolone) A drug used for healing peptic ulcers.

quinestradol An oestrogen. See SEX HORMONES (FEMALE).

Rapitard MC (biphasic insulin preparation) An intermediate-acting insulin preparation.

Rastinon (tolbutamide) A HYPOGLYCAEMIC.

Reasec (diphenoxylate hydrochloride) An ANTIDIARRHOEAL.

Redoxon (ascorbic acid) Vitamin C.

Remnos (nitrazepam) A SLEEPING DRUG.

Retcin (erythromycin) An ANTIBIOTIC.

Rifadin (rifampicin) An ANTIBIOTIC.

rifampicin An ANTIBIOTIC used to treat tuberculosis. Possible side-effects (in addition to those common to the group): loss of appetite, jaundice, orange-red urine, and inefficiency of oral contraception.

Rifinah (rifampicin) An ANTIBIOTIC.

Rimactane (rifampicin) An ANTIBIOTIC.

Rimactazid (rifampicin) An ANTIBIOTIC.

Rimifon (isoniazid) An ANTIBIOTIC.

rimiterol hydrobromide A BRONCHODILATOR.

Rivotril (clonazepam) An ANTI-CONVULSANT.

Rondomycin (methacycline hydrochloride) An ANTIBIOTIC.

Rynacrom (sodium cromoglycate) A drug used for preventing asthma and allergic rhinitis.

Rythmodan (disopyramide) An ANTI-ARRHYTHMIC.

salbutamol A BRONCHODILATOR.

Saluric (chlorothiazide) A DIURETIC.

Sancos* (pholcodine) A COUGH SUPPRESSANT.

Sectral (acebutolol hydrochloride) A BETA-BLOCKER.

SEDATIVES See ANTI-ANXIETY DRUGS.

Semi-Daonil (glibenclamide) A HYPOGLYCAEMIC.

Semitard (insulin zinc suspension) An intermediate-acting insulin preparation.

Senade* (senna) A stimulant LAXATIVE.

senna* A stimulant LAXATIVE. Possible side-effects: abdominal cramps, red-tinged urine.

Senokot* (senna) A stimulant LAXATIVE.

Septrin (co-trimoxazole) An ANTIBIOTIC.

Serc (betahistine hydrochloride) An ANTI-EMETIC.

Serenace (haloperidol) An ANTIPSYCHOTIC.

Serenid (oxazepam) An ANTI-ANXIETY DRUG.

SEX HORMONES (FEMALE) The hormones responsible for development of female secondary sexual characteristics and regulation of menstrual cycle. Sex hormone drugs fall into 2 main categories, oestrogens and progestogens. They are used in treatment of menstrual and menopausal disorders, and as oral contraceptives. Oestrogens may be used for treating cancer of the breast or prostate, progestogens for treating endometriosis. Sex hormones may be taken as tablets, given by injection, or implanted in muscle tissue. Possible side-effects: nausea, weight gain, headache, depression, breast enlargement and tenderness, rashes and skin pigmentation, changes in sexual drive, abnormal blood-clotting causing heart disorders. Oestrogens are not prescribed for anyone with circulatory or liver trouble, and oestrogen treatment must be carefully controlled for people who have had jaundice, diabetes, epilepsy, or heart or kidney disease. Progestogen treatment is not prescribed for people with liver trouble and must be

carefully controlled for anyone who has asthma, epilepsy, or heart or kidney disease.

SEX HORMONES (MALE) Hormones (of which the most powerful is testosterone) responsible for development of male secondary sexual characteristics. Small quantities are also produced in females. As drugs, male sex hormones are given to compensate for hormonal deficiency in hypopituitarism or testicular disorders. They may be used for treating cancer of the breast in women, but synthetic derivatives, the anabolic steroids, which have less marked side-effects and specific anti-oestrogens are often preferable. Anabolic steroids also have a "body building" effect that has led to their (usually illegal) use in competitive sports, for both men and women. Male sex hormones and anabolic steroids can be taken as tablets, given by injection, or implanted in muscle tissue. Possible side-effects: oedema, weight gain, weakness, loss of appetite, drowsiness, nausea. High dose in women may cause cessation of menstruation, enlargement of the clitoris, deepening of the voice, shrinking of the breasts, hairiness, male-pattern baldness. Treatment is inadvisable for people with kidney or liver trouble and must be carefully controlled for anyone suffering from epilepsy or migraine.

Sinemet (levodopa) A drug used for treating Parkinson's disease.

SLEEPING DRUGS The 2 main groups of drugs used for inducing sleep are ANTI-ANXIETY drugs and barbiturates. All such drugs have a sedative effect in low doses and are effective sleeping pills (or potions) in higher doses. Anti-anxiety drugs are more widely used than barbiturates because they are safer, side-effects are less marked, and there is less risk of eventual physical and psychological dependence. Possible side-effects of all types: "hangover", dizziness, dry mouth, and (especially in the elderly) clumsiness and confusion. Sleeping drugs are habit-forming, should be taken for short periods only, and should be discontinued gradually. Broken, restless sleep and vivid dreams may follow withdrawal and may persist for weeks. It is inadvisable to drive, handle dangerous machinery, or drink alcohol until the effects of a sleeping drug have completely worn off.

sodium bicarbonate* An ANTACID. Preparations containing sodium bicarbonate are unsuitable for prolonged use or for anyone on a salt-restricted diet. Possible side-effect: belching.

sodium cromoglycate A drug for preventing attacks of asthma and allergic rhinitis. Normally taken by inhalation, in the form of aerosol spray, powder, or nasal drops. Possible side-effects: throat irritation and cough, chest tightness, breathlessness.

sodium picosulphate* A stimulant LAXATIVE. Possible side-effect: abdominal cramps.

sodium valproate An ANTI-CONVULSANT. Possible side-effect (in addition to those common to the group): temporary loss of hair.

Solprin* (soluble aspirin) An ANALGESIC and ANTIPYRETIC.

Soneryl (butobarbitone) A SLEEPING DRUG.

Sorbitrate (isosorbide dinitrate) A VASODILATOR.

Sotacor (sotalol hydrochloride) A BETA-BLOCKER.

sotalol hydrochloride A BETA-BLOCKER.

Sparine (promazine hydrochloride) An ANTIPSYCHOTIC.

stanozolol An anabolic steroid. See SEX HORMONES (MALE).

Stelazine (trifluoperazine) An ANTIPSYCHOTIC and ANTI-EMETIC.

Stemetil (prochlorperazine) An ANTIPSYCHOTIC and ANTI-EMETIC.

sterculia* A bulk LAXATIVE.

STEROIDS See CORTICO-STEROIDS.

Streptase (streptokinase) A thrombolytic drug. See ANTI-COAGULANTS AND THROMBOLYTICS.

streptokinase A thrombolytic drug, given by injection only. Side-effects: rashes, haemorrhage, fever, allergic reactions. See ANTICOAGULANTS AND THROMBOLYTICS.

streptomycin An ANTIBIOTIC, given only by injection. Possible side-effects (in addition to those common to the group): disturbance of hearing and balance.

Streptotriad (sulphadiazine) An ANTIBIOTIC.

Stromba (stanozolol) A SEX HORMONE (MALE).

Stugeron* (cinnarizine) An ANTIHISTAMINE.

Sudafed (pseudoephedrine hydrochloride) A BRONCHO-DILATOR and DECONGESTANT.

sulphadiazine An ANTIBIOTIC, given only by injection.

sulphadimidine An ANTI-BIOTIC used for urinary-tract infections and given by injection.

sulphamethizole An ANTI-BIOTIC used primarily for urinary-tract infections.

Sulphamezathine (sulpha-dimidine) An ANTIBIOTIC.

Sulphatriad (sulphadiazine) An ANTIBIOTIC.

sulphinpyrazone A drug taken in tablet form, for prevention of gout. Possible side-effects: nausea, abdominal pain.

Surmontil (trimipramine) An ANTIDEPRESSANT.

Sustac (glyceryl trinitrate) A VASODILATOR.

Sustanon 100 (testosterone) A SEX HORMONE (MALE).

Symmetrel (amantadine) A drug used for treating Parkinson's disease and as an ANTIVIRAL.

Synflex (naproxen sodium) An ANALGESIC and ANTI-INFLAMMATORY.

Syraprim (trimethoprim) An ANTIBIOTIC.

Tace (chlorotrianisene) A SEX HORMONE (FEMALE).

Tacitin (benzoctamine hydro-chloride) An ANTI-ANXIETY DRUG.

Tagamet (cimetidine) A drug used for healing peptic ulcers.

talampicillin hydrochloride A broad-spectrum ANTIBIOTIC.

Talpen (talampicillin hydro-chloride) An ANTIBIOTIC.

tamoxifen citrate A CYTO TOXIC.

Tegretol (carbamazepine) An ANTICONVULSANT.

Tenormin (atenolol) A BETA-BLOCKER.

terbutaline sulphate A BRONCHODILATOR.

Terramycin (oxytetracycline) An ANTIBIOTIC.

testosterone A SEX HOR-MONE (MALE).

Tetrabid (tetracycline) An ANTI-BIOTIC.

tetracycline A broad-spectrum ANTIBIOTIC. Must be taken between meals, and not with milk, antacids, or iron preparations. Because it may cause staining of developing teeth, tetracycline should not be taken in pregnancy or given to children under 8.

Tetracyn (tetracycline) An ANTIBIOTIC.

Tetralysal (lymecycline) An ANTIBIOTIC.

Theodrox (aminophylline) A BRONCHODILATOR.

Theograd (theophylline) A BRONCHODILATOR.

theophylline A BRONCHO-DILATOR.

thioridazine An ANTI-PSYCHOTIC.

THROMBOLYTICS See ANTI-COAGULANTS AND THROM-BOLYTICS.

thyroxine A HORMONE taken in tablet form for treatment of hypothyroidism. Possible side-effects: angina, palpitations, muscle cramps, headache, rest-lessness, excitability, flushing,

sweating, diarrhoea, weight loss. Thyroxine is not prescribed for people with heart trouble.

timolol maleate A BETA-BLOCKER.

Tofranil (imipramine hydro-chloride) An ANTIDEPRESSANT.

Tolanase (tolazamide) A HYPO-GLYCAEMIC.

tolazamide A HYPO-GLYCAEMIC.

tolbutamide A HYPO-GLYCAEMIC.

Trancopal (chlormezanone) An ANTI-ANXIETY DRUG.

TRANQUILLIZERS ''Tranquillizer'' describes any drug with a calming or sedative effect. Drugs sometimes described as minor tranquillizers are called ANTI-ANXIETY DRUGS, and drugs sometimes described as major tranquillizers are called ANTI-PSYCHOTICS.

Tranxene (clorazepate dipotas-sium) An ANTI-ANXIETY DRUG.

tranylcypromine A monoamine-oxidase inhibitor ANTIDEPRESSANT.

Trasicor (oxprenolol hydro-chloride) A BETA-BLOCKER.

triamcinolone A CORTICO-STEROID.

triamterene A DIURETIC.

trifluoperazine An ANTI-PSYCHOTIC, also used as an ANTI-EMETIC.

trimethoprim An ANTIBIOTIC used primarily for urinary-tract infections.

trimipramine A tricyclic ANTI-DEPRESSANT.

Trimopan (trimethoprim) An ANTIBIOTIC.

Trinordiol A triphasic oral contraceptive.

Triopaed* (pholcodine) A COUGH SUPPRESSANT

Triplopen (benethamine penicil-lin) An ANTIBIOTIC.

triprolidine hydrochloride* An ANTIHISTAMINE.

Trisequens (oestrogen and progestogen) A preparation for treating menopausal symptoms. See SEX HORMONES (FEMALE).

Tryptizol (amitriptyline) An ANTIDEPRESSANT.

Tuinal (amylobarbitone) A SLEEPING DRUG.

Ubretid (distigmine bromide) A stimulant LAXATIVE.

Ultratard (insulin zinc suspen-sion) A long-acting insulin preparation.

Urolucosil (sulphamethizole) An ANTIBIOTIC.

Utovlan (norethisterone) A SEX HORMONE (FEMALE).

Valium (diazepam) An ANTI-ANXIETY DRUG.

Valoid* (cyclizine) An ANTI-HISTAMINE.

Vancocin (vancomycin) An ANTIBIOTIC.

vancomycin An ANTIBIOTIC. Possible side-effects (in addition to those common to the group): fever, rashes, ringing in the ears.

Vascardin (isosorbide dinitrate) A VASODILATOR.

VASODILATORS Drugs that dilate blood vessels. Most widely used in prevention and treatment of angina, but also for treating heart failure and certain circulat-ory disorders. Vasodilators are taken as tablets, often dissolved beneath the tongue for swift action. Possible side-effects: headache, palpitations, feelings of faintness, nausea, vomiting, diarrhoea, nasal stuffiness.

Vatensol (guanoclor sulphate) An ANTIHYPERTENSIVE.

V-Cil-K (phenoxymethyl-penicillin) An ANTIBIOTIC.

Velosef (cephradine) An ANTI-BIOTIC.

Ventolin (salbutamol) A BRONCHODILATOR.

verapamil hydrochloride An ANTI-ARRHYTHMIC. Possible side-effects: nausea, feelings of faintness.

Vertigon (prochlorperazine) An ANTIPSYCHOTIC.

Vibramycin (doxycycline) An ANTIBIOTIC.

vincristine sulphate A CYTO-TOXIC, given only by injection. Possible side-effects (in addition to those common to the group): odd skin sensations, muscle weakness, constipation, abdominal pain.

Vi-Siblin* (ispaghula husk) A bulk LAXATIVE.

Vita-E (alpha tocopheryl ace-tate) Vitamin E.

VITAMINS Chemicals, essential for good health, that are not man-ufactured by the body, but are present in a normal diet. People whose diet is inadequate or who suffer from digestive-tract or liver disorders may need extra vita-mins. These are generally availa-ble without prescription.

Vitavel A multivitamin prepara-tion.

warfarin An ANTICOAGULANT, taken in tablet form.

Welldorm (dichloralphenazone) A SLEEPING DRUG.

xylometazoline hydrochlor-ide* A DECONGESTANT.

X-Prep* (senna) A stimulant LAXATIVE.

Zarontin (ethosuximide) An ANTICONVULSANT.

Zinamide (pyrazinamide) An ANTIBIOTIC.

Zyloric (allopurinol) A drug used for prevention of gout.

Glossary

A

Abrasion A wound in which the surface of the body (usually the skin) is scraped or worn away, with little or no damage to underlying tissues.

Abscess A localized collection of pus that builds up under pressure and may eventually burst.

Acid reflux The welling up of acidic stomach juices into the lower part of the oesophagus. Acid reflux irritates the lining of the oesophagus and causes heartburn.

Acupuncture A system of treatment in which needles are inserted into the skin and either left or manipulated for several minutes. Acupuncturists are not usually medical doctors, but there is evidence that acupuncture is an effective form of treatment for a number of complaints – particularly for painful conditions such as sciatica.

Acute A term applied to an illness or pain that comes on suddenly. Acute attacks of illness tend to be brief but severe. Compare Chronic.

Acute adrenal failure The sudden failure of the adrenal glands to produce steroid hormones because of a condition such as Addison's disease or because a course of steroid tablets is abruptly stopped. The symptoms are profound weakness, confusion, and even collapse.

Addiction Habitual and irresistible use of a drug (including nicotine or alcohol). An addict's reliance on the addictive drug may cause painful "withdrawal symptoms" if abstinence is attempted. See also Dependence and Tolerance.

Allergen Any substance – for instance, food, animal fur, pollen grain, speck of dust – that is normally harmless but provokes an allergic reaction in susceptible individuals.

Allergy A reaction, marked by any of various symptoms, to an allergen to which previous exposure has made the body sensitive. Allergies usually occur as the result of a misdirected response by the immune system, which usually involves production of antibodies against otherwise harmless substances.

Allopathy The standard form of medical practice in this country. Compare Homeopathy.

Ambylopia Partial or complete blindness without obvious physical cause – for example, the blindness sometimes associated with alcohol poisoning.

Amnesia Partial or complete loss of memory.

Anaesthetic A drug for inducing loss of sensation (and hence pain) in many medical and surgical procedures. Local anaesthetics, used for deadening pain in only one part of the body, may be either given as injections – as, for example, in epidural or spinal injections – or, very occasionally, rubbed or sprayed onto a limited area. General anaesthetics produce unconsciousness and are normally administered by specially trained doctors (anaesthetists). General anaesthetics are given either by inhalation through tubes leading to a mask placed over the patient's face or by injection.

Anaesthetist A doctor who specializes in administering anaesthetics and caring for patients during a surgical operation and immediately afterwards.

Analgesic A painkilling drug. For further information see Drug index.

Anaphylaxis A generalized allergic reaction. Anaphylaxis produces symptoms ranging from mild (flushing, urticaria, and asthma) to severe (such as collapse due to shock).

Aneurysm A swelling that occurs if a blood-vessel wall or the heart wall becomes weakened and balloons outwards as a result of pressure of the blood within it.

Angiography A technique for examining the interior of blood vessels by the injection – usually through a catheter – of a solution visible on X-ray. Passage of the solution can be followed on a television screen simultaneously with a recording on film of a progression of pictures (angiograms).

Anosmia Loss of sense of smell. Sense of taste is also diminished since the two senses are closely related.

Anoxia Lack of oxygen. Anoxic tissues cannot function properly; if completely deprived of oxygen for more than a few minutes, they die. See also Cyanosis and Infarct.

Ante-natal Before birth. The term "ante-natal" is applied to an event or condition relating to pregnancy that occurs during pregnancy. Compare Post-natal and Neonatal.

Antibiotic A drug, usually derived from living organisms, that combats bacterial infection. For further information see Drug index.

Antibodies Complex substances formed by special cells to neutralize or destroy antigens. Antibodies recognize only the antigens that provoke their formation. Their activity fights infection but can be damaging, as in allergies and auto-immune disease.

Anticoagulant A drug that prevents the formation of blood clots. For further information see Drug index.

Anticonvulsant A drug for prevention or relief of fits. For further information see Drug index.

Antidepressant A mood-lifting drug. For further information see Drug index.

Antifungal A drug that combats fungal infections such as thrush. For further information see Drug index.

Antigen Any substance – for example, the cellular protein of a toxic microbe – that can be detected by the body's immune system. Detection of an antigen usually stimulates production of antibodies.

Antihistamine A drug to counteract some types of allergy. For further information see Drug index.

Antiseptic Any substance for killing microbes that is too powerful to be swallowed or injected into the body.

Antiserum Serum rich in antibodies. Animal as well as human blood may be used for obtaining types of antiserum to combat specific types of infection by providing a temporary supply of antibodies.

Antithrombotic A drug that prevents the formation of blood clots. For further information see ANTICOAGULANTS in Drug index.

Antitoxin A substance that neutralizes the effects of a toxin.

Apicectomy A dental procedure used to treat chronic tooth abscesses. Under anaesthetic an incision is made in the gum below the infected tooth, the infected root tip is cut away, and the remaining root of the tooth is filled.

Arteriography Angiography of an artery. The resultant pictures are known as arteriograms.

Artificial insemination A procedure in which seminal fluid is injected into the vagina in order to accomplish conception without sexual intercourse.

Ascites An abnormal collection of fluid within the abdominal cavity due to disease of the heart, liver, and kidney etc.

Aspiration A diagnostic or treatment procedure in which fluid is sucked from a body cavity by means of an instrument

such as a syringe. The cavity may be a natural one (the abdominal cavity, for example) or one due to disease (a kidney cyst, for example).

Ataxia Lack of coordination in body movements due to some form of nerve or brain damage.

Atheroma Fatty tissue that develops in an arterial wall and forms a patch (also called a plaque) that narrows the artery.

Atresia Congenital membranous blockage of a body orifice such as the anus, or complete absence of a portion of a passageway such as the oesophagus. Atresia is life-threatening, but can often be treated soon after birth by surgical removal of the blockage or restoration of the missing passageway.

Atrium One of the 2 smaller chambers of the heart (formerly known as auricles).

Audiometry A test of hearing ability. Audiometry involves the use of special headphones in a soundproof room. The resultant measurements of hearing ability are called audiograms. See also Impedance testing.

Auricle 1. The visible part of the ear (also called the pinna). 2. See Atrium.

Autoimmune A term used to describe a condition in which the body manufactures antibodies against the body itself, causing damage to tissues that the antibodies attack. This defect in the immune system produces symptoms of autoimmune disease (see, for instance, rheumatoid arthritis or pernicious anaemia).

Autopsy Examination of a dead body in order to ascertain the cause of death. Also known as Post mortem.

B

Barium enema An enema containing the metallic chemical barium, which shows up on X-ray pictures. A series of pictures taken while the enema is retained in the bowel reveals the lining of the colon and rectum. The procedure takes about 1 hour. Compare Barium meal and Barium swallow.

Barium meal A palatable liquid containing the metallic chemical barium, which is visible on X-ray. The liquid is drunk, and its progress through the upper part of the digestive tract during the next 2 to 3 hours can be followed visually on a screen simultaneously with the recording on film of a progressive series of X-ray pictures. By the time the barium reaches the colon

it is too diluted to give a clear picture; a barium enema is needed to view lower parts of the intestinal tract.

Barium swallow A palatable liquid containing the metallic chemical barium, which is visible on X-ray. The liquid is drunk and its progress down the oesophagus recorded on a series of X-ray pictures. The procedure, which takes about 10 minutes, is used for detecting oesophageal disease (for example, stricture) where there is no need to follow the passage of barium through the rest of the digestive tract.

Behaviour therapy A form of psychotherapy in which, by means of various techniques, patients are trained to replace undesirable by more desirable habits of behaviour. Behaviour therapists do not normally try to analyse probable reasons for the original development of undesirable behaviour patterns.

Benign A term applied to an abnormal growth, indicating that it will neither spread to surrounding tissues nor recur after removal. Compare Malignant.

Beta-blocker A drug that slows heart activity and thus lowers blood pressure. For further information see Drug index.

Biliary colic Colic in the upper right part of the abdomen, often accompanied by nausea and vomiting. Biliary colic is due to spasm in the muscles of the gallbladder or bile duct, usually provoked by the passage or attempted passage of a gallstone.

Biofeedback A method of controlling an involuntary body function such as blood pressure or temperature by means of a sight or sound signal on a recording instrument wired to the patient. When alerted by the signal to a change in pressure or body temperature, the patient makes an effort to relax; a further signal informs him or her when relaxation has produced the sought-after effect. Patients who train in biofeedback often carry the experience on into daily life.

Biopsy A small piece of tissue removed from anywhere in the body for microscopic analysis. Biopsies are usually done in order to determine whether or not an abnormal growth is malignant.

Blood count A diagnostic test of a specimen of blood in order to determine the numbers of the various cells (red, white, and platelets) within a standard volume. Also known as a cell count.

Blood volume estimation A diagnostic test in which a sample of blood is taken from a vein and then reinjected with a radioactive isotope marker into the vein. After a period of time more blood samples are taken. These are analysed, and from the results the volume of blood in the body is calculated.

Bolus The technical name for a ball of chewed food as it passes from the mouth through the gastrointestinal tract.

Bone graft A piece or pieces of bone – normally taken from somewhere else in the patient's body – packed around a fractured bone to facilitate healing.

Botulism A rare type of food poisoning caused by a bacterium found, usually, in improperly canned or preserved foods. Early symptoms – vomiting, abdominal pains, double vision – begin hours after eating the contaminated substance. Severe breathing difficulties may develop, and risk of death is high.

Bougie A tube or rod-like instrument made of a flexible or rigid material. Bougies are useful for either exploring body passages or dilating over-narrow channels (as, for instance, in cases of oesophageal stricture).

Breech A fetus that is positioned in the womb so that the buttocks rest at the base of the womb.

Bronchodilator A drug for widening bronchial passages. For further information see Drug index.

Bronchoscopy A diagnostic procedure in which a flexible endoscope with a lighting system (a bronchoscope) is passed down the throat in order to examine the air passages (bronchi) of the lungs. Modern bronchoscopes are thin and flexible, and the procedure usually causes little discomfort.

Buffer A substance composed of selected chemicals that acts to neutralize an acid or alkali added to it.

Bypass A term for the surgical construction of a diversion to allow a body fluid such as blood to flow round an obstruction. Compare Shunt.

C

Calculus A hard white, creamish, or brown deposit that forms on teeth surfaces. Calculus is composed of plaque that has become hardened by deposits of calcium compounds, probably from the saliva.

Capsule 1. An oval or cylindrical pill containing a liquid, granular, or powdered drug within a soluble plastic-like coating. 2. The tough fibrous tissue that encloses

an organ or surrounds a joint. A joint capsule is lined with synovial membrane and reinforced by external ligaments.

Carcinogen A cancer-causing substance.

Carcinoma A malignant growth composed of abnormally multiplying surface tissues such as those of the skin, linings of internal organs (the bladder or intestines, for instance), or linings of glands (in the breast or prostate, for instance). Carcinomas, the most common type of cancer, can often be treated successfully if discovered early.

Cardiac catheterization A diagnostic procedure in which a catheter is passed along a blood vessel on into the heart in order to investigate the heart at work. The procedure is done under local anaesthetic at the point of entry of the catheter and is virtually painless.

Cardiac massage A manual technique for stimulating and reviving a stopped heart by rhythmically pressing upon and releasing the lower breastbone.

Cardiogenic A term applied to shock brought on by faulty action of the heart – as a result, for instance, of the heart's inability to work properly because of severe damage from thrombosis.

Cardiomyotomy Surgical cutting of the muscles encircling the entrance to the stomach. Cardiomyotomy is done when the junction between oesophagus and stomach has become severely narrowed by disease. The incision is made in the upper part of the abdomen.

Carrier 1. A person whose body harbours infectious disease-producing organisms without developing symptoms of the disease. Without suffering themselves, carriers spread infectious diseases to other people. 2. A person whose chromosomes bear a gene for some type of hereditary characteristic that he or she may not have but that may be passed on to future generations.

CAT brain scan An abbreviation for "computerized axial tomography" brain scan, a painless diagnostic procedure in which hundreds of X-ray pictures are taken as a camera revolves around the head. The pictures are fed into a computer, which integrates them to reveal structures within the skull.

Catheter A flexible tube for withdrawing fluid (or air) from or squirting fluid into a part of the body such as the bladder or a blood vessel.

Cauterization The destruction of tissue by burning it away with a caustic chemical

or red-hot instrument, or by means of diathermy. Cauterization is most often used for the removal of growths on the skin or mucous membrane such as warts.

Cell The smallest structural unit of body tissue. Every cell consists of a nucleus containing genetic information surrounded by a protein-rich mass known as the cytoplasm. Different body tissues are built up from different types of cell, and there are many billions of cells in a human body.

Cell count See Blood count.

Centrifuge An apparatus for separating heavier substances from lighter ones in a mixture. Separation is achieved through a rapid-spinning process in which gravitational pull is greater on the heavier substances. See, for example, Plasmapheresis.

Cerebral Applying to or associated with the structure or functions of the brain.

Cerebral angiography Angiography of blood vessels that supply the brain. The resultant pictures (cerebral angiograms) can indicate the presence of neurological and circulatory conditions such as tumours and aneurysms.

Chancre An ulcerated, swollen, but painless lump. Most – but not all – chancres are an early symptom of syphilis.

Chiropodist A non-medically qualified specialist in the treatment of minor disorders of the feet.

Chiropractic A system of treatment involving forceful manipulation of joints in order to effect cure. Chiropractors are not usually medically qualified doctors.

Cholecystography A diagnostic procedure for examining the interior of the gallbladder and bile duct. A substance visible on X-ray is taken as a tablet and photographed as it becomes concentrated in the gallbladder and passes down the bile duct. Findings are recorded on a series of pictures (cholecystograms). Cholecystography is usually an outpatient procedure and takes about 30 minutes to perform.

Cholesterol A steroid-like chemical present in some foods, notably animal fats, eggs, and dairy produce. An over-high level of cholesterol in the body is associated with atherosclerosis, and excess cholesterol in the bile may cause gallstones.

Chorea Involuntary body movements of a jerky, complex, but coordinated nature. The cause is brain damage, not a muscular disorder.

Chromosomes The thread-like structures in a living cell that contain the cell's genetic information. Each chromosome is composed of thousands of genes; and all cells in complex organisms, except reproductive cells, contain paired sets of chromosomes (one from each parent). Chromosomes in reproductive cells are not paired.

Chronic A term applied to a condition that has been, or is expected to be, present for a long time. Chronic conditions tend to improve or worsen slowly, and are not necessarily life-threatening. Compare Acute.

Cilia Minute hairs on the surface of mucous membranes such as those lining the trachea and bronchi. The waving movement of cilia propels mucus, dust particles, and bacteria out of the lungs.

Circumcision Surgical removal of the prepuce (foreskin), leaving the tip of the penis harmlessly exposed.

Climacteric See Menopause.

Clinic Any place where patients may be seen or treated by medical personnel.

Clubbing A condition in which fingertips become thickened and nails unnaturally curved. Although a common symptom of disorders such as bronchiectasis and congenital heart disease, clubbing itself is harmless and needs no treatment.

Colic Abdominal pain that comes in waves separated by relatively pain-free intervals. Precise site of pain depends upon the cause. Biliary colic, for example, affects the upper right area of the abdomen, near the gallbladder; the colic of gastroenteritis generally spreads over the whole abdomen; etc.

Colposcope A special microscope with a lens that can be inserted in the vagina to examine the interior. Colposcopy is useful for detection of cervical conditions.

Cone biopsy A surgical procedure in which a cone-shaped portion of cervix is removed for laboratory examination.

Congenital A term used for a disease or condition present at birth.

Congestive A term applied to heart failure when both the left and right sides of the heart are affected.

Contagious A term applied to disease spread by personal contact rather than indirectly as in air or water.

Contusion Injury caused by crushing of body tissues. Bruises are the most familiar examples of contusion.

Convalescence An indefinite period of time during which health continues to improve after active treatment for an illness or injury has ceased. The convalescent period ends when maximum recovery has been achieved.

Coronary Applying to or associated with the structure or functions of the arteries that supply blood to the heart.

Coronary arteriography Angiography of the heart muscle done during cardiac catheterization. The resultant pictures, called coronary arteriograms, can show the location of patches of atheroma, blockage due to thrombosis, etc. in the coronary arteries.

Cryosurgery The use of extreme cold – for example, from liquid or solid gas – to destroy tissues. Cryosurgery, used for freezing away excessive or abnormal tissue not necessarily due to a growth, is an effective treatment in some cases of haemorrhoids, cervical erosions, and certain kinds of brain trouble.

Culture A medical term for growing microbes or living cells on a specially prepared substance (known as the growth medium). The preparation of such organisms on the medium is known as a culture. Cultures are especially useful for identifying disease-producing organisms and testing drugs.

Curettage A procedure involving the removal of a thin layer of skin or internal lining (e.g. from the uterus). The purpose of curettage is either to remove abnormal tissue or obtain a sample of tissue for microscopic analysis.

Cyanosis Blueness of skin resulting from an excessive amount of oxygen-depleted haemoglobin in the blood.

Cyclothymia An inborn tendency to experience repeated swings of mood from elation to depression not directly related to external events. People with cyclothymic temperaments are not necessarily mentally ill.

Cyst 1. Any cavity enclosed by a protective wall of cells or fibrous tissue and containing liquid or semi-liquid material. 2. The prefix "cyst-" often refers specifically to the bladder as in cystitis. 3. An encapsulated protective form assumed by many microbes and parasites.

Cystography A diagnostic procedure in which an X-ray (cystogram) of the bladder is obtained by passing a solution visible on X-ray into the bladder.

Cystoscopy Endoscopy of the bladder by means of a cystoscope passed through the urethra. Cystoscopy is usually done under a general anaesthetic and requires an overnight stay in hospital.

Cytotoxic A drug for destroying body cells, particularly cancerous ones. For further information see Drug index.

D

Defibrillation See Electroversion.

Dehydration A physical condition caused by the loss of an excessive amount of water from the body, often due to severe vomiting or diarrhoea. Easily recognized signs of dehydration are sunken eyes, wrinkled skin, dry mouth, and – in babies – a sunken fontanelle.

Delirium tremens A group of symptoms that may occur if an alcoholic abstains from drinking for a day or so (or even, in rare cases, without abstention). Symptoms range in severity from shaking limbs to hallucinations, often of insects crawling over the sufferer's body.

Denture granuloma A hard, pale lump that may form along the edge of a denture as the result of constant slight irritation and rubbing from an ill-fitting or worn-out denture.

Dependence The need for regular doses of a drug (including nicotine or alcohol) in order to maintain a sense of relative well-being. See also Addiction and Tolerance.

Depot A medical term for the form in which a drug may be administered in order to achieve its effects gradually over an extensive period. Examples of depot drugs designed to seep into the bloodstream by degrees are sex hormones, insulin, and certain kinds of tranquillizer.

Desensitization 1. A process in which sufferers from allergies are repeatedly given small quantities of causative substances (usually by injection) so as to build up resistance to allergic reaction. 2. A similar treatment for phobic people. By repeated exposure to increasingly severe aspects of the thing feared, they may eventually "learn" to tolerate it.

Dialysis A technique for artificial removal of waste products from the body by clearing either the blood (haemodialysis) or the peritoneal cavity (peritoneal dialysis). Dialysis is a means of compensating for the inadequate functioning of diseased kidneys. All artificial kidney machines use some form of dialysis.

Diastole The part of the heart's cycle when the ventricles are relaxing and refilling with blood. Diastolic blood pressure is the lower reading obtained when blood pressure is measured. Compare Systole.

Diathermy The use of high-frequency electric current to heat body tissues. Current passed through a small electrode can burn away the tissues it touches and may be used as a form of bloodless surgery. Applied over a large area, the warmth of diathermy relieves pain.

Dilatation See Dilation.

Dilation The widening of a passageway or body orifice either intentionally, as with a bougie or drug, or by involuntary relaxation of constricting walls or encircling tissue. Also known as dilatation.

Diuretic Any substance that increases urine production, thus reducing fluid content of the body. See also Drug index.

Douche A stream of fluid or gas projected onto part of the body or into a cavity in order to cleanse or provide superficial treatment. Doctors do not generally recommend one very common use of douching: the flushing out of the vagina for hygienic or contraceptive purposes.

Drip The common name for an intravenous infusion. A fluid substance is injected into the body by letting it flow down into a vein from an elevated sterile container; the rate of flow is measured by counting the rate of dripping through a transparent chamber.

Dys- A prefix meaning painful, difficult, and/or abnormal. For example, dysmenorrhoea (painful periods), dysphagia (painful and/or difficult swallowing), dysuria (painful and/or difficult urination).

E

ECG Abbreviation for electrocardiogram. See Electrocardiography.

Echocardiography The use of ultrasound to examine the structure of the heart. The waves are directed at the heart through the chest, with findings recorded graphically on an echocardiogram.

ECT See Electroconvulsive therapy.

EEG See Electroencephalography.

Effusion A collection of fluid in an abnormal space between neighbouring body tissues that are normally in contact – for instance, between the lung and pleura or the meeting of bones within a joint.

Electrocardiography A painless procedure for making a graphic recording (electrocardiogram, abbreviated as ECG) of the electrical impulses that pass through the heart to initiate and control its activity. Small changes occur as the heart beats, and the normal form of these is altered by

heart disease. Electrocardiography is done by means of metal plates that, when placed on body surfaces, pick up and record the electrical changes.

Electrocautery Cauterization by means of an apparatus heated to burning point by electricity.

Electroconvulsive therapy A treatment for depression in which, under a general anaesthetic, an electric current is passed through the brain. Such therapy (known as ECT) is repeated several times at weekly intervals. Drowsiness and some loss of recent memories are possible side-effects of the treatment.

Electroencephalography A painless procedure for recording electrical impulses of the brain. A variety of patterns normally produced by nerve cells are altered in recognizable ways by abnormal conditions such as epilepsy. Electroencephalography is done by placing on the head metal plates that record impulses graphically. The recording is called an electroencephalogram (EEG).

Electrolysis The passing of an electric current through a small area of body tissue. Electrolysis is usually used for removing unwanted body hair.

Electromyography A diagnostic procedure in which metal probes are attached to or inserted into the skin in order to detect the electrical activities of contracting muscles. Such activities are altered in recognizable ways by diseases affecting either muscles or nerves that supply the muscles.

Electroversion A procedure for restoring normal, efficient rhythm to a heart with an irregular beat by passing an electric current through it. Defibrillation is one form of electroversion.

Embolectomy Emergency surgery to remove an embolus that has caused an embolism. A successful embolectomy restores the flow of blood to the deprived tissues.

Embolism The sudden blockage of a blood vessel caused by an impacted embolus (the name for a blood clot or other foreign matter carried along in the blood).

Endoscope An instrument that enables a doctor to look into a body cavity, photograph the interior, and (if desirable) take a sample of tissue or remove a small growth. The basic instrument is a tube equipped with a lighting and lens system. A claw-like attachment can be passed through the tube for cutting. Endoscopes designed for use in certain parts of the

body have special names (cystoscope, bronchoscope, etc.).

Endoscopy Any procedure involving the use of an endoscope. As most generally used, however, the term refers to examination of the oesophagus, stomach, or duodenum. Special names are usually given to endoscopic procedures involving other parts of the body.

Enema A liquid drained into the rectum through a tube or syringe and held for a set time before release by defecation or by being drained away. Enemas are used either for treatment (as in relief of constipation) or for diagnostic purposes (as in a barium enema).

Enzymes Substances in the body necessary for accomplishing chemical changes (for instance, in the burning up of sugar to produce energy or in breaking down food within the intestinal tract). An example of an enzyme is pepsin, which is contained in digestive juices.

Excision biopsy Surgical removal of an entire lump or patch of skin that may be malignant. If microscopic analysis of the excised tissue shows that it is malignant, further treatment in the form of anti-cancer drugs or radiotherapy may be given. See also Biopsy.

Excretion The removal of waste matter from the body by normal processes such as defecation and urination. Compare Secretion.

F

Febrile A term applied to a condition characterized by raised temperature.

Fibre 1. Any body tissue composed mainly of threadlike structures – for example, nerve fibres, muscle fibres, connective tissue. 2. The indigestible components (including chiefly cellulose) of plant-cell walls. Fibrous fruit and vegetables not only relieve constipation but may also reduce the risk of cancer of the colon. Dietary fibre is also known as roughage.

Fibrin An insoluble protein formed in blood as it clots. Fibrin is the substance that unites blood cells so as to close any accidental breach of a blood vessel.

Fistula An abnormal passage leading from a cavity within the body to another cavity or the skin surface.

Fluorosis Mottling of the enamel of teeth seen in people who have grown up in areas where there is excessive fluoride in the water. The quantity of fluoride that is artificially added to water supplies to help prevent tooth decay is insufficient to cause fluorosis.

Follicle 1. A small indentation or pouch-like cavity, such as the indentations containing roots of hairs, on a body surface. 2. An alternative name for a lymph gland.

Fontanelle A soft spot on the scalp of babies due to a gap between bones of the skull. The gap, which allows the skull to change shape during the birth process, closes within 12 to 18 months after birth.

Fulguration The use of diathermy to burn away abnormal tissues such as protruding cancerous growths on the bladder lining or within the rectum.

G

Gammaglobulin A type of blood protein that includes antibodies. Extracted from donated blood, gamma-globulins may be used to prevent or treat infections such as hepatitis.

Gene The smallest unit of inherited information, carrying the code for manufacture of a single protein. Since proteins lead, whether directly or indirectly, to the construction of all body parts and metabolic activities, genes transmit all necessary information for the physical and mental characteristics of every living thing.

Genetic engineering The manipulation of genetic material in an organism so as to alter the normal pattern of inherited characteristics. By means of such engineering bacteria can now be reprogrammed to produce artificial human hormones such as insulin.

Geriatrician A doctor who specializes in geriatrics, the care of the elderly.

Gingivectomy A dental procedure which involves removal of diseased areas of gum. The wound may be covered with a protective dressing, which is left in place for several days while it heals.

Gynaecologist A doctor who specializes in conditions affecting female reproductive organs. Gynaecologists do not treat problems such as breast cancer, but they are usually specialists in obstetrics as well as gynaecology.

H

Haematologist A specialist in the treatment of diseases of the blood, bone marrow, and lymph glands.

Haematuria The medical term for blood in the urine.

Haemodialysis See Dialysis.

Haemoglobin A protein compound in the blood. Haemoglobin carries oxygen from the lungs to body tissues; it is present only in red blood cells and gives blood its characteristic colour.

Haemorrhage A medical term for bleeding, which may be either internal (within a body cavity) or external (from the skin or an orifice).

Hard drugs Drugs, such as heroin and morphine, whose frequent use is likely to lead to self-destructive addiction.

Heaf test A method of determining whether or not a person is immune to tuberculosis (either as a result of vaccination or because of having already had a form of the disease). The forearm is lightly punctured with a ring of marks stained with an extract prepared from TB-causing bacteria; if the marks coalesce into a single red patch within about 3 days, the subject of the test is immune to TB.

Heartburn A burning pain felt behind the breast bone, often beginning at its base and moving upwards. Heartburn is usually due to acid reflux in conditions such as hiatus hernia or during pregnancy.

Hernia A bulge of tissue, such as a portion of the intestines, that protrudes through an abnormal opening between muscles. The opening may be due to a congenital weakness of muscular tissue or to weakness resulting from an external force such as an injury.

Hirsutism Abnormal hairiness, particularly in women.

Histamine A chemical that is released into the body, causing a variety of symptoms, when an allergic reaction occurs. A common symptom is dilation and leakage of small blood vessels, as a result of which the surrounding tissues become swollen and ooze fluid. Another very common symptom is itching.

Homoeopathy Treatment of disease by means of extremely small amounts of specially prepared drugs that would, in larger quantities given to a healthy person, produce the symptoms of the disease itself. Conventional treatment in this country is known as allopathy; doctors who practice homoeopathy are fairly rare.

Hormone A chemical in the bloodstream that controls the activities of certain body organs or tissues. Hormonal effects and parts of body affected differ according to the type of hormone involved. Most hormones are produced by special glands known as endocrine glands; and the higher the concentration of a specific hormone, the more active the function or functions it controls.

Hormone replacement therapy The giving of hormones, in drug form, to replace those which – usually because of damage to an endocrine gland – are no longer made naturally. Hormone replacements, which may be given either by injection or in tablet form, must be taken regularly, usually for life. The most familiar examples of hormone replacement therapy are the treatment of diabetes with insulin and the treatment of menopausal symptoms with oestrogen.

Hydrocortisone A type of steroid. For further information see CORTICO-STEROIDS in Drug index.

Hyper- A prefix meaning "above" or "high", as in hypertension (high blood pressure).

Hyperbaric A term used to describe a pressure greater than normal atmospheric pressure.

Hypo- A prefix meaning "below" or "low", as in hypotension (low blood pressure).

Hypoglycaemia The condition of having an abnormally low level of sugar in the blood. A hypoglycaemic drug is one that lowers the level of blood sugar; for further information see HYPOGLYCAEMICS in Drug index.

Hypovolaemic A term used to describe shock caused by hypovolaemia (loss of fluid from the blood). Hypovolaemic shock may be simply due to severe bleeding, but the volume of blood can also be greatly decreased by oozing from severe burns or by relentless vomiting.

I

Idiopathic A term applied to any disease or symptom with an unknown cause.

Immobilization The fixing of fractured bones or damaged joints in correct position so as to help them heal firmly and to prevent dislocation from occurring. The procedure usually involves the use of slings or plaster of Paris splints, but it sometimes requires an operation in which fractures are repaired by means of metal splints fixed directly to bones. See also Traction.

Immune system A natural bodily mechanism for recognizing and destroying invading microbes or foreign tissues. White blood cells are the basis of the immune system. Different forms of white blood cell can make antibodies or can attack invaders directly. The immune system may itself cause trouble (most commonly, allergies and autoimmune diseases) if it does not work properly; and it also becomes a problem in transplantation of body organs.

Immunity Resistance developed against a disease. Immunity may be achieved naturally (see Immune system) or by some such artificial means as vaccination.

Immunosuppressive A drug that hampers the body's mechanisms for immunity. This is particularly useful in the treatment of autoimmune disease and after organ transplants. For further information see Drug index.

Impaction The prevention of a normal process by a blockage or obstruction. Common examples are an impacted tooth, prevented from growing into its correct position (by an adjacent tooth, for example), and impacted intestinal contents.

Impedance testing A test of hearing ability involving measurements of vibration caused by sound at the eardrum. Sounds are transmitted by means of a special earplug inserted into the ear. See also Audiometry.

Incompetence A medical term applied to a valve (in the circulatory or digestive system, for example) that does not close well enough to prevent leakage.

Incubation period The time lag between the moment of infection and the appearance of symptoms. During this period disease-producing microbes are multiplying but are insufficient in number to cause symptoms or infect other people. Incubation periods range from a few days (for example, in influenza) to months (for example, in certain types of hepatitis).

Infarct An area of body tissue that has died because of a failure of blood supply due to blockage of a blood vessel, usually resulting from thrombosis or embolism.

Inflammation The reaction of body tissue to any form of injury – for example, as the result of a physical blow, infection, or autoimmune disease. The affected tissues become red, swollen, warm to the touch, and painful because of increased blood supply in response to chemical and nervous stimuli from the injured area. The influx of extra blood provides large quantities of white cells to combat possible infection and to remove dead tissue; it

also supplies extra nutrients to encourage repair and rapid healing.

Inoculation Injection into the body of a vaccine (a solution containing weakened or altered strains of a disease-producing organism). The aim is to procure resistance against a disease by stimulating the production of antibodies without causing severe symptoms. "Vaccination" is often used as a synonym for "inoculation".

Insecticide A chemical that kills insects, either selectively or generally.

Insufflation The pumping of a substance such as air or vapour into a body cavity. Insufflation is useful, for example, in investigating causes of infertility; if gas blown into the uterus does not escape into the abdominal cavity, a blockage of fallopian tubes is obviously preventing passage of eggs into the uterus.

Intention tremor Noticeable shaking, especially in the arm, that occurs only after the affected part of the body begins to move. Intention tremor is a symptom of certain nervous-system diseases such as Friedreich's ataxia.

Intravenous Inserted into or present within a vein. Intravenous feeding, for example, is the insertion of nourishment into the bloodstream by means of a drip.

Intravenous pyelography (IVP) A diagnostic procedure, involving the injection into a vein of a solution visible on X-rays, for examining the urinary system by means of a series of pictures known as pyelograms. IVP takes 1–2 hours and is painless, but patients often feel faint for a few minutes after the injection.

Involuntary A term applied generally to any physical activity not subject to conscious control. In particular, muscles not consciously controlled, such as those that propel food through the digestive tract, are known as involuntary muscles.

Irreducible A term applied to a hernia, fractured bone, or dislocated joint that cannot be treated by reduction.

Ischaemia A deficiency in blood supply to part of the body, often as a result of the narrowing or complete blockage of an artery or arteriole.

IVP See Intravenous pyelography.

K

Keratin A hard or horny substance present in skin, hair, nails, and teeth.

Keratosis A condition in which a patch of skin surface or mucous membrane (within the mouth, for instance) becomes

thickened and toughened. Calluses and warts are familiar examples.

L

Laceration A wound with jagged edges caused by tearing of tissue. Laceration may result, for example, from a fall onto broken glass.

Lactation The production and release of milk from the breasts of a woman after giving birth. The period during which suckling continues is also called lactation.

Laparoscopy Examination of the inside of the abdomen by means of a laparoscope (an endoscope) inserted through a small slit made near the navel. Laparoscopy, done under general anaesthetic, involves an overnight stay in hospital.

Laparotomy The cutting open of the abdominal wall in order to do exploratory or surgical work within the abdomen.

Laser beam An intensified, controlled beam of light powerful enough to cut, destroy, or fuse body tissues. Laser beams can be precisely focused for use in delicate operations such as those carried out in eye surgery.

Libido The emotion and drive that underlie sexual desire.

Lipids The fats that circulate in the bloodstream.

Liver failure Inability of the liver to perform its tasks efficiently, causing symptoms such as oedema, excessive bleeding and bruising, confusion, drowsiness, trembling, and hiccupping. Symptoms can sometimes be relieved by changes in diet and by drugs such as antibiotics and diuretics.

Lumbar puncture A procedure for investigating or treating diseases of the nervous system by insertion of a needle between the vertebrae at the base of the spine in order to tap cerebrospinal fluid and – occasionally – inject drugs. Lumbar puncture is done under local anaesthetic and takes about 20 minutes.

Lymph A diluted form of plasma that seeps from blood vessels into tissues and delivers nutrients to local cells. Lymph collects in thin-walled vessels (lymph vessels) and eventually drains back into the circulation, carrying with it waste products from the cells. White blood cells in lymph also help to protect tissues from invasion by microbes.

Lymphangiography A diagnostic procedure for outlining lymph vessels and nodes. Lymphangiography is done by injecting dye under the skin in order to locate the vessels. Once these have been found, a solution visible on X-rays is injected into them, and a series of X-ray pictures (lymphangiograms) reveals progress of the solution as it passes through the lymph system.

Lymph gland A bean-shaped organ at the junction of several lymph vessels. Each of the many lymph glands in the human body contains thousands of white blood cells for combating invading organisms in the lymph as it passes through the gland. A lymph gland may swell if the nearby parts of the body are infected.

Lymphoma A malignant tumour composed of diseased white blood cells. Lymphomas originate in the lymph nodes and often spread to the spleen and bone marrow. All types are rare, and the success of treatment is variable.

M

Malignant A term applied to a cancerous growth indicating it is likely to penetrate the tissues in which it originated and to spread further (metastasize). Because of their pervasive qualities, malignant growths sometimes recur after apparent removal, and complete eradication may be impossible. Compare Benign.

Malnutrition A condition resulting from the lack of essential nutrients. Malnutrition may be due to an inadequate or unbalanced diet or to an inability to digest foods properly. Symptoms vary according to the cause.

Malocclusion A term that dentists apply to the "bite" when upper and lower sets of teeth do not meet effectively as the mouth closes.

Mammography A procedure for detecting breast cancer by means of X-rays directed through the breast on to an external surface sensitive to changes in strength of X-rays as they pass through breast tissue. The photographic results are known as mammograms. Mammography takes only about half an hour and can be done as an out-patient procedure.

Mantoux test A method of determining whether or not a person is immune to tuberculosis (either as a result of vaccination or because of having already had a form of the disease). An extract prepared from TB-causing bacteria is injected into the forearm; if a patch of redness develops within 48 hours, the subject of the test is immune.

Massage Stroking, rubbing, and/or kneading the body in order to relax muscles. Massage sometimes relieves backaches, headaches, and the pain of injuries caused or worsened by muscle tension.

Meconium A greenish-black, mucus-like substance present in the intestines of newborn babies. Meconium is eliminated in the first bowel movement after birth.

Membrane A thin layer of tissue that covers and/or lines each of various organs and cavities in the body.

Menarche The first menstrual period.

Menopause Technically, the end of the final menstrual period. As commonly used, the word denotes the time of life – around the age of 50 – when menopause occurs. The technical term for what is popularly called "change of life" is "climacteric".

Metabolism A collective term for all physical and chemical reactions that occur in the body. The adjective "metabolic" may be applied to any such reaction or series of reactions.

Metastasis A term usually applied either to a malignant growth that develops in one part of the body as a result of the transfer of abnormal cells from elsewhere, or to the process by which such transfer occurs. Cancer that has spread to a different tissue from that in which it originated is said to have metastasized.

Micturating cystography A diagnostic procedure for observing bladder activity during urination by recording the working of the urinary system on an X-ray film known as a micturating cystogram. The procedure is often done at the conclusion of an IVP and is painless. Occasionally, however, a solution visible on X-rays is injected into the bladder by means of a catheter passed through the urethra; this procedure takes about 30 minutes and may involve some discomfort.

Mini-laparotomy Laparotomy through a very small incision adequate for minor procedures such as female sterilization. Mini-laparotomy is done under general anaesthetic and normally involves only a brief hospital stay.

Motor A term applied to nerves that relay commands from the brain to muscles. Areas of the brain that control specific muscle movements are known as motor centres.

Mucous membrane A thin tissue that lines parts of the body such as the mouth or vagina and secretes slimy or watery substances.

Murmur A term applied medically to certain sounds, usually audible only through a stethoscope, caused by changes in blood flow through the heart. A murmur is sometimes – but not always – caused by damaged heart valves or a defect in the heart itself.

Muscle-relaxant A drug that relaxes tense muscles or muscles in spasm. Many anti-anxiety drugs have this facility. For further information see ANTI-ANXIETY DRUGS in Drug index.

Mutation Any deviation from the normal characteristics of an organism resulting from permanent change in genetic make-up. Mutation may occur when a microbe such as a bacterium or virus is being formed or during development of the reproductive cells of a more complex organism. The change can happen without apparent cause or may be due to radiation or certain drugs.

Myelography A diagnostic procedure for X-raying the fluid-filled space around the spinal cord in order to detect disorders such as prolapsed discs or growths on the cord. The basic method involves a lumbar puncture and injection into the space of a solution visible on X-rays, after which the patient is tilted in various ways so as to record the movement of the solution on a series of pictures known as myelograms. Myelography is done under sedation, takes about an hour, and may be uncomfortable.

Myringotomy A surgical procedure in which a small cut is made in the eardrum to release fluid trapped in the middle ear. The operation is usually done under general anaesthetic.

Myxoedema Puffy, thickened skin caused by deposits of mucus-like substances. Myxoedema is a characteristic symptom of hypothyroidism.

N

Naevus A congenital abnormality of the skin. Naevi are varied in appearance; they may, for instance, be dark spots, hairy lumps, or fleshy nodules.

Narcotic Any drug (particularly morphine or a morphine-like drug) that causes extreme drowsiness or loss of consciousness even in moderate quantities.

Nasogastric A term applied to a thin, flexible tube that can be passed through a nostril into the stomach via the throat. Nasogastric tubes are used either for passing nourishment into the digestive tract or for draining away digestive juices (a helpful procedure when intestines are not working properly – as, for example, during the period immediately following an abdominal operation).

Naturopathy A system of treatment that avoids use of conventional medicines and other procedures and concentrates on diet, fresh air, exercise, massage, etc. Naturopaths, who are seldom medically qualified, are most successful at relieving symptoms caused by an unhealthful life style.

Nausea An unpleasant sensation originating in the upper abdomen, chest, or throat, often accompanied with or followed by vomiting.

Neonatal Newborn. The term "neonatal" is applied to any event or condition directly affecting a baby during its first month after birth. Compare Ante-natal and Post-natal.

Neurasthenia A mental state marked by fatigue, a sense of inadequacy, and oversensitivity, often along with such physical symptoms as loss of appetite and insomnia. Neurasthenia is not a psychiatric illness unless symptoms become intense enough to indicate development of actual depression.

Neurologist A doctor who specializes in treating diseases of the brain and nerves as well as nervous-system-related disorders of sense organs and muscles. Neurologists do not do surgery but often work closely with neurosurgeons.

Neurosurgeon A specialist in surgery of the nervous system, principally the brain and spinal cord. Compare Neurologist.

Neurotic Predisposed to over-reactions to mental and emotional stresses, but unlikely to lose contact with reality. Compare Psychotic.

Nystagmus Rapid, involuntary movements of the eyeballs. Nystagmus is an occasional symptom of conditions affecting the brain or eyes.

O

Obstetrician A doctor who specializes in the care of women during and immediately following pregnancy and childbirth.

Obstruction Any blockage of the passageway from one part of the body to another. A common example is blockage of a length of intestine in a hernia. In obstructed labour the fetus cannot pass out of the uterus owing to the disproportion between it and the size of the mother's birth canal.

Occlusion A term that dentists apply to a patient's "bite"; the way in which upper and lower teeth come together as the mouth closes.

Occupational therapy The use of practical tasks such as needlework, pottery, cooking, etc. to help patients – especially victims of serious accidents or psychiatric cases – prepare for daily life at home or at work. Occupational therapy can also help to relieve the tedium for individuals under long-term care in nursing homes or mental hospitals. People who supervise this form of treatment are called occupational therapists.

Oedema The swelling of body tissue due to excess water content. The ankles are a common site. The swollen tissue may "pit" (remain indented) when you press it with your finger.

Oestrogen One of the main sex hormones responsible for female sexual characteristics. In women, oestrogen is produced in the ovaries. In men, small amounts of this hormone are produced in the testes. Artificial oestrogens are an ingredient of many types of contraceptive pill and are also used in hormone-replacement therapy. For further information see SEX HORMONES (FEMALE) in Drug index.

Omentum A membranous flap formed from the peritoneal lining that hangs down from the stomach and covers the front of the intestines.

Oncology The study of tumours, especially with reference to research into the development and treatment of malignant growths (cancers).

Open-brain surgery A procedure in which part of the skull-bone is removed to permit direct operation on the brain. Such surgery is usually done to repair blood-vessel abnormalities or remove tumours. As healing occurs, new bone replaces the removed bone.

Open-heart surgery A procedure in which the heart wall is cut open to permit interior surgery. The incision for open-heart surgery is made along the breast-bone. During the operation blood is diverted through a heart-lung machine, which both circulates it and refreshes it with oxygen.

Ophthalmologist A doctor who specializes in treating eye disease and injuries. Ophthalmologists do not normally supply spectacles. Compare Optician.

Ophthalmoscope An instrument for visually examining the tissues of the interior of the eye by shining a light through the pupil.

Optician A medical or non-medical specialist who examines eyes for visual defects and supplies corrective lenses where necessary. Opticians do not treat eye diseases or injuries. Compare Ophthalmologist.

Organic 1. Derived from a living organism. In general, organic substances are chemically more complex than inorganic substances such as salt and more likely to cause allergic reactions. 2. A term applied to a mental illness with an identifiable physical cause (for example, some forms of brain damage).

Orthodontist A dentist who specializes in orthodontics (correcting teeth irregularities and treating jaw and facial-tissue disorders).

Orthopaedic surgeon A doctor who specializes in conditions affecting muscles, bones, and joints.

Orthoptist A person trained in orthoptics, a system of eye exercises designed to bring squinting eyes into alignment.

Osteoma A benign growth of hard, bony tissue, which needs treatment only if it becomes troublesome – for example, by obstructing the passageway between the external ear and the eardrum. Troublesome osteomas are removed by surgery.

Osteopathy A system of treatment emphasizing massage and manipulation of joints in addition to other kinds of treatment. Osteopaths may or may not be medical doctors.

Osteotomy A surgical procedure involving the cutting and repositioning of bones in order to treat diseased or deformed joints or the bones themselves.

Otoscope An instrument for viewing internal parts of the ear from the outer ear canal through the slightly transparent eardrum in order to diagnose ear disease.

Ovum The female reproductive cell (egg). A human ovum, though so tiny as to be barely visible to the naked eye, is one of the largest of body cells.

P

Paediatrician A doctor who specializes in treating children. Most paediatricians do not normally treat youngsters past the age of puberty.

Papilloma A wart-like or branching growth projecting from a surface such as the skin, a mucous membrane, or the lining of a gland. Papillomas are formed from the over-growth of cells but are rarely malignant.

Paracentesis A diagnostic or therapeutic procedure for draining fluid from part of the body (especially the abdomen). Paracentesis involves puncturing the affected area and may in some cases require a local anaesthetic, but the procedure is usually painless.

Paranoid Suffering from a mental illness characterized by extreme over-sensitivity and a deluded sense of being constantly persecuted.

Patch test The application of potential allergens to small patches of skin in order to determine whether or not the sufferer is sensitive to them.

Pathologist A medical specialist in the study and analysis of diseased body organs and cells. Pathologists normally work in laboratories and have little or no contact with patients.

Peak-flow meter An instrument for determining lung efficiency by measuring how swiftly patients can expel air from their lungs. Peak-flow meters are useful for diagnosing respiratory-tract diseases or for assessing recovery rate during treatment of lung disorders.

Percussion A diagnostic technique for mapping out the area of an organ and ascertaining possible changes in consistency of its tissues by means of short, sharp taps on the overlying skin with the fingers.

Perforation A hole formed in the wall of an organ or passageway such as the digestive tract which occurs as a result of erosion caused by a condition such as duodenal ulcer or appendicitis.

Pericardectomy Surgical removal of the pericardium (the membranous bag enclosing the heart). The incision is made between the ribs. Loss of the pericardium does not impair functioning of the heart.

Pericoronitis Inflammation of the gums around a partially erupted tooth, usually caused by accumulation of food and bacteria within the gap between the gum and the tooth.

Peripheral A term applied to (1) all nerves other than those of the brain and spinal cord; (2) blood vessels that supply the limbs.

Peristalsis The rhythmic, wave-like contraction of digestive-tract muscles that propels food along the tract. Peristaltic action occurs from the moment of

swallowing to the expulsion of waste matter from the rectum as faeces.

Peritoneal dialysis See Dialysis.

Pessary 1. A vaginal suppository. 2. A device inserted into the vagina either to effect contraception or to provide temporary correction for a gynaecological condition such as prolapse of the uterus.

Photophobia The sensation that light is painful to the eyes. Photophobia is a significant symptom of certain nervous-system diseases such as meningitis.

Phototherapy The treatment of disease by exposure to ultra-violet rays for set periods of time over several days or more. Severe jaundice in the newborn and psoriasis in adults are sometimes treated by phototherapy.

Physiotherapy The use of physical measures such as exercise, heat, and massage for treatment of disease. Such conditions as arthritis, lung disease, and the effects of certain types of injury are particularly responsive to physiotherapy, which is carried out by trained medical staff known as physiotherapists.

Placenta The plate-shaped organ that nourishes a baby while it is in the womb, and that also produces hormones responsible for many of the changes in the mother's body during pregnancy. When the baby is born, the placenta is expelled; an expelled placenta is commonly known as the afterbirth.

Plaque (arterial) A patch of atheroma on the inside lining of an artery.

Plaque (dental) Coating on the teeth consisting of mucus, food particles, and bacteria. Plaque builds up rapidly without regular, effective brushing, and leads to tooth and gum diseases.

Plasma The fluid (as opposed to cellular) part of blood. Plasma can be separated from the cells and used as a replacement fluid in the treatment of shock.

Plasmapheresis A procedure in which blood is removed through a vein and spun in a centrifuge to separate plasma from blood cells. The cells along with replacement plasma are then re-injected into the patient's vein. Plasmapheresis takes about 2 hours and, apart from the discomfort of insertion of needles into veins, is virtually painless.

Polyp A short-stalked outgrowth of tissue from the skin or a mucous membrane. Polyps are often caused by inflammation and are rarely malignant.

Polyunsaturated A chemically descriptive term for fats that are thought to be

least likely to encourage the production of arterial plaque when eaten in quantity. Polyunsaturated fats tend to be more liquid than saturated fats and are found mainly in vegetable oils such as sunflower oil and corn oil, and in margarines that contain these oils.

Possetting The regurgitation or "bringing back" of a small amount of milk after a baby has been fed.

Post-coital contraception Prevention of pregnancy by means of measures taken only after intercourse.

Post mortem See Autopsy.

Post-natal After birth. The term "postnatal" is generally applied to events or conditions affecting a baby's family as well as the baby itself during the first weeks after birth. Compare Ante-natal and Neonatal.

Prepuce Another name for the foreskin – the fold of skin that covers the tip (glans) of the penis.

Primary A term applied to the original growth of a malignant tumour from which further growths (metastases) develop. Compare Secondary.

Proctoscopy Endoscopy of the anus and rectum by means of a proctoscope, which is a short, stumpy form of endoscope. The procedure, though uncomfortable, is generally painless.

Prolapse Partial or full slipping of a body organ or structure (the rectum or uterus, for example) from its normal position. Prolapse is usually due to the weakening of surrounding supportive tissues.

Prophylactic A substance or procedure that helps to prevent disease – for example, an antimalarial drug or an immunization injection.

Psychoanalysis A method of treating mental disorders by probing into and analysing both the unconscious and conscious parts of the sufferer's mind.

Psychosomatic The medical term applied to a physical disorder due to an underlying mental or emotional condition. Indigestion is a psychosomatic illness, for example, if entirely caused by nervous tension adversely affecting the digestive processes.

Psychotherapy Any form of nonsurgical treatment for mental disorders by other means than the giving of drugs. Among such means may be discussions, advice, psychoanalysis, etc.

Psychotic Incapable of reasonable behaviour in certain – or in severe cases, all – situations. Unlike neurotic people, psychotics actually lose contact with reality when they are mentally ill.

Puberty The age when children begin to develop adult sexual characteristics, capabilities, and feelings. Puberty usually occurs between the ages of 10 and 14.

Pus A thick fluid, usually yellow or greenish, composed of dead white blood cells, decomposed tissue, and bacteria. Pus is a result of the battle against infection.

R

Radioactive A term defining unstable chemical elements that emit electromagnetic rays and/or charged particles as they decay. These penetrate the body and can be used for either diagnosis or treatment.

Radioactive fibrinogen A radioactive chemical that is incorporated into blood clots so that a clot forming in the body – for example, a deep-vein thrombosis – can be detected on a scan.

Radioactive implant Treatment of a malignant tumour by means of a pellet of radioactive material – for instance, radium – inserted into the tumour. The pellet, usually implanted under general anaesthetic, is left in place for several days and then removed.

Radioactive isotope A radioactive form of a chemical element, which, when introduced into natural body substances, is detectable by specialized equipment. Radioactive isotopes (commonly known as radio-isotopes) are used for locating blood clots, malfunction of thyroid glands, etc. Findings of radio-isotope scans are recorded either in individual photographs or on a screen.

Radiologist A specialist in diagnosis by means of X-ray photographs. Radiologists take and interpret X-rays and report their findings to patients' doctors.

Radiotherapy Treatment of disease by either radioactivity or X-rays. Radiotherapy is mainly used for destroying malignant growths and stopping the spread of abnormal cells.

Radium implant See Radioactive implant.

Reducible A term applied to a hernia, fractured bone, or dislocated joint that can be successfully treated by reduction.

Reduction A medical term for (1) the manipulation into correct position of a dislocated joint or fractured bone; (2) the pushing of a hernia back through its muscular gap.

Referral Transfer of a patient's care, usually temporarily, from one doctor to another doctor who is for some reason particularly capable of dealing with the patient's current problem.

Rehabilitation 1. Restoration of movement and strength to a limb in which a bone or joint has been immobilized after an injury. Such procedures are generally carried out by physiotherapists. 2. Preparation of a patient recovering from an accident or serious illness for a return to domestic and working life. This type of rehabilitation is largely carried out by occupational therapists.

Resection Surgical removal of part of an organ. A resection usually leaves enough of the organ intact for adequate functioning to continue.

Respirator A machine (sometimes called a ventilator) that regularly pumps air in and out of the lungs in order to compensate for the loss of natural respiration.

Respiratory failure Failure of the lungs, which may be either acute or chronic. In either case insufficient oxygen is extracted from the air for the body's needs.

Resuscitation Restoration of respiration and/or circulation by an appropriate emergency method such as cardiac massage.

Retention 1. The medical term for a condition in which a substance that should be excreted is retained in the body. Urinary retention, for example, is the inability to pass urine. 2. A term used in dentistry for the maintenance in correct position of a denture or brace.

Rheumatologist A doctor who specializes in treating diseases that affect the joints. Rheumatologists do not perform operations. Patients who require surgery for joint diseases are referred to orthopaedic surgeons.

S

Sarcoma A malignant tumour composed of diseased connective tissue. Sarcomas originate in bones, cartilage, or fibrous or muscular tissues. All types are rare and tend to be difficult to treat.

Saturated A term applied to fats that are thought to encourage production of arterial plaque when eaten in quantity. Among saturated fats are animal fats, dairy products, and such vegetable oils as coconut and palm oils, which are often used in margarines. Compare Polyunsaturated and Unsaturated.

Scan A diagnostic procedure for viewing a body organ in order to examine some aspect of structure or functioning. Scanning is done by observation of detectable waves – for instance, from ultrasound or X-rays – as they are passed through the appropriate area of the body. Findings may be recorded on a screen or in photographs.

Sclerosant An irritant substance such as phenol sometimes used for treating haemorrhoids and similar conditions. Sclerosants heal by causing the formation of thick scar tissue as a result of prior inflammation.

Screening Blanket testing of a large group of drugs, people, etc. in order to determine whether there is evidence of something amiss among any elements in the group.

Sebum The oily substance produced by sebaceous glands. Sebum spreads out over the skin, helping to keep it supple and moistened.

Secondary A term applied to a malignant growth that develops as a result of spreading (metastasis) from an earlier tumour. Compare Primary.

Secretion The production of a substance – for instance, hormones or lubricating fluids – from special glands or cells. Substances so produced are also known as secretions. Compare Excretion.

Sensory A term applied to nerves or body organs that relay information about sensations – sight, sound, touch, etc. – to the brain. The areas of the brain that receive this information are known as sensory centres.

Sepsis Infection. Infected tissue is sometimes said to be septic. Severe infection may lead to septic shock.

Serum The clear fluid content of blood when separated from all blood cells and clotting substances. Most blood tests are done on this portion of the blood. The term is often used, somewhat loosely, as a synonym for antiserum.

Shock 1. Any mental upset, which may or may not cause a physical reaction such as fainting. 2. A medical emergency in which, for some reason (for example, severe loss of blood), circulation suddenly becomes inefficient. Sufferers become cold and clammy, with rapid, feeble heartbeats and breathing. Vomiting, thirst, and unconsciousness may also occur; and swift medical treatment is essential.

Shunt A term for the surgical construction of a pathway along which fluid flow can be diverted from one vessel to another. Compare Bypass.

Sialography A diagnostic procedure for examining the ducts in a salivary gland. A solution visible on X-rays is injected into the gland, and pictures (sialograms) are taken while the solution is in place. The procedure takes about 30 minutes and is usually painless.

Smear A scraping from a body surface, or a drop of fluid such as blood or pus, that has been smeared on a glass slide in preparation for microscopic examination.

Soft drugs Drugs, such as cannabis or alcohol, whose frequent use does not usually lead to self-destructive addiction.

Spasm An uncontrollable contraction of one or more muscles.

Spastic A person with cerebral palsy, which is a paralysis of muscles, usually caused by congenital brain abnormality. Limb movements of a spastic tend to be weak and/or poorly controlled, but the condition does not worsen with time. As an adjective, "spastic" may also refer to muscle that is permanently in spasm or regularly goes into spasm.

Speculum An instrument for examining the interior of a normally closed body orifice such as the vagina or rectum.

Speech therapy The use of techniques such as practising the articulation of difficult sounds or learning how to control a stammer or stutter. This form of treatment is supervised by specially trained speech therapists.

Sphincter A ring of muscle that narrows or closes off a passageway by contracting. Obvious examples of sphincters are those at the anus and at the opening from the bladder to the urethra.

Spider naevus A skin blemish composed of small red lines that radiate from a central point. Such spider-like blemishes develop because a blood vessel erupts near the surface of the skin and fans out into a circle of blood-filled vessels. Spider naevi appear only on the upper part of the body, and their presence often indicates liver disease.

Splenectomy Surgical removal of the spleen. The incision is made in the upper part of the abdomen. Emergency splenectomy becomes necessary if the spleen is accidentally ruptured; planned splenectomies are usually done as partial treatment for a disease of the blood. The spleen is not essential for life.

Stapedectomy A surgical procedure for restoring hearing by removing a diseased

stirrup bone (stapes) from the middle ear and replacing it with an artificially made substitute. The operation is performed under general anaesthetic.

Stenosis Abnormal narrowing of a necessary passage through (or an opening into or out of) a vital part of the body – as, for example, in mitral stenosis. Compare Incompetence and Atresia.

Sterile 1. Infertile (said of a person of either sex incapable of procreation). 2. Free from contamination by living microbes (as a sterile surgical instrument).

Steroid A name given to a group of chemicals, many of which are normally found in the body. Most steroids are hormones and greatly affect body processes such as the overcoming of inflammation from whatever cause. Steroids given as drugs damp down inflammation and immune reactions.

Stethoscope An instrument for monitoring the activity of various organs, especially the lungs and heart. Internal sounds are picked up by the bell-shaped end, which rests on the body surface while the doctor listens through the ear-pieces for unusual or abnormal sounds that may indicate disease.

Strangulation 1. Prevention of respiration by compression of the throat. 2. Prevention of circulation by compression of blood vessels. This type of strangulation occurs if, for example, a swollen hernia blocks the flow of blood through the muscular gap through which the hernia protrudes. Such hernias are called strangulated hernias.

Streptococcus A group of bacteria responsible for diseases such as bacterial pneumonia, scarlet fever, and rheumatic fever.

Stridor A medical term for the high-pitched, crowing sound of an intaken breath produced by partial blockage of the upper respiratory tract. The cause of the blockage is usually severe inflammation, but occasionally a laryngeal growth.

Suppository A soluble medicated tablet inserted into the rectum or vagina to be either absorbed (in much the same way as a swallowed drug) or to act directly on the surrounding area (as, for example, a glycerine suppository which may be taken for constipation).

Surgery 1. The offices in which – or the hours during which – a doctor or dentist sees patients. 2. Treatment of disease, injury, or deformity by the cutting and/or repair of body tissues.

Suture 1. Thread for sewing up wounds or surgical incisions. Stitches fashioned from the thread are also called sutures, and the stitching process is known as suturing. 2. The interlocking joints that unite the bones of the skull, holding them firmly in place.

Swab A piece of soft material or a stick tipped with cotton wool. Swabs are used for cleaning wounds or body orifices or for taking samples of pus or mucus from on or within the body.

Sympathectomy An operation to inactivate some portion of the sympathetic nervous system (the part of the nervous system that, among other functions, controls the diameter of blood vessels). The nerves are cut or injected with a chemical, causing dilation of the affected blood vessels, with a resultant increase in blood supply to a given part of the body.

Synovectomy Surgical removal of diseased synovial membrane. Synovectomy relieves pain but is not practical if several joints or tendons are affected. The operation is done under general anaesthetic. The type of operation and length of hospital stay depend on the site of the affected synovium.

Synovium A membrane that lines the tough layers surrounding a joint or tendon. Synovial membranes normally produce small amounts of fluid to lubricate – and probably nourish – adjoining surfaces.

Syringe An apparatus for injecting liquids or air into, or withdrawing them from, body cavities or tissues.

Systole The period of contraction of the ventricles of the heart, when blood is forced into the arteries. Systolic blood pressure is the high reading obtained when blood pressure is measured. Compare Diastole.

T

Teratology The study of physical abnormalities which, arising during early fetal life, result in either death of the fetus (abortion) or congenital abnormality.

Testosterone A male sex hormone. For further information see SEX HORMONES (MALE) in Drug index.

Tetany Muscle twitchings and cramps caused by a lack of calcium in the blood. Tetany – which is especially apt to affect the hands, feet, and/or throat muscles – should not be confused with tetanus, a disease that causes similar symptoms for different reasons.

Therapy The technical term for treatment of diseases and disorders. Various types of treatment are identified by appropriate prefixes – for example, radiotherapy, physiotherapy, speech therapy, group therapy.

Thermography A diagnostic procedure for detecting certain conditions – for instance, varicose veins and breast tumours – by focusing a heat-sensitive camera on overlying surfaces of the body. The camera records small variations in temperature on photographs (thermograms); slight alterations in normal temperature patterns indicate the possible existence of underlying problems.

Thoracoscopy Endoscopy of the thorax (chest) by means of a thoracoscope passed through an incision in the chest wall. This is an in-hospital diagnostic procedure done under a local anaesthetic.

Thrombectomy Surgical removal of a thrombus (blood clot). Thrombectomy is most commonly done in the leg; the clot is removed through an incision made in the groin.

Thrombolytic A drug that acts to dissolve blood clots. For further information see ANTICOAGULANTS AND THROMBO-LYTICS in Drug index.

Thrombosis Formation of a blood clot (thrombus) on the lining of a blood vessel or the heart. A thrombus that breaks away and is carried along in the bloodstream is one type of embolus. See Embolism.

Thyroxine A hormone produced by the thyroid gland. Release of thyroxine is controlled by the pituitary gland. Thyroxine is rich in iodine and assists growth, repair, and efficient functioning of the body.

Tinnitus The medical term for buzzing, ringing, or roaring in the ear heard only by the sufferer. The noises may be either intermittent or continuous.

Tissue typing A system of classifying body tissues so as to make the closest possible match between the original and the donated organ in a transplant operation. Success of such operations depends largely upon the matching procedure.

Tolerance A term used medically to characterize a situation in which, because of habitual use of a drug, the body requires increasingly large doses in order to feel the effects. Tolerance may lead to eventual addiction.

Toxin A poisonous substance produced by bacteria, other microbes, and some plants and animals.

Tracheotomy A surgical procedure to open an air passage between the trachea and the front of the neck when the throat or larynx is blocked, or when artifical breathing by means of a respirator must be maintained for several weeks. To keep the air passage open, a tube is inserted. Tracheotomy is an easy operation, which may be done under either local or general anaesthetic.

Traction A treatment for broken legs, broken vertebrae, prolapsed discs, etc., in which damaged parts that have become compressed together are pulled apart and held in the correct position until healed. Compare Immobilization.

Transfusion The transfer of blood or one of its components such as plasma from a donor to a recipient. After blood is taken from the donor, its components can, if necessary, be separated; the blood or its components may be stored under refrigeration for a period before being given to a recipient through a drip.

Trauma Any wound or injury, whether physical or mental.

Tumour A medical term for any swelling – usually applied, however, to swellings due to abnormal multiplication of cells within a tissue.

U

Ulcer An open sore on any external or internal surface of the body. The tissues of an ulcerous area rot away,and pus is likely to ooze from the sore.

Ultrasound High-frequency sound waves, which are absorbed and reflected to different degrees by various body tissues. Ultrasound is useful for both diagnostic and treatment procedures. The reflections may be recorded pictorially to reveal the interior of such organs as the heart (see Echocardiography); and high-powered doses of ultrasound can be used to destroy abnormalities such as bladder stones.

Unsaturated A chemically descriptive term for fats that are thought not to encourage the production of arterial plaque even when eaten in quantity. They include the polyunsaturated fats (see Polyunsaturated) and they are found in most vegetable oils.

Urologist A doctor who specializes in treatment of urinary-tract disorders in both sexes and in conditions affecting male reproductive organs. Compare Gynaecologist.

V

Vaccination See Inoculation.

Vaccine A solution containing a killed or altered strain of a disease-producing organism. Vaccines, usually given by injection, procure resistance against the diseases they cause. See also Inoculation.

Vaginismus A rare condition of women in which sexual intercourse or vaginal examination causes painful muscular contractions that prevent penetration.

Valvotomy Surgery to separate the flaps of a heart valve when they have become fused together by rheumatic heart disease. The operation is done through an incision made either along the centre of the breastbone or alongside a rib.

Vascular A term applied to activities, functions, tissues, etc. directly associated with blood vessels.

Vasoconstrictor Any substance, whether a drug or a chemical naturally produced by the body, that causes blood vessels to narrow. For further information see DECONGESTANTS in Drug index.

Vasodilator Any substance, whether a drug or a chemical produced by the body, that causes blood vessels to widen. For further information see Drug index.

Venereal A term usually applied to disease caused by, or resulting from, some form of sexual contact.

Venography A technique for viewing the interior of a vein by injecting a solution visible on X-ray. Passage of the solution through the vein is recorded on a series of pictures (venograms). Venography is used for detecting conditions such as deep-vein thrombosis.

Ventilator See Respirator.

Ventricle A term for (1) one of the four fluid-filled cavities of the brain; (2) one of the two larger chambers of the heart.

Voluntary A term applied generally to any physical activity subject to conscious control. In particular, such muscles as those that move the arms and legs are known as voluntary muscles.

X

X-rays Rays with a short wavelength that enables them to pass through body tissues. An X-ray photograph resembles a negative of an ordinary photograph, with dense tissues such as bones showing up as white shapes. X-rays with very short wavelengths, which can penetrate tissues deeply enough to destroy them, are used in radiotherapy.

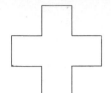

Accidents and emergencies

First aid

The aims of first-aid measures are: to help the patient recover, or at least to prevent the injury or illness from worsening; to organize help; to provide reassurance; and to make the patient as comfortable as possible.

For many minor injuries, first aid may be all that is needed. More serious injuries may require professional medical attention and further treatment. And, sometimes, first aid has to deal with life-threatening injuries, perhaps even involving the resuscitation of someone whose breathing has stopped. Correct and speedy assessment is therefore crucial, and this includes having a sense of self-preservation (there is no point, for instance, in trying to save a person drowning in deep water if you yourself cannot swim). But equally important is knowing the order in which actions should be taken: the priority checklist below serves as an instant guide.

The more knowledge you have immediately to hand, the more useful you will be in an emergency. The pages in this section supply valuable information, but cannot substitute for practical first-aid training.

FIRST-AID INDEX

Priority checklist for life-threatening emergencies

If you have to deal with an emergency on your own, follow these steps *before* arranging professional help. But if possible send someone else for help while you give the emergency treatment.

1 Check breathing. If victim is *choking* (p.803) clear airway. If there is *absence of breathing* (p.802) carry out artificial respiration.

2 If breathing fails to start, check heartbeat. If there is *absence of heartbeat* (p.804), give cardiac massage and alternate with artificial respiration.

3 Carry out measures to deal with *severe bleeding* (p.806).

4 If the victim is unconscious but breathing, place in *recovery position* (p.805).

5 Deal with any *severe burns* (p.808) or *fractures* (p.810).

6 Guard against the onset of *shock* (p.807).

Absence of breathing

If someone's breathing has stopped, emergency action (known as artificial respiration) is needed within three minutes. Common causes of stopped breathing are heart attack, drowning, electric shock (including lightning), poisoning, suffocation by strangling, and choking.

When someone has stopped breathing there is no rise-and-fall chest movement, and the face becomes a bluish-grey colour. *Do not waste time going for help or loosening clothing around the neck (unless strangulation is obviously the cause).* Give artificial respiration, continuing until the patient's breathing assumes a natural rhythm.

GET MEDICAL HELP NOW!

Mouth-to-mouth respiration

The simplest and most effective method of artificial respiration is to breathe into the lungs yourself (expired-air or mouth-to-mouth respiration). Mouth-to-mouth respiration may be given to someone whose breathing, while it is fairly regular, is weak and laboured.

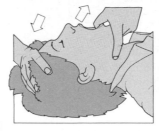
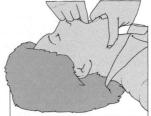

1 Lay the patient face upwards. Support the back of the neck, tip the head well back, and pull the lower jaw forwards and upwards.

2 Sweep around deep inside the patient's mouth with your finger to make sure that nothing is blocking the windpipe. Remove loose false teeth.

How to resuscitate babies and children

The method of restoring breathing in a baby or small child is much the same as that for an adult, except that you will probably find it easier to seal your mouth over both the mouth and nose of the child. Without tipping the child's head back very far (because a child's neck is more fragile than an adult's), blow gentle breaths of air into the lungs, at the rate of 1 breath every 2 seconds.

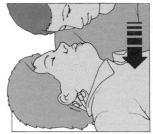
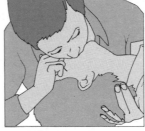
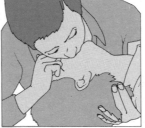

3 Pinch the patient's nostrils closed, then take a deep breath and seal your mouth around the patient's mouth. Blow strongly into the lungs.

4 Remove your mouth. If the chest does not fall as the air is exhaled, sweep your finger around the patient's mouth again to check for blockage.

Mouth-to-nose respiration

Facial injuries may prevent you from breathing easily into the patient's mouth. In these circumstances follow steps 1 and 2 in mouth-to-mouth respiration, then take a deep breath and seal your mouth around the patient's nose, covering the mouth or holding it closed with one hand. Blow strongly into the nose. Remove your mouth and open the patient's mouth with your hand, holding it open so that air can escape. Repeat the whole process as for mouth-to-mouth respiration.

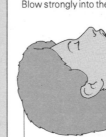
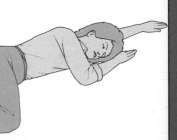

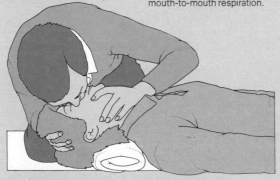

5 Give 4 breaths, then check the heartbeat (p.804) – cardiac massage may be needed in conjunction with artificial respiration.

6 Continue breathing into the patient's mouth at the rate of 1 breath every 5 seconds until the patient's breathing assumes a natural rhythm. Then place in the recovery position (p.805).

Choking

Obstruction of the airway by any object – a piece of food, or a small plaything – is an emergency. If the airway is only partly blocked, a choking person will probably inhale enough air to be able to cough effectively, and as long as the coughing is effective and seems not to lose force you should not offer help. However, if someone is coughing only weakly or is having difficulty in breathing, first aid is needed. A person whose airway is totally blocked will be unable to speak, or cough, or breathe; he or she may look bluish or clutch at the throat, and after a minute or so will become unconscious. If the upper airway is blocked, sweeping a finger round deep inside the mouth may clear it.

Note: Any choking person who has been revived by an abdominal thrust (see step 2 below) should see a doctor. Very occasionally the thrust (known as the Heimlich manoeuvre) can cause damage to internal organs, but you should never be unwilling to use the thrust because of this unlikely eventuality.

GET MEDICAL HELP NOW!

1 Make the patient sit and lean forward, head down between the knees. With the heel of your hand give several hard thumps between the shoulder blades.

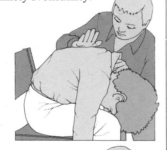

2 If this is not enough, clasp the patient from behind with one fist. Hold your other hand over the fist and quickly thrust hard, inwards and upwards, under the breastbone.

3 This abdominal thrust should shoot the obstruction clear. If it does not, repeat 3 times. If this fails emergency help is vital. If the patient loses consciousness, give mouth-to-mouth respiration (opposite).

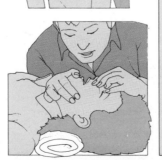

Drowning

In any case of drowning, speed in starting mouth-to-mouth respiration is essential. *Do not* waste time either fetching help or trying to clear the lungs of water. You may need to blow quite hard, but the air you breathe into the patient's chest will bubble through any water in the lungs.

If you are on your own and the patient is lying in shallow water, start resuscitation on the spot. If two or more helpers are available, you may be able to start giving artificial respiration while the helpers are carrying the patient out of the water to safety, and making him or her warm and comfortable.

GET MEDICAL HELP NOW!

1 Start mouth-to-mouth respiration (opposite). Do not stop until the patient is breathing again regularly or until medical help arrives.

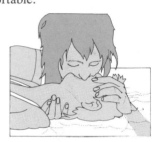

2 Once the patient is breathing naturally, place in the recovery position (p.805), and keep him or her warm.

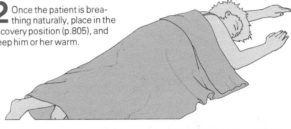

How to revive a choking baby or child

Revive a choking child by sitting down and laying the child face downwards across your knee (a very small child or baby can be held upside down by the ankles).

Give several thumps with the heel of your hand between the child's shoulder blades. Thump more gently than you would if reviving an adult.

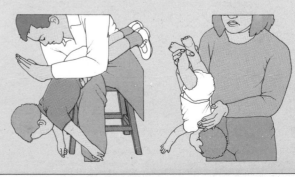

Absence of heartbeat

A heart which has stopped beating (known as a *cardiac arrest* – see p.388) can sometimes be made to start again by a technique called cardiac massage, also called external cardiac compression.

Anyone whose heart has stopped will not be breathing either, so cardiac massage, when needed, must *always* be done in conjunction with artificial respiration.

How to give cardiac massage

Cardiac massage is a skilled technique, which cannot be adequately learned from a book. It must be practised under expert supervision, since if misused it can be dangerous. If cardiac massage has no apparent immediate effect, carry on giving it all the same. *Do not* stop to give details of the emergency when help arrives – hand over to someone else first.

GET MEDICAL HELP NOW!

When to give cardiac massage

DO NOT give cardiac massage to anyone whose heart is beating.
DO NOT give cardiac massage to anyone who is still breathing.
DO NOT give cardiac massage to anyone whose colour is normal, or returns to normal after five breaths of air by mouth-to-mouth respiration.

1 The patient will be unconscious and will not be breathing. Skin colour will be extremely pale, or bluish-grey, especially around the lips.

2 The patient's heart will not be beating, so you will be unable to feel a pulse in the wrist or neck, and you will be un-able to hear a heartbeat when you put your ear to the patient's chest.

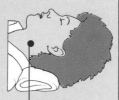

Position of pulse in neck

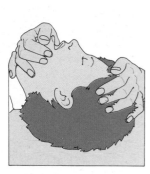

1 If patient is breathing easily, place in recovery position. If not, give mouth-to-mouth respiration (p.802). If breathing does not restart, check for pulse or heartbeat.

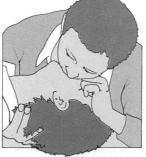

2 If the heart is not beating, give one sharp thump to the patient's chest, to the left of the lower half of the breast bone (this thump is termed the "precordial" thump). Use the side of your hand or a clenched fist, raised about 200mm (8in) above the chest.

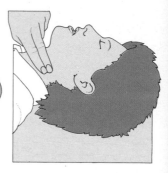

3 Often the thump is enough to start the heart beating again. Check for pulse or heartbeat. If present, re-sume mouth-to-mouth respiration.

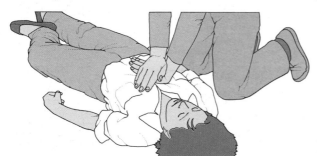

4 If you cannot detect pulse or heartbeat, start cardiac massage. Place the heel *only* of one hand on the lower third of the breast bone and cover with the heel *only* of the other hand.

Rock forwards, keeping your arms straight so that you push the breast bone down smooth-ly but firmly about 35–50mm (1½–2in). Rock backwards to re-lease the chest.

5 Repeat the cardiac mas-sage (step 4) at the rate of 1 compression per second. After every 5 compressions give one breath by mouth-to-mouth respiration.

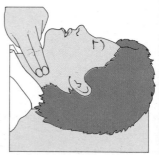

6 Stop cardiac massage as soon as you detect pulse or heartbeat; continue mouth-to-mouth respiration until the patient resumes normal, regu-lar breathing.

Unconsciousness

Unconsciousness not only refers to unrousable coma, but also to a state in which someone is drowsy and confused and does not respond to your presence. It may result from such conditions as: brain damage (e.g. head injury or stroke); loss of blood; lack of oxygen in the blood (e.g. drowning); chemical changes in the blood; or overdose of certain drugs.

Note: If you suspect a possible spinal injury, *do not* place the patient in the recovery position *unless* he or she is vomiting, when you must use the recovery position so that fluids can drain from the mouth; in such cases, try to move the patient without flexing the spine.

GET MEDICAL HELP NOW!

How to treat unconsciousness

When someone loses consciousness, the body's normal reflexes disappear and the muscles may lose their tone and become floppy. The main danger is obstruction of the airway, either because the tongue has become limp and flopped backwards, blocking the airway, or because the patient can no longer cough to clear vomit or other matter from the back of the throat. Even after treating an unconscious person, try not to leave him or her unattended. A person who goes into a coma may stop breathing and the heart may stop.

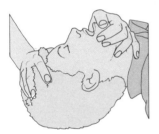

1 Bend the patient's head well back. If the patient is not breathing, start mouth-to-mouth respiration (p.802).

2 If breathing sounds noisy or gurgling, sweep a finger round deep inside the patient's mouth. Remove loose false teeth.

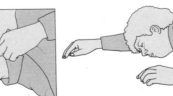

3 Loosen any tight clothing around the patient's neck and chest as soon as normal breathing is established.

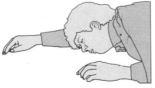

4 Place the patient in the recovery position (see box, right), if possible on a blanket or coat to minimize heat loss. Cover with a blanket or coat and keep a check on the patient.

The recovery position

When you have done everything you can to help the patient (see *Priority checklist*, p.801), you should always place the patient in the recovery position while waiting for help to arrive.

In the recovery position the head faces forwards and downwards so that the patient can breathe freely and fluids can drain easily from the mouth. The bent limbs support the body in a stable and comfortable position, and body weight is evenly distributed.

Note: *Do not* use the recovery position if you suspect a spinal injury *unless* the patient is vomiting (see *Unconsciousness*, left).

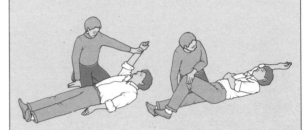

1 Kneeling at the patient's side, straighten the arm and hand nearest to you and place it above the head.

2 Fold the far arm towards you over the chest, and cross the far leg over the near one at the knee.

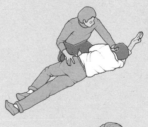

3 Grasping clothing at the hip, pull the patient gently over towards you with one hand, protecting the patient's face with your other hand.

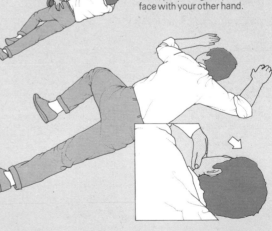

4 Swing out the patient's upper arm and thigh until they form right angles with the body, bent at elbow and knee.

5 Tilt the head well back so that the chin juts forward. Keep the patient warm, and stay close until help arrives.

Severe bleeding

Blood can be lost very rapidly from a severed or torn artery. Severe blood loss can lead to shock and unconsciousness and – if not controlled – may finally prove fatal. If an adult loses more than one litre (about 1¾ pints) of blood, or a child loses as little as one-third that amount, blood loss is considered severe.

The natural response of a damaged blood vessel is to contract, thereby reducing the amount of blood lost. This combines with formation of a blood clot to seal the wound (see *Bleeding and bruising*, p.424). If the blood does not clot for any reason (such as *haemophilia*, p.424, or because the person is taking *anticoagulant* or *antithrombotic* drugs) then bleeding will not stop on its own.

GET MEDICAL HELP NOW!

Stopping severe bleeding

In a minor wound, bleeding usually stops by itself after a short time. In a severe wound, blood may be flowing so freely that it cannot clot before spurting from the body. The aim of first aid for severe bleeding is therefore to stop or slow the flow of blood as quickly as possible.

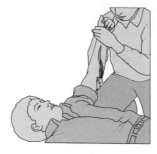

1 Lay the patient down and, if possible, raise the injured part. This will reduce the blood flow to it.

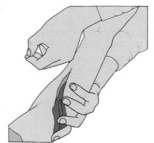

2 Pick out any visible and easily removable foreign bodies, but do not probe for anything embedded within the wound.

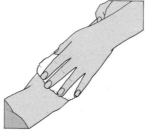

3 Press hard on the wound with a clean pad. If the wound is gaping, hold its edges together firmly. If there is a foreign body in the wound, exert pressure around it, not over it. Maintain this pressure.

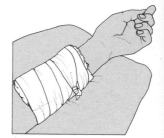

4 Take a firm pad and bind it tightly over the whole wound so that pressure is maintained. If no proper dressing is available, use an item of clothing (scarf, tie).

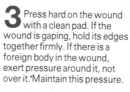

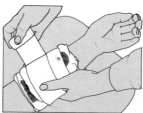

5 If blood oozes through the bandage, do not remove the dressing. Instead put more padding over the wound and bandage tightly.

6 If direct pressure fails to slow down or stop the bleeding, you may be able to control it by pressure on a given pressure point (left).

Arterial pressure points

If direct pressure on the wound proves ineffective, or if the wound is extensive and not suitable for direct pressure, an alternative method of stopping bleeding should be tried. Apply pressure to a major artery, at a point between the wound and the heart where the artery can be compressed against an underlying bone. The most accessible pressure points are the brachial pressure point, which you should use if a wound in the arm does not respond to direct pressure, and the femoral pressure point, which you should use to stem severe bleeding from a wound in the leg.

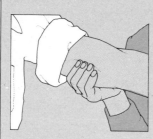

Brachial pressure point
The brachial artery runs along the inner side of the upper arm. Press it against the arm bone with your fingertips at a point between the patient's armpit and elbow in line with the underlying arm muscle.

Femoral pressure point
The femoral artery runs across the groin before going down the leg. Hold the patient's upper thigh with both hands and press hard in the centre of the groin with both thumbs, one thumb beside the other.

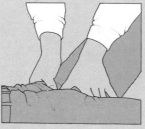

How to deal with a severed limb or digit

If a part of the body is severed, it is vital (besides treating the wound) to get both the patient and the severed part to the casualty department of the nearest hospital immediately. The greater the time lapse, the less chance there is of successfully rejoining the severed part to the body. It is important to keep the part clean, cool, and moist (but *not* wet); if possible put it into a plastic bag and then inside another plastic bag packed tightly with ice. If this is difficult, place the part inside any clean container. Take the container with the patient to the hospital and make sure the casualty staff know of its existence at once.

Head injuries

Head injuries nearly always bleed profusely. If you are treating a superficial head wound, apply a clean pad or handkerchief to the wound with steady pressure.

If the patient has a bad head injury (whether actual or suspected), tie a clean pad *lightly* over the wound. If you apply pressure on the wounded area to stop the bleeding, you may press foreign bodies or broken fragments of skull bone into the brain.

If a clear, straw-coloured fluid (known as *cerebro-spinal* fluid) issues from an ear, place a clean pad over the affected ear, but do not impede free drainage of the fluid. If this fluid flows from the nose, place the patient in the *recovery position* (p.805).

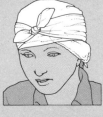

Do not press hard on a severe head wound: you risk pressing bits of broken bone into the tissues around the brain. Cover the injured area lightly with a clean pad and bandage in place.

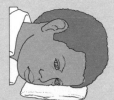

If a clear fluid trickles from an ear, cover the ear with a clean pad and lay the patient on that side to allow free drainage of the fluid from the ear.

Shock

GET MEDICAL HELP NOW!

The patient in shock is usually pale, faint, and sweating, with a weak, rapid pulse and cold, moist skin. He or she may be thirsty and anxious, and may gradually become drowsy, confused, and eventually unconscious. The patient in shock requires immediate first aid and urgent medical attention. (For general information see *Shock*, p.386.)

Note: Shock may be confused with a faint, where the patient complains of dizziness and then rapidly becomes unconscious. Onlookers at the scene of an accident often faint, especially if they are squeamish or emotionally involved with someone who has been injured or killed. However, circumstances usually make it clear whether a person has fainted or is in shock, and someone in a faint will never be unconscious for more than a minute or so. It is safe to ignore a fainting onlooker while you are busy offering first aid to the seriously injured, as long as the fainting person is in the *recovery position* (p.805).

The prevention of shock

Shock can follow any severe injury, particularly if there is a severe burn or copious blood loss. First-aid treatment after *all* severe injuries should therefore include measures to prevent, or at least minimize, shock.

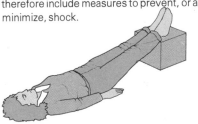

1 Lay the patient down, head low and turned to one side, and legs raised about 300mm (12in). If the patient is unconscious, place in the recovery position (p.805).

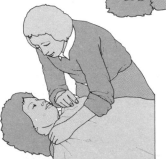

2 Loosen any tight clothing, and prevent heat loss by wrapping in a coat or blanket. Do not use hot-water bottles or electric blankets.

3 Do not give anything to eat or drink. Offer reassurance and make the patient as comfortable as you can.

Electric shock

The shock of an electric current entering and leaving the body can knock someone down, cause unconsciousness, or even stop breathing and heartbeat. The current fans out through the underlying tissues and may cause deep and widespread damage, even though a small mark is all that is visible on the skin.

GET MEDICAL HELP NOW!

Dealing with electric shock

Your first action must be to switch off the current – at the mains if possible – or safely to separate the victim from the source of the current. Until this has been done he or she may be electrically "live" and anyone who comes into contact will also receive a shock. This does not apply to someone who has been struck by lightning – he or she is not "live" and can be given first aid straight away.

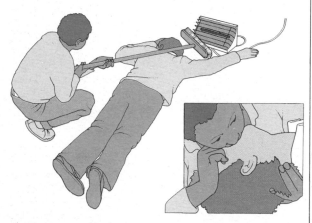

1 Switch off the current, or knock the victim away from the source of electricity with a dry, non-conducting object – a wooden chair or broom.

2 Check breathing. If the victim is not breathing, start mouth-to-mouth respiration (p.802) at once.

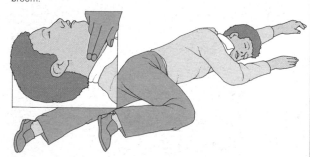

3 If the victim's breathing does not return to normal after 5 breaths, check the heartbeat. Cardiac massage (p.804) may be needed as well as artificial respiration.

4 If the victim is breathing but unconscious, place in the recovery position (p.805). Treat any visible burns (right).

Severe burns

Burns may be caused by dry heat, moist heat (scalds), electricity, friction, or corrosive chemicals. The severity of a burn depends on the area and depth of damage. A severe burn destroys all the layers of the skin, leaving a painless white or charred area.

GET MEDICAL HELP NOW!

Dealing with severe burns

If someone's clothing is on fire, throw the person to the ground with the burning side uppermost. Smother the flames with whatever is to hand, directing them away from the head towards the feet.

Avoid bursting blisters and do not breathe or cough over the burned area. Quickly remove anything constricting (shoes, rings, bracelets, etc) from the burned part. *Do not* dress the burn with anything fluffy such as cotton wool, and *do not* apply lotions or ointments.

Note: Nothing but cold water should be put on the burn. If the skin has been burned by corrosive chemicals, it is vital to put *all* of the affected area under a steady flow of water immediately.

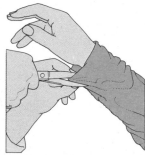

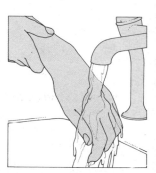

1 Remove at once any clothing that has been soaked in hot fat or boiling water, or corrosive chemicals. Do not remove dry, burned clothing or dry clothing stuck to the burn.

2 Immerse the burned part in cold water for at least 10 minutes. If the burned area is extensive, cover with a clean folded sheet or towel soaked in cold water.

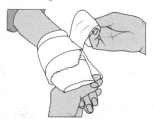

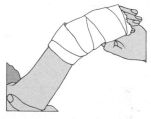

3 Lightly bandage the whole burned area with a clean, dry dressing. If fluid oozes through, cover with another layer. Protect a limb by a clean plastic bag over the bandage.

4 Raise a burned limb to reduce swelling, and give frequent small sips of cold water to combat fluid loss (provided the patient is conscious and not vomiting).

Hypothermia (exposure or chilling)

Body temperature is normally constant at about 37°C (98°F). During prolonged exposure to cold, more body heat may be lost than can easily be replaced, so the body temperature drops. This is known as hypothermia. (For general information see *Hypothermia*, p.723.) If the temperature drops as low as 25°C (77°F) survival is unlikely.

In young, fit people hypothermia occurs after prolonged physical exertion in cold, windy conditions. Once the stores of energy have been used up, the drop in body temperature causes a gradual physical and mental slowing down, which may pass unnoticed. The person becomes increasingly clumsy, unreasonable, and irritable; speech becomes slurred; there is confusion, drowsiness, and eventually unconsciousness, with slow, weak breathing and heartbeat. Hypothermia needs urgent medical attention.

GET MEDICAL HELP NOW!

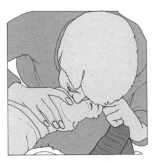
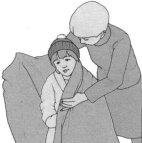
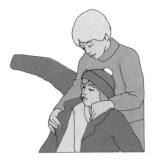
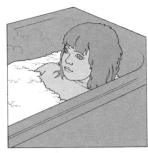

1 If the patient is unconscious, check breathing. If he or she has become very chilled, artificial respiration (p.802) may be necessary.

2 Once breathing is regular, shelter the patient from the cold. If you have to remain outdoors until help arrives, cover the patient's head and insulate from the ground.

3 If possible, change the patient into warm, dry clothes and give sips of warm drinks. *Do not* give alcohol.

4 Once habitation is reached, a healthy adult or older child can be rewarmed gradually in a well-heated room, or more rapidly in a warm bath.

Hypothermia in babies and old people

Babies and old people are especially vulnerable to chilling. They may lose a dangerous amount of body heat in conditions that may not seem particularly cold to an adult – such as an inadequately heated house, for instance.

In old people, hypothermia can easily be mistaken for a stroke or heart attack. A chilled old person should be rewarmed gradually by being taken into warm surroundings, wrapped in a blanket and given warm (*not* hot) drinks. *Do not* use hot-water bottles or electric blankets, which can cause heat to drain away from vital organs towards the surface of the skin, possibly causing shock.

A baby who has become dangerously chilled will be drowsy, floppy, and unable to feed. The hands, feet, and face may be bright pink. Get medical help immediately. Meanwhile, remove the baby's clothing and take him or her into a bed or sleeping bag with you, so that the baby is rewarmed gradually by your body heat.

Frostbite

Frostbite is a serious condition and needs urgent medical attention (for symptoms and general information, see *Frostbite*, p.413). Get the person inside as soon as possible and summon medical help. Meanwhile, shelter the person from the wind, give warm drinks, and cover the frozen part with extra clothing or blankets, or warm it against the body. *Do not* use direct heat and *do not* rub the area. As frostbitten parts warm up, encourage the person to exercise them gently.

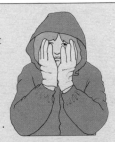

If the face is affected, cover it with dry, gloved hands.

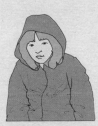
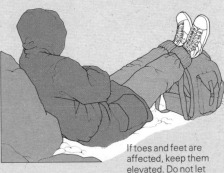

If the hands are affected, tuck them into the person's armpits inside the coat.

If toes and feet are affected, keep them elevated. Do not let the person walk.

Heatstroke

The serious condition of heatstroke usually follows prolonged exposure to very hot or humid conditions, which can upset the body's heat-regulating mechanism so that body temperature rises from a normal value of 37°C (98°F) to 40°C (104°F) or higher. The person is flushed, with hot, dry skin and a strong, rapid pulse. He or she quickly becomes confused or unconscious. Someone who has suffered from heatstroke should always receive medical attention.

GET MEDICAL HELP NOW!

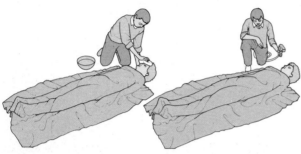

1 Remove clothing and wrap the patient in a cold, wet sheet, or sponge with cold or tepid water.

2 Fan the patient – use your hands, a stiff board, an electric fan, or a hair-dryer set to cold.

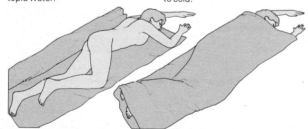

3 When the patient feels cooler to the touch, place him or her in the recovery position (p.805).

4 Cover with a dry sheet and continue to fan. If body temperature starts to rise again, repeat the cooling process.

Fractures and dislocations

Without an *X-ray* it is not always possible to tell if a bone is broken. If in doubt, treat the injury as a fracture. Suspect a fracture or dislocation if the patient cannot move or put weight on the injured part, or if it is very painful or misshapen (see *Fracture* and *Dislocation*, p.534).

GET MEDICAL HELP NOW!

How to treat a fracture or dislocation

Do not try to force back a dislocated joint yourself – this should only be done by a doctor. Take the patient to hospital, unless the injury makes walking impossible. In such cases summon medical help and wait until it arrives.

1 Treat any severe bleeding (p.806). Move the patient as little as possible. Movement may further displace broken bones and damage organs. Cover an open wound with a clean dressing.

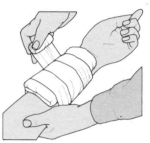

2 Give nothing to eat or drink (a general anaesthetic may have to be given before the bones can be set). Keep the patient warm and watch for signs of shock (p.807).

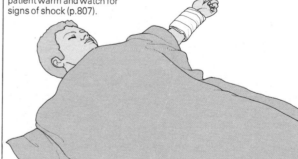

Heat exhaustion

If someone who is not used to very hot conditions neglects to take plenty of extra fluids and salt, excessive sweating can lead to heat exhaustion. The person is exhausted, with pale, clammy skin and may feel sick, dizzy, and faint. The pulse rate and breathing become rapid and headache or muscle cramps may develop. If left untreated, heat exhaustion may develop into *heatstroke* (above).

1 Lay the patient down in a cool, quiet place, with feet raised a little.

2 Loosen any tight clothing and give water to drink, to which 1 teaspoonful of salt has been added for every 1 litre (about 1¾ pints).

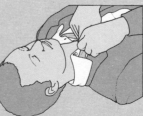

Applying a splint

Splinting is usually only necessary if you have to move the patient, or if there is a long delay before help arrives. The patient will be more comfortable in these circumstances if you immobilize the fractured or dislocated part by splinting it, often to another part of the body. Splinting prevents movement, relieves pain, and stops the injury from worsening. A splint should be rigid and, if possible, long enough to immobilize the joints above and below the injury – an umbrella or padded broom handle will do, or even a tightly rolled newspaper.

Broken arm
If the patient can comfortably hold a broken arm across the chest, apply a splint and hold it in this position with a sling. If the arm cannot be bent, splint it in the straight position and secure it to the side of the body.

What is a splint?
A splint is any sort of material (usually rigid) placed along or around a damaged part of the body to keep it from moving painfully or injuriously. To secure a splint, tie it down in at least 2 places (*not* on or right next to the site of injury) by means of wide strips of cloth (*not* rope or string). Use anything you can lay your hands on – a bandage, tie, scarf, belt, or even a torn-up piece of clothing.

Broken leg
Put padding between the legs and splint the broken leg to the sound one, using a broad band of cloth – a bandage, tie, scarf, or belt. Tie the knots above and below the break on the side of the good limb.

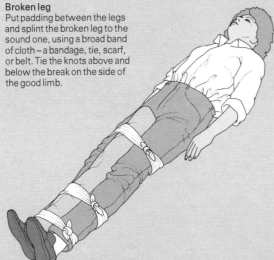

Spinal injuries

If the patient has severe pain in the neck or spine, or develops tingling or loss of feeling or control in the limbs, or suffers any loss of bladder or bowel control, he or she may have a fracture of the spinal column. In such circumstances *do not* move the patient *unless* his or her life is in immediate danger *or* he or she is choking on vomit. Treat the patient where he or she lies.

Chest injuries

If the chest wall is penetrated in an accident, air can enter the chest cavity through the wound. You will be able to hear the noise of air being sucked in as the patient inhales, and see bloodstained bubbles around the wound as he or she exhales. Do *not* remove any object still embedded in the wound, and *do not* give anything to eat or drink after you have dealt with the wound. (See also *Pneumothorax*, p.362.)

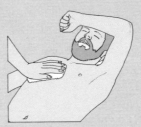

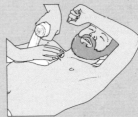

1 Press firmly with a clean pad, held in the palm of your hand, over the site of the wound to make an airtight seal.

2 Cover the entire wound with a large dressing – a cloth or metal foil will do if sterile dressing is unavailable.

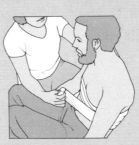

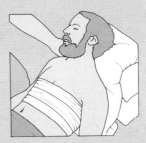

3 Cover the dressing with a thick pad of cotton wool and bandage it firmly, so that the seal remains airtight.

4 Make the patient comfortable, with head and shoulders raised and the body leaning slightly towards the injured side.

Poisoning

Swallowing is the most usual form of poisoning (including *food poisoning*, p.462, and deliberate self-poisoning). Other forms include *bites and stings* (p.814), drugs injected through the skin, inhaled gases (such as vehicle exhaust fumes), and chemicals absorbed through the skin.

GET MEDICAL HELP NOW!

How to deal with a poisoning emergency

In any poisoning emergency, medical help is the most urgent need. Do not try to induce vomiting by giving salt water or by sticking a finger down the patient's throat. If you see chemical burns around the mouth, wash the skin with water, give mouth-to-nose respiration (if needed), and do not give fluids to drink.

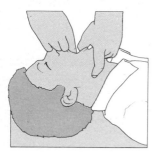

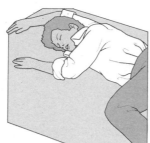

1 If the patient is unconscious, check breathing. If the patient is not breathing, start artificial respiration (p.802) at once.

2 If the patient is unconscious, or conscious but drowsy, place in the recovery position (p.805). Show containers that may have held the poison, and a sample of any vomit, to the doctor.

Common household poisons

The following substances are found in most homes. If swallowed accidentally in excess they may be extremely harmful or possibly even fatal. All such substances should therefore be stored out of the reach of small children.

Alcohol
Cigarettes and tobacco
Aspirin and any other drugs not in child-proof containers
Bleach
Lavatory cleaner
Washing-up liquid
Detergent

Scouring pads
Oven cleaner
Furniture polish
Weedkiller
Grease remover
Insect powder
Paraffin
Paint thinner
Cosmetics

Emergency childbirth

Sometimes a woman's labour proceeds so fast (especially if she is having her second or subsequent baby) that there is not enough time to reach a hospital or for medical help to arrive before the baby is born. If you are the only person present at such a birth, remember that birth is a natural process; interfere as little as possible. The majority of births are *not* life-threatening emergencies.

GET MEDICAL HELP NOW!

Preparing for the birth

Make the room warm, and the mother comfortable with pillows. Put a clean sheet or newspapers underneath her, if possible with a large plastic sheet beneath them. Boil a pair of scissors and a length of string to sterilize them.

If the mother seems distressed or in a lot of pain, be calm and reassuring. As the birth proceeds, there may seem to be a lot of fluid, some of it blood-stained. This is normal.

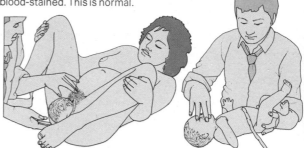

1 When the baby's head is visible in the vagina, birth is imminent. Once the head and shoulders are born, support the baby, but do not pull on the baby or cord.

2 Holding the baby with its head lower than its feet, wipe mucus from both nose and mouth. If breathing does not start within 1 minute of birth, commence artificial respiration (p.802).

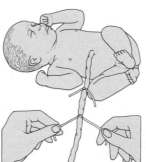

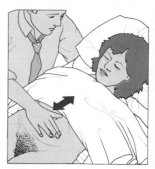

3 Wait until the cord stops pulsating. Then tie a tight knot with the sterilized string 100mm (4in) away from the baby and another knot 50mm (2in) further on. Cut the cord between the two knots.

4 About 10–20 minutes after the birth, the placenta will appear. Do not pull on the cord. If bleeding seems very heavy, massage the abdomen gently every few minutes until medical help arrives.

Foreign body in the eye

Never try to remove anything which is on the pupil of the eye, or which seems to be stuck or embedded in the white of the eye. In such circumstances, do not let the patient rub the eye, but cover it with a soft pad and seek medical help.

If the foreign body is floating on the white of the eye or the inside of the eyelid, try to remove it with the corner of a clean cloth, handkerchief, or paper tissue, as described below. Seek medical help if attempts at removing the object are unsuccessful.

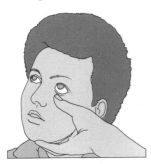 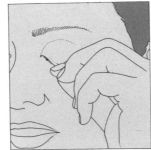

1 Seat the person in a good light. Get him or her to look up while you pull the lower lid gently down. If you can see the foreign body, pick it off with a clean cloth.

2 If you can see nothing, pull the upper lid down and out over the lower lid and let it slide back. This may be enough to dislodge the object.

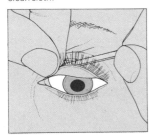 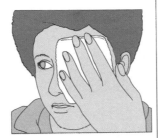

3 If the object remains, ask the person to look down while you place a matchstick across the upper lid and fold the lid up over the match.

4 If you can see the foreign body, pick it off with the cloth. If not, cover the eye with a soft pad and seek medical help right away.

Corrosive chemicals in the eye

Chemicals or corrosive fluids splashed in the eye must be washed out quickly by holding the person's face under a flow of running water. Tilt the head with the injured side downwards so that the chemical is not washed over the uninjured eye. Keep the eyelids apart with your fingers. After a few minutes, cover the eye with a pad and get the person to hospital.

Foreign body in the ear or nose

Children often stuff small objects such as beans or beads into their ears or noses. Do not try to remove these, but take the child to a doctor or hospital casualty department.

Insect in the ear

If an insect becomes lodged in the ear, get the person to tilt his or her head so that the affected side is uppermost. Then float out the insect by pouring tepid water into the ear. Pull the ear lobe gently backwards and upwards to straighten the ear canal while you do this. If you do not succeed in removing the insect, take the person to a doctor.

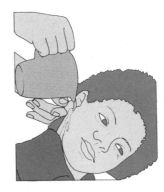

Foreign body in the skin (splinter)

A small splinter projecting from the skin can usually be removed by a gentle pull with a pair of tweezers. To remove a splinter embedded under the skin, slit the skin over one end of the splinter with the tip of a needle that has been sterilized in a flame, and lift up the end of the splinter with the needle tip. The splinter should then be removable with tweezers. If it does not emerge easily, do not probe further with the needle, but take the person to a doctor.

Fish hooks

If the barb of a fish hook becomes embedded in the skin, get a doctor to remove it. Only try to remove it yourself if no medical help is available, and remember to consult a doctor afterwards because of the high risk of infection.

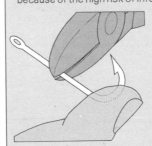 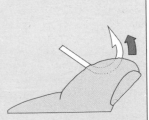

1 Push the hook on through the skin until the barb protrudes; then cut off either the barb or the shank.

2 Draw the hook gently through the skin to remove it. Clean the wound and cover with a dressing.

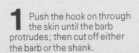

Bites and stings

The injuries that come under this heading are varied, and can range from the mild and almost unnoticed to the extremely serious and probably fatal. Each part of the world has its own dangers; make sure that you and your children are always aware of the poisonous plants and animals in your locality.

Plants and insects

Minor bites and stings: Most insect bites and nettle stings cause only local reddening, itching, and swelling, best relieved by calamine lotion or surgical spirit. Pain and swelling should subside within an hour or two.

Bees and hornets may leave their stings in the skin. Remove a sting by pulling firmly with a pair of tweezers or by scraping it out with a sterilized needle tip.

Poison ivy: A few people are immune to poison ivy, a plant native to North America. However, most people, once they touch the plant, develop a severe allergic reaction the next time they come in contact with it (see *Urticaria*, p.256). The skin should be washed with soap and water straight away to remove the oily substance which causes the reaction. If a rash or blisters develop, calamine lotion or cold compresses may soothe them. If there is a very severe reaction, with widespread rash and raised temperature, seek medical aid.

Poisonous bites: A very severe, generalized reaction may occasionally result after a bite from one of a few species of scorpion and spider, causing nausea, vomiting, and raised temperature. Keep the patient still and transport him or her to hospital immediately, immobilizing the affected part. Though such bites may be poisonous and very painful, they are rarely fatal except to young children.

Stings in the mouth: Stings inside the mouth may cause so much swelling that they interfere with breathing. Seek medical aid urgently and meanwhile give the person ice cubes to suck.

Anaphylactic shock: Occasionally, breathing difficulties or signs of *shock* (p.807) such as pallor, faintness, shallow rapid pulse, and sweating follow a bite or sting. Such a severe allergic reaction, known as *anaphylactic* shock, usually occurs only in people who have been stung previously and become hypersensitive. Treat the shock and get medical help.

Animal bites

Treat superficial bites and scratches as for *cuts and grazes* (opposite). Seek urgent medical aid for any human bites or any deep bites, especially the puncture wounds of a dog bite, which easily become infected and carry the risk of *tetanus* (p.564). An injection may be needed. If you are bitten by *any* animal, domestic or wild, outside Britain, treatment with anti-rabies serum may be needed (see *Rabies*, p.565).

Jellyfish stings

Jellyfish stings are seldom dangerous, though they may cause painful burning and swelling, which are best relieved with calamine lotion or antihistamine cream. The Portuguese Man-of-War (found occasionally in European waters) may cause a more serious reaction, with shortness of breath and fainting. Scrape off the stings, which stick to the skin (use dry sand if available), and get medical help. Place the person in the *recovery position* (p.805) and keep warm while waiting for help to arrive.

Snake bites

In Britain the only poisonous snake is the adder, whose bite is seldom dangerous except for the very old or the very young. In America, poisonous snakes include the rattlesnake, the copperhead, the cottonmouth, and the coral snake. If you are bitten by *any* snake, try and kill it so that it can be identified. If this cannot be done, try and remember as many of the snake's characteristics as possible.

The most common symptoms are pain and swelling at the site of the bite, sometimes spreading throughout the limb. If you have been bitten by an adder, these may be the only symptoms. But a serious snake bite can cause nausea, convulsions, shock, or asphyxiation. Since *any* snake bite carries the risk of tetanus, get emergency medical help.

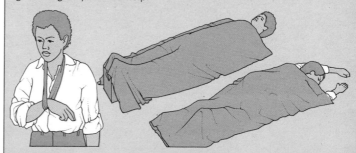

1 Give a mild painkiller and wash around the wound with soap and water. Immobilize the bitten part and keep the patient still.

2 If the patient is pale, sweating, faint, or has difficulty in breathing, lay him or her down with feet raised, and keep warm by covering with a coat or blanket.

3 If the patient feels sick or vomits, place him or her in the recovery position (p.805) to prevent choking.

Cuts and grazes

If blood spurts from a wound or flows so heavily that it cannot be staunched after pressure for several minutes, this is *severe bleeding* (p.806) and is a medical emergency.

Slight bleeding from a cut or graze usually stops spontaneously within a few minutes as the blood clots. If it does not, press a gauze pad firmly over the wound for about two minutes. Any wound that later becomes tender, or inflamed, or is seen to contain pus, should be seen by a doctor.

If the cut is deep, lacerated, or on the face, or if the edges gape so badly that they cannot easily be drawn together with surgical tape, seek medical aid. Such cuts probably need stitching to prevent scarring. A graze with dirt or grit embedded beneath the skin should also be properly cleaned and dressed by a doctor or nurse.

If bleeding from the ear or nose follows a severe blow on the head, the base of the skull may have been fractured. Lay the person on the bleeding side with a pad covering (but not blocking) the ear or nose so that fluid can drain onto it. Seek medical help at once. (If the nose starts bleeding for no apparent reason, there is probably no cause for concern – see *Nosebleed*, p.349.)

Puncture wound: A deep wound caused by something dirty – a nail or a dog's tooth – carries a high risk of infection, because dirt is carried deep into the tissues and the wound bleeds very little to carry it back out. If numbness, tingling, or weakness in a limb follows a deep cut or puncture wound, underlying nerves or tendons may have been damaged. *Antibiotics* and a tetanus injection are advisable for all deep wounds.

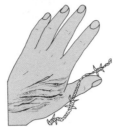

Lacerated wound

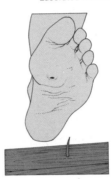

Puncture wound

Bleeding carries dirt out of the wound, so you need only clean around a cut. Wipe from the edges of the wound outwards, using a clean swab of cotton wool for each stroke. Put any antiseptics or other ointments on the cleansing swab, *not* directly on the wound.

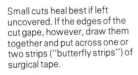

Small cuts heal best if left uncovered. If the edges of the cut gape, however, draw them together and put across one or two strips ("butterfly strips") of surgical tape.

Minor burns and scalds

If a burn or scald damages only the superficial layer of skin over a fairly small area, causing reddening and perhaps blistering, it can be treated at home. (*Severe burns*, p.808, are a medical emergency.) *Sunburn* (p.257) usually comes into the category of a minor burn.

Superficial burns are very painful, so first aid is aimed chiefly at cooling the area to relieve pain. If blisters form over a burn, do not break them; if they are on a part of the skin normally rubbed by clothing, cover them with a padded dressing (see *Blisters*, below). Do not put any cream, grease, or ointment on a burn (except for a large area of mild sunburn, which can be soothed by calamine lotion).

Cooling a burn
Plunge the burned area into cold water, or hold it under a cold running tap for at least 10 minutes, or until the pain stops.

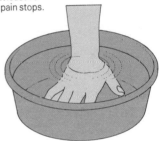

Blisters

Blisters form when the skin is affected by an allergic reaction, or when it is damaged by heat or friction. New skin forms beneath the blister, while the fluid in the blister is gradually absorbed and the outer layer of skin sloughs off.

Do not prick a blister or try to remove the top layer of skin; this will increase soreness and leave the raw skin beneath open to infection.

If a blister is likely to be damaged by further friction, protect it with a padded adhesive dressing. A burst blister should be left uncovered provided there is no risk of infection or further damage by rubbing.

Bruises

Bruises (*contusions*) occur when a fall or blow causes bleeding into the tissues beneath the skin. They normally fade slowly, changing colour as they do so, and disappear without any treatment after about a week. If a bruise does not fade and disappear in this way, or if you notice bruises appearing for no obvious reason, consult your doctor (see *Bleeding and bruising*, p.424).

Bruises on the head or the shin, where the bone is just beneath the skin, may swell considerably. To reduce pain and swelling treat bruises in these places by cooling. Wring out a clean cloth in cold water and lay it over the affected part for about 10 minutes.

Black eye
A bruise near the eye – known as a "black eye" – may swell dramatically. Apply a clean, wet cloth to the area for 10 minutes. If any disturbance of vision follows a blow to the eye, seek medical aid.

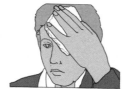

Sprains and strains

If a joint or muscle is wrenched beyond its normal range of movement, the joint is said to be sprained (see *Sprain*, p.532), the muscle strained (see *Pulled muscle*, p.532). The symptoms of both types of injury are the same – pain, swelling, and bruising. A severe sprain may be indistinguishable from a *fracture* (p.810) and should be treated as such.

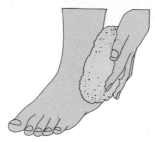

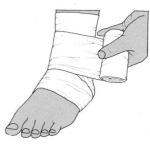

1 Sponge a mild strain or sprain with cold water to reduce pain and swelling.

2 Support the affected joint or muscle with a light bandage, and do not put any weight on it for a day or two.

Home first-aid kit

The list below contains all the items which it is sensible to have together and readily available in the home, especially if you live with young children. A first-aid kit in the car is also advisable.

1 Sterile prepared dressings (a pad attached to a length of bandage – quick and easy to put on in an emergency). Two large, two medium, two small.
2 Several non-adherent (gauze) dressings, dry and paraffin-coated, assorted sizes.
3 One packet of waterproof adhesive dressings (plasters) of various sizes.
4 One roll of rayon porous surgical tape (as an alternative to plasters).
5 Triangular bandages: to make slings or secure dressings.
6 Two standard open-weave (gauze) and one or more crepe bandages.
7 One packet of cotton wool.
8 Calamine lotion: for sunburn, stings, etc.
9 Analgesic tablets (soluble aspirin or paracetamol).
10 Tweezers (blunt ended), scissors, safety pins.
11 Clinical thermometer (or temperature indicator strip).
12 Small mirror.

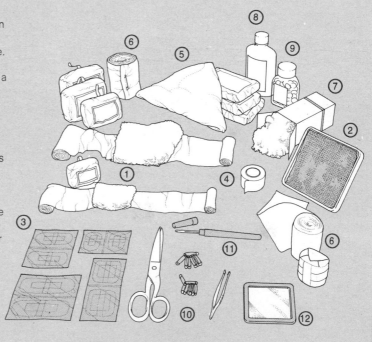

Index

The page numbers in italic type refer to an article or information box on the subject; the page numbers in bold type refer to self-diagnosis symptom charts, found between pages 70 and 232. If you have a symptom that you cannot find in this index, turn to the *Chart-finder* on p.68. For information on a specific drug or drug type look it up in the *Drug index* on p.778. For fast access to first-aid treatment see the *First-aid index* on p.801.

A

Abdomen,
  anatomy of, *58–62*
  swollen, **50**
  see also Acute abdomen
Abdominal migraine, 684
Abdominal pain, **48**
  in children, **93**
  in women, **78**
  recurrent, **49**
Abortion, 715
  incomplete, 593
  see also Miscarriage
Abreaction therapy, 303
Abscess
  anal, 484
  and inflamed diverticulum, 480
  appendix, 478
  breast, *590*
  epidural, *275*
  fallopian tube, 596
  liver, 461
  lung, *364*
  ovary, 596
  tooth, *439–40*
Accidental haemorrhage *see*
  Haemorrhage, accidental
Accidents
  and emergencies, 801–16
  chief causes of death, *42*
  prevention of, 43
Accommodation, of vision, 310, 311
Acetylcholine, 291
Achalasia, *457–8*
Acid reflux, 456
Acne, *708–9*
  visual symptoms, 240
Acne rosacea, 255
Acrocyanosis, *413*
Acrophobia, *300*
Actin, 529
Activity, fitness values of, 17
Acupuncture, *752*
Acute abdomen, *477*
Acute disorders, 788
Acute otitis media, *333–4*
Addiction, *304–7*
  dangers of, *713–4*
  to alcohol, 304–5
  to drugs, 305–7
  to gambling, 307
Addison's disease, *524*
Adenoidectomy *see* Adenoids
Adenoids, *677*
  removal of, *677*
  swollen, 676
Adenoma, 518
ADH *see* Antidiuretic hormone

Adolescents
  emotional problems of, *712–5*
  need for sex education, 715
  physical development of, *706, 707*
  sexual behaviour of, *714–5*
  special problems of, *706–15*
Adrenal failure, acute, *524*
Adrenal glands, 523
  disorders of, *523–4*
Adrenaline
  and tension, 19
  and urticaria, 256
  function of, 523, 524
Aerosol inhalants, 357
AFH protein, raised levels of, 630
Afterbirth *see* Placenta
Ageing process, *716*
  see also Elderly people
Agoraphobia, *300*
Agranulocytosis, *431*
Alactasia, 475
Alcohol
  and chills, 37
  drinking assessment questionnaire, *32*
  effects of, *32–6*
  limiting consumption of, 36–7
  see also Alcoholism
Alcoholic drinks, varying strengths of, 35
Alcoholism, *304–5*
  and Dupuytren's contracture, 542
  and nutritional cardiomyopathy, 400
  and peripheral nerve damage, 283
  in adolescents, 713–4
Aldosterone, 523
  over-production, 524
Aldosteronism, *524*
Allergens, *344–6*, 705
  in the home, 356
Allergic rhinitis, *344–6*, 705
Allergic substances *see* Allergens
Allergies, *705*
  and asthma, 355
  and conjunctivitis, 316
  and drugs, 755
  and urticaria, 255
  infantile, 666
  visual symptoms, 236
Allopathy, 788
Alopecia, areata, *264*
Alternative medicine, *752–3*
Alveoli, 340
Amalgam, silver, 448
Ambulatory peritoneal dialysis, 512

Amblyopia, 788
Amenorrhoea, *583–4*
  and anorexia nervosa, 710
  and cirrhosis of the liver, 487
Amino-acids, excessive, 688
Ammonia, as cause of nappy rash, 650
Ammonia dermatitis, 650
Amnesia *see* Memory, loss of
Amoebic dysentery, *461*
Amniocentesis, 630, *639*
Amniotic fluid, 634
  excessive, 630
  release of, 634
    premature, 632
  sample of for analysis, 639, 647
Amphetamines, effects of, 306
Anaemia, *419–21*
  and leukaemia in children, 682
  during pregnancy, *623*
Anaesthetic, 788
Anaesthetist, 738
Anal fissure, *484*
  and constipation, 474
Anal fistula, *484*
Anal sphincter, 435
Analgesic drugs, 778
Analgesic nephropathy, 513
Anaphylactic shock *see* Shock
Anaphylactoid purpura, *681*
Anaphylaxis, 788
Androgens, 523
Aneurysms, *407–9*
  formation of, 407
  "berry", 407, 408
  "dissecting", 408
  "fusiform", 408
  "saccular", 407, 408
Angina, *376–8*
Angina pectoris *see* Angina
Angio-oedema, 255
  visual symptoms, 236
Angiography *see* Coronary arteriography
Angioma *see* Birthmarks
Angle-closure glaucoma *see* Glaucoma, acute
Animal fur, and allergic rhinitis, 334
Ankle
  painful, **68**
  sprained, 533
  swollen, **69**
Ankylosing spondylitis *see* Spondylitis, ankylosing
Anopheles mosquito, and malaria, 567
Anorexia nervosa, *709–11*
Anosmia *see* Smell, loss of sense
Anoxia, 788
Antacid drugs, 778
Ante-natal care, *743–4*
Ante-partum haemorrhage *see* Haemorrhage, ante-partum
Anterior root *see* Nerve roots
Anterior uveitis *see* Iritis
Anthrax, *565*
Anti-anxiety drugs, 778
Anti-arrhythmic drugs, 778
Antibiotic drugs, *778–9*
Antibodies, 789
Anticancer drugs *see* Cytotoxic drugs

Anticoagulant drugs, 778
Anticonvulsant drugs, 779
Anti-D serum, 627
Antidepressant drugs, 779
Antidiarrhoeals, 779
Antidiuretic hormone (ADH), 515
  deficiency, 517
Anti-emetic drugs, 779
Antifungal drugs, 779
Antigens, 428
Anti-haemophilic globulin, 424
Antihistamine drugs, 779
Antihypertensive drugs, 779
Anti-inflammatory drugs, 779
Antipsychotic drugs, 779
Antipyretic drugs, 779
Antirheumatic drugs *see* Analgesics; Anti-inflammatory drugs
Antiseptic substances, 789
Antiserum, 789
Antisickness drugs *see* Anti-emetic drugs
Antisocial personality *see* Psychopathy
Antispasmodic drugs, 779
Antithrombotic drugs *see* Thrombolytics
Antitoxins, 789
Antiviral drugs, 779
Anus, 435
  disorders of, *483–4*
  see also Imperforate anus
Anvil, ear, 328, 329
Anxiety, **21**, *300*
Anxiolytic drugs *see* Anti-anxiety drugs
Aorta, 371, 403
  coarctation of, 659
  in fetal heart, 656
Aortic incompetence, *399*
Aortic stenosis, *398*
  congenital, *658*
Aortic valve
  disorders of, *398–9*
  replacement, 378
Aperient drugs *see* Laxatives
Aphthous ulcer, *450–1*
Apicectomy, 439
Aplasia, *430–1*
Aplastic anaemia *see* Aplasia
Apocrine sweat glands, development and function of, 707
Appendicectomy *see* Appendix, removal of
Appendicitis, *476–8*
Appendix, 476
  burst, 478
  "grumbling", 478
  removal of, *477*
  Aqueous humour, 308, 309
  Arachnoid membrane, 271
  Areola, 588
  cysts in, 591
Arm, painful, **64**
Arsenic, and peripheral nerve damage, 283
Arterial embolism, *415*
Arteries, 371, 403
  anatomy of, 56
  carotid, 267, 391
  central retinal, 325

Acknowledgements

Illustrators
David Ashby
Giovanni Caselli (*Atlas of the body*)
Helen Cowcher
Nicholas Hall
Shian Hartshorn
Edwina Keene
Kevin Molloy
Andrew Popkiewicz
James Robins
Anne Savage
Sue Smith
Venner Artists

Photographic sources
Dr P B Cotton

Institute of Dermatology, Department
of Medical Illustration

Institute of Child Health

Institute of Neurology

Institute of Ophthalmology, Audio
Visual Department

International General Electric Company
of New York Ltd

King's College Hospital

Maudsley Hospital

The Middlesex Hospital

Dr John L W Parker

St Bartholomew's Hospital,
Department of Medical Illustration

St Mary's Hospital Medical School,
Department of Audio Visual Communication

Sefton Photo Library

Spenco Medical UK Ltd

Dr P Stradling

Dr F Swain

John Watney

Carl Zeiss (Oberkochen) Ltd

Photographic Services
Negs Photographic Services Ltd

**Special thanks to the following
organizations for their help**
Action on Smoking and Health (ASH)
Alcoholics Anonymous
Cancer Research Campaign
Engineering Industry Training Board
J E Hanger & Co Ltd
Migraine Trust
National Society for the Prevention of
Cruelty to Children
Newsweek
OEC Orthopaedic Ltd
Optical Information Council
Vitatron UK Ltd (Medical Division)

Medical and other advisers
Mr M Bridger, The Middlesex Hospital
Dr N Cameron, Institute of Child Health
Mr J F Crewdson, St Thomas's Hospital
Dr E Gambrill
Dr P A Gardiner, Guy's Hospital
Dr L Goldie
Dr A J Gregory
Dr R A Hardman
J Hornby, London Ambulance Service
E Hornsey, Health Education Council
Dr N Johnson, The Middlesex Hospital
Dr M Jones
Dr A Keightley, King's College Hospital
Sister Lacy and the staff of The Middlesex
Hospital Coronary Care Unit
Dr D N Landon, Institute of Neurology
Dr R M Langford, St Bartholomew's Hospital
Dr P Leech
Mr R W Lloyd-Davies, St Thomas's Hospital
Dr K MacLennan, The Middlesex Hospital
Dr M Momen
Prof E N Morris
Dr I H Nicholas, The Middlesex Hospital
M A Parker
Dr J N Pattinson, The Middlesex Hospital
Dr B Peck
Sir Douglas Ranger, The Middlesex Hospital
Dr C Sheppard
Dr S Smail
Dr H Swanton, The Middlesex Hospital
Prof J M Tanner, Institute of Child Health
Dr C Thompson, Maudsley Hospital
Dr C M Thompson
Dr P Vernon
Mr P Watt
Dr R H Whitehouse, Institute of Child Health
Dr C Whiteside, The Middlesex Hospital
Dr P Williams
Dr A J Wing, St Thomas's Hospital
R Wright

**In addition, Dorling Kindersley Ltd
would like to thank the following people**
Hazel Bennington
Susan Berry
Gill Della Casa
Kate Duffield
Sheila Garbutt
Lesley Gilbert
Ann Kramer
Tony Livesey
Julian Mannering
Bridget Morley
Dr Ralph Stebbins
Sybil del Strother

char'i•ty
char'la•tan
char'ley horse
char'lotte
charm'er
char•meuse'
char'nel
chart
char'ter
char•treuse'
char'wom'an
char'y
chase, chased, chas'-
  ing
chas'er
chasm
chas'mal
Chas'sid *pl.* -si'dim,
  also Has'sid, Ha'sid
chas'sis *pl.* -sis
chaste *(pure),* chast'er,
  chast'est
  ♦*chased*
chas'ten
chas•tise', -tised',
  -tis'ing
chas'ti•ty
chas'u•ble
chat, chat'ted, chat'-
  ting
cha•teau' *pl.* -teaux',
  also châ•teau'
chat'e•laine'
chat'tel
chat'ter
chat'ter•box'
chat'ty

chauf 'feur
chau'vin•ism
chau'vin•ist
chau'vin•is'tic
cheap *(inexpensive)*
  ♦*cheep*
cheap'en
cheap'jack'
cheap'skate'
cheat'er
check *(halt, restraint,*
  verification, bank or-
  der, pattern)
  ♦*Czech*
check'a•ble
check'book'
check'er
check'er•board'
check'ered
check'ers
check'mate', -mat'ed,
  -mat'ing
check'-out' *n.*
check'point'
check'room'
check'up' *n.*
Ched'dar *also* ched'-
  dar
cheek'bone'
cheek'y
cheep *(chirp)*
  ♦*cheap*
cheer'ful
cheer'lead'er
cheer'y
cheese'burg'er
cheese'cake'

cheese
chees'y
chee'ta
chef-d'o
  chefs-d'
chef's sala
chem'i•cal
Chemical N
chem'i•lu'm
  cence
che•mise'
chem'ist
chem'is•try
che'mo•syn'th
che'mo•syn•th
che'mo•tax•on
  o•my
che'mo•ther'a•
chem•ur'gic *also*
  chem•ur'gi•cal
chem'ur•gy
che•nille'
cher'ish
che•root'
cher'ry
cher'ry•stone'
cher'ub *pl.* -u•bim'
che•ru'bic
cher'vil
chesh'ire cheese
chess'board'
chess'man'
chest
ches'ter•field'
chest'nut'
chev'a•lier'
chev'i•ot

'ron
w'ing gum
•wink'
w'y
i•an'ti
i•a'ro•scu'ro *pl.*
-ros
ic *(stylish)*
♦*chick, sheik*
Chi•ca'na
Chi•can'er•y
Chi•ca'no *pl.* -nos
chick *(young bird)*
♦*chic*
chick'a•dee'
chick'en
chick'en-heart'ed
chick'en-liv'ered
chick'pea'
chick'weed'
chic'le
chic'o•ry
chide, chid'ed *or* chid,
chid'ed *or* chid *or*
chid'den, chid'ing
chief'ly
chief'tain
chif•fon'
chif'fo•nier'
chig'ger
chi•gnon'
Chi•hua'hua
chil'blain'
child *pl.* chil'dren
child'bear'ing
child'birth'
child'hood'

child'ish
child'like'
Chil'e•an
chil'e con car'ne
  also chil'i con car'ne
chil'i *(pepper)*, *pl.* -ies,
  also chil'e, chil'li *pl.*
  -lies
chill'y *(cold)*
  ♦*chili*
chime, chimed, chim'-
  ing
chim'er
chi•me'ra
chi•mer'i•cal
chim'i•chan'ga
chim'ney *pl.* -neys
chimp
chim'pan•zee'
chin, chinned, chin'-
  ning
chi'na
chi'na•ber'ry
Chi'na•town'
chi'na•ware'
chinch
chin•chil'la
chine
Chi•nese' *pl.* -nese'
chink
chi'no *pl.* -nos
chi•nook'
chin'qua•pin'
chintz'y
chip, chipped, chip'-
  ping
chip'munk'

Chip'pen•dale'
chip'per
chi'ro•man'cy
chi•rop'o•dist
chi•rop'o•dy
chi'ro•prac'tic
chi'ro•prac'tor
chirp'er
chirr *(trill)*
  ♦*churr*
chir'rup
chis'el, -eled *or* -elled,
  -el•ing *or* -el•ling
chi'-square'
chit'chat', -chat'ted,
  -chat'ting
chi'tin *(hornlike sub-
  stance)*
chi'ton *(mollusk)*
chit'ter
chit'ter•lings *also*
  chit'lins, chit'lings
chi•val'ric
chiv'al•rous
chiv'al•ry
chive
chlo'ral
chlo'rate'
chlor'dane' *also*
  chlor'dan'
chlo'ride'
chlo'rin•ate', -at'ed,
  -at'ing
chlo'rine'
chlo'rite'
chlo'ro•form'
chlo'ro•phyll *also*

chlo′ro•phyl
chlo′ro•plast′
chlo•ro′sis
chlor′tet•ra•cy′-
　cline′
chock′-a-block′
chock′-full′
choc′o•late
choice, choic′er,
　choic′est
choir *(singers)*
　♦*quire*
choir′boy′
choke, choked, chok′-
　ing
choke′cher′ry
choke′damp′
choke′hold′
choke′point′
chok′er
chol′er *(anger)*
　♦*collar*
chol′er•a
chol′er•ic
cho•les′ter•ol′
choose, chose, cho′-
　sen, choos′ing
choos′er
choos′y *also* choos′ey
chop, chopped, chop′-
　ping
chop′house′
chop′log′ic
chop′per
chop′py
chop′sticks′
chop su′ey

cho′ral *(of a chorus)*
　♦*coral*
cho•rale′ *(hymn),*
　also cho•ral′
　♦*corral*
chord *(musical tones,*
　line segment)
　♦*cord*
chor′date′
chore
cho•re′a
cho′re•o•graph′
cho′re•og′ra•pher
cho′re•o•graph′ic
cho′re•og′ra•phy
cho′ric
cho′rine′
cho′ri•on′
cho′ris•ter
cho′roid′ *also* cho-
　roi′de•a
chor′tle, -tled, -tling
cho′rus *pl.* -rus•es
cho′rus, -rused *or*
　-russed, -rus•ing *or*
　-rus•sing
cho′sen
chow′der
chow′ mein′
chrism
chris′ten
Chris′ten•dom
Chris′tian
Chris′ti•an′i•ty
Christ′mas
chro′mate′
chro•mat′ic

chro•mat′i•cism
chro′ma•tin
chro′ma•tog′ra•phy
chrome
chro′mic
chro′mite′
chro′mi•um
chro′mo•lith′-
　o•graph′
chro′mo•li•thog′ra-
　phy
chro′mo•so′mal
chro′mo•some′
chro′mo•sphere′
chron′ic
chron′i•cle, -cled,
　-cling
chron′i•cler
chron•o•log′i•cal
　also chron′o•log′ic
chro•nol′o•gist
chro•nol′o•gy
chro•nom′e•ter
chrys′a•lid
chrys′a•lis *pl.* chrys′-
　a•lis•es *or* chry•sal′-
　i•des′
chry•san′the•mum
chub′by
chuck
chuck′le, -led, -ling
chuck′le•head′
chug, chugged, chug′-
　ging
chuk′ka
chum, chummed,
　chum′ming

chum'my
chump
chunk'y
church'go'er
church'war'den
church'yard'
churl'ish
churn'ing
churr *(trill)*
 ♦*chirr*
chute *(trough)*
 ♦*shoot, shute*
chut'ney *pl.* -neys
chutz'pah
chyle
chyme
ci•ca'da
cic'a•trix' *pl.* cic'-
 a•tri'ces
cic'e•ro'ne *pl.* -nes *or*
 -ni
ci'der
ci•gar'
cig'a•rette' *also* cig-
 a•ret'
cig'a•ril'lo *pl.* -los
cil'i•a *sing.* -i•um
cil'i•ar'y
cil'i•ate *also* cil'i•at'-
 ed
cinch
cin•cho'na
cinc'ture, -tured,
 -tur•ing
cin'der
Cin'der•el'la
cin•e•ma

cin'e•ma•go'er
cin'e•mat'ic
cin'e•ma•tize',
 -tized', -tiz'ing
cin'e•ma•tog'ra-
 pher
cin'e•ma•tog'ra-
 phy
ci'né•ma' vé'ri•té'
cin'e•phile'
cin'na•bar'
cin'na•mon
cinque'foil'
ci'pher *also* cy'pher
cir'ca
cir•ca'di•an
cir'cle, -cled, -cling
cir'clet
cir'cuit
cir•cu'i•tous
cir'cuit•ry
cir'cu•lar
cir'cu•lar'i•ty
cir'cu•lar•ize',
 -ized', -iz'ing
cir'cu•late', -lat'ed,
 -lat'ing
cir'cu•la'tion
cir'cu•la'tor
cir'cu•la•to'ry
cir'cum•am'bu•late'
 , -lat'ed, -lat'ing
cir'cum•cise',
 -cised', -cis'ing
cir'cum•ci'sion
cir•cum'fer•ence
cir'cum•flex'

cir•cum'flu•ous
cir'cum•lo•cu'tion
cir'cum•loc'u•to'ry
cir'cum•nav'i•gate',
 -gat'ed, -gat'ing
cir'cum•nav'i•ga'-
 tion
cir'cum•nav'i•ga'-
 tor
cir'cum•po'lar
cir'cum•scribe',
 -scribed', -scrib'ing
cir'cum•scrip'tion
cir'cum•spect'
cir'cum•spec'tion
cir'cum•stance'
cir'cum•stan'tial
cir'cum•stan'ti•ate',
 -at'ed, -at'ing
cir'cum•stan'ti-
 a'tion
cir'cum•vent'
cir'cum•ven'tion
cir'cus
cirque
cir•rho'sis
cir•rhot'ic
cir'ro•cu'mu•lus
cir'ro•stra'tus
cir'rus *pl.* -ri'
cis•lu'nar
cis'tern
cis•ter'nal
cit'a•del
ci•ta'tion
cite *(to quote)*, cit'ed,
 cit'ing

♦*sight, site*
cit′i•fy′, -fied′, -fy′ing
cit′i•zen
cit′i•zen•ry
cit′i•zen•ship′
cit′rate′
cit′ric
cit′ron
cit′ro•nel′la
cit′rus *pl.* -rus•es *or*
-rus
cit′y
cit′y-state′
cit′y•wide′
civ′et
civ′ic
civ′ics
civ′il
ci•vil′ian
ci•vil′i•ty
civ′i•liz′a•ble
civ′i•li•za′tion
civ′i•lize′, -lized′,
-liz′ing
civ′vies *also* civ′ies
clab′ber
clack *(noise)*
♦*claque*
clad, clad, clad′ding
claim′ant
clair•voy′ance
clair•voy′ant
clam, clammed, clam′-
ming
clam′bake′
clam′ber
clam′my

clam′or
clam′or•ous
clamp
clam′shell′
clan
clan•des′tine
clang
clan′gor
clank
clan′nish
clans′man
clap, clapped, clap′-
ping
clap′board
clap′per
clap′trap′
claque *(group)*
♦*clack*
clar′et
clar′i•fi•ca′tion
clar′i•fy′, -fied′, -fy′-
ing
clar′i•net′
clar′i•net′ist *also*
clar′i•net′tist
clar′i•on
clar′i•ty
clash
clasp
class′-con′scious *adj.*
clas′sic
clas′si•cal
clas′si•cism
clas′si•cist
clas′si•cize′, -cized′,
-ciz′ing
clas′si•fi′a•ble

clas′si•fi•ca′tion
clas′si•fi•ca•to′ry
clas′si•fy′, -fied′, -fy′-
ing
class′ism
class′mate′
class′room′
class′y
clat′ter
clause *(words)*
♦*claws*
claus′tro•pho′bi•a
claus′tro•pho′bic
clav′i•chord′
clav′i•cle
cla•vic′u•lar
cla•vier′
claw
clay′ey *or* clay′ish
clean′-cut′
cleanse, cleansed,
cleans′ing
cleans′er
clean′-shav′en
clean′up′ *n.*
clear′ance
clear′-cut′
clear′-eyed′
clear′ing
clear′ing-house′ *also*
clear′ing•house′
clear′-sight′ed
cleat
cleav′age
cleave *(to split)*, cleft
or cleaved *or* clove,
cleft *or* cleaved *or*

clo'ven, cleav'ing
cleave (to adhere),
    cleaved or clove,
    cleaved, cleav'ing
cleav'er
clef
cleft
clem'a•tis
clem'en•cy
clem'ent
clench
cler'gy
cler'gy•man
cler'gy•wom'an
cler'ic
cler'i•cal
cler'i•cal•ism
clerk
clev'er
clew (ball of yarn, cor-
    ner of a sail)
    ♦clue
cli•ché'
click (sound)
    ♦clique
click'er
cli'ent
cli'en•tele'
cliff 'hang'er
cli•mac'ter•ic
cli•mac'tic
cli'mate
cli•mat'ic also cli-
    mat'i•cal
cli'ma•to•log'ic also
    cli'ma•to•log'i•cal
cli'ma•tol'o•gist

cli'ma•tol'o•gy
cli'max'
climb (ascent)
    ♦clime
climb'a•ble
clime (climate)
    ♦climb
clinch'er
cline
cling, clung, cling'ing
cling'stone'
clin'ic
clin'i•cal
cli•ni'cian
clink'er
clip, clipped, clip'ping
clip'board'
clip'per
clip'ping
clique (exclusive
    group)
    ♦click
cliqu'ey also cliqu'y,
    cliqu'ish
clit'o•ral
clit'o•ris
clo•a'ca pl. -cae'
cloak'-and-dag'ger
    adj.
cloak'room'
clob'ber
cloche
clock'wise'
clock'work'
clod'dish
clod'hop'per
clog, clogged, clog'-

ging
cloi'son•né'
clois'ter
clois'tral
clone, cloned, clon'ing
clop, clopped, clop'-
    ping
close, clos'er, clos'est
close (to shut), closed,
    clos'ing
    ♦clothes
closed'-cir'cuit adj.
close'-fist'ed
close'-grained'
close'-mouthed'
close'-out' n.
clos'et
close'-up' n.
clos•trid'i•um pl.
    -i•a
clo'sure (a closing)
    ♦cloture
clot, clot'ted, clot'ting
cloth pl. cloths
cloth'bound'
clothe, clothed or
    clad, cloth'ing
clothes (apparel)
    ♦close
clothes'horse'
clothes'line'
clothes'pin'
cloth'ier
cloth'ing
clo'ture (parliamenta-
    ry procedure), also
    clo'sure

cloud′burst′
cloud′y
clout
clove
clo′ven-hoofed′
clo′ver
clo′ver•leaf′
clown
cloy′ing
club, clubbed, club′-
   bing
club′by
club′foot′
club′foot′ed
club′house′
cluck
clue (to give guiding
   information), clued,
   clue′ing or clu′ing,
   also clew
clump
clum′sy
clunk′y
clus′ter
clutch
clut′ter
Clydes′dale′
coach′man
co′ad•ju′tor
co•ag′u•lant
co•ag′u•lase′
co•ag′u•late′, -lat′ed,
   -lat′ing
co•ag′u•la′tion
co•ag′u•la′tor
coal (fuel)
   ♦kohl

co′a•lesce′, -lesced′,
   -lesc′ing
co′a•les′cence
co′a•les′cent
coal′field′
co•a•li′tion
co′-an′chor
coarse (rough), coars′-
   er, coars′est
   ♦course
coars′en
coast′al
coast′er
coast′land′
coast′line′
coat (garment)
   ♦cote
coat′dress′
co•a′ti pl. -tis
coat′ing
coat of arms pl.
   coats of arms
coat of mail pl. coats
   of mail
coat′room′
coat′tail′
co-au′thor
coax
co•ax′i•al
cob
co′balt′
cob′ble, -bled, -bling
cob′bler
cob′ble•stone′
CO′BOL′ or Co′bol′
co′bra
cob′web′

co′ca
co•caine′ also co-
   cain′
coc′coid′ also coc′cal
coc′cus pl. -ci′
coc′cyx pl. coc•cy′ges
coch′i•neal′
coch′le•a pl. -ae′
cock•ade′
cock′a•ma′mie also
   cock′a•ma′my
cock′-and-bull′
   story
cock′a•too′ pl. -toos′
cock′a•trice′
cock′chaf′er
cock′crow′
cock′er•el
cock′er spaniel
cock′eyed′
cock′fight′
cock′le
cock′le•bur′
cock′le•shell′
cock′ney pl. -neys
cock′pit′
cock′roach′
cocks′comb′
cock′sure′
cock′tail′
cock′y
co′co (palm tree), pl.
   -cos
co′coa (beverage)
co′con•spir′a•tor
co′co•nut′ also co′-
   coa•nut′

co•coon′

cod *pl.* cod *or* cods

co′da

cod′dle, -dled, -dling

code, cod′ed, cod′ing

co•de•fen′dant

co′deine′

co′dex′ *pl.* -di•ces′

cod′fish′ *pl.* -fish′ *or* -fish′es

codg′er

cod′i•cil

cod′i•fi•ca′tion

cod′i•fy′, -fied′, -fy′- ing

cod′ling

cod′-liv′er oil

co′ed′ *or* co′-ed′

co•ed′u•ca′tion *also* co-ed′u•ca′tion

co′ed•u•ca′tion•al

co′ef•fi′cient

coe′la•canth′

coe•len′ter•ate′

co•en′zyme′

co•e′qual

co•e•qual′i•ty

co•erce′, -erced′, -erc′- ing

co•erc′i•ble

co•er′cion

co•er′cive

co•e′val

co′ex•ist′

co′ex•is′tence

co′ex•is′tent

co′ex•tend′

co′ex•ten′sive

cof′fee

coffee house *also* cof′fee•house′

cof′fee•mak′er

cof′fee•pot′

cof′fer

cof′fer•dam′

cof′fin

co′func′tion

cog

co′gen•cy

co′gent

cog′i•ta•ble

cog′i•tate′, -tat′ed, -tat′ing

cog′i•ta′tion

cog′i•ta′tor

co′gnac′

cog′nate′

cog•ni′tion

cog′ni•tive

cog′ni•za•ble

cog′ni•zance

cog′ni•zant

cog•no′men *pl.* -no′- mens *or* -nom′i•na

co′gno•scen′te *pl.* -ti

cog′wheel′

co•hab′it

co•hab′i•tant

co•hab′i•ta′tion

co•here′ *(to stick to- gether)*, -hered′, -her′ing
♦*adhere*

co•her′ence *also* co- her′en•cy

co•her′ent

co•he′sion

co•he′sive

co′hort′

coif•feur′ *(hairdress- er)*

coif•fure′ *(to style hair)*, -fured′, -fur′- ing

coil

coin *(money)*
♦*quoin*

coin′age

co′in•cide′, -cid′ed, -cid′ing

co•in′ci•dence

co•in′ci•dent

co•in′ci•den′tal

co′i′tus *also* co•i′tion

coke *(fuel)*

Coke® *(beverage)*

co′la

col′an•der

cold′-blood′ed

co′le•op′ter•an *also* co′le•op′ter•on

cole′slaw′

co′le•us *pl.* -us•es

col′ic

col′ick•y

col′i•se′um

co•li′tis

col•lab′o•rate′, -rat′- ed, -rat′ing

col•lab′o•ra′tion

col•lab′o•ra′tion-

ism
col•lab′o•ra′tion•ist
col•lab′o•ra′tor
col•lage′
col•la•gen
col•lapse′, -lapsed′,
  -laps′ing
col•laps′i•ble *also*
  col•laps′a•ble
col′lar *(neckpiece)*
  ♦*choler*
col′lar•bone′
col′lard
col•late′, -lat′ed, -lat′-
  ing
col•lat′er•al
col•la′tion
col•la′tor
col′league′
col•lect′
col•lect′i•ble *also*
  col•lect′a•ble
col•lec′tion
col•lec′tive
col•lec′tiv•ism
col•lec′tiv•ist
col•lec′tiv•i•za′tion
col•lec′tiv•ize′,
  -ized′, -iz′ing
col•lec′tor
col′leen′
col′lege
col•le′gi•al′i•ty
col•le′gian
col•le′giate
col′lide′, -lid′ed, -lid′-
  ing

col′lie
col′lier
col′lier•y
col′lin′e•ar
col•li′sion
col′lo•cate′, -cat′ed,
  -cat′ing
col′lo•ca′tion
col•lo′di•on *also*
  col•lo′di•um
col′loid′
col•loi′dal
col•lo′qui•al
col•lo′qui•al•ism
col•lo′qui•um *pl.*
  -qui•ums *or* -qui•a
col′lo•quy
col•lude′, -lud′ed,
  -lud′ing
col•lu′sion
col•lu′sive
co•logne′
Co•lom′bi•an *(na-*
  tive of Colombia)
  ♦*Columbian*
co′lon *(punctuation*
  mark)
co′lon *(intestine), pl.*
  -lons *or* -la
colo′nel *(officer)*
  ♦*kernel*
colo′nel•cy
co•lo′ni•al
co•lo′ni•al•ism
co•lo′ni•al•ist
col′o•nist
col′o•ni•za′tion

col′o•nize′, -nized′,
  -niz′ing
col′o•niz′er
col′on•nade′
col′on•nad′ed
col′o•ny
col′o•phon′
col′or
Col′o•ra′dan
col′or•a′tion
col′or•a•tu′ra
col′or•blind′
col′or•cast′, -cast′ *or*
  -cast′ed, -cast′ing
col′ored
col′or•fast′
col′or•ful
col′or•im′e•ter
col′or•ing
col′or•ist
col′or•i•za′tion
col′or•ize′, -ized′, -iz′-
  ing
col′or•less
co•los′sal
co•los′sus *pl.* -si′ *or*
  -sus•es
colt′ish
Co•lum′bi•an *(of the*
  U.S.)
  ♦*Colombian*
co•lum′bic
col′um•bine′
co•lum′bi•um
Co•lum′bus Day
col′umn
co•lum′nar

col'um•nist
co'ma *pl.* -mas
co'ma•tose'
comb
com•bat' *v.*
com'bat' *n.*
com•bat'ant
com•bat'ive
com•bi•na'tion
com•bine', -bined',
  -bin'ing
com'bine' *n.*
com•bin'er
comb'ings
com'bo *pl.* -bos
com•bus'ti•bil'i•ty
com•bus'ti•ble
com•bus'tion
com•bus'tive
come, came, come,
  com'ing
come'back' *n.*
co•me'di•an
co•me'dic
co•me'di•enne'
com'e•do' *pl.* com'-
  e•dos' *or* com'e•do'-
  nes
come'down' *n.*
com'e•dy
come'ly
come'-on' *n.*
com'er
co•mes'ti•ble
com'et
come'up'pance
com'fit

com'fort
com'fort•a•ble
com'fort•er
com'fy
com'ic
com'i•cal
com'ing-out' *n.*
com'i•trag'e•dy
com'i•ty *pl.* -ties
com'ma
com•mand'
com'man•dant'
com'man•deer'
com•mand'er
commander in chief
  pl. commanders in
  chief
com•mand'ing
com•mand'ment
com•man'do *pl.* -dos
  or -does
com•me'di•a
  dell'ar'te
com•mem'o•rate',
  -rat'ed, -rat'ing
com•mem'o•ra'tion
com•mem'o•ra•tive
com•mem'o•ra'tor
com•mem'o•ra•to'-
  ry
com•mence',
  -menced', -menc'ing
com•mence'ment
com•mend'
com•mend'a•ble
com'men•da'tion
com•men'da•to'ry

com•men'sal
com•men'sal•ism
com•men'su•ra•ble
com•men'su•rate
com'ment'
com'men•tar'y
com'men•tate', -tat'-
  ed, -tat'ing
com'men•ta'tor
com'merce
com•mer'cial
com•mer'cial•ism
com•mer'cial•i•za'-
  tion
com•mer'cial•ize',
  -ized', -iz'ing
com•mer'cial•ly
com•min'gle, -gled,
  -gling
com•mis'er•ate', -at'-
  ed, -at'ing
com•mis'er•a'tion
com•mis'er•a'tive
com•mis'er•a'tor
com'mis•sar'
com'mis•sar'i•at
com'mis•sar'y
com•mis'sion
com•mis'sion•er
com•mit', -mit'ted,
  -mit'ting
com•mit'ment
com•mit'tal
com•mit'tee
com•mix'
com•mix'ture
com•mode'

com•mo'di•ous
com•mod'i•ty
com'mo•dore'
com'mon
com'mon•al•ty
com'mon•er
com'mon-law' *adj.*
com'mon•place'
com'mons
com'mon•sense'
com'mon•weal'
com'mon•wealth'
com•mo'tion
com•mu'nal
com•mu'nal•ism
com•mu'nal•ist
com•mu•nal'i•ty
com•mune' *n.*
com•mune',
  -muned', -mun'ing
com•mu•ni•ca•bil'-
  i•ty
com•mu'ni•ca•ble
com•mu'ni•cant
com•mu'ni•cate',
  -cat'ed, -cat'ing
com•mu•ni•ca'tion
com•mu'ni•ca'tive
com•mu'ni•ca'tor
com•mun'ion
com•mu'ni•qué'
com'mu•nism
Com'mu•nist *also*
  com'mu•nist
com'mu•nis'tic
com•mu'ni•ty
com•mu•ni•za'tion

com'mu•nize',
  -nized', -niz'ing
com'mu•ta'tion
com'mu•ta'tive
com'mu•ta'tor
com•mute', -mut'ed,
  -mut'ing
com•mut'er
com•pact' *adj. & v.*
com'pact' *n.*
com•pac'tor
com•pa'dre
com•pan'ion
com•pan'ion•a•ble
com•pan'ion•ship'
com•pan'ion•way'
com'pa•ny
com•pa•ra•bil'i•ty
com'pa•ra•ble
com•par'a•tive
com•pare', -pared',
  -par'ing
com•par'i•son
com•part'ment
com'part•men'tal•
  ize', -ized', -iz'ing
com'pass
com•pas'sion
com•pas'sion•ate
com•pat•i•bil'i•ty
com•pat'i•ble
com•pa'tri•ot
com•peer'
com•pel', -pelled',
  -pel'ling
com•pen'di•ous
com•pen'di•um *pl.*

  -di•ums *or* -di•a
com'pen•sate', -sat'-
  ed, -sat'ing
com'pen•sa'tion
com'pen•sa'tor
com•pen'sa•to'ry
com•pcte', -pet'ed,
  -pet'ing
com•pe'tence *also*
  com'pe•ten•cy
com'pe•tent
com•pe•ti'tion
com•pet'i•tive
com•pet'i•tor
com'pi•la'tion
com•pile', -piled',
  -pil'ing
com•pla'cen•cy *also*
  com•pla'cence
com•pla'cent *(smug)*
  ♦*complaisant*
com•plain'
com•plain'ant
com•plaint'
com•plai'sance
  (compliance)
  ♦*complacence*
com•plai'sant *(oblig-
  ing)*
  ♦*complacent*
com'ple•ment *(full
  amount)*
  ♦*compliment*
com'ple•men•tar'-
  i•ty
com'ple•men'ta•ry
  (completing)

♦*complimentary*
com•plete′, -plet′ed,
　-plet′ing
com•ple′tion
com•plex′ *adj.*
com′plex′ *n.*
com•plex′ion
com•plex′i•ty
com•pli′ance *also*
　com•pli′an•cy
com•pli′ant
com′pli•cate′, -cat′-
　ed, -cat′ing
com′pli•cat′ed
com′pli•ca′tion
com•plic′it
com•plic′i•ty
com′pli•ment
　(praise)
♦*complement*
com′pli•men′ta•ry
　(flattering)
♦*complementary*
com′plin *also* com′-
　pline
com•ply′, -plied′,
　-ply′ing
com•po′nent
com•port′
com•port′ment
com•pose′, -posed′,
　-pos′ing
com•pos′er
com•pos′ite
com′po•si′tion
com•pos′i•tor
com′post′

com•po′sure
com′pote′
com′pound′ *adj. & n.*
com•pound′ *v.*
com′pre•hend′
com′pre•hend′i•ble
com′pre•hen′si•bil′-
　i•ty
com′pre•hen′si•ble
com′pre•hen′sion
com′pre•hen′sive
com•press′ *n.*
com•press′ *v.*
com•press′i•bil′i•ty
com•press′i•ble
com•pres′sion
com•pres′sive
com•pres′sor
com•prise′, -prised′,
　-pris′ing
com′pro•mise′,
　-mised′, -mis′ing
com′pro•mis′er
com•pul′sion
com•pul′sive
com•pul′so•ry
com•punc′tion
com•put′a•bil′i•ty
com•put′a•ble
com′pu•ta′tion
com•pute′, -put′ed,
　-put′ing
com•put′er
com•put′er•dom
com•put′er•i•za′-
　tion
com•put′er•ize′,

-ized′, -iz′ing
com′rade
Com′sat′
con, conned, con′ning
con•cat′e•nate′,
　-nat′ed, -nat′ing
con•cat′e•na′tion
con•cave′
con•cav′i•ty
con•ceal′
con•ceal′ment
con•cede′, -ced′ed,
　-ced′ing
con•ceit′
con•ceit′ed
con•ceiv′a•bil′i•ty
con•ceiv′a•ble
con•ceive′, -ceived′,
　-ceiv′ing
con•cel′e•brant
con•cel′e•brate′,
　-brat′ed, -brat′ing
con′cen•trate′, -trat′-
　ed, -trat′ing
con′cen•tra′tion
con′cen•tra′tor
con•cen′tric
con′cen•tric′i•ty
con′cept
con•cep′tion
con•cep′tu•al
con•cep′tu•al•ism
con•cep′tu•a•list
con•cep′tu•al•i•za′-
　tion
con•cep′tu•al•ize′,
　-ized′, -iz′ing

con•cern′
con•cern′ing
con′cert n. & adj.
con•cert′ v.
con•cert′ed
con′cert•go′er
con•cer•ti′na
con•cer•ti′no pl. -nos
con′cert•mas′ter
con•cer′to pl. -tos or
  -ti
con•ces′sion
con•ces′sion•aire′
con•ces′sive
conch (mollusk), pl.
  conchs or conch′es
  ♦conk
con•cierge′
con•cil′i•ate′, -at′ed,
  -at′ing
con•cil′i•a′tion
con•cil′i•a′tor
con•cil′i•a•to′ry
con•cise′
con′clave
con•clude′, -clud′ed,
  -clud′ing
con•clu′sion
con•clu′sive
con•clu′so•ry
con•coct′
con•coc′tion
con•com′i•tance
con•com′i•tant
con′cord (harmony)
  ♦Concorde
con•cor′dance

con•cor′dant
con•cor′dat′
Con•corde′ (plane)
  ♦concord
con′course′
con•cres′cence
con•crete′ adj.
con′crete′ n.
con•crete′, -cret′ed,
  -cret′ing
con•cre′tion
con•cu′bine′
con•cu′pis•cence
con•cu′pis•cent
con•cur′, -curred′,
  -cur′ring
con•cur′rence
con•cur′rent
con•cus′sion
con•demn′
con•dem•na′tion
con•dem′na•to′ry
con•dens′a•ble also
  con•dens′i•ble
con•den•sa′tion
con•dense′, -densed′,
  -dens′ing
con•dens′er
con•de•scend′
con•de•scen′sion
con•dign′
con′di•ment
con•di′tion
con•di′tion•al
con•di′tioned
con•di′tion•er
con•di′tion•ing

con•dole′, -doled′,
  -dol′ing
con•do′lence
con′do•min′i•um
con′do•na′tion
con•done′, -doned′,
  -don′ing
con′dor
con•duce′, -duced′,
  -duc′ing
con•du′cive
con′duct′ n.
con•duct′ v.
con•duc′tance
con•duct′i•ble
con•duc′tion
con•duc′tive
con′duc•tiv′i•ty
con•duc′tor
con′duit
cone
con′fab′, -fabbed′,
  -fab′bing
con•fab′u•late′, -lat′-
  ed, -lat′ing
con•fab′u•la′tion
con•fab′u•la′tor
con•fec′tion
con•fec′tion•er′y
con•fed′er•a•cy
con•fed′er•ate′, -at′-
  ed, -at′ing
con•fed′er•a′tion
con•fed′er•a′tive
con•fer′, -ferred′,
  -fer′ring
con′fer•ee′

con•fer•ence
con•fess′
con•fes′sion
con•fes′sion•al
con•fes′sor
con•fet′ti
con′fi•dant′ *(friend)*,
  fem. con′fi•dante′
  ♦*confident*
con•fide′, -fid′ed,
  -fid′ing
con′fi•dence
con′fi•dent *(self-as-
  sured)*
  ♦*confidant*
con′fi•den′tial
con′fi•den′ti•al′i•ty
con•fig′u•ra′tion
con•fig′u•ra′tive
con•fig′ure, -ured,
  -ur•ing
con•fine′, -fined′,
  -fin′ing
con•fine′ment
con•firm′
con′fir•ma′tion
con′fis•cate′, -cat′ed,
  -cat′ing
con′fis•ca′tion
con′fis•ca′tor
con′fla•gra′tion
con′flict′ *n.*
con•flict′ *v.*
con•flic′tive
con′flu•ence *also*
  con′flux
con′flu•ent

con•form′
con•form′a•ble
con′for•ma′tion
con•form′ist
con•form′i•ty *also*
  con•for′mance
con•found′
con•fra•ter′ni•ty
con•frere′
con•front′
con′fron•ta′tion
Con•fu′cian
Con•fu′cian•ism
con•fuse′, -fused′,
  -fus′ing
con•fus′ed•ly
con•fu′sion
con′fu•ta′tion
con•fute′, -fut′ed,
  -fut′ing
con′ga
con•geal′
con•ge•ner
con•gen′ial
con•ge′ni•al′i•ty
con•gen′i•tal
con′ger
con•ge′ries
con•gest′
con•ges′tion
con•ges′tive
con•glom′er•ate′,
  -at′ed, -at′ing
con•glom′er•a′tion
Con•go•lese′ *pl.*
  -lese′
con•grat′u•late′,

  -lat′ed, -lat′ing
con•grat′u•la′tion
con•grat′u•la′tor
con•grat′u•la•to′ry
con′gre•gate′, -gat′-
  ed, -gat′ing
con′gre•ga′tion
con′gre•ga′tion•al
con′gre•ga′tion•al•
  ism
Con′gre•ga′tion•al•
  ist
con′gre•ga′tor
con′gress
con•gres′sion•al
con′gress•man
con′gress•per′son
con′gress•wom′an
con′gru•ence *also*
  con′gru•en•cy
con′gru•ent
con•gru′i•ty
con′gru•ous
con′ic *also* con′i•cal
con′i•fer
co•nif′er•ous
con•jec′tur•al
con•jec′ture, -tured,
  -tur•ing
con•join′
con•joint′
con′ju•gal
con′ju•gate′, -gat′ed,
  -gat′ing
con′ju•ga′tion
con′ju•ga′tor
con•junct′

con•junc′tion

con′junc•ti′va *pl.*
　-vas *or* -vae

con′junc•ti′val

con•junc′tive

con•junc′ti•vi′tis

con•junc′ture

con′ju•ra′tion

con′jure, -jured, -jur-
　ing

con′jur•er *also* con′-
　jur•or

conk *(to hit)*
　♦*conch*

con′nate′

con•nect′

con•nec′tion

con•nec′tive

con•nec′tor

con′ning tower

con•nip′tion

con•niv′ance

con•nive′, -nived′,
　-niv′ing

con′nois•seur′

con′no•ta′tion

con′no•ta′tive

con•note′, -not′ed,
　-not′ing

con•nu′bi•al

con′quer

con′quer•a•ble

con′quer•or

con′quest

con•quis′ta•dor

con•san′guin′e•ous

con′san•guin′i•ty

con′science

con′sci•en′tious

con′scious

con′scious•ness

con′scious•ness-
　rais′ing

con•script′ *n.*

con•script′ *v.*

con•scrip′tion

con′se•crate′, -crat′-
　ed, -crat′ing

con′se•cra′tion

con′se•cra′tor

con•sec′u•tive

con•sen′sus

con•sent′

con′se•quence

con′se•quent

con′se•quen′tial

con•serv′a•ble

con′ser•va′tion

con′ser•va′tion•ist

con•ser′va•tism

con•ser′va•tive

con•ser′va•tor

con•ser′va•to′ry

con•serve′, -served′,
　-serv′ing

con•sid′er

con•sid′er•a•ble

con•sid′er•ate

con•sid′er•a′tion

con•sign′

con′sign•ee′

con•sign′ment

con•sig′nor *also* con-
　sign′er

con•sist′

con•sis′ten•cy *also*
　con•sis′tence

con•sis′tent

con•sis′to′ri•al

con•sis′to•ry

con′sol
　♦*console*

con•sol′a•ble

con′so•la′tion

con•sol′a•to′ry

con•sole′ *n.*

con•sole′, -soled′,
　-sol′ing
　♦*consol*

con•sol′i•date′, -dat′-
　ed, -dat′ing

con•sol′i•da′tion

con•sol′i•da′tor

con′som•mé′

con′so•nance

con′so•nant

con′so•nan′tal

con′sort′ *n.*

con•sort′ *v.*

con•sor′ti•um *pl.*
　-ti•a

con•spec′tus

con•spic′u•ous

con•spir′a•cist

con•spir′a•cy

con•spir′a•tor

con•spir′a•to′ri•al

con•spir′a•to′ri-
　a•list

con•spire′, -spired′,
　-spir′ing

con'sta•ble
con'stab'u•lar'y
con'stan•cy
con'stant
con'stel•la'tion
con'ster•na'tion
con'sti•pate', -pat'-
ed, -pat'ing
con'sti•pa'tion
con•stit'u•en•cy
con•stit'u•ent
con'sti•tute', -tut'ed,
-tut'ing
con'sti•tu'tion
con'sti•tu'tion•al
con'sti•tu'tion•al'-
i•ty
con'sti•tu'tion•al•
ize', -ized', -iz'ing
con'sti•tu'tive
con•strain'
con•straint'
con•strict'
con•stric'tion
con•stric'tive
con•stric'tor
con•struct'
con•struc'tion
con•struc'tive
con•struc'tor *also*
con•struct'er
con•strue', -strued',
-stru'ing
con'sul
con'su•lar
con'su•late
con•sult'

con•sul'tant
con'sul•ta'tion
con•sul'ta•tive
con•sul'tor
con•sum'a•ble
con•sume', -sumed',
-sum'ing
con•sum'er
con•sum'er•ism
con•sum'er•ist
con•sum'mate *adj.*
con'sum•mate',
-mat'ed, -mat'ing
con'sum•ma'tion
con•sump'tion
con•sump'tive
con'tact'
con'tact•or
con•ta'gion
con•ta'gious
con•tain'
con•tain'er
con•tain'er•i•za'-
tion
con•tain'er•ize',
-ized', -iz'ing
con•tain'ment
con•tam'i•nant
con•tam'i•nate',
-nat'ed, -nat'ing
con•tam'i•na'tion
con•tam'i•na'tor
con'tem•plate',
-plat'ed, -plat'ing
con'tem•pla'tion
con•tem'pla•tive
con'tem•pla'tor

con•tem'po•ra'ne-
ous
con•tem'po•rar'y
con•tempt'
con•tempt'i•ble
con•temp'tu•ous
con•tend'
con•tent' *adj. & v.*
con•tent' *n.*
con•tent'ed
con•ten'tion
con•ten'tious
con•tent'ment
con•ter'mi•nous
con'test' *n.*
con•test' *v.*
con•test'a•ble
con•test'ant
con'text
con•tex'tu•al
con•tex'tu•al•ize',
-ized', -iz'ing
con•ti•gu'i•ty
con•tig'u•ous
con'ti•nence
con'ti•nent
con'ti•nen'tal
con•tin'gen•cy
con•tin'gent
con•tin'u•al
con•tin'u•ance
con•tin'u•a'tion
con•tin'ue, -ued,
-u•ing
con•tin'u•er
con'ti•nu'i•ty
con•tin'u•o' *pl.* -os

con•tin′u•ous
con•tin′u•um *pl.*
  -u•a *or* -u•ums
con•tort′
con•tor′tion
con•tor′tion•ist
con•tor′tion•is′tic
con′tour
con′tra•band′
con′tra•bass′
con′tra•bas•soon′
con′tra•cep′tion
con′tra•cep′tive
con•tract′ *n.*
con•tract′ *v.*
con•tract′i•ble
con•trac′tile
con•trac′tion
con′trac•tor
con•trac′tu•al
con′tra•dict′
con′tra•dict′er *also*
  con′tra•dic′tor
con′tra•dic′tion
con′tra•dic′to•ry
con′tra•dis•tinc′-
  tion
con′trail′
con′tral′to *pl.* -tos
con•trap′tion
con′tra•pun′tal
con′tra•pun′tist
con′trar′i•an
con′tra•ri′e•ty
con′trar•i•wise′
con′trar′y
con′trast′ *n.*

con•trast′ *v.*
con′tra•vene′,
  -vened′, -ven′ing
con′tra•ven′tion
con′tre•temps′
con•trib′ute, -ut•ed,
  -ut•ing
con′tri•bu′tion
con•trib′u•tive
con•trib′u•tor
con•trib′u•to′ry
con•trite′
con•tri′tion
con•tri′vance
con•trive′, -trived′,
  -triv′ing
con•triv′ed•ly
con•trol′, -trolled′,
  -trol′ling
con•trol′la•ble
con•trol′ler *also*
  comp•trol′ler
con′tro•ver′sial
con′tro•ver′sy
con′tro•vert′
con′tro•vert′i•ble
con′tu•ma′cious
con′tu•ma•cy
con′tu•me′li•ous
con′tu•me•ly
con•tuse′, -tused′,
  -tus′ing
con•tu′sion
co•nun′drum
con′ur•ba′tion
con′va•lesce′,
  -lesced′, -lesc′ing

con′va•les′cence
con′va•les′cent
con•vect′ *v.*
con•vec′tion
con•vec′tor
con•vene′, -vened′,
  -ven′ing
con•ven′ience
con•ven′ient
con′vent
con•ven′tion
con•ven′tion•al
con•ven′tion•al′i•ty
con•ven′tion•eer′
con•verge′, -verged′,
  -verg′ing
con•ver′gence *also*
  con•ver′gen•cy
con•ver′gent
con•ver′sant
con′ver•sa′tion
con′ver•sa′tion•al
con′ver•sa′tion•al-
  ist
con•verse′ *adj.*
con′verse′ *n.*
con•verse′, -versed′,
  -vers′ing
con•ver′sion
con′vert′ *n.*
con•vert′ *v.*
con•vert′er *also* con-
  ver′tor
con•vert′i•bil′i•ty
con•vert′i•ble
con′vex
con•vex′i•ty

con•vey′
con•vey′ance
con•vey′er *also* con-
  vey′or
con′vict′ *n.*
con•vict′ *v.*
con•vic′tion
con•vince′, -vinced′,
  -vinc′ing
con•vinc′i•ble
con•viv′i•al
con•viv′i•al′i•ty
con′vo•ca′tion
con•voke′, -voked′,
  -vok′ing
con′vo•lute′, -lut′ed,
  -lut′ing
con′vo•lu′tion
con′voy′
con•vulse′, -vulsed′,
  -vuls′ing
con•vul′sion
con•vul′sive
co′ny *also* co′ney *pl.*
  -neys
coo *(murmuring*
  sound), pl. coos
  ♦*coup*
coo *(to make a mur-*
  muring sound),
  cooed, coo′ing
  ♦*coup*
cook′book′
cook′er
cook′er•y
cook′out′
cook′ware′

cook′y *or* cook′ie
cool′ant
cool′er
cool′-head′ed
coo′lie *(laborer), also*
  coo′ly
  ♦*coulee*
cool′ly *(in a cool*
  manner)
  ♦*coulee*
coon′hound′
coon′skin′
coop *(cage)*
  ♦*coupe*
co-op′ *(cooperative)*
coo′per
coo′per•age
co•op′er•ate′, -at′ed,
  -at′ing
co•op′er•a′tion
co•op′er•a•tive
co•op′er•a′tor
co-opt′
co•or′di•nate′, -nat′-
  ed, -nat′ing
co•or′di•na′tion
co•or′di•na′tor
coot
coo′tie
cop, copped, cop′ping
co′pal
co•part′ner
cope, coped, cop′ing
co′pe•pod′
Co•per′ni•can
cop′i•er
co′pi′lot

cop′ing
co′pi•ous
co•pla′nar
co•pol′y•mer
cop′-out′ *n.*
cop′per
cop′per•as
cop′per•head′
cop′per•plate′
cop′per•smith′
cop′pice
cop′ra
copse
cop′ter
cop′u•la
cop′u•lar
cop′u•late′, -lat′ed,
  -lat′ing
cop′u•la′tion
cop′u•la′tive
cop′y, -ied, -y•ing
cop′y•book′
cop′y•cat′
cop′y-ed′it
cop′y•ist
cop′y•read′er
cop′y•right′
cop′y•writ′er
coq au vin′
co′quet•ry
co•quette′
co•quet′tish
co•quille′
co•qui′na
cor′a•cle
cor′al *(marine skele-*
  ton)

♦*choral*
cor'al-bells'
cor'bel
cord *(rope)*
  ♦*chord*
cord'age
cor'dial
cor'dial'i•ty
cor'dil•le'ra
cor'dil•le'ran
cord'ite'
cor'don
cor'do•van
cor'du•roy
cord'wood'
core *(to remove the center)*, cored, cor'-ing
  ♦*corps*
cor'er
co're•spon'dent *(adulterer)*
  ♦*correspondent*
co'ri•an'der
co'ri•um *pl.* -ri•a
cork'er
cork'screw'
cork'y
corm
cor'mo•rant
corn'cob'
corn'crib'
cor'ne•a
cor'ne•al
cor'nc•ous
cor'ner
cor'ner•back'

cor'ner•stone'
cor•net'
cor•net'ist *also* cor-net'tist
corn'field'
corn'flow'er
corn'husk'
cor'nice
corn'meal'
corn'stalk'
corn'starch'
cor'nu•co'pi•a
cor'nu•co'pi•an
corn'y
co•rol'la
cor'ol•lar'y
co•ro'na *pl.* -nas *or* -nae
cor'o•nar'y
cor'o•na'tion
cor'o•ner
cor'o•net'
cor•poc'ra•cy
cor'po•ral
cor'po•rate
cor'po•ra'tion
cor•po're•al
corps *(troops)*
  ♦*core*
corpse *(body)*
cor'pu•lence
cor'pu•lent
cor'pus *pl.* -po•ra
cor'pus•cle
cor•pus'cu•lar
corpus de•lic'ti
cor•ral' *(to capture or*

pen up), -ralled', -ral'ling
  ♦*chorale*
cor•rect'
cor•rec'tion
cor•rec'tion•al
cor•rec'tive
cor're•late', -lat'ed, -lat'ing
cor're•la'tion
cor•rel'a•tive
cor're•spond'
cor're•spon'dencc
cor're•spon'dent *(writer)*
  ♦*corespondent*
cor'ri•dor
cor'ri•gen'dum *pl.* -da
cor•rob'o•rate', -rat'-ed, -rat'ing
cor•rob'o•ra'tion
cor•rob'o•ra'tive
cor•rob'o•ra'tor
cor•rode', -rod'ed, -rod'ing
cor•rod'i•ble *or* cor-ro'si•ble
cor•ro'sion
cor•ro'sive
cor'ru•gate', -gat'ed, -gat'ing
cor'ru•ga'tion
cor•rupt'
cor•rup'ter *or* cor-rup'tor
cor•rupt'i•ble

cor•rup'tion
cor•rup'tive
cor•sage'
cor'sair
cor'set
Cor'si•can
cor•tege'
cor'tex *pl.* -ti•ces *or* -tex•es
cor'ti•cal
cor'ti•sone'
co•run'dum
cor'us•cate', -cat'ed, -cat'ing
cor'us•ca'tion
cor•vette'
cor'vine'
co•ry'za
co•se'cant
co•sign' *(to sign jointly)*
co'sine' *(mathematical function)*
cos•met'ic
cos'me•tol'o•gist
cos'me•tol'o•gy
cos'mic *also* cos'mi•cal
cos•mog'o•ny
cos•mog'ra•phy
cos'mo•log'i•cal
cos•mol'o•gist
cos•mol'o•gy
cos'mo•naut
cos•mop'o•lis
cos'mo•pol'i•tan
cos'mos

co•spon'sor
Cos'sack
cos'set
cost
cos'ta *pl.* -tae
co'star' *also* co'-star'
Cos'ta Ri'can
cost'-ef•fec'tive
cost'-ef•fi'cient
cost'ly
cost'-plus'
cost'-push'
cos'tume, -tumed, -tum•ing
cos'tum•er
cot
co•tan'gent
cote *(shelter)*
♦*coat*
co'te•rie
co•til'lion
cot'tage
cot'tag•er
cot'ter
cot'ton
cot'ton•mouth'
cot'ton•seed'
cot'ton•tail'
cot'ton•wood'
cot'y•le'don
cot'y•le'don•al *also* cot'y•le'do•nous
couch
cou•chette'
cou'gar
cough
could'n't

cou'lee *(ravine)*
♦*coolie, coolly*
cou'lomb'
coun'cil *(assembly)*
♦*counsel*
coun'cil•or *(council member), also* coun'cil•lor
♦*counselor*
coun'sel *(to advise),* -seled *or* -selled, -sel•ing *or* -sel•ling
♦*council*
coun'sel•or *(adviser), also* coun'sel•lor
♦*councilor*
count'a•ble
count'down'
coun'te•nance, -nanced, -nanc•ing
coun'ter *(contrary)*
count'er *(serving table, game piece, one that counts)*
coun'ter•act'
coun'ter•ac'tion
coun'ter•ac'tive
coun'ter•ar'gu•ment
coun'ter•at•tack'
coun'ter•bal'ance n.
coun'ter•bal'ance, -anced, -anc•ing
coun'ter•blow'
coun'ter•claim' n.
coun'ter•claim' v.
coun'ter•clock'wise'

coun'ter•cul'ture

coun'ter•es'pi-
  o•nage'

coun'ter•feit'

coun'ter•foil'

coun'ter•force'

coun'ter•in•tel'li-
  gence

coun'ter•ir'ri•tant

coun'ter•mand'

coun'ter•mea'sure

coun'ter•of•fen'sive

coun'ter•pane'

coun'ter•part'

coun'ter•per'son

coun'ter•point'

coun'ter•poise' *n.*

coun'ter•poise',
  -poised', -pois'ing

coun'ter•pose',
  -posed', -pos'ing

coun'ter•pro•duc'-
  tive

coun'ter•punch'

coun'ter•rev'o•lu'-
  tion

coun'ter•shaft'

coun'ter•sign'

coun'ter•sink',
  -sunk', -sink'ing

coun'ter•spy'

coun'ter•ten'or

coun'ter•top'

coun'ter•weight'

count'ess

count'less

coun'try

coun'try•side'

coun'ty

coup *(masterstroke)*
  ♦*coo*

coup' de grâce' *pl.*
  coups' de grâce'

coup' d'é•tat' *pl.*
  coups' d'é•tat'

coupe *(dessert)*
  ♦*coop*

cou•pé' *(car),* also
  coupe

cou'ple, -pled, -pling

cou'plet

cou'pon'

cour'age

cou•ra'geous

cou'ri•er

course *(to flow),*
  coursed, cours'ing
  ♦*course*

cours'er

course'ware'

court

cour'te•ous

cour'te•san

cour'te•sy

court'house'

court'i•er

court'ly

court'-mar'tial *pl.*
  courts'-mar'tial

court'-mar'tial,
  -tialed *or* -tialled,
  -tial•ing *or* -tial•ling

court'room'

court'ship'

court'yard'

cous'in *(relative)*
  ♦*cozen*

cou•ture'

cou•tu'ri•er

co•va'lence *also* co-
  va'len•cy

co•va'lent

cove

cov'en

cov'e•nant

cov'er

cov'er•age

cov'er•alls'

cov'er•ing

cov'er•let

cov'ert

cov'er-up' *n. also*
  cov'er•up'

cov'et

cov'et•ous

cov'ey *pl.* -eys

cow'ard

cow'ard•ice

cow'bell'

cow'bird'

cow'boy'

cow'catch'er

cow'er

cow'girl'

cow'hand'

cow'herd'

cow'hide'

cow'lick'

cowl'ing

co'work'er

cow'poke'

cow′pox′
cow′punch′er
cow′ry *also* cow′rie
cow′skin′
cow′slip′
cox′comb′
cox′swain′
coy′ly
coy•o′te
coz′en *(to deceive)*
  ♦*cousin*
co′zy *also* co′sy
crab, crabbed, crab′-
  bing
crab′bed *adj.*
crab′by
crab′grass′
crack′brain′
crack′er
crack′er-bar′rel *adj.*
crack′er•jack′
crack′ing
crack′le, -led, -ling
crack′pot′
crack′up′ *n.*
cra′dle, -dled, -dling
cra′dle•song′
crafts′man
craft′y
crag′gy
cram, crammed,
  cram′ming
cramp
cram′pon
cran′ber′ry
crane, craned, cran′-

ing
cra′ni•al
cra•ni•ot′o•my
cra′ni•um *pl.* -ni-
  ums *or* -ni•a
crank′case′
crank′shaft′
crank′y
cran′ny
crap′pie
craps
crap′shoot′er
crap′u•lence
crash′-land′ *v.*
crass
crate, crat′ed, crat′ing
crat′er *(one that*
  crates)
cra′ter *(pit)*
cra•vat′
crave, craved, crav′-
  ing
cra′ven
crav′er
craw′fish′ *pl.* -fish′ *or*
  -fish′es
crawl′y
cray′fish′ *pl.* -fish′ *or*
  -fish′es
cray′on
craze, crazed, craz′ing
cra′zy
creak *(squeaking*
  sound)
  ♦*creek*
creak′y
cream′er

cream′er•y
crease, creased, creas′-
  ing
cre•ate′, -at′ed, -at′-
  ing
cre•a′tion
cre•a′tion•ism
cre•a′tion•ist
cre•a′tive
cre•a•tiv′i•ty
cre•a′tor
crea′ture
crèche
cre′dence
cre•den′tial
cre•den′za
cred′i•bil′i•ty
cred′i•ble
cred′it
cred′it•a•bil′i•ty
cred′it•a•ble
cred′i•tor
cre′do *pl.* -dos
cre•du′li•ty
cred′u•lous
creed
creek *(stream)*
  ♦*creak*
creel
creep, crept, creep′ing
creep′er
creep′y
cre′mate′, -mat′ed,
  -mat′ing
cre•ma′tion
cre′ma′tor
cre′ma•to′ri•um *pl.*

-ri•ums *or* -ri•a

cre'ma•to'ry

crème' de ca•ca•o'

crème' de la crème'

crème' de menthe'

cre'nate' *also* cre'nat'-
ed

Cre'ole'

cre'o•sol'

cre'o•sote'

crepe *also* crêpe

crêpe' de Chine'

crêpe' su•zette'

cre•pus'cu•lar

cres•cen'do *pl.* -dos
or -di

cres'cent

cre'sol'

cress

cres'set

crest'fall'en

Cre•ta'ceous

cre'tin

cre'tin•ism

cre•tonne'

cre•vasse' *(deep
crack)*

crev'ice *(narrow open-
ing)*

crew'-cut' *adj.*

crew'el *(yarn)*
♦*cruel*

crib, cribbed, crib'-
bing

crib'bage

crick

crick'et

cri'er

crime

Cri•me'an

crim'i•nal

crim'i•nal'i•ty

crim'i•no•log'i•cal

crim'i•nol'o•gist

crim'i•nol'o•gy

crimp

crim'son

cringe, cringed, cring'-
ing

crin'kle, -kled, -kling

crin'o•line

crip'ple, -pled, -pling

cri'sis *pl.* -ses'

crisp'er

crisp'y

criss'cross'

cri•te'ri•on *pl.* -ri•a
or -ri•ons

crit'ic

crit'i•cal

crit'i•cal'i•ty

crit'i•cism

crit'i•cize', -cized',
-ciz'ing

cri•tique', -tiqued',
-tiqu'ing

crit'ter

croak

cro•chet', -cheted',
-chet'ing

crock'er•y

croc'o•dile'

croc'o•dil'i•an

cro'cus *pl.* -cus•es *or*

-ci'

croft'er

crois•sant'

Cro-Mag'non

crom'lech

crone

cro'ny

crook'ed

crook'neck'

croon'er

crop, cropped, crop'-
ping

crop'per

cro•quet' *(game)*

cro•quette' *(food)*

cro'sier *also* cro'zier

cross'bar'

cross'beam'

cross'bones'

cross'bow'

cross'breed', -bred',
-breed'ing

cross'check'

cross'-coun'try

cross'court'

cross'cur'rent

cross'cut', -cut', -cut'-
ting

cross'-ex•am'i•na'-
tion

cross'-ex•am'ine,
-ined, -in•ing

cross'-eye'

cross'-eyed'

cross'-fer'ti•li•za'-
tion

cross'-fer'ti•lize',

-lized', -liz'ing
cross'fire'
cross'-grained'
cross'hatch'
cross'-leg'ged
cross'ing
cross'o'ver n.
cross'piece'
cross'-pol'li•nate',
 -nat'ed, -nat'ing
cross'-pol'li•na'tion
cross'-pur'pose
cross'-re•fer',
 -ferred', -fer'ring
cross'-ref 'er•ence
cross'road'
cross'-stitch'
cross'-town'
cross'walk'
cross'wise' also cross'-
 ways'
cross'word' puzzle
crotch'et
crotch'et•y
crouch
croup
crou'pi•er
crou'ton'
crow (bird)
crow, crowed, crow'-
 ing
crow'bar'
crowd
crow'foot' pl. -foots'
 or-feet'
crown'-of-thorns'
crow's'-foot' pl. -feet'

crow's'-nest'
cru'cial
cru'ci•ble
cru'ci•fix'
cru'ci•fix'ion
cru'ci•form'
cru'ci•fy', -fied', -fy'-
 ing
crud'dy
crude, crud'er, crud'-
 est
crude'ly
cru'di•ty
cru'el (merciless, pain-
 ful)
 ♦crewel
cru'el•ty
cru'et
cruise (to sail),
 cruised, cruis'ing
 ♦crews, cruse
cruis'er
crul'ler
crumb
crum'ble, -bled,
 -bling
crum'my
crum'pet
crum•ple, -pled,
 -pling
crunch'y
cru•sade', -sad'ed,
 -sad'ing
cru•sad'er
cruse (jar)
 ♦crews, cruise
crush'a•ble

crus•ta'cean
crus•ta'ceous
crust'y
crutch
crux pl. crux'es or cru'-
 ces
cry, cried, cry'ing
cry'ba•by
cry'o•bi•ol'o•gy
cry'o•gen
cry'o•gen'ic
cry'o•gen'ics
cry•on'ics
cry'o•sur'geon
cry'o•sur'ger•y
cry'o•sur'gi•cal
crypt
crypt•an'a•lyze',
 -lyzed', -lyz'ing
cryp'tic
cryp'to•gram'
cryp'to•graph'
cryp•tog'ra•pher
cryp'to•graph'ic
cryp•tog'ra•phy
cryp•tol'o•gy
crys'tal
crys'tal•line
crys'tal•li•za'tion
crys'tal•lize', -lized',
 -liz'ing
crys'tal•log'ra•pher
crys'tal•log'ra•phy
crys'tal•loid'
cten'o•phore'
Cu'ban
cub'by•hole'

cube, cubed, cub'ing
cu'bic
cu'bi•cal *(cubic)*
cu'bi•cle *(small compartment)*
cub'ism
cub'ist
cu'bit
cuck'old
cuck'old•ry
cuck'oo
cu'cum'ber
cud
cud'dle, -dled, -dling
cud'dle•some
cudg'el, -eled *or* -elled, -el•ing *or* -el•ling
cue *(rod, hint)*
    ♦*queue*
cue *(to hit a ball, signal),* cued, cu'ing
    ♦*queue*
cuff
cui•rass'
cui•sine'
cul'-de-sac' *pl.* -sacs'
cu'li•nar'y
cull
cul'mi•nate', -nat'ed, -nat'ing
cul'mi•na'tion
cu•lottes'
cul'pa•bil'i•ty
cul'pa•ble
cul'prit
cul'tic

cult'ist
cul'ti•va•ble *also* cul'ti•vat'a•ble
cul'ti•vate', -vat'ed, -vat'ing
cul'ti•va'tion
cul'ti•va'tor
cul'tur•al
cul'ture, -tured, -tur-ing
cul'vert
cum'ber
cum'ber•some
cum'brance
cum'brous
cum'in
cum lau'de
cum'mer•bund'
cu'mu•la'tive
cu'mu•lo•nim'bus *pl.* -bus•es *or* -bi'
cu'mu•lous *adj.*
cu'mu•lus *pl.* -li'
cu'ne•i•form'
cun'ning
cup, cupped, cup'ping
cup'board
cup'cake'
cu'pel, -peled *or* -pelled, -pel•ing *or* -pel•ling
cup'ful *pl.* -fuls'
Cu'pid
cu•pid'i•ty
cu'po•la
cu'pric
cu'prous

cur
cur'a•ble
cu•ra're *or* cu•ra'ri
cu'rate
cur'a•tive
cu•ra'tor
curb'ing
curb'side'
curb'stone'
curd
cur'dle, -dled, -dling
cure *(to remedy, preserve),* cured, cur'ing
cu•ré' *(parish priest)*
cure'-all'
cu'ret•tage'
cu•rette' *also* cu•ret'
cur'few
cu'ri•a *pl.* -ae'
cu'rie
cu'ri•o' *pl.* -os'
cu'ri•os'i•ty
cu'ri•ous
cu'ri•um
curl'er
curl'ew
curl'i•cue *also* curl'-y•cue'
curl'ing
curl'y
cur•mudg'eon
cur'rant *(berry)*
    ♦*current*
cur'ren•cy
cur'rent *(prevalent)*
    ♦*currant*
cur'rent *(electric*

charge)
♦*currant*
cur•ric′u•lar
cur•ric′u•lum *pl.* -la *or* -lums
cur′ry, -ried, -ry•ing
cur′ry•comb′
curse, cursed *or* curst, curs′ing
curs′ed *adj. also* curst
curs′er *(one that curs-es)*
♦*cursor*
cur′sive
cur′sor′ *(indicator)*
♦*curser*
cur′so•ry
cur•tail′
cur•tail′ment
cur′tain
curt′ly
curt′sy, -sied, -sy•ing
cur•va′ceous
cur′va•ture
curve, curved, curv′-ing
curv′ed•ly
cur′vet
cur•vi•lin′e•ar
cush′ion
cush′y
cusp
cus′pid
cus′pi•date′
cus′pi•dor′
cuss
cuss′ed *adj.*

cus′tard
cus•to′di•al
cus•to′di•an
cus′to•dy
cus′tom
cus′tom•ar′y
cus′tom-built′
cus′tom•er
cus′tom•house′
cus′tom•ize′, -ized′, -iz′ing
cus′tom-made′
cut, cut, cut′ting
cut′-and-dried′
cu•ta′ne•ous
cut′a•way′
cut′back′
cute, cut′er, cut′est
cute′ly
cu′ti•cle
cut′-in′ *(film shot)*
cu′tin *(waxlike sub-stance)*
cut′lass
cut′ler•y
cut′let
cut′off′ *n.*
cut′out′ *n.*
cut′-rate′
cut′ter
cut′throat′
cut′ting
cut′tle•bone′
cut′tle•fish′ *pl.* -fish′ *or* -fish′es
cut′up′ *n.*
cut′worm′

cy′an *(blue)*
♦*scion*
cy•an′ic
cy′a•nide′, -nid′ed, nid′ing
cy•an′o•gen
cy′a•no′sis
cy′a•not′ic
cy′ber•net′ic
cy′ber•net′ics
cyc′la•mate′
cyc′la•men
cyc′la•mic′ acid
cy′cle, -cled, -cling
cy′clic *also* cy′cli•cal
cy′clist *also* cy′cler
cy′cloid′
cy′clone′
cy•clon′ic
cy′clo•pe′di•a *also* cy′clo•pae′di•a
Cy′clops′ *pl.* Cy•clo′-pes
cy′clo•ram′a
cy′clo•tron′
cyg′net *(swan)*
♦*signet*
cyl′in•der
cy•lin′dri•cal *also* cy•lin′dric
cym′bal *(percussion instrument)*
♦*symbol*
cyn′ic
cyn′i•cal
cyn′i•cism
cy′no•sure′

cy′press
Cyp′ri•an
cyp′ri•noid′
Cyp′ri•ot *also* Cyp′-
ri•ote
Cy•ril′lic
cyst
cys′tic
cys•ti′tis
cy′to•gen′e•sis
cy′to•log′i•cal
cy•tol′o•gist
cy•tol′o•gy
cy′to•plasm
cy′to•plas′mic
cy′to•plast′
cy′to•sine′
czar *also* tsar, tzar
czar′e•vitch
cza•rev′na
cza•ri′na
czar′ism
czar′ist
Czech *(inhabitant)*
♦*check*
Czech′o•slo′vak *also*
Czech′o•slo•va′ki-
an

D

dab, dabbed, dab′bing
dab′ber
dab′ble, -bled, -bling
dab′bler
da ca′po
dace *pl.* dace *or* dac′es

da′cha
dachs′hund′
Da′cron′®
dac′tyl
dac•tyl′ic
Da′da *or* da′da, *also*
Da′da•ism
dad′dy
daddy long′legs′ *pl.*
daddy long′legs′
da′do *pl.* -does
daf′fo•dil
daf′fy
daft
dag′ger
da•guerre′o•type′
dahl′ia
dai′ly
dain′ty
dai′qui•ri *pl.* -ris
dair′y
dair′y•ing
dair′y•maid′
dair′y•man
da′is
dai′sy
Da•ko′tan
dale
dal′li•ance
dal′ly, -lied, -ly•ing
Dal•ma′tian
dam *(barrier, female*
parent)
♦*damn*
dam *(to restrain),*
dammed, dam′ming
♦*damn*

dam′age, -aged, -ag-
ing
dam′as•cene′,
-cened′, -cen′ing
dam′ask
dame
damn *(to condemn)*
♦*dam*
dam′na•ble
dam•na′tion
damned *(condemned)*
♦*dammed*
damp′en
damp′er
dam′sel
dam′sel•fly′
dam′son
dance, danced, danc′-
ing
danc′er
dance′wear′
dan′de•li′on
dan′der
Dan′die Din′mont′
dan′di•fi•ca′tion
dan′di•fy′, -fied′, -fy′-
ing
dan′dle, -dled, -dling
dan′druff
dan′dy
Dane *(native of Den-*
mark)
♦*deign*
dan′ger
dan′ger•ous
dan′gle, -gled, -gling
Dan′ish

dank'ness
dan•seur'
dan•seuse'
daph'ni•a *pl.* -ni•a
dap'per
dap'ple, -pled, -pling
dare, dared, dar'ing
dare'dev'il
dar'er
dare'say'
dar'ing
Dar•jee'ling
dark'en
dark'ness
dark'room'
dar'ling
darn
dar'nel
darn'ing needle
dart
dart'er
dar'tle, -tled, -tling
Dar•win'i•an
Dar'win•ism
dash'board'
dash'er
da•shi'ki
dash'ing
das'tard
da'ta *sing.* -tum
dat'a•ble *or* date'-
   a•ble
date, dat'ed, dat'ing
date'line'
da'tive
daub'er
daugh'ter

daugh'ter-in-law' *pl.*
   daugh'ters-in-law'
daunt'less
dau'phin
dav'en•port'
dav'it
daw
daw'dle, -dled, -dling
dawn
day'book'
day'break'
day'-care' *adj.*
day'dream',
   -dreamed' *or*
   -dreamt', -dream'ing
Day'-Glo'®
day'light'
day'light'-sav'ing
   time
day'long'
day'pack'
day'star'
day'time'
day'-to-day'
day'wear'
daze *(to stun),* dazed,
   daz'ing
   ♦*days*
daz'zle, -zled, -zling
de'-ac'ces'sion
dea'con
dea'con•ry
de•ac'ti•vate', -vat'-
   ed, -vat'ing
de•ac'ti•va'tion
dead'beat'

dead'en
dead'-end' *adj.*
dead'head'
dead'line'
dead'lock'
dead'ly
dead'pan'
dead'wood'
deaf'en
deaf'-mute'
deal, dealt, deal'ing
deal'er
deal'er•ship'
dean'er•y
dear *(beloved)*
   ♦*deer*
dearth
death'bed'
death'blow'
death'less
death'ly
death's'-head'
death'trap'
death'watch'
de•ba'cle
de•bar', -barred',
   -bar'ring
de•bark'
de'bar•ka'tion
de•base', -based',
   -bas'ing
de•base'ment
de•bat'a•ble
de•bate', -bat'ed,
   -bat'ing
de•bauch'
de•bauch'er•y

de•ben'ture
de•bil'i•tate', -tat'ed,
  -tat'ing
de•bil'i•ta'tion
de•bil'i•ta'tive
de•bil'i•ty
deb'it
deb'o•nair' *also* deb'-
  o•naire'
de•bone', -boned',
  -bon'ing
de•brief'
de•bris' *also* dé•bris'
debt'or
de•bug', -bugged',
  -bug'ging
de•bunk'
de•but' *also* dé•but'
deb'u•tante' *also* dé'-
  bu•tante'
dec'ade
dec'a•dence *also* dec'-
  a•den•cy
dec'a•dent
de•caf'fein•ate', -at'-
  ed, -at'ing
dec'a•gon'
dec'a•gram' *or* dek'-
  a•gram'
dec'a•he'dral
dec'a•he'dron *pl.*
  -drons *or* -dra
de'cal'
de•cal'ci•fi•ca'tion
de•cal'ci•fy', -fied',
  -fy'ing
de•cal•co•ma'ni•a

Dec'a•logue' *or* Dec'-
  a•log'
dec'a•me'ter *or* dek'-
  a•me'ter
de•camp'
de•cant'
de'can•ta'tion
de•cant'er
de•cap'i•tate', -tat'-
  ed, -tat'ing
de•cap'i•ta'tion
de•cap'i•ta'tor
de•car'bon•ate', -at'-
  cd, -at'ing
de•cath'lon
de•cay'
de•cease', -ceased',
  -ceas'ing
de•ce'dent
de•ceit'
de•ceit'ful
de•ceive', -ceived',
  -ceiv'ing
de•ceiv'er
de•cel'er•ate', -at'ed,
  -at'ing
de•cel'er•a'tion
De•cem'ber
de'cen•cy
de'cent *(proper)*
  ♦*descent, dissent*
de•cen'tral•i•za'-
  tion
de•cen'tral•ize',
  -ized', -iz'ing
de•cep'tion
de•cep'tive

dec'i•bel
de•cide', -cid'ed,
  -cid'ing
de•cid'u•ous
dec'i•gram'
dec'i•li'ter
de•cil'lion
de•cil'lionth
dec'i•mal
dec'i•mate', -mat'ed,
  -mat'ing
dec'i•ma'tion
dec'i•ma'tor
dec'i•me'ter
de•ci'pher
de•ci'pher•a•ble
de•ci'sion
de•ci'sive
deck'house'
deck'le, -led, -ling
deck'le-edged'
de•claim'
dec'la•ma'tion
de•clam'a•to'ry
de•clar'a•ble
dec'la•ra'tion
de•clar'a•tive
de•clare', -clared',
  -clar'ing
de•clas'si•fi•ca'tion
de•clas'si•fy', -fied',
  -fy'ing
de•claw'
de•clen'sion
dec'li•na'tion
de•cline', -clined',
  -clin'ing

de·cliv'i·ty
dec'o *pl.* dec'os
de·coct'
de·coc'tion
de·code', -cod'ed,
 -cod'ing
de·cod'er
dé'colle·tage'
dé'colle·té'
de'com·mis'sion
de'com·pos'a·ble
de'com·pose',
 -posed', -pos'ing
de'com·po·si'tion
de'com·press'
de'com·pres'sion
de'con·gest'
de'con·tam'i·nate',
 -nat'ed, -nat'ing
de'con·tam'i·na'-
 tion
de'con·trol',
 -trolled', -trol'ling
dé·cor' *also* de'cor'
dec'o·rate', -rat'ed,
 -rat'ing
dec'o·ra'tion
dec'o·ra'tive
dec'o·ra'tor
dec'o·rous
de·co'rum
de'coy'
de·crease' *n.*
de·crease', -creased',
 -creas'ing
de·cree'
dec're·ment

de·crep'it
de·crep'i·tude'
de'cre·scen'do *pl.*
 -dos
de·cre'tal
de·crim'i·nal·i·za'-
 tion
de·crim'i·nal·ize',
 -ized', -iz'ing
de·cry', -cried', -cry'-
 ing
de·crypt'
de·cus'sate', -sat'ed,
 -sat'ing
ded'i·cate', -cat'ed,
 -cat'ing
ded'i·ca'tion
ded'i·ca'tor
de·duce', -duced',
 -duc'ing
de·duc'i·ble
de·duct'
de·duct'i·ble
de·duc'tion
de·duc'tive
deed
dee'jay' *pl.* -jays'
deem
deep'en
Deep'freeze'®
deep'-fry', -fried',
 -fry'ing
deep'-root'ed
deep'-sea' *adj.*
deep'-seat'ed
deer *(animal) pl.* deer
 or deers

♦*dear*
deer'hound'
deer'skin'
deer·stalk'er
de'-es·ca·late', -lat'-
 ed, -lat'ing
de'-es·ca·la'tion
de·face', -faced', -fac'-
 ing
de·face'ment
de fac'to
de·fal'cate', -cat'ed,
 -cat'ing
de·fal·ca'tion
de·fal'ca'tor
def'a·ma'tion
de·fam'a·to'ry
de·fame', -famed',
 -fam'ing
de·fault'
de·feat'
de·feat'ism
de·feat'ist
def'e·cate', -cat'ed,
 -cat'ing
def'e·ca'tion
def'e·ca'tor
de'fect' *n.*
de·fect' *v.*
de·fec'tion
de·fec'tive
de·fec'tor
de·fend'
de·fen'dant
de·fense'
de·fen'si·ble
de·fen'sive

de•fer′, -ferred′, -fer′-
ring
def′er•ence *(respect)*
♦*difference*
def′er•ent
def′er•en′tial
de•fer′ment *also* de-
fer′al
de•fer′ra•ble
de•fer′rer
de•fi′ance
de•fi′ant
de•fi′cien•cy
de•fi′cient
def′i•cit
de•file′, -filed′, -fil′-
ing
de•file′ment
de•fil′er
de•fin′a•ble
de•fine′, -fined′, -fin′-
ing
de•fin′er
def′i•nite *(clear)*
♦*definitive*
def′i•ni′tion
de•fin′i•tive *(final)*
♦*definite*
de•flate′, -flat′ed,
-flat′ing
de•fla′tion
de•fla′tor
de•flect′
de•flect′a•ble
de•flec′tion
de•flec′tive
de•flec′tor

de•fo′li•ant
de•fo′li•ate′, -at′ed,
-at′ing
de•fo′li•a′tion
de•fo′li•a′tor
de•for′est
de•for′es•ta′tion
de•form′
de•for′ma′tion
de•form′i•ty
de•fraud′
de•fray′
de•fray′a•ble
de•fray′al
de•frock′
de•frost′
de•frost′er
deft′ly
de•funct′
de•func′tive
de•fund′
de•fuse′, -fused′, -fus′-
ing
de•fy′, -fied′, -fy′ing
de•gauss′
de•gen′er•a•cy
de•gen′er•ate′, -at′-
ed, -at′ing
de•gen′er•a′tion
de•gen′er•a•tive
de•glu′ti•nate′, -nat′-
ed, -nat′ing
de•glu′ti•na′tion
de′glu•ti′tion
deg′ra•da′tion
de•grade′, -grad′ed,
-grad′ing

de•grad′er
de•grease′, -greased′,
-greas′ing
de•gree′
de•gree′-day′
de•hisce′, -hisced′,
-hisc′ing
de•his′cence
de•his′cent
de•hu′man•i•za′-
tion
de•hu′man•ize′,
-ized′, -iz′ing
de′hu•mid′i•fi•ca′-
tion
de′hu•mid′i•fi′er
de′hu•mid′i•fy′,
-fied′, -fy′ing
de•hy′drate′, -drat′-
ed, -drat′ing
de′hy•dra′tion
de•hy′dra•tor
de•hy′dro•ge•nate′,
-nat′ed, -nat′ing
de•hy′dro•ge•na′-
tion
de•ice′, -iced′, -ic′ing
de•ic′er
de′i•fi•ca′tion
de′i•fy′, -fied′, -fy′ing
deign *(to condescend)*
♦*Dane*
de•i′on•ize′, -ized′,
-iz′ing
de′ism
de′ist
de•is′tic

de'i•ty
dé•jà vu'
de•ject'
de•jec'tion
de ju're
Del'a•war'e•an
de•lay'
de•lec'ta•bil'i•ty
de•lec'ta•ble
de'lec•ta'tion
del'e•gate', -gat'ed,
  -gat'ing
del'e•ga'tion
de•lete', -let'ed, -let'-
  ing
del'e•te'ri•ous
de•le'tion
delft'ware'
del'i pl. -is
de•lib'er•ate', -at'ed,
  -at'ing
de•lib'er•a'tion
de•lib'er•a'tive
del'i•ca•cy
del'i•cate
del'i•ca•tes'sen
de•li'cious
de•light'
de•light'ful
de•lim'it
de•lim'i•ta'tion
de•lin'e•ate', -at'ed,
  -at'ing
de•lin'e•a'tion
de•lin'e•a'tive
de•lin'e•a'tor
de•lin'quen•cy

de•lin'quent
del'i•quesce',
  -quesced', -quesc'ing
del'i•ques'cence
del'i•ques'cent
de•lir'i•ous
de•lir'i•um pl.
  -i•ums or -i•a
de•liv'er
de•liv'er•a•ble
de•liv'er•ance
de•liv'er•y
de•louse', -loused',
  -lous'ing
del•phin'i•um
del'ta
del•ta'ic also del'tic
del'toid
de•lude', -lud'ed,
  -lud'ing
del'uge, -uged, -ug-
  ing
de•lu'sion
de•lu'sive also de•lu'-
  so•ry
de luxe' also de•luxe'
delve, delved, delv'-
  ing
delv'er
de•mag'net•i•za'-
  tion
de•mag'net•ize',
  -ized', -iz'ing
dem'a•gog'ic also
  dem'a•gog'i•cal
dem'a•gogue'
dem'a•gogu'er•y

dem'a•go'gy
de•mand'
de•mand'-pull' adj.
de•mar'cate', -cat'ed,
  -cat'ing
de'mar•ca'tion
de•mar'ca•tor
dé•marche'
de•mean'
de•mean'or
de•ment'ed
de•men'tia
dementia prae'cox'
de•mer'it
de•mesne'
dem'i•god'
dem'i•john'
de•mil'i•ta•ri•za'-
  tion
de•mil'i•ta•rize',
  -rized', -riz'ing
dem'i•mon•daine'
dem'i•monde'
de•min'er•al•ize',
  -lized', -liz'ing
de•min'er•al•i•za'-
  tion
de•mise', -mised',
  -mis'ing
dem'i•tasse'
de•mo'bil•i•za'tion
de•mo'bil•ize',
  -ized', -iz'ing
de•moc'ra•cy
dem'o•crat'
dem'o•crat'ic
de•moc'ra•ti•za'-

tion
de•moc′ra•tize′,
  -tized′, -tiz′ing
de•mod′u•late′, -lat′-
  ed, -lat′ing
de•mod′u•la′tion
de•mod′u•la′tor
de•mog′ra•pher
dem′o•graph′ic *also*
  dem′o•graph′i•cal
dem′o•graph′ics
de•mog′ra•phy
dem•oi•selle′
de•mol′ish
dem′o•li′tion
de′mon
de•mo′ni•ac′ *also*
  de′mo•ni′a•cal
de•mon′ic
de′mon•ol′o•gist
de′mon•ol′o•gy
de•mon′stra•ble
dem′on•strate′,
  -strat′ed, -strat′ing
dem′on•stra′tion
de•mon′stra•tive
dem′on•stra′tor
de•mor′al•i•za′tion
de•mor′al•ize′,
  -ized′, -iz′ing
de•mote′, -mot′ed,
  -mot′ing
de•mo′tion
de•mount′
de•mul′cent
de•mur′ *(to object)*,
  -murred′, -mur′ring

de•mure′ *(modest)*
de•mur′ra•ble
de•mur′rage
de•mur′ral
de•mur′rer
de•mys′ti•fi•ca′tion
de•mys′ti•fy′, -fied′,
  -fy′ing
den
de•na′tion•al•i•za′-
  tion
de•na′tion•al•ize′,
  -ized′, -iz′ing
de•nat′u•ral•i•za′-
  tion
de•nat′u•ral•ize′,
  -ized′, -iz′ing
de•na′tur•ant
de•na′ture, -tured,
  -tur•ing
den′drite′
den•drol′o•gy
den′gue
de•ni′al
de•ni′er *(one who de-*
  nies)
den•ier′ *(yarn gauge)*
den′i•grate′, -grat′ed,
  -grat′ing
den′i•gra′tion
den′i•gra′tor
den′im
de•ni′tri•fi•ca′tion
de•ni′tri•fy′, -fied′,
  -fy′ing
den′i•zen
de•nom′i•nate′,

-nat′ed, -nat′ing
de•nom′i•na′tion
de•nom′i•na′tion-
  al•ism
de•nom′i•na′tive
de•nom′i•na′tor
de′no•ta′tion
de•no′ta•tive
de•note′, -not′ed,
  -not′ing
dé′noue•ment′ *also*
  de′noue•ment′
de•nounce′,
  -nounced′, -nounc′-
  ing
dense, dens′er, dens′-
  est
dense′ly
den′si•ty
dent
den′tal
den′tate′
den•tic′u•late *also*
  den•tic′u•lat′ed
den′ti•frice
den′ti•nal
den′tine′ *also* den′tin
den′tist
den′tist•ry
den•ti′tion
den′ture
de•nude′, -nud′ed,
  -nud′ing
de•num′er•a•ble
de•nun′ci•a′tion
de•ny′, -nied′, -ny′ing
de•o′dor•ant

de•o'dor•ize', -ized',
  -iz'ing
de•o'dor•iz'er
de•ox'i•di•za'tion
de•ox'i•dize',
  -dized', -diz'ing
de•ox'y•gen•ate',
  -at'ed, -at'ing
de•ox'y•ri•bo•nu-
  cle'ic acid
de•part'
de•part'ment
de'part•men'tal
de•par'ture
de•pend'
de•pend'a•bil'i•ty
de•pend'a•ble
de•pend'ence *also*
  de•pend'ance
de•pend'en•cy *also*
  de•pend'an•cy
de•pend'ent *also* de-
  pend'ant
de•per'son•al•i•za'-
  tion
de•pict'
de•pic'tion
de•pil'a•to'ry
de•plane' -planed',
  -plan'ing
de•plet'a•ble
de•plete', -plet'ed,
  -plet'ing
de•ple'tion
de•plor'a•ble
de•plore', -plored',
  -plor'ing

de•ploy'
de•ploy'ment
de•po'lar•i•za'tion
de•po'lar•ize',
  -ized', -iz'ing
de•po'nent
de•pop'u•late', -lat'-
  ed, -lat'ing
de•pop'u•la'tion
de•pop'u•la'tor
de•port'
de'port•ee'
de'por•ta'tion
de•port'ment
de•pos'a•ble
de•pos'al
de•pose', -posed',
  -pos'ing
de•pos'it
dep'o•si'tion
de•pos'i•tor
de•pos'i•to'ry
de'pot
dep'ra•va'tion *(cor-
  ruption)*
  ♦*deprivation*
de•prave', -praved',
  -prav'ing
de•prav'i•ty
dep're•cate', -cat'ed,
  -cat'ing
dep're•ca'tion
dep're•ca'tor
dep're•ca•to'ry *also*
  dep're•ca'tive
de•pre'ci•ate', -at'-
  ed, -at'ing

de•pre'ci•a'tion
de•pre'ci•a'tor
de•pre'ci•a•to'ry
dep're•date', -dat'ed,
  -dat'ing
dep're•da'tion
de•press'
de•pres'sant
de•pres'sion
de•pres'sive
de•pres'sor
dep'ri•va'tion *(loss)*,
  also de•priv'al
  ♦*depravation*
de•prive', -prived',
  -priv'ing
de•pro'gram',
  -grammed' *or*
  -gramed', -gram'-
  ming *or* -gram'ing
de•pro'gram'mer *or*
  de•pro'gram'er
depth
dep'u•ta'tion
de•pute', -put'ed,
  -put'ing
dep'u•tize', -tized',
  -tiz'ing
dep'u•ty
de•rail'
de•rail'ment
de•range', -ranged',
  -rang'ing
de•range'ment
der'by
de•reg'u•late', -lat'-
  ed, -lat'ing

de•reg′u•la′tion
de•reg′u•la′tor
de•reg′u•la•to′ry
der′e•lict
der′e•lic′tion
de•ride′, -rid′ed, -rid′-ing
de•ri′sion
de•ri′sive
de•riv′a•ble
der′i•va′tion
de•riv′a•tive
de•rive′, -rived′, -riv′-ing
der′ma *(skin), also* derm, der′mis
der′ma *(food)*
der′mal
der′ma•ti′tis
der′ma•tol′o•gist
der′ma•tol′o•gy
der′o•gate′, -gat′ed, -gat′ing
der′o•ga′tion
de•rog′a•tive
de•rog′a•to′ry
der′rick
der′ri•ère′ *also* der′-ri•ere′
der′ring-do′
der′rin•ger
der′vish
de•sal′i•nate′, -nat′-ed, -nat′ing
de•sal′i•na′tion
de•sal′i•ni•za′tion
de•sal′in•ize′, -ized′, -iz′ing
de•salt′
des′cant
de•scend′
de•scen′dant *(off-spring)*
de•scen′dent *(de-scending), also* de-scen′dant
de•scend′i•ble *also* de•scend′a•ble
de•scent′ *(downward incline)*
♦*decent, dissent*
de•scram′bler
de•scrib′a•ble
de•scribe′, -scribed′, -scrib′ing
de•scrip′tion
de•scrip′tive
de•scry′, -scried′, -scry′ing
des′e•crate′, -crat′ed, -crat′ing
des′e•cra′tion
de•seg′re•gate′, -gat′-ed, -gat′ing
de′seg•re•ga′tion
de•sen′si•ti•za′tion
de•sen′si•tize′, -tized′, -tiz′ing
des′ert *(barren region)*
de•sert′ *(deserved re-ward)*
♦*dessert*
de•sert′ *(to leave)*
♦*dessert*
de•ser′tion
de•serve′, -served′, -serv′ing
de•serv′ed•ly
des′ic•cant
des′ic•cate′, -cat′ed, -cat′ing
des′ic•ca′tion
des′ic•ca′tive
de•sid′er•a′tum *pl.* -ta
de•sign′
des′ig•nate′, -nat′ed, -nat′ing
des′ig•na′tion
des′ig•na′tive *also* des′ig•na•to′ry
des′ig•na′tor
de•sign′ed•ly
des′ig•nee′
de•sign′er
de•sir′a•bil′i•ty
de•sir′a•ble
de•sire′, -sired′, -sir′-ing
de•sir′er
de•sir′ous
de•sist′
desk
desk′top′
des′o•late′, -lat′ed, -lat′ing
des′o•la′tion
de•spair′
des′per•a′do *pl.* -does *or* -dos
des′per•ate *(hopeless)*

♦*disparate*
des'per•a'tion
des'pi•ca•ble
de•spise', -spised',
  -spis'ing
de•spis'er
de•spite'
de•spoil'
de•spo'li•a'tion
de•spond'
de•spon'den•cy *also*
  de•spon'dence
de•spon'dent
des'pot
des•pot'ic
des'pot•ism
des•sert' *(food)*
  ♦*desert (deserved re-
  ward; to leave)*
des•sert'spoon'
des'ti•na'tion
des'tine, -tined, -tin-
  ing
des'ti•ny
des'ti•tute'
des'ti•tu'tion
de•stroy'
de•stroy'er
de•struct'
de•struc'ti•bil'i•ty
de•struc'ti•ble
de•struc'tion
de•struc'tive
des'ue•tude'
des'ul•to'ry
de•tach'
de•tach'a•ble

de•tach'ment
de•tail'
de•tain'
de•tain'ment
de•tect'
de•tect'a•ble *also*
  de•tect'i•ble
de•tec'tion
de•tec'tive
de•tec'tor
dé•tente'
de•ten'tion
de•ter', -terred', -ter'-
  ring
de•ter'gent
de•te'ri•o•rate', -rat'-
  ed, -rat'ing
de•te'ri•o•ra'tion
de•ter'ment
de•ter'min•a•ble
de•ter'mi•nant
de•ter'mi•nate
de•ter'mi•na'tion
de•ter'mi•na'tive
de•ter'mine, -mined,
  -min•ing
de•ter'min•er
de•ter'min•ism
de•ter'rence
de•ter'rent
de•test'
de•test'a•ble
de'tes•ta'tion
de•throne',
  -throned', -thron'ing
det'o•nate', -nat'ed,
  -nat'ing

det'o•na'tion
det'o•na'tor
de'tour'
de•tox'i•fi•ca'tion
de•tox'i•fy', -fied',
  -fy'ing *also* de•tox'-
  i•cate', -cat'ed, -cat'-
  ing
de•tract'
de•trac'tion
de•trac'tor
de•train'
det'ri•ment
det'ri•men'tal
de•tri'tus
deuce
deuc'ed
de'us ex mach'i•na'
deu•te'ri•um
deu'ter•on
de•val'u•ate', -at'ed,
  -at'ing, *also* de•val'-
  ue, -ued, -u•ing
de•val'u•a'tion
dev'as•tate', -tat'ed,
  -tat'ing
dev'as•ta'tion
de•vel'op
de•vel'op•ment
de•vel'op•men'tal
de'vi•ance
de'vi•ant
de'vi•ate', -at'ed, -at'-
  ing
de'vi•a'tion
de'vi•a'tor
de•vice' *(contrivance)*

♦*devise*

dev'il, -iled *or* -illed,
-il•ing *or* -il•ling

dev'il•fish' *pl.* -fish'
or -fish'es

dev'il•ish

dev'il-may-care'

dev'il•ment

dev'il's-food' cake

dev'il•try *also* dev'il-
ry

de'vi•ous

de•vis'a•ble

de•vise' *(to invent),*
-vised', -vis'ing
♦*device*

de•vi'tal•ize', -ized',
-iz'ing

de•void'

dev'o•lu'tion

de•volve', -volved',
-volv'ing

de•vote', -vot'ed,
-vot'ing

dev'o•tee'

de•vo'tion

de•vour'

de•vout'

dew *(moisture)*
♦*do (what should be
done, party; to
perform), due*

dew'ber'ry

dew'drop'

dew'fall'

dew'lap'

dew'y

dew'y-eyed'

dex•ter'i•ty

dex'ter•ous *also* dex'-
trous

dex'tral

dex'trin *also* dex'trine

dex'trose'

di'a•be'tes

diabetes mel•li'tus

di'a•bet'ic

di'a•bol'ic *also* di'-
a•bol'i•cal

di•ac'e•tyl•mor'-
phine'

di'a•chron'ic

di•ach'ro•ny

di'a•crit'i•cal *also*
di'a•crit'ic

di'a•dem'

di•ag•nose', -nosed',
-nos'ing

di'ag•no'sis *pl.* -ses'

di'ag•nos'tic

di'ag•nos•ti'cian

di•ag'o•nal

di'a•gram',
-grammed' *or*
-gramed', -gram'-
ming *or* -gram'ing

di'a•gram•mat'ic
also di'a•gram•mat'-
i•cal

di'al, -aled *or* -alled,
-al•ing *or* -al•ling

di'a•lect'

di'a•lec'tal

di'a•lec'tic

di'a•lec'ti•cal

di'a•lec•ti'cian

di'al•er

di'a•logue' *also* di'-
a•log'

di•al'y•sis *pl.* -ses'

di'a•lyze', -lyzed',
-lyz'ing

di'a•mag•net'ic

di•am'e•ter

di'a•met'ri•cal *also*
di'a•met'ric

dia'mond

dia'mond•back'

di'a•pa'son

di'a•per

di•aph'a•nous

di'a•pho•re'sis

di'a•pho•ret'ic

di'a•phragm'

di'a•rist

di'ar•rhe'a *also* di'-
ar•rhoe'a

di'a•ry

Di•as'po•ra *also* di-
as'po•ra

di'a•stase'

di'a•sta'sic

di•as'to•le

di'a•stol'ic

di•as'tro•phic

di•as'tro•phism

di'a•ther'my

di'a•tom'

di'a•to•ma'ceous

di'a•tom'ic

di•at'o•mite'

di'a•ton'ic
di'a•tribe'
di•az'e•pam'
di•ba'sic
dib'ble, -bled, -bling
dice *sing.* die
dice, diced, dic'ing
dic'er
di•chlo'ride
di•chot'o•mize',
  -mized', -miz'ing
di•chot'o•mous
di•chot'o•my
di•chro'mate'
di'chro•mat'ic
dick'ens
dick'er
dick'ey *pl.* -eys, *also*
  dick'ie, dick'y
di•cli'nous
di'cot'y•le'don *also*
  di'cot
di'cot•y•le'don•ous
Dic'ta•phone'®
dic'tate', -tat'ed, -tat'-
  ing
dic•ta'tion
dic'ta•tor
dic•ta•to'ri•al
dic•ta'tor•ship'
dic'tion
dic'tion•ar'y
dic'tum *pl.* -ta *or*
  -tums
di•dac'tic *also* di-
  dac'ti•cal
di•dac'ti•cism

did'dle, -dled, -dling
did'n't
di•dym'i•um
die *(to expire),* died,
  dy'ing
  ♦*dye*
die *(to stamp),* died,
  die'ing
  ♦*dye*
die'-hard' *also* die'-
  hard'
di'e•lec'tric
di•er'e•sis *pl.* -ses',
  also di•aer'e•sis
die'sel engine
di'et
di'e•tar'y
di'e•tet'ic
di•eth'yl ether
di'e•ti'tian *also* di'-
  e•ti'cian
dif'fer
dif'fer•ence *(diversi-
  ty)*
  ♦*deference*
dif'fer•ent
dif'fer•en'tial
dif'fer•en'ti•ate',
  -at'ed, -at'ing
dif'fer•en'ti•a'tion
dif'fi•cult'
dif'fi•cul'ty
dif'fi•dence'
dif'fi•dent'
dif•fract'
dif•frac'tion
dif•frac'tive

dif•fuse', -fused',
  -fus'ing
dif•fus'er
dif•fus'i•ble
dif•fu'sion
dif•fu'sive
dig, dug, dig'ging
di•gest' *n.*
di•gest' *v.*
di•gest'i•ble
di•ges'tion
di•ges'tive
dig'ger
dig'gings
dig'it
dig'i•tal
dig'i•tal'is
dig'i•tal•i•za'tion
dig'ni•fy', -fied', -fy'-
  ing
dig'ni•tar'y
dig'ni•ty
di'graph'
di•gress'
di•gres'sion
di•gres'sive
di•he'dral
dike, diked, dik'ing,
  also dyke, dyked,
  dyk'ing
di•lap'i•dat'ed
di•lap'i•da'tion
di•lat'a•ble
dil'a•ta'tion
di•late', -lat'ed, -lat'-
  ing
di•la'tion

di•la′tive
di•la′tor *also* di•lat′-
  er, dil′a•ta′tor
dil′a•to′ry
di•lem′ma
dil′et•tante′ *pl.*
  -tantes′ *or* -tan′ti
dil′et•tan′tism
dil′i•gence
dil′i•gent
dill
dil′ly
dil′ly-dal′ly, -lied,
  -ly•ing
di•lute′, -lut′ed, -lut′-
  ing
di•lu′tion
di•lu′vi•al *also* di•lu′-
  vi•an
dim, dim′mer, dim′-
  mest
dim, dimmed, dim′-
  ming
dime
di•men′sion
di•men′sion•al
dim′er•ous
di•min′ish
di•min′u•en′do *pl.*
  -dos
dim′i•nu′tion
di•min′u•tive
dim′i•ty
dim′mer
di′morph′
di•mor′phic *also* di-
  mor′phous

di•mor′phism
dim′-out′ *n.*
dim′ple, -pled, -pling
dim′wit′
din, dinned, din′ning
di•nar′
dine *(to eat),* dined,
  din′ing
  ♦*dyne*
din′er
di•nette′
ding′bat′
ding′-dong′
din′ghy
din′go *pl.* -goes
din′gus
din′gy
din′ky
din′ner
din′ner•ware′
di′no•saur′
dint
di•oc′e•san
di′o•cese
di′ode′
di′o•ram′a
di′o•rite′
di•ox′ide′
dip, dipped, dip′ping
diph•the′ri•a
diph′the•rit′ic *also*
  diph•ther′ic, diph-
  the′ri•al
diph′thong′
dip′lo•coc′cus *pl.* -ci′
dip′loid′
di•plo′ma

di•plo′ma•cy
dip′lo•mat′
dip′lo•mat′ic
di•plo′ma•tist
di′pole′
dip′per
dip′py
dip′so•ma′ni•a
dip′so•ma′ni•ac
dip′stick′
dip′ter•ous
dip′tych
dire *(disastrous),* dir′-
  er, dir′est
  ♦*dyer*
di•rect′
di•rec′tion
di•rec′tion•al
di•rec′tive
di•rect′ly
di•rec′tor
di•rec′tor•ate
di•rec′tor•ship′
di•rec′to•ry
dirge
dir′i•gi•ble
dirn′dl
dirt′-cheap′
dirt′y
dis′a•bil′i•ty
dis•a′ble, -bled,
  -bling
dis′a•buse′, -bused′,
  -bus′ing
di•sac′cha•ride′
dis′ad•van′tage,
  -taged, -tag•ing

dis′ad′van′taged
dis•ad′van•ta′geous
dis•af•fect′
dis•af•fec′tion
dis•af•fil′i•ate, -at′-
　ed, -at′ing
dis•af•firm′
dis•af•fir′mance *also*
　dis•af′fir•ma′tion
dis•a•gree′
dis•a•gree′a•ble
dis•a•gree′ment
dis•al•low′
dis•al•low′a•ble
dis•ap•pear′
dis•ap•pear′ance
dis•ap•point′
dis•ap•point′ment
dis•ap′pro•ba′tion
dis•ap•prov′al
dis•ap•prove′,
　-proved′, -prov′ing
dis•arm′
dis•ar′ma•ment
dis•arm′ing
dis•ar•range′,
　-ranged′, -rang′ing
dis•ar•ray′
dis•as•sem′ble,
　-bled, -bling
dis•as•sem′bly
dis•as•so′ci•ate′, -at′-
　ed, -at′ing
dis•as•so′ci•a′tion
dis•as′ter
dis•as′trous
dis•a•vow′

dis•a•vow′al
dis•band′
dis•bar′, -barred′,
　-bar′ring
dis•be•lief′
dis•be•lieve′,
　-lieved′, -liev′ing
dis•be•liev′er
dis•bud′, -bud′ded,
　-bud′ding
dis•bur′den
dis•burse′ (*to pay
　out*), -bursed′, -burs′-
　ing
　♦*disperse*
dis•burse′ment *also*
　dis•bur′sal
disc (*record*), *also* disk
dis•card′ *n.*
dis•card′ *v.*
dis•cern′
dis•cern′i•ble
dis•cern′ment
dis•charge′ *n.*
dis•charge′ -charged′,
　-charg′ing
dis•ci′ple
dis′ci•pli•nar′i•an
dis′ci•pli•nar′y
dis′ci•pline, -plined,
　-plin•ing
dis•claim′
dis•close′, -closed′,
　-clos′ing
dis•clo′sure
dis•co′ *pl.* -cos′
dis•cog′ra•pher

dis•cog′ra•phy
dis′coid′
dis•col′or
dis•col′or•a′tion
dis•com•bob′u•late′,
　-lat′ed, -lat′ing
dis•com′fit (*to frus-
　trate*)
　♦*discomfort*
dis•com′fi•ture′
dis•com′fort (*to
　make uneasy*)
　♦*discomfit*
dis•com•mode′,
　-mod′ed, -mod′ing
dis′com•pose′,
　-posed′, -pos′ing
dis′com•po′sure
dis′con•cert′
dis′con•nect′
dis′con•nec′tion
dis•con′so•late′
dis′con•tent′
dis′con•tin′u•ance
dis′con•tin′u•a′tion
dis′con•tin•ue, -ued,
　-u•ing
dis•con′ti•nu′i•ty
dis′con•tin′u•ous
disc′o•phile′
dis•cord′ *n.*
dis•cord′ *v.*
dis•cor′dance *also*
　dis•cor′dan•cy
dis•cor′dant
dis′co•theque′ *also*
　dis′co•thèque′

dis'count'
dis'count'a·ble
dis·coun'te·nance,
　-nanced, -nanc·ing
dis·cour'age, -aged,
　-ag·ing
dis·cour'age·ment
dis'course' *n.*
dis·course',
　-coursed', -cours'ing
dis·cour'te·ous
dis·cour'te·sy
dis·cov'er
dis·cov'er·a·ble
dis·cov'er·y
dis·cred'it
dis·cred'it·a·ble
dis·creet' *(judicious)*
　♦*discrete*
dis·crep'an·cy
dis·crep'ant
dis·crete' *(separate)*
　♦*discreet*
dis·cre'tion
dis·cre'tion·ar'y
dis·crim'i·nate',
　-nat'ed, -nat'ing
dis·crim'i·na'tion
dis·crim'i·na'tive
dis·crim'i·na'tor
dis·crim'i·na·to'ry
dis·cur'sive
dis'cus *(disk)*, *pl.*
　-cus·es
dis·cuss' *(to speak
　about)*
dis·cuss'ant

dis·cuss'i·ble
dis·cus'sion
dis·dain'
dis·dain'ful
dis·ease', -eased',
　-eas'ing
dis'em·bark'
dis·em'bar·ka'tion
dis'em·bar'rass
dis'em·bod'i·ment
dis'em·bod'y, -ied,
　-y·ing
dis'em·bow'el
dis'en·chant'
dis'en·chant'ment
dis'en·cum'ber
dis'en·gage', -gaged',
　-gag'ing
dis'en·gage'ment
dis'en·tan'gle, -gled,
　-gling
dis'es·tab'lish
dis'es·teem'
dis·fa'vor
dis·fig'ure, -ured,
　-ur·ing
dis·fran'chise',
　-chised', -chis'ing,
dis·fran'chise'ment
dis·gorge', -gorged',
　-gorg'ing
dis·grace', -graced',
　-grac'ing
dis·grace'ful
dis·grun'tle, -tled,
　-tling
dis·guise', -guised',

　-guis'ing
dis·gust'
dish
dis'ha·bille' *also* des'-
　ha·bille'
dis'har·mo'ni·ous
dis·har'mo·ny
dish'cloth'
dis·heart'en
di·shev'el, -eled *or*
　-elled, -el·ing *or* -el-
　ling
di·shev'eled
dis·hon'est
dis·hon'es·ty
dis·hon'or
dis·hon'or·a·ble
dish'pan'
dish'rag'
dish'tow'el
dish'wash'er
dish'wa'ter
dis'il·lu'sion
dis'il·lu'sion·ment
dis·in'cli·na'tion
dis'in·cline', -clined',
　-clin'ing
dis'in·fect'
dis'in·fec'tant
dis'in·form'
dis'in·gen'u·ous
dis'in·her'it
dis·in'te·grate',
　-grat'ed, -grat'ing
dis·in'te·gra'tion
dis·in'te·gra'tor
dis'in·ter', -terred',

-ter'ring
dis•in'ter•est
dis•in'ter•est•ed
dis•join'
dis•joint'
dis•junc'tion
dis•junc'tive
disk *(plate), also* disc
disk•ette'
dis•like', -liked', -lik'-
  ing
dis'lo•cate', -cat'ed,
  -cat'ing
dis'lo•ca'tion
dis•lodge', -lodged',
  -lodg'ing
dis•lodge'ment *also*
  dis•lodg'ment
dis•loy'al
dis•loy'al•ty
dis'mal
dis•man'tle, -tled,
  -tling
dis•may'
dis•mem'ber
dis•mem'ber•ment
dis•miss'
dis•miss'al
dis•miss'i•ble
dis•mis'sive
dis•mount'
dis'o•be'di•ence
dis'o•be'di•ent
dis'o•bey'
dis'o•blige', -bliged',
  -blig'ing
dis•or'der

dis•or'der•ly
dis•or'gan•i•za'tion
dis•or'gan•ize',
  -ized', -iz'ing
dis•o'ri•ent'
dis•o'ri•en•ta'tion
dis•own'
dis•par'age, -aged,
  -ag•ing
dis'pa•rate *(separate)*
  ♦*desperate*
dis•par'i•ty
dis•pas'sion•ate
dis•patch' *also* des-
  patch'
dis•patch'er
dis•pel', -pelled', -pel'-
  ling
dis•pen'sa•bil'i•ty
dis•pen'sa•ble
dis•pen'sa•ry
dis'pen•sa'tion
dis•pen'sa•to'ry
dis•pense', -pensed',
  -pens'ing
dis•pens'er
dis•per'sal
dis•perse' *(to scatter),*
  -persed', -pers'ing
  ♦*disburse*
dis•pers'i•ble
dis•per'sion
dis•pir'it
dis•place', -placed',
  -plac'ing
dis•place'a•ble
dis•place'ment

dis•play'
dis•please', -pleased',
  -pleas'ing
dis•pleas'ure
dis•port'
dis•pos'a•bil'i•ty
dis•pos'a•ble
dis•pos'al
dis•pose', -posed',
  -pos'ing
dis'po•si'tion
dis'pos•sess'
dis'pos•ses'sion
dis'pos•ses'sor
dis•proof'
dis'pro•por'tion
dis'pro•por'tion•al
dis'pro•por'tion•ate
dis•prove', -proved',
  -prov'ing
dis•put'a•bil'i•ty
dis•put'a•ble
dis•pu'tant
dis'pu•ta'tion
dis'pu•ta'tious
dis•pute', -put'ed,
  -put'ing
dis•qual'i•fi•ca'tion
dis•qual'i•fy', -fied',
  -fy'ing
dis•qui'et
dis•qui'e•tude'
dis'qui•si'tion
dis're•gard'
dis're•pair'
dis•rep'u•ta•ble
dis're•pute'

dis're•spect'
dis're•spect'ful
dis•robe', -robed',
  -rob'ing
dis•rupt'
dis•rupt'er *also* dis-
  rup'tor
dis•rup'tion
dis•rup'tive
dis•sat'is•fac'tion
dis•sat'is•fac'to•ry
dis•sat'is•fy', -fied',
  -fy'ing
dis•sect'
dis•sec'tion
dis•sec'tor
dis•sem'ble, -bled,
  -bling
dis•sem'i•nate',
  -nat'ed, -nat'ing
dis•sem'i•na'tion
dis•sem'i•na'tor
dis•sen'sion
dis•sent' *(to differ)*
  ♦decent, descent
dis•sent'er
dis'ser•ta'tion
dis•scrv'ice
dis•sev'er
dis'si•dence
dis'si•dent
dis•sim'i•lar
dis•sim'i•lar'i•ty
dis•si•mil'i•tude'
dis•sim'u•late', -lat'-
  ed, -lat'ing
dis•sim'u•la'tion

dis'si•pate', -pat'ed,
  -pat'ing
dis'si•pat'er *also* dis'-
  si•pa'tor
dis'si•pa'tion
dis•so'ci•ate', -at'ed,
  -at'ing
dis•so'ci•a'tion
dis•sol'u•ble
dis'so•lute'
dis'so•lu'tion
dis•solv'a•ble
dis•solve', -solved',
  -solv'ing
dis'so•nance *also*
  dis'so•nan'cy
dis'so•nant
dis•suade', -suad'ed,
  -suad'ing
dis•sua'sion
dis•sua'sive
dis'taff'
dis'tal
dis'tance, -tanced,
  -tanc•ing
dis'tant
dis•taste'
dis•taste'ful
dis•tem'per
dis•tend'
dis•ten'si•ble
dis•ten'tion *also* dis-
  ten'sion
dis•till'
dis'til•late'
dis'til•la'tion
dis•till'er•y

dis•tinct'
dis•tinc'tion
dis•tinc'tive
dis•tin'guish
dis•tin'guish•a•ble
dis•tort'
dis•tor'tion
dis•tract'
dis•trac'tion
dis•traught'
dis•tress'
dis•trib'ute, -ut•ed,
  -ut•ing
dis'tri•bu'tion
dis•trib'u•tive
dis•trib'u•tor
dis'trict
dis•trust'
dis•trust'ful
dis•turb'
dis•tur'bance
di•sul'fide'
dis•un'ion
dis'u•nite', -nit'ed,
  -nit'ing
dis•u'ni•ty
dis•use'
ditch
dith'er
dit'sy
dit'to *pl.* -tos
dit'ty
di•u•ret'ic
di•ur'nal
di'va
di•va'lent
di•van'

dive, dived *or* dove,
   dived, div'ing
dive'-bomb'
div'er
di•verge', -verged',
   -verg'ing
di•ver'gence *also* di-
   ver'gen•cy
di•ver'gent
di'vers *(various)*
di•verse' *(unlike)*
di•ver'si•fi•ca'tion
di•ver'si•fy', -fied',
   -fy'ing
di•ver'sion
di•ver'sion•ar'y
di•ver'si•ty
di•vert'
di•ver'tisse•ment
di•vest'
di•vest'i•ture
di•vid'a•ble
di•vide', -vid'ed,
   -vid'ing
div'i•dend'
di•vid'er
div'i•na'tion
di•vine', -vined',
   -vin'ing
di•vin'er
di•vin'i•ty
di•vis'i•bil'i•ty
di•vis'i•ble
di•vi'sion
di•vi'sive
di•vi'sor
di•vorce', -vorced',

-vorc'ing
di•vor•cée'
div'ot
di•vulge', -vulged',
   -vulg'ing
di•vul'gence
di•vulg'er
div'vy, -vied, -vy•ing
Dix'ie
Dix'ie•land'
diz'zy, -zied, -zy•ing
do *(what should be
   done, party)*, pl. do's
   or dos
   ♦*dew, due*
do *(musical tone)*, pl.
   dos
   ♦*doe, dough*
do *(to perform)*, did,
   done, do'ing, does
   ♦*dew, due*
dob'bin
Do'ber•man pin'-
   scher
do'cent
doc'ile
do•cil'i•ty
dock'age
dock'et
dock'hand'
dock'yard'
doc'tor
doc'tor•al
doc'tor•ate
doc'tri•naire'
doc'trin•al
doc'trine

doc'u•dra'ma
doc'u•ment
doc'u•men'ta•ry
doc'u•men•ta'tion
dod'der
do•dec'a•gon'
do'de•cag'o•nal
do'dec•a•he'dral
do'dec•a•he'dron
   pl. -drons *or* -dra
dodge, dodged, dodg'-
   ing
dodg'er
do'do *pl.* -does *or*
   -dos
doe *(deer)*, *pl.* doe *or*
   does
   ♦*do (musical tone),
   dough*
do'er
doe'skin'
does'n't
doff
dog, dogged, dog'ging
dog'cart'
dog'catch'er
dog'-ear'
dog'fight'
dog'fish' *pl.* -fish' *or*
   -fish'es
dog'ged
dog'ger•el
dog'gy bag *or* dog'gie
   bag
dog'house'
do'gie *also* do'gy
dog'ma

dog•mat′ic
dog′ma•tism
dog′ma•tist
do′-good′er
dog′-tired′
dog′trot′
dog′watch′
dog′wood′
doi′ly
do′-it-your•self′
Dol′by System®
dol′drums
dole, doled, dol′ing
doll
dol′lar
doll′house′
dol′lop
dol′ly
dol′man *(robe)*
dol′men *(monument)*
dol′o•mite′
do′lor
do′lor•ous
dol′phin
dolt′ish
do•main′
dome, domed, dom′-
  ing
do•mes′tic
do•mes′ti•cate′,
  -cat′ed, -cat′ing
do•mes′ti•ca′tion
do′mes•tic′i•ty
dom′i•cile′, -ciled′,
  -cil′ing
dom′i•nance
dom′i•nant

dom′i•nate′, -nat′ed,
  -nat′ing
dom′i•na′tion
dom′i•na′tor
dom′i•neer′
Do•min′i•can
do•min′ion
dom′i•no′ *pl.* -noes′
  or -nos′
don, donned, don′-
  ning
do′nate′, -nat′ed,
  -nat′ing
do•na′tion
do′na•tor
done *(finished)*
  ♦*dun*
don′jon *(tower)*
  ♦*dungeon*
don′key *pl.* -keys
don′ny•brook′
do′nor
do′-noth′ing *adj.*
doo′dad′
doo′dle, -dled, -dling
doo′dle•bug′
doo′hick′ey *pl.* -eys
doom
dooms′day′
door′bell′
door′jamb′
door′keep′er
door′knob′
door′man′
door′mat′
door′nail′
door′step′

door′stop′
door′way′
doo′zy
dope, doped, dop′ing
dop′ey *also* dop′y
dor′man•cy
dor′mant
dor′mer
dor′mi•to′ry
dor′mouse′ *pl.*
  -mice′
dor′sal
do′ry
dos′age
dose, dosed, dos′ing
do•sim′e•ter
dos′si•er′
dot, dot′ted, dot′ting
do′tage
do′tard
dote, dot′ed, dot′ing
dot′-ma′trix
dot′tle
dot′ty
dou′ble, -bled, -bling
dou′ble-bar′reled
dou′ble-breast′ed
dou′ble-check′ *v.*
dou′ble-cross′
dou′ble-deal′er
dou′ble-deal′ing
dou′ble-deck′er
dou′ble-dig′it *adj.*
dou′ble-edged′
dou′ble-en•ten′dre
dou′ble-faced′
dou′ble-head′er

dou′ble-joint′ed
dou′ble•knit′ *adj.*
dou′ble-park′
dou′ble-quick′
dou′ble-reed′
dou′ble-space′,
 -spaced′, -spac′ing
dou′blet
dou′ble-time′,
 -timed′, -tim′ing
dou•bloon′
dou′bly
doubt′ful
doubt′less
douche, douched,
 douch′ing
dough *(bread mixture,
 money)*
 ♦*do (musical tone),
 doe*
dough′boy′
dough′nut′ *also* do′-
 nut′
dough•ty
dough′y
dour′ly
douse *(to extinguish),*
 doused, dous′ing
douse *(to immerse),*
 doused, dous′ing,
 also dowse, dowsed,
 dows′ing
dove′cote′ *also*
 dove′cot′
dove′tail′
dow′a•ger
dow′dy

dow′el, -eled *or* -elled,
 -el•ing *or* -el•ling
dow′er
down′beat′
down′cast′
down′er
down′fall′
down′grade′, -grad′-
 ed, -grad′ing
down′heart′ed
down′hill′
down′load′
down′pour′
down′range′
down′right′
down′scale′
down′shift′
down′side′
down′spin′
down′stage′
down′stairs′
down′stream′
down′swing′
down′time′
down′-to-earth′
down′town′
down′trod′den
down′turn′
down′ward *also*
 down′wards
down′wind′
down′y
dow′ry
dowse *(to divine),*
 dowsed, dows′ing,
 also douse, doused,
 dous′ing

dows′er
dox•ol′o•gy
doze, dozed, doz′ing
doz′en
doz′enth
drab, drab′ber, drab′-
 best
drab′ly
dra•cae′na
dra•co′ni•an *also*
 dra•con′ic
draft•ee′
draft′ing
drafts′man
draft′y
drag, dragged, drag′-
 ging
drag′ger
drag′gle, gled, -gling
drag′net′
drag′on
drag′on•fly′
dra•goon′
drag′ster
drain′age
drain′pipe′
drake
dram
dra′ma
Dram′a•mine′®
dra•mat′ic
dra•mat′ics
dram′a•tis per•so′-
 nae
dram′a•tist
dram′a•ti•za′tion
dram′a•tize′, -tized′,

-tiz′ing
dram′a•tur′gy
drape, draped, drap′-
  ing
drap′er•y
dras′tic
draw, drew, drawn,
  draw′ing
draw′back′
draw′bridge′
draw′er
draw′knife′
drawl
draw′string′
dray′age
dread′ful
dread′locks′
dread′nought′
dream, dreamed or
  dreamt, dream′ing
dream′land′
dream′y
drear′y
dredge, dredged,
  dredg′ing
dregs
drench′er
Dres′den china
dres•sage′
dress′er
dress′ing
dress′mak′er
dress′y
drib′ble, -bled, -bling
drib′let
dri′er (one that dries),
  also dry′er

drift′er
drift′wood′
drill′mas′ter
drink, drank, drunk,
  drink′ing
drink′a•ble
drip, dripped, drip′-
  ping
drip′-dry′ adj.
drip′pings
drip′py
drive, drove, driv′en,
  driv′ing
drive′-in′
driv′el, -eled or -elled,
  -el•ing or -el•ling
driv′er
drive′way′
driz′zle, -zled, -zling
drogue
droll′er•y
drom′e•dar′y
drone, droned, dron′-
  ing
drool
droop (to sag)
  ♦drupe
droop′y
drop, dropped, drop′-
  ping
drop′-kick′ v.
drop′-leaf′ adj.
drop′let
drop′out′ n.
drop′per
drop′pings
drop′sy

dross
drought also drouth
drove (herd)
drov′er
drown
drowse, drowsed,
  drows′ing
drows′y
drub, drubbed, drub′-
  bing
drudge, drudged,
  drudg′ing
drudg′er•y
drudge′work′
drug, drugged, drug′-
  ging
drug′gist
drug′store′
dru′id also Dru′id
drum, drummed,
  drum′ming
drum′beat′
drum′head′
drum′lin
drum′mer
drum′stick′
drunk′ard
drunk′en
dru•pa′ceous
drupe (fruit)
  ♦droop
dry, dri′er or dry′er,
  dri′est or dry′est
dry, dried, dry′ing
dry′ad
dry′-clean′ v.
dry′-dock′ v.

dry'er *(appliance)*
  ♦*drier*
du'al *(double)*
  ♦*duel*
du'al•ism
du'al•ist *(one who be-*
  lieves in dualism)
  ♦*duelist*
du'al•is'tic
du•al'i•ty
dub, dubbed, dub'-
  bing
du•bi'e•ty
du'bi•ous
du'cal
duc'at
duch'ess
duch'y
duck'board'
duck'ling
duck'pin'
duck'weed'
duct *(passage)*
  ♦*ducked*
duc'tile
duc•til'i•ty
dud
dude
dudg'eon
duds
due *(payable)*
  ♦*dew, do (what*
  should be done; to
  perform)
du'el *(to fight)*, -eled
  or -elled, -el•ing or
  -el•ling

♦*dual*
du'el•er *also* du'el•ist
du•et'
duf'fel
duf'fer
du'gong'
dug'out'
duke'dom
dul'cet
dul'ci•mer
dull'ard
dull'ness *also* dul'-
  ness
dul'ly
du'ly
dumb'bell'
dumb'wait'er
dum'-dum *(person)*
dum'dum' bullet
dum'found' *or*
  dumb'found'
dum'my
dump'ling
dump'site'
dump'y
dun *(dull brown)*
  ♦*done*
dun *(to demand pay-*
  ment), dunned, dun'-
  ning
  ♦*done*
dunce
dun'der•head'
dune
dun'ga•ree'
dun'geon *(prison)*
  ♦*donjon*

dung'hill'
dunk
du'o *pl.* -os
du'o•dec'i•mal
du'o•dec'i•mo' *pl.*
  -os'
du'o•de'nal
du'o•de'num *pl.* -na
dupe, duped, dup'ing
dup'er•y
du'ple
du'plex'
du'pli•cate *adj.*
du'pli•cate', -cat'ed,
  -cat'ing
du'pli•ca'tion
du'pli•ca'tor
du•plic'i•ty
du'ra•bil'i•ty
du'ra•ble
du'ra ma'ter
du'rance
du•ra'tion
du•ress'
dur'ing
du'rum
dusk'y
dust'bin'
dust'er
dust'pan'
dust'up'
dust'y
Dutch
du'te•ous
du'ti•a•ble
du'ti•ful
du'ty

du'ty-free' *adj. &*
   adv.
du•vet'
dwarf *pl.* dwarfs *or*
   dwarves
dwarf 'ism
dweeb
dwell, dwelt*or*
   dwelled, dwel'ling
dwin'dle, -dled,
   -dling
dy'ad
dy•ad'ic
dye *(to color),* dyed,
   dye'ing
   ♦*die*
dyed'-in-the-wool'
dy'er *(colorer)*
   ♦*dire*
dye'stuff'
dy'ing *(declining)*
   ♦*dyeing*
dy•nam'ic *also* dy-
   nam'i•cal
dy•nam'ics
dy'na•mism
dy'na•mist
dy'na•mis'tic
dy'na•mite', -mit'ed,
   -mit'ing
dy'na•mo' *pl.* -mos'
dy'na•mo'e•lec'tric
   also dy'na•mo'-
   e•lec'tri•cal
dy'na•mom'e•ter
dy'nast'
dy•nas'tic

dy'nas•ty
dyne *(unit of force)*
   ♦*dine*
Dy•nel'®
dys'en•ter'ic
dys'en•ter'y
dys•func'tion
dys•gen'ic
dys•lec'tic
dys•lex'i•a
dys•lex'ic
dys•pep'sia
dys•pep'tic
dys•pha'sia
dys•pro'si•um
dys•troph'ic
dys'tro•phy *also* dys-
   tro'phi•a

E

each
ea'ger
ea'gle
ea'gle-eyed'
ea'glet
ear'ache'
ear'drum'
eared
ear'flap'
ear'lap'
earl'dom
car'ly
ear'mark'
ear'muff'
earn *(to gain)*
   ♦*urn*

ear'nest
earn'ings
ear'phone'
ear'piece'
ear'plug'
ear'ring
ear'shot'
ear'split'ting
earth'bound'
earth'en
earth'en•ware'
earth'ling
earth'ly *(not spiritual)*
   ♦*earthy*
earth'man'
earth'quake'
earth'shak'ing
earth'ward *also*
   earth'wards
earth'work'
earth'worm'
earth'y *(of the soil,*
   uninhibited)
   ♦*earthly*
ear'wax'
ear'wig'
ease, eased, eas'ing
ea'sel
ease'ment
eas'i•ly
east'bound'
Eas'ter
east'er•ly
east'ern
east'ern•most'
East'er•tide'
east'ward *also* east'-

wards
eas'y
eas'y•go'ing *also*
　eas'y-go'ing
eat, ate, eat'en, eat'ing
eat'a•ble
eat'er•y
eau' de co•logne' *pl.*
　eaux' de co•logne'
eaves'drop',
　-dropped', -drop'-
　ping
eaves'drop'per
ebb
eb'on•ite'
eb'on•y
e•bul'lience
e•bul'lient
eb'ul•li'tion
ec•cen'tric
ec'cen•tric'i•ty
ec•cle'si•as'tic
ec•cle'si•as'ti•cal
ech'e•lon'
e•chid'na
e•chi'no•derm'
ech'o *pl.* -oes
ech'o, -oed, -o•ing
ech'o•lo•ca'tion
é•clair'
é•clat'
e•clec'tic
e•clec'ti•cism
e•clipse', e•clipsed',
　e•clips'ing
e•clip'tic
ec'logue'

ec'o•cide'
ec'o•log'i•cal
e•col'o•gist
e•col'o•gy
e•con'o•met'rics
ec'o•nom'ic
ec'o•nom'i•cal
ec'o•nom'ics
e•con'o•mist
e•con'o•mize ',
　-mized', -miz'ing
e•con'o•miz'er
e•con'o•my
ec'o•spe'cies
ec'o•sys'tem
ec'o•type'
ec'ru
ec'sta•sy
ec•stat'ic
ec'to•derm'
ec'to•plasm'
Ec'ua•dor'i•an
ec'u•men'i•cal
ec'u•men'i•cism
ec'u•men'ism
ec'ze•ma
ec•zem'a•tous
E'dam cheese
ed'dy, died, -dy•ing
e'del•weiss'
e•de'ma *pl.* -mas *or*
　-ma•ta
E'den
e•den'tate'
edge, edged, edg'ing
edge'wise' *also* edge'-
　ways'

edg'y
ed'i•bil'i•ty
ed'i•ble
e'dict'
ed'i•fi•ca'tion
ed'i•fice
ed'i•fy', -fied', -fy'ing
ed'it
e•di'tion *(publication)*
　♦*addition*
ed'i•tor
ed'i•to'ri•al
ed'i•to'ri•al•ize',
　-ized', -iz'ing
ed'i•to'ri•al•iz'er
ed'i•tor•ship'
ed'u•ca•ble
ed'u•cate', -cat'ed,
　-cat'ing
ed'u•ca'tion
ed'u•ca'tion•al
ed'u•ca'tor
e•duce', e•duced',
　e•duc'ing
e•duc'i•ble
eel *pl.* eel *or* eels
e'er *(ever)*
　♦*air, are (metric
　unit), ere, heir*
ee'rie *(weird),* or ee'ry
　♦*aerie*
ee'ri•ly
ef•face', -faced', -fac'·
　ing
ef•fect' *(result)*
　♦*affect*
ef•fec'tive

ef•fec'tive•ly
ef•fec'tu•al
ef•fec'tu•ate', -at'ed,
 -at'ing
ef•fem'i•na•cy
ef•fem'i•nate
ef'fer•ent
ef'fer•vesce',
 -vesced', -vesc'ing
ef'fer•ves'cence
ef'fer•ves'cent
ef•fete'
ef•fi•ca'cious
ef'fi•ca•cy
ef•fi'cien•cy
ef•fi'cient
ef'fi•gy
ef•flo•resce',
 -resced', -resc'ing
ef•flo•res'cence
ef•flo•res'cent
ef'flu•ence
ef'flu•ent
ef•flu'vi•al
ef•flu'vi•um pl. -vi•a
 or -vi•ums
ef'flux'
ef'fort
ef•front'er•y
ef•ful'gence
ef•ful'gent
ef•fuse', -fused', -fus'-
 ing
ef•fu'sion
ef•fu'sive
eft
e•gad'

e•gal'i•tar'i•an
e•gal'i•tar'i•an•ism
egg'beat'er
egg'head'
egg'nog'
egg'plant'
egg'shell'
eg•lan•tine'
e'go pl. e'gos
e'go•cen'tric
e'go•ism
e'go•ist
e'go•is'tic also e'go-
 is'ti•cal
e'go•tism
e'go•tist
e'go•tis'tic also e'go-
 tis'ti•cal
e'go-trip', -tripped',
 -trip'ping
e•gre'gious
e'gress
e'gret
E•gyp'tian
E'gyp•tol'o•gist
E'gyp•tol'o•gy
ei'der
ei'der•down'
eight (number)
 ♦ate
eight•een'
eight•eenth'
eighth
eight'i•eth
eight'y
ein•stein'i•um
ei'ther

e•jac'u•late', -lat'ed,
 -lat'ing
e•jac'u•la'tion
e•jac'u•la'tor
e•ject'
e•jec'tion
e•jec'tor
eke, eked, ek'ing
e•lab'o•rate', rat'ed,
 -rat'ing
e•lab'o•ra'tion
e'land
e•lapse', e•lapsed',
 e•laps'ing
e•las'tic
e•las'tic'i•ty
e•las'ti•cize', -cized',
 -ciz'ing
e•late', e•lat'ed, e•lat'-
 ing
e•la'tion
el'bow
el'bow•room'
eld'er (older person)
el'der (shrub)
el'der•ber'ry
el'der•care'
e•lect'
e•lec'tion
e•lec'tion•eer'
e•lec'tive
e•lec'tor
e•lec'tor•al
e•lec'tor•ate
e•lec'tric or e•lec'tri-
 cal
e•lec•tri'cian

e•lec′tric′i•ty
e•lec′tri•fi•ca′tion
e•lec′tri•fy′, -fied′,
 -fy′ing
e•lec′tro•car′di-
 o•gram′
e•lec′tro•car′di-
 o•graph′
e•lec′tro•chem′i•cal
e•lec′tro•chem′is-
 try
e•lec′tro•cute′, -cut′-
 ed, -cut′ing
e•lec′tro•cu′tion
e•lec′trode′
e•lec′tro•dy•nam′-
 ics
e•lec′tro•dy•na-
 mom′e•ter
e•lec′tro•en•ceph′-
 a•lo•gram′
e•lec′tro•en•ceph′-
 a•lo•graph′
e•lec•trol′y•sis
e•lec′tro•lyte′
e•lec′tro•lyt′ic
e•lec′tro•lyze′,
 -lyzed′, -lyz′ing
e•lec′tro•mag•net′-
 ic
e•lec′tro•mag′net-
 ism
e•lec•trom′e•ter
e•lec′tro•mo′tive
e•lec′tron′
e•lec′tro•neg′a•tive
e•lec•tron′ic

e•lec•tron′ics
e•lec′tro•plate′,
 -plat′ed, -plat′ing
e•lec′tro•pos′i•tive
e•lec′tro•scope′
e•lec′tro•scop′ic
e•lec′tro•shock′
e•lec′tro•stat′ic
e•lec′tro•stat′ics
e•lec′tro•ther′a•py
e•lec′tro•type′,
 -typed′, -typ′ing
e•lec′tro•va′lence
 also e•lec′tro•va′-
 len•cy
e•lec′tro•va′lent
el′ee•mos′y•nar′y
el′e•gance
el′e•gant
el′e•gi′ac
el′e•gize′, -gized′,
 -giz′ing
el′e•gy
el′e•ment
el′e•men′tal
el′e•men′ta•ry
el′e•phant
el′e•phan•ti′a•sis
el′e•phan′tine
el′e•vate′, -vat′ed,
 -vat′ing
el′e•va′tion
el′e•va′tor
e•lev′en
e•lev′enth
elf pl. elves
elf′in

e•lic′it (to draw out)
 ♦illicit
e•lic′i•ta′tion
e•lic′i•tor
e•lide′, e•lid′ed,
 e•lid′ing
el′i•gi•bil′i•ty
el′i•gi•ble
e•lim′i•nate′, -nat′-
 ed, -nat′ing
e•lim′i•na′tion
e•lim′i•na′tor
e•li′sion
e•lite′ or é•lite′
e•lit′ism′ or é•lit′ism′
e•lit′ist or é•lit′ist
e•lix′ir
E•liz′a•be′than
elk pl. elk or elks
elk′hound′
ell
el•lipse′
el•lip′sis pl. -ses′
el•lip′soid′
el′lip•soid′al
el•lip′tic or el•lip′ti-
 cal
elm
el′o•cu′tion
el′o•cu′tion•ar′y
el′o•cu′tion•ist
e•lon′gate′, -gat′ed,
 -gat′ing
e•lon′ga′tion
e•lope′, e•loped′,
 e•lop′ing
e•lope′ment

el'o•quence
el'o•quent
else'where'
e•lu'ci•date', -dat'ed,
  -dat'ing
e•lu'ci•da'tion
e•lu'ci•da'tor
e•lude' *(to avoid),*
  e•lud'ed, e•lud'ing
  ♦*allude*
e•lu'sive *(evasive)*
  ♦*allusive, illusive*
el'ver
E•ly'sian
e•ma'ci•ate', -at'ed,
  -at'ing
e•ma'ci•a'tion
em'a•nate', -nat'ed,
  -nat'ing
em'a•na'tion
em'a•na'tive
e•man'ci•pate', -pat'-
  ed, -pat'ing
e•man'ci•pa'tion
e•man'ci•pa'tor
e•mas'cu•late', -lat'-
  ed, -lat'ing
e•mas'cu•la'tion
e•mas'cu•la'tor
em•balm'
em•bank'
em•bank'ment
em•bar'go *pl.* -goes
em•bark'
em'bar•ka'tion *also*
  em•bark'ment
em•bar'rass

em•bar'rass•ment
em'bas•sy
em•bat'tle, -tled,
  -tling
em•bed', -bed'ded,
  -bed'ding
em•bel'lish
em'ber
em•bez'zle, -zled,
  -zling
em•bez'zle•ment
em•bit'ter
em•blaze', -blazed',
  -blaz'ing
em•bla'zon
em'blem
em'ble•mat'ic *or* em'-
  blem•at'i•cal
em•bod'i•ment
em•bod'y, -ied,
  -y•ing
em•bold'en
em•bol'ic
em'bo•lism
em'bo•lus *pl.* -li'
em'bon•point'
em•bos'om
em•boss'
em'bou•chure'
em•bow'er
em•brace', -braced',
  -brac'ing
em•bra'sure
em•brit'tle, -tled,
  -tling
em•broi'der
em•broi'der•y

em•broil'
em'bry•o' *pl.* -os'
em'bry•o•log'ic *also*
  em'bry•o•log'i•cal
em'bry•ol'o•gist
em'bry•ol'o•gy
em'bry•on'ic
em•cee', -ceed', -cee'-
  ing
e•mend' *(to edit)*
  ♦*amend*
e•men'da'tion
e'men•da'tor
e•men'da•to'ry
em'er•ald
e•merge', e•merged',
  e•merg'ing
e•mer'gence
e•mer'gen•cy
e•mer'gent
e•mer'i•tus
em'er•y
e•met'ic
em'i•grant *(one who
  leaves one's native
  land)*
  ♦*immigrant*
em'i•grate' *(to leave
  one's native land),*
  -grat'ed, -grat'ing
  ♦*immigrate*
em'i•gra'tion *(depar-
  ture from one's na-
  tive land)* ♦
  ♦*immigration*
é'mi•gré'
em'i•nence

em'i•nent
(prominent)
♦*immanent,*
imminent
e•mir' *or* e•meer',
also amir', a•meer'
e•mir'ate
em'is•sar'y
e•mis'sion
e•mis'sive
e•mit', e•mit'ted,
e•mit'ting
e•mit'ter
e•mol'lient
e•mol'u•ment
e•mote', e•mot'ed,
e•mot'ing
e•mo'tion
e•mo'tion•al
e•mo'tion•al•ism
e•mo'tive
em'pa•thet'ic
em•path'ic
em'pa•thize',
-thized', -thiz'ing
em'pa•thy
em'per•or
em'pha•sis *pl.* -ses'
em'pha•size', -sized',
-siz'ing
em•phat'ic
em'phy•se'ma
em'pire'
em•pir'i•cal
em•pir'i•cism
em•pir'i•cist
em•place'ment

em•ploy'
em•ploy'a•ble
em•ploy'ee
em•ploy'er
em•ploy'ment
em•po'ri•um *pl.* -ri-
ums *or* -ri•a
em•pow'er
em'press
emp'ty, -tied, -ty•ing
emp'ty-hand'ed
em'py•re'an
e'mu *pl.* e'mus
em'u•late', -lat'ed,
-lat'ing
em'u•la'tion
em'u•la'tor
em'u•lous
e•mul'si•fi•ca'tion
e•mul'si•fy', -fied',
-fy'ing
e•mul'sion
en•a'ble, -bled, -bling
en•act'
en•act'ment
en•ac'tor
e•nam'el, -eled *or*
-elled, -el'ing *or* -el-
ling
e•nam'el•ware'
en•am'or
en•camp'
en•camp'ment
en•cap'su•late', -lat'-
ed, -lat'ing, *also* in-
cap'su•late'
en•cap'su•la'tion

en•cap'sule, -suled,
-sul•ing
en•case', -cased',
-cas'ing, *also* in-
case'
en•caus'tic
en'ce•phal'ic
en•ceph'a•lit'ic
en•ceph'a•li'tis
en•ceph'a•lo•gram'
en•ceph'a•lo•my'-
e•li'tis
en•ceph'a•lon' *pl.*
-la
en•chain'
en•chant'
en•chant'ment
en•chant'ress
en'chi•la'da
en•ci'pher
en•cir'cle, -cled,
-cling
en'clave'
en•close', -closed',
-clos'ing, *also* in-
close'
en•clo'sure
en•code', -cod'ed,
-cod'ing
en•cod'er
en•co'mi•um *pl.*
-mi•ums *or* -mi•a
en•com'pass
en•core', -cored', -cor'-
ing
en•coun'ter
en•cour'age, -aged,

-ag•ing
en•cour'age•ment
en•croach'
en•croach'ment
en•crust' *also* in•crust'
en'crust•a'tion
en•crypt'
en•cum'ber
en•cum'brance
en•cyc'li•cal
en•cy'clo•pe'di•a *or* en•cy'clo•pae'di•a
en•cy'clo•pe'dic *or* en•cy'clo•pae'dic
end
en•dan'ger
en•dear'
en•dear'ment
en•deav'or
en•dem'ic
end'game'
end'ing
en'dive'
end'less
end'note'
en•do•blast' *also* en'to•blast'
en'do•carp'
en'do•crine
en'do•cri•nol'o•gist
en'do•cri•nol'o•gy
en'do•derm'
en'do•der'mis
en•do•me'tri•um *pl.* -tri•a
en•do•morph'

en'do•mor'phic
en'do•plasm
en•dorse', -dorsed', -dors'ing, *also* in•dorse'
en•dorse'ment
en•dors'er *also* en•dor'sor
en'do•skel'e•ton
en'do•the'li•al
en'do•the'li•um *pl.* -li•a
en'do•ther'mic *also* en'do•ther'mal
en•dow'
en•dow'ment
end'plate'
end'play'
en•due', -dued', -du'-ing, *also* in•due'
en•dur'a•ble
en•dur'ance
en•dure', -dured', -dur'ing
end'wise' *also* end'-ways'
en•e•ma
en'e•my
en'er•get'ic
en'er•gize', -gized', -giz'ing
en'er•giz'er
en'er•gy
en'er•vate', -vat•ed, -vat'ing
en'er•va'tion
en'er•va'tor

en•fee'ble, -bled, -bling
en•fee'ble•ment
en'fi•lade'
en•fold'
en•force', -forced', -forc'ing
en•force'a•ble
en•force'ment
en•forc'er
en•fran'chise', -chised', -chis'ing
en•fran'chise'ment
en•gage', -gaged', -gag'ing
en•gage'ment
en garde'
en•gen'der
en'gine
en'gi•neer'
en'gi•neer'ing
Eng'lish
en•gorge', -gorged', -gorg'ing
en•graft'
en•grave', -graved', -grav'ing
en•grav'er
en•gross'
en•gulf'
en•hance', -hanced', -hanc'ing
en•hance'ment
en•har•mon'ic
e•nig'ma
en'ig•mat'ic *or* en'ig•mat'i•cal

en•join'
en•joy'
en•joy'a•ble
en•joy'ment
en•kin'dle, -dled,
-dling
en•lace', -laced', -lac'-
ing, *also* in•lace'
en•large', -larged',
-larg'ing
en•large'ment
en•larg'er
en•light'en
en•light'en•ment
en•list'
en•list'ment
en•li'ven
en masse'
en•mesh'
en'mi•ty
en•no'ble, -bled,
-bling
en•nui'
e•nor'mi•ty
e•nor'mous
e•nough'
en•plane', -planed',
-plan'ing
en•rage', -raged',
-rag'ing
en•rap'ture, -tured,
-tur•ing
en•rich'
en•rich'ment
en•roll', -rolled', -roll'-
ing, *also* en•rol',
-rolled', -rol'ling

en•roll'ment *or* en-
rol'ment
en route'
en•sconce',
-sconced', -sconc'ing
en•sem'ble
en•shrine', -shrined',
-shrin'ing, *also* in-
shrine'
en•shroud'
en'sign
en'si•lage
en•sile', -siled', -sil'-
ing
en•slave', -slaved',
-slav'ing
en•snare', -snared',
-snar'ing, *also* in-
snare'
en•snarl'
en•sue', -sued', -su'-
ing
en•sure' *(to make cer-
tain)*, -sured', -sur'-
ing
♦assure, insure
en•tab'la•ture'
en•tail'
en•tan'gle, -gled, -gling
en•tan'gle•ment
en•tente'
en'ter
en•ter'ic
en'ter•i'tis
en'ter•prise'
en'ter•pris'ing

en'ter•tain'
en'ter•tain'er
en'ter•tain'ment
en•thrall' *or* in-
thrall'
en•throne',
-throned', -thron'-
ing, *also* in•throne'
en•thuse', -thused',
-thus'ing
en•thu'si•asm
en•thu'si•ast'
en•thu'si•as'tic
en•tice', -ticed', -tic'-
ing
en•tice'ment
en•tire'
en•tire'ty
en•ti'tle, -tled, -tling
en•ti'tle•ment
en'ti•ty
en•tomb'
en'to•mo•log'ic *also*
en'to•mo•log'i•cal
en'to•mol'o•gist
en'to•mol'o•gy
en•tou•rage'
en'tr'acte'
en'trails'
en•train'
en'trance *n.*
en•trance', -tranced',
-tranc'ing
en'trance•way'
en'trant
en•trap', -trapped',
-trap'ping

en•trap′ment
en•treat′ *also* in•treat′
en•treat′y
en′trée *or* en′tree
en•trench′ *or* in•trench′
en′tre nous′
en′tre•pre•neur′
en′tro•py
en•trust′ *or* in•trust′
en′try
en′try•way′
en•twine′, -twined′, -twin′ing, *also* in•twine′
e•nu′mer•ate′, -at′ed, -at′ing
e•nu′mer•a′tion
e•nu′mer•a′tive
e•nu′mer•a′tor
e•nun′ci•ate′, -at′ed, -at′ing
e•nun′ci•a′tion
e•nun′ci•a′tor
en′u•re′sis
en•vel′op v.
en′ve•lope′ n.
en•ven′om
en′vi•a•ble
en′vi•ous
en•vi′ron•ment
en•vi′ron•men′tal•ist
en•vi′rons
en•vis′age, -aged, -ag•ing

en•vi′sion
en′voi *(closing stanza)*, *also* en′voy
en′voy *(diplomat)*
en′vy, -vied, -vy•ing
en•wrap′, -wrapped′, -wrap′ping, *also* in•wrap′
en′zy•mat′ic
en′zyme′
E′o•cene′
e′o•hip′pus
e′o•lith′
E′o•lith′ic
e′on′
e′o•sin
ep′au•let′ *also* ep′au•lette′
é•pée′ *also* e•pee′
e•phed′rine
e•phem′er•al
ep′ic *(poem)*
♦*epoch*
ep′i•can′thic fold
ep′i•cen′ter
ep′i•cure′
ep′i•cu•re′an *also* Ep′i•cu•re′an
ep′i•dem′ic
ep′i•de′mi•ol′o•gist
ep′i•der′mal
ep′i•der′mis
ep′i•glot′tis *pl.* -glot′tis•es *or* -glot′ti•des′
ep′i•gram′
ep′i•gram•mat′ic
ep′i•graph′

ep′i•graph′ic *also* ep′i•graph′i•cal
ep′i•lep′sy
ep′i•lep′tic
ep′i•logue′ *also* ep′i•log′
E•piph′a•ny
ep′i•phyte′
ep′i•phyt′ic
e•pis′co•pa•cy
e•pis′co•pal
E•pis′co•pa′li•an
e•pis′co•pate′
ep′i•sode′
ep′i•sod′ic
e•pis′te•mo•log′i•cal
e•pis′te•mol′o•gy
e•pis′tle
e•pis′to•lar′y
ep′i•taph′
ep′i•the′li•um *pl.* -li•ums *or* -li•a
ep′i•thet′
e•pit′o•me
e•pit′o•mize′, -mized′, -miz′ing
ep′och *(era)*
♦*epic*
ep′och•al
ep′ode′
ep′o•nym′
e•pon′y•mous
ep•ox′y
ep′si•lon′
Ep′som salts
eq′ua•bil′i•ty

eq'ua•ble
e'qual, e'qualed *or*
  e'qualled, e'qualing
  or e'qual•ling
e•qual'i•ty
e'qual•ize', -ized',
  -iz'ing
e'qua•nim'i•ty
e•quate', e•quat'ed,
  e•quat'ing
e•qua'tion
e•qua'tor
e'qua•to'ri•al
eq'uer•ry
e•ques'tri•an
e•ques'tri•enne'
e'qui•an'gu•lar
e'qui•dis'tant
e'qui•lat'er•al
e'qui•lat'er•al•ism
e'qui•lib'ri•um
e'quine'
e'qui•noc'tial
e'qui•nox'
e•quip', e•quipped',
  e•quip'ping
eq'ui•page
e•quip'ment
e'qui•poise'
eq'ui•ta•ble
eq'ui•ta'tion
eq'ui•ty
e•quiv'a•lence *also*
  e•quiv'a•len•cy
e•quiv'a•lent
e•quiv'o•cal
e•quiv'o•cate', -cat'-

ed, -cat'ing
e•quiv'o•ca'tion
e'ra
e•rad'i•ca•ble
e•rad'i•cate', -cat'ed,
  -cat'ing
e•rad'i•ca'tion
e•rad'i•ca'tor
e•ras'a•ble
e•rase', e•rased',
  e•ras'ing
e•ras'er
e•ra'sure
er'bi•um
ere *(before)*
  ♦*air, are (metric
  unit), e'er, heir*
e•rect'
c•rec'tion
e•rec'tor
er'e•mite'
erg
er'go
er'go•nom'ics
er'got
er'mine
e•rode', e•rod'ed,
  e•rod'ing
e•rog'e•nous *also* er'-
  o•gen'ic
e•ro'sion
e•ro'sive
e•rot'ic
e•rot'i•cism
err
er'rand
er'rant

er•rat'ic
er•ra'tum *pl.* -ta
er•ro'ne•ous
er'ror
er'satz'
erst'while'
e•ruct'
e•ruc'ta'tion
er'u•dite'
er'u•di'tion
e•rupt'
e•rup'tion
e•rup'tive
er'y•sip'e•las
e•ryth'ro•blast'
e•ryth'ro•cyte'
e•ryth'ro•my'cin
es'ca•drille'
es'ca•late', -lat'ed,
  -lat'ing
es'ca•la'tion
es'ca•la'tor
es•cap'a•ble
es•ca•pade'
es•cape', -caped',
  -cap'ing
es•cap'ee'
es•cap'ism
es•cap'ist
es•car•got'
es•ca•role'
es•carp'ment
es•chat'o•log'i•cal
es•chew'
es'cort' *n.*
es•cort' *v.*
es'cri•toire'

es'crow
es•cutch'eon
es'ker
Es•ki•mo' *pl.* -mo' *or* -mos'
e•soph'a•ge'al
e•soph'a•gus *pl.* -gi'
es'o•ter'ic
es'o•ter'i•ca
es'o•ter'i•cism
es'pa•drille'
es•pal'ier
es•par'to *pl.* -tos
es•pe'cial
Es'pe•ran'to
es'pi•o•nage'
es'pla•nade'
es•pou'sal
es•pouse', -poused', -pous'ing
es•pres'so *pl.* -sos
es•prit' de corps'
es•py', -pied', -py'ing
es'quire'
es•say' *(to attempt)*
♦ *assay*
es'say *n.*
es'say•is'tic
es'sence
es•sen'tial
es•tab'lish
es•tab'lish•ment
es•tate'
es•teem'
es'ter
es'ti•ma•ble
es'ti•mate', -mat'ed,
-mat'ing
es'ti•ma'tion
es'ti•ma'tor
Es•to'ni•an
es•trange', -tranged', -trang'ing
es'tro•gen
es'tro•gen'ic
es'trous *adj.*
es'trus *n.*
es'tu•ar'y
é'ta•gère' *also* e'ta•gere'
et cet'er•a
etch'ing
e•ter'nal
e•ter'ni•ty
eth'ane'
eth'a•nol'
e'ther
e•the're•al
eth'ic
eth'i•cal
eth'i•cist
eth'ics
E'thi•o'pi•an
eth'nic
eth•nic'i•ty
eth'no•cen'tric
eth'no•cen'trism
eth'no•graph'ic
eth•nog'ra•phy
eth'no•log'ic *also* eth'no•log'i•cal
eth•nol'o•gist
eth•nol'o•gy
e'thos'

eth'yl
eth'yl•ene'
e'ti•o•log'ic *also* e'ti•o•log'i•cal
e'ti•ol'o•gist
e'ti•ol'o•gy
et'i•quette'
E•trus'can
e'tude'
et'y•mo•log'i•cal
et'y•mol'o•gist
et'y•mol'o•gy
eu•ca•lyp'tus *pl.* -tus•es *or* -ti'
Eu'cha•rist
eu'chre
Eu•clid'e•an
eu•gen'ics
eu'lo•gis'tic
eu'lo•gize', -gized', -giz'ing
eu'lo•gy
eu'nuch
eu'phe•mism
eu'phe•mis'tic
eu•pho'ni•ous
eu•pho'ni•um
eu'pho•ny
eu•pho'ri•a
eu•pho'ri•ant
eu•phor'ic
Eur•a'sian
eu•re'ka
Eur'o•cen'tric
eu'ro•cur'ren•cy
Eu'ro•dol'lar
Eur'o•mar'ket

Eu'ro•pe'an

eu•ro'pi•um

Eu•sta'chian tube

eu'tha•na'sia

eu•then'ics

e•vac'u•ate', -at'ed, -at'ing

e•vac'u•a'tion

e•vac'u•a'tor

e•vac'u•ee'

e•vade', e•vad'ed, e•vad'ing

e•val'u•ate', -at'ed, -at'ing

e•val'u•a'tion

ev'a•nes'cence

ev'a•nes'cent

e'van•gel'i•cal *also* e'van•gel'ic

e•van'gel•ism

e•van'gel•ist

e•van'gel•is'tic

e•van'gel•ize', -ized', -iz'ing

e•vap'o•rate', -rat'ed, -rat'ing

e•vap'o•ra'tion

e•vap'o•ra'tor

e•va'sion

e•va'sive

eve

e'ven

eve'ning *(night)*

e'ven•ing *(smoothing)*

eve'ning•wear'

e•vent'

e•vent'ful

e'ven•tide'

e•ven'tu•al

e•ven'tu•al'i•ty

e•ven'tu•ate', -at'ed, -at'ing

ev'er

ev'er•bear'ing

ev'er•bloom'ing

ev'er•glade'

ev'er•green'

ev'er•last'ing

ev'er•more'

e•ver'sion

e•vert'

eve'ry

eve'ry•bod'y

eve'ry•day'

eve'ry•one' *pron.*

eve'ry•place'

eve'ry•thing'

eve'ry•where'

e•vict'

e•vic'tion

e•vic'tor

ev'i•dence, -denced, -denc•ing

ev'i•dent

ev'i•den'tial

e'vil

e'vil•do'er

e'vil-mind'ed

e•vince', e•vinced', e•vinc'ing

e•vin'ci•ble

e•vis'cer•ate', -at'ed, -at'ing

e•vis'cer•a'tion

ev'o•ca'tion

e•voc'a•tive

e•voke', e•voked', e•vok'ing

ev'o•lu'tion

ev'o•lu'tion•ar'y

ev'o•lu'tion•ism

ev'o•lu'tion•ist

e•volve', e•volved', e•volv'ing

ewe *(female sheep)* ♦*yew, you*

ew'er

ex•ac'er•bate', -bat'ed, -bat'ing

ex•ac'er•ba'tion

ex•act'

ex•ac'tion

ex•act'i•tude'

ex•ac'tor

ex•ag'ger•ate', -at'ed, -at'ing

ex•ag'ger•a'tion

ex•ag'ger•a'tor

ex•alt'

ex'al•ta'tion

ex•am'

ex•am'i•na'tion

ex•am'ine, -ined, -in•ing

ex•am'in•er

ex•am'ple

ex•as'per•ate', -at'ed, -at'ing

ex•as'per•a'tion

ex ca•the'dra

ex'ca•vate', -vat'ed,

-vat'ing
ex'ca•va'tion
ex'ca•va'tor
ex•ceed' *(to surpass)*
 ♦*accede*
ex•ceed'ing•ly
ex•cel', -celled', -cel'-
 ling
ex'cel•lence
Ex'cel•len•cy
ex'cel•lent
ex•cel'si•or
ex•cept' *(to exclude)*
 ♦*accept*
ex•cept'ing
ex•cep'tion
ex•cep'tion•al
ex'cerpt'
ex•cess' *(superfluity)*
 ♦*access*
ex•ces'sive
ex•change',
 -changed', -chang'-
 ing
ex•change'a•ble
ex•cheq'uer
ex'cise' *(tax)*
ex•cise' *(to cut)*,
 -cised', -cis'ing
ex•ci'sion
ex•cit'a•bil'i•ty
ex•cit'a•ble
ex'ci•ta'tion
ex•cite', -cit'ed, -cit'-
 ing
ex•cite'ment
ex•claim'

ex'cla•ma'tion
ex•clam'a•to'ry
ex'clave'
ex•clud'a•ble *also*
 ex•clud'i•ble
ex•clude', -clud'ed,
 -clud'ing
ex•clu'sion
ex•clu'sion•ar'y
ex•clu'sive
ex'com•mu'ni•cate',
 -cat'ed, -cat'ing
ex'com•mu'ni•ca'-
 tion
ex'com•mu'ni•ca'-
 tor
ex•co'ri•ate', -at'ed,
 -at'ing
ex•co'ri•a'tion
ex'cre•ment
ex•cres'cence
ex•cres'cent
ex•cre'ta
ex•cre'tal
ex•crete', -cret'ed,
 -cret'ing
ex•cre'tion
ex'cre•to'ry
ex•cru'ci•at'ing
ex'cul•pate', -pat'ed,
 -pat'ing
ex'cul•pa'tion
ex•cul'pa•to'ry
ex•cur'sion
ex•cus'a•ble
ex•cuse', -cused',
 -cus'ing

ex'e•cra•ble
ex'e•crate', -crat'ed,
 -crat'ing
ex'e•cra'tion
ex'e•cra'tor
ex'e•cute', -cut'ed,
 -cut'ing
ex'e•cu'tion
ex'e•cu'tion•er
ex•ec'u•tive
ex•ec'u•tor
ex•ec'u•trix'
ex'e•ge'sis *pl.* -ses
ex•em'plar
ex•em'pla•ry
ex•em'pli•fi•ca'tion
ex•em'pli•fy', -fied',
 -fy'ing
ex•empt'
ex•empt'i•ble
ex•emp'tion
ex'er•cise' *(to exert)*,
 -cised', -cis'ing
 ♦*exorcise*
ex'er•cis'er
ex•ert'
ex•er'tion
ex'e•unt
ex•fo'li•ate', -at'ed,
 -at'ing
ex•fo'li•a'tion
ex'ha•la'tion
ex•halc', -haled', -hal'-
 ing
ex•haust'
ex•haust'i•ble
ex•haus'tion

ex•haus'tive
ex•hib'it
ex'hi•bi'tion
ex'hi•bi'tion•ism
ex'hi•bi'tion•ist
ex'hi•bi'tion•is'tic
ex•hib'i•tor
ex•hil'a•rate', -rat'-
ed, -rat'ing
ex•hil'a•ra'tion
ex•hort'
ex'hor•ta'tion
ex•hor'ta•tive *also*
ex•hor'ta•to'ry
ex'hu•ma'tion
ex•hume', -humed',
-hum'ing
ex'i•gen•cy *also* ex'-
i•gence
ex'i•gent
ex'ile', -iled', -il'ing
ex•ist'
ex•is'tence
ex•is'tent
ex'is•ten'tial
ex'is•ten'tial•ism
ex'is•ten'tial•ist
ex'it
ex li'bris
ex'o•bi•ol'o•gy
ex'o•crine'
ex'o•dus
ex•og'e•nous
ex•on'er•ate', -at'ed,
-at'ing
ex•on'er•a'tion
ex•or'bi•tant

ex'or•cise' *(to expel)*,
-cised', -cis'ing
♦*exercise*
ex'or•cis'er
ex'or•cism
ex'or•cist'
ex'o•skel'e•ton
ex'o•sphere'
ex'o•ther'mic *also*
ex'o•ther'mal
ex•ot'ic
ex•ot'i•ca
ex•pand'
ex•panse'
ex•pan'sion
ex•pan'sion•ism
ex•pan'sion•ist
ex•pan'sive
ex par'te
ex•pa'ti•ate', -at'ed,
-at'ing
ex•pa'ti•a'tion
ex•pa'tri•ate', -at'ed,
-at'ing
ex•pa'tri•a'tion
ex•pect'
ex•pec'tan•cy
ex•pec'tant
ex'pec•ta'tion
ex•pec'to•rant
ex•pec'to•rate', -rat'-
ed, -rat'ing
ex•pec'to•ra'tion
ex•pe'di•en•cy *also*
ex•pe'di•ence
ex•pe'di•ent
ex•pe'di•en'tial

ex'pe•dite', -dit'ed,
-dit'ing
ex'pe•dit'er *also* ex'-
pe•di'tor
ex'pe•di'tion
ex'pe•di'tion•ar'y
ex'pe•di'tious
ex•pel', -pelled', -pel'-
ling
ex•pend'
ex•pend'a•ble
ex•pen'di•ture
ex•pense'
ex•pen'sive
ex•pe'ri•ence,
-enced, -enc•ing
ex•per'i•ment
ex•per'i•men'tal
ex•per'i•men•ta'-
tion
ex'pert'
ex'per•tise'
ex'pi•ate', -at'ed, -at'-
ing
ex'pi•a'tion
ex'pi•a'tor
ex'pi•ra'tion
ex•pire', -pired', -pir'-
ing
ex•plain'
ex•plain'a•ble
ex'pla•na'tion
ex•plan'a•to'ry
ex'ple•tive
ex'pli•ca•ble
ex'pli•cate', -cat'ed,
-cat'ing

ex'pli•ca'tion
ex'pli•ca'tor
ex•plic'it
ex•plode', -plod'ed, -plod'ing
ex'ploit' *n.*
ex•ploit' *v.*
ex•ploit'a•ble
ex'ploi•ta'tion
ex•ploit'a•tive
ex•plo•ra'tion
ex•plor'a•to'ry
ex•plore', -plored', -plor'ing
ex•plor'er
ex•plo'sion
ex•plo'sive
ex•po'nent
ex'po•nen'tial
ex'port' *n.*
ex•port' *v.*
ex•pose', -posed', -pos'ing
ex'po•sé'
ex'po•si'tion
ex•pos'i•tor
ex•pos'i•to'ry
ex' post fac'to
ex•pos'tu•late', -lat'ed, -lat'ing
ex•pos'tu•la'tion
ex•po'sure
ex•pound'
ex•press'
ex•press'i•ble
ex•pres'sion
ex•pres'sion•ism

ex•pres'sion•ist
ex•pres'sion•is'tic
ex•pres'sive
ex•press'way'
ex•pro'pri•ate', -at'ed, -at'ing
ex•pro'pri•a'tion
ex•pro'pri•a'tor
ex•pul'sion
ex•punge', -punged', -pung'ing
ex•pur•gate', -gat'ed, -gat'ing
ex'pur•ga'tion
ex'pur•ga'tor
ex'qui•site
ex'tant *(existing)*
♦*extent*
ex•tem'po•ra'ne•ous
ex•tem'po•rar'y
ex•tem'po•re
ex•tem'po•rize', -rized', -riz'ing
ex•tend'
ex•tend'i•bil'i•ty
ex•tend'i•ble
ex•ten'si•ble
ex•ten'sion
ex•ten'sive
ex•ten'sor
ex•tent' *(size)*
♦*extant*
ex•ten'u•ate', -at'ed, -at'ing
ex•ten'u•a'tion
ex•te'ri•or

ex•ter'mi•nate', -nat'ed, -nat'ing
ex•ter'mi•na'tion
ex•ter'mi•na'tor
ex'tern
ex•ter'nal
ex•ter'nal•i•za'tion
ex•ter'nal•ize', -ized', -izing
ex•tinct'
ex•tinc'tion
ex•tin'guish
ex•tin'guish•er
ex'tir•pate', -pat'ed, -pat'ing
ex'tir•pa'tion
ex'tir•pa'tor
ex•tol', -tolled', -tol'-ling
ex•tol'ler
ex•tort'
ex•tor'tion
ex•tor'tion•ist
ex'tra
ex'tract' *n.*
ex•tract' *v.*
ex•trac'tion
ex•trac'tive
ex•trac'tor
ex'tra•cur•ric'u•lar
ex'tra•dite', -dit'ed, -dit'ing
ex'tra•di'tion
ex'tra•ga•lac'tic
ex'tra•mar'i•tal
ex'tra•ne•ous
ex•traor'di•naire'

ex•traor'di•nar'y
ex•trap'o•late', -lat'-
  ed, -lat'ing
ex•trap'o•la'tion
ex'tra•sen'so•ry
ex'tra•ter•res'tri•al
ex'tra•ter'ri•to'ri•al
ex•trav'a•gance
ex•trav'a•gant
ex•trav'a•gan'za
ex'tra•ve•hic'u•lar
  activity
ex•treme'
ex•trem'ism
ex•trem'ist
ex•trem'i•ty
ex•tri•ca•ble
ex'tri•cate', -cat'ed,
  -cat'ing
ex•tri•ca'tion
ex•trin'sic
ex'tro•ver'sion
ex'tro•ver'sive
ex'tro•vert'
ex•trude', -trud'ed,
  -trud'ing
ex•tru'sion
ex•tru'sive
ex•u'ber•ance
ex•u'ber•ant
ex'u•da'tion
ex•ude', -ud'ed, -ud'-
  ing
ex•ult'
ex•ul'tant
ex•ul•ta'tion
eye (to look), eyed,

eye'ing or ey'ing
  ♦aye, I
eye'ball'
eye'bolt'
eye'brow'
eye'cup'
eyed'ness
eye'drop'per
eye'ful'
eye'glass'
eye'lash'
eye'let (hole)
  ♦islet
eye'lid'
eye'piece'
eye'shot'
eye'sight'
eye'sore'
eye'spot'
eye'stalk'
eye'strain'
eye'tooth'
eye'wash'
eye'wear'
eye'wit'ness

F

fa'ble
fa'bled
fab'ric
fab'ri•cate', -cat'ed,
  -cat'ing
fab'ri•ca'tion
fab'ri•ca'tor
fab'u•late', -lat'ed,
  -lat'ing

fab'u•list
fab'u•lous
fa•çade' also fa•cade'
face, faced, fac'ing
face'down'
face'lift'ing also face'
  -lift'
face'mask'
face'-off' n.
fac'et
fa•ce'tious
face'up'
fa'cial
fac'ile
fa•cil'i•tate', -tat'ed,
  -tat'ing
fa•cil'i•ta'tion
fa•cil'i•ty
fac'ing
fac•sim'i•le
fact'-find'er
fact'-find'ing
fac'tion
fac'tion•al•ism
fac'tious
fac•ti'tious (artificial)
  ♦fictitious
fac'toid
fac'tor
fac'tor•a•ble
fac•to'ri•al
fac'tor•i•za'tion
fac'to•ry
fac•to'tum
fac'tu•al
fac'ul•ty
fad'dish

fad′dist

fade, fad′ed, fad′ing

fade′a•way′

fade′-in′ *n.*

fade′-out′ *n.*

fa′er•ie *also* fa′er•y

fag, fagged, fag′ging

fag′ot *also* fag′got

fag′ot•ing *also* fag′-
got•ing

Fahr′en•heit′

fa•ience′ *also* fa•ï
ence′

fail *(to be unsuccess-
ful)*
 ♦*faille*

faille *(fabric)*
 ♦*fail, file*

fail′-safe′

fail′ure

fain *(gladly)*
 ♦*feign*

faint *(indistinct)*
 ♦*feint*

faint′-heart′ed

fair *(lovely, pale, just)*
 ♦*fare*

fair *(market)*
 ♦*fare*

fair′ground′ *also* fair′-
grounds′

fair′-haired′

fair′ly

fair′-mind′ed

fair′-spo′ken

fair′-trade′, -trad′ed,
 -trad′ing

fair′way′

fair′-weath′er *adj.*

fair′y

fair′y•land′

faith′ful

faith′less

fa•ji′ta

fake, faked, fak′ing

fak′er *(imposter)*
 ♦*fakir*

fak′er•y

fa•kir′ *(beggar)*
 ♦*faker*

fal′con

fal′con•ry

fall, fell, fall′en, fall′-
 ing

fal•la′cious

fal′la•cy

fal′li•bil′i•ty

fal′li•ble

fall′ing-out′ *pl.* fall′-
 ings-out′ *or* fall′ing-
 outs′

Fal•lo′pi•an tube

fall′out′ *n.*

fal′low

false, fals′er, fals′est

false′-heart′ed

false′hood′

fal•set′to *pl.* -tos

fal′si•fi•ca′tion

fal′si•fy′, -fied′, -fy′-
 ing

fal′si•ty

fal′ter

fame, famed, fam′ing

fa•mil′ial

fa•mil′iar

fa•mil′i•ar′i•ty

fa•mil′iar•ize′,
 -ized′, -iz′ing

fam′i•ly

fam′ine

fam′ished

fa′mous

fan, fanned, fan′ning

fa•nat′ic

fa•nat′i•cal

fa•nat′i•cism

fan′cied

fan′ci•er

fan′ci•ful

fan′cy, -cied, -cy•ing

fan′cy-free′

fan′cy•work′

fan•dan′go *pl.* -gos

fan′dom

fan′fare′

fang

fan′light′

fan′tail′

fan•ta′sia

fan′ta•size′, -sized′,
 -siz′ing

fan•tas′tic

fan′ta•sy

fan′ta•sy•land′

far, far′ther *or* fur′-
 ther, far′thest *or* fur′-
 thest

far′ad

far′a•day′

far′a•way′

farce
far•ceur′
far′ci•cal
fare *(charge)*
  ♦*fair*
fare *(to get along),*
  fared, far′ing
  ♦*fair*
fare•well′
far′-fetched′
far′-flung′
fa•ri′na
far′i•na′ceous
farm′er
farm′house′
farm′land′
farm′stead′
farm′yard′
far′o
far′-off′
far′-out′
far•ra′go *pl.* -goes
far′-reach′ing
far′row
far′see′ing
far′-sight′ed
far′ther *(to a greater distance)*
  ♦*further*
far′thest *(to the most distant point)*
  ♦*furthest*
far′thing
far′thin•gale′
fas′ci•a *pl.* -ci•ae′
fas′ci•cle
fas•cic′u•late′ *also*

fas•cic′u•lat′ed
fas′ci•nate′, -nat′ed, -nat′ing
fas′ci•na′tion
fas′ci•na′tor
fas′cism
fas′cist
fash′ion
fash′ion•a•ble
fast′back′
fast′ball′
fas′ten
fas′ten•er
fast′-food′ *adj.*
fas•tid′i•ous
fast′ness
fat, fat′ter, fat′test
fa′tal
fa′tal•ism
fa′tal•ist
fa′tal•is′tic
fa•tal′i•ty
fat′back′
fate *(destiny)*
  ♦*fete*
fat′ed
fate′ful
fa′ther
fa′ther•hood′
fa′ther-in-law′ *pl.* fa′-thers-in-law′
fa′ther•land′
fa′ther•less
fa′ther•ly
fath′om *pl.* -om *or* -oms
fath′om•a•ble

fa•tigue′, -tigued′, -tigu′ing
fat′-sol′u•ble
fat′ten
fat′ty
fa•tu′i•ty
fat′u•ous
fau′cet
fault′find′er
fault′find′ing
fault′y
faun *(deity)*
  ♦*fawn*
fau′na *pl.* -nas *or* -nae′
fauv′ism
faux pas′ *pl.* faux pas′
fa′vor
fa′vor•a•ble
fa′vor•ite
fa′vor•it•ism
fawn *(deer)*
  ♦*faun*
fawn *(to grovel)*
  ♦*faun*
fax *(facsimile)*
  ♦*facts*
faze *(to upset),* fazed, faz′ing
  ♦*phase*
fe′al•ty
fear′ful
fear′less
fear′some
fea′si•bil′i•ty
fea′si•ble
feast

feat (exploit)
 ♦feet
feath'er
feath'er•bed', -bed'-
 ded, -bed'ding
feath'er•brain'
feath'er•stitch'
feath'er•weight'
feath'er•y
fea'ture, -tured, -tur-
 ing
feb'rile
Feb'ru•ar'y
fe'cal
fe'ces also fae'ces
feck'less
fe'cund
fe'cun•date', -dat'ed,
 -dat'ing
fe•cun'di•ty
fed'er•al
fed'er•al•ism
fed'er•al•ist
fed'er•al•i•za'tion
fed'er•al•ize', -ized',
 -iz'ing
fed'er•ate', -at'ed,
 -at'ing
fed'er•a'tion
fe•do'ra
fee
fee'ble
fee'ble-mind'ed
feed, fcd, feed'ing
feed'back'
feed'bag'
feed'er

feel, felt, feel'ing
feel'er
feign (to pretend)
 ♦fain
feint (strategem)
 ♦faint
feist'y
feld'spar' also fel'-
 spar'
fe•lic'i•tate', -tat'ed,
 -tat'ing
fe•lic'i•ta'tion
fe•lic'i•ta'tor
fe•lic'i•tous
fe•lic'i•ty
fe'line
fell
fel'low
fel'low•ship'
fel'ly also fel'loe
fel'on
fe•lo'ni•ous
fel'o•ny
felt'ing
fe'male
fem'i•nine
fem'i•nin'i•ty
fem'i•nism
fem'i•nist
femme fa•tale' pl.
 femmes fa•tales'
fem'o•ral
fe'mur pl. fe'murs or
 fem'o•ra
fen
fence, fenced, fenc'ing
fenc'er

fend
fend'er
fen'es•tra'tion
fen'nel
fe'ral
fer'-de-lance'
fer'ment' n.
fer•ment' v.
fer'men•ta'tion
fer'mi•um
fern'er•y pl. -ies
fern'y
fe•ro'cious
fe•roc'i•ty
fer'ret (animal)
fer'ret (tape), also fer'-
 ret•ing
fer'ric
Fer'ris wheel also
 fer'ris wheel
fer'rite'
fer'ro•al'loy'
fer'ro•mag•net'ic
fer'ro•mag'ne•tism
fer'ro•man'ga•nese'
fer'ro•type'
fer'rous
fer'rule (metal ring)
 ♦ferule
fer'ry, -ried, -ry•ing
fer'ry•boat'
fer'tile
fer•til'i•ty
fer'til•i•za'tion
fer'til•ize', -ized', -iz'-
 ing
fer'til•iz'er

fer'ule *(stick)*
 ♦*ferrule*
fer'ven•cy
fer'vent
fer'vid
fer'vor
fes'tal
fes'ter
fes'ti•val
fes'tive
fes•tiv'i•ty
fes•toon'
fe'tal *also* foe'tal
fetch'ing
fete *(festival), also* fête
 ♦*fate*
fete *(to honor),* fet'ed,
 fet'ing, *also* fête, fêt'-
 ed, fêt'ing
 ♦*fate*
fet'id
fet'ish
fet'ish•ism
fet'ish•ist
fet'lock'
fet'ter
fet'tle
fe'tus *pl.* -tus•es, *also*
 foe'tus
feud
feu'dal
feu'dal•ism
feu'dal•ist
feu'dal•is'tic
feu'da•to'ry
fe'ver
fe'ver•ish

few
fey
fez *pl.* fez'zes
fi'an•cé' *masc.*
fi'an•cée' *fem.*
fi•as'co *pl.* -coes *or*
 -cos
fi'at'
fib, fibbed, fib'bing
fib'ber
fi'ber
fi'ber•board'
Fi'ber•fil' ®
Fi'ber•glas' ®
fi'bril
fib'ril•la'tion
fi'brin
fi•brin'o•gen
fi'broid'
fi•bro'sis
fi'brous
fib'u•la *pl.* -lae' *or*
 -las
fick'le
fic'tion
fic•ti'tious *(imagi-*
 nary)
 ♦*factitious*
fic'tive
fid'dle, -dled, -dling
fid'dler
fid'dle•sticks'
fi•del'i•ty
fidg'et
fidg'et•y
fi•du'ci•ar'y
fie

fief
fief'dom
field'er
field'stone'
field'work'
fiend'ish
fierce, fierc'er, fierc'-
 est
fier'y
fi•es'ta
fife
fif•teen'
fif•teenth'
fifth
fif'ti•eth
fif'ty
fif'ty-fif'ty
fig
fight, fought, fight'ing
fight'er
fig'ment
fig'ur•a'tion
fig'ur•a•tive
fig'ure, -ured, -ur•ing
fig'ure•head'
fig'u•rine'
Fi'ji•an
fil'a•ment
fil'bert
filch'er
file *(collection, tool)*
 ♦*faille*
file *(to catalogue,*
 smooth), filed, fil'ing
 ♦*faille*
fi'let mi•gnon'
fil'i•al

fil'i•bus'ter
fil'i•gree', -greed',
  -gree'ing
fil'ing
Fil'i•pi'no *pl.* -nos
fill'er
fil'let *(ribbon)*
fil•let' *(meat), also* fi-
  let'
fil'let *(to bind),* -let-
  ed, -let•ing
fil•let' *(to bone),*
  -leted', -let'ing, *also*
  fi•let'
fill'-in' *n.*
fill'ing
fil'lip
fil'ly
film'go'er
film'mak'er
film'mak'ing
film'strip'
film'y
fil'ter *(strainer)*
  ♦*philter*
fil'ter•a•bil'i•ty
fil'ter•a•ble *also* fil'-
  tra•ble
filth'y
fil'trate', -trat'ed,
  -trat'ing
fil•tra'tion
fin
fi•na'gle, -gled, -gling
fi'nal
fi•na'le
fi'nal•ist

fi•nal'i•ty
fi'nal•ize', -ized', -iz'-
  ing
fi'nal•ly
fi•nance', -nanced',
  -nanc'ing
fi•nan'cial
fin'an•cier'
finch
find, found, find'ing
find'er
fine, fin'er, fin'est
fine, fined, fin'ing
fine'-drawn'
fine'-grained'
fin'er•y
fi•nesse'
fin'ger
fin'ger•board'
fin'ger•ing
fin'ger•ling
fin'ger•nail'
fin'ger-paint'
fin'ger•print'
finger tip *also* fin'-
  ger•tip'
fin'i•al
fin'i•cal
fin'ick•y
fi'nis
fin'ish
fi'nite'
fin'nan had'die
finned
Finn'ish
fin'ny
fir *(tree)*

  ♦*fur*
fire, fired, fir'ing
fire'arm'
fire'ball'
fire'boat'
fire'box'
fire'brand'
fire'break'
fire'brick'
fire'bug'
fire'crack'er
fire'damp'
fire'dog'
fire'fight'er
fire'fly'
fire'guard'
fire'house'
fire'light'
fire'man
fire'place'
fire'plug'
fire'pow'er
fire'proof '
fire'side'
fire'storm'
fire'trap'
fire'wa'ter
fire'weed'
fire'wood'
fire'works'
fir'ing
fir'kin
fir'ma•ment
firm'ly
first'-born'
first'-class' *adj. &*
  adv.

first′hand′
first′-rate′
first′-string′
firth
fis′cal
fish *pl.* fish *or* fish′es
fish′bowl′
fish′er *(one that fish-es)*
 ♦*fissure*
fish′er•man
fish′er•y
fish′eye′
fish′hook′
fish′meal′
fish′net′
fish′pond′
fish′tail′
fish′wife′
fish′y
fis′sile
fis′sion
fis′sion•a•ble
fis′sure *(crack)*
 ♦*fisher*
fist′ful′ *pl.* -fuls′
fist′i•cuffs′
fis′tu•la *pl.* -las *or* -lae′
fis′tu•lous
fit, fit′ter, fit′test
fit, fit′ted *or* fit, fit′-ting
fit′ful
five′-and-dime′ *n.*
five′-and-ten′ *n.*
five′fold′

fix′a•ble
fix′ate′, -at′ed, -at′ing
fix•a′tion
fix′a•tive
fixed
fix′ed•ly
fix′ings
fix′ture
fizz
fiz′zle, -zled, -zling
fjord *or* fiord
flab′ber•gast′
flab′by
flac′cid
flack *(press agent)*
 ♦*flak*
flac′on
flag, flagged, flag′ging
flag′el•lant
flag′el•late′, -lat′ed, -lat′ing
flag′el•la′tion
fla•gel′lum *pl.* -la
flag′eo•let′
flag′ging
flag′on
flag′pole′
fla′gran•cy *also* fla′-grance
fla′grant
flag′ship′
flag′staff′
flag′stick′
flag′stone′
flail
flair *(knack)*
 ♦*flare*

flak *(artillery, criti-cism)*
 ♦*flack*
flake, flaked, flak′ing
flak′y
flam•bé′, -béed′, -bé′-ing
flam•boy′ance *also* flam•boy′an•cy
flam•boy′ant
flame, flamed, flam′-ing
fla•men′co
flame′out′ *n.*
flam′ing
fla•min′go *pl.* -gos *or* -goes
flam′ma•bil′i•ty
flam′ma•ble
flange
flan′ken
flank′er•back′
flan′nel
flan′nel•ette′
flap, flapped, flap′-ping
flap′jack′
flap′per
flare *(to flame)*, flared, flar′ing
 ♦*flair*
flare′-up′ *n.*
flash′back′ *n.*
flash′cube′
flash′light′
flash′y
flask

flat, flat′ter, flat′test
flat, flat′ted, flat′ting
flat′bed′
flat′boat′
flat′bread′
flat′car′
flat′fish′ *pl.* -fish′ *or*
　-fish′es
flat′foot′ *(fallen arch),*
　pl. -feet′
flat′foot′ *(policeman),*
　pl. -foots′
flat′foot′ed
flat′i′ron
flat′ten
flat′ter
flat′ter•y
flat′top′
flat′u•lence
flat′u•lent
flat′ware′
flat′worm′
flaunt *(to show off)*
　♦*flout*
flau′tist
fla′vor
flaw′less
flax′en
flax′seed′
flay′er
flea *(insect)*
　♦*flee*
flea′-bit•ten
fleck
fledge, fledged,
　fledg′ing
fledg′ling *also* fledge′-

ling
flee *(to run),* fled, flee′-
　ing
　♦*flea*
fleece, fleeced, fleec′-
　ing
fleec′y
fleet′ing
Flem′ing
Flem′ish
flesh′ly *(of the body,*
　physical)
flesh′y *(of flesh,*
　plump)
fleur′-de-lis′ *pl.*
　fleurs′-de-lis′, *or*
　fleur′-de-lys′ *pl.*
　fleurs′-de-lys′
flex′i•bil′i•ty
flex′i•ble
flex′ion *also* flec′tion
flex•og′ra•phy
flex′or *(muscle)*
　♦*flexure*
flex′time′
flex′ure *(bend)*
　♦*flexor*
flib′ber•ti•gib′bet
flick′er
fli′er *also* fly′er
flight′less
flight′wor′thy
flight′y
flim′flam′,
　-flammed′, -flam′-
　ming
flim′sy

flinch
fling, flung, fling′ing
flint′lock′
flint′y
flip, flipped, flip′ping
flip′-flop′
flip′pan•cy
flip′pant
flip′per
flirt
flir•ta′tion
flir•ta′tious
flit, flit′ted, flit′ting
float′er
float′ing
flock
floe *(ice mass)*
　♦*flow*
flog, flogged, flog′ging
flog′ger
flood′gate′
flood′light′, -light′ed
　or -lit′, -light′ing
flood′wa′ter
floor′board′
floor′ing
floor′-through′
floor′walk′er
flop, flopped, flop′-
　ping
flop′house′
flop′py
flo′ra *pl.* -ras *or* -rae′
flo′ral
Flor′en•tine′
flo•res′cence
flo′ret

flo′ri•cul′ture
flor′id
flo′rist
floss′y
flo•ta′tion *also* floa-
 ta′tion
flo•til′la
flot′sam
flounce, flounced,
 flounc′ing
floun′der
flour *(powder)*
 ♦*flower*
flour′ish
flour′y *(covered with
 flour)*
 ♦*flowery*
flout *(to scoff)*
 ♦*flaunt*
flow *(stream)*
 ♦*floe*
flow′er *(blossom)*
 ♦*flour*
flow′er•pot′
flow′er•y *(like flow-
 ers, fancy)*
 ♦*floury*
flu *(influenza)*
 ♦*flew, flue*
fluc′tu•ate′, -at′ed,
 -at′ing
fluc′tu•a′tion
flue *(pipe)*
 ♦*flew, flu*
flu′en•cy
flu′ent
fluff ′y

flu′id
flu•id′ics
flu•id′i•ty
flu′id•ize′, -ized′, -iz′-
 ing
fluke
fluke *(blade, stroke of
 luck)*
fluke *(fish), pl.* fluke
fluk′y
flume
flum′mer•y
flum′mox
flunk
flunk′out′
flun′ky *also* flun′key
 pl. -keys
flu•o•resce′, -resced′,
 resc′ing
flu•o•res′cence
flu•o•res′cent
fluor′i•date′, -dat′ed,
 -dat′ing
fluor′i•da′tion
flu′o•ride′
flu′o•rine′
fluor′ite′
flu′o•ro•car′bon
fluor′o•scope′
fluor′o•scop′ic
flu′o•ros′co•py
flur′ry, -ried, -ry•ing
flush
flush•om′e•ter
flus′ter
flute, flut′ed, flut′ing
flut′ist

flut′ter
flu′vi•al
flux
fly *(to move through
 air)*, flew, flown, fly′-
 ing
fly *(to hit a baseball)*,
 flied, flied, fly′ing
fly′a•way′
fly′blown′
fly′boat′
fly′bridge′
fly′by′ *pl.* -bys′
fly′-by-night′
fly′catch′er
fly′ing
fly′leaf ′
fly′pa′per
fly′sheet′
fly′speck′
fly′trap′
fly′weight′
fly′wheel′
f ′-num′ber
foal
foam′y
fob, fobbed, fob′bing
fo′cal
fo′cus *pl.* -cus•es *or*
 -ci′
fo′cus, -cused *or*
 -cussed, -cus•ing *or*
 -cus•sing
fod′der
foe
fog, fogged, fog′ging
fog′gy

fog'horn'
fo'gy *also* fo'gey *pl.*
  -geys
foi'ble
foil
foist
fold'a•way'
fold'er
fol'de•rol'
fold'up'
fo'li•age
fo'li•ate', -at'ed, -at'-
  ing
fo'li•a'tion
fo'lic acid
fo'li•o' *pl.* -os'
fo'li•um *pl.* -li•a
folk *pl.* folk *or* folks
folk'lore'
folk'lor'ist
folk'sy
folk'way'
fol'li•cle
fol'low
fol'low•er
fol'low-through' *n.*
fol'low-up' *n.*
fol'ly
fo•ment'
fo'men•ta'tion
fond
fon'dant
fon'dle, -dled, -dling
fond'ness
fon•due' *also* fon•du'
font
food'stuff'

fool'er•y
fool'har'dy
fool'ish
fool'proof'
fools'cap'
foot *pl.* feet
foot'age
foot'-and-mouth'
  disease
foot'ball'
foot'bath'
foot'board'
foot'bridge'
foot'-can'dle
foot'fall'
foot'gear'
foot'hill'
foot'hold'
foot'ing
foot'less
foot'lights'
foot'ling
foot'lock'er
foot'long'
foot'loose'
foot'man
foot'note'
foot'path'
foot'-pound'
foot'print'
foot'rest'
foot'sore'
foot'step'
foot'stool'
foot'wear'
foot'work'
fop'per•y

fop'pish
for *prep. & conj.*
  ♦*fore, four*
for'age, -aged, -ag•ing
for'ag•er
fo•ra'men *pl.* -ram'-
  i•na *or* -ra'mens
for'as•much' as
for'ay'
for•bear' *(to refrain),*
  -bore', -borne',
  -bear'ing
  ♦*forebear*
for•bid', -bade' *or*
  -bad', -bid'den *or*
  -bid', -bid'ding
force, forced, forc'ing
force'a•ble
force'ful
force'meat'
for'ceps *pl.* -ceps
for'ci•ble
ford
fore *(at or toward the*
  front)
  ♦*for, four*
fore'-and-aft' *adj.*
fore•arm'*v.*
fore'arm' *n.*
fore'bear' *(ancestor),*
  also forebear
fore•bode', -bod'ed,
  -bod'ing
fore'brain'
fore'cast', -cast' *or*
  -cast'ed, -cast'ing

fore'cas•tle
fore•close', -closed',
  -clos'ing
fore•clo'sure
fore'court'
fore•doom'
fore'fa'ther
fore'fin'ger
fore'foot'
fore'front'
fore•go' *(to precede)*,
  -went', -gone', -go'-
  ing, -goes
  ♦*forgo*
fore'ground'
fore'hand'
fore'head'
for'eign
fore•knowl'edge
fore'leg'
fore'limb'
fore'lock'
fore'man
fore'mast
fore'most'
fore'name'
fore'noon'
fo•ren'sic
fore'or•dain'
fore'part'
fore'quar'ter
fore'run'ner
fore'sail
fore•see', -saw',
  -seen', -see'ing
fore•see'a•ble
fore•shad'ow

fore'shore'
fore•short'en
fore'sight'
fore'skin'
for'est
fore•stall'
for'est•ry
fore•taste' -tast'ed,
  -tast'ing
fore•tell', -told', -tell'-
  ing
fore'thought'
fore•to'ken
for•ev'er
for•ev'er•more'
for•ev'er•ness
fore•warn'
fore'wing'
fore'word' *(preface)*
  ♦*forward*
for'feit
for'fei•ture'
for•gath'er *also* fore-
  gath'er
forge, forged, forg'ing
forg'er
forg'er•y
for•get', -got', -got'-
  ten *or* -got', -get'ting
for•get'ful
for•get'-me-not'
for•get'ta•ble
for•get'ter
for•giv'a•ble
for•give', -gave', -giv'-
  en, -giv'ing
for•go' *(to relinquish)*,

-went', -gone', -go'-
  ing, -goes
  ♦*forego*
for•go'er
fork'•ful *pl.* fork'fuls
  or forks'ful
for•lorn'
form
for'mal
for•mal'de•hyde'
for'mal•ism
for'mal•ist
for'mal•is'tic
for•mal'i•ty
for'mal•ize', -ized',
  -iz'ing
for'mal•ly *(in a for-
  mal manner)*
  ♦*formerly*
for'mal•wear'
for'mat
for•ma'tion
for'ma•tive
form'er *(one that
  forms)*
for'mer *(earlier)*
for'mer•ly *(once)*
  ♦*formally*
form'fit'ting
For•mi'ca®
for'mic acid
for'mi•da•bil'i•ty
for'mi•da•ble
for'mu•la *pl.* -las *or*
  -lae'
for'mu•la'ic
for'mu•lar•ize',

-ized', -iz'ing
for'mu•late', -lat'ed,
  -lat'ing
for'mu•la'tion
for'mu•la'tor
for'ni•cate', -cat'ed,
  -cat'ing
for'ni•ca'tion
for•sake', -sook',
  -sak'en, -sak'ing
for•sooth'
for•swear', -swore',
  -sworn', -swear'ing,
  also fore•swear'
for•syth'i•a
fort *(fortified place)*
forte *(strong point)*
for•te' *(musical direc-*
  tion)
forth *(forward)*
  ◆*fourth*
forth•com'ing
forth'right'
forth•with'
for'ti•eth
for'ti•fi•ca'tion
for'ti•fy', -fied', -fy'-
  ing
for•tis'si•mo' *pl.*
  -mos'
for'ti•tude'
fort'night'
FOR'TRAN'
for'tress
for•tu'i•tous
for•tu'i•ty
for'tu•nate

for'tune
for'tune•tell'er
for'tune•tell'ing
for'ty
for'ty-five'
for'ty-nin'er
fo'rum *pl.* -rums *or*
  -ra
for'ward *(toward the*
  front), also for'wards
  ◆*foreword*
fos'sil
fos'sil•ize', -ized', -iz'-
  ing
fos'ter
foul *(offensive)*
  ◆*fowl*
fou•lard'
foul'-mouthed'
foul'-up' *n.*
foun•da'tion
found'er *n.*
foun'der *v.*
found'ling
foun'dry
fount
foun'tain
foun'tain•head'
four *(number)*
  ◆*for, fore*
four'-di•men'sion-
  al
four'-flush'er
four'fold'
four'hand'ed
Four'-H' Club
four'-in-hand'

four'-leaf ' clover
four'-o'clock' *(plant)*
four'-post'er
four'score'
four'some
four'square'
four•teen'
four•teenth'
fourth *(number)*
  ◆*forth*
fo've•a *pl.* -ae'
fowl *(bird), pl.* fowl *or*
  fowls
  ◆*foul*
foxed
fox'glove'
fox'hole'
fox'hound'
fox'trot', -trot'ted,
  -trot'ting
fox'y
foy'er
fra'cas
frac'tion
frac'tion•al
frac'tion•al•ize',
  -ized', -iz'ing
frac'tion•ate', -at'ed,
  -at'ing
frac'tious
frac'ture, -tured, -tur-
  ing
frag'ile
fra•gil'i•ty
frag'ment
frag'men•tar'y
frag'men•ta'tion

fra′grance
fra′grant
frail′ty
frame, framed, fram-
  ing
fram′er
frame′-up′ *n.*
frame′work′
franc *(money)*
  ♦*frank*
fran′chise′, -chised′,
  -chis′ing
fran′chi•see′
fran′chis′er
Fran•cis′can
fran′ci•um
fran′gi•ble
fran′gi•pan′i
frank *(straightforward)*
  ♦*franc*
Frank′en•stein′
frank′furt•er
frank′in•cense′
fran′tic
frap•pé′
fra•ter′nal
fra•ter′nal•ism
fra•ter′ni•ty
frat′er•ni•za′tion
frat′er•nize′, -nized′,
  -niz′ing
frat′ri•cid′al
frat′ri•cide′
Frau *pl.* Frau′en
fraud′u•lence
fraud′u•lent
fraught

Fräu′lein′ *pl.* -lein′
fray
fraz′zle, -zled, -zling
freak′ish
freck′le, -led, -ling
free, fre′er, fre′est
free, freed, free′ing
free′bie *also* free′bee
free′board′
free′boot′er
free′born′
free′dom
free′-for-all′
free′form′
free′hand′
free′hand′ed
free′hold′
free′-lance′ *adj.*
free′-lance′, -lanced′,
  -lanc′ing
free′-lanc′er *or* free
  lance
free′load′
free′load′er
free′man
free′ma′son
free′ma′son•ry
free′sia
free′-soil′
free′stand′ing
free′stone′
free′think′er
free′think′ing
free′-throw′ line
free′way′
free′wheel′ing
free′will′ *adj.*

freeze *(to chill)*, froze,
  fro′zen, freez′ing
  ♦*frieze*
freeze′-dry′, -dried′,
  -dry′ing
freez′er
freight′age
freight′er
French
French′-Ca•na′di-
  an
fre•net′ic *also* fre-
  net′i•cal
fren′zied
fren′zy
Fre′on′®
fre′quence
fre′quen•cy
fre′quent *adj.*
fre•quent′ *v.*
fre•quen′ta•tive
fres′co *pl.* -coes *or*
  -cos
fresh′en
fresh′et
fresh′man
fresh′wa′ter
fret, fret′ted, fret′ting
fret′work′
Freu′di•an
fri′a•bil′i•ty
fri′a•ble
fri′ar *(monk)*
  ♦*fryer*
fric′as•see′
fric′a•tive
fric′tion

Fri′day
friend′ly
friend′ship′
frieze *(ornament)*
  ♦*freeze*
frig′ate
fright′en
fright′ful
frig′id
fri•gid′i•ty
fri•jol′ *pl.* -jo′les, *also*
  fri•jo′le
frill′y
fringe, fringed, fring′-
  ing
Fris′bee®
frisk′y
fris•son′
frit′il•lar′y
frit′ter
fri•vol′i•ty
friv′o•lous
frizz
friz′zle, -zled, -zling
friz′zy
fro
frock
frog′gy
frog′man′
frol′ic, -icked, -ick-
  ing
frol′ick•er
frol′ic•some
from
frond
front′age
fron′tal

fron•tier′
fron•tiers′man
fron′tis•piece′
front′-page′ -paged′,
  -pag′ing
front′-run′ner
frost′bite′, -bit′, -bit′-
  ten, -bit′ing
frost′ed
frost′ing
frost′y
froth′y
frown
frow′zy *also* frow′sy
fro′zen
fruc′tose′
fru′gal
fru•gal′i•ty
fruit *pl.* fruit *or* fruits
fruit•ar′i•an
fruit′cake′
fruit′ful
fru•i′tion
fruit′less
fruit′y
frump′ish
frump′y
frus′trate′, -trat′ed,
  -trat′ing
frus•tra′tion
frus′tum *pl.* -tums *or*
  -ta
fry, fried, fry′ing
fry′er *(one that fries)*,
  also fri′er
  ♦*friar*
f ′-stop′

fuch′sia
fud′dle, -dled, -dling
fud′dy-dud′dy
fudge, fudged, fudg′-
  ing
fu′el, fu′eled *or* -elled,
  -el′ing *or* -el′ling
fu′gal
fu′gi•tive
fugue
füh′rer *also* fueh′rer
ful′crum *pl.* -crums *or*
  -cra
ful•fill′ *also* ful•fil′,
  -filled′, -fill′ing
ful•fill′ment
full′back′
full′-blood′ed
full′-blown′
full′bod′ied
full′er
full′-fash′ioned
full′-fledged′
full′-length′
full′ness *also* ful′ness
full′-scale′
full′-size′ *adj., also*
  full′-sized′
full′-time′ *adj. & adv.*
ful′ly
ful′mi•nate′, -nat′ed,
  -nat′ing
ful′mi•na′tion
ful′mi•na′tor
ful′some
fum′ble, -bled, -bling
fume, fumed, fum′ing

fu′mi•gate′, -gat′ed,
  -gat′ing
fu′mi•ga′tion
fu′mi•ga′tor
fun
func′tion
func′tion•al
func′tion•al•ism
func′tion•ar′y
fund
fun′da•men′tal
fun′da•men′tal•ism
fun′da•men′tal•ist
fu′ner•al
fu′ner•ar′y
fu•ne′re•al
fun′gal
fun′gi•cide′
fun′gous (of a fungus)
fun′gus (plant), pl. -gi′
  or -gus•es
fu•nic′u•lar
funk′y
fun′nel
fun′ny
fur (pelt)
  ♦fir
fur′be•low′
fur′bish
Fu′ries
fu′ri•ous
furl
fur′long′
fur′lough
fur′nace
fur′nish
fur′nish•ings

fur′ni•ture
fur′ror′
furred
fur′ri•er
fur′ring
fur′row
fur′ry (like fur)
  ♦fury
fur′ther (more)
  ♦farther
fur′ther•ance
fur′ther•more′
fur′ther•most′
fur′thest (to the great-
  est degree)
  ♦farthest
fur′tive
fu′ry (rage)
  ♦furry
furze (shrub)
  ♦firs, furs
fuse (lighting device,
  circuit breaker)
  ♦fuze
fuse (to melt, blend)
  fused, fus′ing
  ♦fuze
fu•see′ also fu•zee′
fu′se•lage′
fu′sel oil
fus′i•ble
fu′sil•lade′
fu′sion
fuss′-budg′et
fuss′y
fus′tian
fus′ty

fu′tile
fu•til′i•ty
fu′ton
fu′ture
fu′tur•ism
fu′tur•ist
fu′tur•is′tic
fu•tu′ri•ty
fu•tu•rol′o•gy
fuze (detonator), also
  fuse
fuzz′y
fuzz′y•head′ed

G

gab, gabbed, gab′bing
gab′ar•dine′
gab′ber
gab′ble, -bled, -bling
gab′by
gab′fest′
ga′ble
gad, gad′ded, gad′ding
gad′a•bout′
gad′fly′
gadg′et
gadg′a•teer′
gadg′et•ry
gad′o•lin′i•um
Gael (Celt)
  ♦gale
Gael′ic
gaff (hook)
gaffe (error)
gag, gagged, gag′ging
ga′ga′

gage *(pledge)*
♦*gauge*
gag'gle
gag'man'
gag'ster
gai'e•ty
gai'ly
gain'ful
gain•say', -said', -say'-
ing
gait *(motion)*
♦*gate*
gai'ter
ga'la
ga•lac'tic
gal'an•tine'
gal'ax•y
gale *(wind)*
♦*Gael*
ga•le'na
Gal'i•le'an *also* Gal'-
i•lae'an
gall
gal'lant
gal'lant•ry
gall'blad'der
gal'le•on
gal'ler•i'a
gal'ler•y
gal'ley *pl.* -leys
Gal'lic
gal'li•mau'fry
gal'li•na'ceous
gall'ing
gal'li•um
gal'li•vant'
gal'lon

gal'lop
gal'lows
gall'stone'
ga•lore'
ga•losh'
ga•lumph'
gal•van'ic
gal'va•nism
gal'va•ni•za'tion
gal'va•nize', -nized',
-niz'ing
gal'va•nom'e•ter
gam'bit
gam'ble *(to bet)*,
-bled, -bling
gam'bol *(to play)*,
-boled *or* -bolled,
-bol•ing *or* -bol•ling
game, gam'er, gam'est
game, gamed, gam'ing
game'cock'
game'keep'er
games'man
games'man•ship'
gam'ete'
ga•me'to•cyte'
gam'in
gam'ma
gam'mon
gam'ut
gam'y
gan'der
gang *(group)*
♦*gangue*
gang'bus'ter
gan'gling *also* gan'gly
gan'gli•on *pl.* -gli•a

or -gli•ons
gang'plank'
gang'punch'
gan'grene'
gan'gre•nous
gang'ster
gangue *(rock), also*
gang
gang'way'
gan'net
gant'let *(track), also*
gaunt'let
gan'try
gap, gapped, gap'ping
gape, gaped, gap'ing
gar
ga•rage', -raged', -rag'-
ing
garb
gar'bage
gar'ble, -bled, -bling
gar•çon'
gar'den
gar'den•er
gar•de'nia
gar'fish' *pl.* -fish' *or*
-fish'es
gar•gan'tu•an
gar'gle, -gled, -gling
gar'goyle'
gar'ish
gar'land
gar'lic
gar'lick•y
gar'ment
gar'ner
gar'net

gar'nish
gar'nish•ee', -eed',
  -ee'ing
gar'nish•ment
gar'ni•ture
gar'ret
gar'ri•son
gar•rote', -rot'ed,
  -rot'ing, or gar•rotte'-
  , -rot'ted, -rot'ting
gar•ru'li•ty
gar'ru•lous
gar'ter
gas pl. gas'es or gas'scs
gas, gassed, gas'sing
gas'e•ous
gash
gas'ket
gas'light
gas'o•hol'
gas'o•line'
gasp
gas'ser
gas'sy
gas'tric
gas•tri'tis
gas'tro•en'ter•i'tis
gas'tro•in•tes'ti•nal
gas•tro•nom'ic also
  gas'tro•nom'i•cal
gas•tron'o•my
gas'tro•pod'
gas•trop'o•dan also
  gas•trop'o•dous
gas'tru•la pl. -las or
  -lae'
gas'works'

gate (opening)
  ♦gait
gate'crash'er
gate'fold'
gate'house'
gate'keep'er
gate'post'
gate'way'
gath'er
gath'er•ing
Gat'or•ade'®
gauche (awkward)
  ♦gouache
gau'che•rie'
gaud'y
gauge (scale)
  ♦gage
gauge (to measure),
  gauged, gaug'ing
  ♦gage
gaunt
gaunt'let (glove), also
  gant'let
gauss pl. gauss or
  gauss'es
gauze
gauz'y
gav'el
ga'vi•al
ga•votte'
gawk'y
gay
gay'ness
gaze, gazed, gaz'ing
ga•ze'bo pl. -bos or
  -boes
ga•zelle'

ga•zette'
gaz'et•teer'
gear'box
gear'ing
gear'shift'
gear'wheel'
geck'o pl. -os or -oes
gee'zer
ge•fil'te fish
Gei'ger counter
gei'sha pl. -sha or
  -shas
gel (jelly)
  ♦jell
gel'a•tin also gel'-
  a•tine
ge•lat'i•nous
ge•la'to pl. -ti
geld'ing
gel'id
Gem'i•ni'
gem'o•log'i•cal
gem•ol'o•gist
gem•ol'o•gy or gem-
  mol'o•gy
gems'bok'
gem'stone'
gen'darme'
gen'der
gene
ge'ne•a•log'i•cal
ge'ne•al'o•gist
ge'ne•al'o•gy
gen'er•al
gen'er•al•ist
gen'er•al'i•ty
gen'er•al•i•za'tion

gen'er•al•ize', -ized', -iz'ing
gen'er•al•ly
gen'er•al-pur'pose *adj.*
gen'er•al•ship'
gen'er•ate', -at'ed, -at'ing
gen'er•a'tion
gen'er•a'tive
gen'er•a'tor
ge•ner'ic
gen'er•os'i•ty
gen'er•ous
gen'e•sis *pl.* -ses'
gen•et'
ge•net'ic *also* ge•net'i•cal
ge•net'i•cist
ge•net'ics
gen'ial
ge'ni•al'i•ty
ge'nie
gen'i•tal
gen'i•ta'li•a
gen'i•tals
gen'i•tive
gen'i•tor
gen'i•to•u'ri•nar'y
gen'ius *(gifted person),* *pl.* -ius•es
  ♦*genus*
gen'o•cid'al
gen'o•cide'
Gen'o•ese' *pl.* -ese'
gen'o•type'
gen'o•typ'ic

gen're
gent
gen•teel'
gen'tian
Gen'tile
gen•til'i•ty
gen'tle
gen'tle•folk' *also* gen'tle•folks'
gen'tle•man
gen'tle•per'son
gen'tle•wom'an
gen'tri•fi•ca'tion
gen'tri•fy', -fied', -fy'ing
gen'try
gen•u•flect'
gen•u•flec'tion
gen•u•ine
ge'nus *(classification),* *pl.* gen'er•a
  ♦*genius*
ge'o•cen'tric
ge'o•chem'is•try
ge'o•chro•nol'o•gy
ge'o•code'
ge•ode'
ge'o•des'ic
ge•od'e•sy
ge'o•det'ic *also* ge'o•det'i•cal
ge•og'ra•pher
ge'o•graph'ic *also* ge'o•graph'i•cal
ge•og'ra•phy
ge'o•log'ic *also* ge'o•log'i•cal

ge•ol'o•gist
ge•ol'o•gy
ge'o•mag•net'ic
ge'o•mag'ne•tism
ge•om'e•ter
ge'o•met'ric *also* ge'o•met'ri•cal
ge•om'e•tri'cian *also* ge•om'e•ter
ge'o•met'ri•cize', -cized', -ciz'ing
ge•om'e•try
ge'o•mor'phic
ge'o•mor'pho•log'ic *also* ge'o•mor'pho•log'i•cal
ge'o•mor•phol'o•gy
ge'o•phys'i•cal
ge'o•phys'i•cist
ge'o•phys'ics
ge'o•po•lit'i•cal
ge'o•pol'i•tics
Geor•gette' crepe
Geor'gian
ge'o•tac'tic
ge'o•tax'is
ge'o•ther'mal *also* ge'o•ther'mic
ge'o•tro'pic
ge•ot'ro•pism
ge•ra'ni•um
ger'bil
ger'i•at'ric
ger'i•at'rics
germ
Ger'man
ger•mane'

Ger•man'ic
ger•ma'ni•um
ger'mi•cid'al
ger'mi•cide'
ger'mi•nal
ger'mi•nant
ger'mi•nate', -nat'ed,
  -nat'ing
ger'mi•na'tion
germ'y
ger'on•toc'ra•cy
ge•ron'to•log'i•cal
  also ge•ron'to•log'ic
ger'on•tol'o•gy
ger'ry•man'der
ger'und
ge•run'dive
ges'so
ge•stalt' pl. -stalts' or
  -stalt'en, or Ge•stalt'
Ge•sta'po
ges'tate', -tat'ed, -tat'-
  ing
ges•ta'tion
ges•tic'u•late', -lat'-
  ed, -lat'ing
ges•tic'u•la'tion
ges•tic'u•la'tor
ges'ture, -tured, -tur-
  ing
get, got, got or got'ten,
  get'ting
get'a•ble also get'ta-
  ble
get'a•way' n.
get'ter
get'-to•geth'er n.

get'-up' n.
get'-up'-and-go' n.
gew'•gaw'
gey'ser
Gha•na•ian also
  Gha'ni•an
ghast'ly
gher'kin
ghet'to pl. -tos or
  -toes
ghost'ly
ghost'write', -wrote',
  -writ'ten, -writ'ing
ghost'writ'er
ghoul'ish
GI pl. GIs or GI's
gi'ant
gi'ant•ess
gib'ber
gib'ber•ish
gib'bet, -bet•ed or
  -bet•ted, -bet•ing or
  -bet•ting
gib'bon
gib'bous
gibe (to taunt), gibed,
  gib'ing, also jibe,
  jibed, jib'ing
gib'let
gid'dy
gid'dy•ap'
gift'ed
gift'ware'
gig, gigged, gig'ging
gig'a•bit'
gig'a•byte'
gi•gan'tic

gi•gan'tism
gig'a•watt'
gig'gle, -gled, -gling
gig'ot
gigue
Gi'la monster
gild (to cover with
  gold), gild'ed or gilt,
  gild'ing
  ♦guild
gill
gil'ly•flow'er
gilt (layer of gold)
  ♦guilt
gilt'-edged' also gilt'
  -edge'
gim'bals
gim'crack'
gim'let
gim'mick
gim'mick•ry
gim'mick•y
gimp'y
gin, ginned, gin'ning
gin'ger
gin'ger•bread'
gin'ger•root'
gin'ger•snap'
ging'ham
gin•gi'val
gin'gi•vi'tis
gink'go pl. -goes, also
  ging'ko pl. -koes
gin'seng'
gi•raffe'
gird, gird'ed or girt,
  gird'ing

gird'er
gir'dle, -dled, -dling
girl'friend' *also* girl
  friend
girl'ish
girth
gis'mo *pl.* -mos, *also*
  giz'mo
gist *(essence)*
  ♦*jest*
give, gave, giv'en, giv'-
  ing
give'-and-take' *n.*
give'a•way' *n.*
give'back' *n.*
giv'en
giz'zard
gla•cé'
gla'cial
gla'cier *(ice)*
  ♦*glazier*
gla•ci•ol'o•gy
glad, glad'der, glad'-
  dest
glad'den
glade
glad'-hand' *n.*
glad'i•a'tor
glad'i•a•to'ri•al
glad'i•o'lus *pl.* -li' *or*
  -lus•es
glam'or•i•za'tion
glam'or•ize', -ized',
  -iz'ing, *also* glam'-
  our•ize'
glam'or•ous *also*
  glam'our•ous

glam'our *also* glam'or
glance, glanced, glanc'-
  ing
gland
glan'ders
glan'du•lar
glare, glared, glar'ing
glas'nost
glass'ful' *pl.* -fuls'
glass•ine'
glass'ware'
glass'work'
glass'y
glau•co'ma
glau•co'ma•tous
glaze, glazed, glaz'ing
glaz'er *(one that
  glazes)*
gla'zier *(glass worker)*
  ♦*glacier*
gleam
glean
glee'ful
glen
glib, glib'ber, glib'best
glide, glid'ed, glid'ing
glid'er
glim'mer
glimpse, glimpsed,
  glimps'ing
glint
glis•sade', -sad'ed,
  -sad'ing
glis•san'do *pl.* -dı *or*
  -dos
glis'ten
glis'ter

glitch
glit'ter
glit'te•ra'ti
gloam'ing
gloat
glob
glob'al
glo'bate' *also* glo'bat'-
  ed
globe'fish' *pl.* -fish'
  or -fish'es
globe'trot'ter
glob'u•lar
glob'ule
glob'u•lin
glock'en•spiel'
gloom'y
glo'ri•fi•ca'tion
glo'ri•fy', -fied', -fy'-
  ing
glo'ri•ous
glo'ry, -ried, -ry•ing
glos'sa•ry
gloss'y
glot'tal
glot'tis *pl.* -tis•es *or*
  -ti•des'
glove, gloved, glov'ing
glov'er
glow'er
glow'ing
glow'worm'
glox•in'i•a
glu'cose'
glue, glued, glu'ing
glum, glum'mer,
  glum'mest

glut, glut'ted, glut'ting
glu'ten
glu'te•nous *(of glu-ten)*
 ♦*glutinous*
glu'te•us *pl.* -te•i'
glu'ti•nous *(adhesive)*
 ♦*glutenous*
glut'ton
glut'ton•ous
glut'ton•y
glyc'er•in
glyc'er•ol'
gly'co•gen
gly'co•gen'ic
gly'col'
glyph
G'-man'
gnarl
gnash
gnat
gnaw *(to chew)*,
 gnawed, gnawed *or*
 gnawn, gnaw'ing
 ♦*naw*
gneiss *(rock)*
 ♦*nice*
gneiss'ic *also* gneiss'-oid', gneiss'ose'
gnoc'chi
gnome
gno'mon
gnu *(antelope)*
 ♦*knew, new*
go, went, gone, go'ing,
 goes
go *pl.* goes

go'a
goad
go'-a•head'
goal'ie
goal'keep'er
goat•ee'
goat'skin'
gob
gob'ble, -bled, -bling
gob'ble•dy•gook'
 also gob'ble•de-gook'
go'-be•tween' *n.*
gob'let
gob'lin
go'-cart'
god'child'
god'daugh'ter
god'dess
god'fa'ther
god'for•sak'en
god'head'
god'hood'
god'less
god'like'
god'moth'er
god'par'ent
god'send'
god'son'
God'speed'
go'fer *(errand runner)*
 also go'-fer
 ♦*gopher*
go'-get'ter
gog'gle, -gled, -gling
go'ing
goi'ter *also* goi'tre

gold'brick'
gold'en
gold'en•rod'
gold'-filled'
gold'finch'
gold'fish' *pl.* -fish' *or*
 -fish'es
gold'smith'
golf'er
Go•li'ath
go'nad'
gon'do•la
gon'do•lier'
gon'er
gon'fa•lon'
gong
gon'o•coc'cus *pl.* -ci'
gon'or•rhe'a
gon'or•rhe'al *also*
 gon'or•rhe'ic
goo'ber
good, bet'ter, best
good-by' *or* good-bye'
good'-for-noth'ing
good'heart'ed
good'-hu'mored
good'-look'ing
good'ly
good'-na'tured
good'ness
goods
Good Sa•mar'i•tan
good'-sized'
good'-tem'pered
good will *also* good'-will'
good'y-good'y

goo′ey
goof′y
goo′gol′
goo′gol•plex′
gook
goon
goose *pl.* geese
goose′ber′ry
goose′neck′
goose′-step′,
  -stepped′, -step′ping
go′pher *(animal)*
  ♦*gofer*
gore, gored, gor′ing
gorge, gorged, gorg′-
  ing
gor′geous
Gor′gon•zo′la
go•ril′la *(animal)*
  ♦*guerilla*
gorse
gor′y
gos′hawk′
gos′ling
gos′pel
gos′sa•mer
gos′sip
Goth′ic
gouache *(painting)*
  ♦*gauche*
Gou′da
gouge, gouged, goug′-
  ing
gou′lash
gourd
gour′mand
gour•met′

gout′y
gov′ern
gov′ern•a•ble
gov′ern•ance
gov′ern•ess
gov′ern•ment
gov′er•nor
governor general *pl.*
  governors general
gown
grab, grabbed, grab′-
  bing
grab′ber
grace, graced, grac′ing
grace′ful
Grac′es
gra′cious
grack′le
grad
gra′date′, -dat′ed,
  -dat′ing
gra•da′tion
grade, grad′ed, grad′-
  ing
gra′di•ent
grad′u•al
grad′u•al•ism
grad′u•al•ist
grad′u•ate′, -at′ed,
  -at′ing
grad′u•a′tion
graf•fi′tist
graf•fi′to *pl.* -ti
graft
gra′ham
grail *also* Grail
grain′y

gram′-at′om
gram′i•ci′din
gram′mar
gram•mar′i•an
gram•mat′i•cal
gram′-mo•lec′u•lar
  weight
gram′o•phone′
gram′pus *pl.* -pus•es
gran′a•ry
gran′dam′ *also* gran′-
  dame′
grand′aunt′
grand′child′
grand′dad′
grand′dad′dy *also*
  gran′dad′dy
grand′daugh′ter
gran•dee′
gran′deur
grand′fa′ther
gran•dil′o•quence
gran•dil′o•quent
gran′di•ose′
gran′di•os′i•ty
grand′ma′
grand′moth′er
grand′neph′ew
grand′niece′
grand′pa′
grand′par′ent
grand′sire′
grand′son′
grand′stand′
grand′un′cle
grange
gran′ite

gran'ny *or* gran'nie
gra•no'la
grant•ee'
gran'tor
gran'u•lar
gran'u•lar'i•ty
gran'u•late', -lat'ed,
-lat'ing
gran'u•la'tion
gran'ule
grape'fruit'
grape'shot'
grape'vine'
graph'eme'
graph'ic *also* graph'-
i•cal
graph'ics
graph'ite'
gra•phit'ic
grap'nel
grap'ple, -pled, -pling
grasp'ing
grass'hop'per
grass'land'
grass'roots'
grass'y
grate *(framework)*,
♦ *great*
grate *(to rub)*, grat'ed,
grat'ing
♦*great*
grat'er *(one that
grates)*
♦*greater*
grat'i•fi•ca'tion
grat'i•fy, -fied', -fy'-
ing

grat'is
grat'i•tude'
gra•tu'i•tous
gra•tu'i•ty
grave, grav'er, grav'-
est
grave, graved, grav'-
en, grav'ing
grave'dig'ger
grav'el, -eled *or*
-elled, -el•ing *or* -el-
ling
grave'side'
grave'site'
grave'stone'
grave'yard'
grav'id
gra•vim'e•ter
grav'i•met'ric *also*
grav'i•met'ri•cal
grav'i•tate', -tat'ed,
-tat'ing
grav'i•ta'tion
grav'i•ton'
grav'i•ty
gra•vure'
gra'vy
gray *also* grey
gray'beard'
gray'mail'
gray'ling *pl.* -ling *or*
-lings
graze, grazed, graz'ing
grease, greased, greas'-
ing
greas'y
great *(large)*

♦*grate*
great'-aunt'
great'coat'
great'er *(larger)*
♦*grater*
great'-grand'child'
great'-grand'daugh'-
ter
great'-grand'fa'ther
great'-grand'moth'-
er
great'-grand'par'ent
great'-grand'son'
great'heart'ed
great'-neph'ew
great'-niece'
great'-un'cle
grebe
Gre'cian
Grec'o-Ro'man
greed'y
Greek
green'back'
green'belt'
green'er•y
green'-eyed'
green'gage'
green'gro'cer
green'horn'
green'house'
green'ing
green'mail'
green'mar'ket
green'room'
greens'keep'er
green'sward'
green'way'

green'wood'
greet'ing
gre•gar'i•ous
grem'lin
gre•nade'
gren'a•dier'
gren'a•dine'
grey'hound'
grid'dle, -dled, -dling
grid'dle•cake'
grid'i'ron
grid'lock'
grief
griev'ance
grieve, grieved, griev'-
 ing
griev'ous
grif'fin *also* grif'fon,
 gryph'on
grill *(utensil)*
grille *(grating)*, *also*
 grill
grill'room'
grill'work'
grim, grim'mer, grim'-
 mest
grim'ace, -aced, -ac-
 ing
grime
grim'y
grin, grinned, grin'-
 ning
grind, ground, grind'-
 ing
grind'er
grind'stone'
grin'go *pl.* -gos

grip *(to grasp)*,
 gripped, grip'ping
gripe *(to complain)*,
 griped, grip'ing
grippe *(influenza)*,
 also grip
gris'ly *(gruesome)*
 ♦*gristly, grizzly*
grist
gris'tle
gris•tly *(fatty)*
 ♦*grisly, grizzly*
grist'mill'
grit, grit'ted, grit'ting
grits
grit'ty
griz'zle, -zled, -zling
griz'zly *(bear)*
 ♦*grisly, gristly*
groan *(to complain)*
 ♦*grown*
groats
gro'cer
gro'cer•y
grog
grog'gy
grog'ram
groin
grom'met
groom
grooms'man
groove, grooved,
 groov'ing
groov'y
grope, groped, grop'-
 ing
gros'beak'

gros'grain'
gross'ly
gro•tesque'
grot'to *pl.* -toes *or*
 -tos
grouch'y
ground'break'er
ground'break'ing
ground'less
ground'nut'
ground'out'
ground'side'
grounds'keep'er
ground'stroke'
ground'work'
group'er *pl.* -per *or*
 -pers
group'ie
group'ing
grouse *pl.* grouse
grouse, groused,
 grous'ing
grout
grove
grov'el, -eled *or*
 -elled, -el•ing *or* -el-
 ling
grow, grew, grown,
 grow'ing
growl
grown'-up'
growth
grub, grubbed, grub'-
 bing
grub'by
grub'stake'
grudge, grudged,

grud'ging
gru'el
gru'el·ing
grue'some *also* grew'-
   some
gruff 'ly
gruff 'ness
grum'ble, -bled,
   -bling
grump'y
grun'ion
grunt
Gru•yère'
gua•ca•mo'le
gua•na'co *pl.* -cos
gua'nine'
gua'no *pl.* -nos
guar'an•tee' *(to se-*
   cure), -teed', -tee'ing
   ♦*guaranty*
guar'an•tor'
guar'an•ty *(pledge)*
   ♦*guarantee*
guard'ed
guard'house'
guard'i•an
guard'rail'
guard'room'
guards'man
Gua•te•ma'lan
gua'va
gu'ber•na•to'ri•al
gudg'eon
Guern'sey *pl.* -seys
guer•ril'la *(soldier),*
   or gue•ril'la
   ♦*gorilla*

guess'work'
guest *(visitor)*
   ♦*guessed*
guest'house'
guff
guf•faw'
guid'ance
guide, guid'ed, guid'-
   ing
guide'book'
guide'line'
guide'post'
gui'don'
guild *(association)*
   ♦*gild*
guild'hall'
guile'ful
guile'less
guil'lo•tine', -tined',
   -tin'ing
guilt *(remorse)*
   ♦*gilt*
guilt'y
guimpe
guin'ea
guise *(appearance)*
   ♦*guys*
gui•tar'
gui•tar'ist
gu'lag
gulch
gulf 'weed'
gull
gul'let
gul'li•bil'i•ty
gul'li•ble
gull'wing'

gul'ly
gulp
gum, gummed, gum'-
   ming
gum ar'a•bic
gum'ball'
gum'bo *pl.* -bos
gum'boil'
gum'drop'
gum'my
gump'tion
gum'shoe'
gum'wood'
gun, gunned, gun'ning
gun'boat'
gun'cot'ton
gun'fight'
gun'fire'
gun'lock'
gun'man
gun'met'al
gun'ner
gun'ner•y
gun'ny
gun'play'
gun'pow'der
gun'run'ner
gun'shot'
gun'-shy'
gun'sling'er
gun'smith'
gun'wale *also* gun'nel
gup'py
gur'gle, -gled, -gling
gu'ru
gush'er
gush'y

gus'set

gus'ta•to'ry

gus'to *pl.* -toes

gust'y

gut, gut'ted, gut'ting

guts'y

gut'ta-per'cha

gut'ter

gut'ter•snipe'

gut'tur•al

guy

guz'zle, -zled, -zling

gym•na'si•um *pl.*
　-si•ums *or* -si•a

gym'nast'

gym•nas'tics

gym•no'sperm'

gy'ne•co•log'i•cal
　also gy'ne•co•log'ic

gy'ne•col'o•gist

gy'ne•col'o•gy

gyp, gypped, gyp'ping,
　also gip, gipped, gip'-
　ping

gyp'sum

Gyp'sy *also* Gip'sy

gy'rate', -rat'ed, -rat'-
　ing

gy•ra'tion

gy'ra'tor

gy'ra•to'ry

gyr'fal'con

gy'ro *pl.* -ros

gy'ro•com'pass

gy'ro•scope'

gy'ro•scop'ic

gy'ro•sta'bi•liz'er

H

ha'be•as cor'pus

hab'er•dash'er

hab'er•dash'er•y

hab'it

hab'i•ta•bil'i•ty

hab'it•a•ble

hab'i•tat'

hab'i•ta'tion

hab'it-form'ing

ha•bit'u•al

ha•bit'u•ate', -at'ed,
　-at'ing

ha•bit'u•a'tion

hab'i•tude'

ha•bit'u•é'

ha'ci•en'da

hack'er

hack'ie

hack'le

hack'ney *pl.* -neys

hack'neyed

hack'saw'

had'dock *pl.* -dock *or*
　-docks

Ha'des

haf'ni•um

haft

hag

hag'fish' *pl.* -fish *or*
　-fish'es

hag'gard

hag'gis

hag'gle, -gled, -gling

hag'i•og'ra•pher

hag'i•o•graph'ic
　also hag'i•o•graph'-
　i•cal

hag'i•og'ra•phy

hai'ku *pl.* -ku

hail *(precipitation,*
　shout)
　♦hale

hail'stone'

hail'storm'

hair *(threadlike*
　growth)
　♦hare

hair'breadth'

hair'brush'

hair'cloth'

hair'cut'

hair'do' *pl.* -dos'

hair'dress'er

hair'dress'ing

hair'line'

hair'pin'

hair'-rais'ing

hairs'breadth' *or*
　hair's'-breadth', *also*
　hair'breadth'

hair'split'ting

hair'spring'

hair'-trig'ger *adj.*

hair'y *(covered with*
　hair)
　♦harry

Hai'tian

hake *pl.* hake *or* hakes

ha•la'tion

hal'berd

hal'cy•on

hale *(healthy),* hal'er,
 hal'est
 ♦*(hail)*
hale *(to compel),*
 haled, hal'ing
 ♦*hail*
half *pl.* halves
half'-and-half'
half 'back'
half'-baked'
half'-breed'
half'-caste'
half 'cocked'
half 'heart'ed
half'-hour'
half'-life'
half'-line'
half'-mast'
half'-moon'
half'-slip'
half'-staff'
half'-tim'bered *also*
 half'-tim'ber
half 'tone'
half'-track'
half'-truth'
half 'way'
half'-wit'
half'-wit'ted
hal'i•but *pl.* -but *or*
 -buts
hal'ide'
hal'ite'
hal'i•to'sis
hall *(corridor)*
 ♦*haul*
hal'le•lu'jah

hall'mark'
hal•loo', -looed', -loo'-
 ing
hal'low
Hal'low•een' *also*
 Hal'low•e'en'
hal•lu'ci•nate', -nat'-
 ed, -nat'ing
hal•lu'ci•na'tion
hal•lu'ci•na•to'ry
hal•lu'cin•o•gen
hal•lu'cin•o•gen'ic
hall'way'
ha'lo *pl.* -los *or* -loes
hal'o•gen
hal'o•phyte'
hal'o•phyt'ic
hal'ter
halt'ing
halve *(to divide into
 two parts),* halved,
 halv'ing
 ♦*have*
hal'yard
ham, hammed, ham'-
 ming
ham'burg'er
ham'let
ham'mer
ham'mer•head'
ham'mock
ham'per
ham'ster
ham'string', -strung',
 -string'ing
hand'bag'
hand'ball'

hand'bill'
hand'book'
hand'breadth' *also*
 hand's'-breath' *or*
 hand's' breath'
hand'car'
hand'cart'
hand'clasp'
hand'cuff'
hand'ful' *pl.* -fuls'
hand'gun'
hand'i•cap' -capped',
 -cap'ping
hand'i•cap'per
hand'i•craft'
hand'i•work'
hand'ker•chief
han'dle, -dled, -dling
han'dle•bar'
hand'made' *(pre-
 pared by hand)*
hand'maid' *(attend-
 ant), also* hand'-
 maid'en
hand'-me-down'
hand'-off' *n.*
hand'out' *n.*
hand'-pick'
hand'rail'
hand'shake'
hand'some
 (good-looking)
 ♦*hansom*
hand'spring'
hand'stand'
hand'-to-hand' *adj.*
hand'-to-mouth' *adj.*

hand'work'
hand'writ'ing
hand'y
hand'y•man'
hang, hung or hanged,
  hang'ing'
han'gar (shed)
  ♦hanger
hang'dog'
hang'er (device for
  hanging something)
  ♦hangar
hang'er-on' pl. hang'-
  ers-on'
hang'nail'
hang'out' n.
hang'o'ver
hang'-up' n.
hank
han'ker
han'ky-pan'ky
han'som (carriage)
  ♦handsome
hap•haz'ard
hap'less
hap'loid'
hap'pen
hap'pen•ing
hap'pen•stance'
hap'py
hap'py-go-luck'y
ha'ra-ki'ri
ha•rangue',
  -rangued', -rangu'ing
ha•rass'
ha•rass'ment
har'bin•ger

har'bor
har'bor•mas'ter
hard'back'
hard'ball'
hard'-bit'ten
hard'board'
hard'-boiled'
hard'-core' adj., also
  hard'core'
hard'-edge' adj.
hard'en
hard'hat' adj.
hard'head'ed
hard'heart'ed
har•di•hood
hard'-line' adj., also
  hard'line'
hard'-lin'er
hard'ly
hard'ness
hard'pan'
hard'-shell' also
  hard'-shelled'
hard'ship'
hard'tack'
hard'top'
hard'ware'
hard'wood'
har'dy
hare (animal)
  ♦hair
hare'brained'
hare'lip'
hare'lipped'
har'em
har'i•cot'
hark

har'le•quin
har'lot
harm'ful
har•mon'ic
har•mon'i•ca
har•mon'ics
har•mo'ni•ous
har•mo'ni•um
har'mo•nize',
  -nized', -niz'ing
har'mo•ny
har'ness
harp'ist
har•poon'
harp'si•chord'
har'py
har'que•bus
har'ri•dan
har'ri•er (hawk,
  hound)
  ♦hairier
har'row
har'row•ing
har•rumph'
har'ry (to disturb),
  -ried, -ry•ing
  ♦hairy
harsh'ly
hart (deer), pl. harts or
  hart
  ♦heart
har'te•beest'
har'um-scar'um
har'vest
has'-been'
ha'sen•pfef'fer
hash

hash'ish' *also* hash'-
  eesh'
hasp
has'sle, -sled, -sling
has'sock
haste
has'ten
hast'y
hat'box'
hatch'back'
hatch'er•y
hatch'et
hatch'way'
hate, hat'ed, hat'ing
hate'ful
ha'tred
hau'berk
haugh'ty
haul *(to drag)*
  ♦*hall*
haul'age
haunch
haunt'ed
haut'boy'
hau•teur'
have, had, hav'ing,
  has
  ♦*halve*
ha'ven
have'-not' *n.*
hav'er•sack'
hav'oc
Ha•wai'ian
hawk'er
hawk'-eyed'
hawks'bill'
hawk'-weed'

haw'ser
haw'thorn'
hay *(grass)*
  ♦*hey*
hay'fork'
hay'loft'
hay'mow'
hay'rack'
hay'ride'
hay'seed'
hay'stack'
hay'wire'
haz'ard
haz'ard•ous
haze, hazed, haz'ing
ha'zel
ha'zel•nut'
haz'y
H'-bomb'
he
head'ache'
head'band'
head'board'
head'cheese'
head'dress'
head'first'
head'gear'
head'-hunt'er
head'-hunt'ing
head'ing
head'land
head'light'
head'line', -lined',
  -lin'ing
head'lin'er
head'lock'
head'long'

head'mas'ter
head'mis'tress
head'-on'
head'phone'
head'piece'
head'quar'ters
head'rest'
head'room'
head'set'
head'shot'
head'stall'
head'stand'
head'stock'
head'stone'
head'strong'
head'wait'er
head'wa'ters
head'way'
head'work'
head'y
heal *(to cure)*
  ♦*heel, he'll*
health'y
heap'ing
hear *(to listen to)*,
  heard, hear'ing
  ♦*here*
hear'ing
hear'ing-im•paired'
heark'en *also* hark'en
hear'say'
hearse
heart *(organ)*
  ♦*hart*
heart'ache'
heart'beat'
heart'break'

heart'bro'ken
heart'burn'
heart'en
heart'felt'
hearth'stone'
heart'land'
heart'less
heart'-rend'ing
hearts'ease' *also*
  heart's'-ease'
heart'sick'
heart'strings'
heart'-to-heart'
heart'wood'
heart'y
heat'er
heath
hea'then *pl.* -thens *or*
  -then
heath'er
heave, heaved *or*
  hove, heav'ing
heav'en
heav'en•ward *also*
  heav'en•wards
heav'y
heav'y-dut'y
heav'y-foot'ed
heav'y-hand'ed
heav'y-heart'ed
heav'y•set'
heav'y•weight'
He•bra'ic *also* He-
  bra'i•cal
He'brew
heck'le, -led, -ling
hec'tare'

hec'tic
hec'to•gram'
hec'to•graph'
hec'to•li'ter
hec'to•me'ter
hec'tor
hedge, hedged, hedg-
  ing
hedge'hog'
hedge'hop', -hopped',
  -hop'ping
hedge'row'
he'don•ism
he'don•ist
he'don•is'tic
hee'bie-jee'bies
heed *(attention)*
  ♦*he'd*
heed'less
hee'haw'
heel *(part of the foot,*
  a tilting)
  ♦*heal, he'll*
heft'y
he•gem'o•ny
heif'er
height'en
hei'nous
heir *(inheritor)*
  ♦*air, are (metric*
  unit), e'er, ere
heir apparent *pl.*
  heirs apparent
heir'ess
heir'loom'
heir presumptive *pl.*
  heirs presumptive

heist
hel'i•borne'
hel'i•cal
hel'i•con'
hel'i•cop'ter
he'li•o•cen'tric
he'li•o•cen•tric'i•ty
he'li•o•graph'
he'li•og'raph•er
he'li•og'raph•y
he'li•o•trope'
he'li•ot'ro•pism
hel'i•pad'
hel'i•port'
he'li•um
he'lix *pl.* he'lix•es *or*
  hel'i•ces'
hell'-bent'
hell'cat'
hel'le•bore'
Hel•len'ic
Hel'le•nism
hell'gram•mite'
hell'hole'
hel'lion
hel•lo', -loed', -lo'ing
hel•lo' *pl.* -los
helm
hel'met
helms'man
hel'ot
hel'ot•ry
help'er
help'ful
help'ing
help'less
help'mate'

help'meet'
hel'ter-skel'ter
helve
hem, hemmed, hem'-
    ming
he'-man'
hem'a•tite'
he'ma•to•log'i•cal
he'ma•tol'o•gist
he'ma•tol'o•gy
heme
hem'i•sphere'
hem'i•spher'ic *also*
    hem'i•spher'i•cal
hem'lock'
he'mo•glo'bin
he'mo•phil'i•a
he'mo•phil'i•ac'
hem'or•rhage,
    -rhaged, -rhag•ing
hem'or•rhag'ic
hem'or•rhoid'
he'mo•sta'sis *pl.* -ses
he'mo•stat'
he'mo•stat'ic
hemp
hem'stitch'
hen'bane'
hence'forth' *also*
    hence•for'ward
hench'man
hen'na
hen'peck'
hen'ry -ries *or* -rys
hep'a•rin
he•pat'i•ca
hep'a•ti'tis

Hep'ple•white'
hep'ta•gon'
hep•tag'o•nal
hep•tam'e•ter
hep•tath'lon
her
her'ald
he•ral'dic
her'ald•ry
her•ba'ceous
herb'age
herb'al
herb'al•ist
her•bar'i•um *pl.*
    -i•ums *or* -i•a
her'bi•cid'al
her'bi•cide'
her'bi•vore'
her•biv'o•rous
her'cu•le'an
Her'cu•les'
herd *(group)*
    ♦*heard*
herds'man
here *(at this place)*
    ♦*hear*
here'a•bout' *also*
    here'a•bouts'
here•af 'ter
here•by'
he•red'i•tar'i•an-
    ism
he•red'i•tar'y
he•red'i•ty
Here'ford
here•in'
here'in•af 'ter

here•of '
here•on'
her'e•sy
her'e•tic
he•ret'i•cal
here•to'
here'to•fore'
here•un'to
here'up•on'
here•with'
her'i•ta•ble
her'i•tage
her•maph'ro•dite'
her•maph'ro•dit'ic
her•met'ic *also* her-
    met'i•cal
her'mit
her'mit•age
hcr'ni•a *pl.* -ni•as *or*
    -ni•ae'
he'ro *pl.* -roes
he•ro'ic *also* he•ro'-
    i•cal
her'o•in *(narcotic)*
her'o•ine *(female
    character)*
her'o•ism
her'on
her'pes'
her•pet'ic
her'pe•tol'o•gist
her'pe•tol'o•gy
her'ring *pl.* -ring *or*
    -rings
her'ring•bone'
hers
her•self '

hertz *(unit)*
♦*hurts*
hes'i•tan•cy
hes'i•tant
hes'i•tate', -tat'ed,
-tat'ing
hes'i•tat'er
hes'i•ta'tion
het'er•o•chro'mo-
some'
het'er•o•dox'
het'er•o•dox'y
het'er•o•dyne',
-dyned', -dyn'ing
het'er•og'a•mous
het'er•o•ge•ne'i•ty
het'er•o•ge'ne•ous
also het'er•og'-
e•nous
het'er•ol'o•gous
het'er•o•mor'phic
het'er•o•nym'
het'er•o•sex'ism
het'er•o•sex'u•al
het'er•o•sex'u•al'-
i•ty
heu•ris'tic
hew *(to cut)*, hewed,
hewn *or* hewed,
hew'ing
♦*hue*
hex
hex'a•chlo'ro-
phene'
hex'a•gon'
hex•ag'o•nal
hex'a•gram'

hex'a•he'dral
hex'a•he'dron *pl.*
-drons *or* -dra
hex•am'e•ter
hex'ane'
hex'a•pod'
hey *interj.*
♦*hay*
hey'day'
hi *interj.*
♦*hie, high*
hi•a'tus *pl.* -tus•es *or*
-tus
hi•ba'chi -*chis*
hi'ber•nate', -nat'ed,
-nat'ing
hi'ber•na'tion
hi'ber•na'tor
hi•bis'cus
hic'cup, -cupped,
-cup'ping, *also* hic'-
cough
hick
hick'o•ry
hi•dal'go *pl.* -gos
hide, hid, hid'den *or*
hid, hid'ing
hide'-and-seek'
hide'a•way'
hide'bound'
hid'e•ous
hide'-out' *n.*
hie *(to hasten)*, hied,
hie'ing *or* hy'ing
♦*hi, high*
hi'er•ar'chi•cal *also*
hi'er•ar'chic

hi'er•ar•chize',
-chized', -chiz'ing
hi'er•ar'chy
hi'er•o•glyph'ic *adj.*,
also hi'er•o•glyph'-
i•cal
hi'er•o•glyph'ic *n.*,
also hi'er•o•glyph'
hi'-fi'
high *(tall)*
♦*hi, hie*
high'ball'
high'born'
high'boy'
high'bred'
high'brow'
high'chair'
high'-class'
high'er-up'
high'fa•lu'tin *or* hi'-
fa•lu'tin
high'-fi•del'i•ty *adj.*
high'fli'er
high'-flown'
high'-grade' *adj.*
high'hand'ed
high'-hat', -hat'ted,
-hat'ting
high jinks *also* hi'-
jinks'
high'land
high'land•er
high'light', -light'ed,
-light'ing
high'-mind'ed
high'ness
high'-oc'tane'

high′-pitched′
high′-pres′sure,
　-sured, -sur•ing
high′-rise′
high′road′
high′-school′ *adj.*
high′-sound′ing
high′-spir′it•ed
high′-strung′
high′tail′
high′-ten′sion
high′-test′
high′-toned′
high′-wa′ter mark
high′way′
high′way′man
hi′jack′
hike, hiked, hik′ing
hik′er
hi•lar′i•ous
hi•lar′i•ty
hill′bil′ly
hill′crest′
hill′ock
hill′side′
hill′top′
hilt
him *pron.*
　♦hymn
him•self′
hin′der
Hin′di
hind′most′ *also* hin′-
　der•most′
hind′quar′ter
hin′drance
hind′sight′

Hin′du
Hin′du•ism
hinge, hinged, hing′-
　ing
hint
hin′ter•land′
hip, hip′per, hip′pest
hip′bone′
hip′-hug′gers
hip′pie *also* hip′py
hip′po *pl.* -pos
Hip′po•crat′ic oath
hip′po•drome′
hip′po•pot′a•mus
　pl. -mus•es *or* -mi′
hip′ster•ism
hire, hired, hir′ing
hire′ling
hir′sute′
his
His•pan′ic
His′pa•nism
His′pa•nist
His•pa′no *pl.* -nos
His•pa′no-
hiss
his′ta•mine′
his′ta•min′ic
his′to•log′i•cal
his•tol′o•gist
his•tol′o•gy
his•tol′y•sis
his′to•lyt′ic
his•to′ri•an
his•tor′ic *(famous)*
his•tor′i•cal *(con-
　cerned with history)*

his•tor′i•cize′,
　-cized′, -ciz′ing
his′to•ried
his•to′ri•og′ra•pher
his•to′ri•og′ra•phy
his′to•ry
his′tri•on′ic *also* his′-
　tri•on′i•cal
his′tri•on′ics
hit, hit, hit′ting
hit′-and-run′
hitch′hike′, -hiked′,
　-hik′ing
hitch′hik′er
hith′er
hith′er•to′
hit′-or-miss′ *adj.*
hit′ter
hive, hived, hiv′ing
hives
ho *interj.*
　♦hoe
hoa′gie
hoar
hoard *(cache)*
　♦horde
hoar′frost′
hoarse *(grating),*
　hoars′er, hoars′est
　♦horse
hoar′y
hoax
hob′ble, -bled, -bling
hob′by
hob′by•horse′
hob′by•ist
hob′gob′lin

hob′nail′

hob′nob′, -nobbed′,
  -nob′bing

ho′bo *pl.* -boes *or* -bos

hock

hock′ey

ho′cus-po′cus

hod

hodge′podge′

hoe *(to weed),* hoed,
  hoe′ing
  ♦*ho*

hoe′cake′

hoc′-down′

hog, hogged, hog′ging

hog′back′

hogs′head′

hog′-tie′, -tied′, -ty′-
  ing *or* -tie′ing, *also*
  hog′tie′

hog′wash′

hoist′er

hoi′ty-toi′ty

ho′kum

hold, held, hold′ing

hold′er

hold′out′ *n.*

hold′o′ver *n.*

hold′up′ *n.*

hole *(cavity)*
  ♦*whole*

hole *(to puncture),*
  holed, hol′ing
  ♦*whole*

hole′y *(having holes)*
  ♦*holy, wholly*

hol′i•day′

ho′li•er-than-thou′
  adj.

ho′li•ness

ho′lism

ho•lis′tic

hol′lan•daise′ sauce

Hol′land•er

hol′ler

hol′low

hol′ly

hol′ly•hock′

Hol′ly•wood′

hol′mi•um

hol′o•caust′

Hol′o•cene′

hol′o•gram′

hol′o•graph′

hol′o•graph′ic *also*
  hol′o•graph′i•cal

ho•log′ra•phy

Hol′stein

hol′ster

ho′ly *(sacred)*
  ♦*wholly*

ho′ly•stone′

hom′age

hom′bre

Hom′burg *also* hom′-
  burg′

home, homed, hom′-
  ing

home′bod′y

home′bred′

home′-brew′

home′build′er

home′buy′er

home′com′ing

home′land′

home′ly

home′made′

home′mak′er

ho′me•o•path′ *also*
  ho′me•op′a•thist

ho′me•o•path′ic

ho′me•op′a•thy

ho′me•o•sta′sis

ho′me•o•stat′ic

home′own′er

hom′er

Ho•mer′ic

home′room′

home′sick′

home′spun′

home′stead′

home′stretch′

home′ward *also*
  home′wards

home′work′

home′y, hom′i•er,
  hom′i•est, *also*
  hom′y

hom′i•cid′al

hom′i•cide′

hom′i•let′ic *also*
  hom′i•let′i•cal

hom′i•ly

hom′ing pigeon

hom′i•nid′

hom′i•noid′

hom′i•ny

ho′mo•ge•ne′i•ty

ho′mo•ge′ne•ous

ho•mog′en•i•za′-
  tion

ho•mog'en•ize',
-ized', -iz'ing
ho•mog'en•iz'er
hom'o•graph'
ho•mol'o•gous
hom'o•logue' *also*
hom'o•log'
ho•mol'o•gy
hom'o•nym'
hom'o•nym'ic
ho•mon'y•mous
hom'o•phone'
hom'o•phon'ic
ho•moph'o•ny
ho•mop'ter•ous
Ho'mo sa'pi•ens'
ho'mo•sex'u•al
ho'mo•sex'u•al'i•ty
ho•mun'cu•lus
hon'cho *pl.* -chos
hon'cho, -choed,
-cho•ing
Hon•du'ran
hone, honed, hon'ing
hon'est
hon'es•ty
hon'ey *pl.* -eys
hon'ey•bee'
hon'ey•comb'
hon'ey•dew'
hon'eyed
hon'ey•moon'
hon'ey•suck'le
honk'er
hon'ky-tonk'
hon'or
hon'or•a•ble

hon'o•rar'i•um *pl.*
-i•ums *or* -i•a
hon'or•ar'y
hon'or•if'ic
hood'ed
hood'lum
hood'wink'
hoo'ey
hoof *pl.* hooves *or*
hoofs
hoo'kah
hook'-and-lad'der
truck
hook'up' *n.*
hook'worm'
hook'y
hoo'li•gan
hoop *(circle)*
♦*whoop*
hoop'la'
hoo'poe
hoose'gow'
Hoo'sier
hoot
hoot'en•an'ny
hop, hopped, hop'ping
hope, hoped, hop'ing
hope'ful
hope'less•ness
hop'per
hop'sack'ing
hop'scotch'
horde *(throng)*
♦*hoard*
hore'hound'
ho•ri'zon
hor'i•zon'tal

hor•mon'al *also* hor-
mon'ic
hor'mone'
horn'bill'
horn'blende'
horn'book'
horned
hor'net
horn'pipe'
hor'o•loge'
hor'o•log'ic *also* hor'-
o•log'i•cal
ho•rol'o•gy
hor'o•scope'
ho•ros'co•py
hor•ren'dous
hor'ri•ble
hor'rid
hor•rif'ic
hor'ri•fy', -fied', -fy'-
ing
hor'ror
hors d'oeuvre' *pl.*
hors d'oeuvres' *or*
hors d'oeuvre'
horse *(animal)*
♦*hoarse*
horse *(to play rough-
ly)*, horsed, hors'ing
♦*hoarse*
horse'back'
horse'car'
horse'feath'ers
horse'flesh'
horse'fly'
horse'hair'
horse'hide'

horse'laugh'
horse'man
horse'man•ship'
horse'play'
horse'pow'er
horse'rad'ish
horse'shoe'
horse'tail'
horse'whip',
  -whipped', -whip'-
  ping
horse'wom'an
hors'y *also* hors'ey
hor'ta•tive
hor'ta•to'ry
hor'ti•cul'tur•al
hor'ti•cul'ture
hor'ti•cul'tur•ist
ho•san'na
hose *pl.* hose *or* hos'es
hose, hosed, hos'ing
ho'sier•y
hos'pice
hos'pi•ta•ble
hos'pi•tal
hos'pi•tal'i•ty
hos'pi•tal•i•za'tion
hos'pi•tal•ize',
  -ized', -iz'ing
host
hos'tage
hos'tel *(lodging)*
  ♦*hostile*
host'ess
hos'tile *(antagonistic)*
  ♦*hostel*
hos•til'i•ty

hos'tler
hot, hot'ter, hot'test
hot'bed'
hot'-blood'ed
hotch'potch'
hot'-dog', -dogged',
  -dog'ging
ho•tel'
ho'te•lier'
hot'foot' *pl.* -foots'
hot'head'ed
hot'house'
hot'shot'
hound
hound's'-tooth'
  check
hour *(time)*
  ♦*our*
hour'glass'
hour'long'
hour'ly
house, housed, hous'-
  ing
house'boat'
house'break'ing
house'bro'ken
house'coat'
house'dress'
house'fly'
house'guest'
house'hold'
house'hus'band
house'keep'er
house'maid'
house'moth'er
house'paint'er
house'plant'

house'top'
house'warm'ing
house'wife'
house'work'
hous'ing
hov'el
hov'er
Hov'er•craft'®
how'dah
how'dy
how•ev'er
how'it•zer
howl'er
howl'ing
how'so•ev'er
hoy'den
hub'bub'
hub'cap'
hu'bris
huck'le•ber'ry
huck'ster
hud'dle, -dled, -dling
hue *(color, outcry)*
  ♦*hew*
huff'y
hug, hugged, hug'ging
huge, hug'er, hug'est
hug'ger
hug'ger•mug'ger *or*
  hug'ger-mug'ger
Hu'gue•not'
hu'la
hulk'ing
hull
hul'la•ba•loo'
hum, hummed, hum'-
  ming

hu′man
hu•mane′
hu′man•ism
hu′man•ist
hu′man•is′tic
hu•man′i•tar′i•an
hu•man′i•tar′i•an•ism
hu•man′i•ty
hu′man•i•za′tion
hu′man•ize′, -ized′, -iz′ing
hu′man•kind′
hu′man•ly
hu′man•oid′
hum′ble, -bled, -bling
hum′bug′, -bugged′, -bug′ging
hum′bug′ger
hum′ding′er
hum′drum′
hu′mer•al
hu′mer•us (bone), pl. -mer•i′
♦humorous
hu′mid
hu•mid′i•fi•ca′tion
hu•mid′i•fi′er
hu•mid′i•fy′, -fied′, -fy′ing
hu•mid′i•ty
hu′mi•dor′
hu•mil′i•ate′, -at′ed, -at′ing
hu•mil′i•a′tion
hu•mil′i•ty
hum′ming•bird′

hum′mock
hu′mor
hu′mor•esque′
hu′mor•ist
hu′mor•ous (funny)
♦humerus
hump′back′
humph
hu′mus
hunch′back′
hunch′backed′
hun′dred pl. -dred or -dreds
hun′dredth
hun′dred•weight′ pl. -weight′ or -weights′
Hun′gar′i•an
hun′ger
hun′gry
hunk
hun′ker
hun′ky-do′ry
hunt′er
hunt′ing
hunts′man
hur′dle (to jump over), -dled, -dling
♦hurtle
hur′dy-gur′dy
hurl′er
hur′ly-bur′ly
hur•rah′ also hoo-ray′, hur•ray′
hur′ri•cane′
hur′ry, -ried, -ry•ing
hurt, hurt, hurt′ing
hur′tle (to throw),

-tled, -tling
♦hurdle
hus′band
hus′band•ry
hush′-hush′
hush′pup′py
husk′er
husk′y (hoarse, burly)
hus′ky (dog)
hus•sar′
hus′sy
hus′tle, -tled, -tling
hut
hutch
hy′a•cinth
hy′a•line
hy′a•lite′
hy′brid
hy′brid•ism
hy′brid•i•za′tion
hy′brid•ize′, -ized′, -iz′ing
hy•dran′ge•a
hy′drant
hy′drate′, -drat′ed, -drat′ing
hy•dra′tion
hy′dra•tor
hy•drau′lic
hy•drau′lics
hy′dra•zine′
hy′dride′
hy′dro•car′bon
hy′dro•ce•phal′ic
hy′dro•ceph′a•lus
hy′dro•chlo′ric acid
hy′dro•cor′ti•sone′

hy′dro•dy•nam′ic
hy′dro•dy•nam′ics
hy′dro•e•lec′tric
hy′dro•e•lec•tric′-
i•ty
hy′dro•flu•or′ic
acid
hy′dro•foil′
hy′dro•gen
hy′dro•gen•ate′, -at′-
ed, -at′ing
hy′dro•gen•a′tion
hy•drog′e•nous
hy•drog′ra•pher
hy•drog′ra•phy
hy′dro•log′ic
hy•drol′o•gist
hy•drol′o•gy
hy•drol′y•sis
hy′dro•lyt′ic
hy′dro•lyze′, -lyzed′,
-lyz′ing
hy•drom′e•ter
hy′dro•pho′bi•a
hy′dro•plane′
hy′dro•pon′ics
hy′dro•pow′er
hy′dro•sphere′
hy′dro•stat′ic *also*
hy′dro•stat′i•cal
hy′dro•stat′ics
hy′dro•ther′a•py
hy•drot′ro•pism
hy′drous
hy•drox′ide′
hy•drox′yl
hy•e′na *also* hy•ae′na

hy′giene′
hy′gi•en′ic
hy•gien′ist
hy′grom′e•ter
hy′gro•met′ric
hy•grom′e•try
hy′gro•scope′
hy′gro•scop′ic
hy′men
hy•me•ne′al
hymn *(song)*
♦him
hym′nal
hym′no•dy
hy′oid′
hype, hyped, hyp′ing
hy′per•ac′id
hy′per•ac•id′i•ty
hy′per•ac′tive
hy•per′bo•la *(curve)*
hy•per′bo•le *(exag-
geration)*
hy′per•bol′ic
hy′per•bo′re•an
hy′per•crit′i•cal
(overcritical)
♦hypocritical
hy′per•gly•ce′mi•a
hy′per•o′pi•a
hy′per•re′al•ism
hy′per•sen′si•tive
hy′per•son′ic
hy′per•ten′sion
hy′per•text′
hy′per•thy′roid
hy′per•thy′roid•ism
hy′per•ven′ti•la′-

tion
hy′phen
hy′phen•ate′, -at′ed,
-at′ing
hy′phen•a′tion
hyp•no′sis *pl.* -ses′
hyp•no•ther′a•py
hyp•not′ic
hyp′no•tism
hyp′no•tist
hyp′no•tize′, -tized′,
-tiz′ing
hy′po *pl.* -pos
hy′po•chon′dri•a
hy′po•chon′dri•ac′
hy•poc′ri•sy
hyp′o•crite′
hyp′o•crit′i•cal *(in-
sincere)*
♦hypercritical
hy′po•der′mic
hy′po•der′mis *also*
hy′po•derm′
hy′po•gly•ce′mi•a
hy′pot′e•nuse′
hy′po•thal′a•mus
hy•poth′e•cate′,
-cat′ed, -cat′ing
hy•poth′e•sis *pl.*
-ses′
hy•poth′e•size′,
-sized′, -siz′ing
hy′po•thet′i•cal *also*
hy′po•thet′ic
hy′po•thy′roid•ism
hy′rax′ *pl.* -rax′es *or*
-ra•ces

hys'sop
hys'ter•ec'to•my
hys'ter•e'sis *pl.* -ses'
hys•ter'i•a
hys•ter'ic
hys•ter'i•cal
hys•ter'ics

I

i'amb'
i•am'bic
i'bex'
i'bis
ice, iced, ic'ing
ice'berg'
ice'boat'
ice'bound'
ice'box'
ice'break•er'
ice'-cream' cone
Ice'land•er
Ice•land'ic
ice'mak'er
ice'man'
ice'scape'
ice'-skate', -skat'ed,
   -skat'ing
ich•neu'mon
ich'thy•o•log'ic *also*
   ich'thy•o•log'i•cal
ich'thy•ol'o•gist
ich'thy•ol'o•gy
ich'thy•o•saur' *also*
   ich'thy•o•sau'rus *pl.*
   -sau'ri'
i'ci•cle

ic'ing
i'con *also* i'kon
i•con'o•clasm
i•con'o•clast'
i•con'o•clas'tic
ic'y
id
i•de'a
i•de'al
i•de'al•ism
i•de'al•ist
i•de'al•is'tic
i•de'al•i•za'tion
i•de'al•ize', -ized',
   -iz'ing
i•de•ate', -at'ed, -at'-
   ing
i'de•a'tion
i•dée fixe' *pl.* i•dées
   fixes'
i•den'ti•cal
i•den'ti•fi'a•ble
i•den'ti•fi•ca'tion
i•den'ti•fy', -fied',
   -fy'ing
i•den'ti•ty
id'e•o•gram' *also* id'-
   e•o•graph'
i'de•o•log'i•cal
i'de•ol'o•gy
ides
id' est'
id'i•o•cy
id'i•om
id'i•o•mat'ic
id'i•o•syn'cra•sy
id'i•o•syn•crat'ic

id'i•ot
id'i•ot'ic
i'dle *(to move lazily)*,
   i'dled, i'dling
   ♦*idol, idyll*
i'dol *(image)*
   ♦*idle, idyll*
i•dol'a•ter
i•dol'a•trous
i•dol'a•try
i'dol•ize', -ized', -iz'-
   ing
i'dyll *(poem)*, *also*
   i'dyl
   ♦*idle, idol*
i•dyl'lic
if
ig'loo *pl.* -loos
ig'ne•ous
ig•nite', -nit'ed, -nit'-
   ing
ig•ni'tion
ig•no'ble
ig'no•min'i•ous
ig'no•min'y
ig'no•ra'mus
ig'no•rance
ig'no•rant
ig•nore', -nored',
   -nor'ing
i•gua'na
il'e•ac'
il'e•al
il'e•i'tis
il'e•um *(intestine)*, *pl.*
   -e•a
   ♦*ilium*

Il'i•ad
il'i•um *(bone), pl.* -i•a
  ♦*ileum*
ilk
ill, worse, worst
ill'-ad•vised'
ill'-bred'
il•le'gal
il•le•gal'i•ty
il•leg'i•bil'i•ty
il•leg'i•ble
il'le•git'i•ma•cy
il'le•git'i•mate
ill'-fat'ed
ill'-fa'vored
ill'-got'ten
ill'-hu'mored
il•lib'er•al
il•lic'it *(unlawful)*
  ♦*elicit*
il•lim'it•a•ble
Il'li•nois'an
il•liq'uid
il•lit'er•a•cy
il•lit'er•ate
ill'-man'nered
ill'-na'tured
ill'ness
il•log'i•cal
ill'-o'mened
ill'-starred'
ill'-tem'pered
ill'-timed'
ill'-treat'
il•lu'mi•nate', -nat'-
  ed, -nat'ing
il•lu'mi•na'tion

il•lu'mi•na'tor
il•lu'mine, -mined,
  -min•ing
ill'-use' *n., also* ill'-us'-
  age
ill'-use', -used', -us'-
  ing
il•lu'sion *(misconcep-
  tion)*
  ♦*allusion*
il•lu'sion•ist
il•lu'sive *(deceptive)*
  ♦*allusive, elusive*
il•lu'so•ry
il'lus•trate', -trat'ed,
  -trat'ing
il'lus•tra'tion
il•lus'tra•tive
il'lus•tra'tor
il•lus'tri•ous
il'ly
im'age, -aged, -ag•ing
im'age•ry
i•mag'i•na•ble
i•mag'i•nar'y
i•mag'i•na'tion
i•mag'i•na•tive
i•mag'ine, -ined, -in•
  ing
i•ma'go *pl.* -goes *or*
  -gi•nes
im•bal'ance
im'be•cile
im'be•cil'i•ty
im•bibe', -bibed',
  -bib'ing
im•bro'glio *pl.* -glios

im•brue', -brued',
  -bru'ing
im•bue', -bued', -bu'-
  ing
im'i•tate', -tat'ed,
  -tat'ing
im'i•ta'tion
im'i•ta'tive
im'i•ta'tor
im•mac'u•late
im'ma•nent *(within)*
  ♦*eminent, imminent*
im•ma•te'ri•al
im'ma•ture'
im'ma•tur'i•ty
im•meas'ur•a•ble
im•me'di•a•cy
im•me'di•ate
im•me•mo'ri•al
im•mense'
im•men'si•ty
im•merse', -mersed',
  -mers'ing
im•mer'sion
im'mi•grant
im'mi•grate', -grat'-
  ed, -grat'ing
im'mi•gra'tion
im'mi•nence
im'mi•nent *(impend-
  ing)*
  ♦*eminent, immanent*
im•mo'bile
im'mo•bil'i•ty
im•mo'bi•li•za'tion
im•mo'bi•lize',
  -lized', -liz'ing

im•mod′er•ate
im•mod′er•a′tion
im•mod′est
im•mod′es•ty
im′mo•late′, -lat′ed,
  -lat′ing
im′mo•la′tion
im′mo•la′tor
im•mor′al
im′mor•al′i•ty
im•mor′tal
im′mor•tal′i•ty
im•mor′tal•ize′,
  -ized′, -iz′ing
im•mov′a•bil′i•ty
im•mov′a•ble
im•mune′
im•mu′ni•ty
im′mu•ni•za′tion
im′mu•nize′, -nized′,
  -niz′ing
im′mu•nol′o•gist
im′mu•nol′o•gy
im•mure′, -mured′,
  -mur′ing
im•mu′ta•bil′i•ty
im•mu′ta•ble
imp
im′pact′ n.
im•pact′ v.
im•pact′ed
im•pac′tion
im•pair′
im•pair′ment
im•pa′la
im•pale′, -paled′,
  -pal′ing

im•pal′pa•ble
im•pan′el, -eled or
  -elled, -el•ing or -el-
  ling
im•part′
im•par′tial
im•par′ti•al′i•ty
im•pass′a•ble (im-
  possible to cross)
♦impassible
im′passe
im•pas′si•ble (un-
  feeling)
♦impassable
im•pas′sioned
im•pas′sive
im′pas•siv′i•ty
im•pa′tience
im•pa′tient
im•peach′
im•peach′ment
im•peach′a•ble
im•pec′ca•bil′i•ty
im•pec′ca•ble
im′pe•cu′ni•ous
im•pe′dance
im•pede′, -ped′ed,
  -ped′ing
im•ped′i•ment
im•ped′i•men′ta
im•pel′, -pelled′, -pel′-
  ling
im•pend′ing
im•pen′e•tra•bil′-
  i•ty
im•pen′e•tra•ble
im•pen′i•tence

im•pen′i•tent
im•per′a•tive
im′per•cep′ti•bil′-
  i•ty
im′per•cep′ti•ble
im′per•cep′tive
im•per′fect
im•per•fec′tion
im′per•fec′tive
im•per′fo•rate
im•pe′ri•al
im•pe′ri•al•ism
im•pe′ri•al•ist
im•pe′ri•al•is′tic
im•per′il, -iled or
  -illed, -il•ing or -il-
  ling
im•pe′ri•ous
im•per′ish•a•bil′-
  i•ty
im•per′ish•a•ble
im•per′ma•nence
im•per′ma•nent
im•per′me•a•ble
im•per′son•al
im•per′son•al′i•ty
im•per′son•ate′, -at′-
  ed, -at′ing
im•per′son•a′tion
im•per′son•a′tor
im•per′ti•nence
im•per′ti•nent
im′per•turb′a•bil′-
  i•ty
im′per•turb′a•ble
im•per′vi•ous
im′pe•ti′go

im·pet'u·os'i·ty
im·pet'u·ous
im·pe'tus *pl.* -tus·es
im·pi'e·ty
im·pinge', -pinged',
-ping'ing
im·pi'ous
imp'ish
im·pla'ca·bil'i·ty
im·pla'ca·ble
im·plant' *n.*
im·plant' *v.*
im·plan·ta'tion
im·plau'si·bil'i·ty
im·plau'si·ble
im'ple·ment
im'ple·men·ta'tion
im'pli·cate', -cat'ed,
-cat'ing
im'pli·ca'tion
im·plic'it
im·plied'
im·plode', -plod'ed,
-plod'ing
im·plore', -plored',
-plor'ing
im·plo'sion
im·plo'sive
im·ply', -plied', -ply'-
ing
im'po·lite'
im·pol'i·tic
im·pon'der·a·ble
im'port' *n.*
im·port' *v.*
im·por'tance
im·por'tant

im'por·ta'tion
im·port'er
im·por'tu·nate
im'por·tune',
-tuned', -tun'ing
im'por·tu'ni·ty
im·pose', -posed',
-pos'ing
im'po·si'tion
im·pos'si·bil'i·ty
im·pos'si·ble
im'post'
im·pos'tor
im·pos'ture
im'po·tence
im'po·tent
im·pound'
im·pov'er·ish
im·prac'ti·ca·bil'-
i·ty
im·prac'ti·ca·ble
im·prac'ti·cal
im'pre·cate', -cat'ed,
-cat'ing
im'pre·ca'tion
im'pre·ca'tor
im'pre·ca·to'ry
im'pre·cise'
im'pre·ci'sion
im·preg'na·ble
im·preg'nate', -nat'-
ed, -nat'ing
im'preg·na'tion
im'preg·na'tor
im'pre·sa'ri·o' *pl.*
-os'
im·press' *n.*

im·press' *v.*
im·pres'sion
im·pres'sion·a·bil'-
i·ty
im·pres'sion·a·ble
im·pres'sion·ism
im·pres'sion·ist
im·pres'sion·ist'ic
im·pres'sive
im'pri·ma'tur'
im'print' *n.*
im·print' *v.*
im·pris'on
im·pris'on·ment
im·prob'a·bil'i·ty
im·prob'a·ble
im·promp'tu
im·prop'er
im'pro·pri'e·ty
im·prove', -proved',
-prov'ing
im·prove'ment
im·prov'i·dence
im·prov'i·dent
im·prov'i·sa'tion
im'pro·vise', -vised',
-vis'ing
im·pru'dence
im·pru'dent
im'pu·dence
im'pu·dent
im·pugn'
im'pulse'
im·pul'sion
im·pul'sive
im·pu'ni·ty
im·pure'

im•pu′ri•ty
im•put′a•ble
im′pu•ta′tion
im•pute′, -put′ed,
    -put′ing
in *(within)*
    ♦*inn*
in′a•bil′i•ty
in′ ab•sen′tia
in′ac•ces′si•ble
in•ac′cu•ra•cy
in•ac′cu•rate
in•ac′tion
in•ac′tive
in′ac•tiv′i•ty
in•ad′e•qua•cy
in•ad′e•quate
in′ad•mis′si•bil′i•ty
in′ad•mis′si•ble
in′ad•ver′tence
in′ad•ver′tent
in′ad•vis′a•bil′i•ty
in′ad•vis′a•ble
in•al′ien•a•ble
in•ane′
in•an′i•mate
in•an′i•ty
in•ap′pli•ca•bil′i•ty
in•ap′pli•ca•ble
in′ap•pre′cia•ble
in′ap•pro′pri•ate
in•arch′
in•ar•tic′u•late
in′as•much′ as
in′at•ten′tion
in′at•ten′tive
in•au′di•ble

in•au′gu•ral
in•au′gu•rate′, -rat′-
    ed, -rat′ing
in•au′gu•ra′tion
in•au′gu•ra′tor
in′aus•pi′cious
in′au•then′tic
in′-be•tween′ *adj.* &
    n.
in′board′
in′born′
in′bound′
in′breed′, -bred′,
    -breed′ing
In′ca *pl.* -ca *or* -cas
in•cal′cu•la•bil′i•ty
in•cal′cu•la•ble
In′can
in′can•des′cence
in′can•des′cent
in•can•ta′tion
in•ca′pa•bil′i•ty
in•ca′pa•ble
in′ca•pac′i•tant
in′ca•pac′i•tate′,
    -tat′ed, -tat′ing
in′ca•pac′i•ta′tion
in′ca•pac′i•ty
in•car′cer•ate′, -at′-
    ed, -at′ing
in•car′cer•a′tion
in•car′cer•a′tor
in•car′nate′, -nat′ed,
    -nat′ing
in′car•na′tion
in•cau′tious
in′cen•di•ar′y

in′cense′ *n.*
in•cense′, -censed′,
    -cens′ing
in•cen′tive
in•cep′tion
in•cep′tive
in•cer′ti•tude′
in•ces′sant
in′cest′
in•ces′tu•ous
in•cho′ate
inch′worm′
in′ci•dence
in′ci•dent
in′ci•den′tal
in•cin′er•ate′, -at′ed,
    -at′ing
in•cin′er•a′tion
in•cin′er•a′tor
in•cip′i•en•cy *also*
    in•cip′i•ence
in•cip′i•ent
in•cise′, -cised′, -cis′-
    ing
in•ci′sion
in•ci′sive
in•ci′sor
in•cite′ *(to provoke)*,
    -cit′ed, -cit′ing
    ♦*insight*
in•cite′ment
in•clem′en•cy
in•clem′ent
in′cli•na′tion
in•cline′, -clined′,
    -clin′ing
in′cli•nom′e•ter

in•clude′, -clud′ed,
-clud′ing
in•clu′sion
in•clu′sive
in′cog•ni′to
in′co•her′ence *also*
in′co•her′en•cy
in′co•her′ent
in′com•bus′ti•ble
in′come′
in′com′ing
in′com•men′su•ra-
ble
in′com•men′su•rate
in′com•mode′,
-mod′ed, -mod′ing
in′com•mo′di•ous
in′com•mu′ni•ca-
ble
in′com•mu′ni•ca′-
do
in′com•mu′ni•ca′-
tive
in•com′pa•ra•ble
in′com•pat′i•bil′-
i•ty
in′com•pat′i•ble
in•com′pe•tence
also in•com′pe•ten-
cy
in•com′pe•tent
in′com•plete′
in′com•pre•hen′si-
bil′i•ty
in′com•pre•hen′si-
ble
in•com′pre•hen′-

sion
in′com•press′i•bil′-
i•ty
in′com•press′i•ble
in′con•ceiv′a•bil′-
i•ty
in′con•ceiv′a•ble
in′con•clu′sive
in′con•gru′ent
in′con•gru′i•ty
in′con•gru′ous
in•con′se•quent
in•con′se•quen′tial
in′con•sid′er•a•ble
in′con•sid′er•ate
in′con•sis′ten•cy
in′con•sis′tent
in′con•sol′a•bil′i•ty
in′con•sol′a•ble
in•con′so•nant
in′con•spic′u•ous
in•con′stan•cy
in•con′stant
in′con•test′a•bil′-
i•ty
in′con•test′a•ble
in•con′ti•nence
in•con′ti•nent
in•con′tro•vert′-
i•bil′i•ty
in•con′tro•vert′-
i•ble
in′con•ven′ience,
-ienced, -ienc•ing
in′con•ven′ient
in′con•vert′i•bil′-
i•ty

in′con•vert′i•ble
in•cor′po•rate′, -rat′-
ed, -rat′ing
in•cor′po•ra′tion
in•cor′po•ra′tor
in′cor•po′re•al
in′cor•rect′
in′cor•ri•gi•bil′i•ty
in•cor′ri•gi•ble
in′cor•rupt′i•bil′-
i•ty
in′cor•rupt′i•ble
in•creas′a•ble
in′crease′ *n.*
in•crease′, -creased′,
-creas′ing
in•cred′i•bil′i•ty
in•cred′i•ble *(unbe-*
lievable)
♦*incredulous*
in•cre•du′li•ty
in•cred′u•lous *(skep-*
tical)
♦*incredible*
in′cre•ment
in•crim′i•nate′, -nat′-
ed, -nat′ing
in•crim′i•na′tion
in•crim′i•na′tor
in•crim′i•na•to′ry
in′cu•bate′, -bat′ed,
-bat′ing
in′cu•ba′tion
in′cu•ba′tor
in′cu•bus *pl.* -bus•es
or -bi′
in•cul′cate′, -cat′ed,

-cat'ing
in'cul•ca'tion
in•cul•ca'tor
in•cul'pa•ble
in•cul'pate', -pat'ed,
-pat'ing
in•cum'ben•cy
in•cum'bent
in'cu•nab'u•lum *pl.*
-la
in•cur', -curred', -cur'-
ring
in•cur'a•ble
in•cu'ri•ous
in•cur'sion
in'cus *pl.* in•cu'des
in•debt'ed
in•de'cen•cy
in•de'cent
in•de•ci'pher•a•bil'-
i•ty
in•de•ci'pher•a•ble
in'de•ci'sion
in'de•ci'sive
in•dec'o•rous
in•deed'
in•de•fat'i•ga•bil'-
i•ty
in•de•fat'i•ga•ble
in'de•fen'si•bil'i•ty
in'de•fen'si•ble
in'de•fin'a•ble
in•def'i•nite
in•de•his'cence
in•de•his'cent
in•del'i•bil'i•ty
in•del'i•ble

in•del'i•ca•cy
in•del'i•cate
in•dem'ni•fi•ca'-
tion
in•dem'ni•fy', -fied',
-fy'ing
in•dem'ni•ty
in'dent'
in'den•ta'tion
in•den'tion
in•den'ture, -tured,
-tur•ing
in'de•pend'ence
in'de•pend'ent
in'-depth'
in•de•scrib'a•bil'-
i•ty
in•de•scrib'a•ble
in•de•struc'ti•bil'-
i•ty
in•de•struc'ti•ble
in•de•ter'min•a•ble
in•de•ter'mi•na•cy
in•de•ter'mi•nate
in•de•ter'mi•na'-
tion
in'dex' *pl.* -dex'es or
-di•ces'
In'di•a ink
In'di•an
In'di•an'i•an
in'di•cate', -cat'ed,
-cat'ing
in'di•ca'tion
in•dic'a•tive
in'di•ca'tor
in•dict' *(to accuse)*

♦*indite*
in•dict'er *also* in-
dict'or
in•dif'fer•ence
in•dif'fer•ent
in'di•gence
in•dig'e•nous
in'di•gent
in'di•gest'i•bil'i•ty
in'di•gest'i•ble
in'di•ges'tion
in•dig'nant
in'dig•na'tion
in•dig'ni•ty
in'di•go' *pl.* -gos' or
-goes'
in'di•rect'
in'di•rec'tion
in'dis•cern'ible
in'dis•creet' *(impru-
dent)*
in'dis•crete' *(unified)*
in'dis•cre'tion
in'dis•crim'i•nate
in'dis•pen'sa•bil'-
i•ty
in'dis•pen'sa•ble
in'dis•pose', -posed',
-pos'ing
in•dis'po•si'tion
in'dis•put'a•ble
in'dis•sol'u•bil'i•ty
in'dis•sol'u•ble
in•dis'tinct'
in'dis•tin'guish-
a•bil'i•ty
in'dis•tin'guish-

a•ble
in•dite′ (to compose),
  -dit′ed, -dit′ing
  ♦indict
in′di•um
in′di•vid′u•al
in′di•vid′u•al•ism
in′di•vid′u•al•ist
in′di•vid′u•al•is′tic
in′di•vid′u•al′i•ty
in′di•vid′u•al•ize′,
  -ized′, -iz′ing
in′di•vis′i•bil′i•ty
in′di•vis′i•ble
In′do•chi′nese′ pl.
  -nese′
in•doc′tri•nate′,
  -nat′ed, -nat′ing
in•doc′tri•na′tion
In′do-Eu′ro•pe′an
in′do•lence
in′do•lent
in•dom′i•ta•ble
In′do•ne′sian
in′door′
in•doors′
in•drawn′
in•du′bi•ta•ble
in•duce′, -duced′,
  -duc′ing
in•duce′ment
in•duct′
in•duc′tance
in′duc•tee′
in•duc′tion
in•duc′tive
in•duc′tor

in•dulge′, -dulged′,
  -dulg′ing
in•dul′gence
in•dul′gent
in•dus′tri•al
in•dus′tri•al•ism
in•dus′tri•al•ist
in•dus′tri•al•i•za′-
  tion
in•dus′tri•al•ize′,
  -ized′, -iz′ing
in•dus′tri•ous
in′dus•try
in′dus•try•wide′
in•e′bri•ate′, -at′ed,
  -at′ing
in•e′bri•a′tion
in•ed′i•ble
in•ed′u•ca•ble
in•ef′fa•bil′i•ty
in•ef′fa•ble
in′ef•face′a•bil′i•ty
in′ef•face′a•ble
in′ef•fec′tive
in′ef•fec′tu•al
in′ef•fi′cien•cy
in′ef•fi′cient
in•e′gal′i•tar′i•an
in•e•las′tic
in•el′e•gance
in•el′e•gant
in•el′i•gi•bil′i•ty
in•el′i•gi•ble
in′e•luc′ta•bil′i•ty
in′e•luc′ta•ble
in•ept′
in•ep′ti•tude′

in•e•qual′i•ty
in•eq′ui•ta•ble
in•eq′ui•ty (injustice)
  ♦iniquity
in•ert′
in•er′tia
in•er′tial
in′es•cap′a•ble
in•es′ti•ma•ble
in•ev′i•ta•bil′i•ty
in•ev′i•ta•ble
in′ex•act′
in′ex•cus′a•ble
in′ex•haust′i•bil′-
  i•ty
in′ex•haust′i•ble
in•ex′o•ra•ble
in′ex•pen′sive
in′ex•pe′ri•ence
in′ex•pe′ri•enced
in•ex′pert′
in•ex′pli•ca•bil′i•ty
in•ex′pli•ca•ble
in′ex•press′i•bil′-
  i•ty
in′ex•press′i•ble
in′ex•pres′sive
in′ex•tin′guish-
  a•ble
in′ex•tri•ca•bil′i•ty
in′ex•tri•ca•ble
in•fal′li•bil′i•ty
in•fal′li•ble
in′fa•mous
in′fa•my
in′fan•cy
in′fant

in•fan'ti•cide'
in'fan•tile'
in'fan•til•ism
in'fan•try
in'fan•try•man
in•fat'u•ate', -at'ed,
  -at'ing
in•fat'u•a'tion
in•fect'
in•fec'tion
in•fec'tious
in•fec'tive
in'fe•lic'i•tous
in'fe•lic'i•ty
in•fer', -ferred', -fer'-
  ring
in•fer'a•ble
in'fer•ence
in'fer•en'tial
in•fe'ri•or
in•fe'ri•or'i•ty
in•fer'nal
in•fer'no pl. -nos
in•fer'tile
in'fer•til'i•ty
in•fest'
in'fes•ta'tion
in'fi•del'
in'fi•del'i•ty
in'field'
in'fight'ing
in'fil•trate', -trat'ed,
  -trat'ing
in'fil•tra'tion
in'fi•nite
in'fin•i•tes'i•mal
in•fin'i•tive

in•fin'i•ty
in•firm'
in•fir'ma•ry
in•fir'mi•ty
in•fix' n.
in•fix' v.
in•flame', -flamed',
  -flam'ing
in•flam'ma•ble
in'flam•ma'tion
in•flam'ma•to'ry
in•flat'a•ble
in•flate', -flat'ed,
  -flat'ing
in•fla'tion
in•fla'tion•ar'y
in•flect'
in•flec'tion
in•flec'tor
in•flex'i•bil'i•ty
in•flex'i•ble
in•flict'
in•flic'tion
in'flo•res'cence
in'flo•res'cent
in'flu•ence, -enced,
  -enc•ing
in'flu•en'tial
in'flu•en'za
in'flux'
in•form'
in•for'mal
in'for•mal'i•ty
in•for'mant
in'for•ma'tion
in•for'ma•tive
in•formed'

in•frac'tion
in'fra•hu'man
in'fra•red'
in'fra•son'ic
in'fra•struc'ture
in•fre'quence also
  in•fre'quen•cy
in•fre'quent
in•fringe', -fringed',
  -fring'ing
in•fringe'ment
in•fu'ri•ate', -at'ed,
  -at'ing
in•fuse', -fused', -fus'-
  ing
in•fus'i•ble
in•fu'sion
in•gen'ious (clever)
  ♦ingenuous
in'gé•nue'
in'ge•nu'i•ty
in•gen'u•ous (inno-
  cent)
  ♦ingenious
in•gest'
in•ges'tion
in•glo'ri•ous
in'got
in'grain'
in'grate'
in•gra'ti•ate', -at'ed
  -at'ing
in•gra'ti•a'tion
in•grat'i•tude'
in•gre'di•ent
in'gress'
in'-group'

in'grown'
in'gui•nal
in•hab'it
in•hab'it•a•bil'i•ty
in•hab'it•a•ble
in•hab'i•tan•cy
in•hab'i•tant
in•ha'lant
in'ha•la'tion
in'ha•la'tor
in•hale', -haled', -hal'-
　ing
in'har•mo'ni•ous
in•here', -hered',
　-her'ing
in•her'ence
in•her'ent
in•her'it
in•her'it•a•ble
in•her'i•tance
in•her'i•tor
in•hib'it
in'hi•bi'tion
in•hib'i•tor
in•hib'i•to'ry
in•hos'pi•ta•ble
in'-house' adj.
in•hu'man
in'hu•mane'
in'hu•man'i•ty
in•im'i•cal
in•im'i•ta•bil'i•ty
in•im'i•ta•ble
in•iq'ui•tous
in•iq'ui•ty (sin)
　♦inequity
in•i'tial, -tialed or

-tialled, -tial•ing or
　-tial•ling
in•i'ti•ate', -at'ed,
　-at'ing
in•i'ti•a'tion
in•i'ti•a•tive
in•i'ti•a'tor
in•ject'
in•jec'tant
in•jec'tion
in•jec'tor
in'ju•di'cious
in•junc'tion
in•jure, -jured, -jur-
　ing
in•ju'ri•ous
in'ju•ry
in•jus'tice
ink'blot'
ink'horn'
ink'ling
ink'stand'
ink'well'
ink'y
in'laid'
in'land
in'-law'
in'lay' n.
in•lay', -laid', -lay'ing
in'let'
in'mate'
in me'di•as' res'
in' me•mo'ri•am
in'-mi'grant
in'-mi'grate, -grat-
　ed, -grat•ing
in'-mi•gra'tion

in'most'
inn (hotel)
　♦in
in'nards
in•nate'
in'ner
in'ner-cit'y adj.
in'ner•most'
in'ner•sole'
in'ner•spring'
in•ner'vate', -vat'ed,
　-vat'ing
in'ning
inn'keep'er
in'no•cence
in'no•cent
in•noc'u•ous
in'no•vate', -vat'ed,
　-vat'ing
in'no•va'tion
in'no•va'tive
in'no•va'tor
in•nu•en'do pl. -does
in•nu'mer•a•ble
in•nu'mer•ate
in•oc'u•late', -lat'ed,
　-lat'ing
in•oc'u•la'tion
in•of•fen'sive
in•op'er•a•ble
in•op'er•a•tive
in•op'por•tune'
in•or'di•nate
in•or•gan'ic
in•pa'tient
in'put'
in'quest'

in•qui'e•tude'
in•quire', -quired',
  -quir'ing
in•quir'y
in'qui•si'tion
in•quis'i•tive
in•quis'i•tor
in•quis'i•to'ri•al
in'road'
in'rush'
in'sa•lu'bri•ous
in•sane'
in•san'i•ty
in•sa'tia•bil'i•ty
in•sa'tia•ble
in•sa'ti•ate
in'scape'
in•scribe', -scribed',
  -scrib'ing
in•scrip'tion
in•scru'ta•bil'i•ty
in•scru'ta•ble
in'seam'
in'sect'
in•sec'ti•cide'
in•sec'ti•vore'
in'sec•tiv'o•rous
in•se•cure'
in•se•cu'ri•ty
in•sem'i•nate', -nat'-
  ed, -nat'ing
in•sem'i•na'tion
in•sem'i•na'tor
in•sen'sate'
in•sen'si•bil'i•ty
in•sen'si•ble
in•sen'si•tive

in•sen'si•tiv'i•ty
in•sen'tience
in•sen'tient
in•sep'a•ra•bil'i•ty
in•sep'a•ra•ble
in•sert' v.
in'sert' n.
in•ser'tion
in•set', -set, -set'ting
in'set' n.
in'shore'
in•side'
in•sid'er
in•sid'i•ous
in'sight' (understand-
  ing)
  ♦incite
in•sig'ni•a pl. -ni•a
  or -ni•as, also in-
  sig'ne
in'sig•nif'i•cance
in'sig•nif'i•cant
in•sin•cere'
in'sin•cer'i•ty
in•sin'u•ate', -at'ed,
  -at'ing
in•sin'u•a'tion
in•sin'u•a'tor
in•sip'id
in•sist'
in•sis'tence also in-
  sis'ten•cy
in•sis'tent
in'so•bri'e•ty
in'so•far'
in'sole'
in'so•lence

in'so•lent
in•sol'u•bil'i•ty
in•sol'u•ble
in•sol'ven•cy
in•sol'vent
in•som'ni•a
in•som'ni•ac'
in'so•much'
in•sou'ci•ance
in•sou'ci•ant
in•spect'
in•spec'tion
in•spec'tor
in'spi•ra'tion
in'spi•ra'tion•al
in•spire', -spired',
  -spir'ing
in•spir'it
in•sta•bil'i•ty
in•stall' also in•stal',
  -stalled', -stall'ing
in'stal•la'tion
in•stall'ment
In'sta•mat'ic®
in'stance, -stanced,
  -stanc•ing
in'stant
in•stan•ta'ne•ous
in•stead'
in'step'
in'sti•gate', -gat'ed,
  -gat'ing
in'sti•ga'tion
in'sti•ga'tor
in•still'
in'stil•la'tion
in'stinct'

in•stinc'tive
in•stinc'tu•al
in'sti•tute', -tut'ed,
    -tut'ing
in'sti•tu'tion
in'sti•tu'tion•al-
    i•za'tion
in'sti•tu'tion•al
in'sti•tu'tion•al-
    ize', -ized', -iz'ing
in'sti•tu'tor
in•struct'
in•struc'tion
in•struc'tive
in•struc'tor
in'stru•ment
in'stru•men'tal
in'stru•men'tal•ist
in'stru•men•tal'i•ty
in'stru•men•ta'tion
in'sub•or'di•nate
in'sub•or'di•na'tion
in'sub•stan'tial
in'sub•stan'ti•al'-
    i•ty
in•suf'fer•a•ble
in'suf•fi'cien•cy
in'suf•fi'cient
in'su•lar
in'su•lar'i•ty
in'su•late', -lat'ed,
    -lat'ing
in'su•la'tion
in'su•la'tor
in'su•lin
in•sult' n.
in•sult' v.

in•su'per•a•bil'i•ty
in•su'per•a•ble
in'sup•port'a•ble
in•sur'a•ble
in•sur'ance
in•sure' *(to protect
    with insurance, guar-
    antee),* -sured', -sur'-
    ing
    ♦*assure, ensure*
in•sur'gence
in•sur'gen•cy
in•sur'gent
in'sur•mount'a•ble
in'sur•rec'tion
in'sur•rec'tion•ist
in•tact'
in•ta'glio *pl.* -glios
in'take'
in•tan'gi•bil'i•ty
in•tan'gi•ble
in'te•ger
in'te•gral
in'te•grate', -grat'ed,
    -grat'ing
in'te•gra'tion
in'te•gra'tive
in'te•gra'tor
in•teg'ri•ty
in•teg'u•ment
in'tel•lect'
in'tel•lec'tu•al
in'tel•lec'tu•al•i•za'-
    tion
in'tel•lec'tu•al•ize',
    -ized', -iz'ing
in•tel'li•gence

in•tel'li•gent
in•tel'li•gent'si•a
in•tel'li•gi•bil'i•ty
in•tel'li•gi•ble
in•tem'per•ance
in•tem'per•ate
in•tend'
in•tense'
in•ten'si•fi•ca'tion
in•ten'si•fi'er
in•ten'si•fy', -fied',
    -fy'ing
in•ten'si•ty
in•ten'sive
in•tent'
in•ten'tion
in•ten'tion•al
in•ter', -terred', -ter'-
    ring
in'ter•act'
in'ter•ac'tion
in'ter•ac'tive
in'ter•a'gen•cy
in'ter a'li•a
in'ter•breed', -bred',
    -breed'ing
in'ter'ca•lar'y
in•ter'ca•late', -lat'-
    ed, -lat'ing
in•ter'ca•la'tion
in'ter•cede', -ced'ed,
    -ced'ing
in'ter•cel'lu•lar
in'ter•cept'
in'ter•cep'tion
in'ter•cep'tive
in'ter•cep'tor *also*

in'ter•cept'er
in'ter•ces'sion
in'ter•ces'sor
in'ter•ces'so•ry
in'ter•change' *n.*
in'ter•change',
    -changed', -chang'-
    ing
in'ter•change'a•ble
in'ter•cit'y
in'ter•col•le'giate
in'ter•com'
in'ter•com•mu'ni-
    cate', -cat'ed, -cat'-
    ing
in'ter•con•nect'
in'ter•con'ti•nen'tal
in'ter•cos'tal
in'ter•course'
in'ter•cul'tur•al
in'ter•de•nom'i•na'-
    tion•al
in'ter•de'part•men'-
    tal
in'ter•de•pend'ence
in'ter•de•pend'ent
in'ter•dict'
in'ter•dic'tion
in'ter•dic'tor
in'ter•dis'ci•pli•
    nar'y
in'ter•est
in'ter•face', -faced',
    -fac'ing
in'ter•faith'
in'ter•fere', -fered',
    -fer'ing

in'ter•fer'ence
in'ter•fer'on'
in'ter•ga•lac'tic
in'ter•im
in•te'ri•or
in'ter•ject'
in'ter•jec'tion
in'ter•jec'tor
in'ter•lace', -laced',
    -lac'ing
in'ter•lard'
in'ter•leaf'
in'ter•leave',
    -leaved', -leav'ing
in'ter•line', -lined',
    -lin'ing
in'ter•lin'e•ar
in'ter•link'
in'ter•lock'
in'ter•loc'u•tor
in'ter•loc'u•to'ry
in'ter•lope', -loped',
    -lop'ing
in'ter•lude'
in'ter•lu'nar
in'ter•mar'riage
in'ter•mar'ry, -ried,
    -ry•ing
in'ter•me'di•ar'y
in'ter•me'di•ate
in•ter'ment
in'ter•mez'zo *pl.*
    -zos *or* -zi
in•ter'mi•na•ble
in'ter•min'gle, -gled,
    -gling
in'ter•mis'sion

in'ter•mit', -mit'ted,
    -mit'ting
in'ter•mit'tence
in'ter•mit'tent
in'ter•mix'
in'ter•mix'ture
in'tern' *also* in'terne'
in•ter'nal
in•ter'nal-com•bus'-
    tion engine
in•ter'nal•i•za'tion
in•ter'nal•ize',
    -ized', -iz'ing
in'ter•na'tion•al
in'ter•na'tion•al•
    ism
in'ter•na'tion•al•ist
in'ter•na'tion•al•
    i•za'tion
in'ter•na'tion•al•
    ize', -ized', -iz'ing
in'ter•nec'ine'
in'tern•ee'
in•ter'nist
in•tern'ment
in'ter•per'son•al
in'ter•plan'e•tar'y
in'ter•play'
in•ter'po•late', -lat'-
    ed, -lat'ing
in•ter'po•la'tion
in•ter'po•la'tor
in'ter•pose', -posed',
    -pos'ing
in'ter•po•si'tion
in•ter'pret
in•ter'pret•a•bil'-

i•ty
in•ter•pret•a•ble
in•ter'pre•ta'tion
in•ter'pre•ta'tive
  also in•ter'pre•tive
in•ter'pret•er
in'ter•ra'cial
in'ter•reg'nal
in'ter•reg'num *pl.*
  -nums *or* -na
in'ter•re•late', -lat'-
  ed, -lat'ing
in'ter•re•la'tion
in'ter•re•la'tion-
  ship'
in•ter'ro•gate', -gat'-
  ed, -gat'ing
in•ter'ro•ga'tion
in•ter•rog'a•tive
in•ter'ro•ga'tor
in•ter•rog'a•to'ry
in'ter•rupt'
in'ter•rupt'er *also* in'-
  ter•rup'tor
in'ter•rup'tion
in'ter•scho•las'tic
in'ter•sect'
in'ter•sec'tion
in'ter•sperse',
  -spersed', -spers'ing
in'ter•sper'sion
in'ter•state' *(between
  states)*
  ◆intrastate
in'ter•stel'lar
in•ter'stice *pl.* -sti-
  ces'

in'ter•sti'tial
in'ter•twine',
  -twined', -twin'ing
in'ter•ur'ban
in'ter•val
in'ter•vene', -vened',
  -ven'ing
in'ter•ven'tion
in'ter•ven'tion•ism
in'ter•ven'tion•ist
in'ter•view'
in'ter•weave',
  -wove', -wov'en,
  weav'ing
in•tes'ta•cy
in•tes'tate'
in•tes'ti•nal
in•tes'tine
in'ti•ma•cy
in'ti•mate *adj. & n.*
in'ti•mate', -mat'ed,
  -mat'ing
in'ti•ma'tion
in•tim'i•date', -dat'-
  ed, -dat'ing
in•tim'i•da'tion
in•tim'i•da'tor
in'to
in•tol'er•a•bil'i•ty
in•tol'er•a•ble
in•tol'er•ance
in•tol'er•ant
in'to•na'tion
in•tone', -toned',
  -ton'ing
in to'to
in•tox'i•cant

in•tox'i•cate', -cat'-
  ed, -cat'ing
in•tox'i•ca'tion
in•tox'i•ca'tor
in'tra•cel'lu•lar
in'trac•ta•bil'i•ty
in•trac'ta•ble
in'tra•mu'ral
in•tran'si•gence
in•tran'si•gent
in•tran'si•tive
in'tra•state' *(within a
  state)*
  ◆interstate
in'tra•u'ter•ine
in'tra•ve'nous
in•trep'id
in'tre•pid'i•ty
in'tri•ca•cy
in'tri•cate
in•trigue' *n.*
in•trigue', -trigued',
  -trigu'ing
in•trin'sic
in'tro•duce', -duced',
  -duc'ing
in'tro•duc'tion
in'tro•duc'to•ry
In'tro•it *also* In'tro'it
in'tro•spec'tion
in'tro•spec'tive
in'tro•ver'sion
in'tro•vert'
in•trude', -trud'ed,
  -trud'ing
in•tru'sion
in•tru'sive

in•tu'it
in'tu•i'tion
in•tu'i•tive
in'u•lin
in'un•date', -dat'ed,
　-dat'ing
in'un•da'tion
in'un•da'tor
in•ure', -ured', -ur'-
　ing, also en•ure'
in•vade', -vad'ed,
　-vad'ing
in'va•lid (ill)
in•val'id (null)
in•val'i•date', -dat'-
　ed, -dat'ing
in•val'i•da'tion
in•val'i•da'tor
in•val'u•a•ble
in•var'i•a•bil'i•ty
in•var'i•a•ble
in•var'i•ance
in•var'i•ant
in•va'sion
in•va'sive
in•vec'tive
in•veigh'
in•vei'gle, -gled,
　-gling
in•vent'
in•ven'tion
in•ven'tive
in•ven'tor
in'ven•to'ry, -ried,
　-ry•ing
in•verse'
in•ver'sion

in•vert'
in•ver'te•brate
in•vest'
in•ves'ti•gate', -gat'-
　ed, -gat'ing
in•ves'ti•ga'tion
in•ves'ti•ga'tive also
　in•ves'ti•ga•to'ry
in•ves'ti•ga'tor
in•ves'ti•ture'
in•vest'ment
in•ves'tor
in•vet'er•a•cy
in•vet'er•ate
in•vid'i•ous
in•vig'o•rate', -rat'-
　ed, -rat'ing
in•vig'o•ra'tion
in•vin'ci•bil'i•ty
in•vin'ci•ble
in•vi'o•la•bil'i•ty
in•vi'o•la•ble
in•vi'o•late
in•vis'i•bil'i•ty
in•vis'i•ble
in'vi•ta'tion
in•vite', -vit'ed, -vit'-
　ing
in'vo•ca'tion
in•voice', -voiced',
　-voic'ing
in•voke', -voked',
　-vok'ing
in•vol'un•tar'y
in'vo•lu'tion
in•volve', -volved',
　-volv'ing

in•volve'ment
in•vul'ner•a•bil'-
　i•ty
in•vul'ner•a•ble
in'ward also in'wards
in'ward•ly
i'o•dide'
i'o•dine'
i'o•dize', -dized',
　-diz'ing
i'on
i•on'ic
i'on•i•za'tion
i'on•ize', -ized', -iz'-
　ing
i•on'o•sphere'
i•o'ta
IOU pl. IOU's or
　IOUs
I'o•wan
ip'e•cac'
ip'so fac'to
I•ra'ni•an
I•raq'i pl. I•raq'i or
　I•raq'is
i•ras'ci•bil'i•ty
i•ras'ci•ble
i•rate'
ire
ir'i•des'cence
ir'i•des'cent
i•rid'i•um
i'ris pl. i'ris•es or i'ri•des'
I'rish
irk'some
i'ron

i'ron•bound'
i'ron•clad'
i•ron'ic *also* i•ron'-
  i•cal
i'ron•ing
i'ron•stone'
i'ron•ware'
i'ron•wood'
i'ron•work'
i'ron•works'
i'ro•ny
ir•ra'di•ate', -at'ed,
  -at'ing
ir•ra'di•a'tion
ir•ra'di•a'tor
ir•ra'tion•al
ir•ra'tion•al'i•ty
ir're•claim'a•ble
ir•rec'on•cil'a•ble
ir're•cov'er•a•ble
ir're•deem'a•ble
ir're•duc'i•ble
ir•ref'u•ta•bil'i•ty
ir•ref'u•ta•ble
ir•reg'u•lar
ir•reg'u•lar'i•ty
ir•rel'e•vance
ir•rel'e•vant
ir're•lig'ious
ir're•me'di•a•ble
ir're•mov'a•ble
ir•rep'a•ra•ble
ir're•place'a•ble
ir're•pres'si•bil'i•ty
ir're•pres'si•ble
ir're•proach'a•ble
ir're•sist'i•bil'i•ty

ir're•sist'i•ble
ir•res'o•lute'
ir're•spec'tive
ir're•spon'si•bil'-
  i•ty
ir're•spon'si•ble
ir•re•triev'a•ble
ir•rev'er•ence
ir•rev'er•ent
ir're•vers'i•bil'i•ty
ir're•vers'i•ble
ir•rev'o•ca•bil'i•ty
ir•rev'o•ca•ble
ir'ri•gate', -gat'ed,
  -gat'ing
ir'ri•ga'tion
ir'ri•ga'tor
ir'ri•ta•bil'i•ty
ir'ri•ta•ble
ir'ri•tant
ir'ri•tate', -tat'ed,
  -tat'ing
ir'ri•ta'tion
ir'ri•ta'tor
ir•rupt'
ir•rup'tion
ir•rup'tive
is
is'chi•um *pl.* -chi•a
i'sin•glass'
Is'lam
Is•lam'ic
is'land
isle *(island)*
  ♦*aisle, I'll*
is'let *(small island)*
  ♦*eyelet*

is'n't
i'so•bar'
i'so•bar'ic
i'so•gam'ete'
i'so•gon'ic *also* i•sog'-
  o•nal
i'so•late', -lat'ed, -lat'-
  ing
i•so•la'tion
i'so•la'tion•ism
i'so•la'tion•ist
i'so•la'tor
i'so•mer
i'so•mer'ic
i•som'er•ism
i'so•met'ric *also*
  i'so•met'ri•cal
i'so•mor'phic
i'so•mor'phism
i'so•mor'phous
i'so•oc'tane
i'so•prene'
i'so•pro'pyl alcohol
i•sos'ce•les'
i'so•therm'
i'so•ther'mal
i'so•tope'
i'so•top'ic
i'so•trop'ic
i•sot'ro•py *also*
  i•sot'ro•pism
Is•rae'li *pl.* -rael'i *or*
  -rael'is
Is'ra•el•ite'
is'su•ance
is'sue, -sued, -su•ing
isth'mi•an

isth'mus *pl.* -mus•es
  or -mi'
it
I•tal'ian
i•tal'ic
i•tal'i•ci•za'tion
i•tal'i•cize', -cized',
  -ciz'ing
itch'y
i'tem
i'tem•i•za'tion
i'tem•ize', -ized', -iz'-
  ing
it'er•ate', -at'ed, -at'-
  ing
it'er•a'tion
it'er•a'tive
i•tin'er•ant
i•tin'er•ar'y
its *pron.*
it's *contraction*
it•self'
i'vied
i'vo•ry
i'vy

J

jab, jabbed, jab'bing
jab'ber
jab•ot'
jac'a•ran'da
jack'al
jack'a•napes'
jack'ass'
jack'boot'
jack'daw'

jack'et
jack'ham'mer
jack'-in-the-box' *pl.*
  jack'-in-the-box'es
  or jacks'-in-the-box'
jack'-in-the-pul'pit
jack'knife', -knifed',
  -knif'ing
jack'-of-all'-trades'
  pl. jacks'-of-
  all'-trades'
jack'-o'-lan'tern
jack'pot'
jack'rab'bit
jack'screw'
jack'straw'
jac'quard' *also* Jac'-
  quard'
Ja•cuz'zi®
jad'ed
jade'ite'
jag, jag•ged, jag'ging
jag'uar'
jai' a•lai'
jail'bird'
jail'break'
jail'er *also* jail'or
jail'house'
ja'la•pe'ño *pl.* -ños
ja•lop'y
ja'lou•sie *(shutter)*
  ♦*jealousy*
jam *(preserves)*
  ♦*jamb*
jam *(to wedge)*,
  jammed, jam'ming
  ♦*jamb*

Ja•mai'can
jamb *(door post)*
  ♦*jam*
jam'bo•ree'
jam'-pack' *v.*
jam'-up' *n.*
jan'gle, -gled, -gling
jan'i•tor
Jan'u•ar'y
ja•pan', -panned',
  -pan'ning
Jap'a•nese' *pl.* -nese'
jape, japed, jap'ing
jap'er•y
ja•pon'i•ca
jar, jarred, jar'ring
jar'di•nière'
jar'ful' *pl.* -fuls'
jar'gon
Jarls'berg
jas'mine *also* jes'sa-
  mine
jas'per
jaun'dice
jaun'diced
jaunt
jaun'ty
Jav'a•nese' *pl.* -nese'
jave'lin
jaw'bone', -boned',
  -bon'ing
jaw'break'er
Jay'cee'
jay'hawk'er
jay'vee'
jay'walk'
jazz'y

jeal'ous
jeal'ous•y *(suspicion)*
 ♦*jalousie*
jeans
jeep
jeer
Je•ho'vah
je•june'
je•ju'num *pl.* -na
jell *(to congeal)*
 ♦*gel*
jel'lied
jel'li•fy', -fied', -fy'-
 ing
Jell'-O®
jel'ly, -lied, -ly•ing
jel'ly•bean'
jel'ly•fish' *pl.* -fish'
 or -fish'es
jen'net
jen'ny
jeop'ard•ize', -ized',
 -iz'ing
jeop'ard•y
jer'e•mi'ad
jerk
jer'kin
jerk'wa'ter
jerk'y
jer'ry•build', -built',
 -build'ing
jer'sey *pl.* -seys
Je•ru'sa•lem
 artichoke
jest *(joke)*
 ♦*gist*
Jes'u•it

jet, jet'ted, jet'ting
jet'fight'er
jet'lin'er
jet'pack'
jet'port'
jet'-pro•pelled'
jet'sam
jet'ti•son
jet'ty
jew'el, -eled *or* -elled,
 -el•ing *or* -el•ling
jew'el•ry
jew'el•weed'
Jew'ish
Jew'ry
jew's'-harp' *also*
 jews"-harp'
jez'e•bel'
jib, jibbed, jib'bing
jibe *(to shift a sail,
 agree)*, jibed, jib'ing
 ♦*gibe*
jif'fy
jig, jigged, jig'ging
jig'ger
jig'gle, -gled, -gling
jig'saw'
jilt
jim'my, -mied, -my-
 ing
jim'son•weed'
jin'gle, -gled, -gling
jin'go *pl.* -goes
jin'go•ish
jin'go•ism
jin'go•ist
jin'go•is'tic

jin'ni *pl.* jinn
jin•rik'sha *or* jin-
 rick'sha
jinx
jit'ney *pl.* -neys
jit'ter
jit'ter•bug', -bugged',
 -bug'ging
jit'ter•y
jive
job, jobbed, job'bing
job'ber
job'ber•y
job'hold'er
jock'ey
jock'ey *pl.* -eys
jock'strap'
jo•cose'
jo•cos'i•ty
joc'u•lar
joc'u•lar'i•ty
joc'und
jo•cun'di•ty
jodh'purs
jog, jogged, jog'ging
jog'ger
jog'gle, -gled, -gling
john'ny•cake'
John'ny-come'-late'
 ly
joie de vi'vre
join'er
join'er•y
joint'ed
joint'er
join'ture
joist

joke, joked, jok'ing
jok'er
joke'ster
jol'li•fi•ca'tion
jol'li•ty
jol'ly
jolt
jon'quil
Jor•da'ni•an
josh
jos'tle, -tled, -tling
jot, jot'ted, jot'ting
joule
jounce, jounced,
  jounc'ing
jour'nal
jour'nal•ese'
jour'nal•ism
jour'nal•ist
jour'nal•is'tic
jour'ney pl. -neys
jour'ney•man
joust
jo'vi•al
jo'vi•al'i•ty
jowl
jowl'y
joy'ful
joy'ous
ju'bi•lance
ju'bi•lant
ju'bi•la'tion
ju'bi•lee'
Ju•da'ic also Ju•da'-
  i•cal
Ju'da•ism
Ju'das

judge, judged, judg'-
  ing
judge advocate pl.
  judge advocates
judge'ship'
judg'ment also judge'-
  ment
judg•men'tal
ju'di•ca•ble
ju'di•ca•to'ry
ju'di•ca•ture'
ju•di'cial (of the law)
  ♦judicious
ju•di'ci•ar'y
ju•di'cious (wise)
  ♦judicial
ju'do
jug
jug'ger•naut'
jug'gle, -gled, -gling
jug'gler
jug'u•lar
juice, juiced, juic'ing
juic'er
juic'y
ju•jit'su also ju•jut'-
  su, jiu•jit'su, jiu•jut'-
  su
ju'jube'
juke box
ju'lep
Jul'ian calendar
ju'li•enne'
Ju•ly'
jum'ble, -bled, -bling
jum'bo pl. -bos

jump'er
jump'-start'
jump'y
jun'co pl. -cos
junc'tion
junc'ture
June
jun'gle
jun'ior
ju'ni•per
junk
jun'ket
jun'ket•eer'
junk'ie also junk'y
jun'ta
Ju'pi•ter
ju•rid'i•cal
ju•ris•dic'tion
ju'ris•pru'dence
ju'rist
ju'ror
ju'ry
just
jus'tice
jus'ti•fi'a•ble
jus'ti•fi•ca'tion
jus'ti•fy,' -fied', -fy'-
  ing
just'ly
jut, jut'ted, jut'ting
jute
ju've•nile'
ju've•nil'i•ty
jux'ta•pose', -posed'
  -pos'ing
jux'ta•po•si'tion

K

ka•bob'
ka•bu'ki
Kai'ser
kale
ka•lei'do•scope'
ka•lei'do•scop'ic
ka'mi•ka'ze
kan'ga•roo' *pl.* -roos'
Kan'san
ka'o•lin *also* ka'-
  o•line
ka'pok'
kap'pa
ka•put'
kar'a•kul
kar'at *(measure), also*
  car'at
  ♦*caret, carrot*
ka•ra'te
kar'ma
ka'sha
ka'ty•did'
kay'ak'
ka•zoo' *pl.* -zoos'
ke•bab' *also* ke•bob'
ked'ger•ee'
kcel'boat'
keel'haul'
keen'ly
keep, kept, keep'ing
keep'er
keep'sake'
keg
kelp

kel'vin
ken, kenned *or* kent,
  ken'ning
ken'nel
ke'no
Ken•tuck'i•an
kep'i *pl.* -is
ker'a•tin
ke•rat'i•nous
ker'chief
ker'nel *(grain)*
  ♦*colonel*
ker'o•sene' *also* ker'-
  o•sine'
kes'trel
ketch
ketch'up *also* catch'-
  up, cat'sup
ket'tle
ket'tle•drum'
key *(implement, is-
land)*
  ♦*cay, quay*
key'board'
key'hole'
key'note', -not'ed,
  -not'ing
key'pad'
key'stone'
key'stroke'
key'word' *also* key
  word
khak'i *pl.* -is
khan
kib•butz' *pl.* -but-
  zim'
kib'itz

ki'bosh'
kick'back' *n.*
kick'box'ing
kick'off' *n.*
kid, kid'ded, kid'ding
kid'com'
kid'dy *also* kid'die
kid'nap', -naped' *or*
  -napped', -nap'ing
  or -nap'ping
kid'nap'er *or* kid'nap'-
  per
kid'ney *pl.* -neys
kid'skin'
kill *(to slay)*
  ♦*kiln*
kill'deer' *pl.* -deer' *or*
  -deers'
kil'li•fish' *pl.* -fish' *or*
  -fish'es
kill'joy'
kiln *(oven)*
  ♦*kill*
ki'lo *pl.* -los
kil'o•bar'
ki'lo•bit'
ki'lo•byte'
ki'lo•cy'cle
kil'o•gram'
kil'o•gram'-me'ter
ki'lo•hertz'
kil'o•meg'a•bit
kil'o•meg'a•cy'cle
kil'o•me'ter
kil'o•met'ric
kil'o•ton'
kil'o•watt'

kil'o•watt'-hour'
kilt
kil'ter
ki•mo'no *pl.* -nos
kin
kin'der•gar'ten
kind'heart'ed
kin'dle, -dled, -dling
kin'dling
kind'ly
kind'ness
kin'dred
kin'e•mat'ics
kin'e•scope'
ki•ne'sics
kin'es•the'sia
ki•net'ic
ki•net'ics
king'bird'
king'bolt'
king'dom
king'fish'er
kin'folk' *also* kins'-
    folk', kin'folks'
king'pin'
king'-size' *also* king'-
    sized'
kink'a•jou'
kink'y
kin'ship'
kins'man
kins'wom'an
ki•osk'
kip'per
kirsch
kis'met
kiss'-and-tell'

kiss'er
kit
kitch'en
kitch'en•ette'
kitch'en•ware'
kite, kit'ed, kit'ing
kith
kitsch
kit'ten
kit'ty
kit'ty-cor'nered
ki'wi
Klans'man
Kleen'ex'®
klep•toc'ra•cy
klep'to•ma'ni•a
klep'to•ma'ni•ac'
klieg light
klutz
knack
knack'wurst' *also*
    knock'wurst'
knap'sack'
knave *(rogue)*
    ♦*nave*
knav'er•y
knav'ish
knead *(to mix)*
    ♦*need*
knee'board'
knee'cap'
knee'-deep'
knee'-high'
knee'hole'
kneel, knelt *or*
    kneeled, kneel'ing
knee'-length'

knee'pad'
knell
knick'er•bock'ers
knick'ers
knick'knack'
knife *pl.* knives
knife, knifed, knif'ing
knife'-edge'
knife'point'
knight *(soldier)*
    ♦*night*
knight'hood'
knish
knit *(to intertwine*
    yarn), knit *or* knit'-
    ted, knit'ting
    ♦*nit*
knob'by
knock'a•bout'
knock'down' *adj. &*
    n.
knock'-knee'
knock'-kneed'
knock'off' *n.*
knock'out' *n.*
knoll
knot *(to tie),* knot'ted,
    knot'ting
    ♦*not*
knot'hole'
knot'ty
know *(to perceive),*
    knew, known, know'-
    ing
    ♦*no*
know'-how'
know'-it-all'

knowl'edge
knowl'edge•a•ble
know'-noth'ing
knuck'le, -led, -ling
knuck'le•bone'
knurl
KO *pl.* KO's
KO, KO'd, KO'ing
ko•a'la
Ko'di•ak bear
kohl *(cosmetic)*
　♦*coal*
kohl•ra'bi *pl.* -bies
kook'a•bur'ra
kook'y
Ko•ran'
Ko•re'an
ko'sher
kow'tow'
kraal
krill
Kru'ger•rand'
kryp'ton'
ku'dos'
Ku' Klux' Klan'
küm'mel
kum'quat'
kung' fu'
kwash'i•or'kor
ky'mo•graph'
Kyr'i•e'

L

la'bel, -beled *or*
　-belled, -bel•ing *or*
　-bel•ling

la'bel•er *or* la'bel•ler
la'bi•al
la'bi•um *pl.* -bi•a
la'bor
lab'o•ra•to'ry
la•bo'ri•ous
la'bor•ite'
la'bor•sav'ing
Lab'ra•dor
　retriever
la•bur'num
lab'y•rinth'
lab'y•rin'thine'
lac *(resin)*
　♦*lack*
lace, laced, lac'ing
lac'er•ate', -at'ed, -at'-
　ing
lac'er•a'tion
lac'er•a'tive
lace'wing'
lach'ry•mal
lach'ry•mose'
lack *(deficiency)*
　♦*lac*
lack'a•dai'si•cal
lack'ey *pl.* -eys
lack'lus'ter
la•con'ic
lac'quer
la•crosse'
lac'ta•ry
lac'tase'
lac'tate', -tat'ed, -tat'-
　ing
lac'ta'tion
lac'te•al

lac'tic
lac•tif'er•ous
lac'to•ba•cil'lus *pl.*
　-li'
lac'tose'
la•cu'na *pl.* -nae *or*
　-nas
lac'y
lad
lad'der
lade *(to load)*, lad'ed,
　lad'en *or* lad'ed, lad'-
　ing
　♦*laid*
la'dle, -dled, -dling
la'dy
la'dy•bird'
la'dy•bug'
la'dy•fin'ger
la'dy•love'
lady in waiting *pl.*
　ladies in waiting
la'dy-kill'er
la'dy•like'
la'dy•ship'
la'dy's-slip'per
la'e•trile'
Laf 'fer curve
lag, lagged, lag'ging
la'ger
lag'gard
la•gniappe'
la•goon'
la'ic *also* la'i•cal
lair
laird
lais'sez faire'

la'i•ty
lake
lake'front'
lake'side
lam *(to thrash, escape)*, lammed, lam'ming
 ♦*lamb*
la'ma *(monk)*
 ♦*llama*
La•maze'
lamb *(young sheep)*
 ♦*lam*
lam•baste', -bast'ed, -bast'ing
lamb'da
lam'ben•cy
lam'bent
lamb'skin'
lame *(disabled)*, lam'er, lam'est
lame *(to cripple)*, lamed, lam'ing
la•mé' *(metallic fabric)*
la•mel'la *pl.* -lae' *or* -las
la•mel'late'
lam'el•la'tion
la•ment'
lam'en•ta•ble
lam'en•ta'tion
lam'i•na *pl.* -nae' *or* -nas
lam'i•nar *also* lam'i•nal
lam'i•nate', -nat'ed,

-nat'ing
lam'i•na'tion
lam'i•na'tor
lamp'black'
lamp'light'
lam•poon'
lam•poon'er *also* lam•poon'ist
lam•poon'er•y
lamp'post'
lam'prey' *pl.* -preys
lamp'shade'
la•na•i' *pl.* -is'
Lan•cas'tri•an
lance, lanced, lanc'ing
lance'let
lan'cet
lan'dau
land'fall'
land'form'
land'-grant' *adj.*
land'hold'er
land'ing
land'la'dy
land'locked'
land'lord'
land'lub'ber
land'mark'
land'own'er
land'-poor' *adj.*
land'scape', -scaped', -scap'ing
land'scap'ist
land'slide'
land'ward *also* land'wards
lane *(road)*

♦*lain*
lan'guage
lan'guid
lan'guish
lan'guor
lank'y
lan'o•lin
lan'tern
lan'tha•nide'
lan'tha•num
lan'yard
Lao *pl.* Lao *or* Laos, *also* La•o'tian
lap *(to fold)*, lapped, lap'ping
 ♦*Lapp*
la•pel'
lap'i•dar'i•an
lap'i•dar'y
lap'in
lap'is
lap'is laz'u•li
Lapp *(native of Lapland)*
 ♦*lap*
lap'per
lap'pet
lapse, lapsed, laps'ing
lap'wing'
lar'board
lar'ce•nous
lar'ce•ny
larch
lard
lar'der
large, larg'er, larg'est
large'ly

large'mouth' bass
large-scale'
lar•gess' *also* lar-
  gesse'
larg'ish
lar'go *pl.* -gos
lar'i•at
lark'spur
lar'rup
lar'va *pl.* -vae
lar'val
la•ryn'ge•al *also* la-
  ryn'gal
lar'yn•gi'tis
la•ryn'go•scope'
lar'ynx *pl.* la•ryn'ges
  or lar'ynx•es
la•sa'gna *also* la•sa'-
  gne
las•civ'i•ous
la'ser
lash'ing
lass
las'sie
las'si•tude'
las'so *pl.* -sos *or* -soes
Las'tex®
last'ing
latch'key'
latch'string'
late, lat'er, lat'est
late'com'er
la•teen'
late'ly
la'ten•cy
la'tent
lat'er•al

la'tex' *pl.* -ti•ces *or*
  -tex'es
lath *(narrow strip), pl.*
  laths
lathe *(shaping ma-*
  chine)
lathe *(to shape),*
  lathed, lath'ing
lath'er
lath'er•y *adj.*
Lat'in
La•ti'na
Lat'in-A•mer'i•can
La•ti'no *pl.* -nos
lat'i•tude'
lat'i•tu'din•al
lat'i•tu'di•nar'i•an
lat'i•tu'di•nar'i•an-
  ism
lat'ke
la•trine'
lat'ter
lat'ter-day'
Lat'ter-day' Saints
lat'tice
lat'tice•work'
Lat'vi•an
laud'a•bil'i•ty
laud'a•ble
lau'da•num
laud'a•to'ry
laugh'a•ble
laugh'ing•stock'
laugh'ter
launch'er
laun'der
laun'dress

Laun'dro•mat'®
laun'dry
laun'dry•man'
laun'dry•wom'an
lau're•ate
lau'rel
la'va
lav'a•liere'
lav'a•to'ry
lave, laved, lav'ing
lav'en•der
lav'ish
law'-a•bid'ing
law'break'er
law'ful
law'giv'er
law'less
law'mak'er
lawn
law•ren'ci•um
law'suit'
law'yer
lax'a•tive
lax'i•ty
lay *(to place),* laid, lay'-
  ing
  ♦*lei*
lay *(secular)*
  ♦*lei*
lay *(ballad)*
  ♦*lei*
lay'a•way' *n.*
lay'er
lay•ette'
lay'man
lay'off' *n.*
lay'out' *n.*

lay'o'ver *n.*

lay'-up' *n.*

laze, lazed, laz'ing

la'zy

la'zy•bones'

lea *(meadow)*
 ♦*lee*

leach *(to percolate away)*
 ♦*leech*

lead *(element)*
 ♦*led*

lead *(to guide),* led, lead'ing
 ♦*lied (song)*

lead'en

lead'er *(guide)*
 ♦*lieder*

lead'er•ship'

lead'-in' *n.*

lead'ing

lead'off' *adj. & n.*

lead'-time'

leaf *(plant part), pl.* leaves
 ♦*lief*

leaf'hop'per

leaf'let

leaf'stalk'

leaf'y

league, leagued, leagu- ing

leak *(escape)*
 ♦*leek*

leak'age

leak'y

lean *(thin)*

lien

lean *(to incline),* leaned *or* leant, lean'- ing
 ♦*lien*

lean'-to' *pl.* -tos'

leap, leaped *or* leapt, leap'ing

leap'frog', -frogged', -frog'ging

learn, learned *or* learnt, learn'ing

learn'ed *adj.*

lease, leased, leas'ing

lease'back'

lease'hold'

leash

least'wise'

lcath'er

leath'er•neck'

leath'er•work'

leath'er•y

leave, left, leav'ing

leaved *adj.*

leav'en

leave'-tak'ing

leav'ings

Leb'a•nese' *pl.* -nese'

lech'er

lech'er•ous

lech'er•y

lec'i•thin

lec'tern

lec'tor

lec'ture, -tured, -tur- ing

lec'tur•er

ledge

ledg'er

lee *(shelter)*
 ♦*lea*

leech *(blood-sucker, parasite)*
 ♦*leach*

leek *(plant)*
 ♦*leak*

leer'y

lees

lee'ward

lee'way'

left'-hand' *adj.*

left'-hand'ed

left'-hand'er

left'ish

left'ist

left'most'

left'o'ver *adj.*

left'o'vers

left'-wing' *adj.*

left'y

leg, legged, leg'ging

leg'a•cy

le'gal

le'gal•ism

le'gal•ist

le'gal•is'tic

le•gal'i•ty

le'gal•i•za'tion

le'gal•ize', -ized', -iz'- ing

leg'ate

leg'a•tee'

le•ga'tion

le•ga'to *pl.* -tos

leg'end
leg•en•dar'y
leg'end•ry
leg'er•de•main'
leg'ged
leg'ging
leg'gy
leg'horn'
leg•i•bil'i•ty
leg'i•ble
le'gion
le'gion•ar'y
le'gion•naire'
leg'is•late', -lat'ed,
   -lat'ing
leg'is•la'tion
leg'is•la'tive
leg'is•la'tor
leg'is•la'ture
le•git'
le•git'i•ma•cy
le•git'i•mate
le•git'i•mize',
   -mized', -miz'ing
leg'man'
leg'-of-mut'ton
leg'ume'
le•gu'mi•nous
leg'work'
lei (garland)
   ◆lay
lei'sure
lei'sured
lei'sure•wear'
leit'mo•tif' also leit'-
   mo•tiv'
lem'ma pl. -mas or

ma•ta
lem'ming
lem'on
lem'on•ade'
le'mur
lend, lent, lend'ing
lend'a•ble
length'en
length'way'
length'wise'
length'y
le'ni•en•cy also le'-
   ni•ence
le'ni•ent
Len'in•ist
len'i•tive
lens
lens'man
Lent'en
len'til
len'to
Le'o
le'o•nine'
leop'ard
le'o•tard'
lep'er
lep'i•dop'ter•ist
lep're•chaun'
lep'ro•sy
lep'rous
lep'ton'
les'bi•an
les'bi•an•ism
le'sion
less
les•see'
less'en (to decrease)

◆lesson
less'er (smaller)
   ◆lessor
les'son (instruction)
   ◆lessen
les'sor (landlord)
   ◆lesser
lest
let, let, let'ting
let'down' n.
le'thal
le•thal'i•ty
le•thar'gic
leth'ar•gy
let'ter
let'ter•box'
let'ter•head'
let'ter•ing
let'ter•man'
let'ter-per'fect
let'ter•press'
let'tuce
let'up' n.
leu'co•plast'
leu•ke'mi•a
leu'ko•cyte' also leu'-
   co•cyte'
le•va'tor pl. lev'a•to'-
   res
lev'ee (embankment)
   ◆levy
lev'el, -eled or -elled,
   -el•ing or -el•ling
lev'el•er also lev'el-
   ler
lev'el•head'ed
lev'er

lev′er•age, -aged,
-ag•ing

le•vi′a•than

Le′vi′s′®

lev′i•tate′, -tat′ed,
-tat′ing

lev′i•ta′tion

lev′i•ta′tor

lev′i•ty

lev′y (to tax), -ied,
-y•ing
♦*levee*

lewd′ly

lex′i•cal

lex′i•cog′ra•pher

lex′i•co•graph′ic
also lex′i•co•graph′-
i•cal

lex′i•cog′ra•phy

lex′i•con′

lex′is *pl.* -lex′es

li′a•bil′i•ty

li′a•ble (responsible)
♦*libel*

li•aise′, -aised, -ais′-
ing

li′ai•son′

li•an′a *also* li•ane′

li′ar (one who lies)
♦*lyre*

li•ba′tion

li′bel (to defame),
-beled *or* -belled,
-bel•ing *or* -bel•ling
♦*liable*

li′bel•ous

lib′er•al

lib′er•al•ism

lib′er•al′i•ty

lib′er•al•i•za′tion

lib′er•al•ize′, -ized′,
-iz′ing

lib′er•ate′, -at′ed, -at′-
ing

lib′er•a′tion

lib′er•a′tion•ist

lib′er•a′tor

lib′er•tar′i•an

lib′er•tine′

lib′er•ty

li•bid′i•nal

li•bid′i•nous

li•bi′do *pl.* -dos

Li′bra

li•brar′i•an

li′brar•y

li•bret′tist

li•bret′to *pl.* -tos *or*
-ti

Lib′y•an

li′cens•a•ble

li′cense, -censed,
-cens•ing

li′cen•see′

li′cen•sure′

li•cen′ti•ate

li•cen′tious

li′chen (plant)
♦*liken*

lic′it

lick′e•ty-split′

lick′ing

lic′o•rice

lid

lie (to recline), lay,
lain, ly′ing
♦*lye*

lie (to deceive), lied,
ly′ing
♦*lye*

lied (song), *pl.* lie′der
♦*lead (to guide)*

lief (readily)
♦*leaf*

liege

lien (claim)
♦*lean*

lieu

lieu•ten′an•cy

lieu•ten′ant

life *pl.* lives

life′blood′

life′boat′

life′guard′

life′less

life′like′

life line *also* life′line′

life′long′

life′sav′er

Life Saver®

life′-size′ *also*
life′-sized′

life′style′ *also*
life′-style′, life′ style′

life′time′

life′work′

lift′off′ *n.*

lig′a•ment

lig′a•ture

light, light′ed *or* lit,
light′ing

light'en
light'er
light'face'
light'faced'
light'-fin'gered
light'-foot'ed
light'head'ed
light'heart'ed
light'house'
light'ing
light'ness
light'ning
light'ship'
light'some
light'weight'
light'-year'
lig'ne•ous
lig'nin
lig'nite'
lig'ro•in
lik'a•ble *also* like'-
a•ble
like, liked, lik'ing
like'li•hood'
like'ly
like'-mind'ed
lik'en *(to compare)*
♦*lichen*
like'ness
like'wise
lik'ing
li'lac
Lil'li•pu'tian
lilt
lil'y
lily of the valley *pl.*
lil'ies of the valley

lil'y-white'
li'ma bean
limb *(appendage)*
♦*limn*
lim'ber
lim'bo *pl.* -bos
Lim'burg'er cheese
lime'ade'
lime'light'
lim'er•ick
lime'stone'
lim'it
lim'it•a•ble
lim'i•ta'tion
lim'it•ed
limn *(to draw)*
♦*limb*
lim'ner
li'mo•nite'
lim'ou•sine'
lim'pet
lim'pid
lim•pid'i•ty
limp'ly
lim'y
lin'age *(number of
lines)*
♦*lineage*
linch'pin'
lin'den
line, lined, lin'ing
lin'e•age *(ancestry)*
♦*linage*
lin'e•al
lin'e•a•ment
lin'e•ar
line'back'er

line'man
lin'en
lin'er
lines'man
line'-up' *n., also* line'-
up'
ling *pl.* ling *or* lings
lin'ger
lin'ge•rie'
lin'go *pl.* -goes
lin'gua fran'ca
lin'gual
lin•gui'ne *also* lin-
gui'ni
lin'guist
lin•guis'tic
lin•guis'tics
lin'i•ment
lin'ing
link'age
links *(golf course)*
♦*lynx*
lin'net
li•no'le•um
Li'no•type'®
lin'seed'
lint
lin'tel
li'on
li'on•ess
li'on•heart'ed
li'on•i•za'tion
li'on•ize', -ized', -iz'-
ing
lip
lip'ase'
lip'id *also* lip'ide'

lip'oid' *also* li•poi'dal

lip'-read', -read', -read'ing

lip'stick'

lip'synch'

liq'ue•fac'tion

liq'ue•fy', -fied', -fy'-ing

li•queur'

liq'uid

liq'ui•date', -dat'ed, -dat'ing

liq'ui•da'tion

li•quid'i•ty

liq'uor

li'ra *pl.* -re *or* -ras

lisle

lisp

lis'some

lis'ten

lis'ten•er•ship'

list'ing

list'less

lit'a•ny

li'tchi *also* li'chee, ly'-chee

li'ter

lit'er•a•cy

lit'er•al *(verbatim)*
♦*littoral*

lit'er•al•ism

lit'er•ar'y

lit'er•ate

lit'er•a'ti

lit'er•a•ture'

lithe, lith'er, lith'est

lithe'some

lith'i•um

lith'o•graph'

li•thog'ra•pher

lith'o•graph'ic *also* lith'o•graph'i•cal

li•thog'ra•phy

li•thol'o•gy

lith'o•sphere'

Lith'u•a'ni•an

lit'i•gant

lit'i•gate', -gat'ed, -gat'ing

lit'i•ga'tion

lit'i•ga'tor

li•ti'gious

lit'mus

lit'ter

lit'ter•bug'

lit'ter•mate'

lit'tle, lit'tler *or* less, lit'tlest *or* least

lit'tle•neck'

lit'to•ral *(coastal region)*
♦*literal*

li•tur'gi•cal

lit'ur•gy

liv'a•ble *also* live'-a•ble

live, lived, liv'ing

live'-in' *adj.*

live'li•hood'

live'long'

live'ly

li'ven

liv'er

liv'er•ied

liv'er•wort'

liv'er•wurst'

liv'er•y

live'stock'

liv'id

liv'ing

liz'ard

lla'ma *(animal)*
♦*lama*

lla'no *pl.* -nos

lo *interj.*
♦*low*

load *(weight)*
♦*lode*

load'ed

loaf *pl.* loaves

loaf, loafed, loaf'ing, loafs

loaf'er

loam'y

loan *(money, borrowing)*
♦*lone*

loan'-word' *also* loan'word'

loath *(reluctant)*

loathe *(to detest)*, loathed, loath'ing

loath'some

lob, lobbed, lob'bing

lo'bar

lob'by, -bied, -by•ing

lob'by•ist

lobe

lobed

lo•be'li•a

lob'lol'ly

lo•bot'o•my
lob'ster
lo'cal
lo•cale'
lo•cal'i•ty
lo'cal•i•za'tion
lo'cal•ize', -ized', -iz'-
  ing
lo'cate', -cat'ed, -cat'-
  ing
lo•ca'tion
loc'a•tive
lo'ca'tor
loch *(lake)*
lock *(mechanism,*
  strand of hair)
lock'er
lock'et
lock'jaw'
lock'out' *n.*
lock'smith'
lock'up' *n.*
lo'co *pl.* -cos
lo'co•mo'tion
lo'co•mo'tive
lo'co•weed'
lo'cus *pl.* -ci'
lo'cust
lo•cu'tion
lode *(ore deposit)*
  ♦*load*
lode'star'
lode'stone'
lodge, lodged, lodg'-
  ing
lodg'ment *also* lodge'-
  ment

lo'ess
loft
loft'y
log, logged, log'ging
lo'gan•ber'ry
log'a•rithm'
log'a•rith'mic *also*
  log'a•rith'mi•cal
log'book'
loge
log'ger
log'ger•head'
log'gi•a
log'ging
log'ic
log'i•cal
lo•gi'cian
lo•gis'tic *also* lo•gis'-
  ti•cal
lo•gis'tics
log'jam'
lo'go *pl.* -gos
lo•gom'a•chy *pl.*
  -chies
log'or•rhe'a
lo'go•type'
log'roll'ing
lo'gy
loin'cloth'
loi'ter
loll
lol'la•pa•loo'za
lol'li•pop' *also* lol'ly-
  pop'
lone *(solitary)*
  ♦*loan*
lone'ly

lon'er
lone'some
long'boat'
long'bow'
long'-dis'tance *adj.*
lon•gev'i•ty
long'hair'
long'haired'
long'hand'
long'horn'
long'ing
lon'gi•tude'
lon'gi•tu'di•nal
long'leaf ' pine
long'-lived'
long'neck'
long'-play'ing
long'-range'
long'shore'man
long'-sight'ed
long'-stand'ing
long'-suf 'fer•ing
long'-term'
long'time'
long'-wind'ed
loo'fah *or* luf 'fa
look'ing glass
look'out' *n.*
look'-up'
loom
loon'y
loop *(circular or oval*
  figure)
  ♦*loupe*
loop'hole'
loose, loos'er, loos'est
loose'-joint'ed

loose'-leaf'
loos'en
loot *(spoils)*
 ♦*lute*
lop, lopped, lop'ping
lope, loped, lop'ing
lop'-eared'
lop'sid'ed
lo•qua'cious
lo•quac'i•ty
lo'ran'
lord'ly
lord'ship'
lore
lor•gnette'
lor'ry
lose, lost, los'ing
loss
lost
lot
lo'tion
lot'ter•y
lot'to
lo'tus *pl.* -tus•es
loud'ly
loud'mouth'
loud'mouthed'
loud'speak'er
lounge, lounged,
 loung'ing
lounge'wear'
loupe *(magnifying
 glass)*
 ♦*loop*
louse *pl.* lice
louse, loused, lous'ing
lous'y

lout'ish
lou'ver *also* lou'vre
lov'a•ble *also* love'-
 a•ble
love, loved, lov'ing
love'bird'
love'less
love'lorn'
love'ly
lov'er
love'sick'
love'y-dove'y
lov'ing
low *(having little
 height)*
 ♦*lo*
low *(to moo)*
 ♦*lo*
low'born'
low'boy'
low'brow'
low'-down' *adj.*
low'down' *n.*
low'er *(below)*
low'er *(to scowl), also*
 lour
low'er-case', -cased',
 -cas'ing
low'er-class' *adj.*
low'er•most'
low'-key'
low'-keyed'
low'land
low'ly
low'-mind'ed
low'-pres'sure *adj.*
low'-rise'

low'-test' *adj.*
lox *(smoked salmon)*
 ♦*locks*
loy'al
loy'al•ist
loy'al•ty
loz'enge
lu•au'
lub'ber
lu'bri•cant
lu'bri•cate', -cat'ed,
 -cat'ing
lu'bri•ca'tion
lu'bri•ca'tor
lu•bri'cious
lu'cent
lu'cid
lu•cid'i•ty
Lu'ci•fer
Lu'cite'®
luck'y
lu'cra•tive
lu'cre
lu'di•crous
lug, lugged, lug'ging
lug'gage
lu•gu'bri•ous
luke'warm'
lull
lull'a•by'
lum•ba'go
lum'bar *(of the back)*
lum'ber *(wood)*
lum'ber *(to move
 heavily)*
lum'ber•jack'
lum'ber•yard'

lu'men *pl.* -mens *or*
-mi•na
lu'mi•nance
lu'mi•nar'y
lu'mi•nes'cence
lu'mi•nes'cent
lu'min•ism
lu'mi•nos'i•ty
lu'mi•nous
lum'mox
lump'y
lu'na•cy
lu'nar
lu'nar•scape'
lu'na•tic
lunch'eon
lunch'eon•ette'
lunch'meat'
lunch'room'
lunch'time'
lu•nette'
lunge, lunged, lung'-
ing
lung'fish' *pl.* -fish' *or*
-fish'es
lu'pine *also* lu'pin
lu'pus
lurch
lure, lured, lur'ing
lu'rid
lurk
lus'cious
lus'cious•ness
lush
lust
lus'ter
lus'ter•less

lus'trous
lust'y
lute *(musical instru-*
ment)
♦*loot*
lu•te'ti•um *also* lu-
te'ci•um
Lu'ther•an
lux•u'ri•ance
lux•u'ri•ant
lux•u'ri•ate', -at'ed,
-at'ing
lux•u'ri•ous
lux'u•ry
ly•ce'um
Ly'cra®
lye *(chemical)*
♦*lie*
lymph
lym•phat'ic
lym'pho•cyte'
lym'phoid'
lynch
lynx *(cat)*
♦*links*
lyre *(harp)*
♦*liar*
lyre'bird'
lyr'ic
lyr'i•cal
lyr'i•cism
lyr'i•cist
lyr'i•cize', -cized',
-ciz'ing
ly•ser'gic ac'id di'-
eth•yl•am'ide'

ly'sin
ly'sine'

M

ma•ca'bre
mac•ad'am
mac•a•da'mi•a nut
mac•ad'am•ize',
-ized', -iz'ing
mac'a•ro'ni *pl.* -ni
mac'a•roon'
ma•caw'
mace
mac'er•ate, -at'ed,
-at'ing
mac'er•a'tion
mac'er•a'tor *also*
mac'er•at'er
ma•chet'e
Mach'i•a•vel'li•an
mach'i•na'tion
ma•chine', -chined',
-chin'ing
ma•chine'-gun',
-gunned', -gun'ning
ma•chine'-read'-
a•ble
ma•chin'er•y
ma•chin'ist
ma•chis'mo
Mach number
ma'cho *pl.* -chos
mack'er•el *pl.* -el *or*
-els
mack'i•naw'
mack'in•tosh' *(rain-*

coat), also mac'in-
tosh'
♦McIntosh
mac'ra•mé'
mac'ro' pl. -ros'
mac'ro•bi•ot'ics
mac'ro•cosm
mac'ro•cos'mic
mac'ro•ec'o•nom'-
ics
ma•crog'ra•phy
mac'ro•mol'e•cule
ma'cron'
mac'ro•scop'ic also
mac'ro•scop'i•cal
mac'u•la pl. -lae'
mac'u•lar
mac'u•late', -lat'ed,
-lat'ing
mac'u•la'tion
mad, mad'der, mad'-
dest
Mad'am pl. Mes-
dames'
Mad'ame pl. Mes-
dames'
mad'cap'
mad'den
mad'der
Ma•dei'ra
Mad'e•moi•selle' pl.
Mes'de•moi•selles'
made'-to-or'der
made'-up' adj.
mad'house'
mad'man'
mad'ness

Ma•don'na
ma'dras
mad'ri•gal
ma'dri•lène' also
ma'dri•lene'
mael'strom
mae'nad'
maes'tro pl. -tros
Ma'fi•a
Ma'fi•o'so' pl. -si'
mag'a•zine'
ma•gen'ta
mag'got
Ma'gi'
mag'ic
mag'i•cal
ma•gi'cian
mag'is•te'ri•al
mag'is•tra•cy
mag'is•trate'
mag'ma pl. mag'ma'-
ta or mag'mas
mag'na cum lau'de
mag'na•nim'i•ty
mag•nan'i•mous
mag'nate' (influential
person)
♦magnet
mag•ne'sia
mag•ne'si•um
mag'net (something
that attracts)
♦magnate
mag'net'ic
mag'net•ism
mag'net•ite'
mag'net•i•za'tion

mag'net•ize', -ized',
-iz'ing
mag•ne'to pl. -tos
mag'ne•tom'e•ter
mag•ne'to•sphere'
mag'ne•tron'
mag'ni•fi•ca'tion
mag•nif'i•cence
mag•nif'i•cent
(splendid)
♦munificent
mag•nif'i•er
mag'ni•fy', -fied', -fy'-
ing
mag•nil'o•quence
mag•nil'o•quent
mag'ni•tude'
mag•no'lia
mag'num
mag'num o'pus
mag'pie
Mag'yar
ma•ha•ra'jah or ma'-
ha•ra'ja
ma•ha•ra'ni or ma'-
ha•ra'nee
ma•hat'ma
mah'jong' also mah'-
jongg'
ma•hog'a•ny
maid (girl, servant)
♦made
maid'en
maid'en•hair'
maid'en•hood'
maid of honor pl.
maids of honor

maid′ser′vant
mail *(postal material,*
  armor)
  ♦*male*
mail′bag′
mail′boat′
mail′box′
mail′man′
mail′-or′der house
mail′room′
maim
main *(principal)*
  ♦*mane*
main′land′
main′line′, -lined′,
  -lin′ing
main′mast
main′sail′
main′sheet′
main′spring′
main′stay′
main′stream′
main•tain′
main′te•nance
main′top′
main top′mast
maî′tre d′hô•tel′ *pl.*
  maî′tres d′hô•tel′
maize *(grain)*
  ♦*maze*
ma•jes′tic
maj′es•ty
ma•jol′i•ca
ma′jor
ma′jor-do′mo *pl.*
  -mos
ma′jor•ette′

ma•jor′i•tar′i•an
ma•jor′i•ty
ma′jor-league′ *adj.*
ma′jor-med′i•cal
  adj.
ma•jus′cule
make, made, mak′ing
make′-be•lieve′ *n. &*
  adj.
make′-do′ *adj. & n.*
make′-or-break′ *adj.*
make′o′ver *n.*
make′-read′y *n.*
make′shift′
make′-up′ *n., also*
  make′up′
make′-work′
mal′a•chite′
mal′ad•just′ed
mal′ad•just′ment
mal′a•droit′
mal′a•dy
Mal•a•gas′y *pl.* -gas′y
  or -gas′ies
mal•aise′
mal′a•mute′ *or* mal′-
  e•mute′
mal′a•prop′
mal′a•prop•ism
mal′a•pro•pos′
ma•lar′i•a
ma•lar′i•al *also* ma-
  lar′i•an, ma•lar′-
  i•ous
ma•lar′key *also* ma-
  lar′ky
Ma′lay

Ma•lay′an
mal′con•tent′
male *(masculine)*
  ♦*mail*
mal′e•dic′tion
mal′e•fac′tion
mal′e•fac′tor
ma•lef′ic
ma•lef′i•cent
ma•lev′o•lence
ma•lev′o•lent
mal•fea′sance
mal•fea′sant
mal′for•ma′tion
mal•formed′
mal•func′tion
mal′ice
ma•li′cious
ma•lign′
ma•lig′nan•cy
ma•lig′nant
ma•lig′ni•ty
ma•lin′ger
mall *(promenade)*
  ♦*maul*
mal′lard
mal′le•a•bil′i•ty
mal′le•a•ble
mal′let
mal′le•us *pl.* -le•i′
mal′low
malm′sey *pl.* -seys
mal•nour′ished
mal′nu•tri′tion
mal′oc•clu′sion
mal•o′dor
mal•o′dor•ous

mal•prac'tice
mal'prac•ti'tion•er
malt
mal'tase'
malt'ed milk
Mal•tese' *pl.* -tese'
mal'tose'
mal•treat'
ma'ma *also* mam'ma
mam'ba *(snake)*
mam'bo *(dance),* pl.
  -bos
mam'mal
mam•ma'li•an
mam'ma•ry
mam'mo•gram'
mam•mog'ra•phy
mam'moth
mam'my
man *pl.* men
man, manned, man'-
  ning, mans
man'a•cle, -cled,
  -cling
man'age, -aged, -ag-
  ing
man'age•a•bil'i•ty
man'age•a•ble
man'age•ment
man'ag•er
man'a•ge'ri•al
man'-at-arms' *pl.*
  men'-at-arms'
Man•chu'ri•an
man•da'mus
man'da•rin
man'date', -dat'ed,

-dat'ing
man'da•to'ry
man'di•ble
man'do•lin'
man'drake'
man'drel *(spindle),* or
  man'dril
man'drill *(baboon)*
mane *(hair)*
  ♦*main*
man'-eat'er
man'-eat'ing
ma•neu'ver
ma•neu'ver•a•bil'-
  i•ty
ma•neu'ver•a•ble
man'ful
man'ga•nese'
mange
man'ger
man'gle, -gled, -gling
man'go *pl.* -goes *or*
  -gos
man'grove'
man'gy
man'han'dle, -dled,
  -dling
Man•hat'tan
man'hole'
man'hood'
man'-hour' *pl.*
  man'-hours'
man'hunt'
ma'ni•a
ma'ni•ac'
ma•ni'a•cal
man'ic

man'ic-de•pres'sive
man'i•cot'ti
man'i•cure', -cured',
  -cur'ing
man'i•cur'ist
man'i•fest'
man'i•fes•ta'tion
man'i•fes'to *pl.* -toes
  or -tos
man'i•fold
man'i•kin *(dwarf),* or
  man'ni•kin
  ♦*mannequin*
Ma•nil'a paper
man'i•oc' *also* man'-
  i•o'ca
man'i•ple
ma•nip'u•la•ble
ma•nip'u•late', -lat'-
  ed, -lat'ing
ma•nip'u•la'tion
ma•nip'u•la'tive
ma•nip'u•la'tor
man'kind'
man'ly
man'made'
man'na
man'ne•quin *(model)*
  ♦*manikin*
man'ner *(behavior)*
  ♦*manor*
man'nered
man'ner•ism
man'ner•ly
man'nish
man'-of-war' *pl.*
  men'-of-war'

ma•nom'e•ter
man'or *(estate)*
  ♦*manner*
ma•no'ri•al
ma•no'ri•al•ism
man'pow'er
man•qué'
man'sard
manse
man'ser'vant *pl.*
  men'ser'vants
man'sion
man'-sized' *also*
  man'-size'
man'slaugh'ter
man'ta
man'-tai'lored
man'tel *(shelf), also*
  man'tle
man'tel•piece' *also*
  man'tle•piece'
man'tic
man•til'la
man'tis
man•tis'sa
man'tle *(to cloak),*
  -tled, -tling
  ♦*mantel*
man'tra
man'trap'
man'u•al
man'u•fac'to•ry
man'u•fac'ture,
  -tured, -tur•ing
man'u•fac'tur•er
man'u•mis'sion
man'u•mit', -mit'ted,

-mit'ting
ma•nure'
man'u•script'
Manx
Manx cat *or* manx
  cat
man'y, more, most
Mao'ist
Mao'ri *pl.* -ri *or* -ris
map, mapped, map'-
  ping
ma'ple
mar, marred, mar'ring
mar'a•bou'
ma•ra'ca
mar'a•schi'no
mar'a•thon'
mar'a•thon'er
ma•raud'
mar'ble, -bled, -bling
mar'ble•ize', -ized',
  -iz'ing
march *(journey, bor-*
  der)
March *(month)*
mar'chion•ess
Mar'di gras'
mare *(female horse)*
ma're *(region of the*
  moon), pl. -ri•a
mar'ga•rine'
mar'ga•ri'ta
mar'gin
mar'gin•al
mar'gi•na'li•a
mar'gue•rite'
mar'i•gold'

mar'i•jua'na *or* mar-
  i•hua'na
ma•rim'ba
ma•ri'na
mar'i•nade'
mar'i•nate', -nat'ed,
  -nat'ing
ma•rine'
mar'i•ner
mar'i•o•nette'
mar'i•po'sa
mar'i•tal
mar'i•time'
mar'jo•ram
marked
mark'ed•ly
mark'er
mar'ket
mar'ket•a•ble
mar'ket•eer'
mar'ket•place'
mark'ing
marks'man
marks'man•ship'
mark'up' *n.*
marl
mar'lin *(fish)*
mar'line *(rope)*
mar'line•spike'
mar'ma•lade'
mar•mo're•al
mar'mo•set'
mar'mot
ma•roon'
mar•quee' *(tent, en-*
  trance)
  ♦*marquis, marquise*

mar′que•try *also*
  mar′que•terie

mar′quis *(nobleman)*,
  pl. -quis *or* -quis•es
  ♦*marquee, marquise*

mar•quise′ *(noble-
  woman, ring)*
  ♦*marquee, marquis*

mar′qui•sette′

mar′riage

mar′riage•a•ble

mar′ried

mar′row

mar′row•bone′

mar′ry, -ried, -ry•ing

Mars

mar•sa′la

marsh

mar′shal *(to orga-
  nize)*, -shaled *or*
  -shalled, -shal•ing *or*
  -shal•ling
  ♦*martial*

marsh′land′

marsh′mal′low

marsh′y

mar•su′pi•al

mart

mar′ten *(animal)*
  ♦*martin*

mar′tial *(warlike)*
  ♦*marshall*

Mar′tian

mar′tin *(bird)*
  ♦*marten*

mar′ti•net′

mar′tin•gale′

mar•ti′ni *pl.* -nis

mar′tyr

mar′tyr•dom

mar′vel, -veled *or*
  -velled, -vel•ing *or*
  -vel•ling

mar′vel•ous *also*
  mar′vel•lous

Marx′i•an

Marx′ism

Marx′ist

mar′zi•pan′

mas•car′a

mas′cot

mas′cu•line

mas′cu•lin′i•ty

ma′ser

mash′ie

mask *(covering)*
  ♦*masque*

mas′o•chism

mas′o•chist

mas′o•chis′tic

ma′son

Ma•son′ic

Ma′son•ite′®

Mason jar

ma′son•ry

masque *(drama)*, *also*
  mask

mas′quer•ade′, -ad′-
  ed, -ad′ing

mass *(matter)*

Mass *(Eucharist cere-
  mony)*, *also* mass

mas′sa•cre, -cred,
  -cring

mas•sage′, saged′,
  -sag′ing

mas•seur′

mas•seuse′

mas•sif ′ *(mountain)*

mas′sive *(large)*

mass′-pro•duce′,
  -duced′, -duc′ing

mast

mas•tec′to•my

mas′ter

mas′ter-at-arms′ *pl.*
  mas′ters-at-arms′

mas′ter•ful

mas′ter•ly

mas′ter•mind′

mas′ter•piece′

mas′ter•stroke′

mas′ter•work′

mas′ter•y

mast′head′

mas′tic

mas′ti•cate′, -cat′ed,
  -cat′ing

mas′ti•ca′tion

mas′ti•ca′tor

mas′tiff

mas′to•don

mas′toid′

mas′toid•i′tis

mas′tur•bate′, -bat′-
  ed, -bat′ing

mas′tur•ba′tion

mat *(to cover, tangle,
  or border)*, mat′ted,
  mat′ting
  ♦*matte*

mat'a•dor'
match'book'
match'box'
match'less
match'lock'
match'mak'er
match'mak'ing
match'stick'
match'up' *n.*
mate, mat'ed, mat'ing
ma'ter
ma•te'ri•al *(sub-
    stance)*
    ♦*materiel*
ma•te'ri•al•ism
ma•te'ri•al•ist
ma•te'ri•al•is'tic
ma•te'ri•al•i•za'-
    tion
ma•te'ri•al•ize',
    -ized', -iz'ing
ma•te'ri•el' *(equip-
    ment),* or ma•té'ri•
    el'
    ♦*material*
ma•ter'nal
ma•ter'ni•ty
math'e•mat'i•cal
    also math'e•mat'ic
math'e•ma•ti'cian
math'e•mat'ics
mat'i•nee' *or* mat'-
    i•née'
mat'ins
ma'tri•arch'
ma'tri•ar'chal
ma'tri•ar'chy

mat'ri•ci'dal
mat'ri•cide'
ma•tric'u•late', -lat'-
    ed, -lat'ing
ma•tric'u•la'tion
mat'ri•lin'e•age
mat'ri•lin'e•al
mat'ri•mo'ni•al
mat'ri•mo'ny
ma'trix *pl.* -tri•ces' *or*
    -trix•es
ma'tron
matron of honor *pl.*
    matrons of honor
mat'ter
mat'ter-of-fact' *adj.*
mat'ting
mat'tock
mat'tress
mat'u•rate', -rat'ed,
    -rat'ing
mat'u•ra'tion
mat'u•ra'tive
ma•ture', tured', -tur'-
    ing
ma•tur'i•ty
mat'zo *pl.* -zoth' *or*
    -zos *or* -zot'
maud'lin
maul *(hammer), also*
    mall
maun'der
Mau•ri•ta'ni•an
Mau•ri'ti•an
mau'so•le'um *pl.* -le'-
    ums *or* -le'a
mauve

mav'er•ick
maw
mawk'ish
max'i *pl.* -is
max•il'la *pl.* -lae *or*
    -las
max'il•lar
max'il•lar'y
max'im
max'i•mal
max'i•mi•za'tion
max'i•mize',
    -mized', -miz'ing
max'i•mum *pl.*
    -mums *or* -ma
may *auxiliary, past
    tense* might
May *(month)*
Ma'ya *pl.* -ya *or* -yas
Ma'yan
may'be
may'day' *(signal)*
May Day *(May 1)*
may'flow'er
may'fly'
may'hem'
may'on•naise'
may'or
may'or•al
may'or•al•ty
May'pole' *also* may'-
    pole'
maze *(labyrinth)*
    ♦*maize*
ma•zur'ka
Mc•Car'thy•ism
Mc'In•tosh' (apple)

♦*mackintosh*
me *pron.*
　♦*mi*
mead *(beverage, meadow)*
　♦*meed*
mead'ow
mead'ow•lark'
mea'ger *also* mea'gre
meal'time'
meal'y-mouthed'
mean *(low)*
　♦*mien*
mean *(midpoint)*
　♦*mien*
mean *(to signify),* meant, mean'ing
　♦*mien*
me•an'der
mean'ing•ful
mean'ing•less
mean'time'
mean'while'
mea'sles
mea'sly
meas'ur•a•ble
meas'ure, -ured, -ur•ing
meas'ure•ment
meat *(food)*
　♦*meet, mete*
meat'ball'
meat'pack'ing
meat'y
mec'ca
me•chan'ic
me•chan'i•cal

me•chan'ics
mech'a•nism
mech'a•nis'tic
mech'a•ni•za'tion
mech'a•nize', -nized', -niz'ing
med'al *(award)*
　♦*meddle*
me•dal'lion
med'dle *(to interfere),* -dled, -dling
　♦*medal*
med'dle•some
me'di•al
me'di•an
me'di•ate', -at'ed, -at'ing
me'di•a'tion
me'di•a'tor
med'ic
Med'i•caid' *also* med'i•caid'
med'i•cal
me•dic'a•ment
Med'i•care' *also* med'i•care'
med'i•cate', -cat'ed, -cat'ing
med'i•ca'tion
me•dic'i•nal
med'i•cine
med'i•co' *pl.* -cos'
me'di•e'val *also* me'di•ae'val
me'di•e'val•ist *also* me'di•ae'val•ist
me'di•o'cre

me'di•oc'ri•ty
med'i•tate', -tat'ed, -tat'ing
med'i•ta'tion
med'i•ta'tive
med'i•ta'tor
me'di•um *pl.* -di•a *or* -di•ums
med'ley *pl.* -leys
me•dul'la *pl.* -las *or* -lae
medulla ob'lon•ga'-ta *pl.* medulla ob'-lon•ga'tas *or* medullae ob'lon•ga'-tae
me•dul'lar *also* med'-ul•lar'y
meed *(reward)*
　♦*mead*
meek'ly
meer'schaum
meet *(fitting)*
　♦*meat, mete*
meet *(to come upon),* met, meet'ing
　♦*meat, mete*
meg'a•bit'
meg'a•buck'
meg'a•byte'
meg'a•cy'cle
meg'a•death'
meg'a•hertz'
meg'a•lith'
meg'a•lith'ic
meg'a•lo•ma'ni•a
meg'a•lo•ma'ni•ac'

meg'a•lop'o•lis
meg'a•phone'
meg'a•spore'
meg'a•ton'
me'grim
mei•o'sis *pl.* -ses'
mei•ot'ic
Meis'sen
mel'a•mine'
mel'an•cho'li•a
mel'an•chol'ic
mel'an•chol'y
Mel'a•ne'sian
mé•lange' *also* me-
   lange'
mel'a•nin
mel'a•no'ma *pl.*
   -mas *or* -ma•ta
Mel'ba toast
meld
me•lee' *also* mê•lée'
mel'io•rate', -rat'ed,
   -rat'ing
mel'io•ra'tion
mel•lif'lu•ous
mel'low
me•lo'de•on
me•lod'ic
me•lo'di•ous
mel'o•dra'ma
mel'o•dra•mat'ic
mel'o•dy
mel'on
melt'down'
melt'ing point
mem'ber
mem'ber•ship'

mem'brane'
mem'bra•nous
me•men'to *pl.* -tos *or*
   -toes
mem'o *pl.* -os
mem'oir'
mem'o•ra•bil'i•a
mem'o•ra•ble
mem'o•ran'dum *pl.*
   -dums *or* -da
me•mo'ri•al
me•mo'ri•al•i•za'-
   tion
me•mo'ri•al•ize',
   -ized', -iz'ing
mem'o•ri•za'tion
mem'o•rize', -rized',
   -riz'ing
mem'o•ry
men'ace, -aced, -ac-
   ing
mé•nage'
me•nag'er•ie
mend
men•da'cious
men•dac'i•ty
men'de•le'vi•um
men'di•cant
mend'ing
men•ha'den *pl.* -den
   or -dens
me'ni•al
men'in•gi'tis
me•ninx *pl.* me•nin'-
   ges
me•nis'cal *also* me-
   nis'cate', me•nis'-

coid', men'is•coi'dal
me•nis'cus *pl.* -ci' *or*
   -cus•es
men'o•paus'al
men'o•pause'
men'sal
men'ses
men'stru•al
men'stru•ate', -at'ed,
   -at'ing
men'stru•a'tion
men'su•ra•bil'i•ty
men'su•ra•ble
men'su•ra'tion
men'su•ra'tive
men'tal
men•tal'i•ty
men•ta'tion
men'thol'
men'tho•lat'ed
men'tion
men'tor
men'u
me•ow'
Meph'i•stoph'e•les'
me•phit'ic *also* me-
   phit'i•cal
me•phi'tis
mer'can•tile'
mer'can•til•ism
mer'can•til'ist
mer'ce•nar'y
mer'cer
mer'cer•ize', -ized',
   -iz'ing
mer'chan•dise',
   -dised', -dis'ing

mer'chan•dis'er
mer'chant
mer'ci•ful
mer'ci•less
mer•cu'ri•al
mer•cu'ri•al•ism
mer•cu'ric
Mer•cu'ro•
	chrome'®
mer•cu'rous
mer'cu•ry (element)
Mer'cu•ry (god, plan-
	et)
mer'cy
mere superl. mer'est
mer•e•tri'cious
mer•gan'ser
merge, merged, merg'-
	ing
merg'er
me•rid'i•an
me•ringue'
me•ri'no pl. -nos
mer'it
mer'i•toc'ra•cy
mer'it•o•crat'
mer'i•to'ri•ous
mer•lot'
mer'maid'
mer'man'
mer'ri•ment
mer'ry
mer'ry-go-round'
mer'ry•mak'er
mer'ry•mak'ing
Mer•thi'o•late'®
me'sa

mes•cal'
mes'ca•line'
mes'en•ter'ic
mes'en•ter'y also
	mes'en•ter'i•um pl.
	-i•a
mesh'work'
mes'mer•ism
mes'mer•ize', -ized',
	-iz'ing
mes'o•derm'
Mes'o•lith'ic
mes'on'
Mes'o•po•ta'mi•an
mes'o•sphere'
mes'o•spher'ic
Mes'o•zo'ic
mes•quite'
mess
mes'sage
mes'sen•ger
Mes•si'ah
mes'si•an'ic
mess'y
met'a•bol'ic
me•tab'o•lism
me•tab'o•lize',
	-lized', -liz'ing
met'a•car'pal
met'a•car'pus
met'al (element)
	♦mettle
me•tal'lic
met'al•loid'
met'al•lur'gic also
	met'al•lur'gi•cal
met'al•lur'gist

met'al•lur'gy
met'al•work'
met'a•mor'phic also
	met'a•mor'phous
met'a•mor'phism
met'a•mor'phose',
	-phosed', -phos'ing
met'a•mor•pho•sis
	pl. -ses'
met'a•phase'
met'a•phor'
met'a•phor'ic also
	met'a•phor'i•cal
met'a•phys'i•cal
met'a•phy•si'cian
met'a•phys'ics
me•tas'ta•sis pl. -ses'
me•tas'ta•size',
	-sized', -siz'ing
met'a•tar'sal
met'a•tar'sus pl. -si'
met'a•zo'an
mete (to distribute),
	met'ed, met'ing
	♦meat, meet
me•tem'psy•cho'sis
	pl. -ses'
me'te•or
me'te•or'ic
me'te•or•ite'
me'te•or•oid'
me'te•or'o•log'i•cal
me'te•or•ol'o•gist
me'te•or•ol'o•gy
me'ter
meth'a•done'
	hydrochloride

meth'ane'
meth'a•nol'
me•thinks'
meth'od
me•thod'i•cal *also*
  me•thod'ic
Meth'od•ist
meth'od•o•log'i•cal
meth'od•ol'o•gy
meth'yl
meth'yl•at'ed
me•tic'u•lous
mé•tier'
met'o•nym'
me•ton'y•my
met'ric
met'ri•cal
met'ri•ca'tion
met'ri•fi•ca'tion
met'ri•fy', -fied', -fy'-
  ing
met'ro *pl.* -ros
me•trol'o•gy
met'ro•nome'
met'ro•nom'ic
me•trop'o•lis *pl.*
  -lis•es
met'ro•pol'i•tan
met'tle *(spirit)*
  ♦*metal*
mewl *(to cry)*
  ♦*mule*
mews *(street)*
  ♦*muse, Muse*
Mex'i•can
me•zu'zah, *also* me-
  zu'za

mez'za•nine'
mez'zo *pl.* -zos
mez'zo-so•pran'o *pl.*
  -os
mez'zo•tint'
mho *(electrical unit)*,
  pl. mhos
  ♦*mow*
mi *(musical tone)*
  ♦*me*
mi•as'ma *pl.* -mas *or*
  -ma•ta
mi•as'mal *also* mi'-
  as•mat'ic, mi•as'mic
mi'ca
mi'crobe'
mi'cro•bi•cide'
mi'cro•bi•o•log'-
  i•cal *also* mi'cro-
  bi'o•log'ic
mi'cro•bi•ol'o•gist
mi'cro•bi•ol'o•gy
mi'cro•chip'
mi'cro•cir'cuit
mi'cro•com•put'er
mi'cro•cosm
mi'cro•cos'mic *also*
  mi'cro•cos'mi•cal
mi'cro•ec'o•nom'-
  ics
mi'cro•fiche'
mi'cro•film'
Mi'cro•groove'®
mi•crom'e•ter
mi•crom'e•try
mi'cron' *pl.* -crons *or*
  -cra, *also* mi'kron'

  pl. -krons' *or* -kra
Mi'cro•ne'sian
mi'cro•nu'cle•us *pl.*
  -cle•i' *or* -cle•us•es
mi'cro•or'gan•ism
mi'cro•phone'
mi'cro•pho'to-
  graph'
mi'cro•pho•tog'ra-
  phy
mi'cro•proc'es•sor
mi'cro•scope'
mi'cro•scop'ic *also*
  mi'cro•scop'i•cal
mi•cros'co•pist
mi•cros'co•py
mi'cro•sur'ger•y
mi'cro•wave'
mid'air'
Mi'das touch
mid'course'
mid'day
mid'dle
mid'dle-aged' *adj.*
mid'dle•brow'
mid'dle-class' *adj.*
mid'dle•man'
mid'dle•weight'
mid'dling
mid'dy *(blouse)*
  ♦*midi*
midge
mid'get
mid'i *(skirt), pl.* -is
  ♦*middy*
mid'land
mid'lev'el

mid′life′
mid′morn′ing
mid′most′
mid′night′
mid′point′
mid′range′
mid′rib′
mid′riff ′
mid′sec′tion
mid′ship′man
midst
mid′stream′
mid′sum′mer
mid′term′
mid′town′
mid′way′
mid′week′
mid′wife′
mid′wife′ry
mid′win′ter
mid′year′
mien *(bearing)*
  ♦*mean*
miff
might *(power)*
  ♦*mite*
might′y
mi′gnon•ette′
mi′graine′
mi′grant
mi′grate′, -grat′ed,
  -grat′ing
mi•gra′tion
mi′gra•to′ry
mi•ka′do *pl.* -dos
mike, miked, mik′ing
mil *(unit of length)*

  ♦*mill*
mi•la′dy
milch
mil′dew
mild′ly
mile′age
mile′post′
mil′er
mile′stone′
mi•lieu′
mil′i•tan•cy
mil′i•tant
mil′i•tar′i•a
mil′i•ta•rism
mil′i•ta•rist
mil′i•ta•ris′tic
mil′i•ta•rize′,
  -rized′, -riz′ing
mil′i•tar′y
mil′i•tate′, -tat′ed,
  -tat′ing
mi•li′tia
milk′maid′
milk′man′
milk′sop′
milk′weed′
milk′y
Milk′y Way
mill *(grinder, money)*
  ♦*mil*
mill′age
mill′dam′
mil′le•nar′i•an
mil′le•nar′y *(thou-
  sand)*
  ♦*millinery*
mil•len′ni•al

mil•len′ni•um *pl.*
  -ni•ums *or* -ni•a
mil′let
mil′liard
mil′li•gram′
mil′li•li′ter
mil′li•me′ter
mil′li•ner
mil′li•ner′y *(hats)*
  ♦*millenary*
mill′ing
mil′lion *pl.* -lion *or*
  -lions
mil′lion•aire′
mil′lionth
mil′li•pede′ *or* mil′-
  le•pede′
mill′race′
mill′stone′
mill′stream′
mi•lord′
milque′toast′
milt
mime, mimed, mim′-
  ing
mim′e•o•graph′
mi•me′sis
mi•met′ic
mim′ic, -icked, -ick-
  ing
mim′ick•er
mim′ic•ry
mi•mo′sa
min′a•ret′
min′a•to′ry
mince, minced, minc′-
  ing

mince′meat′
mind *(intelligence, to heed)*
　♦*mined*
mind′-al′ter•ing
mind′-blow′ing
mind′ful
mind′less
mind′scape′
mine, mined, min′ing
mine *pron.*
mine′field′
min′er *(one that mines)*
　♦*minor*
min′er•al
min′er•a•log′i•cal
min′er•al′o•gist
min′er•al′o•gy
min′e•stro′ne
mine′work′er
min′gle, -gled, -gling
min′i *pl.* -is
min′i•a•ture
min′i•a•tur′i•za′-
　tion
min′i•a•tur•ize′,
　-ized′, -iz′ing
min′i•bar′
min′i•bus′
min′i•cab′
min′i•cam′
min′i•com•put′er
min′im
min′i•mal′
min′i•mal•ism
min′i•mal•ist

min′i•mal•ize′,
　-ized′, -iz′ing
min′i•mi•za′tion
min′i•mize′, -mized′,
　-miz′ing
min′i•mum *pl.*
　-mums *or* -ma
min′ing
min′ion
min′i•se′ries
min′i•skirt′
min′is•ter
min′is•te′ri•al
min′is•trant
min′is•tra′tion
min′is•try
min′i•van′
mink *pl.* mink *or*
　minks
Min′ne•so′tan
min′now *pl.* -now *or*
　-nows
mi′nor *(smaller)*
　♦*miner*
mi•nor′i•ty
mi′nor-league′ *adj.*
Min′o•taur′
min′strel
min′strel•sy
mint′age
mint′mark′
min′u•end′
min′u•et′
mi′nus
mi•nus′cu•lar
min•us•cule′ *also*
　min•is•cule′

mi•nute′ *(small)*
min′ute *(unit of time)*
mi•nute′ly *(on a
　small scale)*
min′ute•ly *(once a
　minute)*
min′ute•man′
mi•nu′ti•a *pl.* -ti•ae′
minx
Mi′o•cene′
mir′a•cle
mi•rac′u•lous
mi•rage′
mire, mired, mir′ing
mir′ror
mirth′ful
mis′ad•ven′ture
mis′al•li′ance
mis′al•lo•cate′, -cat′-
　ed, -cat′ing
mis′an•thrope′ *also*
　mis•an′thro•pist
mis′an•throp′ic *also*
　mis•an•throp′i•cal
mis•an′thro•py
mis′ap•pli•ca′tion
mis′ap•ply′, -plied′,
　-ply′ing
mis′ap•pre•hend′
mis′ap•pre•hen′-
　sion
mis′ap•pro′pri•ate′,
　-at′ed, -at′ing
mis′ap•pro′pri•
　a′tion
mis′be•got′ten
mis′be•have′,

-haved', -hav'ing
mis•be•hav'ior
mis•cal'cu•late',
  -lat'ed, -lat'ing
mis•cal•cu•la'tion
mis•call'
mis•car'riage
mis•car'ry, -ried, -ry•
  ing
mis•cast', -cast',
  -cast'ing
mis•ce•ge•na'tion
mis•cel•la'ne•ous
mis•cel•la'ny
mis•chance'
mis'chief
mis•chie•vous
mis•ci•bil'i•ty
mis•ci•ble
mis•com•mu'ni•ca'-
  tion
mis•con•ceive',
  -ceived', -ceiv'ing
mis•con•cep'tion
mis•con'duct
mis•con•struc'tion
mis•con•strue',
  -strued', -stru'ing
mis•count' n.
mis•count' v.
mis'cre•ant
mis•deal' n.
mis•deal', -dealt',
  -deal'ing
mis•deed'
mis•de•mean'or
mis•di•rect'

mis•do'ing
mi'ser
mis'er•a•ble
mis'er•y
mis•fea'sance
mis•fea'sor
mis•fire', -fired', -fir'-
  ing
mis'fit'
mis•for'tune
mis•giv'ing
mis•gov'ern
mis•guid'ance
mis•guide', -guid'ed,
  -guid'ing
mis•han'dle, -dled,
  -dling
mis'hap'
mis•hear', -heard',
  -hear'ing
mish'mash'
mis•in•form'
mis•in•for•ma'tion
mis•in•ter'pret
mis•in•ter'pre•ta'-
  tion
mis•judge', -judged',
  -judg'ing
mis•judg'ment
mis•lay', -laid', -lay'-
  ing
mis•lead', -led',
  -lead'ing
mis•man'age, -aged,
  -ag•ing
mis•man'age•ment
mis•match'

mis•name', -named',
  -nam'ing
mis•no'mer
mi•sog'a•my
mi•sog'y•nist
mi•sog'y•nous
mi•sog'y•ny
mis•place', -placed',
  -plac'ing
mis•play'
mis'print' n.
mis•print' v.
mis•pri'sion
mis•pro•nounce',
  -nounced', -nounc'-
  ing
mis•pro•nun'ci-
  a'tion
mis•quo•ta'tion
mis•quote', -quot'ed,
  -quot'ing
mis•read', -read',
  -read'ing
mis•rep•re•sent'
mis•rep•re•sen•ta'-
  tion
mis•rule', -ruled',
  -rul'ing
miss
mis'sal *(prayer book)*
  ♦*missile*
mis•shape', -shaped',
  -shap'ing
mis•shap'en
mis'sile *(weapon)*
  ♦*missal*
mis'sile•ry *also* mis'-

sil•ry
miss'ing
mis'sion
mis'sion•ar'y
Mis'sis•sip'pi•an
mis'sive
Mis•sou'ri•an
mis•speak', -spoke',
-spo'ken, -speak'ing
mis•spell', -spelled'
or -spelt', -spell'ing
mis•spend', -spent',
-spend'ing
mis•state', -stat'ed,
-stat'ing
mis•step'
mist
mis•tak'a•ble
mis•take', -took',
-tak'en, -tak'ing
Mis'ter
mis•time', -timed',
-tim'ing
mis'tle•toe'
mis'tral
mis•treat'
mis•treat'ment
mis'tress
mis•tri'al
mis•trust'
mist'y
mis'un•der•stand',
-stood', -stand'ing
mis•use', -used', -us'-
ing
mite *(organism, small
amount)*

♦*might*
mi'ter
mit'i•gate', -gat'ed,
-gat'ing
mit'i•ga'tion
mit'i•ga'tor
mi'to•chon'dri•on
pl. -dri•a
mi'to'sis
mi•tot'ic
mitt
mit'ten
mixed
mix'er
mix'ture
mix'-up' *n.*
miz'zen *or* miz'en
miz'zen•mast *or*
miz'en•mast
mne•mon'ic
moan *(sound)*
♦*mown*
moat *(ditch)*
♦*mote*
mob, mobbed, mob'-
bing
mo'bile
mo•bil'i•ty
mo'bi•li•za'tion
mo'bi•lize', -lized',
-liz'ing
Mö'bi•us strip
mob'ster
moc'ca•sin
mo'cha
mock'er•y
mock'-he•ro'ic

mock'ing•bird'
mock'up' *n., also*
mock'-up'
mod
mo'dal
mo•dal'i•ty
mode
mod'el
mo'dem
mod'er•ate', -at'ed,
-at'ing
mod'er•a'tion
mod'e•ra'to *pl.* -tos
mod'er•a'tor
mod'ern
mo•derne'
mod'ern•ism
mod'ern•ist
mod'ern•ist'ic
mod'ern•i•za'tion
mod'ern•ize', -ized',
-iz'ing
mod'est
mod'es•ty
mod'i•cum
mod'i•fi•ca'tion
mod'i•fi'er
mod'i•fy', -fied', -fy'-
ing
mod'ish
mod'u•lar
mod'u•lar'i•ty
mod'u•late', -lat'ed,
-lat'ing
mod'u•la'tion
mod'u•la'tive *also*
mod'u•la•to'ry

mod'u•la'tor
mod'ule
mo'gul *(magnate)*
Mo'gul *(Indian Moslem)*
mo'hair'
Mo•ham'med•an
moi'e•ty
moil
moi•ré' *also* moire
moist
mois'ten
mois'ture
mo'lar
mo•las'ses
mold'a•ble
mold'ing
mold'y
mo•lec'u•lar
mol'e•cule'
mole'hill'
mole'skin'
mo•lest'
mo'les•ta'tion
moll
mol'li•fi'a•ble
mol'li•fi•ca'tion
mol'li•fy', -fied', -fy'-
  ing
mol'lusk *also* mol'-
  lusc
mol'ly
mol'ly•cod'dle,
  -dled, -dling
molt
mol'ten
mo•lyb'de•num

mom
mo'ment
mo'men•tar'i•ly
mo'men•tar'y
mo•men'tous
mo•men'tum *pl.* -ta
  or -tums
Mon'a•can
mo'nad'
mo•nad'ic *also* mo-
  nad'i•cal
mon'arch
mon•ar'chic *also*
  mon•ar'chi•cal
mon'ar•chism
mon'ar•chist
mon'ar•chis'tic
mon'ar•chy
mon•as•te'ri•al
mon'as•ter'y
mo•nas'tic
mo•nas'ti•cism
mon'a•tom'ic
mon•au'ral
mon'a•zite'
Mon'day
mon'e•ta•rism
mon'e•ta•rist
mon'e•tar'y
mon'ey *pl.* -eys *or* -ies
mon'ey•bag'
mon'ey•chang'er
mon'eyed *also* mon'-
  ied
mon'ey•grub'ber
mon'ey•lend'er
mon'ey•mak'er

mon'ey•mak'ing
mon'ger
Mon'gol
Mon•go'li•an
Mon'gol•oid'
mon'goose' *pl.* -goos'-
  es
mon'grel
mon'i•ker *or* mon'-
  ick•er
mo'nism
mo'nist
mo•nis'tic
mo•ni'tion
mon'i•tor
mon'i•to'ry
mon'key *pl.* -keys
mon'key•shine'
monk'ish
monks'hood'
mon'o•chro•mat'ic
  also mon'o•chro'ic
mon'o•chro'ma-
  tism
mon'o•chrome'
mon'o•chro'mic
mon'o•cle
mon'o•cot'y•le'don
  also mon'o•cot'
mon'o•cot'y•le'-
  don•ous
mo•noc'u•lar
mon'o•cul'ture
mo•nod'ic
mon'o•dist
mon'o•dy
mo•nog'a•mist

mo•nog′a•mous
mo•nog′a•my
mon′o•glot′
mon′o•gram′,
  -grammed′ or
  -gramed′, -gram′-
  ming or -gram′ing
mon′o•graph′
mo•nog′ra•pher
mon′o•graph′ic
mon′o•lith′
mon′o•lith′ic
mo•nol′o•gist
mon′o•logue′
mon′o•ma′ni•a
mon′o•ma′ni•ac′
mon′o•ma•ni′a•cal
mon′o•mer
mo•no′mi•al
mon′o•nu′cle•o′sis
mon′o•phon′ic
mon′o•plane′
mo•nop′o•list
mo•nop′o•lis′tic
mo•nop′o•li•za′-
  tion
mo•nop′o•lize′,
  -lized′, -liz′ing
mo•nop′o•ly
mon′o•rail′
mon′o•so′di•um
  glu′ta•mate′
mon′o•syl•lab′ic
mon′o•syl′la•ble
mon′o•the•ism
mon′o•the′ist
mon′o•the•is′tic

mon′o•tone′
mo•not′o•nous
mo•not′o•ny
Mon′o•type′®
mon•ox′ide′
Mon•sieur′ pl. Mes′-
  sieurs
Mon•si′gnor also
  mon•si′gnor
mon•soon′
mon′ster
mon′strance
mon•stros′i•ty
mon′strous
mon•tage′
Mon•tan′an
mon•tane′
month′ly
mon′u•ment
mon′u•men′tal
moo, mooed, moo′ing
moo pl. moos
mooch′er
mood′y
moon′beam′
moon′calf′
moon′child′
moon′light′, -light′-
  ed, -light′ing
moon′lit′
moon′scape′
moon′shine′,
  -shined′, -shin′ing
moon′stone′
moon′struck′ also
  moon′strick′en
moon′walk′

moon′y
moor (open land)
moor (to secure)
Moor (North African)
moor′age
Moor′ish
moose (animal), pl.
  moose
  ♦mousse
moot
mop, mopped, mop′-
  ping
mope, moped, mop′-
  ing
mo′ped′ (bike)
mop′pet
mo•raine′
mor′al
mo•rale′
mor′al•ist
mor′al•is′tic
mo•ral′i•ty
mor′al•i•za′tion
mor′al•ize′, -ized′,
  -iz′ing
mo•rass′
mor′a•to′ri•um pl.
  -ri•ums or -ri•a
mo′ray
mor′bid
mor•bid′i•ty
mor•da′cious
mor•dac′i•ty
mor′dan•cy
mor′dant (caustic)
mor′dent (melodic or-
  nament)

more *superl.* most
mo•rel′
more•o′ver
mo′res
mor•ga•nat′ic
morgue
mor′i•bund′
Mor′mon
morn *(morning)*
  ♦*mourn*
morn′ing *(dawn)*
  ♦*mourning*
morn′ing-glo′ry
Mo•roc′can
mo•roc′co *(leather)*,
  pl. -cos
mo′ron′
mo•ron′ic
mo•rose′
mor′pheme′
Mor′phe•us
mor′phine′
mor′pho•log′i•cal
  also mor′pho•log′ic
mor•phol′o•gist
mor•phol′o•gy
mor′row
Morse code
mor′sel
mor′tal
mor•tal′i•ty
mor′tar
mor′tar•board′
mort′gage, -gaged,
  -gag•ing
mort′ga•gee′
mort′ga•gor′

mor•ti′cian
mor′ti•fi•ca′tion
mor′ti•fy′, -fied′, -fy′-
  ing
mor′tise, -tised, -tis-
  ing, *also* mor′tice,
  -ticed, -tic•ing
mor′tu•ar′y
mo•sa′ic
mo′sey, -seyed, -sey-
  ing, -seys
Mos′lem
mosque
mos•qui′to *pl.* -toes
  or -tos
moss′back′
moss′y
most′ly
mote *(speck)*
  ♦*moat*
mo•tel′
mo•tet′
moth *pl.* moths
moth′ball′ *n.*
moth′-ball′ *v.*
moth′-eat′en
moth′er
moth′er•hood′
moth′er-in-law′ *pl.*
  moth′ers-in-law
moth′er•land′
moth′er•ly
moth′er-of-pearl′
mo•tif′ *(design), also*
  mo′tive
mo′tile
mo•til′i•ty

mo′tion
mo′tion•less
mo′ti•vate′, -vat′ed,
  -vat′ing
mo′ti•va′tion
mo′tive *(reason, im-*
  pulse)
  ♦*motif*
mot′ley
mo′tor
mo′tor•bike′
mo′tor•boat′
mo′tor•cade′
mo′tor•car′
mo′tor•cy′cle, -cled,
  -cling
mo′tor•cy′clist
mo′tor•ist
mo′tor•i•za′tion
mo′tor•ize′, -ized′,
  -iz′ing
mot′tle, -tled, -tling
mot′to *pl.* -toes *or*
  -tos
mound
mount′a•ble
moun′tain
moun′tain•eer′
moun′tain•ous
moun′tain•side′
moun′te•bank′
mount′ing
mourn *(to grieve)*
  ♦*morn*
mourn′ing *(grief)*
  ♦*morning*
mouse *pl.* mice

mouse, moused,
  mous'ing
mouse'trap'
mousse *(dessert)*
  ♦*moose*
mousse•line'
mous'y
mouth *pl.* mouths
mouth'ful' *pl.* -fuls'
mouth'piece'
mouth'wash'
mouth'wa•ter•ing
mou'ton' *(sheepskin)*
  ♦*mutton*
mov'a•ble *also*
  move'a•ble
move, moved, mov'-
  ing
move'ment
mov'er
mov'ie
mov'ie•mak'er
mow *(to cut down),*
  mowed, mowed *or*
  mown, mow'ing
  ♦*mho*
moz'za•rel'la
much, more, most
mu'ci•lage
mu'ci•lag'i•nous
muck'rake', -raked',
  -rak'ing
mu'cous *adj., also*
  mu'cose'
mu'cus *n.*
mud'dle, -dled, -dling
mud'dle-head'ed

mud'dy, -died, -dy-
  ing
mud'guard'
mud'sling'er
mud'sling'ing
muff
muf'fin
muf'fle, -fled, -fling
muf'fler
muf'ti
mug, mugged, mug'-
  ging
mug'ger
mug'gy
muk'luk'
mu•lat'to *pl.* -tos *or*
  -toes
mul'ber'ry
mulch *(covering)*
mulct *(penalty)*
mule *(animal, slipper)*
  ♦*mewl*
mule'skin'ner
mu'le•teer'
mul'ish
mull
mul'lein
mul'let *pl.* -let *or* -lets
mul'li•gan
mul'li•ga•taw'ny
mul'lion
mul'ti•col'ored
mul'ti•di•men'-
  sion•al
mul'ti•eth'nic
mul'ti•far'i•ous
mul'ti•form'

mul'ti•gen'er-
  a'tion•al
mul'ti•lat'er•al
Mul'ti•lith'®
mul'ti•me'di•a
mul•ti•mil•lion-
  aire'
mul'ti•na'tion•al
mul'ti•pack'
mul'ti•ple
mul'ti•ple-choice'
  adj.
multiple scle•ro'sis
mul'ti•plex'
mul'ti•pli•cand'
mul'ti•pli•ca'tion
mul'ti•pli•ca'tive
mul'ti•plic'i•ty
mul'ti•pli'er
mul'ti•ply', -plied',
  -ply'ing
mul'ti•pronged'
mul'ti•pur'pose
mul'ti•stage'
mul'ti•tude'
mul'ti•tu'di•nous
mul'ti•va'lent
mum'ble, -bled,
  -bling
mum'ble•ty-peg'
mum'bo jum'bo
mum'mer
mum'mer•y
mum'mi•fi•ca'tion
mum'mi•fy', -fied',
  -fy'ing
mum'my

mumps
munch
mun•dane′
mu•nic′i•pal
mu•nic′i•pal′i•ty
mu•nif′i•cence
mu•nif′i•cent (gen-
  erous)
  ♦magnificent
mu•ni′tions
mu′ral
mu′ral•ist
mur′der
mur′der•er
mur′der•ous
mu′rex′ pl. -ri•ces′ or
  -rex′es
murk′y
mur′mur
mur′rain
mus′ca•tel′
mus′cle (to force),
  -cled, -cling
  ♦mussel, muzzle
mus′cle-bound′
mus′co•vite′
mus′cu•lar
muscular dys′tro-
  phy
mus′cu•lar′i•ty
mus′cu•la•ture′
muse (to ponder),
  mused, mus′ing
  ♦mews
Muse (goddess)
  ♦mews
mu•se′um

mu•se′um•go′er
mush′room′
mush′y
mu′sic
mu′si•cal (of music)
mu′si•cale′ (concert)
mu•si′cian
mu•si′cian•ship′
mu′si•col′o•gist
mu′si•col′o•gy
musk
mus′kel•lunge′ pl.
  -lunge′ or -lung′es
mus′ket
mus′ket•eer′
mus′ket•ry
musk′mel′on
musk′rat′
Mus′lim
mus′lin
muss
mus′sel (shellfish)
  ♦muscle, muzzle
must
mus′tache′ also
  mous′tache′
mus•ta′chio pl.
  -chios
mus′tang′
mus′tard (plant)
  ♦mustered
mus′ter
must′y
mu′ta•bil′i•ty
mu′ta•ble
mu′tant
mu•tate′, -tat′ed, -tat′-

  ing
mu•ta′tion
mu′ta•tive
mute, mut′er, mut′est
mute, mut′ed, mut′ing
mu′ti•late′, -lat′ed,
  -lat′ing
mu′ti•la′tion
mu′ti•la′tor
mu′ti•neer′
mu′ti•nous
mu′ti•ny, -nied, -ny-
  ing
mutt
mut′ter
mut′ton (sheep)
  ♦mouton
mu′tu•al
mu′tu•al′i•ty
muu′muu′
muz′zle (to restrain),
  -zled, -zling
  ♦muscle, mussel
my
my′as•the′ni•a
my•ce′li•um pl. -li•a
my′co•log′i•cal also
  my′co•log′ic
my•col′o•gist
my•col′o•gy
my•co′sis pl. -ses′
my′e•lin also my′-
  e•line
my′na or my′nah
my′o•car′di•al
my′o•car′di•um
my•o′pi•a

my•op'ic
myr'i•ad
myr'mi•don'
myrrh
myr'tle
my•self'
mys•te'ri•ous
mys'ter•y
mys'tic
mys'ti•cal
mys'ti•cism
mys'ti•fi•ca'tion
mys'ti•fy', -fied', -fy'-
ing
mys•tique'
myth'i•cal
myth'o•log'i•cal
also myth'o•log'ic
my•thol'o•gist
my•thol'o•gy

N

nab, nabbed, nab'bing
na'bob'
na•celle'
na'cre
na'cre•ous
na'dir
nag, nagged, nag'ging
nag'ger
nai'ad pl. -a•des' or
-ads
nail
na•ive' or na•îve',
also na•if' or na•îf'
na'ive•té' or na'îve-

té'
na'ked
nam'a•ble also name'-
a•ble
nam'by-pam'by
name, named, nam'-
ing
name'less
name•ly
name'sake'
name'tag'
name'tape'
nan•keen'
nan'ny
nap, napped, nap'ping
na'palm'
nape
na'per•y
naph'tha
naph'tha•lene'
nap'kin
na•po'le•on (pastry)
Na•po'le•on'ic
nap'time'
nar'cis•sism
nar'cis•sist
nar'cis•sis'tic
nar•cis'sus pl. -sus•es
or -si'
nar'co•dol'lar
nar•co'sis
nar•cot'ic
nard
nar'rate', -rat'ed, -rat'-
ing
nar•ra'tion
nar'ra•tive

nar'ra'tor also nar'-
rat'er
nar'row
nar'row•back'
nar'row•cast', -cast',
-cast'ing
nar'row-gauge' also
nar'row-gauged'
nar'row-mind'ed
nar'whal
nar'y
na'sal
na•sal'i•ty
nas'cence
nas'cent
na•stur'tium
nas'ty
na'tal
na'tion
na'tion•al
na'tion•al•ism
na'tion•al•ist
na'tion•al•is'tic
na'tion•al•i•ty
na'tion•al•i•za'tion
na'tion•al•ize',
-ized', -iz'ing
na'tion•wide'
na'tive
na'tive-born' adj.
na•tiv'i•ty
nat'ty
nat'u•ral
nat'u•ral•ism
nat'u•ral•ist
nat'u•ral•is'tic
nat'u•ral•i•za'tion

nat′u•ral•ize′, -ized′,
 -iz′ing
nat′u•ral•ly
na′ture
naught *also* nought
naugh′ty
nau•se•a
nau′se•ate′, -at′ed,
 -at′ing
nau′seous *(causing
 sickness)*
nau′ti•cal
nau′ti•lus *pl.* -lus•es
 or -li′
na′val *(nautical)*
 ♦*navel*
nave *(part of a
 church)*
 ♦*knave*
na′vel *(bellybutton)*
 ♦*naval*
nav′i•ga•bil′i•ty
nav′i•ga•ble
nav′i•gate′, -gat′ed,
 -gat′ing
nav′i•ga′tion
nav′i•ga′tor
na′vy
nay *(no)*
 ♦*née, neigh*
nay′say′, -said′, -say′-
 ing
nay′say′er
Na′zi *pl.* -zis
Na′zism *also* Na′zi-
 ism
Ne•an′der•thal′

Ne′a•pol′i•tan
neap tide
near′by′
near′ly
near′sight′ed
neat′ly
neat′s′-foot′ oil
neb′bish
Ne•bras′kan
neb′u•la *pl.* -lae′ *or*
 -las
neb′u•lar
neb′u•los′i•ty
neb′u•lous
nec′es•sar′i•ly
nec′es•sar′y
ne•ces′si•tate′, -tat′-
 ed, -tat′ing
ne•ces′si•ta′tion
ne•ces′si•tous
ne•ces′si•ty
neck′band′
neck′er•chief
neck′lace
neck′line′
neck′piece′
neck′tie′
neck′wear′
ne•crol′o•gy
nec′ro•man′cer
nec′ro•man′cy
ne•crop′o•lis *pl.* -lis-
 es *or* -leis′
nec′tar
nec′tar•ine′
née *(born), also* nee
 ♦*nay, neigh*

need *(requirement)*
 ♦*knead, kneed*
nee′dle, -dled, -dling
nee′dle•craft′
nee′dle•fish′ *pl.* -fish′
 or -fish′es
nee′dle•point′
need′less
nee′dle•work′
need′n′t
need′y
ne′er′-do-well′
ne•far′i•ous
ne•gate′, -gat′ed, -gat′-
 ing
ne•ga′tion
neg′a•tive, -tived,
 -tiv′ing
neg′a•tiv•ism
neg′a•tiv•ist
neg′a•tiv•is′tic
ne•glect′
ne•glect′ful
neg′li•gee′ *also* neg′-
 li•gée′
neg′li•gence
neg′li•gent
neg′li•gi•bil′i•ty
neg′li•gi•ble
ne•go′tia•bil′i•ty
ne•go′tia•ble
ne•go′ti•ate′, -at′ed,
 -at′ing
ne•go′ti•a′tion
ne•go′ti•a′tor
Ne′gro *pl.* -groes
Ne′groid′

neigh *(horse's cry)*
 ♦*nay, née*
neigh'bor
neigh'bor•hood'
neigh'bor•ly
nei'ther *(not either)*
 ♦*nether*
nek'ton
nek•ton'ic
nel'son
nem'a•to•cyst'
nem'a•tode'
Nem'bu•tal'®
nem'e•sis *pl.* -ses'
ne'o•clas'sic *also* ne'-
 o•clas'si•cal
ne'o•clas'si•cism
ne'o•clas'si•cist
ne'o•co•lo'ni•al•ist
ne'o•con•ser'va-
 tism
ne'o•dym'i•um
ne'o•fas'cism
ne'o•im•pres'sion-
 ism
ne'o•im•pres'sion-
 ist
ne'o•lib'er•al•ism
Ne'o•lith'ic
ne•ol'o•gism
ne'o•my'cin
ne'on'
ne'o•na'tal
ne'o•nate'
Ne'o-Na'zi
ne'o•phyte'
ne'o•plasm

ne'o•prene'
Nep'al•ese' *pl.* -ese'
ne•pen'the
neph'ew
neph'rite'
ne•phri'tis
nep'o•tism
nep'o•tis'tic *also*
 nep'o•tis'ti•cal
Nep'tune'
nep•tu'ni•um
ner•va'tion
nerve'-rack'ing *also*
 nerve'-wrack'ing
nerv'ous
nerv'y
nes'tle, -tled, -tling
nest'ling *(young bird)*
net, net'ted, net'ting
net'back'
neth'er *(below)*
 ♦*neither*
neth'er•most'
net'su•ke'
net'ting
net'tle, -tled, -tling
net'tle•some
net'work'
net'work'ing
Neuf'châ•tel'
neu'ral
neu•ral'gia
neu•ral'gic
neu•ras•the'ni•a
neu•ri'tis
neu'ro•bi•ol'o•gy

neu'ro•chem'is•try
neu'ro•log'i•cal
neu•rol'o•gist
neu•rol'o•gy
neu'ron'
neu'ro•pa•thol'o•gy
neu•rop'ter•an
neu•ro'sis *pl.* -ses'
neu•rot'ic
neu'ter
neu'tral
neu'tral•ism
neu'tral•ist
neu•tral'i•ty
neu'tral•i•za'tion
neu'tral•ize', -ized',
 -iz'ing
neu•tri'no *pl.* -nos
neu'tron'
Ne•vad'an
nev'er
nev'er•more'
nev'er•the•less'
ne'void'
ne'vus *pl.* -vi'
new *(recent)*
 ♦*gnu, knew*
new'born'
new'com'er
new'el
New Eng'land•er
new'fan'gled
New'found•land•er
New Hamp'shir•ite'
New Jer'sey•ite'
new'ly-wed' *also*
 new'ly•wed'

New Mex'i•can
news'boy'
news'cast'
news'gath'er•ing
news'let'ter
news'mak'er
news'man'
news'pa'per
news'print'
news'reel'
news'stand'
news'wor'thy
news'y
newt
new'ton
New York'er
next
nex'us *pl.* -us *or* -us-
   es
ni'a•cin
nib
nib'ble, -bled, -bling
Nic'a•ra'guan
nice *(pleasing),* nic'er,
   nic'est
   ♦*gneiss*
ni'ce•ty
niche *(recess)*
nick *(notch)*
nick'el
nick'el•o'de•on
nick'name', -named',
   -nam'ing
nic'o•tine'
nic'o•tin'ic
niece
nif'ty

Ni•ger'i•an
nig'gard•ly
nig'gling
nigh
night *(darkness)*
   ♦*knight*
night'cap'
night'clothes'
night'club'
night'dress'
night'fall'
night'gown'
night'hawk'
night'in•gale'
night'mare'
night'rid'er
night'shade'
night'shirt'
night'spot'
night'stick'
night'time'
ni'hil•ism
ni'hil•ist
ni'hil•is'tic
nil
nim'ble
nim'bo•stra'tus
nim'bus *pl.* -bi' *or*
   -bus•es
nin'com•poop'
nine'pin'
nine•teen'
nine•teenth'
nine'ti•eth
nine'ty
nin'ja
nin'ny

ninth
ni•o'bi•um
nip, nipped, nip'ping
nip'per
nip'ple
nip'py
nir•va'na
Ni•sei' *pl.* -sei' *or*
   -seis'
nit *(insect egg)*
   ♦*knit*
ni'ter
nit'-pick'
ni'trate', -trat'ed,
   -trat'ing
ni•tra'tion
ni'tric
ni'tride'
ni'tri•fi•ca'tion
ni'tri•fy', -fied', -fy'-
   ing
ni'trite'
ni'tro•bac•te'ri•a
ni'tro•ben'zene'
ni'tro•cel'lu•lose'
ni'tro•gen
ni•trog'e•nous
ni'tro•glyc'er•in *also*
   ni'tro•glyc'er•ine
ni'trous
nit'ty-grit'ty
nit'wit'
nix
no *pl.* noes
no•bel'i•um
No•bel' Prize
no•bil'i•ty

no'ble
no'ble•man
no•blesse' o•blige'
no'ble•wom'an
no'bod'y
noc•tur'nal
noc'turne'
nod, nod'ded, nod'-
　ding
nod'al
nod'der
node
nod'u•lar
nod'ule
No•ël' *also* No•el'
no'-fault' *adj.*
nog'gin
no'-hit'ter
noise, noised, nois'ing
noise'less
noise'mak'er
noi'some
nois'y
no'mad'
no'mad'ic
nom' de plume'
no'men•cla'ture
nom'i•nal
nom'i•nate', -nat'ed,
　-nat'ing
nom'i•na'tion
nom'i•na'tive
nom'i•na'tor
nom'i•nee'
non'age
non'a•ge•nar'i•an
non'ag•gres'sion

non'a•gon'
non'al•co•hol'ic
non'a•ligned'
non'as•sess'a•ble
nonce
non'cha•lance'
non'cha•lant'
non'com'
non'com•bat'ant
non'com•mis'-
　sioned officer
non'com•mit'tal
non'com•pet'i•tive
non'com•pli'ance
non'con•duc'tor
non'con•form'ist
non'con•form'i•ty
non'de•nom'i•na'-
　tion•al
non'de•script'
none *(not one)*
　♦*nun*
non•en'ti•ty
none'such'
none'the•less'
non'-Eu•clid'e•an
non'ex•ist'ence
non'ex•ist'ent
non•fea'sance
non•fer'rous
non•fic'tion
non•flam'ma•ble
　(not easily burned)
　♦*flammable,*
　inflammable
no•nil'lion
no•nil'lionth

non'in•ter•ven'tion
non'in•ter•ven'-
　tion•ist
non•ju'ror
non•mem'ber
non•met'al
non'me•tal'lic
non'ne•go'tia•ble
non'ob•jec'tive
no-non'sense' *adj.*
non'pa•reil'
non•par'ti•san
non•plus', -plused' *or*
　-plussed', -plus'ing
　or -plus'sing
non'pre•scrip'tion
non'pro•duc'tive
non•prof'it
non'pro•lif'er•
　a'tion
non're•cov'er•a•ble
non'rep•re•sen'ta'-
　tion•al
non'res'i•dent
non're•sis'tant
non're•stric'tive
non'sched'uled
non'sec•tar'i•an
non'sense'
non•sen'si•cal
non se'qui•tur
non'sked'
non'skid'
non•smok'er
non•smok'ing
non'stan'dard
non'stop'

non'sup•port'
non•un'ion
non•ver'bal
non•vi'o•lence
non•vi'o•lent
noo'dle
nook
noon'day'
no one *also* no'-one'
noon'tide'
noon'time'
noose
no'-par' *adj.*
nor
Nor'dic
norm
nor'mal
nor'mal•cy
nor•mal'i•ty
nor'mal•i•za'tion
nor'mal•ize', -ized',
  -iz'ing
nor'ma•tive
Norse *pl.* Norse
Norse'man
North A•mer'i•can
north'bound'
North Car'o•lin'-
  i•an
North Da•ko'tan
north•east'
north•east'er
north•east'er•ly
north•east'ern
north•east'ward *also*
  north•east'wards
north'er•ly

north'ern
north'ern•er
north'ern•most'
north'land'
north'-north•east'
north'-north•west'
north'ward *also*
  north'wards
north•west'
north•west'er•ly
north•west'ern
north•west'ward
  also north•west'-
  wards
Nor•we'gian
nose, nosed, nos'ing
nose'bleed'
nose'-dive', -dived'
  or -dove', -div'ing
nose'gay'
nose'piece'
nosh
no'-show' *n.*
nos•tal'gi•a
nos•tal'gic
nos'tril
nos'trum
nos'y *also* nos'ey
not *(in no way)*
  ♦knot
no'ta be'ne
no'ta•bil'i•ty
no'ta•ble
no'ta•ri•za'tion
no'ta•rize', -rized',
  -riz'ing
no'ta•ry

notary public *pl.*
  notaries public
no•ta'tion
notch
note, not'ed, not'ing
note'book'
note'wor'thy
noth'ing
noth'ing•ness
no'tice, -ticed, -tic-
  ing
no'tice•a•ble
no'ti•fi•ca'tion
no'ti•fy', -fied', -fy'-
  ing
no'tion
no'to•chord'
no'to•ri'e•ty
no•to'ri•ous
no'-trump'
not'with•stand'ing
nou'gat
noun
nour'ish
nour'ish•ment
nou'veau riche' *pl.*
  nou'veaux riches'
no'va *pl.* -vae *or* -vas
No'va Sco'tian
nov'el
nov'el•ette'
nov'el•ist
nov'el•is'tic
no•vel'la *pl.* -las *or*
  -le
nov'el•ty
No•vem'ber

no•ve'na *pl.* -nas *or*
-nae
nov'ice
no•vi'ti•ate
now'a•days'
no'way' *also* no'ways'
no'where'
no'wise'
nox'ious
noz'zle
nu'ance'
nub'bin
nub'ble
nu'bile
nu'cle•ar
nu'cle•ase'
nu'cle•ate', -at'ed,
-at'ing
nu'cle•a'tion
nu•cle'ic acid
nu•cle'o•lar
nu•cle'o•lus *pl.* -li'
nu'cle•on'
nu'cle•on'ic
nu'cle•on'ics
nu'cle•o•pro'tein
nu'cle•o•side'
nu'cle•o•tide'
nu'cle•us *pl.* -cle•i'
nude
nudge, nudged, nudg'-
ing
nud'ism
nud'ist
nu'di•ty
nug'get
nui'sance

nuke
null
nul'li•fi•ca'tion
nul'li•fi'er
nul'li•fy', -fied', -fy'-
ing
nul'li•ty
numb *(insensible)*,
numb'er, numb'est
num'ber *(integer,*
symbol, quantity)
num'ber•less
numb'ness
nu'mer•a•ble
nu'mer•al
nu'mer•ate', -at'ed,
-at'ing
nu'mer•a'tion
nu'mer•a'tor
nu•mer'i•cal *also*
nu•mer'ic
nu'mer•o•log'i•cal
nu'mer•ol'o•gist
nu'mer•ol'o•gy
nu'mer•ous
nu'mis•mat'ic
nu'mis•mat'ics
nu•mis'ma•tist
num'skull' *also*
numb'skull'
nun *(religious sister)*
♦*none*
nun'ci•o' *pl.* -os'
nun'ner•y
nup'tial
nurse, nursed, nurs'-
ing

nurse'maid' *also*
nurs'er•y•maid'
nurs'er•y
nurs'er•y•man
nurs'ling
nur'ture, -tured, -tur-
ing
nut'crack'er
nut'hatch'
nut'meat'
nut'meg'
nu'tri•a
nu'tri•ent
nu'tri•ment
nu'tri•men'tal
nu•tri'tion
nu•tri'tion•al
nu•tri'tion•ist
nu'tri•tive
nut'shell'
nut'ty
nuz'zle, -zled, -zling
ny'lon'
nymph
nym•phet'
nym'pho•ma'ni•a
nym'pho•ma'ni•ac'

O

oaf *pl.* oafs
oak'en
oa'kum
oar *(pole)*
♦*o'er, or, ore*
oar'lock'

oars'man
oars'wom'an
o•a'sis *pl.* -ses'
oat'en
oath *pl.* oaths
oat'meal'
ob'du•ra•cy
ob'du•rate
o•be'di•ence
o•be'di•ent
o•bei'sance
o•bei'sant
ob'e•lisk
o•bese'
o•be'si•ty
o•bey'
ob'fus•cate', -cat'ed,
  -cat'ing
ob'fus•ca'tion
o'bi *pl.* o'bis
o'bit
o'bi•ter dic'tum *pl.*
  o'bi•ter dic'ta
o•bit'u•ar'y
ob'ject *n.*
ob•ject' *v.*
ob•jec'tion
ob•jec'tion•a•ble
ob•jec'tive
ob'jec•tiv'i•ty
ob•jec'tor
o'blast
ob'late'
ob•la'tion
ob'li•gate', -gat'ed,
  -gat'ing
ob'li•ga'tion

ob'li•ga'tor
o•blig'a'to•ry
o•blige', o•bliged',
  o•blig'ing
o•blique'
o•bliq'ui•ty
o•blit'er•ate', -at'ed,
  -at'ing
o•blit'er•a'tion
o•blit'er•a'tor
o•bliv'i•on
o•bliv'i•ous
ob'long'
ob'lo•quy
ob•nox'ious
o'boe
o'bo•ist
ob•scene'
ob•scen'i•ty
ob•scur'ant
ob•scur'ant•ism
ob•scure', -scur'er,
  -scur'est
ob•scure', -scured',
  -scur'ing
ob•scu'ri•ty
ob•se'qui•ous
ob'se•quy
ob•serv'a•ble
ob•ser'vance
ob•ser'vant
ob'ser•va'tion
ob•ser'va•to'ry
ob•serve', -served',
  -serv'ing
ob•sess'
ob•ses'sion

ob•ses'sive
ob•sid'i•an
ob'so•les'cence
ob'so•les'cent
ob'so•lete'
ob'sta•cle
ob•stet'ric *also* ob-
  stet'ri•cal
ob•ste•tri'cian
ob•stet'rics
ob'sti•na•cy
ob'sti•nate
ob•strep'er•ous
ob•struct'
ob•struct'er *also* ob-
  struc'tor
ob•struc'tion
ob•struc'tion•ism
ob•struc'tion•ist
ob•struc'tive
ob•tain'
ob•tain'a•ble
ob•trude', -trud'ed,
  -trud'ing
ob•tru'sion
ob•tru'sive
ob•tuse'
ob•verse' *adj.*
ob'verse' *n.*
ob•ver'sion
ob•vert'
ob'vi•ate', -at'ed, -at'-
  ing
ob'vi•a'tion
ob'vi•a'tor
ob'vi•ous
oc'a•ri'na

oc•ca'sion
oc•ca'sion•al
oc•ci•dent *also* Oc'-
  ci•dent
oc•ci•den'tal *or* Oc'-
  ci•den'tal
oc•cip'i•tal
oc•clude', -clud'ed,
  -clud'ing
oc•clu'sion
oc•clu'sive
oc•cult'
oc•cul'ta'tion
oc•cult'ism
oc•cult'ist
oc'cu•pan•cy
oc'cu•pant
oc'cu•pa'tion
oc'cu•pa'tion•al
oc'cu•pi'er
oc'cu•py', -pied', -py'-
  ing
oc•cur', -curred',
  -cur'ring
oc•cur'rence
oc•cur'rent
o'cean
o'cean•front'
o'ce•an'ic
o'cean•og'ra•pher
o'cean•o•graph'ic
  also o'cean•o•graph'-
  i•cal
o'cean•og'ra•phy
oc'e•lot'
o'cher *or* o'chre
o'clock'

o'co•ti'llo *pl.* -llos
oc'ta•gon'
oc•tag'o•nal
oc•ta•he'dral
oc•ta•he'dron *pl.*
  -drons *or* -dra
oc'tane'
oc'tant
oc'tave
oc•ta'vo *pl.* -vos
oc•tet'
oc•til'lion
Oc•to'ber
oc'to•ge•nar'i•an
oc'to•pus *pl.* -pus•es
  or -pi'
oc'u•lar
oc'u•list
o'da•lisque' *also*
  o'da•lisk'
odd'ball'
odd'i•ty
odd'ment
odds
odds'mak'er
ode *(poem)*
  ♦*owed*
o'di•ous
o'di•um
o•dom'e•ter
o'dor
o'dor•if'er•ous
o'dor•ous
od'ys•sey *(journey),*
  pl. -seys
Od'ys•sey *(epic)*
oed'i•pal *also* Oed'-

  i•pal
Oed'i•pus complex
o'er *(over)*
  ♦*oar, or, ore*
of
of'fal *(refuse)*
  ♦*awful*
off'beat'
off'-Broad'way'
off'-col'or
of•fend'
of•fense' *(violation)*
of'fense' *(attacking)*
of•fen'sive
of'fer
of'fer•er *also* of'fer-
  or
of'fer•to'ry
off'hand'
of'fice
of'fice•hold'er
of'fi•cer
of•fi'cial *(authorized)*
  ♦*officious*
of•fi'cial•dom
of•fi'ci•ant
of•fi'ci•ate', -at'ed,
  -at'ing
of•fi'ci•a'tor
of•fi'cious *(meddle-
  some)*
  ♦*official*
off'ing
off'-line'
off'peak'
off'set', -set", -set'ting
off'shoot'

off 'shore'
off 'side'
off 'spring'
off '-stage'
off '-the-rec'ord *adj.*
off '-the-wall' *adj.*
off '-track'
off '-white'
oft
of 'ten
of 'ten•times' *also*
  oft'times'
o'gee'
o'gle, o'gled, o'gling
o'gre
oh *(exclamation)*
  ♦*owe*
O•hi'o•an
ohm
ohm'me'ter
oil'cloth'
oil'skin'
oil'stone'
oil'y
oint'ment
O.K. *or* OK *or*
  o•kay' *pl.* O.K.'s *or*
  OK's *or* o•kays'
O.K. *or* OK *or*
  o•kay', O.K.'d *or*
  OK'd *or* o•kayed',
  O.K.'ing *or* OK'ing
  or o•kay'ing
o•ka'pi *pl.* -pi *or* -pis
O'kla•ho'man
o'kra
old'en

old'-fash'ioned *adj.*
old'-line'
old'ster
old'-time'
old'-tim'er
old'-world' *also*
  Old'-World'
o'le•ag'i•nous
o'le•an'der
o'le•fin
o•le'ic
o'le•o•mar'ga•rine
o'le•o•res'in
ol•fac'to•ry
ol'i•garch'
ol'i•gar'chic *also* ol'-
  i•gar'chi•cal
ol'i•gar'chy
Ol'i•go•cene'
ol'i•gop'o•ly
o'li•o' *pl.* -os
ol'ive
ol'i•vine'
O•lym'pi•ad'
O•lym'pi•an
O•lym'pic
om'buds•man
o•me'ga
om'e•let *also* om'-
  e•lette
o'men
om'i•nous
o•mis'sion
o•mit', o•mit'ted,
  o•mit'ting
om'ni•bus' *pl.*
  -bus'es

om•nip'o•tence *also*
  om•nip'o•ten•cy
om•nip'o•tent
om'ni•pres'ence
om'ni•pres'ent
om•nis'cience *also*
  om•nis'cien•cy
om•nis'cient
om'ni•vore'
om•niv'o•rous
on•board' *adj.*
once'-o'ver
on'com'ing
one *(single)*
  ♦*won*
one'-lin'er
one'-on-one'
on'er•ous
one•self '
one'-sid'ed
one'time'
one'-to-one'
one'-track'
one-up'man•ship'
one'-way'
on'go'ing
on'ion
on'ion•skin'
on'-line' *adj.*
on'look'er
on'ly
on'o•mat'o•poe'ia
on'o•mat'o•poe'ic
  also on'o•mat'o•po-
  et'ic
on'rush'
on'set'

on'shore'
on'side'
on'slaught'
on'to'
on•to•log'i•cal
on•tol'o•gy
o'nus
on'ward *also* on'-
wards
on'yx
oo'dles
oo'long'
oomph
ooze, oozed, ooz'ing
ooz'y
o•pac'i•ty
o'pal
o'pal•es'cence
o'pal•es'cent
o•paque'
op art
op-ed' page
o'pen
o'pen-air'
o'pen-and-shut' *adj.*
o'pen-end'
o'pen-end'ed
o'pen•er
o'pen-eyed'
o'pen•hand'ed
o'pen-heart' *adj.*
o'pen•heart'ed
o'pen-hearth'
o'pen•ing
o'pen-mind'ed
o'pen•work'
op'er•a

op'er•a•bil'i•ty
op'er•a•ble
op'er•and
op'er•ate', -at•ed, -at'-
ing
op'er•at'ic
op'er•a'tion
op'er•a'tion•al
op'er•a•tive
op'er•a'tor
op'e•ret'ta
o•phid'i•an
oph•thal'mic
oph•thal'mo•log'ic
also oph•thal'mo-
log'i•cal
oph'thal•mol'o•gist
oph'thal•mol'o•gy
o'pi•ate', -at•ed, -at'-
ing
o•pine', o•pined',
o•pin'ing
o•pin'ion
o•pin'ion•at•ed
o'pi•um
o•pos'sum *pl.* -sum
or -sums, *also* pos'-
sum
op•po'nent
op'por•tune'
op'por•tun'ism
op'por•tun'ist
op'por•tun•is'tic
op'por•tu'ni•ty
op•pos'a•ble
op•pose', -posed',
-pos'ing

op'po•site
op'po•si'tion
op•press'
op•pres'sion
op•pres'sive
op•pres'sor
op•pro'bri•ous
op•pro'bri•um
opt
op'tic
op'ti•cal
op•ti'cian
op'tics
op'ti•mal
op'ti•mism
op'ti•mist
op'ti•mis'tic
op'ti•mi•za'tion
op'ti•mize', -mized',
-miz'ing
op'ti•mum *pl.* -ma *or*
-mums
op'tion
op'tion•al
op•tom'e•trist
op•tom'e•try
op'u•lence *also* op'-
u•len•cy
op'u•lent
o'pus *pl.* op'er•a *or*
o'pus•es
or *conj.*
♦*oar, o'er, ore*
or'a•cle *(seer)*
♦*auricle*
o•rac'u•lar
o'ral *(spoken)*

♦*aural*
or′ange
or′ange•ade′
o•rang′u•tan′ *also*
  o•rang′ou•tan′
o•rate′, o•rat′ed,
  o•rat′ing
o•ra′tion
or′a•tor
or′a•tor′i•cal
or′a•to′ri•o′ *pl.* -os′
or′a•to′ry
orb
or•bic′u•lar
or′bit
or′bit•al
or′bit•eer′
or′chard
or′ches•tra
or•ches′tral
or′ches•trate′, -trat′-
  ed, -trat′ing
or′ches•tra′tion
or′chid
or•dain′
or•deal′
or′der
or′der•ly
or′di•nal
or′di•nance *(com-
  mand)*
  ♦*ordnance*
or′di•nar′i•ly
or′di•nar′y
or′di•nate
or′di•na′tion
ord′nance *(military*

supplies)
  ♦*ordinance*
Or′do•vi′cian
or′dure
ore *(mineral)*
  ♦*oar, o′er, or*
o•reg′a•no
Or′e•go′ni•an
or′gan
or′gan•dy *also* or′-
  gan•die
or′gan•elle′
or•gan′ic
or•gan′i•cism
or′gan•ism
or′gan•is′mal *also*
  or′gan•is′mic
or′gan•ist
or′gan•i•za′tion
or′gan•ize′, -ized′,
  -iz′ing
or•gan′za
or′gasm
or′gi•as′tic
or′gy
o′ri•el
o′ri•ent *(to align)*
O′ri•ent *(Asia)*
o′ri•en′tal *also* O′ri-
  en′tal
o′ri•en•ta′tion
or′i•fice
o′ri•ga′mi
or′i•gin
o•rig′i•nal
o•rig′i•nal•ism
o•rig′i•nal′i•ty

o•rig′i•nate′, -nat′ed,
  -nat′ing
o•rig′i•na′tion
o•rig′i•na′tor
o′ri•ole′
Or′lon′®
or′mo•lu′
or′na•ment
or′na•men′tal
or′na•men•ta′tion
or•nate′
or′ner•y
or•ni•tho•log′ic *also*
  or′ni•tho•log′i•cal
or′ni•thol′o•gist
or′ni•thol′o•gy
o′ro•tund′
or′phan
or′phan•age
or′pi•ment
or′ris•root′
or•thi′con′
or′tho•clase′
or′tho•don′tia
or′tho•don′tic
or′tho•don′tist
or′tho•dox′
or′tho•dox′y
or•thog′o•nal
or′tho•graph′ic
or•thog′ra•phy
or′tho•pe′dic
or′tho•pe′dics
or′tho•pe′dist
o′ryx *pl.* o′ryx•es *or*
  o′ryx
Os′car

os'cil•late' *(to swing
  back and forth)*, -lat'-
  ed, -lat'ing
  ♦*osculate*
os'cil•la'tion
os'cil•la'tor
os'cil•la•to'ry
os•cil'lo•scope'
os•cil'lo•scop'ic
os'cine
os'cu•late' *(to kiss)*,
  -lat'ed, -lat'ing
  ♦*oscillate*
os'cu•la'tion
o'sier
os'mi•um
os•mo'sis
os•mot'ic
os'prey *pl.* -preys
os'se•ous
os'si•fi•ca'tion
os'si•fy', -fied', -fy'-
  ing
os•ten'si•ble
os'ten•ta'tion
os'ten•ta'tious
os'te•o•path'
os'te•o•path'ic
os'te•op'a•thy
os'tra•cism
os'tra•cize', -cized',
  -ciz'ing
os'trich
Os'tro•goth'
oth'er
oth'er•wise'
oth'er•world'ly

o'ti•ose'
o'to•lar'yn•gol'o•gy
o•tol'o•gy
ot'ter *pl.* -ter *or* -ters
ot'to•man *pl.* -mans
ou'bli•ette'
ouch
ought *auxiliary*
  ♦*aught*
ounce
our *pron.*
  ♦*hour*
ours *pron.*
  ♦*hours*
our•self'
our•selves'
oust'er
out'-and-out' *adj.*
out'back'
out•bal'ance, -anced,
  -anc•ing
out•bid', -bid', -bid'-
  den *or* -bid', -bid'-
  ding
out'board'
out'bound'
out'break'
out'build'ing
out'burst'
out'cast'
out•class'
out'come'
out'crop', -cropped',
  -crop'ping
out'cry'
out•dat'ed
out•dis'tance,

-tanced, -tanc•ing
out•do', -did', -done',
  -do'ing, -does
out'door'
out•doors'
out•doors'y
out'er
out'er•most'
out'er•wear'
out•face', -faced',
  -fac'ing
out'field'
out•fit', -fit'ted, -fit'-
  ting
out'fit'ter
out•flank'
out'flow'
out•fox'
out'go' *pl.* -goes'
out•go', -went',
  -gone', -go'ing, -goes
out•grow', -grew',
  -grown', -grow'ing
out'growth'
out•guess'
out•gun', -gunned',
  -gun'ning
out'house'
out'ing
out'land'er
out•land'ish
out•last'
out'law'
out'lay'
out'let'
out'line', -lined', -lin'-
  ing

out•live', -lived', -liv'-
ing
out'look'
out'ly'ing
out'ma•neu'ver
out•match'
out'-mi'grate, -grat-
ed, -grat•ing
out'-mi•gra'tion
out•mod'ed
out•num'ber
out'-of-date' adj.
out•pace', -paced',
-pac'ing
out'pa'tient
out•place', -placed',
-plac'ing
out'play'
out'post'
out'pour'ing
out'put'
out•rage', -raged',
-rag'ing
out•ra'geous
out•rank'
out•reach'
out'rid'er
out'rig'ger
out'right'
out•run', -ran', -run',
-run'ning
out•sell', -sold', -sell'-
ing
out'set'
out•shine', -shone',
-shin'ing
out•side'

out•sid'er
out•size' also out'-
sized'
out'skirts'
out•smart'
out•spo'ken
out'spread' adj.
out'spread' n.
out•spread', -spread',
-spread'ing
out'stand'ing
out'sta'tion
out'stay'
out•stretch'
out•strip', -stripped',
-strip'ping
out•vote', -vot'ed,
-vot'ing
out'ward also out'-
wards
out•wear', -wore',
-worn', -wear'ing
out•weigh'
out•wit', -wit'ted,
-wit'ting
out'work' n.
out•work' v.
ou'zel
o'val
o•var'i•an also
o•var'i•al
o'va•ry
o'vate'
o•va'tion
ov'en
ov'en•bird'
ov'en•ware'

o'ver
o'ver•a•bun'dance
o'ver•a•bun'dant
o'ver•a•chieve',
-chieved', -chiev'ing
o'ver•act'
o'ver•age' adj.
o'ver•age n.
o'ver•all' also
o'ver-all'
o'ver•alls'
o'ver•am•bi'tious
o'ver•anx'ious
o'ver•arm'
o'ver•awe', -awed',
-aw'ing
o'ver•bal'ance,
-anced, -anc•ing
o'ver•bear'ing
o'ver•bid' n.
o'ver•bid', -bid',
-bid'den or -bid',
-bid'ding
o'ver•bite'
o'ver•blown'
o'ver•board'
o'ver•book'
o'ver•bur'den
o'ver•call' n.
o'ver•call' v.
o'ver•cap'i•tal•ize',
-ized', -iz'ing
o'ver•cast' adj. & n.
o'ver•cast', -cast'ed,
-cast'ing
o'ver•charge' n.
o'ver•charge',

-charged', -charg'ing
o'ver•coat'
o'ver•come', -came',
　-come', -com'ing
o'ver•com'pen•sate',
　-sat'ed, -sat'ing
o'ver•com'pen•sa'-
　tion
o'ver•con'fi•dence
o'ver•de•vel'op
o'ver•do' *(to do to
　excess)*, -did',
　-done', -do'ing,
　-does
　♦*overdue*
o'ver•dose' *n.*
o'ver•dose', -dosed',
　-dos'ing
o'ver•draft'
o'ver•draw', -drew',
　-drawn', -draw'ing
o'ver•dress'
o'ver•drive' *n.*
o'ver•drive', -drove',
　-driv'en, -driv'ing
o'ver•due' *(unpaid,
　past due)*
　♦*overdo*
o'ver•ea'ger
o'ver•eat', -ate', -eat'-
　ing
o'ver•ed'u•cate',
　-cat'ed, -cat'ing
o'ver•em'pha•sis
o'ver•es'ti•mate',
　-mat'ed, -mat'ing
o'ver•es'ti•ma'tion

o'ver•ex•ert'
o'ver•ex•er'tion
o'ver•ex•pose',
　-posed', -pos'ing
o'ver•ex•po'sure
o'ver•ex•tend'
o'ver•ex•ten'sion
o'ver•flow' *n.*
o'ver•flow' *v.*
o'ver•grow', -grew',
　-grown', -grow'ing
o'ver•growth'
o'ver•hand'
o'ver•hang' *n.*
o'ver•hang', -hung',
　-hang'ing
o'ver•haul' *n.*
o'ver•haul' *v.*
o'ver•head' *adj. & n.*
o'ver•head' *adv.*
o'ver•hear', -heard',
　-hear'ing
o'ver•heat'
o'ver•in•dulge',
　-dulged', -dulg'ing
o'ver•in•dul'gence
o'ver•in•dul'gent
o'ver•joyed'
o'ver•kill'
o'ver•land'
o'ver•lap' *n.*
o'ver•lap', -lapped',
　-lap'ping
o'ver•lay' *n.*
o'ver•lay', -laid', -lay'-
　ing
o'ver•leap', -leaped'

or -leapt', -leap'ing
o'ver•lie', -lay',
　-lain', -lay'ing
o'ver•load' *n.*
o'ver•load' *v.*
o'ver•long'
o'ver•look' *n.*
o'ver•look' *v.*
o'ver•lord'
o'ver•ly
o'ver•mas'ter
o'ver•match' *n.*
o'ver•match' *v.*
o'ver•much'
o'ver•night' *adj.*
o'ver•night' *adv.*
o'ver•pass' *n.*
o'ver•pass', -passed'
　or -past', -pass'ing
o'ver•pay', -paid',
　-pay'ing
o'ver•pay'ment
o'ver•play'
o'ver•pop'u•la'tion
o'ver•pow'er
o'ver•price', -priced'
　-pric'ing
o'ver•print' *n.*
o'ver•print' *v.*
o'ver•pro•duce',
　-duced', -duc'ing
o'ver•pro•duc'tion
o'ver•pro•tec'tive
o'ver•qual'i•fied
o'ver•rate', -rat'ed,
　-rat'ing
o'ver•reach'

o'ver•re•act'
o'ver•re•ac'tion
o'ver•ride', -rode',
  -rid'den, -rid'ing
o'ver•rule', -ruled',
  -rul'ing
o'ver•run' n.
o'ver•run', -ran',
  -run', -run'ning
o'ver•seas' (abroad)
  ♦oversees
o'ver•see', -saw',
  -seen', -see'ing
o'ver•se'er
o'ver•sell', -sold',
  -sell'ing
o'ver•shad'ow
o'ver•shirt'
o'ver•shoe'
o'ver•shoot', -shot',
  -shoot'ing
o'ver•shot' adj.
o'ver•sight'
o'ver•sim'pli•fi•ca'-
  tion
o'ver•sim'pli•fy',
  -fied', -fy'ing
o'ver•size' adj., also
  o'ver•sized'
o'ver•size' n.
o'ver•skirt'
o'ver•sleep', -slept',
  -sleep'ing
o'ver•staff'
o'ver•state', -stat'ed,
  -stat'ing
o'ver•stay'

o'ver•step',
  -stepped', -step'ping
o'ver•stock'
o'ver•stuff'
o'ver•sub•scribe',
  -scribed', -scrib'ing
o'ver•sub•scrip'tion
o•vert'
o'ver•take', -took',
  -tak'en, -tak'ing
o'ver•tax'
o'ver-the-count'er
  adj.
o'ver•throw' n.
o'ver•throw',
  -threw', -thrown',
  -throw'ing
o'ver•time'
o'ver•tone'
o'ver•top', -topped',
  -top'ping
o'ver•trick'
o'ver•trump'
o'ver•ture'
o'ver•turn' n.
o'ver•turn' v.
o'ver•use', -used',
  -us'ing
o'ver•view'
o'ver•ween'ing
o'ver•weigh'
o'ver•weight'
o'ver•whelm'
o'ver•work' n.
o'ver•work' v.
o'ver•wrought'
o'ver•zeal'ous

o'vi•duct'
o'vine'
o'vi•par'i•ty
o•vip'a•rous
o'vi•pos'i•tor
o'void' also o•voi'dal
o'vo•vi•vip'a•rous
o'vu•lar
o'vu•late', -lat'ed,
  -lat'ing
o'vu•la'tion
o'vule
o'vum pl. o'va
owe (to be indebted),
  owed, ow'ing
  ♦oh
owl'et
owl'ish
own'er
own'er•ship'
ox pl. ox'en
ox•al'ic acid
ox'al•is
ox'blood' red
ox'bow'
ox'eye'
ox'ford
ox'i•dant
ox'i•da'tion
ox'i•da'tive
ox'ide'
ox'i•di•za'tion
ox'i•dize', -dized',
  -diz'ing
ox'lip'
Ox•o'ni•an
ox'tail'

ox'y•a•cet'y•lene
ox'y•gen
ox'y•gen•ate', -at'ed,
-at'ing
ox'y•gen•a'tion
ox'y•gen'ic *also* ox-
yg'e•nous
ox'y•mo'ron' *pl.* -ra
o'yez'
oys'ter
o'zone'
o•zo'no•sphere'

P

pab'u•lum
pace, paced, pac'ing
pace'mak'er
pace'set'ter
pace'set'ting
pach'y•derm'
pach'y•san'dra
pa•cif'ic
pac'i•fi•ca'tion
pac'i•fi'er
pac'i•fism
pac'i•fist
pac'i•fy', -fied', -fy'-
ing
pack'age, -aged, -ag-
ing
pack'er
pack'et
pack'ing
pack'sack'
pack'sad'dle
pact *(treaty)*

♦*packed*
pad, pad'ded, pad'-
ding
pad'dle, -dled, -dling
pad'dle•fish' *pl.*
-fish' *or* -fish'es
pad'dock
pad'dy
pad'lock'
pa'dre
pae'an *(song)*
♦*peon*
pa•el'la
pa'gan
pa'gan•ism
page, paged, pag'ing
pag'eant
pag'eant•ry
page'boy'
pag'er
pag'i•nate', -nat'ed,
-nat'ing
pag'i•na'tion
pa•go'da
pail *(bucket)*
♦*pale*
pain *(suffering)*
♦*pane*
pain'ful
pain'kill'er
pain'kill'ing
pain'less
pains'tak'ing
paint'brush'
paint'er
paint'ing
pair *(set of two)*

♦*pare, pear*
pais'ley
pa•ja'mas
Pak'i•stan'i *pl.* -stan'-
is *or* -stan'i
pal, palled, pal'ling
pal'ace
pal'a•din
pal'an•quin'
pal'at•a•bil'i•ty
pal'at•a•ble
pal'a•tal
pal'ate *(roof of the
mouth)*
♦*palette, pallet*
pa•la'tial
pa•lat'i•nate'
pal'a•tine'
pa•lav'er
pale *(wan),* pal'er, pal'-
est
♦*pail*
pale *(picket)*
♦*pail*
pale *(to blanch, fence
in),* paled, pal'ing
♦*pail*
pale'face'
Pa'le•o•cene'
pa'le•og'ra•pher
pa'le•o•graph'ic *also*
pa'le•o•graph'i•cal
pa'le•og'ra•phy
Pa'le•o•lith'ic
pa'le•on•tol'o•gist
pa'le•on•tol'o•gy
Pa'le•o•zo'ic

Pal·es·tin'i·an

pal'ette *(board for paint)*
♦*palate, pallet*

pal'frey *pl.* -freys

pal'i·mo'ny

pal'imp·sest'

pal'in·drome'

pal'ing

pal'i·node'

pal'i·sade'

pall *(coffin cover)*
♦*pawl*

pall *(to grow dull)*
♦*pawl*

pal·la'di·um

pall'bear'er

pal'let *(tool, bed)*
♦*palate, palette*

pal'li·ate', -at'ed, -at'-
ing

pal'li·a'tion

pal'li·a'tive

pal'lid

pal'lor

palm

pal'mate' *also* pal'-
mat'ed

pal·met'to *pl.* -tos *or*
-toes

palm'ist *also* palm'is-
ter

palm'is·try

palm'y

pal'o·mi'no *pl.* -nos

palp

pal·pa·bil'i·ty

pal'pa·ble

pal'pate' *(to examine
by touch),* -pat'ed,
-pat'ing

pal'pi·tate' *(to
throb),* -tat'ed, -tat'-
ing

pal'pi·ta'tion

pal'sied

pal'sy

pal'ter

pal'try *(petty)*
♦*poultry*

pam'pa *pl.* -pas

pam'per

pam'phlet

pam'phlet·eer'

pan *(to wash, cook,
move a camera),*
panned, pan'ning

Pan *(god)*

pan·a·ce'a

pa·nache'

Pan·a·ma'ni·an

Pan'-A·mer'i·can

pan'a·tel'a

pan'-broil'

pan'cake' *(griddle
cake)*

Pan'-Cake' Make'-
Up'®

pan'chro·mat'ic

pan'cre·as

pan'cre·at'ic

pan'da

pan·dem'ic

pan·de·mo'ni·um

pan'der

Pan·do'ra's box

pan·dow'dy

pane *(sheet of glass)*
♦*pain*

pan'e·gyr'ic

pan'e·gyr'i·cal

pan'e·gyr'ist

pan'el, -eled *or* -elled,
-el·ing *or* -el·ling

pan'el·ist

pan'-fry', -fried', -fry'-
ing

pang

pan·go'lin

pan'gram

pan'han·dle, -dled,
-dling

pan'ic, -icked, -ick-
ing

pan'ick·y

pan'i·cle

pan'ic-strick'en

pan'nier

pan'o·ply

pan'o·ram'a

pan'o·ram'ic

pan'pipe'

pan'sy

pant

pan'ta·lets' *also* pan'-
ta·lettes'

pan'ta·loons'

pan'the·ism

pan'the·ist

pan'the·is'tic *also*
pan'the·is'ti·cal

pan'the•on'
pan'ther
pant'ies
pan'to•mime',
  -mimed', -mim'ing
pan'try
pants
pant'suit' *also* pants
  suit
pant'y•hose' *pl.*
  -hose'
pant'y•waist'
pan'zer
pap
pa'pa
pa'pa•cy
pa'pal
pa'pa•raz'zo *pl.* -zi
pa'paw' *also* paw'-
  paw'
pa•pa'ya
pa'per
pa'per•back'
pa'per•board'
pa'per•bound'
pa'per•boy'
pa'per•girl'
pa'per•hang'er
pa'per•knife'
pa'per•weight'
pa'per•work'
pa'pier-mâ•ché'
pa•pil'la *pl.* -lae
pap'il•lar'y
pa'pist
pa•poose'
pa•pri'ka

Pap'u•an New
  Guin'e•an
pa•py'rus *pl.* -rus•es
  or -ri'
par
par'a•ble
pa•rab'o•la
par'a•bol'ic *also* par-
  a•bol'i•cal
par'a•chute', -chut'-
  ed, -chut'ing
par'a•chut'ist
pa•rade', -rad'ed,
  -rad'ing
par'a•digm'
par'a•dise'
par'a•dox'
par'a•dox'i•cal
par'af•fin
par'a•gon'
par'a•graph'
Par'a•guay'an
par'a•keet'
par•al'de•hyde'
par'a•le'gal
par'al•lax'
par'al•lel', -leled' *or*
  -lelled', -lel•ing' *or*
  -lcl'ling
par'al•lel'e•pi'ped
par'al•lel•ism
par'al•lel'o•gram'
pa•ral'y•sis *pl.* -ses'
pa•ra•lyt'ic
pa•ra•lyze', -lyzed',
  -lyz'ing
par•a•me'ci•um *pl.*

  -ci•a *or* -ci•ums
par'a•med'ic
par'a•med'i•cal
pa•ram'e•ter *(con-*
  stant, limit)
  ♦*perimeter*
par'a•mil'i•tar'y
par'a•mount'
par'a•mour'
par'a•noi'a
par'a•noi'ac'
par'a•noid'
par'a•pet
par'a•pher•na'lia
par'a•phrase',
  -phrased', -phras'ing
par'a•ple'gi•a
par'a•ple'gic
par'a•pro•fes'sion-
  al
par'a•psy•chol'o•gy
par'a•site'
par'a•sit'ic *also* par-
  a•sit'i•cal
par'a•sit•ism
par'a•sit•ize', -ized',
  -iz'ing
par'a•sol'
par'a•sym'pa•thet'-
  ic nervous system
par'a•thi'on
par'a•thy'roid'
  gland
par'a•troop'er
par'a•troops'
par'a•ty'phoid'
  fever

par'boil'
par'cel *(to divide)*,
  -celed *or* -celled,
  -cel•ing *or* -cel•ling
  ♦*partial*
parch
Par•chee'si®
parch'ment
par'don
par'don•a•ble
pare *(to peel)*, pared,
  par'ing
  ♦*pair, pear*
par'e•gor'ic
pa•ren'chy•ma
par'ent
par•ent'age
pa•ren'tal
pa•ren'the•sis *pl.*
  -ses'
par'en•thet'i•cal
  also par'en•thet'ic
par'ent•hood'
par'ent•ing
pa•re'sis
pa•ret'ic
par' ex'cel•lence'
par•fait'
pa•ri'ah
pa•ri'e•tal
par'i-mu'tu•el
par'ish *(adminstrative*
  unit)
  ♦*perish*
pa•rish'ion•er
Pa•ri'sian

par'i•ty
par'ka
Par'kin•son's
  disease
park'land'
park'way'
par'lance
par'lay' *(bet)*
par'ley *(discussion)*,
  pl. -leys
par'lia•ment
par'lia•men•tar'-
  i•an
par'lia•men'ta•ry
par'lor
par'lous
Par'me•san'
pa•ro'chi•al
pa•ro'chi•al•ism
par'o•dy, -died, -dy•
  ing
pa•role', -roled', -rol'-
  ing
pa•rol'ee'
pa•rot'id gland
par'ox•ysm
par'ox•ys'mal
par•quet', -queted',
  -quet'ing
par'quet•ry
par'ri•cid'al
par'ri•cide'
par'rot
par'ry, -ried, -ry•ing
parse, parsed, pars'ing
par'sec'
par•si•mo'ni•ous

par•si'mo•ny
pars'ley
pars'nip'
par'son
par'son•age
Par'sons table
par•take', -took',
  -tak'en, -tak'ing
part'ed
par•terre'
par'tial *(incomplete)*
  ♦*parcel*
par'ti•al'i•ty
par•tic'i•pance
par•tic'i•pant
par•tic'i•pate', -pat'-
  ed, -pat'ing
par•tic'i•pa'tion
par•tic'i•pa'tor
par'ti•cip'i•al
par'ti•ci'ple
par'ti•cle
par'ti-col'ored
par•tic'u•lar
par•tic'u•lar'i•ty
par•tic'u•lar•i•za'-
  tion
par•tic'u•lar•ize',
  -ized', -iz'ing
par•tic'u•lar•ly
part'ing
par'ti•san
par'tite'
par•ti'tion
part'ly
part'ner
part'ner•ship'

par'tridge
part'-time' *adj.*
par•tu'ri•en•cy
par•tu'ri•ent
par•tu•ri'tion
par'ty
par'ty•go'er
par've•nu'
PAS•CAL'
pas'chal
pas' de deux' *pl.* pas'
　de deux'
pa'sha
pasque'flow'er
pass'a•ble *(capable of
　being passed)*
　♦*possible*
pas'sage
pas'sage•way'
pas'sant
pass'book'
pas•sé'
pas'sen•ger
pas'ser-by' *pl.* pas'-
　sers-by', *also* pas'-
　ser•by'
pas'ser•ine'
pas'si•ble *(sensitive)*
　♦*passable*
pas'sim
pass'ing
pas'sion
pas'sion•ate
pas'sion•flow'er
pas'sion•less
pas'sive
pas•siv'i•ty

pass'key'
Pass'o'ver
pass'port'
pass'-through' *n.*
pass'word'
past *(ago)*
　♦*passed*
pas'ta
paste, past'ed, past'-
　ing
paste'board'
pas•tel'
pas•tel'ist
pas'tern
paste'-up' *n.*
pas'teur•i•za'tion
pas'teur•ize', -ized',
　-iz'ing
pas•tiche'
pas•tille'
pas'time'
pas'tor
pas'tor•al
pas'tor•al•ize, -ized',
　-iz'ing
pas'tor•ate
pas•tra'mi
pas'try
pas'tur•age
pas'ture, -tured, -tur-
　ing
past'y *(pale)*
pas'ty *(pie)*
pat, pat'ted, pat'ting
patch'ou•li *pl.* -lis,
　also patch'ou•ly,
　pach'ou•li *pl.* -lis

patch'work'
pate *(head)*
pâ•té' *(meat paste)*
　♦*patty*
pâ•té' de foie gras'
pa•tel'la *pl.* -lae
pa•tel'lar *also* pa•tel'-
　late
pat'en
pat'ent
pat'ent•ee'
pa'ter•fa•mil'i•as
pa•ter'nal
pa•ter'nal•ism
pa•ter'nal•is'tic
pa•ter'ni•ty
pa'ter•nos'ter
path *pl.* paths
pa•thet'ic
path'find'er
path'o•gen
path'o•gen'ic
path'o•log'i•cal
pa•thol'o•gist
pa•thol'o•gy
pa'thos'
path'way'
pa'tience
pa'tient
pat'i•na
pat'i•o' *pl.* -os'
pa'tis•se•rie'
pat'ois' *pl.* -ois'
pa'tri•arch
pa'tri•ar'chal
pa'tri•ar'chy
pa•tri'cian

pat′ri•cid′al
pat′ri•cide′
pat′ri•lin′e•age
pat′ri•lin′e•al
pat′ri•mo′ni•al
pat′ri•mo′ny
pa′tri•ot
pa′tri•ot′ic
pa′tri•ot•ism
pa•trol′, -trolled′,
 -trol′ling
pa•trol′man
pa′tron
pa′tron•age
pa′tron•ize′, -ized′,
 -iz′ing
pa′tron•ess
pat′ro•nym′ic
pa•troon′
pat′sy
pat′ter
pat′tern
pat′tern•mak′er
pat′ty *(small cake or
 pie)*
 ♦*pâté*
pau′ci•ty
paunch′y
pau′per•ism
pau′per•i•za′tion
pau′per•ize′, -ized′,
 -iz′ing
pause *(to stop briefly)*,
 paused, paus′ing
 ♦*paws*
pa•vane′ *also* pa-
 van′

pave, paved, pav′ing
pave′ment
pa•vil′ion
paw
pawl *(hinged device)*
 ♦*pall*
pawn′bro′ker
pawn′shop′
pay, paid, pay′ing
pay′a•ble
pay′back′
pay′check′
pay′day′
pay•ee′
pay′load′
pay′mas′ter
pay′ment
pay′off′ *n.*
pay•o′la
pay′roll′
pea
peace *(calm)*
 ♦*piece*
peace′a•ble
peace′ful
peace′keep′er
peace′mak′er
peace′nik
peace′time′
peach′y
pea′cock′
pea′fowl′ *pl.* -fowl′ *or*
 -fowls′
pea′hen′
peak *(point)*
 ♦*peek, pique*
peaked *(pointed)*

peak′ed *(pale)*
peal *(ringing)*
 ♦*peel*
pea′nut′
pear *(fruit)*
 ♦*pair, pare*
pearl *(gem)*
 ♦*purl*
pearl′y
peas′ant
peas′ant•ry
pea′shoot′er
peat
pea′vey *pl.* -veys, *also*
 pea′vy
peb′ble, -bled, -bling
peb′bly
pe•can′
pec′ca•dil′lo *pl.* -loes
 or -los
pec′ca•ry
peck
peck′ing order
pec′tic *also* pec′tin-
 ous
pec′tin
pec′to•ral
pec′u•late′, -lat′ed,
 -lat′ing
pec′u•la′tion
pec′u•la′tor
pe•cu′liar
pe•cu′li•ar′i•ty
pe•cu′ni•ar′y
ped′a•gog′ic *also*
 ped′a•gog′i•cal
ped′a•gogue′

ped'a•go'gy
ped'al (to operate a
   foot lever), -aled or
   alled, -al•ing or -al-
   ling
   ♦peddle
ped'al•er
ped'ant
pe•dan'tic
ped'ant•ry
ped'dle (to sell),
   -dled, -dling
   ♦pedal
ped'es•tal
pe•des'tri•an
pe'di•at'ric
pe'di•a•tri'cian
pe'di•at'rics
ped'i•cure', -cured',
   -cur'ing
ped'i•cur'ist
ped'i•gree'
ped'i•greed'
ped'i•ment
pe•dom'e•ter
ped'o•phile'
ped'o•phil'i•a
peek (brief look)
   ♦peak, pique
peek'a•boo'
peel (skin, rind)
   ♦peal
peen
peep'hole'
peep'ing Tom
peep'show' also peep
   show

peer (nobleman)
   ♦pier
peer (to look)
   ♦pier
peer'age
peer'less
peeve, peeved, peev'-
   ing
pee'vish
pee'wee (small thing)
   ♦pewee
peg, pegged, peg'ging
peg'board'
peg'ma•tite'
pei•gnoir'
pe•jo'ra•tive
Pe'king•ese' pl. -ese',
   also Pe'kin•ese'
pe'koe (tea)
   ♦picot
pel'age
pe•lag'ic
pelf
pel'i•can
pe•lisse'
pel•lag'ra
pel•lag'rous
pel'let
pell'-mell' also pell'-
   mell'
pel•lu'cid
pelt
pel'vic
pel'vis pl. -vis•es or
   -ves'
pem'mi•can
pen (to confine),

penned or pent, pen'-
   ning
pen (to write), penned,
   pen'ning
pe'nal
pe'nal•ize', -ized',
   -iz'ing
pen'al•ty
pen'ance
pen'chant
pen'cil, -ciled or
   -cilled, -cil•ing or
   -cil•ling
pen'dant n., also pen'-
   dent
pen'dent adj., also
   pen'dant
pend'ing
pen'du•lar
pen'du•lous
pen'du•lum
pen'e•tra•bil'i•ty
pen'e•tra•ble
pen'e•trate', -trat'ed,
   -trat'ing
pen'e•tra'tion
pen'e•tra'tive
pen'guin
pen'i•cil'lin
pen•in'su•la
pen•in'su•lar
pe'nis pl. -nis•es or
   -nes'
pen'i•tence
pen'i•tent
pen'i•ten'tial
pen'i•ten'tia•ry

pen'knife'
pen'man
pen'man•ship'
pen name also pen'-
  name'
pen'nant
pen'ne pl. n.
pen'ni•less
pen'non
Penn'syl•va'nian
pen'ny (British coin),
  pl. pen'nies or pence
pen'ny (U.S. coin), pl.
  -nies
pen'ny-pinch'ing
pen'ny•roy'al
pen'ny•weight'
pen'ny-wise'
pen'ny•worth'
pe•nol'o•gist
pe•nol'o•gy
pen'sion
pen'sive
pen'ta•cle
pen'tad'
pen'ta•gon'
pen•tag'o•nal
pen•tam'e•ter
pen'tane'
Pen'ta•teuch'
pen•tath'lon
pen'ta•ton'ic scale
Pen'te•cost'
Pen'te•cos'tal
pent'house'
pen'to•bar'bi•tal
  sodium

pent'-up' adj.
pe•nu'che also pe-
  nu'chi
pe'nult'
pe•nul'ti•mate
pe•num'bra pl. -brae
  or -bras
pe•nu'ri•ous
pen'u•ry
pe'on (laborer)
  ♦paean
pe'on•age
pe'o•ny
peo'ple pl. -ple or
  -ples
peo'ple, -pled, -pling
pep, pepped, pep'ping
pep'lum
pep'per
pep'per-and-salt'
  adj.
pep'per•corn'
pep'per•mint'
pep'per•o'ni
pep'per•y
pep'py
pep'sin
pep'tic
pep'tide' also pep'tid
pep'tone'
per'e•stroi'ka
per'ad•ven'ture
per•am'bu•late',
  -lat'ed, -lat'ing
per•am'bu•la'tion
per•am'bu•la'tor
per•am'bu•la•to'ry

per an'num
per•cale'
per cap'i•ta
per•ceiv'a•ble
per•ceive', -ceived',
  -ceiv'ing
per•cent' also per
  cent'
per•cent'age
per•cen'tile'
per•cep'ti•bil'i•ty
per•cep'ti•ble
per•cep'tion
per•cep'tive
per•cep'tu•al
perch (fish), pl. perch
  or perch'es
perch (roost)
per'chance
per•cip'i•ence
per•cip'i•en•cy
per•cip'i•ent
per'co•late', -lat'ed,
  -lat'ing
per'co•la'tion
per'co•la'tor
per•cus'sion
per•cus'sion•ist
per•cus'sive
per di'em
per•di'tion
per'e•gri•nate', -nat'-
  ed, -nat'ing
per'e•gri•na'tion
per'e•grine
per•emp'to•ry
per•en'ni•al
per'e•stroi'ka

per'fect *adj. & n.*
per•fect' *v.*
per•fect'i•ble
per•fec'tion
per•fec'tion•ism
per•fec'tion•ist
per'fect•ly
per•fec'to *pl.* -tos
per•fer'vid
per•fid'i•ous
per'fi•dy
per'fo•rate', -rat'ed,
   -rat'ing
per'fo•ra'tion
per'fo•ra'tor
per•force'
per•form'
per•form'ance
per•fume' *n.*
per•fume', -fumed',
   -fum'ing
per•fum'er•y
per•func'to•ry
per'go•la
per•haps'
per'i•car'di•al
per'i•car'di•um *pl.*
   -di•a
per'i•gee
per'i•he'li•on *pl.* -li•
   a
per'il
per'il•ous
pe•rim'e•ter *(bound-*
   ary)
   ♦*parameter*
pe'ri•od

pe'ri•od'ic
pe'ri•od'i•cal
pe'ri•o•dic'i•ty
per'i•o•don'tal
per'i•pa•tet'ic
pe•riph'er•al
pe•riph'er•y
per'i•scope'
per'ish *(to die)*
   ♦*parish*
per'ish•a•ble
per'i•stal'sis *pl.* -ses'
per'i•stal'tic
per'i•to•ne'al
per'i•to•ne'um *pl.*
   -ne'a, *also* per'i•to-
   nae'um *pl.* -nae'a
per'i•to•ni'tis
per'i•wig'
per'i•win'kle
per'jure, -jured, -jur-
   ing
per'ju•ry
perk'y
per'ma•frost'
per'ma•nence
per'ma•nen•cy
per'ma•nent
per•man'ga•nate'
per'me•a•bil'i•ty
per'me•a•ble
per'me•ate', -at'ed,
   -at'ing
per'me•a'tion
per•mis'si•ble
per•mis'sion
per•mis'sive

per'mit *n.*
per•mit', -mit'ted,
   -mit'ting
per•mit'ter
per•mu•ta'tion
per•mute', -mut'ed,
   -mut'ing
per•ni'cious
per'o•ra'tion
per•ox'ide', -id'ed,
   -id'ing
per•pen•dic'u•lar
per'pe•trate', -trat'-
   ed, -trat'ing
per'pe•tra'tion
per'pe•tra'tor
per•pet'u•al
per•pet'u•ate', -at'-
   ed, -at'ing
per•pet'u•a'tion
per•pet'u•a'tor
per•pe•tu'i•ty
per•plex'
per•plex'i•ty
per•qui•site *(benefit)*
   ♦*prerequisite*
per se'
per'se•cute' *(to ha-*
   rass), -cut'ed, -cut'-
   ing
   ♦*prosecute*
per'se•cu'tor
per•se•ver'ance
per•se•vere', -vered',
   -ver'ing
Per'sian
per•sim'mon

per•sist′
per•sist′ence *also*
  per•sist′en•cy
per•sist′ent
per•snick′e•ty
per′son
per•so′na *pl.* -nae *or*
  -nas
per′son•a•ble
per′son•age
per′son•al *(private)*
  ♦*personnel*
per′son•al′i•ty *(char-*
  acter)
  ♦*personalty*
per′son•al•ize′,
  -ized′, -iz′ing
per′son•al•ty *(prop-*
  erty)
  ♦*personality*
per•so′na non gra′-
  ta *pl.* per•so′nae
  non gra′tae
per•son′i•fi•ca′tion
per•son′i•fy′, -fied′,
  -fy′ing
per′son•nel′ *(employ-*
  ees)
  ♦*personal*
per•spec′tive *(view)*
  ♦*prospective*
per′spi•ca′cious
per′spi•cac′i•ty
per′spi•cu′i•ty
per•spic′u•ous
per′spi•ra′tion
per•spire′, -spired′,

-spir′ing
per•suad′a•ble
per•suade′, -suad′ed,
  -suad′ing
per•sua′si•ble
per•sua′sion
per•sua′sive
pert
per•tain′
per′ti•na′cious
per′ti•nac′i•ty
per′ti•nence *also* per′-
  ti•nen•cy
per′ti•nent
per•turb′
per′tur•ba′tion
pe•ruke′
pe•rus′a•ble
pe•rus′al
pe•ruse′, -rused′,
  -rus′ing
pe•rus′er
Pe•ru′vi•an
per•vade′, -vad′ed,
  -vad′ing
per•va′sion
per•va′sive
per•verse′
per•ver′sion
per•ver′si•ty
per′vert′ *n.*
per•vert′ *v.*
per•vert′ed
per′vi•ous
pe•se′ta
pes′ky
pe•so′ *pl.* -sos

pes′si•mism
pes′si•mist
pes′si•mis′tic
pest
pes′ter
pest′hole′
pes′ti•cide′
pes•tif′er•ous
pes′ti•lence
pes′ti•lent *also* pes′-
  ti•len′tial
pes′tle
pes′to *pl.* -tos
pet, pet′ted, pet′ting
pet′al
pet′aled *also* pet′alled
pe•tard′
pet′cock′
pe′ter
pet′i•ole′
pet′it *(lesser)*
  ♦*petty*
pe•tite′ *(small)*
pet′it four′ *pl.* pet′its
  fours′ *or* pet′it fours′
pe•ti′tion
pet′it point′
pet′rel *(sea bird)*
  ♦*petrol*
pet′ri•fac′tion
pet′ri•fy′, -fied′, -fy′-
  ing
pet′ro•chem′i•cal
pet′ro•dol′lar
pe•trog′ra•phy
pet′rol *(gasoline)*
  ♦*petrel*

pet′ro•la′tum
pe•tro′le•um
pet′ro•log′ic *also* pet′-
  ro•log′i•cal
pe•trol′o•gy
pet′ti•coat′
pet′ti•fog′ger
pet′tish
pet′ty *(small)*
  ♦*petit*
pet′u•lance
pet′u•lant
pe•tu′nia
pew
pe′wee *(bird), also*
  pee′wee
pe′wit′
pew′ter
pe•yo′te
pha′e•ton
pha•lanx′ *pl.* pha′-
  lanx′es *or* pha•lan′-
  ges
phal′a•rope′
phal′lic
phal′lus *pl.* -li′ *or*
  -lus•es
phan′tasm
phan•tas′ma•go′ri•
  a *also* phan•tas′ma-
  go′ry
phan•tas′mal *also*
  phan•tas′mic
phan′tom
Phar′aoh *also* phar′-
  aoh
phar′i•sa′ic *also*

phar′i•sa′i•cal
phar′i•see
phar′ma•ceu′ti•cal
  also phar′ma•ceu′tic
phar′ma•ceu′tics
phar′ma•cist
phar′ma•col′o•gy
phar′ma•co•poe′ia
phar′ma•cy
pha•ryn′ge•al
phar′ynx *pl.* pha•ryn′-
  ges *or* phar′ynx•es
phase *(to progress in*
  stages), phased,
  phas′ing
  ♦*faze*
phase′down′ *n.*
phase′-in′
pheas′ant *pl.* -ants *or*
  -ant
phe′no•bar′bi•tal
phe′nol′
phe′nol•phthal′ein′
phe•nom′e•nal
phe•nom′e•non′ *pl.*
  -na *or* -nons′
phe′no•type′
phe′no•typ′ic
phen′yl
Phi′ Be′ta Kap′pa
Phil′a•del′phi•an
phi•lan′der
phil′an•throp′ic
phi•lan′thro•pist
phi•lan′thro•py
phil′a•tel′ic
phi•lat′e•list

phi•lat′e•ly
phil′har•mon′ic
Phil′ip•pine′
Phil′is•tine′
phil′o•den′dron *pl.*
  -drons *or* -dra
phi•lol′o•gist
phi•lol′o•gy
phi•los′o•pher
phil′o•soph′i•cal
  also phil′o•soph′ic
phi•los′o•phize′,
  -phized′, -phiz′ing
phi•los′o•phy
phil′ter *(potion), also*
  phil′tre
  ♦*filter*
phle•bi′tis
phle•bot′o•my
phlegm
phleg•mat′ic
phlo′em′
phlox *pl.* phlox *or*
  phlox′es
pho′bi•a
pho′bic
phoe′be
Phoe•ni′cian
phoe′nix
phone, phoned, phon′-
  ing
pho′neme′
pho•ne′mic
pho•net′ic
pho•net′i•cal
pho•ne•ti′cian
pho•net′ics

phon'ic
pho'no•graph'
pho'no•graph'ic
pho•nog'ra•phy
pho•nol'o•gy
pho'non'
pho'ny *also* pho'ney
  pl. -neys
phos'gene'
phos'phate'
phos'phat'ic
phos'phor
phos'pho•resce',
  -resced', -resc'ing
phos'pho•res'cence
phos'pho•res'cent
phos•pho'ric
phos'pho•rous *(of
  phosphorus)*
phos'pho•rus *(ele-
  ment)*
pho'to *pl.* -tos
pho'to•cell'
pho'to•cop'i•er
pho'to•cop'y, -ied,
  -y•ing
pho'to•e•lec'tric
  also pho'to•e•lec'-
  tri•cal
pho'to•e•lec'tron
pho'to•en•grave',
  -graved', -grav'ing
pho'to•fin'ish
pho'to•flash'
pho'to•flood'
pho'to•gen'ic
pho'to•graph'

pho•tog'ra•pher
pho'to•graph'ic
pho•tog'ra•phy
pho'to•gra•vure'
pho'to•jour'na•lism
pho'to•me•chan'-
  i•cal
pho•tom'e•ter
pho•tom'e•try
pho'to•mi'cro-
  graph'
pho'to•mon•tage'
pho'ton'
pho'ton'ic
pho'to•re•cep'tive
pho'to•re•cep'tor
pho'to•sen'si•tive
pho'to•sen'si•tiv'-
  i•ty
pho'to•sen'si•tize',
  -tized', -tiz'ing
pho'to•sphere'
Pho'to•stat'®
pho'to•syn'the•sis
pho'to•syn'the•size',
  -sized', -siz'ing
pho'to•syn•thet'ic
pho•tot'ro•pism
phras'al
phrase, phrased,
  phras'ing
phra'se•ol'o•gy
phre•nol'o•gist
phre•nol'o•gy
phy•lac'ter•y
phy'lum *pl.* -la
phys'ic *(to act as a*

cathartic), -icked,
  -ick•ing
  ♦*physique, psychic*
phys'i•cal
phy•si'cian
phys'i•cist
phys'ics
phys'i•og•nom'ic
  also phys'i•og•nom'-
  i•cal
phys'i•og'no•my
phys'i•o•log'i•cal
phys'i•ol'o•gist
phys'i•ol'o•gy
phys'i•o•ther'-
  a•peu'tic
phys'i•o•ther'a•py
phy•sique' *(body)*
  ♦*physic, psychic*
pi *(Greek letter),* pl.
  pis
  ♦*pie*
pi *(jumbled type),* pl.
  pis, *also* pie
pi'a ma'ter
pi'a•nis'si•mo' *pl.*
  -mos'
pi'an•ist
pi•an'o *pl.* -os
pi•an'o•for'te
pi•az'za *pl.* -zas *or*
  -ze
pi'ca *(type size)*
  ♦*pika*
pic'a•dor' *pl.* pic'-
  a•dors' *or* pic'a•do'-
  res

pic′a•resque′
pic′a•yune′
pic′ca•lil′li pl. -lis
pic′co•lo′ pl. -los′
pick′ax′ also pick′axe′
pick′er•el pl. -el or
   -els
pick′et
pick′le, -led, -ling
pick′lock′
pick′-me-up′
pick′pock′et
pick′up′ n.
pic′nic, -nicked,
   -nick•ing
pic′nick•er
pi′cot (loop)
   ♦pekoe
pic′ric acid
Pict (Britannic tribes-
   man)
   ♦picked
pic′to•gram′
pic′to•graph′
pic′to•graph′ic
pic•tog′ra•phy
pic•to′ri•al
pic•to′ri•al•ize′,
   -ized′, -iz′ing
pic′ture, -tured, -tur-
   ing
pic′tur•esque′
pid′dle, -dled, -dling
pidg′in (language)
   ♦pigeon
pie (pastry)
   ♦pi

pie′bald′
piece (to join parts of),
   pieced, piec′ing
   ♦peace
piece′meal′
piece′work′
pied
pied-à-terre′ pl.
   pieds-à-terre′
pied′mont′
pier (wharf)
   ♦peer
pierce, pierced, pierc′-
   ing
pi′e•tism
pi′e•ty
pi•e′zo•e•lec′tric
pi•e′zo•e•lec′tric′-
   i•ty
pif′fle, -fled, -fling
pig
pi′geon (bird)
   ♦pidgin
pi′geon•hole′,
   -holed′, -hol′ing
pi′geon-toed′
pig′gish
pig′gy•back′
pig′head′ed
pig′let
pig′ment
pig′men•ta′tion
pig′nut′
pig′pen′
pig′skin′

pig′sty′
pig′tail′
pi′ka (animal)
   ♦pica
pike (fish), pl. pike or
   pikes
pik′er
pike′staff′ pl. -staves′
pi•laf′ or pi•laff′
pi′las′ter
pil′chard
pile, piled, pil′ing
pil′fer
pil′fer•age
pil′grim
pil′grim•age, -aged,
   -ag•ing
pil′lage, -laged, -lag-
   ing
pil′lar
pill′box′
pil′lion
pil′lo•ry, -ried, -ry-
   ing
pil′low
pil′low•case′
pi′lot
pi′lot•house′
pi′ma cotton
pi•mien′to pl. -tos,
   also pi•men′to
pim′per•nel′
pim′ple
pim′pled also pim′ply
pin, pinned, pin′ning
pi′ña co•la′da
pin′a•fore′

pi•ña′ta
pin′ball′
pince-nez′ *pl.* -nez′
pin′cers *also* pinch′-
  ers
pinch′beck′
pinch′-hit′, -hit′, -hit′-
  ting
pin′cush′ion
pine, pined, pin′ing
pin′e•al
pine′ap′ple
pine′land′
pine′wood′
pin′feath′er
ping
Ping′-Pong′®
pin′head′
pin′hole′
pin′ion *(wing, gear-
  wheel)*
  ♦*piñon*
pink′eye′
pink′ie *also* pink′y
pin′nace
pin′na•cle
pin′nate′
pi′noch′le *or* pi′noc′le
pi′ñon *(tree), also* pin′-
  yon′
  ♦*pinion*
pin′point′
pin′prick′
pin′set′ter
pin′stripe′
pin′to *pl.* -tos *or* -toes

pint′size′ *also* pint′-
  sized′
pin′up′ *n. & adj.*
pin′wale′
pin′wheel′
pin′worm′
pin′y *also* pine′y
Pin′yin′ *or* pin′yin′
pi′o•neer′
pi′ous
pip, pipped, pip′ping
pipe, piped, pip′ing
pipe′line′
pi•pette′ *(glass tube)*
  ♦*pipit*
pip′it *(bird)*
  ♦*pipette*
pip′kin
pip′pin
pip′-squeak′
pi′quan•cy
pi′quant
pique *(to provoke)*,
  piqued, piqu′ing
  ♦*peak, peek*
pi•qué′ *(fabric)*
pi•quet′ *(card game)*,
  also pic•quet′
pi′ra•cy
pi•ra′nha *also* pi•ra′-
  ña
pi′rate, -rat•ed, -rat-
  ing
pi•rat′i•cal
pir′ou•ette′, -et′ted,
  -et′ting
pis′ca•to′ri•al *also*

pis′ca•to′ry
Pi′sces
pi′scine′
pis′mire′
pis•ta′chi•o′ *pl.* -os′
pis′til *(flower part)*
pis′tol *(gun)*
pis′tol-whip′,
  -whipped′, -whip′-
  ping
pis′ton
pit, pit′ted, pit′ting
pit′a•pat′, -pat′ted,
  -pat′ting
pitch′-black′
pitch′blende′
pitch′-dark′
pitch′er
pitch′fork′
pitch′out′
pit′e•ous
pit′fall′
pith′e•can′thro•pus
pith′y
pit′i•a•ble
pit′i•ful
pit′i•less
pi′ton′
pit′tance
pit′ter-pat′ter
pi•tu′i•tar′y
pit′y, -ied, -y•ing
piv′ot
piv′ot•al
pix′el
pix′y *or* pix′ie
piz′za

piz•zazz′
piz′ze•ri′a
piz′zi•ca′to *pl.* -tos
plac′ard′
pla′cate, -cat′ed, -cat′-
  ing
pla•ca′tion
pla′ca•to′ry
place *(to set)*, placed,
  plac′ing
  ♦*plaice*
pla•ce′bo *pl.* -bos *or*
  -boes
place′-kick′ *v.*
place′ment
pla•cen′ta *pl.* -tas *or*
  -tae
pla•cen′tal
plac′er
plac′id
pla•cid′i•ty
plack′et
pla′gia•rism
pla′gia•rist
pla′gia•rize′, -rized′,
  -riz′ing
pla′gi•o•clase′
plague, plagued,
  plagu′ing
plaice *(fish)*, *pl.* plaice
  or plaic′es
  ♦*place*
plaid
plain *(clear)*
  ♦*plane*
plain *(level region)*
  ♦*plane*

plain′chant′
plain′clothes′ man
  also plain′clothes′-
  man
plains′man
plain′song′
plaint
plain′tiff *(complain-*
  ant)
plain′tive *(mournful)*
plait *(braid)*
  ♦*plat, plate*
plan, planned, plan′-
  ning
pla′nar *(flat)*
  ♦*planer*
pla•nar′i•an
pla•nar′i•ty
plane *(surface, air-*
  plane, tool, tree)
  ♦*plain*
plane *(to smooth,*
  soar), planed, plan′-
  ing
  ♦*plain*
plan′et
plan′e•tar′i•um *pl.*
  -i•ums *or* -i•a
plan′e•tar′y
plan′e•toid′
plan′e•tol′o•gy
plank′ing
plank′ton
plank•ton′ic
plan′ner
plan′tain
plan′tar *(of the sole of*

  the foot)
  ♦*planter*
plan•ta′tion
plant′er *(container,*
  tool, one that plants)
  ♦*plantar*
plant′let
plaque
plash
plas′ma *also* plasm
plas•mat′ic *also* plas′-
  mic
plas•mo′di•um *pl.*
  -di•a
plas′ter
plas′ter•board′
plaster of Par′is
plas′ter•work′
plas′tic
plas•tic′i•ty
plas′tid
plas•tique′
plas′tron
plat *(to braid)*, plat′-
  ted, plat′ting
  ♦*plait, plate*
plate *(to coat)*, plat′ed,
  plat′ing
  ♦*plait, plat*
pla•teau′ *pl.* -teaus′
  or -teaux′
plate′ful′ *pl.* -fuls′
plate′let
plat′en
plat′form′
plat′ing
plat′i•num

plat′i•tude′

plat′i•tu′di•nous

Pla•ton′ic

Pla′to•nism

pla•toon′

plat′ter

plat′y pl. -ys or -ies

plat′y•pus pl. -pus•es

plau′dit

plau′si•bil′i•ty

plau′si•ble

pla′ya

play′a•ble

play′-act′

play′back′ n.

play′bill′

play′book′

play′boy′

play′-by-play′

play′er

play′fel′low

play′ful

play′go′er

play′ground′

play′house′

play′let′

play′mate′

play′-off′ n.

play′pen′

play′room′

play′thing′

play′wright′

pla′za

plea

plea′-bar′gain v.

plead, plead′ed or pled, plead′ing

pleas′ant

pleas′ant•ry

please, pleased, pleas′-ing

pleas′ur•a•ble

pleas′ure, -ured, -ur-ing

pleat

plebe

ple•be′ian

pleb′i•scite′

plec′trum pl. -trums or -tra

pledge, pledged, pledg′ing

pledg•ee′

Pleis′to•cene′

ple′na•ry

plen′i•po•ten′ti•ar′-y

plen′i•tude

plen′te•ous

plen′ti•ful

plen′ty

ple′si•o•sau′rus pl. -sau′ri, also ple′si-o•saur′

pleth′o•ra

ple•tho′ric

pleu′ra pl. -rae′

pleu′ral

pleu′ri•sy

Plex′i•glas′®

plex′us pl. -us or -us-es

pli′a•bil′i•ty

pli′a•ble

pli′an•cy

pli′ant

pli′cate′ also pli′cat-ed

pli•é′ pl. pli•és′

pli′ers

plight

plinth

Pli′o•cene′

plis•sé′

plod, plod′ded, plod′-ding

plod′der

plop, plopped, plop′-ping

plot, plot′ted, plot′ting

plot′ter

plov′er

plow also plough

plow′man

plow′share′

ploy

pluck′y

plug, plugged, plug′-ging

plug′-ug′ly

plum (fruit)
♦plumb

plum′age

plumb (weight)
♦plum

plumb′er

plumb′ing

plume, plumed, plum′-ing

plum′met

plump′ness

plum'y
plun'der
plunge, plunged,
　plung'ing
plunk
plu•per'fect
plu'ral
plu'ral•ism
plu'ral•ist
plu•ral'i•ty
plus
plush
Plu'to
plu•toc'ra•cy
plu'to•crat'
plu'to•crat'ic
plu•tog'ra•phy
plu•to'ni•um
plu'vi•al *also* plu'vi•
　an
plu'vi•al
ply, plied, ply'ing
ply'wood'
pneu•mat'ic
pneu•mo'nia
pneu•mon'ic
poach'er
pock'et
pock'et•book'
pock'et•ful' *pl.* pock'-
　et•fuls' *or* pock'ets-
　ful'
pock'et•knife'
pock'mark'
pod
po•di'a•trist
po•di'a•try

po'di•um *pl.* -di•a *or*
　-di•ums
po'em
po'e•sy
po'et
po'et•as'ter
po•et'ic *also* po•et'-
　i•cal
poet lau're•ate *pl.*
　poets lau're•ate *or*
　poet lau're•ates
po'et•ry
po'go stick
po•grom'
poi
poign'ance *also*
　poign'an•cy
poign'ant
poin•set'ti•a
point'blank'
pointe
point'er
poin'til•lism
poin'til•list
point'less
poise, poised, pois'ing
poi'son
poi'son•ous
poke, poked, pok'ing
poke'ber'ry
pok'er
pok'er•faced'
poke'weed'
po'key *(jail),* pl. -keys
pok'y *(slow), also*
　poke'y
po'lar

Po•lar'is
po•lar'i•ty
po'lar•i•za'tion
po'lar•ize', -ized', -iz'-
　ing
Po'lar•oid'®
pole *(axis point, rod)*
　♦*poll*
pole *(to propel with a*
　pole), poled, pol'ing
　♦*poll*
Pole *(inhabitant of*
　Poland)
　♦*poll*
pole'ax' *or* pole'axe'
pole'cat'
po•lem'ic *n.*
po•lem'ic *also* po-
　lem'i•cal
po•lem'i•cist *also*
　po•lem'ist
po•len'ta
pole'star'
pole'-vault' *v.*
pole'-vault'er
po•lice' *pl.* -lice'
po•lice', -liced', -lic'-
　ing
po•lice'man
po•lice'wom'an
pol'i•clin'ic *(outpa-*
　tient department)
　♦*polyclinic*
pol'i•cy
pol'i•cy•hold'er
po•li'o'
po'li•o•my'e•li'tis

pol'ish *(shine)*
Po'lish *(of Poland)*
pol'it•bu'ro
po•lite', -lit'er, -lit'est
pol'i•tic *(shrewd)*
 ♦*politick*
po•lit'i•cal
pol'i•ti'cian
pol'i•tick' *(to talk
 politics)*
 ♦*politic*
po•lit'i•co' *pl.* -cos'
pol'i•tics
pol'i•ty
pol'ka
poll *(election)*
 ♦*pole, Pole*
pol'len
pol'li•nate', -nat'ed,
 -nat'ing
pol'li•na'tion
pol'li•na'tor
pol'li•wog' *also* pol'-
 ly•wog'
poll'ster
poll'tak'er
pol•lut'ant
pol•lute', -lut'ed, -lut'-
 ing
pol•lu'tion
Pol'ly•an'na
po'lo
pol'o•naise'
po•lo'ni•um
pol'ter•geist'
pol•troon'
pol'y•an'drous

pol'y•an'dry
pol'y•cen'tric
pol'y•chro•mat'ic
pol'y•chrome'
pol'y•clin'ic *(hospi-
 tal)*
 ♦*policlinic*
pol'y•es'ter
pol'y•eth'yl•ene'
po•lyg'a•mist
po•lyg'a•mous
po•lyg'a•my
pol'y•glot'
pol'y•gon'
po•lyg'o•nal
pol'y•graph'
pol'y•he'dral
pol'y•he'dron *pl.*
 -drons *or* -dra
pol'y•mer
pol'y•mer'ic
po•lym'er•i•za'tion
pol'y•mer•ize',
 -ized', -iz'ing
pol'y•mor'phism
Pol'y•ne'sian
pol'y•no'mi•al
pol'yp
pol'y•phon'ic
po•lyph'o•ny
pol'y•rhythm
pol'y•sac'cha•ride'
 also pol'y•sac'cha-
 rid, pol'y•sac'cha-
 rose'
pol'y•sty'rene
pol'y•syl•lab'ic

pol'y•syl'la•ble
pol'y•tech'nic
pol'y•the'ism
pol'y•the'ist
pol'y•the•is'tic
pol'y•un•sat'u•rat'-
 ed
pol'y•u're•thane'
pol'y•va'lence
pol'y•va'lent
pol'y•vi'nyl
po•made'
po'man'der
pome'gran'ate
pom'mel
pomp
pom'pa•dour'
pom'pa•no' *pl.* -no'
 or -nos'
pom'pon' *also* pom'-
 pom'
pom•pos'i•ty
pom'pous
pon'cho *pl.* -chos
pond
pon'der
pon'der•o'sa pine
pon'der•ous
pone
pon•gee'
pon'iard
pons *pl.* pon'tes
pon'tiff
pon•tif'i•cal
pon•tif'i•cate', -cat'-
 ed, -cat'ing
pon•tif'i•ca'tor

pon•toon'
po'ny
po'ny•tail'
Pon'zi scheme
pooch
poo'dle
pooh'-pooh' v.
pool'room'
pool'side'
poop
poor'house'
poor'ly
pop, popped, pop'ping
pop art
pop'corn'
pope
pop'er•y
pop'eyed'
pop'gun'
pop'in•jay'
pop'ish
pop'lar (tree)
♦popular
pop'lin
pop'o'ver
pop'per
pop'py
pop'py•cock'
pop'u•lace (masses)
♦populous
pop'u•lar (well-liked)
♦poplar
pop'u•lar'i•ty
pop'u•lar•i•za'tion
pop'u•lar•ize',
-ized', -iz'ing
pop'u•late', -lat'ed,

-lat'ing
pop'u•la'tion
pop'u•lism
pop'u•list
pop'u•lous (thickly
settled)
♦populace
por'ce•lain
porch
por'cine'
por'cu•pine'
pore (opening)
♦pour
pore (to study), pored,
por'ing
♦pour
por'gy pl. -gy or -gies
pork'er
pork'pie'
por•nog'ra•pher
por'no•graph'ic
por•nog'ra•phy
po•ros'i•ty
po'rous
por'phy•ry
por'poise
por'ridge
por'rin•ger
port
port'a•bil'i•ty
port'a•ble
port'age, -aged, -ag-
ing
por'tal
por'tal-to-por'tal
adj.
port•cul'lis

porte'-co•chère' or
porte'-co•chere'
por•tend'
por'tent'
por•ten'tous
por'ter
por'ter•house'
port•fo'li•o pl. -os
port'hole'
por'ti•co' pl. -coes' or
-cos'
por•tière' or por•
tiere'
por'tion
port'ly
port•man'teau pl.
-teaus or -teaux
por'trait
por'trait•ist
por'trai•ture'
por•tray'
por•tray'al
port'side'
Por'tu•guese' pl.
-guese'
pose, posed, pos'ing
pos'er (one who poses,
baffling question)
po•seur' (affected per-
son)
posh
pos•it
po•si'tion
pos'i•tive
pos'i•tiv•ism
pos'i•tiv•ist
pos'i•tron'

pos'se
pos•sess'
pos•ses'sion
pos•ses'sive
pos•ses'sor
pos•si•bil'i•ty
pos•si•ble
post'age
post'al
post'box'
post-card *also* post'-
   card'
post•date', -dat'ed,
   -dat'ing
post•doc'tor•al
post'er
pos•te'ri•or
pos•ter'i•ty
pos'tern
post•grad'u•ate
post'haste'
post'hu•mous
post'hyp•not'ic
   suggestion
pos•til'ion *also* pos-
   til'lion
post'im•pres'sion-
   ism
post'im•pres'sion-
   ist
post'in•dus'tri•al
post'man
post'mark'
post'mas'ter
postmaster general
   pl. postmasters
   general

post'me•rid'i•an *(in
   the afternoon)*
post' me•rid'i•em
   (after twelve noon)
post•mod'ern
post•mod'ern•ism
post•mod'ern•ist
post•mor'tem
post•na'sal
post•na'tal
post•op'er•a•tive
post•or'bi•tal
post'paid'
post•par'tum
post•pone', -poned',
   -pon'ing
post•pone'ment
post'script'
pos'tu•lant
pos'tu•late', -lat'ed,
   -lat'ing
pos'tu•la'tion
pos'tu•la'tor
pos'tur•al
pos'ture, -tured, -tur-
   ing
post'war'
po'sy
pot, pot'ted, pot'ting
po'ta•ble
po•tage'
pot'ash
po•tas'si•um
po•ta'tion
po•ta'to *pl.* -toes
pot-au-feu'
pot'bel'lied

pot'bel'ly
pot'boil'er
po'ten•cy
po'tent
po'ten•tate'
po•ten'tial
po•ten'ti•al'i•ty
po•ten'ti•om'e•ter
poth'er
pot'herb'
pot'hole'
pot'hook'
po'tion
pot'latch'
pot'luck'
pot'pie'
pot'pour•ri' *pl.* -ris'
pot'sherd' *also* pot'-
   shard'
pot'tage
pot'ted
pot'ter
pot'ter•y
pouch
pouf
poul'tice
poul'try *(fowl)*
   ♦*paltry*
pounce, pounced,
   pounc'ing
pound *(weight), pl.*
   pound *or* pounds
pound *(to hammer)*
pound'age
pound'-fool'ish *adj.*
pour *(to flow)*
   ♦*poor*

pour•boire'
pousse'-ca•fé'
pout *(sulky expression)*
pout *(fish)*, *pl.* pout *or* pouts
pov'er•ty
pow'der
pow'der•y
pow'er
pow'er•boat'
pow'er•ful
pow'er•house'
pow'er•less
pow'wow'
pox *(disease)*
 ♦*pocks*
prac'ti•ca•bil'i•ty
prac'ti•ca•ble *(possible)*
prac'ti•cal *(useful, sensible)*
prac'ti•cal'i•ty
prac'ti•cal•ly
prac'tice, -ticed, -ticing
prac•ti'tio•ner
prae'tor
prae•to'ri•an
prag•mat'ic
prag'ma•tism
prag'ma•tist
prai'rie
praise, praised, prais'ing
praise'wor'thy
pra'line'

pram
prance, pranced, pranc'ing
prank'ster
pra'se•o•dym'i•um
prate, prat'ed, prat'ing
prat'fall'
prat'tle, -tled, -tling
prawn
pray *(to implore)*
 ♦*prey*
pray'er *(one who prays)*
prayer *(petition)*
preach'er
pre'ad•ap•ta'tion
pre'ad•o•les'cence
pre'ad•o•les'cent
pre•am'ble
pre•am'pli•fi'er
pre•ar•range',
 -ranged', -rang'ing
Pre•cam'bri•an
pre•car'i•ous
pre•cau'tion
pre•cau'tion•ar'y
pre•cede' *(to come or go before)*, -ced'ed, -ced'ing
 ♦*proceed*
prec'e•dence
prec'e•dent *(prior example)*
 ♦*president*
pre'cept'
pre•cep'tor

pre•cep'tor•ship'
pre•ces'sion *(precedence, axial movement)*
 ♦*processional*
pre'cinct'
pre'cious
prec'i•pice
pre•cip'i•tance
pre•cip'i•tant
pre•cip'i•tate *(hasty)*
 ♦*precipitous*
pre•cip'i•tate' *(to hurl downward)*, -tat'ed, -tat'ing
pre•cip'i•ta'tion
pre•cip'i•ta'tor
pre•cip'i•tous *(steep)*
 ♦*precipitate*
pré•cis' *(summary)*,
 pl. -cis'
pre•cise' *(definite)*
pre•ci'sion
pre•clude', -clud'ed, -clud'ing
pre•clu'sion
pre•clu'sive
pre•co'cious
pre•coc'i•ty
pre'cog•ni'tion
pre•cog'ni•tive
pre'-Co•lum'bi•an
pre'con•ceive',
 -ceived', -ceiv'ing
pre'con•cep'tion
pre'con•di'tion
pre•cook'

pre·cur'sor
pre·cur'so·ry
pre·cut', -cut', -cut'-
  ting
pre·da'cious or pre-
  da'ceous
pre·date', -dat'ed,
  -dat'ing
pred'a·tor
pred'a·to·ry
pre·de·cease',
  -ceased', -ceas'ing
pred'e·ces'sor
pre·des'ig·nate',
  -nat'ed, -nat'ing
pre·des'ti·na'tion
pre·des'tine, -tined,
  -tin·ing
pre·de·ter'mi·na'-
  tion
pre·de·ter'mine,
  -mined, -min·ing
pred'i·ca·ble
pre·dic'a·ment
pred'i·cate', -cat'ed,
  -cat'ing
pred'i·ca'tion
pred'i·ca'tive
pre·dict'
pre·dict'a·bil'i·ty
pre·dict'a·ble
pre·dic'tion
pre·dic'tor
pred'i·lec'tion
pre·dis·pos'al
pre·dis·pose',
  -posed', -pos'ing

pre·dis·po·si'tion
pre·dom'i·nance
pre·dom'i·nant
pre·dom'i·nate',
  -nat'ed, -nat'ing
pre·dom'i·na'tion
pre·dom'i·na'tor
pre·em'i·nence or
  pre·em'i·nence
pre·em'i·nent or
  pre·em'i·nent
pre·empt' or pre-
  empt'
pre·emp'tion or pre-
  emp'tion
pre·emp'tive or pre-
  emp'tive
pre·emp'tor or pre-
  emp'tor
pre·emp'to·ry or
  pre·emp'to·ry
preen
pre'-ex·ist' or pre'ex-
  ist'
pre'fab'
pre·fab'ri·cate',
  -cat'ed, -cat'ing
pre·fab'ri·ca'tion
pre·fab'ri·ca'tor
pref'ace, -aced, -ac-
  ing
pref'a·to·ry
pre'fect' also prae'-
  fect'
pre'fec'ture
pre·fer', -ferred', -fer'-
  ring

pref'er·a·ble
pref'er·ence
pref'er·en'tial
pre·fer'ment
pre·fig'ure, -ured,
  -ur·ing
pre'fix' n.
pre·fix' v.
pre'flight'
pre·fron'tal
  lobotomy
preg'nan·cy
preg'nant
pre'heat'
pre·hen'sile
pre'his·tor'ic also
  pre'his·tor'i·cal
pre'his'to·ry
pre·judge', -judged',
  -judg'ing
prej'u·dice, -diced,
  -dic·ing
prej'u·di'cial
prel'a·cy
prel'ate
pre·law'
pre·lim'i·nar'y
pre·lit'er·ate
prel'ude', -ud'ed, -ud'·
  ing
pre·lu'sive
pre·mar'i·tal
pre'ma·ture'
pre'med'
pre·med'i·cal
pre·med'i·tate', -tat'-
  ed, -tat'ing

pre•med′i•ta′tion
pre•med′i•ta′tive
pre•med′i•ta′tor
pre′mier (*first in importance*)
pre•mier′ (*prime minister*)
pre•mière′ (*first presentation*)
prem′ise, -ised, -is-ing
pre′mi•um
pre′mix′
pre•mod′ern
pre•mo′lar
pre′mo•ni′tion
pre•na′tal
pre•nup′tial
pre•oc′cu•pa′tion
pre•oc′cu•py′, -pied′, -py′ing
pre′or•dain′
prep, prepped, prep′-ping
pre•pack′age, -aged, -ag•ing
prep′a•ra′tion
pre•par′a•to′ry
pre•pare′, -pared′, -par′ing
pre•par′ed•ness
pre•pay′, -paid′, -pay′-ing
pre•pay′ment
pre•pon′der•ance
pre•pon′der•ant
pre•pon′der•ate′,

-at′ed, -at′ing
prep′o•si′tion
prep′o•si′tion•al
pre′pos•sess′
pre′pos•ses′sion
pre•pos′ter•ous
prep′pie or prep′py
pre•pro′gram′, -grammed′ or -gramed′, -gram′-ming or -gram′ing
pre′puce′
pre-Raph′a•el•ite′
pre′re•lease′, -leased′, -leas′ing
pre•req′ui•site (*prior requirement*)
♦perquisite
pre•rog′a•tive
pres′age n.
pre•sage′, -saged′, -sag′ing
pres′by•ter
Pres′by•te′ri•an
pres′by•ter′y
pre′school′
pre′sci•ence
pre′sci•ent
pre•scribe′ (*to order, enjoin*), -scribed′, -scrib′ing
♦proscribe
pre′script′
pre•scrip′tion
pre•scrip′tive
pres′ence
pres′ent n. & adj.

pre•sent′ v.
pre•sent′a•ble
pres′en•ta′tion
pres′ent-day′ adj.
pre•sen′ti•ment (*premonition*)
♦presentment
pres′ent•ly
pre•sent′ment (*presentation*)
♦presentiment
pres′er•va′tion
pre•serv′a•tive
pres′er•va′tor
pre•serve′, -served′, -serv′ing
pre′shrunk′
pre•side′, -sid′ed, -sid′ing
pres′i•den•cy
pres′i•dent (*chief executive*)
♦precedent
pres′i•dent-e•lect′
pres′i•den′tial
pre•sid′i•um pl. -i•a or -i•ums
pre•soak′
pre•sort′
press′ing
press′man
press′room′
press′run′
pres′sure, -sured, -sur•ing
pres′sur•i•za′tion
pres′sur•ize′, -ized′,

-iz'ing
press'work'
pres'ti·dig'i·ta'tion
pres'ti·dig'i·ta'tor
pres·tige'
pres·tig'ious
pres'to *pl.* -tos
pre·sum'a·ble
pre·sume', -sumed',
-sum'ing
pre·sum'ed·ly
pre·sump'tion
pre·sump'tive
pre·sump'tu·ous
pre'sup·pose',
-posed', -pos'ing
pre'sup·po·si'tion
pre'teen'
pre·tcnd'
pre·tend'er
pre'tense'
pre·ten'sion
pre·ten'tious
pret'er·it *or* pret'er-
ite
pre·term'
pre'ter·nat'u·ral
pre'test' *n.*
pre·test' *v.*
pre'text'
pre·tri'al
pret'ti·fy', -fied', -fy'-
ing
pret'ty, -tied, -ty·ing
pret'zel
pre·vail'
prev'a·lence

prev'a·lent
pre·var'i·cate', -cat'-
ed, -cat'ing
pre·var'i·ca'tion
pre·var'i·ca'tor
pre·vent'
pre·vent'a·ble *also*
pre·vent'i·ble
pre·ven'tion
pre·ven'tive *also*
pre·ven'ta·tive
pre'view' *also* pre'-
vue', -vued', -vu'ing
pre'vi·ous
pre·vi'sion
pre'vo·cal'ic
pre'vo·ca'tion·al
pre'war'
pre'washed'
prey *(victim)*
   ♦*pray*
price, priced, pric'ing
price'-fix'ing
prick'le, -led, -ling
prick'ly
pride, prid'ed, prid'-
ing
prie·dieu' *pl.* -dieus'
or -dieux'
pri'er *(one that pries),*
also pry'er
   ♦*prior*
priest
priest'hood'
prig'gish
prim, prim'mer, prim'-
mest

pri'ma·cy
pri'ma don'na *pl.*
pri'ma don'nas
pri'mal
pri·mar'i·ly
pri'mar'y
pri'mate'
pri'ma·ve'ra
prime, primed, prim'-
ing
prim'er
pri·me'val
prim'i·tive
pri'mo·gen'i·tor
pri'mo·gen'i·ture'
pri·mor'di·al
primp
prim'rose'
prince'ly
prin'cess
prin'ci·pal *(foremost)*
   ♦*principle*
prin'ci·pal'i·ty
prin'ci·ple *(rule, law)*
   ♦*principal*
prin'ci·pled
print'a·ble
print'er
print'ing
print'-out' *n.*
pri'or *(before)*
   ♦*prier*
pri'or *(monk)*
   ♦*prier*
pri·or'i·tize', -tized',
-tiz'ing
pri·or'i·ty

pri′or•y
prism
pris′mat′ic
pris′on
pris′on•er
pris′sy
pris′tine′
pri′va•cy
pri′vate
pri′va•teer′
pri•va′tion
priv′et
priv′i•lege, -leged,
  -leg•ing
priv′y
prix′ fixe′ pl. prix′
  fixes′
prize, prized, priz′ing
prize′fight′
prize′fight′er
prize′fight′ing
pro pl. pros
pro•ac′tive
prob′a•bil′i•ty
prob′a•ble
pro′bate′, -bat′ed,
  -bat′ing
pro•ba′tion
pro•ba′tion•ar′y
pro•ba′tion•er
pro′ba•tive
probe, probed, prob′-
  ing
pro•bi•ty
prob′lem
prob′lem•at′i•cal
  also prob′lem•at′ic

pro bo′no
pro•bos′cis pl. -cis•es
  or -cides′
pro•ce′dur•al
pro•ce′dure
pro•ceed′ (to go for-
  ward)
  ♦precede
pro•ceed′ings
pro′ceeds′
proc′ess′
pro•ces′sion (parade)
  ♦precession
pro•ces′sion•al
pro•claim′
proc′la•ma′tion
pro•cliv′i•ty
pro•con′sul
pro•con′su•lar
pro•con′su•late
pro•cras′ti•nate′,
  -nat′ed, -nat′ing
pro•cras′ti•na′tion
pro•cras′ti•na′tor
pro•cre•ate′, -at′ed,
  -at′ing
pro•cre•a′tion
pro•cre•a′tive
pro•cre•a′tor
pro•crus′te•an
proc′to•log′ic also
  proc′to•log′i•cal
proc•tol′o•gist
proc•tol′o•gy
proc′tor
proc′u•ra′tor
pro•cure′, -cured′,

  -cur′ing
pro•cure′ment
prod, prod′ded, prod′-
  ding
prod′der
prod′i•gal
prod′i•gal′i•ty
pro•di′gious
prod′i•gy
pro′duce n.
pro•duce′, -duced′,
  -duc′ing
pro•duc′er
pro•duc′i•ble
prod′uct
pro•duc′tion
pro•duc′tive
pro′duc•tiv′i•ty
pro′em′
prof ′a•na′tion
pro•fane′, -faned′,
  -fan′ing
pro•fan′i•ty
pro•fess′
pro•fes′sion
pro•fes′sion•al
pro•fes′sion•al•ism
pro•fes′sor
pro′fes•so′ri•al
prof′fer
pro•fi′cien•cy
pro•fi′cient
pro′file′, -filed′, -fil′-
  ing
prof′it (gain)
  ♦prophet
prof′it•a•bil′i•ty

prof′it•a•ble
prof′i•teer′
prof′li•ga•cy
prof′li•gate
pro for′ma
pro•found′
pro•fun′di•ty
pro•fuse′
pro•fu′sion
pro•gen′i•tor
prog′e•ny
pro•ges′ter•one′
prog•no′sis *pl.* -ses′
prog•nos′tic
prog•nos′ti•cate′,
  -cat′ed, -cat′ing
prog•nos′ti•ca′tion
prog•nos′ti•ca′tor
pro′gram′, -grammed′
  or -gramed′, -gram′-
  ming *or* -gram′ing
pro′gram•mat′ic
pro′gram′mer *or* pro′-
  gram′er
prog′ress′ *n.*
pro•gress′ *v.*
pro•gres′sion
pro•gres′sive
pro•hib′it
pro′hi•bi′tion
pro•hib′i•tive *also*
  pro•hib′i•to′ry
proj•ect′ *n.*
pro•ject′ *v.*
pro•jec′tile
pro•jec′tion
pro•jec′tion•ist

pro•jec′tor
pro•le•tar′i•an
pro•le•tar′i•at
pro•lif′er•ate′, -at′-
  ed, -at′ing
pro•lif′er•a′tion
pro•lif′ic
pro•lix′
pro•lix′i•ty
pro′logue′
pro•long′
pro′lon•ga′tion
prom
prom′e•nade′, -nad′-
  ed, -nad′ing
pro•me′thi•um
prom′i•nence
prom′i•nent
pro•mis′cu•i•ty
pro•mis′cu•ous
prom′ise, -ised, -is-
  ing
prom′is•so′ry
prom′on•to′ry
pro•mote′, -mot′ed,
  -mot′ing
pro•mo′tion
pro•mo′tion•al
prompt′book′
prompt′er
prom′ul•gate′, -gat′-
  ed, -gat′ing
prom′ul•ga′tion
prom′ul•ga′tor
prone′ness
prong′horn′ *pl.*
  -horn′ *or* -horns′

pro•nom′i•nal
pro′noun′
pro•nounce′,
  -nounced′, -nounc′-
  ing
pro•nounce′a•ble
pro•nounce′ment
pron′to
pro•nun′ci•a′tion
proof′read′, -read′,
  -read′ing
prop, propped, prop′-
  ping
prop′a•gan′da
prop′a•gan′dist
prop′a•gan•dize′,
  -dized′, -diz′ing
prop′a•gate′, -gat′ed,
  -gat′ing
prop′a•ga′tor
pro′pane′
pro•pel′, -pelled′,
  -pel′ling
pro•pel′lant *also*
  pro•pel′lent
pro•pel′ler *also* pro-
  pel′lor
pro•pen′si•ty
prop′er
prop′er•tied
prop′er•ty
pro′phase′
proph′e•cy *(predic-
  tion)*
proph′e•sy′ *(to pre-
  dict)*, -sied′, -sy′ing
proph′et *(seer)*

◆*profit*
pro•phet′ic
pro′phy•lac′tic
pro•pin′qui•ty
pro•pi′ti•ate′, -at′ed, -at′ing
pro•pi′ti•a′tion
pro•pi′ti•a′tor
pro•pi′ti•a•to′ry
pro•pi′tious
pro•po′nent
pro•por′tion
pro•por′tion•al
pro•por′tion•al′i•ty
pro•por′tion•ate
pro•pos′al
pro•pose′, -posed′, -pos′ing
prop′o•si′tion
pro•pound′
pro•pri′e•tar′y
pro•pri′e•tor
pro•pri′e•tor•ship′
pro•pri′e•ty
pro•pul′sion
pro•pul′sive
pro′pyl•ene′
pro ra′ta
pro•rate′, -rat′ed, -rat′ing
pro•ra′tion
pro′ro•ga′tion
pro•rogue′, -rogued′, -rogu′ing
pro•sa′ic
pro•sce′ni•um *pl.* -ni•ums *or* -ni•a

pro•scribe′ *(to forbid),* -scribed′, -scrib′ing
◆*prescribe*
pro•scrip′tion
pro•scrip′tive
prose
pros′e•cute′ *(to try by law),* -cut′ed, -cut′ing
◆*persecute*
pros′e•cu′tion
pros′e•cu′tor
pros′e•lyte′
pros′e•ly•tize′, -tized′, -tiz′ing
pro•sod′ic
pros′o•dy
pros′pect′
pro•spec′tive
pros•pec′tor
pro•spec′tus
pros′per
pros•per′i•ty
pros′per•ous
pros′tate′ *(gland)*
◆*prostrate*
pros•the′sis *pl.* -ses′
pros•thet′ic
pros•thet′ics
pros′ti•tute′, -tut′ed, -tut′ing
pros′ti•tu′tion
pros′ti•tu′tor
pros′trate′ *(to throw down flat),* -trat′ed, -trat′ing

◆*prostate*
pros•tra′tion
pros′tra′tor
pro′tac•tin′i•um
pro•tag′o•nist
pro′te•an
pro•tect′
pro•tec′tion
pro•tec′tion•ism
pro•tec′tive
pro•tec′tor *also* pro•tect′er
pro•tec′tor•ate
pro′té•gé′ *masc.*
pro′té•gée′ *fem.*
pro′tein
pro tem′po•re
pro′te•ol′y•sis
pro′test′ *n.*
pro•test′ *v.*
Prot′es•tant
Prot′es•tant•ism
prot′es•ta′tion
pro′to•col′
pro′ton′
pro′to•plasm
pro′to•plas′mic *also* pro′to•plas′mal, pro′to•plas•mat′ic
pro′to•typ′al *also* pro′to•typ′i•cal
pro′to•type′
pro′to•zo′an *adj.,* *also* pro′to•zo′ic
pro′to•zo′an *pl.* -zo′ans *or* -zo′a
pro•tract′

pro•trac'tile *also*
  pro•tract'i•ble
pro•trac'tion
pro•trac'tive
pro•trac'tor
pro•trude', -trud'ed,
  -trud'ing
pro•tru'sion
pro•tru'sive
pro•tu'ber•ance
pro•tu'ber•ant
proud'ly
prov•a•bil'i•ty
prov'a•ble
prove, proved, proved
  or prov'en, prov'ing
prov'e•nance
Pro'ven•çal'
prov'en•der
pro•ve'nience
prov'erb'
pro•ver'bi•al
pro•vide', -vid'ed,
  -vid'ing
pro•vid'er
prov'i•dence
prov'i•dent
prov'i•den'tial
prov'ince
pro•vin'cial
pro•vin'cial•ism
pro•vin'ci•al'i•ty
pro•vi'sion
pro•vi'sion•al
pro•vi'so *pl.* -sos *or*
  -soes
pro•vi'so•ry

prov'o•ca'tion
pro•voc'a•tive
pro•voke', -voked',
  -vok'ing
pro'vo•lo'ne
pro'vost'
prow
prow'ess
prowl'er
prox'i•mal
prox'•i•mate
prox•im'i•ty
prox'y
prude
pru'dence
pru'dent
pru•den'tial
prud'er•y
prud'ish
prune, pruned, prun'-
  ing
pru'ri•ence
pru'ri•ent
Prus'sian
prus'sic acid
pry, pried, pry'ing
psalm'ist
psalm'o•dy
Psal'ter *also* psal'ter
psal'ter•y
pseu'do
pseu'do•nym'
pseu•don'y•mous
pseu'do•po'di•um
  pl. -di•a, *also* pseu'-
  do•pod'
pshaw

psit'ta•co'sis
pso•ri'a•sis
psy'che
psy'che•del'ic
psy'chi•at'ric
psy•chi'a•trist
psy•chi'a•try
psy'chic *(of the*
  mind), also psy'chi•
  cal
  ♦physic, physique
psy'chi•cal•ly
psy'cho *pl.* -chos
psy'cho•a•nal'y•sis
psy'cho•an'a•lyst
psy'cho•an'a•lyt'ic
  also psy'cho•an'-
  a•lyt'i•cal
psy'cho•an'a•lyze',
  -lyzed', -lyz'ing
psy'cho•bi•ol'o•gy
psy'cho•dra'ma
psy'cho•his'to•ry
psy'cho•log'i•cal
psy•chol'o•gist
psy•chol'o•gy
psy'cho•met'rics
psy'cho•path'
psy'cho•path'ic
psy•cho'sis *pl.* -ses'
psy'cho•so•mat'ic
psy'cho•ther'a•peu'-
  tic
psy'cho•ther'a•pist
psy'cho•ther'a•py
psy•chot'ic
ptar'mi•gan *pl.* -gan

or -gans
pte•rid'o•phyte'
pter'o•dac'tyl
pter'o•saur'
pto'maine' *also* pto'-
　main'
pty'a•lin
pub
pu'ber•ty
pu•bes'cence
pu•bes'cent
pu'bic
pu'bis *pl.* -bes'
pub'lic
pub'lic-ad•dress'
　system
pub'li•can
pub'li•ca'tion
pub'li•cist
pub•lic'i•ty
pub'li•cize', -cized',
　-ciz'ing
pub'lic•ly
pub'lic-spir'i•ted
pub'lish
pub'lish•a•ble
pub'lish•er
puce
puck *(hockey disk)*
Puck *(sprite)*
puck'er
pud'ding
pud'dle, -dled, -dling
pudg'y
pueb'lo *pl.* -los
pu'cr•ile
pu'er•il'i•ty

pu•er'per•al
Puer'to Ri'can
puff 'ball'
puff 'er
puf 'fin
puff 'y
pug
pu'gi•lism
pu'gi•list
pu'gi•lis'tic
pug•na'cious
pug•nac'i•ty
puis'sance
puis'sant
pul'chri•tude'
pul'chri•tu'di•nous
pule, puled, pul'ing
Pul'it•zer Prize
pull'back' *n.*
pul'let
pul'ley *pl.* -leys
Pull'man
pull'out' *n.*
pull'o'ver *n.*
pull'-up' *n.*
pul'mo•nar'y
pul'pit
pulp'wood'
pulp'y
pul'sar'
pul'sate', -sat'ed, -sat'-
　ing
pul•sa'tion
pulse, pulsed, puls'ing
pul'ver•i•za'tion
pul'ver•ize', -ized',
　-iz'ing

pu'ma
pum'ice, -iced, -ic-
　ing
pum'mel, -meled *or*
　-melled, -mel•ing *or*
　-mel•ling
pump'er
pum'per•nick'el
pump'kin
pump'kin•seed'
pun, punned, pun'-
　ning
punch'-drunk'
pun'cheon
punch'y
punc•til'i•o' *pl.* -os'
punc•til'i•ous
punc'tu•al
punc'tu•al'i•ty
punc'tu•ate', -at'ed,
　-at'ing
punc'tu•a'tion
punc'tu•a'tor
punc'ture, -tured,
　-tur•ing
pun'dit
pun'gen•cy
pun'gent
pun'ish
pun'ish•a•ble
pun'ish•ment
pu'ni•tive
punk
pun'ster
punt'er
pu'ny
pup

pu'pa *pl.* -pae *or* -pas

pu'pal *(of a pupa)*
♦*pupil*

pu'pate', -pat'ed,
-pat'ing

pu•pa'tion

pu'pil *(student)*
♦*pupal*

pup'pet

pup'pet•eer'

pup'pet•ry

pup'py

pur'blind'

pur'chas•a•ble

pur'chase, -chased,
-chas•ing

pure, pur'er, pur'est

pure'bred

pu•rée'

pure'ly

pur•ga'tion

pur'ga•tive

pur'ga•to'ri•al

pur'ga•to'ry

purge, purged, purg'-
ing

pu'ri•fi•ca'tion

pu•rif'i•ca•to'ry

pu'ri•fi'er

pu'ri•fy', -fied', -fy'-
ing

Pu'rim

pur'ism

pur'ist

Pu'ri•tan *also* pu'ri-
tan

pu'ri•tan'i•cal

Pu'ri•tan•ism *also*
pu'ri•tan•ism

pu'ri•ty

purl *(to ripple, knit)*
♦*pearl*

pur'lieu

pur•loin'

pur'ple

pur'plish

pur'port' *n.*

pur•port' *v.*

pur'pose, -posed,
-pos•ing

pur'pose•ful

purr

purse, pursed, purs'-
ing

purs'er

pur•su'a•ble

pur•su'ance

pur•su'ant

pur•sue', -sued', -su'-
ing

pur•suit'

pur'sui•vant

pu'ru•lence

pu'ru•lent

pur•vey'

pur•vey'ance

pur•vey'or

pur'view'

pus

push'back'

push'-but'ton *adj.*

push'cart'

push'er

push'o'ver *n.*

push'pin'

push'up' *n.*

push'y

pu'sil•la•nim'i•ty

pu'sil•lan'i•mous

puss'y *(cat)*

pus'sy *(full of pus)*

puss'y•foot'

pus'tule'

put *(to place),* put,
put'ting
♦*putt*

pu'ta•tive

put'-down' *n.*

put'off' *n.*

put'-on' *n. & adj.*

put'out' *n.*

pu'tre•fac'tion

pu'tre•fac'tive

pu'tre•fy', -fied', -fy'-
ing

pu'trid

pu•trid'i•ty

putsch

putt *(to hit a golf
ball),* put'ted, put'-
ting
♦*put*

put•tee'

putt'er *(golf club)*

put'ter *(to occupy one-
self aimlessly)*

put'ty, -tied, -ty•ing

put'-up' *adj.*

puz'zle, -zled, -zling

puz'zle•ment

Pyg•ma'lion

pyg′my *also* pig′my
py′lon′
py′or•rhe′a *also* py′-
    or•rhoe′a
pyr′a•mid
py•ram′i•dal
pyre
py•re′thrum
py•ret′ic
Py′rex′®
pyr′i•dine′
pyr′i•dox′ine′ *also*
    pyr′i•dox′in
py′rite′
py•ri′tes *pl.* -tes
py′ro•ma′ni•a
py′ro•ma′ni•ac′
py′ro•tech′nic *also*
    py′ro•tech′ni•cal
py′ro•tech′nics
Py•thag′o•re′an
py′thon′
pyx *also* pix

Q

quack′er•y
quad
quad•ran′gle
quad′rant
quad′ra•phon′ic
quad′rate′
quad•rat′ic
quad•ren′ni•al
quad′ri•ceps′
quad′ri•lat′er•al
qua•drille′

quad•ril′lion
quad•ril′lionth
quad′ri•par′tite′
quad′ri•phon′ic *also*
    quad′ro•phon′ic
quad′ri•ple′gi•a
quad′ri•ple′gic
quad•roon′
quad•ru•ped′
quad•ru′ple, -pled,
    -pling
quad•ru′plet
quad•ru′pli•cate′,
    -cat′ed, -cat′ing
quad•ru′pli•ca′tion
quaff
quag′gy
quag′mire′
qua′hog′
quail *pl.* quail *or*
    quails
quaint′ly
quake, quaked, quak′-
    ing
quake′proof ′
Quak′er
quak′y
qual′i•fi•ca′tion
qual′i•fi′er
qual′i•fy′, -fied′, -fy′-
    ing
qual′i•ta′tive
qual′i•ty
qualm
quan′da•ry
quant
quan′tal

quan′tic
quan′ti•fi•ca′tion
quan′ti•fy′, -fied′,
    -fy′ing
quan′ti•ta′tive
quan′ti•ty
quan′tum *pl.* -ta
quar′an•tine′,
    -tined′, -tin′ing
quark
quar′rel, -reled *or*
    -relled, -rel′ing *or*
    -rel•ling
quar′rel•er *or* quar′-
    rel•ler
quar′rel•some
quar′ry, -ried, -ry•ing
quart
quar′ter
quar′ter•back′
quar′ter-deck′
quar′ter•fi′nal
quar′ter-hour′ *also*
    quarter hour
quar′ter•ly
quar′ter•mas′ter
quar′tern
quar′ter•staff ′ *pl.*
    -staves
quar•tet′ *also* quar•
    tette′
quar′to *pl.* -tos
quartz *(mineral)*
    ♦*quarts*
quartz′ite′
qua′sar′
quash

qua'si'
qua'si'-stel'lar
  object
qua'ter•nar'y *(in fours)*
Qua'ter•nar'y *(geologic period)*
quat'rain'
quat're•foil'
qua'ver
quay *(wharf)*
  ♦*cay, key*
quea'sy
queen'ly
queer'ly
quell
quench'a•ble
que•nelle'
quer'u•lous
que'ry, -ried, -ry•ing
quest
ques'tion
ques'tion•a•ble
ques'tion•naire'
queue *(line)*
  ♦*cue*
quib'ble, -bled, -bling
quiche
quick'en
quick'-freeze',
  -froze', -fro'zen,
  -freez'ing
quick'ie
quick'lime'
quick'sand'
quick'sil'ver
quick'step'

quick'-tem'pered
quick'-wit'ted
quid *(money)*, pl. quid
  or quids
quid' pro quo'
qui•es'cence
qui•es'cent
qui'et
qui'e•tude'
qui•e'tus
quill
quill'work'
quilt'ing
quince
qui'nine'
quin•quen'ni•al
quin'sy
quint
quin'tal
quin•tes'sence
quin'tes•sen'tial
quin•tet' *also* quin-
  tette'
quin•til'lion
quin•til'lionth
quin•tu'ple, -pled,
  -pling
quin•tu'plet
quip, quipped, quip'-
  ping
quip'ster
quire *(sheets of paper)*
  ♦*choir*
quirk'y
quis'ling
quit, quit *or* quit'ted,
  quit'ting

quit'claim'
quite
quit'rent'
quit'tance
quit'ter
quiv'er
qui vive'
quix•ot'ic *also* quix-
  ot'i•cal
quiz, quizzed, quiz'-
  zing
quiz pl. quiz'zes
quiz'zi•cal
quiz'zi•cal'i•ty
quoin *(corner)*
  ♦*coin*
quoit
quon'dam
quo'rum
quo'ta
quot'a•ble
quo•ta'tion
quote, quot'ed, quot'-
  ing
quoth
quo•tid'i•an
quo'tient

R

rab'bet *(groove)*
  ♦*rabbit*
rab'bi pl. -bis
rab'bin•ate
rab•bin'i•cal *also*
  rab•bin'ic
rab'bit *(animal)*, pl.

-bit *or* -bits
♦*rabbet*
rab′ble
rab′ble-rous′er
Rab′e•lai′si•an
rab′id
ra•bid′i•ty
ra′bies
rac•coon′ *pl.* -coons′
  or -coon′
race, raced, rac′ing
race′car′
race′course′
race′horse′
ra•ceme′
rac′er
race′track′
race′-walk′
race′way′
ra′cial
ra′cism
rac′ist
rack *(framework)*
  ♦*wrack*
rack′et *(bat),* also *rac′-
  quet*
rack′et *(noise)*
rack′et•eer′
rac′on•teur′
rac′quet•ball′
rac′y
ra′dar′
ra′dar•scope′
ra′di•al
ra′di•an
ra′di•ance *also* ra′di-
  an•cy

ra′di•ant
ra′di•ate′, -at′ed, -at′-
  ing
ra′di•a′tion
ra′di•a′tive
ra′di•a′tor
rad′i•cal
rad′i•cal•ism
rad′i•cal•i•za′tion
rad′i•cal•ize′, -ized′,
  -iz-′ing
rad′i•cand′
ra•dic′chi•o′ *pl.*
  -chi•os′
ra′di•o′ *pl.* -os
ra′di•o′, -oed′, -o′ing
ra′di•o•ac′tive
ra′di•o•ac•tiv′i•ty
ra′di•o•car′bon
ra′di•o•chem′i•cal
ra′di•o•chem′is•try
ra′di•o•gram′
ra′di•o•graph′
ra′di•og′ra•pher
ra′di•og′ra•phic
ra′di•og′ra•phy
ra′di•o•i′so•tope′
ra′di•o•lar′i•an
ra′di•o•log′i•cal
ra′di•ol′o•gist
ra′di•ol′o•gy
ra′di•om′e•ter
ra′di•o•met′ric
ra′di•om′e•try
ra′di•o•phone′
ra′di•opho′to-
  graph′ *also* ra′di-

o•pho′to
ra′di•o•pho•tog′ra-
  phy
ra′di•o•scop′ic *also*
  ra′di•o•scop′i•cal
ra′di•os′co•py
ra′di•o•sen′si•tive
ra′di•o•tel′e•graph′
ra′di•o•tel′e•graph′-
  ic
ra′di•o•te•leg′ra-
  phy
ra′di•o•tel′e•phone′
ra′di•o•tel′e•phon′-
  ic
ra′di•o•te•leph′-
  o•ny
ra′di•o•ther′a•py
rad′ish
ra′di•um
ra′di•us *pl.* -di•i′ *or*
  -di•us•es
ra′dix *pl.* rad′i•ces′ *or*
  ra′dix•es
ra′don′
raf′fi•a
raff′ish
raf′fle, -fled, -fling
raft
raf′ter
rag, ragged, rag′ging
ra′ga
rag′a•muf′fin
rage, raged, rag′ing
rag′ged
rag′ged•y
rag′lan

ra•gout'
rag'tag'
rag'time'
rag'weed'
rah
raid'er
rail'car'
rail'ing
rail'ler•y
rail'road'
rail'way'
rai'ment
rain *(precipitation)*
  ♦*reign, rein*
rain'bow'
rain'coat'
rain'drop'
rain'fall'
rain'mak'er
rain'mak'ing
rain'out'
rain'spout'
rain'storm'
rain'wat'er
rain'wear'
rain'y
raise *(to lift)*, raised,
  rais'ing
  ♦*rays, raze*
rais'er *(one that rais-
  es)*
  ♦*razor*
rai'sin
rai'son d'ê'tre
ra'jah *or* ra'ja
rake, raked, rak'ing
rake'-off' *n.*

rak'ish
ral'ly, -lied, -ly•ing
ram, rammed, ram'-
  ming
ram'ble, -bled, -bling
ram•bunc'tious
ram'e•kin *also* ram'-
  e•quin
ram'ie
ram'i•fi•ca'tion
ram'i•fy', -fied', -fy'-
  ing
ram'jet'
ra'mose'
ramp
ram'page', -paged',
  -pag'ing
ram'pan•cy
ram'pant
ram'part
ram'rod'
ram'shack'le
ranch'er
ran•che'ro *pl.* -ros
ran'cho *pl.* -chos
ran'cid
ran•cid'i•ty
ran'cor
ran'cor•ous
ran'dom
ran'dom•i•za'tion
ran'dom•ize', -ized',
  -iz'ing
range, ranged, rang'-
  ing
rang'er
rang'y

ra'ni *pl.* -nis, *also* ra'-
  nee
rank'ing
ran'kle, -kled, -kling
ran'sack'
ran'som
rant
rap *(to knock)*, rapped,
  rap'ping
  ♦*wrap*
ra•pa'cious
ra•pac'i•ty
rape, raped, rap'ing
rap'id
rap'id-fire'
ra•pid'i•ty
ra'pi•er
rap'ine
rap'ist
rap•pel', -pelled',
  -pel'ling
rap•port'
rap'proche•ment'
rap•scal'lion
rapt *(enchanted)*
  ♦*rapped, wrapped*
rap•to'ri•al
rap'ture
rap'tur•ous
ra'ra a'vis *pl.* ra'ra
  a'vis•es *or* ra'rae
  a'ves
rare, rar'er, rar'est
rare'bit
rare'-earth' element
rar'e•fac'tion
rar'e•fy', -fied', -fy'-

ing
rar′ing
rar′i•ty
ras′cal
ras•cal′i•ty
rash′er
rasp′ber′ry
rasp′y
rat, rat′ted, rat′ting
rat′a•bil′i•ty
rat′a•ble
ra′ta•touille′
ratch′et
rate, rat′ed, rat′ing
rate′mak′ing
rath′er
rat′i•fi•ca′tion
rat′i•fy′, -fied′, -fy′ing
ra′tio *pl.* -tios
ra′ti•oc′i•nate′, -nat′-
ed, -nat′ing
ra′ti•oc′i•na′tion
ra′ti•oc′i•na′tor
ra′tion
ra′tion•al *adj.*
ra′tion•ale′ *n.*
ra′tion•al•ism
ra′tion•al•ist
ra′tion•al•is′tic
ra′tion•al′i•ty
ra′tion•al•i•za′tion
ra′tion•al•ize′,
-ized′, -iz′ing
rat′ite′
rat′line *also* rat′lin
rat•tan′
rat′ter

rat′tle, -tled, -tling
rat′tle-brained′
rat′tler
rat′tle•snake′
rat′tle•trap′
rat′ty
rau′cous
rav′age, -aged, -ag-
ing
rave, raved, rav′ing
rav′el, -eled *or* -elled,
-el•ing *or* -el•ling
ra′ven
rav′en•ing
rav′en•ous
ra•vine′
rav′i•o′li
rav′ish
rav′ish•ing
raw′boned′
raw′hide′
ray *(beam, fish)*
  ♦*re*
ray′on′
raze *(to demolish),*
razed, raz′ing
  ♦*raise, rays*
ra′zor *(cutting instru-
ment)*
  ♦*raiser*
ra′zor•back′
ra′zor-blade′
raz′zle-daz′zle
razz′ma•tazz′
re *(musical tone)*
  ♦*ray*
re *(concerning)*

  ♦*ray*
reach
re•act′
re•ac′tance
re•ac′tant
re•ac′tion
re•ac′tion•ar′y
re•ac′ti•vate′, -vat′-
ed, -vat′ing
re•ac′tive
re•ac′tor
read *(to peruse),* read,
read′ing
  ♦*reed*
read′a•bil′i•ty
read′a•ble
read′er
read′er•ship′
read′i•ly
read′ing
re′ad•just′
re′ad•just′ment
read′-out′ *n.*
read′y, -ied, -y•ing
read′y-made′
re′af•firm′
re′af•fir•ma′tion
re•a′gent
re′al *(actual)*
  ♦*reel*
re′al-es•tate′ *adj.*
re′al•ism
re′al•ist
re′al•is′tic
re•al′i•ty *(actuality)*
  ♦*realty*
re′al•iz′a•ble

re•al•i•za'tion
re'al•ize', -ized', -iz'-
  ing
re'al•ly
realm
re'al-time' *adj.*
Re'al•tor
re'al•ty *(property)*
  ♦*reality*
ream'er
reap'er
re'ap•por'tion
re'ap•por'tion-
  ment
re'ap•prais'al
re•arm'
re•ar'ma•ment
rear'most'
re'ar•range',
  -ranged', -rang'ing
rear'view' mirror
rear'ward *also* rear'-
  wards
rea'son
rea'son•a•bil'i•ty
rea'son•a•ble
re•as•sur'ance
re•as•sure', -sured',
  -sur'ing
re'bate', -bat'ed, -bat'-
  ing
reb'el *n.*
re•bel', -belled', -bel'-
  ling
re•bel'lion
re•bel'lious
re•bind', -bound',

-bind'ing
re•birth'
re•born'
re'bound' *n.*
re•bound' *v.*
re•broad'cast', -cast'
  or -cast'ed, -cast'ing
re•buff'
re•build', -built',
  -build'ing
re•buke', -buked',
  -buk'ing
re'bus *pl.* -bus•es
re•but', -but'ted, -but'-
  ting
re•but'tal
re•cal'ci•trance *also*
  re•cal'ci•tran•cy
re•cal'ci•trant
re•call'
re•call'a•ble
re•cant'
re'can•ta'tion
re'cap' *(tire, summa-*
  ry)
re•cap' *(to rebond a*
  tire), -capped', -cap'-
  ping
re'cap' *(to summa-*
  rize), -capped', -cap'-
  ping
re'ca•pit'u•late',
  -lat'ed, -lat'ing
re'ca•pit'u•la'tion
re'ca•pit'u•la'tive
  also re•ca•pit'u•la-
  to'ry

re•cap'ture, -tured,
  -tur•ing
re'cast' *n.*
re•cast', -cast', -cast'-
  ing
re•cede' *(to ebb),*
  -ced'ed, -ced'ing
re-cede' *(to cede*
  back), -ced'ed, -ced'-
  ing
re•ceipt'
re•ceiv'a•ble
re•ceive', -ceived',
  -ceiv'ing
re•ceiv'er•ship'
re'cent
re•cep'ta•cle
re•cep'tion
re•cep'tion•ist
re•cep'tive
re'cep•tiv'i•ty
re•cep'tor
re'cess'
re•ces'sion *(with-*
  drawal)
re-ces'sion *(restora-*
  tion)
re•ces'sion•al
re•ces'sive
re'charge' *n.*
re•charge', -charged',
  charging
re•cher'ché'
re•cid'i•vism
re•cid'i•vist
re•cid'i•vis'tic
rec'i•pe

re•cip′i•ent
re•cip′ro•cal
re•cip′ro•cate′, -cat′-
　ed, -cat′ing
re•cip′ro•ca′tion
re•cip′ro•ca′tive
re•cip′ro•ca′tor
rec′i•proc′i•ty
re•cit′al
rec′i•ta′tion
rec′i•ta•tive adj.
rec′i•ta•tive n.
re•cite′, -cit′ed, -cit′-
　ing
reck′less
reck′on
re•claim′ (to make
　usable)
re-claim′ (to claim
　again)
re•claim′a•ble
re•claim′ant
rec′la•ma′tion
re•cline′, -clined′,
　-clin′ing
re•clin′er
re•cluse′
re•clu′sive
rec′og•ni′tion
rec′og•niz′a•ble
re•cog′ni•zance
re•cog′ni•zant
rec′og•nize′, -nized′,
　-niz′ing
re•coil′
rec•ol•lect′ (to re-
　member)

re′-col•lect′ (to col-
　lect again)
rec′ol•lec′tion
　(memory)
re′-col•lec′tion (new
　collection)
rec′ol•lec′tive
re•com′bi•nant
re′com•bi•na′tion
rec′om•mend′
rec′om•mend′a•ble
rec′om•men•da′-
　tion
rec′om•pense′,
　-pensed, -pens′ing
re′com•pose′,
　-posed′, -pos′ing
rec′on•cil′a•ble
rec′on•cile′, -ciled′,
　-cil′ing
rec′on•cil′i•a′tion
rec′on•cil′i•a•to′ry
rec′on•dite′
re•con′di•tion
re•con′nais•sance
re′con•noi′ter
re′con•sid′er
re′con•sid′er•a′tion
re′con•sti•tute′, -tut′-
　ed, -tut′ing
re′con•struct′
re′con•struc′tion
rec′ord n.
re•cord′ v.
re•cord′er
re•cord′ing
re•count′ (to narrate)

re-count′ (to count
　again)
re•coup′
re•cov′er (to regain)
re-cov′er (to cover
　anew)
re•cov′er•a•ble
re•cov′er•y
rec′re•ant
rec′re•ate′ (to re-
　fresh), -at′ed, -at′ing
re′-cre•ate′ (to create
　anew), -at′ed, -at′ing
rec′re•a′tion (refresh-
　ment)
re′-cre•a′tion (new
　creation)
rec′re•a′tion•al
re•crim′i•nate′, -nat′-
　ed, -nat′ing
re•crim′i•na′tion
re•crim′i•na′tor
re•crim′i•na•to′ry
re′cru•desce′,
　-desced′, -desc′ing
re′cru•des′cence
re′cru•des′cent
re•cruit′
re•cruit′ment
rec′tal
rec′tan′gle
rec•tan′gu•lar
rec•tan′gu•lar′i•ty
rec′ti•fi′a•ble
rec′ti•fi•ca′tion
rec′ti•fi′er
rec′ti•fy′, -fied′, -fy′-

ing
rec'ti·lin'e·ar
rec'ti·tude'
rec'to *pl.* -tos
rec'tor
rec'tor·ate
rec·to'ri·al
rec'to·ry
rec'tum *pl.* -tums *or*
  -ta
re·cum'bence
re·cum'bent
re·cu'per·ate', -at'-
  ed, -at'ing
re·cu'per·a'tion
re·cu'per·a'tive *also*
  re·cu'per·a·to'ry
re·cur', -curred', -cur'-
  ring
re·cur'rence
re·cur'rent
re·cuse', -cused',
  -cus'ing
re·cy'cle, -cled, -cling
red *(blood-colored),*
  red'der, red'dest
  ◆*read (past tense)*
re·dact'
re·dac'tion
re·dac'tor
red'bird'
red'-blood'ed
red'breast'
red'cap'
red'coat'
red'den
red'dish

re·dec'o·rate', -rat'-
  ed, -rat'ing
re·dec'o·ra'tion
re·deem'
re·deem'a·ble
re'de·liv'er
re·demp'tion
re'de·vel'op
re'de·vel'op·ment
red'-hand'ed
red'head'
red'-hot'
red'in·gote'
re'di·rect'
re'dis·trib'ute, -ut-
  ed, -ut'ing
re·dis'trict
red'-let'ter *adj.*
red'neck'
re'do', -did', -done',
  -do'ing, -does
red'o·lence *also* red'-
  o·len·cy
red'o·lent
re·dou'ble, -bled,
  -bling
re·doubt'
re·doubt'a·ble
re·dound'
re·dress'
re·dress'er *also* re-
  dres'sor
red'start'
re·duce', -duced',
  -duc'ing
re·duc'i·bil'i·ty
re·duc'i·ble

re·duc'ti·o' ad ab-
  sur'dum
re·duc'tion
re·duc'tion·ism
re·duc'tive
re·dun'dan·cy
re·dun'dant
re·du'pli·cate', -cat'-
  ed, -cat'ing
re·du'pli·ca'tion
re·du'pli·ca'tive
re·dux'
red'wing'
red'wood'
re-ech'o, -oed, -o·ing
reed *(grass, musical
  instrument)*
  ◆*read*
re-ed'u·cate', -cat'ed,
  -cat'ing
re-ed'u·ca'tion
reef
reek *(to smell)*
  ◆*wreak*
reel *(spool, whirling,
  dance)*
  ◆*real*
re'-e·lect' *or* re'-
  e·lect'
re'-e·lec'tion *or* re'-
  e·lec'tion
re'-en·act'
re'-en·act'ment
re-en'ter *or* re·en'ter
re-en'trance *or* re·en'-
  trance
re-en'try *or* re·en'try

re•es•tab′lish
reeve *(bailiff, bird)*
reeve *(to fasten a rope)*, reeved or rove, reev′ing
re′-ex•am′i•na′tion *or* re′ex•am′i•na′tion
re′-ex•am′ine, -ined, -in•ing, *or* re′ex•am′-ine
re•fec′tion
re•fec′to•ry
re•fer′, -ferred′, -fer′-ring
ref′er•a•ble
ref′e•ree′
ref′er•ence
ref′er•en′dum *pl.* -dums *or* -da
re•fer′ent
ref′er•en′tial
re•fer′ral
re•fer′rer
re′fill′ *n.*
re•fill′ *v.*
re•fi′nance, -nanced, -nanc•ing
re•fine′, -fined′, -fin′-ing
re•fine′ment
re•fin′er•y
re•fin′ish
re•fit′, -fit′ted, -fit′-ting
re•flect′
re•flec′tance

re•flec′tion
re•flec′tive
re•flec′tor
re′flex′ *adj. & n.*
re•flex′ *v.*
re•flex′ive
re•for′est
re′for•es•ta′tion
re•form′ *(to improve)*
re-form′ *(to form again)*
ref′or•ma′tion
re•for′ma•tive
re•for′ma•to•ry
re•form′er
re•fract′
re•frac′tion
re•frac′tive
re′frac•tiv′i•ty
re•frac′tor
re•frac′to•ry
re•frain′
re•fresh′
re•fresh′er
re•fresh′ment
re•frig′er•ant
re•frig′er•ate′, -at′-ed, -at′ing
re•frig′er•a′tion
re•frig′er•a′tor
re•fu′el
ref′uge
ref′u•gee′
re•ful′gence *also* re•ful′gen•cy
re•ful′gent
re′fund′ *n.*

re•fund′ *v.*
re•fund′a•ble
re•fut′a•bly
re•fur′bish
re•fus′al
ref′use *(trash)*
re•fuse′ *(to decline)*, -fused′, -fus′ing
re•fuse′nik
re•fut′a•bil′i•ty
re•fut′a•ble
ref′u•ta′tion *also* re•fu′tal
re•fute′, -fut′ed, -fut′-ing
re•gain′
re′gal *(royal)*
re•gale′ *(to delight)*, -galed′, -gal′ing
re•ga′lia
re•gard′
re•gard′ing
re•gard′less
re•gat′ta
re′gen•cy
re•gen′er•ate′, -at′-ed, -at′ing
re•gen′er•a′tion
re•gen′er•a′tive
re•gen′er•a′tor
re′gent
reg′i•cid′al
reg′i•cide′
re•gime′
reg′i•men
reg′i•ment
reg′i•men′tal

reg'i•men•ta'tion
re'gion
re'gion•al
re'gion•al•ism
reg'is•ter *(record)*
 ♦*registrar*
reg'is•tered
reg'is•trant
reg'is•trar' *(officer)*
 ♦*register*
reg'is•tra'tion
reg'is•try
reg'nant
re•gress' *n.*
re•gress' *v.*
re•gres'sion
re•gres'sive
re•gret', -gret'ted,
 gret'ting
re•gret'ful•ly
re•gret'ta•ble
re•group'
reg'u•lar
reg'u•lar'i•ty
reg'u•lar•ize', -ized',
 -iz'ing
reg'u•late', -lat'ed,
 -lat'ing
reg'u•la'tion
reg'u•la'tive
reg'u•la'tor
reg'u•la•to'ry
re•gur'gi•tate', -tat'-
 ed, -tat'ing
re•gur'gi•ta'tion
re'ha•bil'i•tate', -tat'-
 ed, -tat'ing

re'ha•bil'i•ta'tion
re'ha•bil'i•ta'tive
re'hash' *n.*
re•hash' *v.*
re•hear', -heard',
 -hear'ing
re•hears'al
re•hearse', -hearsed',
 -hears'ing
re•house', -housed',
 -hous'ing
Reich
reign *(sovereignty)*
 ♦*rain, rein*
reign *(to rule)*
 ♦*rain, rein*
re'im•burse',
 -bursed', -burs'ing
re'im•burse'ment
rein *(strap)*
 ♦*rain, reign*
rein *(to hold back)*
 ♦*rain, reign*
re'in•car'nate', -nat'-
 ed, -nat'ing
re'in•car•na'tion
rein'deer' *pl.* -deer' *or*
 -deers'
re'in•forc'a•ble
re'in•force', -forced',
 -forc'ing
re'in•force'ment
re'in•state', -stat'ed,
 -stat'ing
re'in•state'ment
re'in•sure', -sured',
 -sur'ing

re'in•vest'
re•is'sue, -sued, -su-
 ing
re•it'er•ate', -at'ed,
 -at'ing
re•it'er•a'tion
re•it'er•a'tive
re•ject' *n.*
re•ject' *v.*
re•ject'er *also* re•jec'-
 tor
re•jec'tion
re•joice', -joiced',
 -joic'ing
re•join' *(to respond)*
re-join' *(to reunite)*
re•join'der
re•ju've•nate', -nat'-
 ed, -nat'ing
re•ju've•na'tion
re•ju've•na'tor
re•lapse' *n.*
re•lapse', -lapsed',
 -laps'ing
re•late', -lat'ed, -lat'-
 ing
re•lat'er *also* re•la'tor
re•la'tion
re•la'tion•ship'
rel'a•tive
rel'a•tiv'i•ty
re•lax'
re•lax'ant
re•lax•a'tion
re'lay' *(to pass along)*,
 -laid' *or* -layed', -lay'-
 ing

re•lay' *(to lay again),*
-laid', -lay'ing

re•leas'a•ble

re•lease' *(to set free),*
-leased', -leas'ing

re'-lease' *(to lease
again),* -leased',
-leas'ing

rel'e•gate', -gat'ed,
-gat'ing

rel'e•ga'tion

re•lent'

re•lent'less

rel'e•vance *also* rel'-
e•van•cy

rel'e•vant

re•li'a•bil'i•ty

re•li'a•ble

re•li'ance

re•li'ant

rel'ic

re•lief '

re•liev'a•ble

re•lieve', -lieved',
-liev'ing

re•lig'ion

re•lig'i•os'i•ty

re•lig'ious

re•line', -lined', -lin'-
ing

re•lin'quish

rel'i•quar'y

rel'ish

re•live', -lived', -liv'-
ing

re•lo•cate', -cat'ed,
-cat'ing

re•lo•ca'tion

re•luc'tance *also* re-
luc'tan•cy

re•luc'tant

re•ly', -lied', -ly'ing

re•main'

re•main'der

re•mains'

re•make', -made',
-mak'ing

re•mand'

re•mark'

re•mark'a•ble

re•mar'ry, -ried, -ry-
ing

re•me'di•al

rem'e•dy, -died, -dy-
ing

re•mem'ber

re•mem'ber•a•ble

re•mem'brance

re•mind'

re•mind'er

rem'i•nisce',
-nisced', -nisc'ing

rem'i•nis'cence

rem'i•nis'cent

re•miss'

re•mis'si•bil'i•ty

re•mis'si•ble

re•mis'sion

re•mit', -mit'ted,
-mit'ting

re•mit'tal

re•mit'tance

re•mit'tent

re•mit'ter

rem'nant

re•mod'el

re•mon'strance

re•mon'strant

re•mon'strate',
-strat'ed, -strat'ing

re'mon•stra'tion

re•mon'stra•tive

re•mon'stra'tor

rem'o•ra

re•morse'

re•morse'ful

re•mote', -mot'er,
-mot'est

re•mount'

re•mov'a•bil'-
i•ty

re•mu'ner•a•ble

re•mu'ner•ate', -at'-
ed, -at'ing

re•mu'ner•a'tion

re•mu'ner•a'tive

re•mu'ner•a'tor

ren'ais•sance' *(re-
birth)*
♦renascence

re'nal

re•nas'cence *(renais-
sance)*

re•nas'cent

rend, rent *or* rend'ed,
rend'ing

ren'der

ren'dez•vous' *pl.*
  -vous'
ren•di'tion
ren'e•gade'
re•nege', -neged',
  -neg'ing
re•new'
re•new'a•ble
re•new'al
ren'net
ren'nin
re•nounce',
  -nounced', -nounc'-
  ing
ren'o•vate', -vat'ed,
  -vat'ing
ren'o•va'tion
ren'o•va'tor
re•nown'
re•nowned'
rent'al
re•num'ber
re•nun'ci•a'tion
re•nun'ci•a'tive
re•nun'ci•a•to'ry
re•o'pen
re•or'der
re•or'gan•i•za'tion
re•or'gan•ize',
  -ized', -iz'ing
rep *(ribbed fabric),*
  also repp
rep *(representative)*
re•pack'age, -aged,
  -ag•ing
re•pair'
re•pair'a•ble

re•pair'man'
rep'a•ra•bil'i•ty
rep'a•ra•ble
rep'a•ra'tion
re•par'a•tive *also*
  re•par'a•to'ry
rep'ar•tee'
re•past'
re•pa'tri•ate', -at'ed,
  -at'ing
re•pa'tri•a'tion
re•pay', -paid', -pay'-
  ing
re•pay'a•ble
re•pay'ment
re•peal'
re•peat'
re•pel', -pelled', -pel'-
  ling
re•pel'lcnce *also* re-
  pel'len•cy
re•pel'lent
re•pent'
re•pen'tance
re•pen'tant
re'per•cus'sion
re'per•cus'sive
rep'er•toire' *(group*
  of works), also rep'-
  er•to'ry
rep'er•to'ry *(theatri-*
  cal company)
rep'e•ti'tion
rep'e•ti'tious
re•pet'i•tive
re•phrase', -phrased',
  -phras'ing

re•pine', -pined',
  -pin'ing
re•place', -placed',
  -plac'ing
re•place'a•ble
re•place'ment
re'plant' *n.*
re•plant' *v.*
re'play' *n.*
re•play' *v.*
re•plen'ish
re•plen'ish•ment
re•plete'
re•ple'tion
rep'li•ca
rep'li•cate', -cat'ed,
  -cat'ing
rep'li•ca'tion
re•ply', -plied', -ply'-
  ing
re•port'
re•port'a•ble
re'port•age'
re•port'ed•ly
re•port'er
re•pos'al
re•pose', -posed',
  -pos'ing
re•pos'i•to'ry
re•pos•sess'
re•pos•ses'sion
rep're•hend'
rep're•hen'si•bil'-
  i•ty
rep're•hen'si•ble
rep're•hen'sion
rep're•sent'

rep′re•sen•ta′tion

rep′re•sen•ta′tion-al

rep′re•sen′ta•tive

re•press′

re•press′i•ble

re•pres′sion

re•pres′sive

re•pres′sor

re•priev′a•ble

re•prieve′, -prieved′, -priev′ing

rep′ri•mand′

re′print′ n.

re•print′ v.

re•pris′al

re•prise′

re•proach′

re•proach′ful

rep′ro•bate′

rep′ro•ba′tion

re′pro•duce′, -duced′, -duc′ing

re′pro•duc′er

re′pro•duc′i•ble

re′pro•duc′tion

re′pro•duc′tive

re′pro•graph′ics

re•proof′

re•prove′, -proved′, -prov′ing

rep′tile

rep•til′i•an

re•pub′lic

re•pub′li•can

re•pub′li•can•ism

re•pub′li•ca′tion

re•pub′lish

re•pu′di•ate′, -at′ed, -at′ing

re•pu′di•a′tion

re•pu′di•a′tor

re•pug′nance

re•pug′nant

re•pulse′, -pulsed′, -puls′ing

re•pul′sion

re•pul′sive

rep′u•ta•bil′i•ty

rep′u•ta•ble

rep′u•ta′tion

re•pute′, -put′ed, -put′ing

re•quest′

re′qui•em

re•quire′, -quired′, -quir′ing

re•quire′ment

req′ui•site

req′ui•si′tion

re•quit′al

re•quite′, -quit′ed, -quit′ing

re•route′, -rout′ed, -rout′ing

re′run′ n.

re•run′, -ran′, -run′-ning

re′sale′

re•scind′

re•scind′a•ble

re•scis′sion

res′cue, -cued, -cu•ing

re•search′

re•sec′tion

re•sem′blance

re•sem′ble, -bled, -bling

re•sent′

re•sent′ful

re•sent′ment

res′er•va′tion

re•serve′, -served′, -serv′ing

re•serv′ist

res′er•voir′

re•set′, -set′, -set′ting

re•shuf′fle, -fled, -fling

re•side′, -sid′ed, -sid′-ing

res′i•dence

res′i•den•cy

res′i•dent

res′i•den′tial

re•sid′u•al

re•sid′u•ar′y

res′i•due′

re•sign′ (to give up)

re-sign′ (to sign anew)

res′ig•na′tion

re•sil′ience also re-sil′ien•cy

re•sil′ient

res′in

res′in•ous

re•sist′

re•sis′tance

re•sis′tant

re•sist′er (one that re-sists)

re•sis′tor *(electrical device)*
re•sol′u•ble
res′o•lute′
res′o•lu′tion
re•solv′a•bil′i•ty
re•solv′a•ble
re•solve′, -solved′, -solv′ing
res′o•nance
res′o•nant
res′o•nate′, -nat′ed, -nat′ing
res′o•na′tion
res′o•na′tor
re•sort′
re•sound′
re′source′
re•source′ful
re•spect′
re•spect′a•bil′i•ty
re•spect′a•ble
re•spect′ful
re•spect′ful•ly *(deferentially)*
♦*respectively*
re•spec′tive
re•spec′tive•ly *(in order)*
♦*respectfully*
re•spell′, -spelled′ or -spelt,′ -spell′ing
res′pi•ra′tion
res′pi•ra′tor
res′pi•ra•to′ry
re•spire′, -spired′, -spir′ing

res′pite
re•splen′dence or re•splen′den•cy
re•splen′dent
re•spond′
re•spon′dent
re•sponse′
re•spon•si•bil′i•ty
re•spon′si•ble
re•spon′sive
rest *(quiet, remainder)*
♦*wrest*
re•state′, -stat′ed, -stat′ing
re•state′ment
res′tau•rant
res′tau•ra•teur′
rest′ful
res′ti•tu′tion
res′tive
rest′less
re•stock′
res′to•ra′tion
re•stor′a•tive
re•store′, -stored′, -stor′ing
re•strain′
re•straint′
re•strict′
re•stric′tion
re•stric′tive
re•sult′
re•sul′tant
re•sume′ *(to begin again)*, -sumed′, -sum′ing
rés′u•mé′ *(summary)*

re•sump′tion
re•sur′gence
re•sur′gent
res′ur•rect′
res′ur•rec′tion
re•sur•vey′ *n.*
re′sur•vey′ *v.*
re•sus′ci•tate′, -tat′ed, -tat′ing
re•sus′ci•ta′tion
re•sus′ci•ta′tive
re•sus′ci•ta′tor
re′tail′
re•tain′
re•take′ *n.*
re•take′, -took′, -tak′en, -tak′ing
re•tal′i•ate′, -at′ed, -at′ing
re•tal′i•a′tion
re•tal′i•a•to′ry
re•tard′
re•tar′dant
re•tar′date′
re′tar•da′tion
retch *(to vomit)*
♦*wretch*
re•tell′, -told′, -tell′ing
re•ten′tion
re•ten′tive
re•think′, -thought -think′ing
ret′i•cence
ret′i•cent
re•tic′u•lar
re•tic′u•late

re•tic'u•la'tion
ret'i•cule'
ret'i•na *pl.* -nas *or*
　-nae'
ret'i•nal
ret'i•nue'
re•tire', -tired', -tir'-
　ing
re•tire'ment
re•tool'
re•tort'
re•touch'
re•trace', -traced',
　-trac'ing
re•trace'a•ble
re•tract'
re•tract'a•ble *also*
　re•tract'i•ble
re•trac'tile
re•trac'tion
re•trac'tor
re'tread' *n.*
re•tread' *(to fit a new*
　tire tread), -tread'ed,
　-tread'ing
re-tread' *(to tread*
　again), -trod, -trod'-
　den, -tread'ing
re•treat'
re•trench'
re•trench'ment
re•tri'al
ret'ri•bu'tion
re•trib'u•tive *also*
　re•trib'u•to'ry
re•triev'a•ble
re•triev'al

re•trieve', -trieved',
　-triev'ing
ret'ro•ac'tive
ret'ro•grade'
ret'ro•gress'
ret'ro•gres'sion
ret'ro•gres'sive
ret'ro•rock'et
ret'ro•spect'
ret'ro•spec'tion
ret'ro•spec'tive
re•turn'
re•turn'a•ble
re•turn•ee'
re•un'ion
re'u•nite', -nit'ed,
　-nit'ing
re'up•hol'ster
rev, revved, rev'ving
re•val'u•a'tion
re•vamp'
re•veal'
rev'eil•le
rev'el, -eled *or* -elled,
　-el•ing *or* -el•ling
rev'e•la'tion
rev'el•er
rev'el•ry
re•venge', -venged',
　-veng'ing
rev'e•nue
re•verb'
re•ver'ber•ant'
re•ver'ber•ate', -at'-
　ed, -at'ing
re•ver'ber•a'tion
re•vere', -vered', -ver'-

　ing
rev'er•ence
rev'er•end
rev'er•ent
rev'er•en'tial
rev'er•ie
re•ver'sal
re•verse', -versed',
　-vers'ing
re•vers'i•bil'i•ty
re•vers'i•ble
re•ver'sion
re•vert'
re•vert'i•ble
re•view' *(examina-*
　tion)
　♦*revue*
re•vile', -viled', -vil'-
　ing
re•vis'a•ble
re•vise', -vised', -vis'-
　ing
re•vis'er *also* re•vi'-
　sor
re•vi'sion
re•vi'sion•ism
re•vi'sion•ist
re•vis'it
re•vi'tal•i•za'tion
re•vi'tal•ize', -ized',
　-iz'ing
re•viv'al
re•viv'al•ist
re•vive', -vived', -viv'-
　ing
re•viv'i•fy', -fied',
　-fy'ing

rev'o•ca•bil'i•ty
rev'o•ca•ble
rev'o•ca'tion
re•voke', -voked',
  -vok'ing
re•volt'
rev'o•lu'tion
rev'o•lu'tion•ar'y
rev'o•lu'tion•ist
rev'o•lu'tion•ize',
  -ized', -iz'ing
re•volv'a•ble
re•volve', -volved',
  -volv'ing
re•volv'er
re•vue' (musical
  show)
  ♦review
re•vul'sion
re•ward'
re'wind' n.
re•wind', -wound',
  -wind'ing
re•wire', -wired',
  -wir'ing
re•word'
re•work'
re'write' n.
re•write', -wrote',
  -writ'ten, -writ'ing
re•zone', -zoned',
  -zon'ing
rhap•sod'ic also
  rhap•sod'i•cal
rhap'so•dist
rhap'so•dize',
  -dized', -diz'ing

rhap'so•dy
rhe'a
rhe'ni•um
rhe'o•stat'
rhe'sus monkey
rhet'o•ric
rhe•tor'i•cal
rhet'o•ri'cian
rheum (mucus)
  ♦room
rheu•mat'ic
rheu'ma•tism
rheu'ma•toid'
rheum'y (full of
  rheum)
  ♦roomy
rhine'stone'
rhi'no pl. -nos
rhi•noc'er•os pl. -os
  or -os•es
rhi'zoid'
rhi•zoi'dal
rhi'zome'
rho (Greek letter)
  ♦roe, row (series,
  boat trip)
Rhode Is'land•er
Rho•de'sian
rho'di•um
rho'do•den'dron
rhom'bic
rhom'boid'
rhom•boi'dal
rhom'bus pl. -bus•es
  or -bi'
rhu'barb'
rhyme (to compose

verse), rhymed,
rhym'ing, also rime,
rimed, rim'ing
rhyme'ster also rime'-
ster
rhythm
rhyth'mi•cal also
  rhyth'mic
ri•al'to
ri•a'ta also re•a'ta
rib, ribbed, rib'bing
rib'ald
rib'ald•ry
rib'bon
ri'bo•fla'vin
ri'bo•nu'cle•ic acid
ri'bose'
ri•bo•so'mal
ri'bo•some
rice, riced, ric'ing
ric'er
rich'es
rich'ly
Rich'ter scale
rick'ets
rick'et•y
rick'rack'
ric'o•chet', -cheted'
  or -chet'ted, -chet'-
  ing or -chetting
ri•cot'ta
rid, rid or rid'ded, rid'-
  ding
rid'dance
rid'dle, -dled, -dling
ride, rode, rid'den,
  rid'ing

rid'er
ridge, ridged, ridg'ing
rid'i•cule', -culed',
   -cul'ing
ri•dic'u•lous
rid'ing
rife, rif'er, rif'est
rif'fle *(to shuffle)*,
   -fled, -fling
   ♦*rifle*
riff'raff'
ri'fle *(to plunder, cut
   grooves)*, -fled, -fling
   ♦*riffle*
rift
rig, rigged, rig'ging
rig'a•to'ni
rig'ger *(one who rigs)*
   ♦*rigor*
right *(correct, not left)*
   ♦*rite, write*
right'-an'gled
right'eous
right'ful
right'-hand' *adj.*
right'-hand'ed
right'ish
right'ist
right'ly
right'-on' *adj.*
right'-wing' *adj.*
rig'id
ri•gid'i•ty
rig'ma•role *also* rig'-
   a•ma•role
rig'or *(severity)*
   ♦*rigger*

rigor mor'tis
rig'or•ous
rile, riled, ril'ing
rim, rimmed, rim'-
   ming
rime *(to cover with
   frost)*, rimed, rim'ing
   ♦*rhyme*
rim'y
rind
ring *(circle)*
   ♦*wring*
ring *(encircle)*, ringed,
   ring'ing
   ♦*wring*
ring *(to sound)*, rang,
   rung, ring'ing
   ♦*wring*
ring'er
ring'lead'er
ring'let
ring'mas'ter
ring'-necked'
   pheasant
ring'side'
ring'tail'
ring'-tailed'
ring'worm'
rink
rinse, rinsed, rins'ing
ri'ot
ri'ot•ous
rip, ripped, rip'ping
ri•par'i•an
rip'cord'
ripe, rip'er, rip'est
rip'en

rip'-off' *n.*
ri•poste', -post'ed,
   -post'ing
rip'per
rip'ple, -pled, -pling
rip'ply
rip'-roar'ing *also*
   rip'-roar'i•ous
rise, rose, ris'en, ris'-
   ing
ris'er
ris'i•bil'i•ty
ris'i•ble
risk'y *(dangerous)*
   ♦*risqué*
ri•sot'to
ris•qué' *(suggestive)*
   ♦*risky*
ris'sole
ri'tar•dan'do
rite *(ceremony)*
   ♦*right, write*
rit'u•al
rit'u•al•is'tic
ritz'y
ri'val, -valed, -val•ing
ri'val•rous
ri'val•ry
rive, rived, rived *or*
   riv'en, riv'ing
riv'er
riv'er•bed'
riv'er•boat'
riv'er•side'
riv'ct
riv'u•let
roach *(fish) pl.* roach

or roach'es
road *(way)*
 ♦*rode, rowed*
road'bed'
road'block
road'house'
road'ie
road'run'ner
road'side'
road'stead'
road'ster
road'way'
road'work'
roam
roan
roar'ing
roast'er
rob, robbed, rob'bing
rob'ber
rob'ber•y
robe, robed, rob'ing
rob'in
ro'bot
ro•bot'ics
ro•bust'
ro•bus'tious
roc *(legendary bird)*
rock *(stone, swaying motion)*
rock'-bound'
rock'er
rock'et
rock'et•eer'
rock'et•ry
rock'fish' *pl.* -fish' *or* -fish'es
rock' 'n' roll' *also*

rock'-and-roll'
rock'-ribbed'
rock'y
ro•co'co
rod
ro'dent
ro'de•o' *pl.* -os'
roe *(fish eggs, deer)*
 ♦*rho, row (series, boat trip)*
roe'buck'
roent'gen
rog'er *interj.*
rogue
Rogue'fort cheese
rogu'er•y
rogu'ish
roil *(to muddy)*
 ♦*royal*
rois'ter
rois'ter•ous
role *(part), also* rôle
roll *(list, bread)*
roll *(to revolve)*
roll'a•way'
roll'back' *n.*
roll'er
rol'ler•drome'
roll'er-skate', -skat'- ed, -skat'ing
rol'lick
rol'lick•ing
roll'-on' *adj.*
roll'out'
roll'o'ver
Ro'lo•dex' ®
ro'ly-po'ly

ro•maine
ro'man *(type)*
Ro'man *(of Rome)*
ro•mance' *(story)*
Ro•mance' *(languages)*
Ro'man•esque'
Roman numeral
ro•man'tic
ro•man'ti•cism
ro•man'ti•cist
ro•man'ti•cize', -cized', -ciz'ing
Rom'a•ny *pl.* -ny *or* -nies
Ro'me•o' *pl.* -os'
romp'ers
ron'do *pl.* -dos
rood *(cross)*
 ♦*rude, rued*
roof'ing
rook'er•y
rook'ie
room *(space)*
 ♦*rheum*
room'er *(lodger)*
 ♦*rumor*
room•ette'
room'ful' *pl.* -fuls
room'mate'
room'y *(spacious)*
 ♦*rheumy*
roost'er
root *(plant part, origin)*
 ♦*route*
root *(to dig, cheer)*

♦*route*
root′stock′
rope, roped, rop′ing
rop′y
Roque′fort
Ror′schach test
ro′sa•ry
rose *(flower)*
ro•sé′ *(wine)*
ro′se•ate
rose′bud′
rose′bush′
rose′-col′ored
rose′mar′y
ro•sette′
rose′wood′
Rosh′ Ha•sha′nah
　　also Rosh′ Ha•sha′-
　　na, Rosh′ Ha•sho′-
　　na, Rosh′ Ha•sho′-
　　nah
Ro′si•cru′cian
ros′in
ros′ter
ros′trum *pl.* -trums *or*
　　-tra
ros′y
rot, rot′ted, rot′ting
Ro•tar′i•an
ro′ta•ry
ro′tate′, -tat′ed, -tat′-
　　ing
ro•ta′tion
ro′ta•tive
ro′ta′tor
ro′ta•to′ry
rote *(repetition)*

♦*wrote*
ro′ti•fer
ro•tis′se•rie
ro′to•gra•vure′
ro′tor
rot′ten
ro•tund′
ro•tun′da
ro•tun′di•ty
rou•é′
rouge, rouged, roug′-
　　ing
rough *(uneven)*
♦*ruff*
rough′age
rough′-and-read′y
　　adj.
rough′-and-tum′ble
　　adj.
rough′en
rough′hew′ -hewed′
　　or -hewn′, -hew′ing
rough′house′,
　　-housed′, -hous′ing
rough′neck′
rough′rid′er
rough′shod′
rou•lade′
rou•lette′
round′a•bout′
round′ed
roun′del
roun′de•lay′
round′house′
round′ly′
round′-shoul′dered
round′-the-clock′

round′-trip′ *adj.*
round′up′ *n.*
round′worm′
rouse, roused, rous′-
　　ing
roust′a•bout′
rout *(retreat)*
rout *(to defeat, search)*
route *(way)*
♦*root*
rou•tine′
roux *(thickener)*
♦*rue*
rove, roved, rov′ing
row *(series, boat trip)*
♦*rho, roe*
row *(quarrel)*
row′an
row′boat′
row′dy
row′el
roy′al *(regal)*
♦*roil*
roy′al•ist
roy′al•ty
rub, rubbed, rub′bing
rub′ber
rub′ber•ize′, -ized′,
　　-iz′ing
rub′ber•neck′
rub′ber-stamp′ *v.*
rub′ber•y
rub′bing
rub′bish
rub′ble
rub′down′ *n.*
rube

ru•bel′la
ru′bi•cund
ru•bid′i•um
rub′out′
ru′bric
ru′by
ruche
ruck′sack′
ruck′us
rud′der
rud′dy
rude *(impolite)*, rud′-
  er, rud′est
  ♦*rood, rued*
ru′di•ment
ru′di•men′ta•ry
rue *(to feel regret for)*,
  rued, ru′ing
  ♦*roux*
rue′ful
ruff *(collar)*
  ♦*rough*
ruf′fi•an
ruf′fle, -fled, -fling
rug
Rug′by
rug′ged
ru′in *(destruction)*
  ♦*rune*
ru′in•a′tion
ru′in•ous
rule, ruled, rul′ing
rul′er
ru′ly
rum
Ru•ma′ni•an *also*

Ro•ma′ni•an, Rou-
  ma′ni•an
rum′ba *also* rhum′ba
rum′ble, -bled, -bling
rum•bus′tious
ru′mi•nant
ru′mi•nate′, -nat′ed,
  -nat′ing
ru′mi•na′tion
ru′mi•na′tive
ru′mi•na′tor
rum′mage, -maged,
  -mag•ing
rum′my
ru′mor *(gossip)*
  ♦*roomer*
ru′mor•mon′ger
rump
rum′ple, -pled, -pling
rum′pus
rum′run′ner
run, ran, run, run′ning
run′a•bout′
run′-a•round′
run′a•way′
run′back′ *n.*
run′-down′ *n. & adj.*
rune *(Germanic alpha-
  betic character)*
  ♦*ruin*
rung *(step)*
  ♦*wrung*
run′ic
run′-in′ *n.*
run′let
run′nel

run′ner
run′ner-up′
run′ning
run′ny
run′-off′ *n.*
run′-of-the-mill′ *adj.*
run′-on′ *n. & adj.*
runt
run′-through′ *n.*
run′way′
rup′ture, -tured, -tur-
  ing
ru′ral
ruse
rush′er
rush′-hour′ *adj.*
rus′set
Rus′sian
rust
rus′tic
rus′ti•cate′, -cat′ed,
  -cat′ing
rus′ti•ca′tion
rus′ti•ca′tor
rus•tic′i•ty
rus′tle, -tled, -tling
rus′tler
rust′proof′
rust′y
rut, rut′ted, rut′ting
ru′ta•ba′ga
ru•the′ni•um
ruth′less
rut′ty
ry′a
rye *(grain, whiskey)*
  ♦*wry*

S

Sab'bath
sab•bat'i•cal
sa'ber
sa'ber-toothed' tiger
sa'ble
sa•bot'
sab'o•tage', -taged',
  -tag'ing
sab'o•teur'
sac (pouch)
  ♦sack
sac'cha•rin n.
sac'cha•rine adj.
sac'er•do'tal
sa'chem
sa•chet' (perfume)
  ♦sashay
sack (bag, loot, wine)
  ♦sac
sack (to fire, loot)
  ♦sac
sack'cloth'
sack'ing
sac'ra•ment
sac'ra•men'tal
sa'cred
sac'ri•flce', -ficed',
  -fic'ing
sac'ri•fi'cial
sac'ri•lege
sac'ri•le'gious
sac'ris•tan
sac'ris•ty
sac'ro•il'i•ac'

sac'ro•sanct'
sa'crum pl. -cra
sad, sad'der, sad'dest
sad'den
sad'dle, -dled, -dling
sad'dle•bag'
sad'dle•bow'
sad'dle•cloth'
sad'dler
sad'i'ron
sa'dism
sa'dist
sa•dis'tic
sa•fa'ri pl. -ris
safe, saf'er, saf'est
safe'-con'duct n.
safe'crack'er
safe'-de•pos'it box.
safe'guard'
safe'keep'ing
safe'ty
saf'flow'er
saf'fron
sag, sagged, sag'ging
sa'ga
sa•ga'cious
sa•gac'i•ty
sag'a•more'
sage, sag'er, sag'est
sage'brush'
Sag'it•ta'ri•us
sa'go pl. -gos
sa•gua'ro pl. -ros,
  also sa•hua'ro
sa'hib
said
sail (canvas)

♦sale
sail'boat'
sail'cloth'
sail'fish' pl. -fish' or
  -fish'es
sail'ing
sail'or
saint'ed
saint'hood'
saint'ly
sake (purpose)
sa'ke (liquor), also sa'-
  ki
sa•laam'
sal'a•bil'i•ty
sal'a•ble also sale'-
  a•ble
sa•la'cious
sa•lac'i•ty
sal'ad
sal'a•man'der
sa•la'mi pl. -mis
sal am•mo'ni•ac'
sal'a•ried
sal'a•ry
sale (exchange, bar-
  gain)
  ♦sail
sales'clerk'
sales'man
sales'man•ship'
sales'per'son
sales'room'
sales'wom'an
sal'i•cyl'ic acid
sa'li•ence also sa'li-
  en•cy

sa′li•ent
sa′line′
sa•lin′i•ty
sa•li′va
sal′i•var′y
sal′i•vate′, -vat′ed,
-vat′ing
sal′i•va′tion
sal′low
sal′ly, -lied, -ly•ing
sal′ma•gun′di
salm′on pl. -on or
-ons
sal′mo•nel′la pl. -nel′-
lae, -nel′las, or -nel′-
la
sa•lon′ (room, assem-
blage)
sa•loon′ (tavern)
sa•loon′keep′er
salt′box′
salt′cel′lar
sal•tine′
salt′pe′ter
salt′shak′er
salt′-wa′ter adj.
salt′works′
salt′y
sa•lu′bri•ous
sa•lu′ki pl. -kis
sal′u•tar′y
sal′u•ta′tion
sa•lu′ta•to′ri•an
sa•lu′ta•to′ry
sa•lute′, -lut′ed, -lut′-
ing
sal′va•ble

sal′vage, -vaged,
-vag•ing
sal′vage•a•ble
sal•vag′er
sal•va′tion
salve, salved, salv′ing
sal′ver
sal′vi•a
sal′vo pl. -vos or
-voes
sam′a•ra
Sa•mar′i•tan
sa•mar′i•um
sam′ba
sam•bu′ca
same
same′ness
sam′i•sen′
Sa•mo′an
sam′o•var′
Sam′o•yed′ also
Sam′o•yede′
sam′pan′
sam′ple, -pled, -pling
sam′pler
sam′u•rai′ pl. -rai′ or
-rais′
san′a•to′ri•um
(chronic-treatment
or recuperative hos-
pital), pl. -ri•ums or
-ri•a
♦sanatorium
sanc′ti•fi•ca′tion
sanc′ti•fy′, -fied′, -fy′-
ing
sanc′ti•mo′ni•ous

sanc′ti•mo′ny
sanc′tion
sanc′ti•ty
sanc′tu•ar′y
sanc′tum pl. -tums or
-ta
san′dal
san′dal•wood′
san′da•rac′
sand′bag′, -bagged′,
-bag′ging
sand′bar′
sand′blast′
sand′box′
sand′er
sand′hog′
sand′lot′
sand′man′
sand′pa′per
sand′pi′per
sand′stone′
sand′storm′
sand′wich
sand′y
sane (rational), san′er,
san′est
♦seine
San′for•ized′®
sang-froid′
san•gri′a
san′gui•nar′y
san′guine
san′i•tar′i•um
(health resort), pl.
-i•ums or -i•a
♦sanatorium
san′i•tar′y

san'i•ta'tion
san'i•tize', -tized', -tiz'ing
san'i•ty
san'sei' pl. -sei' or -seis'
San'skrit'
sans ser'if
San'ta Claus'
sap, sapped, sap'ping
sa'pi•ence
sa'pi•ent
sap'ling
sap'o•dil'la
sap'phire
sap'py
sap'ro•phyte'
sap'ro•phyt'ic
sap'suck'er
sap'wood'
sa•ran' also Sa•ran'®
sar'casm'
sar•cas'tic
sar•co'ma pl. -ma•ta or -mas
sar•coph'a•gus pl. -gi' or -gus•es
sard
sar•dine'
Sar•din'i•an
sar•don'ic
sar•gas'so
sa'ri pl. -ris
sa•rong'
sar'sa•pa•ril'la
sar•to'ri•al
sash

sa•shay' (to strut)
♦sachet
sass
sas'sa•fras'
sas'sy
Sa'tan
sa•tan'ic or sa•tan'i•cal
sa'tay
satch'el
sate, sat'ed, sat'ing
sa•teen'
sat'el•lite'
sa'ti•a•bil'i•ty
sa'ti•a•ble
sa'ti•ate', -at'ed, -at'ing
sa'ti•a'tion
sa•ti'e•ty
sat'in
sat'in•wood'
sat'in•y
sat'ire
sa•tir'i•cal or sa•tir'ic
sat'i•rist
sat'i•rize', -rized', -riz'ing
sat'is•fac'tion
sat'is•fac'to•ry
sat'is•fi'er
sat'is•fy', -fied', -fy'ing
sa'trap'
sa'tra•py
sat'u•ra•ble
sat'u•rate', -rat'ed,

-rat'ing
sat'u•ra'tion
sat'u•ra'tor
Sat'ur•day'
Sat'urn
sat'ur•na'li•a
sat'ur•nine'
sat'yr
sa'ty•ri'a•sis
sauce, sauced, sauc'ing
sauce'boat'
sauce'pan'
sauce'pot'
sau'cer
sau'cy
Sau'di A•ra'bi•an
sau'er•bra'ten
sauer'kraut'
sau'na
saun'ter
sau'ri•an
sau'sage
sau•té', -téed', -té'ing
sau•terne' or Sau•terne'
sav'a•ble also save'a•ble
sav'age, -aged, -ag•ing
sav'age•ry
sa•van'na also sa•van'nah
sa•vant'
save, saved, sav'ing
sav'ior also sav'iour
sa'voir-faire'

sa'vor
sa'vor•y
sav'vy, -vied, -vy•ing
saw, sawed, sawed or
  sawn, saw'ing
saw'bones' pl.
  -bones' or -bones'es
saw'buck'
saw'dust'
sawed'-off' adj.
saw'fish' pl. -fish' or
  -fish'es
saw'horse'
saw'mill'
saw'-toothed'
saw'yer
sax'horn'
sax'i•frage
sax'o•phone'
sax'o•phon'ist
say, said, say'ing
say'-so' pl. -sos'
scab, scabbed, scab'-
  bing
scab'bard
scab'by
sca'bies
scab'rous
scads
scaf 'fold
scaf 'fold•ing
sca'lar
scal'a•wag' also scal'-
  ly•wag'
scald
scale, scaled, scal'ing
sca'lene'

scal'lion
scal'lop also es•cal'-
  lop
scal'pel
scalp'er
scal'y
scamp
scam'per
scam'pi
scan, scanned, scan'-
  ning
scan'dal
scan'dal•ize', -ized',
  -iz'ing
scan'dal•mon'ger
scan'dal•ous
Scan'di•na'vi•an
scan'di•um
scan'ner
scan'sion
scant'ling
scant'y
scape'goat'
scape'grace'
scap'u•la pl. -las or
  -lae'
scap'u•lar
scar, scarred, scar'ring
scar'ab
scarce, scarc'er, scarc'-
  est
scar'ci•ty
scare, scared, scar'ing
scare'crow'
scarf pl. scarfs or
  scarves
scar'let

scarp
scar'y
scat, scat'ted, scat'ting
scathe, scathed, scath'-
  ing
scat'o•log'i•cal
sca•tol'o•gy
scat'ter
scat'ter•brain'
scat'ter•brained'
scat'ter•shot'
scav'enge, -enged,
  -eng•ing
sce•nar'i•o' pl. -os'
sce•nar'ist
scene (view)
  ♦seen
scen'er•y
sce'nic
scent (odor)
  ♦cent, sent
scep'ter
sched'ule, -uled, -ul•
  ing
sche'ma pl. -ma•ta
sche•mat'ic
scheme, schemed,
  schem'ing
scher•zan'do pl. -dos
scher'zo pl. -zos or -zi
Schick test
schism
schis•mat'ic
schist
schis'tose' also schis'-
  tous
schiz'oid'

schiz′o•phre′ni•a
schiz′o•phren′ic
schle•miel′
schlep, schlepped,
 schlep′ping
schli•ma′zel
schlock
schmaltz
schmo *pl.* schmoes,
 also schmoe
schnapps
schnau′zer
schnit′zel
schnook
schol′ar
schol′ar•ship′
scho•las′tic
scho•las′ti•cism
school′book′
school′boy′
school′child′
school′girl′
school′house′
school′ing
school′marm′
school′mas′ter
school′mate′
school′mis′tress
school′room′
school′teach′er
school′yard′
schoo′ner
schot′tische
schuss
schwa
sci•at′ic
sci•at′i•ca

sci′ence
sci′en•tif′ic
sci′en•tism
sci′en•tist
sci′en•tol′o•gy
scim′i•tar
scin•til′la
scin′til•late′, -lat′ed,
 -lat′ing
scin′til•la′tion
sci′on *also* ci′on
scis′sile
scis′sion
scis′sors
scle′ra
scle•ro′sis *pl.* -ses′
scle•rot′ic
scoff
scoff′law′
scold′ing
sconce
scone
scoop
scoot′er
scope
sco•pol′a•mine′
scor•bu′tic
scorch
score, scored, scor′ing
score′card′
sco′ri•a *pl.* -ri•ae′
scorn′ful
Scor′pi•o′
scor′pi•on
Scot
scotch *(to stifle)*
Scotch *(people, whis-*

key)
sco′ter
scot′-free′
sco′tia
Scots′man
Scot′tie
Scot′tish
scoun′drel
scourge, scourged,
 scourg′ing
scout′ing
scout′mas′ter
scow
scowl
scrab′ble *(to grope),*
 -bled, -bling
Scrab′ble® *(game)*
scrag′gly
scrag′gy
scram, scrammed,
 scram′ming
scram′ble, -bled,
 -bling
scrap, scrapped,
 scrap′ping
scrap′book′
scrape, scraped,
 scrap′ing
scrap′per
scrap′ple
scrap′py
scratch′board′
scratch′proof
scratch′y
scrawl
scraw′ny
scream′er

screech'ing

screed

screen'ing

screen'play'

screen'-test' *v.*

screen'writ'er

screw'ball'

screw'driv'er

screw'y

scrib'al

scrib'ble, -bled, -bling

scribe, scribed, scrib'-
ing

scrim

scrim'mage, -maged,
-mag•ing

scrimp

scrim'shaw'

scrip *(paper money)*

script *(writing, text)*

scrip'tur•al

Scrip'ture

script'writ'er

scriv'en•er

scrod

scrof'u•la

scrof'u•lous

scroll'work'

Scrooge

scro'tal

scro'tum *pl.* -ta *or*
-tums

scrounge, scrounged,
scroung'ing

scroung'y

scrub, scrubbed,
scrub'bing

scrub'ber

scrub'by

scrub'wom'an

scruff

scruf'fy

scrump'tious

scrunch

scru'ple, -pled, -pling

scru'pu•los'i•ty

scru'pu•lous

scru'ti•nize', -nized',
-niz'ing

scru'ti•ny

scu'ba

scud, scud'ded, scud'-
ding

scuff

scuf'fle, -fled, -fling

scull *(oar)*

♦*skull*

scul'ler•y

scul'lion

sculpt

sculp'tor

sculp'tress

sculp'tur•al

sculp'ture, -tured,
-tur•ing

scum

scup *pl.* scup *or* scups

scup'per

scup'per•nong'

scurf'y

scur•ril'i•ty

scur'ri•lous

scur'ry, -ried, -ry•ing

scur'vy

scut'tle, -tled, -tling

scut'tle•butt'

scut'work'

scythe, scythed, scyth'-
ing

sea *(water)*

♦*see, si*

Sea'bee'

sea'board'

sea'borne'

sea'coast'

sea'far'er

sea'far'ing

sea'food'

sea'go'ing

seal'er

seal'ing wax

seal'skin'

Sea'ly•ham' terrier

seam *(junction)*

♦*seem*

sea'man *(sailor)*

♦*semen*

sea'man•ship'

seam'stress

seam'y

sé'ance'

sea'plane'

sea'port'

sear *(to dry up)*

♦*seer, sere*

search'light'

sea'scape'

sea'shell'

sea'shore'

sea'sick'

sea'side'

sea′son
sea′son•a•ble
sea′son•al
sea′son•ing
seat′back′
seat′ing
seat′mate′
sea′ward *also* sea′-
wards
sea′way′
sea′weed′
sea′wor′thy
se•ba′ceous
se′cant
se•cede′, -ced′ed,
-ced′ing
se•ces′sion
se•ces′sion•ist
se•clude′, -clud′ed,
-clud′ing
se•clu′sion
se•clu′sive
sec′ond
sec′ond•ar′y
sec′ond-class′ *adj. &
adv.*
sec′ond-de•gree′
burn
sec′ond-guess′ *v.*
sec′ond•hand′ *adj. &
adv.*
second hand *(time-
piece part)*
sec′ond-rate′ *adj.*
se′cre•cy
se′cret *(concealed)*
♦*secrete*

se′cret *(something
kept hidden)*
♦*secrete*
sec′re•tar′i•al
sec′re•tar′i•at
sec′re•tar′y
sec′re•tar′y-gen′er-
al *pl.* sec′re•tar′ies-
gen′er•al
se•crete′ *(to exude a
substance, hide),*
-cret′ed, -cret′ing
♦*secret*
se•cre′tion
se•cre•tive
se•cre′tor
se•cre′to•ry
sect
sec•tar′i•an
sec•tar′i•an•ism
sec′tile
sec′tion
sec′tion•al
sec′tion•al•ism
sec′tion•al•ist
sec′tor
sec•to′ri•al
sec′u•lar
sec′u•lar•ism
sec′u•lar•ist
sec′u•lar•i•ty
sec′u•lar•i•za′tion
sec′u•lar•ize′, -ized′,
-iz′ing
se•cur′a•ble
se•cure′, -cur′er, -cur′-
est

se•cure′, -cured′,
-cur′ing
se•cu′ri•ty
se•dan′
se•date′, -dat′ed,
-dat′ing
se•da′tion
sed′a•tive
sed′en•tar′y
Se′der *pl.* Se′ders *or*
Se•dar′im
sedge
sed′i•ment
sed′i•men′ta•ry
sed′i•men•ta′tion
se•di′tion
se•di′tious
se•duce′, -duced′,
-duc′ing
se•duce′a•ble *also*
se•duc′i•ble
se•duc′tion
se•duc′tive
se•duc′tress
se•du′li•ty
sed′u•lous
se′dum
see *(bishopric)*
♦*sea, si*
see *(to perceive),* saw,
seen, see′ing
♦*sea, si*
seed *(plant part),* pl.
seeds *or* seed
♦*cede*
seed′case′
seed′ling

seed'y
seek, sought, seek'ing
seem *(to appear)*
 ♦*seam*
seem'ly
seep'age
seer *(prophet)*
 ♦*sear, sere*
seer'suck'er
see'saw'
seethe, seethed, seeth'-
 ing
see'-through' *adj.*
seg'ment
seg•men'tal
seg'men•ta'tion
seg•ment'ed
se'go *pl.* -gos
seg're•gate', -gat'ed,
 -gat'ing
seg're•ga'tion
seg're•ga'tion•ist
seg're•ga'tor
seign'ior
sei•gnio'ri•al
seine *(to fish with a
 net),* seined, sein'ing
 ♦*sane*
seis'mic
seis'mo•gram'
seis'mo•graph'
seis•mog'ra•pher
seis'mo•graph'ic
seis•mog'ra•phy
seis'mo•log'ic *also*
 seis'mo•log'i•cal
seis•mol'o•gist

seis•mol'o•gy
seis•mom'e•ter
seiz'a•ble
seize, seized, seiz'ing
sei'zure
sel'dom
se•lect'
se•lec'tion
se•lec'tive
se'lec•tiv'i•ty
se•lect'man
se•lec'tor
se•le'ni•um
self *pl.* selves
self'-ab•sorbed'
self'-ad•dressed'
self'-as•sur'ance
self'-as•sured'
self'-cen'tered
self'-con•fessed'
self'-con'fi•dence
self'-con'fi•dent
self'-con'scious
self'-con•tained'
self'-con•trol'
self'-con•trolled'
self'-de•feat'ing
self'-de•fense'
self'-de•ni'al
self'-de•ny'ing
self'-de•struct'
self'-de•struc'tive
self'-de•ter'mi•na'-
 tion
self'-dis'ci•pline
self'-ed'u•cat'ed
self'-ef•fac'ing

self'-em•ployed'
self'-es•teem'
self'-ev'i•dent
self'-ex•plan'a•to'-
 ry
self'-ex•pres'sion
self'-gov'ern•ing
self'-gov'ern•ment
self'-im•por'tance
self'-im•por'tant
self'-im•prove'-
 ment
self'-in•dul'gence
self'-in•dul'gent
self'-in'ter•est
self'ish
self'-knowl'edge
self'less
self'-made'
self'-pit'y
self'-por'trait
self'-pos•sessed'
self'-pos•ses'sion
self'-pres'er•va'tion
self'-re•li'ance
self'-re•li'ant
self'-re•spect'
self'-re•straint'
self'-right'eous
self'-rule'
self'-sac'ri•fice'
self'same'
self'-sat'is•fac'tion
self'-sat'is•fied'
self'-seek'ing
self'-serv'ice *adj.*
self'-start'er

self'-styled'
self'-suf•fi'cien•cy
self'-suf•fi'cient
self'-sup•port'
self'-sup•port'ing
self'-sus•tain'ing
self'-taught'
self'-will'
self'-willed'
self'-wind'ing
sell *(to exchange for money)*, sold, sell'-ing
　♦*cell*
sell'back'
sell'er *(vender)*
　♦*cellar*
sell'off '
sell'out' *n.*
selt'zer
sel'vage *also* sel'vedge
se•man'tic
se•man'ti•cist
se•man'tics
sem'a•phore',
　-phored', -phor'ing
sem'blance
se'men *(sperm)*
　♦*seaman*
se•mes'ter
sem'i•an'nu•al
　(twice a year)
　♦*biannual, biennial, biyearly, semiyearly*
sem'i•au'to•mat'ic
sem'i•cir'cle
scm'i•cir'cu•lar

sem'i•clas'si•cal
sem'i•co'lon
sem'i•con•duc'tor
sem'i•de•tached'
sem'i•dry'
sem'i•fi'nal
sem'i•fi'nal•ist
sem'i•for'mal
sem'i•gloss'
sem'i•month'ly
　(twice a month)
　♦*bimonthly*
sem'i•nal
sem'i•nar'
sem'i•nar'i•an
sem'i•nar'y
sem'i•of•fi'cial
sem'i•pre'cious
sem'i•pri'vate
sem'i•pro•fes'sion-al
sem'i•skilled'
sem'i•sol'id
Sem'ite'
Se•mit'ic
sem'i•tone'
sem'i•ton'ic
sem'i•trans•par'ent
sem'i•trop'i•cal
sem'i•vow'el
sem'i•week'ly *(twice a week)*
　♦*biweekly*
sem'i•year'ly *(twice a year)*
　♦*biannual, biennial, biyearly, semiannual*

sem'o•li•na
sen *pl.* sen
sen'ate *also* Sen'ate
sen'a•tor
sen'a•to'ri•al
send, sent, send'ing
send'off ' *n.*
se'nile'
se•nil'i•ty
sen'ior
sen•ior'i•ty
sen'na
se•ñor' *pl.* -ño'res
se•ño'ra
se•ño•ri'ta
sen'sate' *also* sen'sat-ed
sen•sa'tion
sen•sa'tion•al
sen•sa'tion•al•ism
sen•sa'tion•al•ist
sen•sa'tion•al•ize',
　-ized', -iz'ing
sense *(to perceive)*,
　sensed, sens'ing
　♦*cents*
sense'less
sen'si•bil'i•ty
sen'si•ble
sen'si•tive
sen'si•tiv'i•ty
sen'si•ti•za'tion
sen'si•tize', -tized',
　-tiz'ing
sen'sor
sen'so•ry
sen'su•al

sen'su•al•ist
sen'su•al•is'tic
sen'su•al'i•ty
sen'su•ous
sen'tence, -tenced,
  -tenc•ing
sen•ten'tial
sen•ten'tious
sen'tience
sen'tient
sen'ti•ment
sen'ti•men'tal
sen'ti•men'tal•ism
sen'ti•men'tal•ist
sen'ti•men•tal'i•ty
sen'ti•men'tal•ize',
  -ized', -iz'ing
sen'ti•nel
sen'try
se'pal
sep'a•ra•ble
sep'a•ra•rate, -rat'ed,
  -rat'ing
sep'a•ra'tion
sep'a•ra•tism
sep'a•ra•tist
sep'a•ra'tor
se'pi•a
sep'sis
sep'tal
Sep•tem'ber
sep•ten'ni•al
sep•tet' *also* sep-
  tette'
sep'tic
sep'ti•ce•mi•a
sep•til'lion

sep•til'lionth
sep'tu•a•ge•nar'-
  i•an
Sep'tu•a•ges'i•ma
sep'tu•a•gint'
sep'tum *pl.* -ta
sep'ul•cher
se•pul'chral
se'quel
se'quence
se•quen'tial
se•ques'ter
se•ques'trate', -trat'-
  ed, -trat'ing
se'ques•tra'tion
se'ques•tra'tor
se'quin
se•quoi'a
se•ra'glio *pl.* -glios
se•ra'pe *also* sa•ra'pe
ser'aph *pl.* -a•phim *or*
  -aphs
se•raph'ic
Serb
Ser'bi•an
Ser'bo-Cro•a'tian
sere *(withered)*
  ♦*sear, seer*
ser'e•nade', -nad'ed,
  -nad'ing
ser'en•dip'i•tous
ser'en•dip'i•ty
se•rene'
se•ren'i•ty
serf *(laborer)*
  ♦*surf*
serf'dom

serge *(cloth)*
  ♦*surge*
ser'gean•cy
ser'geant
se'ri•al *(of or in a se-*
  ries)
  ♦*cereal*
se'ri•al•i•za'tion
se'ri•al•ize', -ized',
  -iz'ing
se'ri•a'tim
ser'i•cul'ture
se'ries *pl.* -ries
ser'if
ser'i•graph'
se•rig'ra•phy
se•ri•o•com'ic
se'ri•ous
ser'mon
ser'mon•ize', -ized',
  -iz'ing
ser'o•log'ic *also* ser'-
  o•log'i•cal
se•rol'o•gist
se•rol'o•gy
ser'pent
ser'pen•tine'
ser'rate' *also* ser'rat'-
  ed
ser•ra'tion
ser'ried
se'rum *pl.* -rums *or*
  -ra
ser'vant
serve, served, serv'ing
serv'i•bar'
serv'ice, -iced, -ic•ing

serv′ice•a•bil′i•ty
serv′ice•a•ble
serv′ice•man′
serv′ice•per′son
ser′vile
ser•vil′i•ty
ser′vi•tor
ser′vi•tude′
ser′vo•mech′a•nism
ses′a•me
ses′qui•cen•ten′ni•al
ses′sile
ses′sion *(meeting)*
 ♦*cession*
ses•tet′
set, set, set′ing
se′ta *pl.* -tae′
set′back′ *n.*
set′off′ *n.*
set•tee′
set′ter
set′ting
set′tle, -tled, -tling
set′tle•ment
set′-to′ *pl.* -tos′
set′up′ *n.*
sev′en
sev′en•fold′
sev′en•teen′
sev′en•teenth′
sev′enth
sev′en•ti•eth
sev′en•ty
sev′en-up′
sev′er
sev′er•al

sev′er•al•fold′
sev′er•ance
se•vere′, -ver′er, -ver′-
 est
se•ver′i•ty
Sè′vres
sew *(to stitch),* sewed,
 sewn *or* sewed, sew′-
 ing
 ♦*so, sow (to scatter)*
sew′age
sew′er
sew′er•age
sex′a•ge•nar′i•an
sex′ism
sex′ist
sex′tant
sex•tet′
sex•til′lion
sex•til′lionth
sex′ton
sex•tu′ple, -pled,
 -pling
sex•tu′plet
sex′u•al
sex′u•al′i•ty
shab′by
shack
shack′le, -led, -ling
shad *pl.* shad *or* shads
shade, shad′ed, shad′-
 ing
shad′ow
shad′ow•box′
shad′y
shaft′ing
shag′bark′

shag′gy
shah
shak′a•ble *also*
 shake′a•ble
shake, shook, shak′en,
 shak′ing
shake′down′ *n. &*
 adj.
shake′out′ *n.*
shak′er *(one that*
 shakes)
Shak′er *(member of a*
 religious sect)
Shake•spear′e•an *or*
 Shake•spear′i•an
shake′up′ *n.*
shak′o *pl.* -os *or* -oes,
 also shack′o
shak′y
shale
shall *past tense* should
shal•lot′
shal′low
sha•lom′
sham, shammed,
 sham′ming
sha′man
sha′man•ism
sham′ble, -bled,
 -bling
shame, shamed,
 sham′ing
shame′faced′
shame′ful
shame′less
sham•poo′ *pl.* -poos′
sham′rock′

sha′mus
shang•hai′ *(to kid-
nap)*, -haied′, -hai′-
ing
shank
shan•tung′
shan′ty *(shack)*
♦*chantey*
shan′ty•town′
shape, shaped, shap′-
ing
shape′less
shape′ly
shape′up′ *n.*
shard *also* sherd
share, shared, shar′ing
share′crop′per
share′hold′er
shark′skin′
sharp′en
sharp′er
sharp′-eyed′
sharp′ie
sharp′shoot′er
sharp′-tongued′
Shas′ta daisy
shat′ter
shat′ter•proof′
glass
shave, shaved, shaved
or shav′en, shav′ing
shav′er
Sha′vi•an
shawl
shay
she
sheaf *pl.* sheaves

shear *(to clip)*,
sheared, sheared *or*
shorn, shear′ing
♦*sheer*
shears
sheath *pl.* sheaths
sheathe, sheathed,
sheath′ing
sheave, sheaved,
sheav′ing
she•bang′
shed, shed, shed′ding
shed′der
sheen
sheep *pl.* sheep
sheep′fold′
sheep′herd′er
sheep′ish
sheep′skin′
sheer *(thin)*
♦*shear*
sheer *(to swerve)*
♦*shear*
sheet′-fed′
sheet′ing
sheik *(Arab leader)*,
also sheikh
♦*chic*
sheik′dom
shek′el
shelf *pl.* shelves
shel•lac′, -lacked′,
-lack′ing
shell′bark′
shell′fire′
shell′fish′ *pl.* -fish′ *or*
-fish′es

shell′proof′
shell′-shocked′
shel′ter
shel′tie *also* shel′ty
shelve, shelved, shelv′-
ing
she•nan′i•gans
shep′herd
Sher′a•ton
sher′bet
sher′iff
sher′ry
Shet′land
shib′bo•leth
shield
shift′less
shift′y
shill
shil•le′lagh *also* shil-
la′lah
shil′ling
shil′ly-shal′ly, -lied,
-ly•ing
shim
shim′mer
shim′my, -mied,
-my•ing
shin, shinned, shin′-
ning
shin′bone′
shin′dig′
shine, shone *or*
shined, shin′ing
shin′er
shin′gle, -gled, -gling
shin′ny, -nied, -ny-
ing

shin'plas'ter
Shin'to also Shin'to-ism
shin'y
ship, shipped, ship'-ping
ship'board'
ship'build'er
ship'build'ing
ship'load'
ship'mas'ter
ship'mate'
ship'ment
ship'per
ship'ping
ship'shape'
ship'side'
ship'wreck'
ship'yard'
shire
shirk
shirr
shirt'ing
shirt'tail'
shirt'waist'
shish' ke•bab' also
  shish' ke•bob',
  shish' ka•bob'
shiv'er
shiv'er•y
shoal
shoat also shote
shock
shock'ing
shock'proof'
shod'dy
shoe *(to cover the*

foot), shod, shod *or*
  shod'den, shoe'ing
  ♦*shoo*
shoe'horn'
shoe'lace'
shoe'mak'er
shoe'mak'ing
shoe'string'
shoe'tree'
sho'far' *pl.* sho'fars'
  or sho•froth'
sho'gun'
shoo *interj.*
  ♦*shoe*
shoo *(to scare away)*,
  shooed, shoo'ing
  ♦*shoe*
shoo'fly' pie
shoo'-in' *n.*
shook-up' *adj.*
shoot *(to fire a weap-on)*, shot, shoot'ing
  ♦*chute*
shoot'down'
shoot'-out' *n.,* also
  shoot'out'
shop, shopped, shop'-ping
shop'keep'er
shop'lift'
shop'lift'er
shop'per
shop'talk'
shop'worn'
sho'ran'
shore, shored, shor'-ing

shore'front'
shore'line'
short'age
short'bread'
short'cake'
short'change',
  -changed', -chang'-ing
short'-cir'cuit *v.*
short'com'ing
short'en
short'en•ing
short'fall'
short'hand'
short'-hand'ed
short'horn'
short'-lived'
short'ly
short'-or'der *adj.*
short'sight'ed
short'stop'
short'-tem'pered
short'-wave' *adj.*
short'-wind'ed
shot *pl.* shots *or* shot
shot'gun'
shot'-put'
shot'-put'ter
shoul'der
shout'er
shove, shoved, shov'-ing
shov'el, -eled *or*
  -elled, -el•ing *or* -el-ling
show, showed, shown
  or showed, show'ing

show'boat'
show'case'
show'down'
show'er
show'girl'
show'man
show'man•ship'
show'off' *n.*
show'piece'
show'time'
show'y
shrap'nel *pl.* -nel
shred, shred'ded *or*
 shred, shred'ding
shred'der
shrew
shrewd'ly
shrew'ish
shriek'er
shrift
shrike
shrill'ness
shril'ly
shrimp *pl.* shrimp *or*
 shrimps
shrine
shrink, shrank *or*
 shrunk, shrunk *or*
 shrunk'en, shrink'-
 ing
shrink'a•ble
shrink'age
shrink'-pack'age,
 -aged, -ag•ing
shrink'-wrap',
 -wrapped', -wrap'-
 ping

shrive, shrove *or*
 shrived, shriv'en *or*
 shrived, shriv'ing
shriv'el, -eled *or*
 -elled, -el•ing *or* -el-
 ling
shroud
Shrove'tide'
shrub'ber•y
shrub'by
shrug, shrugged,
 shrug'ging
shuck
shucks
shud'der
shuf'fle, -fled, -fling
shuf'fle•board'
shun, shunned, shun'-
 ning
shun'ner
shun'pike'
shunt
shunt'-wound'
shush
shut, shut, shut'ting
shut'down' *n.*
shut'eye'
shut-in' *adj.*
shut'-in' *n.*
shut'off' *n.*
shut'out' *n.*
shut'ter
shut'ter•bug'
shut'tle, -tled, -tling
shut'tle•cock'
shut'tle•craft'
shy, shi'er *or* shy'er,

shi'est *or* shy'est
shy, shied, shy'ing
shy'lock' *also* Shy'-
 lock'
shy'ly
shy'ster
si *(musical tone)*
 ♦*sea, see*
Si'a•mese' *pl.* -mese'
Si•be'ri•an
sib'i•lance *also* sib'-
 i•lan•cy
sib'i•lant
sib'ling
sib'yl
sic *(thus)*
 ♦*sick*
sic *(to urge on)*, sicced,
 sic'cing, *also* sick
Si•cil'ian
sick *(ill)*
 ♦*sick*
sick'bay'
sick'bed'
sick'en
sick'en•ing
sick'le
sick'ly
sick'ness
sick'-out' *n.*
sick'room'
side, sid'ed, sid'ing
side'arm' *adj.*
side'board'
side'burns'
side'car'
side'kick'

side'light'
side'line', -lined',
  -lin'ing
side'long'
side'man'
si•de're•al
side'sad'dle
side'split'ting
side'step', -stepped',
  -step'ping
side'swipe', -swiped',
  -swip'ing
side'track'
side'walk'
side'ward *also* side'-
  wards
side'ways' *also* side'-
  way', side'wise'
side'-wheel'er
side'wind'er
sid'ing
si'dle, -dled, -dling
siege
si•en'na
si•er'ra
si•es'ta
sieve, sieved, siev'ing
sift'er
sift'ings
sigh
sight *(vision)*
  ♦*cite*
sight'ed
sight'less
sight'line'
sight'-read', -read',
  -read'ing

sight'see'ing
sight'se'er
sig'ma
sign *(indication)*
  ♦*sine*
sig'nal, -naled *or*
  -nalled, -nal•ing *or*
  -nal•ling
sig'nal•er *also* sig'-
  nal•ler
sig'nal•ize', -ized',
  -iz'ing
sig'nal•ly
sig'na•to'ry
sig'na•ture
sign'board'
sig'net *(seal)*
  ♦*cygnet*
sig•nif 'i•cance
sig•nif 'i•cant
sig•ni•fi•ca'tion
sig•ni•fy', -fied', -fy'-
  ing
si•gnor' *pl.* -gno'ri *or*
  -gnors'
si•gno'ra *pl.* -re *or*
  -ras
si•gno're *pl.* -ri
si'gno•ri'na *pl.* -ne *or*
  -nas
sign'post'
si'lage
si'lence, -lenced,
  -lenc•ing
si'lent
sil'hou•ette', -et'ted,
  -et'ting

sil'i•ca
sil'i•cate'
si•li'ceous
sil'i•con *(element)*
sil'i•cone' *(polymer)*
sil'i•co'sis
silk'en
silk'-screen' *v.*
silk'-stock'ing *adj.*
silk'worm'
silk'y
sill
sil'ly
si'lo *pl.* -los
silt
Si•lu'ri•an
sil'ver
sil'ver•fish' *pl.* -fish'
  or -fish'es
sil'ver•smith'
sil'ver-tongued'
sil'ver•ware'
sil'ver•y
sim'i•an
sim'i•lar
sim'i•lar'i•ty
sim'i•le
si•mil'i•tude'
sim'mer
si'mon-pure'
sim'o•ny
sim•pa'ti•co'
sim'per
sim'ple
sim'ple-mind'ed
sim'ple•ton
sim•plic'i•ty

sim′pli•fi•ca′tion
sim′pli•fi′er
sim′pli•fy′, -fied′, -fy′-
  ing
sim′ply
sim′u•late′, -lat′ed,
  -lat′ing
sim′u•la′tion
sim′u•la′tive
sim′u•la′tor
si′mul•cast′, -cast′ed,
  -cast′ing
si′mul•ta•ne′i•ty
si′mul•ta′ne•ous
sin, sinned, sin′ning
since
sin•cere′, -cer′er,
  -cer′est
sin•cer′i•ty
sine *(mathematical*
  function)
  ♦*sign*
si′ne•cure′
si′ne•cur•ist
si′ne di′e
si′ne qua non′
sin′ew
sin′ew•y
sin′ful
sing, sang *or* sung,
  sung, sing′ing,
singe, singed, singe′-
  ing
sing′er
Sin′gha•lese′ *pl.*
  -lese′, *also* Sin′ha-
  lese′

sin′gle, -gled, -gling
sin′gle-breast′ed
sin′gle-en′try *adj.*
sin′gle-hand′ed
sin′gle-mind′ed
sin′gle-space′,
  -spaced′, -spac′ing
sin′gle•ton
sin′gly
sing′song′
sin′gu•lar
sin′gu•lar′i•ty
sin′is•ter
sin′is•tral
sink, sank *or* sunk,
  sunk *or* sunk′en,
  sink′ing
sink′a•ble
sink′hole′
sin′ner
Si•nol′o•gist
Si•nol′o•gy
sin′u•os′i•ty
sin′u•ous
si′nus
si′nus•i′tis
sip, sipped, sip′ping
si′phon *also* sy′phon
si′phon•al *also* si-
  phon′ic
sir
sire, sired, sir′ing
si′ren
sir′loin′
si•roc′co *pl.* -cos, *also*
  sci•roc′co
si′sal

sis′si•fied′
sis′sy
sis′ter
sis′ter•hood′
sis′ter-in-law′ *pl.* sis′-
  ters-in-law′
sit, sat, sit′ting
si•tar′
sit′com′ *also* sit′-com′
sit′-down′ *n. & adj.*
site *(location)*
  ♦*cite, sight*
sit′-in′ *n.*
sit′ter
sit′ting
sit′u•ate′, -at′ed, -at′-
  ing
sit′u•a′tion
sit′-up′ *n.*
sitz bath
six′-gun′
six′-pack′
six′pence
six′pen•ny
six′-shoot′er
six′teen′
six′teenth′
sixth
six′ti•eth
six′ty
six′ty-fourth′ note
siz′a•ble *also* size′-
  a•ble
size, sized, siz′ing
siz′zle, -zled, -zling
skate, skat′ed, skat′ing
skate′board′

skeet
skein
skel'e•tal
skel'e•ton
skep'tic *also* scep'tic
skep'ti•cal
skep'ti•cism
sketch'book'
sketch'pad'
sketch'y
skew'bald'
skew'er
ski *pl.* skis
ski, skied, ski'ing
skid, skid'ded, skid'-
  ding
skiff
skilled
skil'let
skill'ful
skim, skimmed, skim'-
  ming
skim'mer
skimp'y
skin, skinned, skin'-
  ning
skin'-deep'
skin'-dive', -dived',
  -div'ing
skin'flint'
skink
skin'ner
skin'ny
skin'tight'
skip, skipped, skip'-
  ping
skip'per

skirl
skir'mish
skirt
skit
skit'ter
skit'ter•y
skit'tish
skit'tles
skiv'vy
skosh
skulk
skull *(head bones)*
  ♦*scull*
skull'cap'
skull•dug'ger•y *also*
  skul•dug'ger•y
skunk
sky, skied, sky'ing
sky'box'
sky'dive', -dived',
  -div'ing
Skye terrier
sky'-high'
sky'jack'
Sky'lab'
sky'lark'
sky'light'
sky'line'
sky'rock'et
sky'scrap'er
Sky'train'®
sky'ward *also* sky'-
  wards
sky'way'
sky'writ'er
sky'writ'ing
slab

slack'en
slag
slake, slaked, slak'ing
sla'lom
slam, slammed, slam'-
  ming
slam'-dunk'
slan'der
slan'der•ous
slang'y
slant
slant'wise'
slap, slapped, slap'-
  ping
slap'hap'py
slap'stick'
slash
slat
slate, slat'ed, slat'ing
slath'er
slat'ted
slat'tern
slaugh'ter
slaugh'ter•house'
Slav
slave, slaved, slav'ing
slave'hold'er
slav'er•y
Slav'ic
slav'ish
slaw
slay *(to kill),* slew,
  slain, slay'ing
  ♦*sleigh*
slea'zy
sled, sled'ded, sled'-
  ding

sledge, sledged, sledg'-
  ing
sledge'ham'mer
sleek
sleep, slept, sleep'ing
sleep'o'ver
sleep'walk
sleep'walk'er
sleep'y
sleep'y•head'
sleet
sleeve, sleeved, sleev'-
  ing
sleigh *(vehicle)*
  ♦*slay*
sleight *(dexterity,
  trick)*
  ♦*slight*
slen'der
slen'der•ize', -ized',
  -iz'•ing
sleuth'hound'
slew *(large number),
  also* slue
  ♦*slough (swamp)*
slice, sliced, slic'ing
slice'a•ble
slick'en
slick'er
slide, slid, slid'ing
slight *(thin, scant)*
  ♦*sleight*
slight *(to ignore,
  shirk)*
  ♦*sleight*
slight'ly
slim, slim'mer, slim'-

mest
slim, slimmed, slim'-
  ming
slime
slim'y
sling, slung, sling'ing
sling'shot'
slink, slunk, slink'ing
slink'y
slip, slipped, slip'ping
slip'case'
slip'cov'er
slip'knot'
slip'-on' *n.*
slip'o'ver
slip'page
slip'per
slip'per•y
slip'shod'
slip'stitch'
slip'stream'
slip'-up' *n.*
slit, slit, slit'ting
slith'er
sliv'er
sliv'o•vitz
slob'ber
sloe *(fruit)*
  ♦*slow*
sloe'-eyed'
slog, slogged, slog'ging
slo'gan
sloop
slop, slopped, slop'-
  ping
slope, sloped, slop'ing
slop'py

slosh
slot, slot'ted, slot'ting
sloth'ful
slouch
slough *(swamp), also*
  slew
  ♦*slue*
slough *(dead tissue)*
Slo'vak'
slov'en
Slo'vene'
slov'en•ly
slow *(not quick)*
  ♦*sloe*
slow'down' *n.*
slow'-mo'tion *adj.*
slow'poke'
slow'wit'ted
sludge
sludg'y
slue *(to twist)*, slued,
  slu'ing, *also* slew
  ♦*slough (swamp)*
slug, slugged, slug'ging
slug'fest'
slug'gard
slug'ger
slug'gish
sluice, sluiced, sluic'-
  ing
slum, slummed, slum'-
  ming
slum'ber
slum'ber•ous
slum'lord'
slump
slur, slurred, slur'ring

slurp
slur'ry
slush'y
slut'tish
sly, sli'er *or* sly'er, sli'-
   est *or* sly'est
smack'-dab'
smack'ing
small'-mind'ed
small'pox'
small'time'
smart al'eck
smart'-al'eck•y
smart'en
smash'ing
smash'up' *n.*
smat'ter
smear'y
smell, smelled *or*
   smelt, smell'ing
smell'y
smelt *(fish), pl.* smelts
   or smelt
smelt *(to melt)*
smelt'er *also* smelt'-
   er•y
smid'gen *also* smid'-
   geon, smid'gin
smi'lax'
smile, smiled, smil'-
   ing
smirch
smirk
smite, smote, smit'ten
   or smote, smit'ing
smith
smith'er•ecns'

smith'y
smock'ing
smog
smog'gy
smoke, smoked,
   smok'ing
smoke'house'
smoke'less
smoke'stack'
smok'y
smol'der *also*
   smoul'der
smooch
smooth'bore'
smooth'en
smor'gas•bord'
smoth'er
smudge, smudged,
   smudg'ing
smudg'y
smug, smug'ger,
   smug'gest
smug'gle, -gled, -gling
smug'gler
smut'ty
snack
snaf'fle, -fled, -fling
sna•fu' *pl.* -fus
snag, snagged, snag'-
   ging
snag'gle•tooth'
snail
snake, snaked, snak'-
   ing
snake'bitc'
snake'root'
snake'skin'

snak'y
snap, snapped, snap'-
   ping
snap'drag'on
snap'per
snap'pish
snap'py
snap'shot'
snare, snared, snar'ing
snarl
snatch'er
snaz'zy
sneak'ers
sneak'y
sneer
sneeze sneezed, sneez'-
   ing
snick'er
snide, snid'er, snid'est
sniff
snif'fle, -fled, -fling
snif'ter
snig'ger
snip, snipped, snip'-
   ping
snipe *pl.* snipe *or*
   snipes
snipe, sniped, snip'ing
snip'er
snip'pet
snip'pet•y
snip'py
snit
snitch
sniv'el, -eled *or* -ellcd.
   -el•ing *or* -el•ling
snob'ber•y

snob'bish
snob'bism
snood
snook'er
snoop'y
snoot'y
snooze, snoozed, snooz'ing
snore, snored, snor'ing
snor'kel
snort
snout
snow'ball'
snow'bird'
snow'blind' *also* snow'blind'ed
snow'bound'
snow'cap'
snow'capped'
snow'drift'
snow'drop'
snow'fall'
snow'flake'
snow'man'
snow'mo•bile'
snow'plow'
snow'shoe'
snow'storm'
snow'suit'
snow'-white' *adj.*
snow'y
snub, snubbed, snub'bing
snub'-nosed'
snuff 'box'
snuf 'fle, -fled, -fling

snug, snug'ger, snug'gest
snug'ger•y
snug'gle, -gled, -gling
so *(thus)*
♦*sew, sow (to scatter)*
soak'age
so'-and-so' *pl.* -sos'
soap'box'
soap'stone'
soap'suds'
soap'wort'
soap'y
soar *(to fly)*
♦*sore*
so•a've
sob, sobbed, sob'bing
so'ber
so•bri'e•ty
so'bri•quet'
so'-called' *adj.*
soc'cer
so'cia•bil'i•ty
so'cia•ble
so'cial
so'cial•ism
so'cial•ist
so'cial•is'tic
so'cial•ite'
so'cial•i•za'tion
so'cial•ize', -ized', -iz'ing
so•ci'e•tal
so•ci'e•ty
so'ci•o•bi•ol'o•gy
so'ci•o•ec'o•nom'ic
so'ci•o•log'ic *also*

so'ci•o•log'i•cal
so'ci•ol'o•gist
so'ci•ol'o•gy
sock *pl.* socks *or* sox
sock'et
sock'eye' salmon
So•crat'ic
sod, sod'ded, sod'ding
so'da
so•dal'i•ty
sod'den
so'di•um
so'di•um-va'por lamp
Sod'om *or* sod'om
sod'om•y
so•ev'er
so'fa
soft'ball'
soft'-boiled'
soft'cov'er
sof 'ten
sof 'ten•er
soft'heart'ed
soft'ly
soft'-ped'al, -aled *or* -alled, -al•ing *or* -al•ling
soft'-shell' *also* soft'-shelled'
soft'-shoe'
soft'-soap'
soft'-spo'ken
soft'ware'
soft'wood'
soft'y
sog'gy

soi•gne' *also* soi-
gnée'
soil'age
soi•ree' *also* soi•rée'
so'journ
sol *(musical tone)*
♦*Sol, sole, soul*
Sol *(the sun)*
♦*sol, sole, soul*
sol'ace, -aced, -ac•ing
so'lar
so•lar'i•um *pl.* -i•a
or -i•ums
sol'der
sol'dier
sole *(single)*
♦*sol, Sol, soul*
sole *(shoe bottom)*
♦*sol, Sol, soul*
sole *(fish), pl.* sole or
soles
♦*sol, Sol, soul*
sole *(to put a sole on),*
soled, sol'ing
♦*sol, Sol, soul*
sol'e•cism
sol'emn
so•lem'ni•ty
sol'em•ni•za'tion
sol'em•nize', -nized',
-niz'ing
so'le•noid'
so•lic'it
so•lic'i•ta'tion
so•lic'i•tor
so•lic'i•tous
so•lic'i•tude'

sol'id
sol'i•dar'i•ty
so•lid'i•fi•ca'tion
so•lid'i•fy', -fied',
-fy'ing
so•lid'i•ty
sol'id-state' *adj.*
so•lil'o•quist
so•lil'o•quize',
-quized', -quiz'ing
so•lil'o•quy
sol'ip•sism
sol'ip•sist
sol'ip•sis'tic
sol'i•taire'
sol'i•tar'y
sol'i•tude'
so'lo *pl.* -los
so'lo•ist
Sol'o•mon
Sol'o•mon'ic
sol'stice
sol'u•bil'i•ty
sol'u•ble
sol'ute'
so•lu'tion
solv'a•bil'i•ty
solv'a•ble
solve, solved, solv'ing
sol'ven•cy
sol'vent
So•ma'li *pl.* -li or -lis
so•mat'ic
som'ber
som•bre'ro *pl.* -ros
some *(a few)*
♦*sum*

some'bod'y
some'day'
some'how'
some'one'
some'place'
som'er•sault'
some'thing
some'time'
some'times'
some'way' *also* some'-
ways'
some'what'
some'where'
som'me•lier'
som•nam'bu•late',
-lat'ed, -lat'ing
som•nam'bu•lism
som•nam'bu•list
som•nam'bu•lis'tic
also som•nam'bu-
lar
som•nif'er•ous
som'no•lence
som'no•lent
son *(offspring)*
♦*sun*
so'nar'
so•na'ta
song'bird'
song'fest'
song'ster
song'stress
song'writ'er
son'ic
son'-in-law' *pl.*
sons'-in-law'
son'net

son'net•eer'
son'ny *(boy)*
  ♦*sunny*
so•nor'i•ty
so•no'rous
soon
soot
sooth *(truth)*
soothe *(to calm),*
  soothed, sooth'ing
sooth'say'er
soot'y
sop, sopped, sop'ping
soph'ism
soph'ist
so•phis'tic *or* so-
  phis'ti•cal
so•phis'ti•cate', -cat'-
  ed, -cat'ing
so•phis'ti•ca'tion
so•phis'ti•ca'tor
soph'is•try
soph'o•more'
soph'o•mor'ic
so'po•rif'ic
sop'ping
sop'py
so•pran'o *pl.* -os
sor'cer•er
sor'cer•y
sor'did
sore *(painful),* sor'er,
  sor'est
  ♦*soar*
sore'head'
sore'ly
sor'ghum

so•ror'i•ty
sor'rel
sor'row
sor'row•ful
sor'ry
sor•ta'tion
sort'er
sor'tie
so'-so'
sot
sot'tish
sot'to vo'ce
sou
sou•brette'
souf•flé'
sough
soul *(entity)*
  ♦*sol, Sol, sole*
soul'ful
soul'-search'ing
sound'ing
sound'proof'
sound'track'
soup
soup'spoon'
soup'y
source
sour'dough'
sour'puss'
sou'sa•phone'
souse, soused, sous'-
  ing
South Af'ri•can
South A•mer'i•can
south'bound'
South Car'o•lin'-
  i•an

South Da•ko'tan
south•east'
south•east'er
south•east'er•ly
south•east'ern
south•east'ward *also*
  south•east'wards
south'er•ly
south'ern
south'ern•er
south'ern•most'
south'paw'
south'-south•east'
south'-south•west'
south'ward *also*
  south'wards
south•west'
south•west'er
south•west'er•ly
south•west'ern
south•west'ward
  also south•west'-
  wards
sou've•nir'
sov'er•eign
sov'er•eign•ty
so'vi•et'
sow *(to scatter),*
  sowed, sown *or*
  sowed, sow'ing
  ♦*sew, so*
sow *(pig)*
soy'bean'
spa
space, spaced, spac'-
  ing
space'craft' *pl.* -craft'

space'man'
space'port'
space'ship'
space'-time'
spac'ing
spa'cious
Spack'le®, -led, -ling
spade, spad'ed, spad'-
    ing
spade'work'
spa'dix pl. -di•ces'
spa•ghet'ti
span, spanned, span'-
    ning
span'gle, -gled, -gling
Span'iard
span'iel
Span'ish
Span'ish-A•mer'-
    i•can
spank'er
spank'ing
span'ner
spar, sparred, spar'-
    ring
spare, spar'er, spar'est
spare, spared, spar'ing
spare'ribs'
spark
spar'kle, -kled, -kling
spar'kler
spar'row
sparse, spars'er, spars'-
    est
Spar'tan
spasm
spas•mod'ic

spas'tic
spat (gaiter, quarrel)
spat (larval oyster), pl.
    spat or spats
spat (to quarrel,
    spawn), spat'ted,
    spat'ting
spate
spathe
spa'tial
spat'ter
spat'u•la
spat'u•lar
spav'in
spav'incd
spawn
spay
speak, spoke, spok'en,
    speak'ing
speak'eas'y
speak'er
speak'er•phone'
spear'head'
spear'mint'
spe'cial
spe'cial•ist
spe'ci•al'i•ty (char-
    acteristic)
    ♦specialty
spe'cial•i•za'tion
spe'cial•ize', -ized',
    -iz'ing
spe'cial•ty (distinc-
    tive quality)
    ♦speciality
spe'cie (coin)
spe'cies (kind), pl.

    -cies
spe•cif'ic
spec'i•fi•ca'tion
spec'i•fy', -fied', -fy'-
    ing
spec'i•men
spe'cious
speck'le, led, -ling
specs
spec'ta•cle
spec•tac'u•lar
spec'ta•tor
spec'ter
spec'tral
spec'tro•gram'
spec'tro•graph'
spec'tro•graph'ic
spec•trog'ra•phy
spec•trom'e•ter
spec'tro•met'ric
spec•trom'e•try
spec'tro•scope'
spec'tro•scop'ic also
    spec'tro•scop'i•cal
spec•tros'co•py
spec'trum pl. -tra or
    -trums
spec'u•late', -lat'ed,
    -lat'ing
spec'u•la'tion
spec'u•la'tive
spec'u•la'tor
speech'less
speech'mak'er
speech'mak'ing
speech'writ'er
speed, sped or speed'-

ed, speed'ing
speed'boat'
speed'er
speed•om'e•ter
speed'-read', -read',
  -read'ing
speed'ster
speed•up' *n.*
speed'way'
speed'well'
speed'y
spell, spelled *or* spelt,
  spell'ing
spell'bind', -bound',
  -bind'ing
spell'er
spe•lun'ker
spe•lunk'ing
spend, spent, spend'-
  ing
spend'thrift'
Spen•se'ri•an
  sonnet
sperm
sper'ma•ce'ti
sper•mat'ic
sper•mat'o•gen'-
  e•sis
sper'ma•to•ge•net'-
  ic
sper•ma'to•phyte'
sper•mat'o•phyt'ic
sper•ma'to•zoid
sper•ma'to•zo'on
  pl. -zo'a
spew
sphag'num

sphe'noid
sphe•noi'dal
sphere
sphe•ric'i•ty
sphe'roid'
sphinc'ter
sphinx *pl.* sphinx'es
  or sphin'ges
sphyg'mo•ma•nom'-
  e•ter *also* sphyg-
  mom'e•ter
spice, spiced, spic'ing
spick'-and-span' *adj.*
spic'u•lar *also* spic'-
  u•late
spic'ule *also* spic'u•la
  pl. -lae'
spic'y
spi'der
spi'der•y
spiel
spiff
spif'fy
spig'ot
spike, spiked, spik'ing
spike'nard'
spik'y
spill, spilled *or* spilt,
  spill'ing
spill'age
spill'o•ver
spill'way'
spin, spun, spin'ning
spin'ach
spi'nal
spin'dle, -dled, -dling
spin'dly

spine'less
spin'et
spin'na•ker
spin'ner
spin'ner•et'
spin'ning
spin'-off' *n.*
spin'ster
spin'y
spir'a•cle
spi'ral, -raled *or*
  -ralled, -ral•ing *or*
  -ral•ling
spire
spi•ril'lum *pl.* -la
spir'it
spir'it•ed
spir'it•less
spir'i•tu•al
spir'i•tu•al•ism
spir'i•tu•al•ist
spir'i•tu•al•is'tic
spir'i•tu•al'i•ty
spir'i•tu•ous
spi'ro•chet'al
spi'ro•chete'
spi'ro•gy'ra
spit *(to eject from the
  mouth),* spat *or* spit,
  spit'ting
spit *(to place on a
  rod),* spit'ted, spit'-
  ting
spite, spit'ed, spit'ing
spite'ful
spit'fire'
spit'tle

spit•toon′
splash′down′
splash′y
splat′ter
splay′foot′
splay′foot′ed
spleen
splen′did
splen•dif′er•ous
splen′dor
splice, spliced, splic′-
  ing
splint
splin′ter
splin′ter•y
split, split, split′ting
split′-lev′el
split′ting
splotch′y
splurge, splurged,
  splurg′ing
splut′ter
Spode
spoil, spoiled or
  spoilt, spoil′ing
spoil′age
spoil′sport′
spoke, spoked, spok′-
  ing
spo′ken
spoke′shave′
spokes′man
spokes′per′son
spokes′wom′an
spo′li•a′tion
spo′li•a′tor
spon•da′ic

spon′dee′
sponge, sponged,
  spong′ing
spon′gy
spon′sor
spon′sor•ship′
spon•ta•ne′i•ty
spon•ta′ne•ous
spoof
spook′y
spool
spoon
spoon′bill′
spoon′er•ism
spoon′-fed′
spoon′ful′ *pl.* -fuls′
spoor *(animal track)*
  ♦*spore*
spo•rad′ic
spo•ran′gi•al
spo•ran′gi•um *pl.*
  -gi•a
spore *(reproductive or-*
gan)
  ♦*spoor*
spor′ran
sport′ing
spor′tive
sports′man
sports′man•ship′
sports′wear′
sports′wom′an
sports′writ′er
sport′y
spot, spot′ted, spot′-
  ting
spot′-check′ *v.*

spot′less
spot′light′, -light′ed
  or -lit′, -light′ing
spot′ter
spot′ty
spou′sal
spouse
spout
sprain
sprat
sprawl
spray′er
spread, spread,
  spread′ing
spread′-ea′gle, -gled,
  -gling
spread′sheet′
spree
sprig, sprigged, sprig′-
  ging
spright′ly
spring, sprang or
  sprung, sprung,
  spring′ing
spring′board′
spring′bok′ *pl.* -bok′
  or -boks′
spring′tide′
spring′time′
spring′y
sprin′kle, -kled, -kling
sprin′kler
sprint′er
sprit
sprite
spritz
spritz′er

sprock'et

sprout

spruce *(neat)*, spruc'-
er, spruc'est

spruce *(tree)*

spruce *(to neaten)*,
spruced, spruc'ing

spry, spri'er *or* spry'-
er, spri'est *or* spry'-
est

spud

spume, spumed,
spum'ing

spu•mo'ne *also* spu-
mo'ni

spunk'y

spur, spurred, spur'-
ring

spurge

spu'ri•ous

spurn

spurt

sput'nik

sput'ter

spu'tum *pl.* -ta

spy, spied, spy'ing

spy'glass'

squab *pl.* squabs *or*
squab

squab'ble, -bled,
-bling

squad'ron

squal'id

squall

squal'or

squan'der

square, squar'er,

squar'est

square, squared,
squar'ing

square'-dance',
-danced', -danc'ing

square'-rigged'

square'-rig'ger

square'shoot'er

squash'y

squat, squat'ter,
squat'test

squat, squat'ted *or*
squat, squat'ting

squat'ter

squaw

squawk

squeak'y

squeal'er

squea'mish

squee'gee'

squeeze, squeezed,
squeez'ing

squelch'er

squib

squid *pl.* squids *or*
squid

squig'gle, -gled, -gling

squinch

squint'er

squint'-eyed'

squire, squired, squir'-
ing

squire'ar•chy *or*
squir'ar•chy

squirm'y

squir'rel

squirt

squish'y

stab, stabbed, stab'-
bing

sta'bile

sta•bil'i•ty

sta'bi•li•za'tion

sta'bi•lize', -lized',
-liz'ing

sta'ble, -bled, -bling

stac•ca'to *pl.* -tos *or*
-ti

stack

sta'di•um *pl.* -di•a *or*
-di•ums

staff *pl.* staffs *or*
staves

stag

stage, staged, stag'ing

stage'coach'

stage'craft'

stage'hand'

stage'-man'age,
-aged, -ag•ing

stage'-struck'

stag•fla'tion

stag'ger

stag'ing

stag'nan•cy

stag'nant

stag'nate', -nat'ed,
-nat'ing

stag•na'tion

stag'y

staid *(sedate)*
♦*stayed*

stained'-glass' *adj.*

stain'less

stair *(steps)*
♦*stare*
stair'case'
stair'way'
stair'well'
stake *(to mark limits,*
gamble), staked,
stak'ing
♦*steak*
stake'hold'er
sta•lac'tite' *(down-*
ward deposit)
sta•lag'mite' *(upward*
deposit)
stale, stal'er, stal'est
stale, staled, stal'ing
stale'mate', -mat'ed,
-mat'ing
Sta'lin•ist
stalk'er
stalk'ing-horse'
stall
stal'lion
stal'wart
sta'men
stam'i•na
stam'mer
stamp
stam•pede', -ped'ed,
-ped'ing
stance
stanch *(to check)*
♦*staunch*
stan'chion
stand, stood, stand'-
ing
stan'dard

stan'dard-bear'er
stan'dard•i•za'tion
stan'dard•ize',
-ized', -iz'ing
stand'by' *pl.* -bys'
stand•ee'
stand'-in' *n.*
stand'ing
stand'-off' *n.*
stand•off'ish
stand'out' *n.*
stand'pipe'
stand'point'
stand'still'
stand'up' *adj., also*
stand'-up'
stan'nic
stan'nous
stan'za
sta•pes' *pl.* sta'pes' *or*
sta'pe•des'
staph'y•lo•coc'cal
staph'y•lo•coc'cus
pl. -ci'
sta'ple, -pled, -pling
sta'pler
star, starred, star'ring
star'board
star'burst'
starch'y
star'dom
star'dust'
stare *(to gaze fixedly),*
stared, star'ing
♦*stair*
star'fish' *pl.* -fish' *or*
-fish'es

star'gaze', -gazed',
-gaz'ing
star'gaz'er
stark'ly
star'let
star'light'
star'ling
star'lit'
star'-of-Beth'le-
hem'
star'ry
star'ry-eyed'
star'struck'
start'er
star'tle, -tled, -tling
star•va'tion
starve, starved, starv'-
ing
starve'ling
stash
sta'sis *pl.* -ses'
state, stat'ed, stat'ing
state'hood'
state'let
state'ly
state'ment
state'room'
state'side'
states'man
states'man•ship'
state'wide'
stat'ic
stat'ics
sta'tion
sta'tion•ar'y *(unmov-*
ing)
♦*stationery*

sta'tion•er
sta'tion•er'y *(paper)*
  ♦*stationary*
sta'tion•mas'ter
stat'ism
sta•tis'tic
sta•tis'ti•cal
stat•is•ti'cian
sta•tis'tics
sta'tor
stat'u•ar'y
stat'ue
stat'u•esque'
stat'u•ette'
stat'ure
stat'us
status quo'
stat•ute
stat'u•to'ry
staunch *(firm)*
  ♦*stanch*
stave, staved *or* stove,
  stav'ing
stay
stead'fast'
stead'y, -ied, -y•ing
steak *(meat)*
  ♦*stake*
steak tar'tare'
steal *(to rob)*, stole,
  stol'en, steal'ing
  ♦*steel*
stealth'y
steam'boat'
steam'er
steam'rol'ler
steam'ship'

steam'y
ste'a•tite'
steed
steel *(metal)*
  ♦*steal*
steel'work'
steel'work'er
steel'y
steel'yard'
steen'bok' *also* stein'-
  bok'
steep'en
stee'ple
stee'ple•chase'
stee'ple•jack'
steer'age
steers'man
steg'o•saur' *also* steg'-
  o•sau'rus
stein
ste'le *pl.* -les *or* -lae
stel'lar
stem, stemmed, stem'-
  ming
stem'less
stem'ware
stem'-wind'er
stem'-wind'ing *adj.*
stench
sten'cil, -ciled *or*
  -cilled, -cil•ing *or*
  cil•ling
sten'o *pl.* -os
ste•nog'ra•pher
sten'o•graph'ic *also*
  sten'o•graph'i•cal
ste•nog'ra•phy

sten'o•type' *(short-*
  hand symbol)
Sten'o•type'® *(pho-*
  netic keyboard
  machine)
sten•to'ri•an
step *(to walk)*,
  stepped, step'ping
  ♦*steppe*
step'broth'er
step'child'
step'daugh'ter
step'-down' *adj. & n.*
step'fam'i•ly
step'fa'ther
step'-in' *adj. & n.*
step'lad'der
step'moth'er
step'par'ent
steppe *(plain)*
  ♦*step*
step'ping•stone'
step'sib'ling
step'sis'ter
step'son'
step'-up' *adj. & n.*
step'wise'
ste're•o' *pl.* -os'
ster'e•o•phon'ic
ster'e•op'ti•con'
ster'e•o•scope'
ster'e•o•scop'ic
ster'e•os'co•py
ster'e•o•tape',
  -taped', -tap'ing
ster'e•o•type',
  -typed', -typ'ing

ster'e•o•typ'ic *also*
  ster'e•o•typ'i•cal
ster'e•o•ty'py
ster'ile
ste•ril'i•ty
ster'il•i•za'tion
ster'il•ize', -ized', -iz'-
  ing
ster'ling
stern
ster'num *pl.* -na *or*
  -nums
stern'wheel'er
ster'oid'
ster'ol'
stet, stet'ted, stet'ting
steth'o•scope'
steth'o•scop'ic *also*
  steth'o•scop'i•cal
ste•thos'co•py
Stet'son®
ste've•dore'
stew
stew'ard
stew'ard•ess
stib'nite'
stick, stuck, stick'ing
stick'er
stick'le, -led, -ling
stick'le•back'
stick'ler
stick'pin'
stick-to'-it•ive•ness
stick'um
stick'up' *n.*
stick'y
stiff'en

stiff'en•er
stiff'-necked'
sti'fle, -fled, -fling
stig'ma *pl.* stig•ma'ta
  or stig'mas
stig•mat'ic
stig'ma•tism
stig'ma•ti•za'tion
stig'ma•tize', -tized',
  -tiz'ing
stile *(steps, window-
  frame part)*
  ♦*style*
sti•let'to *pl.* -tos *or*
  -toes
still'birth'
still'born'
still'-life' *adj.*
still'ness
stilt'ed
Stil'ton cheese
stim'u•lant
stim'u•late', -lat'ed,
  -lat'ing
stim'u•lat'er *also*
  stim'u•la'tor
stim'u•la'tion
stim'u•la'tive
stim'u•lus *pl.* -li'
sting, stung, sting'ing
sting'ray'
stin'gy
stink, stank *or* stunk,
  stunk, stink'ing
stink'pot'
stink'weed'
stint

sti'pend'
stip'ple, -pled, -pling
stip'u•late', -lat'ed,
  -lat'ing
stip'u•la'tion
stip'u•la'tor
stir, stirred, stir'ring
stir'rer
stir'rup
stir'rup-cup'
stitch'er•y
stitch'ing
sto'a *pl.* -ae' *or* -as
stoat
stock•ade'
stock'bro'ker
stock'hold'er
stock'i•net' *also*
  stock'i•nette'
stock'ing
stock'man
stock'own'er
stock'pile', -piled',
  -pil'ing
stock'room'
stock'y
stock'yard'
stodg'y
sto'gy *or* sto'gie
sto'ic
sto'i•cal
sto'i•cism
stoke, stoked, stok'ing
stole
stol'id
sto•lid'i•ty
sto'ma *pl.* -ma•ta *or*

-mas
stom'ach
stom'ach•ache'
stom'ach•er
stomp
stone, stoned, ston'ing
stone'cut'ter
stone'-deaf' *adj.*
stone'ma'son
stone'wall'
stone'ware'
stone'work'
ston'y
stooge
stool
stoop *(bending, stair-
case)*
 ♦*stoup*
stop, stopped, stop'-
ping
stop'cock'
stop'gap'
stop'light'
stop'o'ver
stop'page
stop'per
stop'watch'
stor'age
store, stored, stor'ing
store'-bought' *adj.*
store'front'
store'house'
store'keep'er
store'room'
store'wide'
sto'ried
stork

storm'y
sto'ry
sto'ry•book'
sto'ry•tell'er
stoup *(basin)*
 ♦*stoop*
stout'heart'ed
stove'pipe'
stove'top'
stow'age
stow'a•way' *n.*
stra•bis'mus
strad'dle, -dled,
 -dling
Strad'i•var'i•us
strafe, strafed,
 straf'ing
strag'gle, -gled, -gling
strag'gly
straight *(direct)*
 ♦*strait*
straight'-arm' *v.*
straight'a•way'
straight'edge'
straight'en *(to make
 straight)*
 ♦*straiten*
straight•for'ward
 also straight•for'-
 wards
straight'way'
strain'er
strait *(water)*
 ♦*straight*
strait'en *(to restrict)*
 ♦*straighten*
strait'jack'et

strait'-laced'
strand'ed
strange, strang'er,
 strang'est
stran'gle, -gled, -gling
stran'gler
stran'gu•late', -lat'-
 ed, -lat'ing
stran'gu•la'tion
strap, strapped, strap'-
 ping
strap'hang'er
strat'a•gem
stra•te'gic
strat'e•gist
strat'e•gy
strat'i•fi•ca'tion
strat'i•fy', -fied', -fy'-
 ing
stra'to•cu'mu•lus
 pl. -li'
strat'o•sphere'
strat'o•spher'ic
stra'tum *pl.* -ta *or*
 -tums
stra'tus *pl.* -ti
straw'ber'ry
straw'-hat' *adj.*
stray
streak'y
stream'er
stream'line', -lined',
 -lin'ing
street'car'
street'scape'
street'walk'er
strength'en

stren'u•ous
strep'to•coc'cal
strep'to•coc'cus *pl.*
　-ci'
strep'to•my'cin
stress
stress'ful
stretch'a•ble
stretch'er
stretch'er-bear'er
stretch'y
streu'sel
strew, strewed, strewn
　or strewed, strew'ing
stri'a *pl.* -ae'
stri'ate' *also* stri'at'ed
stri•a'tion
strick'en
strict'ly
stric'ture
stride, strode, strid'-
　den, strid'ing
stri'dence *also* stri'-
　den•cy
stri'dent
strife
strike, struck, struck
　or strick'en, strik'ing
strike'bound'
strike'break'er
strike'out' *n.*
strike'o'ver *n.*
strik'er
strik'ing
string, strung, string'-
　ing
strin'gen•cy

strin'gent
string'er
string'y
strip, stripped, strip'-
　ping
stripe, striped, strip'-
　ing
strip'ling
strip'-mine', -mined',
　-min'ing
strip'search'
strip'y
strive, strove, striv'en
　or strived, striv'ing
strobe
strob'o•scope'
strob'o•scop'ic
stro'gan•off'
stroke, stroked, strok'-
　ing
stroll'er
strong'-arm' *adj. & v.*
strong'box'
strong'hold'
strong'-mind'ed
strong'point'
stron'ti•um
strop, stropped, strop'-
　ping
stro'phe
struc'tur•al
struc'tur•al•ism
struc'tur•al•ist
struc'ture, -tured,
　-tur•ing
stru'del
strug'gle, -gled, -gling

strum, strummed,
　strum'ming
strum'mer
strum'pet
strut, strut'ted, strut'-
　ting
strych'nine'
stub, stubbed, stub'-
　bing
stub'ble
stub'born
stub'by
stuc'co *pl.* -coes *or*
　-cos
stuck'-up' *adj.*
stud, stud'ded, stud'-
　ding
stud'book'
stu'dent
stu'di•o *pl.* -os
stu'di•ous
stud'y, -ied, -y•ing
stuff'ing
stuff'y
stul'ti•fi•ca'tion
stul'ti•fy', -fied', -fy'-
　ing
stum'ble, -bled, -bling
stum'ble•bum'
stump
stun, stunned, stun'-
　ning
stunt
stunt'man'
stunt'wom'an
stu'pe•fac'tion
stu'pe•fy', -fied', -fy'-

ing
stu•pen′dous
stu′pid
stu•pid′i•ty
stu′por
stu′por•ous
stur′dy
stur′geon
stut′ter
sty *(enclosure), pl.*
sties
sty *(inflammation), pl.*
sties *or* styes
style *(to design),*
styled, styl′ing
♦*stile*
styl′ish
styl′ist
sty•lis′tic
styl′ize′, -ized′, -iz′ing
sty′lus *pl.* -lus•es *or*
-li′
sty′mie, -mied, -mie-
ing, *also* sty′my,
-mied, -my•ing
styp′tic *also* styp′ti-
cal
sty′rene
Sty′ro•foam′®
suave, suav′er, suav′-
est
suav′i•ty
sub, subbed, sub′bing
sub•al′tern
sub′a•tom′ic
sub′base′ment
sub′cen′ter

sub′class′
sub′com•mit′tee
sub•con′scious
sub•con′ti•nent
sub•con′tract′
sub′con•trac′tor
sub′cu•ta′ne•ous
sub′deb′u•tante′
sub′di•vide′, -vid′ed,
-vid′ing
sub′di•vi′sion
sub•dom′i•nant
sub•due′, -dued′, -du′-
ing
sub′e•qua•to′ri•al
sub•fam′i•ly
sub′ge′nus *pl.* -gen′-
er•a
sub′group′
sub′head′
sub′hu′man
sub•ja′cent
sub′ject *adj. & n.*
sub•ject′ *v.*
sub•jec′tion
sub•jec′tive
sub•jec′tiv•ism
sub′jec•tiv′i•ty
sub•join′
sub•ju•gate′, -gat′ed,
-gat′ing
sub′ju•ga′tion
sub′ju•ga′tor
sub•junc′tive
sub′king′dom
sub′lease′ *n.*
sub′lease′, -leased′,

-leas′ing
sub′let′ *n.*
sub•let′, -let′, -let′ting
sub′li•mate′, -mat′-
ed, -mat′ing
sub′li•ma′tion
sub•lime′
sub•lim′i•nal
sub•lim′i•ty
sub•lit′er•ate
sub′ma•chine′ gun
sub′ma•rine′
sub•merge′,
-merged′, -merg′ing
sub•mer′gence
sub•mer′gi•bil′i•ty
sub•mer′gi•ble
sub•merse′, -mersed′,
-mers′ing
sub•mers′i•ble
sub•mer′sion
sub′mi′cro•scop′ic
sub•mis′sion
sub•mis′sive
sub•mit′, -mit′ted,
-mit′ting
sub•mit′tal
sub′nor′mal
sub′or′der
sub•or′di•nate′,
-nat′ed, -nat′ing
sub•or′di•na′tion
sub•orn′
sub′or•na′tion
sub′par′
sub′phy•lum′
sub′plot′

sub•poe'na
sub ro'sa
sub•rou•tine'
sub•scribe', -scribed',
 -scrib'ing
sub'script'
sub•scrip'tion
sub•sec'tion
sub•se•quence'
sub•se•quent
sub•ser'vi•ence
sub•ser'vi•ent
sub'set'
sub•side', -sid'ed,
 -sid'ing
sub•si'dence
sub•sid'i•ar'y
sub•si•dize', -dized',
 -diz'ing
sub'si•dy
sub•sist'
sub•sis'tence
sub'soil'
sub•son'ic
sub'spe'cies
sub'stance
sub'stan'dard
sub•stan'tial
sub•stan'ti•al'i•ty
sub•stan'ti•ate', -at'-
 ed, -at'ing
sub•stan'ti•a'tion
sub'stan•tive
sub'sta'tion
sub'sti•tut'a•bil'it•y
sub'sti•tut'a•ble
sub'sti•tute', -tut'ed,

-tut'ing
sub'sti•tu'tion
sub'sti•tu'tive
sub'stra'tive
sub'stra'tum *pl.* -ta
 or -tums
sub'struc'ture
sub•sum'a•ble
sub•sume', -sumed',
 -sum'ing
sub'sys'tem
sub•ten'ant
sub•tend'
sub'ter•fuge'
sub'ter•ra'ne•an
sub'text'
sub'ti'tle
sub'tle
sub'tle•ty
sub'tly
sub'ton'ic
sub'to'tal
sub•tract'
sub•trac'tion
sub•trac'tive
sub'tra•hend'
sub'trop'i•cal
sub'trop'ics
sub'urb'
sub•ur'ban
sub•ur'ban•ite'
sub•ur'bi•a
sub•ver'sion
sub•ver'sive
sub•vert'
sub'way'
suc•ceed'

suc•cess'
suc•cess'ful
suc•ces'sion
suc•ces'sive
suc•ces'sor
suc•cinct'
suc'cor *(relief)*
 ♦*sucker*
suc'co•tash'
Suc'coth *also* Suk'-
 koth
suc'cu•lence *also*
 suc'cu•len•cy
suc'cu•lent
suc•cumb'
such'like'
suck'er *(dupe, lolli-
 pop)*
 ♦*succor*
suck'le, -led, -ling
su'crose'
suc'tion
Su'da•nese' *pl.*
 -nese'
sud'den
suds'y
sue, sued, su'ing
suede *also* suède
su'et
suf'fer
suf'fer•a•ble
suf'fer•ance
suf•fice', -ficed', -fic'-
 ing
suf•fi'cien•cy
suf•fi'cient
suf'fix'

suf•fo•cate', -cat'ed,
-cat'ing
suf'fo•ca'tion
suf'frage
suf'fra•gette'
suf'fra•gist
suf•fuse', -fused',
-fus'ing
suf•fu'sion
sug'ar
sug'ar-coat' v.
sug'ar•plum'
sug'ar•y
sug•gest'
sug•gest'•bil'i•ty
sug•gest'i•ble
sug•ges'tion
sug•ges'tive
su•i•cid'al
su•i•cide'
suit (garments, cards,
legal action)
♦suite (set of furni-
ture)
suit'a•bil'ity
suit'a•ble
suit'case'
suite (retinue, set)
♦sweet
suite (set of furniture)
♦suit
suit'ing
suit'or
su'ki•ya'ki
sul'fa drug
sul'fa•nil'a•mide'
sul'fate'

sul'fide'
sul'fite'
sul•fon'a•mide'
sul'fur also sul'phur
sul•fu'ric
sul'fur•ous
sulk'y
sul'len
sul'ly, -lied, -ly•ing
sul'tan
sul•tan'a
sul'tan•ate'
sul'try
sum (to add, review),
summed, sum'ming
♦some
su'mac' also su'mach'
sum'ma cum lau'de
sum•ma'ri•ly
sum'ma•ri•za'tion
sum'ma•rize',
-rized', -riz'ing
sum'ma•ry (conden-
sation)
♦summery
sum•ma'tion
sum'mer
sum'mer•house'
sum'mer•time'
sum'mer•y (of sum-
mer)
♦summary
sum'mit
sum'mon
sum'mons pl. -mons-
es
sump

sump'tu•ar'y
(regulating expenses)
sump'tu•ous (lavish)
sun (star)
♦son
sun (to bask in the
sun), sunned, sun'-
ning
sun'bathe', -bathed',
-bath'ing
sun'bath'er
sun'beam'
sun'bon'net
sun'burn', -burned'
or -burnt', -burn'ing
sun'burst'
sun'dae (ice cream)
Sun'day' (Sabbath)
sun'der
sun'di'al
sun'down'
sun'dress'
sun'dries
sun'dry
sun'fish' pl. -fish' or
-fish'es
sun'flow'er
sun'glass'es
sunk'en
sun'light'
sun'lit'
sun'ny (full of sun-
light, cheerful)
♦sonny
sun'rise'
sun'room'
sun'set'

sun'shade'
sun'shine'
sun'spot'
sun'stroke'
sun'struck'
sun'tan'
sun'tanned'
sun'up'
sup, supped, sup'ping
su'per
su'per•a•bun'dance
su'per•a•bun'dant
su'per•an'nu•at'ed
su•perb'
su'per•charge',
  -charged', -charg'ing
su'per•cil'i•ar'y
su'per•cil'i•ous
su'per•con'duc•tiv'-
  i•ty
su'per•con•duc'tor
su'per•e'go
su'per•er'o•ga'tion
su'per•e•rog'a•to'ry
su'per•fi'cial
su'per•fi'ci•al'i•ty
su'per•fine'
su'per•flu•id'i•ty
su'per•flu'i•ty
su•per'flu•ous
su'per•heat'
su'per•high'
  frequency
su'per•high'way'
su'per•hu'man
su'per•im•pose',
  -posed', -pos'ing

su'per•im'po•si'-
  tion
su'per•in•tend'
su'per•in•ten'dence
su'per•in•ten'dent
su•pe'ri•or
su•pe'ri•or'i•ty
su•per'la•tive
su'per•man'
su'per•mar'ket
su•per'nal
su'per•nat'u•ral
su'per•no'va pl. -vae'
  or -vas
su'per•nu'mer•ar'y
su'per•pow'er
su'per•sat'u•rate',
  -rat'ed, -rat'ing
su'per•sav'er
su'per•scribe',
  -scribed', -scrib'ing
su'per•script'
su'per•scrip'tion
su'per•sede', -sed'ed,
  -sed'ing
su'per•son'ic
su'per•star'
su'per•sti'tion
su'per•sti'tious
su'per•store'
su'per•struc'ture
su'per•ton'ic
su'per•vise', -vised',
  -vis'ing
su'per•vi'sion
su'per•vi'sor
su'per•vi'so•ry

su•pine'
sup'per
sup'per•time
sup•plant'
sup'ple
sup'ple•ment
sup'ple•men'ta•ry
  also sup'ple•men'tal
sup'pli•ant
sup'pli•cant
sup'pli•cate', -cat'ed,
  -cat'ing
sup'pli•ca'tion
sup•pli'er
sup•ply', -plied', -ply'-
  ing
sup•port'
sup•port'a•ble
sup•por'tive
sup•pos'a•ble
sup•pose', -posed',
  -pos'ing
sup•pos'ed•ly
sup'po•si'tion
sup•pos'i•to'ry
sup•press'
sup•press'er also
  sup•pres'sor
sup•press'i•ble
sup•pres'sion
sup•pres'sive
sup'pu•rate', -rat'ed,
  -rat'ing
sup'pu•ra'tion
su'pra•re'nal
su•prem'a•cist
su•prem'a•cy

su•preme′
sur′cease′
sur′charge′, -charged′, -charg′ing
sur′cin′gle
sur′coat′
surd
sure, sur′er, sur′est
sure′-fire′
sure′-foot′ed
sure′ly
sure′ty
surf *(waves)*
  ♦*serf*
sur′face, -faced, -fac-ing
sur•fac′tant
surf ′board′
sur′feit
surf ′er
surf ′ing
surge *(to billow)*, surged, surg′ing
sur′geon
Surgeon General *pl.* Surgeons General
sur′ger•y
sur′gi•cal
sur′ly
sur•mise′, -mised′, -mis′ing
sur•mount′
sur•mount′a•ble
sur′name′, -named′, -nam′ing
sur•pass′
sur′plice *(robe)*

sur′plus *(excess)*
sur′print′
sur•prise′, -prised′, -pris′ing
sur•re′al
sur•re′al•ism
sur•re′al•ist
sur•re′al•is′tic
sur•ren′der
sur′rep•ti′tious
sur′rey *pl.* -reys
sur′ro•ga•cy
sur′ro•gate
sur•round′
sur•round′ings
sur′tax′
sur•veil′lance
sur′vey′ *n.*
sur•vey′ *v.*
sur•vey′ing
sur•vey′or
sur•viv′al
sur•viv′al•ist
sur•vive′, -vived′, -viv′ing
sur•vi′vor
sus•cep′ti•bil′i•ty
sus•cep′ti•ble
sus•cep′tive
sus•pect′ *n. & adj.*
sus•pect′ *v.*
sus•pend′
sus•pend′er
sus•pense′
sus•pen′sion
sus•pi′cion
sus•pi′cious

sus•tain′
sus•tain′a•ble
sus′te•nance
su′tra
sut′tee′
su′ture, -tured, -tur-ing
su′ze•rain
su′ze•rain•ty
svelte, svelt′er, svelt′-est
Sven•ga′li *pl.* -lis
swab, swabbed, swab′-bing, *also* swob, swobbed, swob′bing
swad′dle, -dled, -dling
swag
swage, swaged, swag′-ing
swag′ger
swain
swal′low
swal′low•tail′
swal′low-tailed′
swa′mi *pl.* -mis
swamp′land′
swamp′y
swan
swank *also* swank′y
swan′s′-down′ *also* swans′down′
swap, swapped, swap′-ping, *also* swop, swopped, swop′ping
sward *(turf)*
  ♦*sword*

swarm
swarth'y
swash'buck'ler
swash'buck'ling
swas'ti•ka
swat, swat'ted, swat'-
  ting
swatch
swath *(stroke width),*
  also swathe
swathe *(to wrap),*
  swathed, swath'ing
swat'ter
sway'back'
swear, swore, sworn,
  swear'ing
swear'word'
sweat, sweat'ed *or*
  sweat, sweat'ing
sweat'band'
sweat'er
sweat'shop'
sweat'y
Swede
Swed'ish
sweep, swept, sweep'-
  ing
sweep'stakes' *pl.*
  -stakes', *also* sweep'-
  stake'
sweet *(sugary)*
  ♦suite *(retinue, set)*
sweet'bread'
sweet'bri'er *also*
  sweet'bri'ar
sweet'en
sweet'en•er

sweet'heart'
sweet'meat'
swell, swelled, swelled
  or swol'len, swel'ling
swel'ter
swept'back'
swerve, swerved,
  swerv'ing
swift'ly
swig, swigged, swig'-
  ging
swill
swim, swam, swum,
  swim'ming
swim'mer
swim'mer•et'
swim'suit'
swim'wear'
swin'dle, -dled, -dling
swine *pl.* swine
swine'herd'
swing, swung, swing'-
  ing
swin'ish
swipe, swiped, swip'-
  ing
swirl
swish
Swiss
Swiss cheese
switch'blade'
switch'board'
switch'man
switch'o'ver'
switch'yard'
swiv'el, -eled *or*
  -elled, -el•ing *or* -el-

ling
swiz'zle stick
swoon
swoop
sword *(weapon)*
  ♦sward
sword'fish' *pl.* -fish
  or -fish'es
sword'play'
swords'man
sword'tail'
syb'a•rite *also* Syb'-
  a•rite
syb'a•rit'ic *also* syb'-
  a•rit'i•cal
syc'a•more'
syc'o•phan'cy
syc'o•phant
syc'o•phan'tic *also*
  syc'o•phan'ti•cal
syl•lab'ic
syl•lab'i•cate', -cat'-
  ed, -cat'ing, *also* syl-
  lab'i•fy', -fied', -fy'-
  ing
syl•lab'i•ca'tion
syl'la•ble
syl'la•bub' *also* sil'la-
  bub'
syl'la•bus *pl.* -bus•es
  or -bi'
syl'lo•gism
syl'lo•gis'tic
sylph
syl'van
sym'bi•o'sis
sym'bi•ot'ic

sym′bol *(sign)*
♦*cymbal*
sym•bol′ic *also* sym-
bol′i•cal
sym′bol•ism
sym′bol•ist
sym′bol•i•za′tion
sym′bol•ize′, -ized′,
-iz′ing
sym•bol′o•gy
sym•met′ric *also*
sym•met′ri•cal
sym′me•try
sym′pa•thet′ic
sym′pa•thize′,
-thized′, -thiz′ing
sym′pa•thy
sym•phon′ic
sym′pho•ny
sym•po′si•um *pl.*
-si•ums *or* -si•a
symp′tom
symp′to•mat′ic
syn′a•gogue′ *also*
syn′a•gog′
syn′apse′
syn•ap′sis *pl.* -ses′
syn′chro•cy′clo-
tron′
syn′chro•ni•za′tion
syn′chro•nize′,
-nized′, -niz′ing
syn′chro•nous
syn′chro•tron′
syn•cli′nal
syn′cline′
syn′co•pate′, -pat′ed,

-pat′ing
syn′co•pa′tion
syn′co•pa′tor
syn′co•pe
syn′cre•tism
syn′cre•tis′tic
syn′dic
syn′di•cate′, -cat•ed,
-cat•ing
syn′di•ca′tion
syn′drome′
syn′er•get′ic *also*
syn•er′gic
syn′er•gism *also* syn′-
er•gy
syn′er•gis′tic
syn′od
syn′o•nym′
syn•on′y•mous
syn•on′y•my
syn•op′sis *pl.* -ses′
sy•nop′tic *also* sy-
nop′ti•cal
syn•tac′tic *also* syn-
tac′ti•cal
syn′tax′
syn′the•sis *pl.* -ses′
syn′the•size′, -sized′,
-siz′ing
syn•thet′ic *also* syn-
thet′i•cal
syph′i•lis
syph′i•lit′ic
Syr′i•an
sy•ringe′
syr′inx *pl.* sy•rin′ges′
or syr′inx•es

syr′up *also* sir′up
syr′up•y
sys′tem
sys′tem•at′ic *also*
sys′tem•at′i•cal
sys′tem•a•ti•za′tion
sys′tem•a•tize′,
-tized′, -tiz′ing
sys•tem′ic
sys′to•le
sys•tol′ic

T

tab, tabbed, tab′bing
tab′ard
Ta•bas′co®
tab•bou′leh
tab′by
tab′er•na′cle
ta′ble, -bled, -bling
tab•leau′ *pl.* -leaux′
or -leaus′
ta′ble•cloth′
ta′ble d′hôte′ *pl.* ta′-
bles d′hôte′
ta′ble•hop′,
-hopped′, -hop′ing
ta′ble•land′
ta′ble•spoon′ *pl.*
-fuls′
tab′let
ta′ble•top′
ta′ble•ware′
tab′loid′
ta•boo′ *pl.* -boos′,
also ta•bu′ *pl.* -bus′

ta•boo', -booed',
-boo'ing, *also* ta•bu',
-bued, -bu'ing
ta'bor
tab'u•lar
tab'u•la ra'sa
tab'u•late', -lat'ed,
-lat'ing
tab'u•la'tion
tab'u•la'tor
ta'cet (*musical direc-
tion*)
♦*tacit*
ta•chom'e•ter
tach'o•met'ric
tac'it (*unspoken, im-
plied*)
♦*tacet*
tac'i•turn
tac'i•tur'ni•ty
tack
tack'le, -led, -ling
tack'y
ta'co *pl.* -cos
tac'o•nite'
tact (*diplomacy*)
♦*tacked*
tact'ful
tac'tic
tac'ti•cal
tac'ti•cian
tac'tics
tac'tile
tact'less
tad'pole'
taf 'fe•ta
taf 'fy

tag, tagged, tag'ging
Ta•hi'tian
tai'ga
tail (*hind part*)
♦*tale*
tail (*to follow*)
♦*tale*
tail'back'
tail'board'
tail'gate', -gat'ed,
-gat'ing
tail'light'
tai'lor
tai'lor-made'
tail'piece'
tail'pipe'
tail'race'
tail'spin'
taint
take, took, tak'en, tak'-
ing
take'a•way' *adj.* & *n.*
take'down' *adj.* & *n.*
take'-home' pay
take'off' *n.*
take'o'ver *n.* & *adj.*,
also take'-o'ver
talc
tal'cum
tale (*report*)
♦*tail*
tale'bear'er
tal'ent
tale'tell'er
tale'tell'ing
tal'is•man
tal'is•man'ic

talk'a•tive
talk'back'
talk'ie (*film*)
♦*talky*
talk'ing-to' *pl.* -tos
talk'y (*talkative*)
♦*talkie*
tall
tal'low
tal'ly, -lied, -ly•ing
tal'ly•ho' *pl.* -hos'
Tal'mud'
Tal•mu'dic *also* Tal-
mu'di•cal
tal'on
ta'lus (*anklebone*), *pl.*
-li'
ta'lus (*debris*), *pl.*
-lus•es
tam
ta•ma'le
tam'a•rack'
tam'a•rind'
tam'a•risk'
tam'bour'
tam'bou•rine'
tame, tam'er, tam'est
tame, tamed, tam'ing
Tam'ma•ny
tam'-o'-shan'ter
tamp
tamp'er (*neutron re-
flector*)
tam'per (*to interfere*)
tam'pon'
tan, tan'ner, tan'nest
tan, tanned, tan'ning

tan'a•ger
tan'bark'
tan'dem
tang
tan'ge•lo' *pl.* -los'
tan'gent
tan•gen'tial
tan'ger•ine'
tan'gi•bil'i•ty
tan'gi•ble
tan'gle, -gled, -gling
tan'go *pl.* -gos
tan'go, -goed, -go•ing
tang'y
tank'ard
tank'er
tan'ner
tan'ner•y
tan'nic
tan'nin
tan'ning
tan'sy
tan'ta•lite'
tan'ta•li•za'tion
tan'ta•lize', -lized',
  -liz'ing
tan'ta•lum
tan'ta•lus
tan'ta•mount'
tan'trum
Tao'ism
Tao'ist
tap, tapped, tap'ping
ta'pa
tap'-dance', -danced',
  -danc'ing
tape, taped, tap'ing

ta'per *(candle)*
  ♦*tapir*
ta'per *(to diminish)*
  ♦*tapir*
tape'-re•cord' *v.*
tap'es•try
tape'worm'
tap'i•o'ca
ta'pir *(animal)*
  ♦*taper*
tap'room'
tap'root'
taps
tap'ster
tar, tarred, tar'ring
tar'an•tel'la
ta•ran'tu•la
tar'dy
tare *(plant, weight)*
  ♦*tear (to split)*
tar'get
tar'get•a•ble
tar'iff
tar'la•tan
tar'mac'
tar'nish
ta'ro *(plant),* pl. -ros
tar'ot *(card)*
tarp
tar'pa'per
tar•pau'lin
tar'pon *pl.* -pon *or*
  -pons
tar'ra•gon'
tar'ry, -ried, -ry•ing
tar'sal
tar'si•er

tar'sus *pl.* -si'
tart
tar'tan
tar'tar *(acid com-
  pound, deposit, bad-
  tempered person)*
Tar'tar *(Mongol), also*
  Ta'tar
tar•tar'ic
tar'tar•ous
tar'tar sauce *also* tar'-
  tare sauce
tart'ness
task'mas'ter
Tas•ma'ni•an
tas'sel, -seled *or*
  -selled, -sel•ing *or*
  -sel•ling
taste, tast'ed, tast'ing
taste'ful *(showing
  good taste)*
  ♦*tasty*
taste'less
tast'y *(savory)*
  ♦*tasteful*
tat, tat'ted, tat'ting
tat'ter
tat'ter•de•mal'ion
tat'tle, -tled, -tling
tat'tler
tat'tle•tale'
tat•too' *pl.* -toos'
tat•too', -tooed', -too'-
  ing
taunt
taupe *(brownish gray)*
  ♦*tope*

Tau′rus
taut *(tight)*
 ♦*taught*
tau′to•log′i•cal *also*
 tau′to•log′ic
tau•tol′o•gy
tav′ern
taw
taw′dry
taw′ny
tax *(levy)*
 ♦*tacks*
tax′a•bil′i•ty
tax′a•ble
tax•a′tion
tax′-de•duct′i•ble
tax′-ex•empt′
tax′i *pl.* -is *or* -ies
tax′i, -ied, -i•ing *or*
 -y•ing
tax′i•cab′
tax′i•der′mist
tax′i•der′my
tax′i•me′ter
tax′ing
tax′i•way′
tax′o•nom′ic *also*
 tax′o•nom′i•cal
tax•on′o•mist
tax•on′o•my
tax′pay′er
T′-bone′
tea *(beverage)*
 ♦*tee, ti*
tea′cart′
teach, taught, teach′-
 ing

teach′a•ble
teach′er
teach′-in′ *n.*
teach′ing
tea′cup′
tea′cup′ful′ *pl.* -fuls′
tea′house′
teak
tea′ket′tle
teal *pl.* teal *or* teals
team *(group)*
 ♦*teem*
team′mate′
team′ster
team′work′
tea′pot′
tear *(to split),* tore,
 torn, tear′ing
 ♦*tare*
tear *(to cry),* teared,
 tear′ing
 ♦*tier*
tear′drop′
tear′ful
tear′-jerk′er
tea′room′
tear′stain′
tear′y-eyed′
tease, teased, teas′ing
tea′sel
teas′er
tea′spoon′
tea′spoon•ful′ *pl.*
 -fuls′
teat
tea′time′
tech•ne′ti•um

tech′ne•tron′ic
tech′nic
tech′ni•cal
tech′ni•cal′i•ty
tech•ni′cian
Tech′ni•col′or®
tech•nique′
tech•noc′ra•cy
tech′no•crat′
tech′no•crat′ic
tech′no•log′i•cal
 also tech′no•log′ic
tech•nol′o•gist
tech•nol′o•gy
tec•ton′ic
ted′dy bear *also* Ted′-
 dy bear
te′di•ous
te′di•um
tee *(golf peg)*
 ♦*tea, ti*
teem *(to abound)*
 ♦*team*
teen′-age′ *also*
 teen′-aged′
teen′-ag′er
teens
tee′ny *also* teen′sy
teen′y•bop′per
tee′off′ *n.*
tee′ter
tee′ter-tot′ter
teethe, teethed, teeth′-
 ing
tee′to′tal•er′ *or* tee′-
 to′tal•ler
Tef′lon′®

teg'u•ment
tek'tite'
tel'e•cam'er•a
tel'e•cast', -cast' or
  -cast'ed, -cast'ing
tel'e•com•mu'ni•
  cate', -cat'ed, -cat'-
  ing
tel'e•com•mu'ni•
  ca'tion
tel'e•dra'ma
tel'e•gen'ic
tel'e•gram'
tel'e•graph'
te•leg'ra•pher also
  te•leg'ra•phist
tel'e•graph'ic also
  tel'e•graph'i•cal
te•leg'ra•phy
tel'e•ki•ne'sis
tel'e•ki•net'ic
tel'e•mar'ket•ing
te•lem'e•ter
tel'e•met'ric also tel'-
  e•met'ri•cal
te•lem'e•try
tel'e•o•log'i•cal
tel'e•ol'o•gy
tel'e•path'ic
te•lep'a•thist
te•lep'a•thy
tel'e•phone',
  -phoned', -phon'ing
tel'e•phon'ic
te•leph'o•ny
tel'e•pho'to pl. -tos
tel'e•pho'to•graph'

tel'e•pho'to•graph'-
  ic
tel'e•pho•tog'ra-
  phy
tel'e•play'
tel'e•print'er
Tel'e•Promp'Ter®
tel'e•scope', -scoped',
  -scop'ing
tel'e•scop'ic
tel'e•text'
tel'e•thon'
Tel'e•type'®,
  -typed', -typ'ing
tel'e•type'writ'er
tel'e•vise', -vised',
  -vis'ing
tel'e•vi'sion
tel'ex'
tell, told, tell'ing
tell'tale'
tel'lu•ride'
tel•lu'ri•um
te'lo•phase'
Tel'star'
te•mer'i•ty
tem'per
tem'per•a
tem'per•a•ment
tem'per•a•men'tal
tem'per•ance
tem'per•ate
tem'per•a•ture
tem'pered
tem'pest
tem•pes'tu•ous
Tem'plar

tem'plate also tem'-
  plet
tem'ple
tem'po pl. -pos or -pi
tem'po•ral
tem'po•ral'i•ty
tem'po•rar'y
tem'po•ri•za'tion
tem'po•rize', -rized',
  -riz'ing
temp•ta'tion
tempt'ing
tempt'ress
tem'pu•ra
ten
ten'a•bil'i•ty
ten'a•ble
te•na'cious
te•nac'i•ty
ten'an•cy
ten'ant
tend
ten'den•cy
ten•den'tious
ten'der *(soft)*
ten'der *(to offer)*
tend'er *(one who
  tends, boat)*
ten'der•foot' pl.
  -foots' or -feet'
ten'der•heart'ed
ten'der•ize', -ized',
  -iz'ing
ten'der•iz'er
ten'der•loin'
ten'don
ten'dril

ten'e•ment
ten'et
ten'fold'
Ten'nes•se'an
ten'nis
ten'on
ten'or
ten'pin'
tense, tens'er, tens'est
tense, tensed, tens'ing
ten'sile
ten•sil'i•ty
ten'sion
tent
ten'ta•cle
ten•tac'u•lar
ten'ta•tive
ten'ter
ten'ter•hook'
tenth
ten'u•ous
ten'ure
ten'ured
te'pee *also* tee'pee
tep'id
te•pid'i•ty
te•qui'la
ter'bi•um
ter'cen•ten'ar•y *also*
  ter'cen•ten'ni•al
ter'i•ya'ki
term
ter'ma•gant
ter'mi•na•ble
ter'mi•nal
ter'mi•nate', -nat'ed,
  -nat'ing

ter'mi•na'tion
ter'mi•na'tive
ter'mi•na'tor
ter'mi•no•log'i•cal
ter'mi•nol'o•gist
ter'mi•nol'o•gy
ter'mi•nus *pl.* -nus-
  es *or* -ni'
ter'mite'
tern *(bird)*
  ♦*turn*
ter'na•ry
Terp•sich'o•re
terp'si•cho•re'an
ter'race, -raced, -rac-
  ing
ter'ra cot'ta
ter'ra-cot'ta *adj.*
ter'ra fir'ma
ter•rain'
ter'ra•pin
ter•rar'i•um *pl.*
  -i•ums *or* -i•a
ter•raz'zo
ter•res'tri•al
ter'ri•ble
ter'ri•er
ter•rif'ic
ter'ri•fy', -fied', -fy'-
  ing
ter'ri•to'ri•al
ter'ri•to•ri•al'i•ty
ter'ri•to'ry
ter'ror
ter'ror•ism
ter'ror•ist
ter'ror•i•za'tion

ter'ror•ize', -ized',
  -iz'ing
ter'ry
terse, ters'er, ters'est
ter'tian
ter'ti•ar'y *(third)*
Ter'ti•ar'y *(geologic
  period)*
ter'za ri'ma *pl.* ter'ze
  ri'me
tes'sel•late', -lat'ed,
  -lat'ing
tes'sel•la'tion
test
tes'ta *pl.* -tae'
tes'ta•cy
tes'ta•ment
tes'tate'
tes'ta'tor
tes•ta'trix
tes'ter *(canopy)*
test'er *(one that tests)*
tes'ti•cle
tes'ti•fy', -fied', -fy'-
  ing
tes'ti•mo'ni•al
tes'ti•mo'ny
tes'ti•ness
tes'tis *pl.* -tes'
tes•tos'ter•one'
tes'ty
tet'a•nal
te•tan'ic
tet'a•nus
tête'-à-tête'
teth'er
teth'er•ball'

tet′ra
tet′ra•chlo′ride′
tet′ra•cy′cline′
tet′rad′
tet′ra•eth′yl lead
  also tet′ra•eth′yl•
  lead′
tet′ra•he′dral
tet′ra•he′dron pl.
  -drons or -dra
te•tram′e•ter
tet′rarch′
tet′rar′chy also tet′-
  rar′chate′
tet′ra•va′lent
Teu′ton
Teu•ton′ic
Tex′an
text′book′
tex′tile′
tex′tu•al
tex′tur•al
tex′ture
tex′tured
tex′tur•ize′, -ized′,
  -iz′ing
Thai pl. Thai
tha•lam′ic
thal′a•mus pl. -mi′
tha•las′sic
Tha•li′a
tha•lid′o•mide′
thal′li•um
thal′lo•phyte′
than
thane
thank′ful

thank′less
thanks′giv′ing
that pl. those
thatch
thaw
the article
  ♦*thee*
the′a•ter also the′-
  a•tre
the′a•ter•go′er
the′a•ter-in-the-
  round′ pl. the′-
  a•ters-in-the-round′
the•at′ri•cal also
  the•at′ric
the•at′ri•cal′i•ty
the•at′rics
the′ca pl. -cae′
thee pron.
  ♦*the*
theft
their pron.
  ♦*there, they're*
theirs
the′ism
the′ist
the•is′tic also the•is′-
  ti•cal
them
the•mat′ic
theme
them•selves′
then
thence•forth′
thence•for′ward also
  thence•for′wards
the•oc′ra•cy

the′o•crat′
the′o•crat′ic also the′-
  o•crat′i•cal
the′o•lo′gi•an
the′o•log′i•cal also
  the′o•log′ic
the•ol′o•gy
the′o•rem
the′o•ret′i•cal also
  the′o•ret′ic
the′o•re•ti′cian
the′o•rist
the′o•ri•za′tion
the′o•rize′, -rized′,
  -riz′ing
the′o•ry
the′o•soph′i•cal
the•os′o•phist
the•os′o•phy
ther′a•peu′tic also
  ther′a•pcu′ti•cal
ther′a•peu′tics
ther′a•pist
ther′a•py
there (at that place)
  ♦*their, they're*
there′a•bout′ also
  there′a•bouts′
there•af′ter
there•at′
there•by′
there•for′ (for that)
there•fore′ (hence)
there•from′
there•in′
there′in•af′ter
there•of′

there•on'
there•to'
there'to•fore'
there'un•der
there'un•to'
there'up•on'
there•with'
there•with•al'
ther'mal *also* ther'-
  mic
therm'i'on
ther'mo•cou'ple
ther'mo•dy•nam'ic
ther'mo•dy•nam'ics
ther'mo•e•lec'tric
  also ther'mo•e•lec'-
  tri•cal
ther'mo•e•lec'tric'-
  i•ty
ther'mo•graph'
ther•mom'e•ter
ther'mo•met'ric
ther•mom'e•try
ther'mo•nu'cle•ar
ther'mo•plas'tic
Ther'mos® bottle
ther'mo•set'ting
ther'mo•sphere'
ther'mo•stat'
the•sau'rus *pl.* -rus-
  es
the'sis *pl.* -ses'
Thes'pi•an *also* thes'-
  pi•an
they
thi'a•mine *also* thi'-
  a•min

thick'en
thick'et
thick'head'ed
thick'ness
thick'set'
thick'-skinned'
thick'-wit'ted
thief *pl.* thieves
thieve, thieved, thiev'-
  ing
thiev'er•y
thiev'ish
thigh'bone'
thim'ble
thim'ble•ful' *pl.*
  -fuls'
thim'ble•rig'
thin, thin'ner, thin'-
  nest
thine
thing'a•ma•bob'
thing'a•ma•jig'
think, thought, think'-
  ing
think'a•ble
thin'ner
thin'-skinned'
thi•o•pen'tal
  sodium
third'-class' *adj. &*
  adv.
third'-de•gree' burn
thirst'•y
thir'teen'
thir'teenth'
thir'ti•eth
thir'ty

thir'ty-sec'ond note
this *pl.* these
this'tle
this'tle•down'
thith'er
thith'er•to'
thith'er•ward
thole'pin'
thong
Thor
tho•rac'ic
tho•rax' *pl.* -rax'es *or*
  -ra•ces'
tho'ri•um
thorn'y
thor'ough
thor'ough•bred'
thor'ough•fare'
thor'ough•go'ing
thou
though
thought'ful
thought'less
thou'sand
thou'sandth
thrall'dom *also* thral'-
  dom
thrash'ing
thread'bare'
thread'y
threat'en
three'-base' hit
three'-D' *or* 3-D
three'-deck'er
three'-di•men'sion-
  al
three'fold'

three'-piece'
three'-ply'
three'-ring' circus
three'score'
three'some
thren'o•dy
thresh'old'
thrice
thrift'y
thrill'er
thrive, throve or
　thrived, thrived or
　thriv'en, thriv'ing
throat'y
throb, throbbed,
　throb'bing
throe (pang)
　♦throw
throm'bin
throm•bo'sis pl. -ses'
throm'bus pl. -bi'
throne (ceremonial
　chair)
　♦thrown
throng
throt'tle, -tled, -tling
through (by way of)
　♦threw
through•out'
throw (to hurl), threw,
　thrown, throw'ing
　♦throe
throw'a•way' n. &
　adj.
throw'back' n.
thrum, thrummed,
　thrum'ming

thrush
thrust, thrust, thrust'-
　ing
thru'way' also
　through'way'
thud, thud'ded, thud'-
　ding
thug
thu'li•um
thumb'hole'
thumb'-in'dex v.
thumb'nail'
thumb'nut'
thumb'screw'
thumb'tack'
thump'ing
thun'der
thun'der•bird'
thun'der•bolt'
thun'der•clap'
thun'der•cloud'
thun'der•head'
thun'der•ous
thun'der•show'er
thun'der•stone'
thun'der•storm'
thun'der•struck'
thu'ri•ble
Thurs'day
thus
thwack
thwart
thy
thyme (herb)
　♦time
thy'mic
thy'mus

thy'roid'
thy•rox'in also thy-
　rox'ine'
thy•self'
ti (musical tone)
　♦tea, tee
ti•ar'a
Ti•bet'an
tib'i•a pl. -i•ae' or
　-i•as
tib'i•al
tic (spasm)
tick (sound, mark, in-
　sect, casing)
tick'er
tick'et
tick'ing
tick'le, -led, -ling
tick'ler
tick'lish
tick'tack'toe' also
　tick'-tack'-toe'
tid'al
tid'bit'
tid'dly•winks'
tide (to rise and fall),
　tid'ed, tid'ing
　♦tied
tide'land'
tide'mark'
tide'wa'ter
tide'way'
tid'ings
ti'dy, -died, -dy•ing
tie, tied, ty'ing
tie'back'
tie'break'er

tie′-dye′, -dyed′, -dye′-
  ing
tie′-in′ n.
tier (row)
  ♦tear (to cry)
tierce
tie′-up′ n.
tiff
Tif′fa•ny glass
ti′ger
ti′ger-eye′
tight′en
tight′fist′ed
tight′lipped′
tight′rope′
tights
tight′wad′
ti′gress
til′de
tile, tiled, til′ing
till′a•ble
till′age
till′er
tilt
tilth
tim′bale
tim′ber (trees)
  ♦timbre
tim′ber•land′
tim′ber•line′
tim′bre (quality of
  sound)
  ♦timber
time (to clock), timed,
  tim′ing
  ♦thyme
time′card′

time′-con•sum′ing
time′-hon′ored
time′keep′er
time′-lapse′ adj.
time′less
time′ly
time′-out′ n., also
  time out
time′piece′
tim′er
time′sav′ing
time′serv′er
time′-shar′ing
time′ta′ble
time′worn′
tim′id
ti•mid′i•ty
tim′ing
tim′or•ous
tim′o•thy
tim′pa•ni also tym′-
  pa•ni
tim′pa•nist
tin, tinned, tin′ning
tinc′ture
tin′der
tin′der•box′
tine
tin′foil′
tinge, tinged, tinge′ing
  or ting′ing
tin′gle, -gled, -gling
tin′gly
tin′horn′
tink′er
tin′kle, -kled, -kling
tin′ny

tin′-plate′, -plat′ed,
  -pla′ting
tin′sel
tin′smith′
tint
tin′tin•nab′u•la′-
  tion
tin′type′
tin′work′
ti′ny
tip, tipped, tip′ping
tip′-off′ n.
tip′per
tip′pet
tip′ple, -pled, -pling
tip′ster
tip′sy
tip′toe′, -toed′, -toe′-
  ing
tip′top′
ti′rade′
tire, tired, tir′ing
tire′less
tire′some
′tis
ti•sane′
tis′sue
tit
ti′tan (giant)
Ti′tan (god)
ti•tan′ic
ti•ta′ni•um
tithe, tithed, tith′ing
ti′tian
tit′il•late′, -lat′ed,
  -lat′ing
tit′il•la′tion

tit'il•la'tive
tit'lark
ti'tle, -tled, -tling
tit'mouse'
ti•tra'tion
tit'ter
tit'tle
tit'tle-tat'tle, -tled,
  -tling
tit'u•lar
tiz'zy
to (toward)
  ♦too, two
toad (amphibian ani-
  mal)
  ♦toed, towed
toad'fish', pl. -fish' or
  -fish'es
toad'stool'
toad'y, -ied, -y•ing
toast'er
toast'mas'ter
to•bac'co pl. -cos or
  -coes
to•bac'co•nist
to•bog'gan
to•bog'gan•ist
to'by also To'by
toc•ca'ta
toc'sin (alarm)
  ♦toxin
to•day' also to-day'
tod'dle, -dled, -dling
tod'dler
tod'dy
to-do' pl. -dos'
toe (foot digit)

♦tow
toed (having toes)
  ♦toad, towed
toe'hold'
toe'nail'
tof'fee
tog, togged, tog'ging
to'ga
to•geth'er
to•geth'er•ness
tog'gle
togs
toil (labor)
toile (fabric)
toi'let
toi'let•ry
toi•lette'
To•kay'
to'ken
to'ken•ism
Tol'ec'
tol'er•a•bil'i•ty
tol'er•a•ble
tol'er•ance
tol'er•ant
tol'er•ate', -at'ed, -at'-
  ing
tol'er•a'tion
tol'er•a'tive
tol'er•a'tor
toll'booth'
toll'gate'
tol'lu•ene'
tom'a•hawk'
tom•al'ley pl. -leys
to•ma'to pl. -toes
tomb

tom'boy'
tomb'stone'
tom'cat'
tom'cod' pl. -cod' or
  -cods'
tome
tom'fool'
tom•fool'er•y
tom'my•rot'
to•mor'row
tom'tit'
tom'-tom'
ton (weight)
  ♦tun
to'nal
to•nal'i•ty
tone, toned, ton'ing
ton'er
tongs
tongue, tongued,
  tongu'ing
tongue'-in-cheek'
tongue'-lash'ing
tongue'-tied'
ton'ic
to•night' also to-
  night'
ton'nage
ton•neau'
ton'sil
ton'sil•lec'to•my
ton'sil•li'tis
ton•so'ri•al
ton'sure, -sured, -sur-
  ing
ton'tine'
too (also)

♦*to, two*
tool *(implement)*
♦*tulle*
tool′box′
tool′ing
toot
tooth *pl.* teeth
tooth′ache′
tooth′brush′
toothed
tooth′less
tooth′paste′
tooth′pick′
tooth′pow′der
tooth′some
tooth′y
top, topped, top′ping
to′paz′
top′coat′
top′-drawer′ *adj.*
tope *(to drink)*, toped,
   top′ing
♦*taupe*
top′flight′ *adj.*
top•gal′lant
top′-heav′y
to′pi•ar′y
top′ic
top′i•cal
top′i•cal′i•ty
top′knot′
top′less
top′mast
top′most′
top′notch′
to•pog′ra•pher
top′o•graph′ic *also*

top′o•graph′i•cal
to•pog′ra•phy
top′o•log′ic *also* top′-
   o•log′i•cal
to•pol′o•gist
to•pol′o•gy
top′per
top′ping
top′ple, -pled, -pling
top′sail
top′-se′cret *adj.*
top′side′
top′soil′
top′spin′
top′stitch′
top′sy-tur′vy
toque
to′rah
torch′bear′er
tor′e•a•dor′
to•re′ro *pl.* -ros
tor′ment′ *n.*
tor•ment′ *v.*
tor•men′tor *also* tor-
   ment′er
tor•na′do *pl.* -does *or*
   -dos
tor•pe′do *pl.* -does
tor•pe′do, -doed,
   -do•ing
tor′pid
tor′por
torque
tor′rent
tor•ren′tial
tor′rid
tor′sion

tor′so *pl.* -sos *or* -si′
tort *(civil wrong)*
torte *(cake)*
tor•til′la
tor′toise
tor′toise•shell′
tor′tu•ous *(winding)*
♦*torturous*
tor′ture, -tured, -tur-
   ing
tor′tur•ous *(painful)*
♦*tortuous*
To′ry
toss′up′ *n.*
tos•ta′da
tot, tot′ted, tot′ting
to′tal, -taled *or*
   -talled, -tal•ing *or*
   -tal•ling
to•tal′i•tar′i•an
to•tal′i•tar′i•an-
   ism
to•tal′i•ty
to′tal•iz′er
tote, tot′ed, tot′ing
to′tem
to•tem′ic
tot′ter
tou′can′
touch′-and-go′ *adj.*
touch′back′ *n.*
touch′down′ *n.*
tou•ché′
touched
touch′-me-not′
touch′stone′
Touch′-Tone′®

touch'-type', -typed',
-typ'ing
touch'up' n.
touch'y
tough (strong)
♦tuff
tough'en
tough'-mind'ed
tou•pee'
tour' de force'
tour'ism
tour'ist
tour'ma•line
tour'na•ment
tour'ne•dos' pl. -dos'
tour'ney pl. -neys
tour'ni•quet
tou'sle, -sled, -sling
tout'er
tow (dragging, flax)
♦toe
tow (to pull)
♦toe
tow'age
to•ward also to-
wards
tow'el, -eled or -elled,
-el•ing or -el•ling
tow'er
tow'head'
tow'head'ed
tow'hee
tow'line'
town'ie
towns'folk
town'ship'

towns'man
towns'peo'ple
towns'wom'an
tow'path'
tow'rope'
tox•e'mi•a
tox•e'mic
tox'ic
tox'i•cant
tox•ic'i•ty
tox'i•co•log'i•cal
tox'i•col'o•gist
tox'i•col'o•gy
tox'in (poison)
♦tocsin
toy
trace, traced, trac'ing
trace'a•ble
trac'er•y
tra•che•a pl. -ae' or
-as
tra'che•al
tra'che•ot'o•my
tra•cho'ma
trac'ing
track (path)
♦tract
track'age
tract (region, pam-
phlet)
♦track
trac'ta•bil'i•ty
trac'ta•ble
trac'tion
trac'tor
trade, trad'ed, trad'-
ing

trade'-in' n.
trade'mark'
trade'off' n., also
trade'-off'
trades'man
trades'peo'ple
tra•di'tion
tra•di'tion•al
tra•di'tion•al•ism
tra•di'tion•al•ist
tra•di'tion•al•is'tic
tra•duce', -duced',
-duc'ing
traf'fic, -ficked,
-fick•ing
traf'fick•er
tra•ge'di•an
tra•ge'di•enne'
trag'e•dy
trag'ic also trag'i•cal
trag'i•com'c•dy
trag'i•com'ic also
trag'i•com'i•cal
trail'blaz'er
trail'blaz'ing
trail'er
train•ee'
train'er
train'load'
train'man
traipse, traipsed,
traips'ing
trait
trai'tor
trai'tor•ous
tra•jec'to•ry
tram'mel, -meled or

-melled, -mel•ing *or*
-mel•ling
tramp
tram'ple, -pled, -pling
tram'po•line'
tram'way'
trance
tran'quil
tran'quil•i•za'tion
tran'quil•ize', -ized',
　-iz'ing, *also* tran'-
　quil•lize', -lized',
　-liz'ing
tran'quil•iz'er
tran•quil'li•ty *or*
　tran•quil'i•ty
tran'quil•ly
trans•act'
trans•ac'tion
trans•ac'tor
trans•al'pine'
trans'at•lan'tic
tran•scend'
tran•scen'dent
tran'scen•den'tal
tran'scen•den'tal-
　ism
tran'scen•den'tal-
　ist
tran'scen•ti•nen'tal
tran•scribe',
　-scribed', -scrib'ing
tran'script'
tran•scrip'tion
tran'sept'
trans'fer *n.*
trans•fer', -ferred',

-fer'ring
trans•fer'a•bil'i•ty
trans•fer'a•ble
trans•fer'al *also*
　trans•fer'ral
trans•fer'ence
trans'fer•or'
trans'fig•u•ra'tion
trans•fig'ure, -ured,
　-ur•ing
trans•fi'nite'
trans•fix'
trans'form' *n.*
trans•form' *v.*
trans'for•ma'tion
trans'for•ma'tion•al
trans•for'ma•tive
trans•form'er
trans•fuse', -fused',
　-fus'ing
trans•fu'sion
trans•gress'
trans•gres'sion
trans•gres'sor
tran'sience *also* tran'-
　sien•cy
tran'sient
tran•sis'tor
tran•sis'tor•ize',
　-ized', -iz'ing
tran'sit
tran•si'tion
tran•si'tion•al
tran'si•tive
tran'si•to'ry
trans•lat'a•ble
trans•late', -lat'ed,

-lat'ing
trans•la'tion
trans•la'tor
trans•lit'er•ate', -at'-
　ed, -at'ing
trans•lit'er•a'tion
trans•lu'cence *also*
　trans•lu'cen•cy
trans•lu'cent
trans•mi'grate',
　-grat'ed, -grat'ing
trans'mi•gra'tion
trans•mis'si•bil'i•ty
trans•mis'si•ble
trans•mis'sion
trans•mit', -mit'ted,
　-mit'ting
trans•mit'ta•ble
trans•mit'tal
trans•mit'ter
trans•mut'a•bil'i•ty
trans•mut'a•ble
trans'mu•ta'tion
trans•mute', -mut'-
　ed, -mut'ing
trans'o•ce•an'ic
tran'som
tran•son'ic
trans•pa•cif'ic
trans•par'en•cy *also*
　trans•par'ence
trans•par'ent
tran'spi•ra'tion
tran•spire', -spired',
　-spir'ing
trans'plant' *n.*
trans•plant' *v.*

trans'plan•ta'tion
trans•po'lar
trans'port' n.
trans•port' v.
trans•port'a•bil'i•ty
trans•port'a•ble
trans'por•ta'tion
trans•pos'a•ble
trans•pose', -posed', -pos'ing
trans'po•si'tion
trans•sex'u•al
trans•ship', -shipped', -ship'ping, also tran•ship'
trans•ship'ment
tran'sub•stan'ti•ate', -at'ed, -at'ing
tran'sub•stan'ti•a'tion
trans'u•ran'ic
trans•ver'sal
trans•verse'
trans•ves'tite'
trap, trapped, trap'ping
tra•peze'
tra•pe'zi•um pl. -zi•ums or -zi•a
trap'e•zoid'
trap'e•zoi'dal
trap'per
trap'pings
Trap'pist
trap'shoot'ing
trash'y
trat'to•ri'a

trau'ma pl. -mas or -ma•ta
trau•mat'ic
trau'ma•tize', -tized', -tiz'ing
tra•vail' (toil, anguish)
trav'el (to journey), -eled or -elled, -el•ing or -el•ling
trav'el•er also trav'el•ler
trav'e•logue' also trav'e•log'
tra•ver'sal
trav'erse adj.
tra•verse', -versed', -vers'ing
trav'er•tine'
trav'es•ty, -tied, -ty•ing
tra•vois' pl. -vois' or -vois'es
trawl'er
tray (flat receptacle)
♦trey
treach'er•ous
treach'er•y
trea'cle
tread, trod, trod'den or trod, tread'ing
tread'le, -led, -ling
tread'mill'
trea'son
trea'son•a•ble
trea'son•ous
treas'ure, -ured, -ur-

ing
treas'ur•er
treas'ure-trove'
treas'ur•y
treat'a•ble
trea'tise
treat'ment
trea'ty
treb'le, -led, -ling
treb'ly
tree, treed, tree'ing
tre'foil'
tree'top'
trek, trekked, trek'king
trel'lis
trem'ble, -bled, -bling
tre•men'dous
trem'o•lo' pl. -los'
trem'or
trem'u•lous
trench'an•cy
trench'ant
trench'er•man
trend'y
tre•pan', panned', -pan'ning
trep'a•na'tion
tre•pang'
treph'i•na'tion
tre•phine', -phined', -phin'ing
trep'i•da'tion
tres'pass
tres'pass•er
tress
tres'tle

trey *(three)*
♦*tray*
tri•ad′
tri•ad′ic
tri•age′
tri′al
tri′an′•gle
tri•an′gu•lar
tri•an′gu•late′, -lat′-
ed, -lat′ing
tri•an′gu•la′tion
Tri•as′sic
tri•ath′lete
tri•ath′lon
trib′al
tribe
tribes′man
trib′u•la′tion
tri•bu′nal
trib′une′
trib′u•tar′y
trib′ute
trice
tri′ceps′
tri•cer′a•tops′
tri•chi′na *pl.* -nae *or*
-nas
trich′i•no′sis
tri•chi′nous
trick′er•y
trick′le, -led, -ling
trick′ster
trick′y
tri•clin′ic
tri′col′or
tri′col′ored
tri′corn *also* tri′corne′

tri′cot
tri•cus′pid *also* tri-
cus′pi•dal
tri′cy′cle
tri′dent
tried
tri•en′ni•al
tri′fle, -fled, -fling
tri•fo′cal
tri•fo′li•ate *also* tri-
fo′li•at′ed
tri•fur′cate *also* tri′-
fur•cat′ed
trig, trigged, trig′ging
trig•ger
trig′ger-hap′py
trig′o•no•met′ric
also trig′o•no•met′-
ri•cal
trig′o•nom′e•try
tri•lat′er•al•ism
trill
tril′lion
tril′lionth
tril′li•um
tri′lo•bite′
tril•o•gy
trim, trim′mer, trim′-
mest
trim, trimmed, trim′-
ming
tri•mes′ter
trim′mer
tri•mor′phic *also* tri-
mor′phous
tri′nal
trine

Trin′i•tar′i•an
tri•ni′tro•tol′u•ene′
trin′i•ty
trin′ket
tri•no′mi•al
tri′o *pl.* -os
tri′ode′
tri•ox′ide′
trip, tripped, trip′ping
tri•par′tite′
tripe
tri′ple, -pled, -pling
trip′let
tri′plex′
trip′li•cate′, -cat′ed,
-cat′ing
trip′li•ca′tion
tri′ply
tri′pod′
trip′tych
tri′reme′
tri•sect′
tri′sec′tion
tri′sec′tor
trite, trit′er, trit′est
trit′i•um
tri′ton
tri′umph
tri•um′phal
tri•um′phal•ism
tri•um′phant
tri•um′vir *pl.* -virs *or*
-vi•ri′
tri•um′vi•ral
tri•um′vi•rate′
tri′une′
tri•va′lent

triv'et
triv'i•a
triv'i•al
triv'i•al'i•ty
tri•week'ly
tro'che (lozenge)
tro'chee (metrical
　foot)
trog'lo•dyte'
troi'ka
Tro'jan
troll
trol'ley pl. -leys, also
　trol'ly
trol'lop
trom•bone'
trom•bon'ist
tromp
troop (soldiers)
　♦troupe
troop'er (soldier)
　♦trouper
troop'ship'
trope
tro'phy
trop'ic
trop'i•cal
tro'pism
tro'po•sphere'
trot, trot'ted, trot'ting
troth
trot'ter
trou'ba•dour'
troub'le, -led, -ling
troub'le•mak'er
troub'le-shoot'er
troub'le•some

trough
trounce, trounced,
　trounc'ing
troupe (actors)
　♦troop
troup'er (actor)
　♦trooper
trou'sers
trous'seau pl. -seaux
　or -seaus
trout pl. trout or
　trouts
trow'el, -eled or
　-elled, -el•ing or -el-
　ling
troy
tru'an•cy
tru'ant
truce
truck'age
truck'er
truck'le, -led, -ling
truck'load'
truck'man
truc'u•lence
truc'u•lent
trudge, trudged,
　trudg'ing
true, tru'er, tru'est
true, trued, tru'ing or
　true'ing
true'blue' n.
true'-blue' adj.
true'love'
truf'fle
tru'ism
tru'ly

trump'er•y
trum'pet
trum'pet•er
trun'cate', -cat'ed,
　-cat'ing
trun'ca'tion
trun'cheon
trun'dle, -dled, -dling
trunk
truss'ing
trust'bust'er
trus•tee' (guardian)
　♦trusty
trus•tee'ship'
trust'wor'thy
trust'y (dependable)
　♦trustee
truth pl. truths
truth'ful
try, tried, try'ing
try'out' n.
try•pan'o•some'
tryst
tset'se fly
T'-shirt' also tee shirt
T'-square'
tsu•na'mi
tu'a•ta'ra
tub, tubbed, tub'bing
tu'ba
tub'by
tube
tube'less tire
tu'ber
tu'ber•cle
tu•ber'cu•lar
tu•ber'cu•lin

tu·ber′cu·loid′
tu·ber′cu·lo′sis
tu·ber′cu·lous
tube′rose′
tu′ber·os′i·ty *pl.*
  -ties
tu′ber·ous
tub′ing
tu′bu·lar
tu′bule
tuck′er
Tu′dor
Tues′day
tu′fa
tuff *(rock)*
  ♦*tough*
tuf′fet
tuft
tug, tugged, tug′ging
tug′boat′
tug′ger
tu·i′tion
tu′la·re′mi·a
tu′lip
tulle *(net)*
  ♦*tool*
tum′ble, -bled, -bling
tum′ble-down′ *adj.*
tum′bler
tum′ble·weed′
tum′brel *also* tum′bril
tu′me·fac′tion
tu′me·fy′, -fied′, -fy′-
  ing
tu′mer·ic
tu·mes′cence
tu·mes′cent

tu′mid
tu·mid′i·ty
tum′my
tu′mor
tu′mult
tu·mul′tu·ous
tu′mu·lus *pl.* -li′
tun *(cask)*
  ♦*ton*
tu′na *pl.* -na *or* -nas
tun′a·ble *also* tune′-
  a·ble
tun′dra
tune, tuned, tun′ing
tune′ful
tune′less
tun′er
tune′-up′ *n.*
tung′sten
tu′nic
Tu·ni′sian
tun′nel, -neled *or*
  -nelled, -nel·ing *or*
  -nel·ling
tu′pe·lo′ *pl.* -los′
tur′ban *(headdress)*
  ♦*turbine*
tur′bid
tur′bine *(engine)*
  ♦*turban*
tur′bo·charg′er
tur′bo·e·lec′tric
tur′bo·jet′
tur′bo·prop′
tur′bot *pl.* -bot *or*
  -bots
tur′bu·lence

tur′bu·lent
tu·reen′
turf
tur′gid
tur·gid′i·ty
Turk
tur′key *pl.* -keys
Tur′kic
Turk′ish
tur′moil
turn *(to rotate)*
  ♦*tern*
turn′a·bout′
turn′a·round′ *n.*
turn′buck·le
turn′coat′
tur′nip
turn′key *pl.* -keys
turn′off′ *n.*
turn′out′ *n.*
turn′o′ver *n.*
turn′pike′
turn′stile′
turn′ta′ble
tur′pen·tine′
tur′pi·tude′
tur′quoise′
tur′ret
tur′ret·ed
tur′tle
tur′tle·back′
tur′tle·dove′
tur′tle·neck′
tusk
tus′sah
tus′sle, -sled, -sling
tus′sock

tu'te•lage
tu'te•lar'y
tu'tor
tu•to'ri•al
tut'ti *pl.* -tis
tut'ti-frut'ti
tu'tu
tux•e'do *pl.* -dos
TV Dinner®
twad'dle, -dled,
  -dling
twain
twang
tweak
tweed'y
tweet'er
tweez'ers
twelfth
Twelfth'-night'
twelve'month
twelve'-tone'
twen'ti•eth
twen'ty
twen'ty-one'
twice
twid'dle, -dled, -dling
twig'gy
twi'light'
twill
twilled
twin
twine, twined, twin'-
  ing
twinge, twinged,
  twing'ing
twi'night'
twin'jet'

twin'kle, -kled, -kling
twin'-screw' *adj.*
twirl'ing
twist'a•ble
twist'er
twit, twit'ted, twit'ting
twitch
twit'ter
twixt
two *(number)*
  ♦*to, too*
two'-bag'ger
two'-bit' *adj.*
two'-by-four'
two'-di•men'sion•al
two'-edged'
two'-faced'
two'-fist'ed
two'fold'
two'-hand'ed
two'-ply'
two'-seat'er
two'some
two'-step'
two'-time', -timed',
  -tim'ing
two'-tim'er
two'-way'
two'-wheel'er
ty•coon'
tyke *also* tike
tym•pan'ic *also* tym'-
  pa•nal
tym'pa•nist
tym'pa•num *pl.* -na
  or -nums, *also* tim'-
  pa•num

type, typed, typ'ing
type'cast', -cast',
  -cast'ing
type'face'
type'script'
type'set'ter
type'set'ting
type'write', -wrote',
  -writ'ten, -writ'ing
type'writ'er
ty'phoid'
ty'phoon
ty'phous *adj.*
ty'phus *n.*
typ'i•cal *also* typ'ic
typ'i•cal'i•ty
typ'i•fi•ca'tion
typ'i•fy', -fied', -fy'-
  ing
typ'ist
ty'po *pl.* -os
ty•pog'ra•pher
ty•po•graph'i•cal
  also ty'po•graph'ic
ty•pog'ra•phy
ty•pol'o•gy *pl.* -gies
ty•ran'ni•cal *also* ty-
  ran'nic
tyr'an•nize', -nized',
  -niz'ing
ty•ran'no•saur' *also*
  ty•ran'no•saur'us
tyr'an•nous
tyr'an•ny
ty'rant
ty'ro *pl.* -ros, *also* ti'ro
ty'ro•sine'

U

u•biq′ui•tous
u•biq′ui•ty
U′-boat′
ud′der
u•dom′e•ter
ug′ly
u•kase′
uke
U•krain′i•an
u′ku•le′le
ul′cer
ul′cer•ate′, -at′ed,
 -at′ing
ul′cer•a′tion
ul′cer•a′tive
ul′cer•ous
ul′na pl. -nae′ or -nas
ul′nar
ul′ster
ul•te′ri•or
ul′ti•ma
ul′ti•mate
ul′ti•ma′tum pl.
 -tums or -ta
ul′ti•mo′
ul′tra
ul′tra•con•ser′va-
 tive
ul′tra•high′
ul′tra•light′ adj.
ul′tra•light′ n.
ul′tra•ma•rine′
ul′tra•mi′cro•scope′
ul′tra•mod′ern

ul′tra•pas•teur•ize′,
 -ized′, -iz′ing
ul′tra•son′ic
ul′tra•son′ics
Ul′tra•suede′®
ul′tra•vi′o•let
ul′u•late′, -lat′ed,
 -lat′ing
ul′u•la′tion
U•lys′ses
um′bel
um′ber
um•bil′i•cal
um•bil′i•cus pl. -ci′
um′bra pl. -brae
um′brage
um•brel′la
u′mi•ak
um′laut′
um•pire′, -pired′, -pir′-
 ing
ump•teen′
ump•teenth′
un′a•bashed′
un′a•bash′ed•ly
un•a′ble
un′a•bridged′
un•ac′cent•ed
un′ac•cept′a•ble
un′ac•com′pa•nied
un′ac•count′a•ble
un′ac•cus′tomed
un′a•chiev′a•ble
un′ac•knowl′edged
un′ac•quaint′ed
un′a•dopt′a•ble
un′a•dorned′

un′a•dul′ter•at′ed
un′ad•ven′tur•ous
un•ad′ver•tised′
un′ad•vised′
un′ad•vis′ed•ly
un′af•fect′ed
un′af•ford′a•ble
un′a•fraid′
un•aid′ed
un•al′ien•a•ble
un′a•ligned′
un′al•loyed′
un•al′ter•a•ble
un′am•big′u•ous
un′am•bi′tious
un′-A•mer′i•can
u′na•nim′i•ty
u•nan′i•mous
un′an•swer•a•ble
un′an•tic′i•pat′ed
un′ap•peal′ing
un′ap•pre′ci•at′ed
un′ap•proach′a•ble
un′ap•proved′
un•apt′
un•armed′
un′a•shamed′
un•asked′
un′as•sail′a•ble
un′as•sem′bled
un′as•sist′ed
un′as•sum′ing
un′at•tached′
un′at•tain′a•ble
un′at•test′ed
un′a•vail′a•ble
un′a•vail′ing

un′a•void′a•ble
un′a•ware′
un′a•wares′
un•bal′anced
un•bar′, -barred′,
  -bar′ring
un•bear′a•ble
un•beat′a•ble
un•beat′en
un′be•com′ing
un′be•knownst′
un′be•lief′
un′be•liev′a•ble
un′be•liev′er
un•bend′, -bent′,
  -bend′ing
un•bi′ased
un•bid′den
un•bind′, -bound′,
  -bind′ing
un•blem′ished
un•blessed′ *also* un-
  blest′
un•blink′ing
un•blush′ing
un•bolt′
un•born′
un•bos′om
un•bound′ed
un•bowed′
un•bri′dled
un•bro′ken
un•buck′le, -led,
  -ling
un•bur′den
un•but′ton
un•called′-for′

un•can′ny
un•cap′, -capped′,
  -cap′ping
un•car′ing
un•ceas′ing
un•cer′e•mo′ni•ous
un•cer′tain
un•cer′tain•ty
un•chain′
un•change′a•ble
un′char•ac•ter•is′-
  tic
un•char′i•ta•ble
un•chart′ed
un•chaste′
un•chris′tian
un′cial *also* Un′cial
un′ci•form′
un•cir′cum•cised′
un•civ′il
un•civ′i•lized′
un•clad′
un•clasp′
un•clas′si•fied′
un′cle
un•clean′
un•clear′
un•clench′
un•cloak′
un•clog′, -clogged′,
  -clog′ging
un•close′, -closed′,
  -clos′ing
un•clothe′, -clothed′
  or -clad′, -cloth′ing
un•coil′
un•com′fort•a•ble

un•com•mit′ted
un•com′mon
un′com•mu′ni•ca′-
  tive
un•com′pen•sat′ed
un′com•plain′ing
un′com•pli•men′-
  ta•ry
un′com•pro•mis′-
  ing
un′con•cern′
un′con•cerned′
un′con•di′tion•al
un′con•di′tioned
un′con•nect′ed
un′con•quer•a•ble
un′con•scion•a•ble
un•con′scious
un′con•sid′ered
un′con•sol′i•dat′ed
un′con•sti•tu′tion-
  al
un′con•sti•tu′tion-
  al′i•ty
un′con•tam′i•nat′-
  ed
un′con•trol′la•ble
un′con•ven′tion•al
un′con•ven′tion•al′-
  i•ty
un′con•vinc′ing
un•cooked′
un′co•op′er•a•tive
un′co•or′di•nat′ed
un•cork′
un•count′ed
un•cou′ple, -pled,

-pling
un•couth'
un•cov'er
un•crit'i•cal
un'cross'
unc'tion
unc'tu•os'i•ty
unc'tu•ous
un•curl'
un•cut'
un•daunt'ed
un•de•cid'ed
un•de•clared'
un•de•feat'ed
un•de•mon'stra-
tive
un•de•ni'a•ble
un•de•pend'a•ble
un'der
un'der•a•chieve',
-chieved', -chiev'ing
un'der•act'
un'der•age'
un'der•arm'
un'der•bel'ly
un'der•bid', -bid',
-bid'ding
un'der•brush'
un'der•buy',
-bought', -buy'ing
un'der•cap'i•tal-
ize', -ized', -iz'ing
un'der•car'riage
un'der•charge' n.
un'der•charge',
-charged', -charg'ing
un'der•class'man

un'der•clothes' also
un'der•cloth'ing
un'der•coat'
un'der•cov'er
un'der•cur'rent
un'der•cut', -cut',
-cut'ting
un'der•de•vel'oped
un'der•dog'
un'der•done'
un'der•drawers'
un'der•dressed'
un'der•es'ti•mate',
-mat'ed, -mat'ing
un'der•es'ti•ma'-
tion
un'der•ex•pose',
-posed', -pos'ing
un'der•ex•po'sure
un'der•feed', -fed',
-feed'ing
un'der•foot'
un'der•gar'ment
un'der•gird', -gird'ed
or girt, -gird'ing
un'der•go', -went',
-gone', -go'ing, -goes
un'der•grad'u•ate
un'der•ground'
un'der•growth'
un'der•hand'
un'der•hand'ed
un'der•lay' n.
un'der•lay', -laid',
-lay'ing
un'der•lie', -lay',
-lain', -ly'ing

un'der•line', -lined',
-lin'ing
un'der•ling
un'der•mine',
-mined', -min'ing
un'der•most'
un'der•neath'
un'der•nour'ish
un'der•nour'ished
un'der•pants'
un'der•pass'
un'der•pay', -paid',
-pay'ing
un'der•pin'ning
un'der•play'
un'der•priv'i•leged
un'der•pro•duc'-
tion
un'der•rate', -rat'ed,
-rat'ing
un'der•score',
-scored', -scor'ing
un'der•sea' adj.
un'der•sea' also un'-
der•seas'
un'der•sec're•tar'y
un'der•sell', -sold',
-sell'ing
un'der•shirt'
un'der•shoot', -shot',
-shoot'ing
un'der•shot' adj.
un'der•side'
un'der•signed'
un'der•sized' also
un'der•size'
un'der•skirt'

un′der•slung′
un′der•staffed′
un′der•stand′, -stood′, -stand′ing
un′der•stand′a•ble
un′der•state′, -stat′ed, -stat′ing
un′der•state′ment
un′der•stud′y, -ied, -y•ing
un′der•take′, -took′, -tak′en, -tak′ing
un′der•tak′er
un′der•tak′ing n.
un′der-the-count′er adj.
un′der•tone′
un′der•tow′
un′der•val′ue, -ued, -u•ing
un′der•wa′ter adj.
un′der•wat′er adv.
un′der•wear′
un′der•weight′
un′der•world′
un′der•write′, -wrote′, -writ′ten, -writ′ing
un′der•writ′er
un′de•served′
un′de•serv′ed•ly
un′de•sir′a•ble
un′de•ter′mined
un′dies
un•dig′ni•fied′
un′dis•crim′i•nat′-ing

un′dis•tin′guished
un′dis•turbed′
un•do′ *(to reverse),* -did′, -done′, -do′-ing, -does
♦*undue*
un•doc′u•ment′ed
un•doubt′ed
un•dress′
un•due′ *(excessive)*
♦*undo*
un′du•lant
un′du•late′, -lat′ed, -lat′ing
un′du•la′tion
un•du′ly
un•dy′ing
un•earned′
un•earth′
un•earth′ly
un•eas′y
un•ed′u•cat′ed
un′e•mo′tion•al
un′em•ploy′a•ble
un′em•ployed′
un′em•ploy′ment
un•e′qual
un•e′qualed *also* un-e′qualled
un′e•quiv′o•cal
un•err′ing
un•es•sen′tial
un•e′ven
un′e•vent′ful
un′ex•am′pled
un′ex•cep′tion-a•ble

un′ex•cep′tion•al
un′ex•pect′ed
un•fail′ing
un•fair′
un•faith′ful
un′fa•mil′iar
un′fa•mil′i•ar′i•ty
un•fash′ion•a•ble
un•fas′ten
un•fath′om•a•ble
un•fa′vor•a•ble
un•feel′ing
un•feigned′
un•fet′tered
un•fin′ished
un•fit′
un•flap′pa•ble
un•fledged′
un•flinch′ing
un•fold′
un′fore•seen′
un′for•get′ta•ble
un•formed′
un•for′tu•nate
un•found′ed
un′fre•quent′ed
un•friend′ly
un•frock′
un•fruit′ful
un•furl′
un•gain′ly
un•glued′
un•god′ly
un•gov′ern•a•ble
un•gra′cious
un′gram•mat′i•cal
un•grate′ful

un•guard'ed
un'guent
un'gu•late
un•hal'lowed
un•hand'
un•hap'py
un•har'ness
un•health'y
un•heard'
un•heard'-of '
un•hes'i•tat'ing
un•hinge', -hinged',
  -hing'ing
un•hitch'
un•ho'ly
un•hook'
un•horse', -horsed',
  -hors'ing
u'ni•cam'er•al
u'ni•cel'lu•lar
u'ni•corn'
u'ni•cy'cle
un'i•den'ti•fied'
u'ni•di•rec'tion•al
u'ni•fi•ca'tion
u'ni•form'
u'ni•form'i•ty
u'ni•fy', -fied', -fy'ing
u'ni•lat'er•al
un'i•mag'in•a•ble
un'i•mag'i•na•tive
un'im•peach'a•ble
un'im•por'tance
un'im•por'tant
un'im•proved'
un'in•formed'
un'in•hab'it•ed

un'in•hib'i•ted
un'in•spired'
un'in•tel'li•gent
un'in•tel'li•gi•ble
un'in•tend'ed
un'in•ten'tion•al
un'in•ter•est•ed
un'in•vit'ed
un'ion
un'ion•ism
un'ion•ist
un'ion•i•za'tion
un'ion•ize', -ized',
  -iz'ing
u•nique'
u'ni•sex'
u'ni•son
u'nit
u'ni•tard'
U'ni•tar'i•an
u'ni•tar'y
u•nite', -nit'ed, -nit'-
  ing
u'ni•ty
U'ni•vac'®
u'ni•va'lent
u'ni•valve'
u'ni•ver'sal
u'ni•ver'sal•is'tic
u'ni•ver•sal'i•ty
u'ni•verse'
u'ni•ver'si•ty
un•just'
un•jus'ti•fi'a•ble
un•kempt'
un•kind'
un•know'a•ble

un•know'ing
un•known'
un•lace', -laced', -lac'-
  ing
un•lad'y•like'
un•latch'
un•law'ful
un•lead'ed
un•learn', learned',
  -learn'ing
un•learn'ed *adj.*
un•leash'
un•leav'ened
un•less'
un•let'tered
un•li'censed
un•like'
un•like'ly
un•lim'ber
un•lim'it•ed
un•list'ed
un•load'
un•lock'
un•looked'-for'
un•loose', -loosed',
  -loos'ing
un•loos'en
un•love'ly
un•luck'y
un•made'
un•man'age•a•ble
un•man'ly
un•manned'
un•man'nered
un•man'ner•ly
un•marked'
un•mar'ried

un·mask'
un·men'tion·a·ble
un·mer'ci·ful
un·mind'ful
un'mis·tak·a·ble
un·mit'i·gat'ed
un·mor'al
un·mo'ti·va'ted
un·nat'u·ral
un·nec'es·sar'y
un·nerve', -nerved',
  -nerv'ing
un·num'bered
un'ob·struct'ed
un'ob·tru'sive
un·oc'cu·pied'
un'of·fi'cial
un'op·posed'
un·or'gan·ized'
un·or'tho·dox'
un·pack'
un·paid'
un·pal'a·ta·ble
un·par'al·leled'
un·pin', -pinned',
  -pin'ning
un·planned'
un·pleas'ant
un·plug', -plugged',
  -plug'ging
un·pop'u·lar
un'pop·u·lar'i·ty
un·prec'e·dent'ed
un'pre·dict'a·ble
un·prej'u·diced
un'pre·med'i·tat'ed
un'pre·pared'

un'pre·pos·sess'ing
un'pre·ten'tious
un·prin'ci·pled
un·print'a·ble
un'pro·duc'tive
un'pro·fes'sion·al
un·prof'it·a·ble
un'pro·tect'ed
un'pro·voked'
un·qual'i·fied'
un·ques'tion·a·ble
un·ques'tioned
un·quote', -quot'ed,
  -quot'ing
un·rav'el, -eled or
  -elled, -el·ing or -el-
  ling
un·read'
un·read'a·ble
un·read'y
un·re'al
un're·al·is'tic
un·rea'son·a·ble
un're·con·struct'ed
un·reel'
un're·gen'er·ate
un're·hearsed'
un're·lent'ing
un're·li'a·bil'i·ty
un're·li'a·ble
un're·mark'a·ble
un're·mit'ting
un're·quit'ed
un're·served'
un're·serv'ed·ly
un're·spon'sive
un·rest'

un're·strained'
un·ripe'
un·ri'valed
un·roll'
un·ruf'fled
un·ru'ly
un·sad'dle, -dled,
  -dling
un·safe'
un·salt'ed
un·san'i·tar'y
un·sat'is·fac'to·ry
un·sat'u·rat'ed
un·sa'vor·y
un·scathed'
un·schooled'
un'sci·en·tif'ic
un·scram'ble, -bled,
  -bling
un·screw'
un·scru'pu·lous
un·seal'
un·sea'son·a·ble
un·sea'soned
un·seat'
un·seem'ly
un·seen'
un·sel'fish
un·set'tle, -tled,
  -tling
un·shack'le, -led,
  -ling
un·shak'a·ble
un·shak'en
un·sheathe',
  -sheathed', -sheath'-
  ing

un•shod′
un•sight′ly
un•skilled′
un•skill′ful
un•snap′, -snapped′,
  -snap′ping
un•snarl′
un•so′cia•bil′i•ty
un•so′cia•ble
un′so•lic′it•ed
un′so•phis′ti•cat′ed
un•sound′
un•spar′ing
un•speak′a•ble
un•sports′man•like′
un•sta′ble
un•stead′y
un•stop′, -stopped′,
  -stop′ping
un•stressed′
un•string′, -strung′,
  -string′ing
un•struc′tured
un•stud′ied
un′sub•stan′tial
un′suc•cess′ful
un•suit′a•bil′i•ty
un•suit′a•ble
un•sul′lied
un•sung′
un′sur•passed′
un′sus•pect′ed
un′sus•pect′ing
un′sym•pa•thet′ic
un•tan′gle, -gled,
  -gling
un•ten′a•ble

un•think′a•ble
un•think′ing
un•ti′dy
un•tie′, -tied′, -ty′ing
un•til′
un•time′ly
un•tir′ing
un′to
un•told′
un•touch′a•ble
un•to′ward′
un•tried′
un•trou′bled
un•true′
un•truth′
un•truth′ful
un•tu′tored
un•twine′, -twined′,
  -twin′ing
un•twist′
un•used′
un•u′su•al
un•ut′ter•a•ble
un•var′nished
un•veil′
un•voiced′
un•war′i•ly
un•war′rant•ed
un•war′y
un•wel′come
un•well′
un•whole′some
un•wield′y
un•will′ing
un•wind′, -wound′,
  -wind′ing
un•wise′, -wis′er,

  -wis′est
un•wit′ting
un•wont′ed
un•work′a•ble
un•world′ly
un•worn′
un•wor′thy
un•wrap′, -wrapped′,
  -wrap′ing
un•writ′ten
un•yield′ing
un•yoke′, -yoked′,
  -yok′ing
un•zip′, -zipped′,
  -zip′ping
up′-and-com′ing
U•pan′i•shad′
up′beat′
up•braid′
up′bring′ing
up′com′ing
up′coun′try *adj. & n.*
up•coun′try *adv.*
up•date′ *n.*
up•date′, -dat′ed,
  -dat′ing
up′draft′
up•end′
up•grade′, -grad′ed,
  -grad′ing
up•heav′al
up′hill′
up•hold′, -held′,
  -hold′ing
up•hol′ster
up•hol′ster•y
up′keep′

up'land
up'lift' *adj. & n.*
up•lift' *v.*
up'load'
up'mar'ket
up•on'
up'per
up'per-case', -cased',
  -cas'ing
up'per-class'
up'per•class'man
up'per•cut'
up'per•most'
up'pi•ty
up•raise', -raised',
  -rais'ing
up'right'
up'ris'ing
up'riv'er
up'roar'
up•roar'i•ous
up'root'
up'scale'
up'set' *n.*
up'set', -set', -set'ting
up'shot'
up'side'-down'
up'stage' *adj. & adv.*
up•stage', -staged',
  -stag'ing
up'stairs' *adj. & n.*
up'stairs' *adv.*
up•stand'ing
up'start'
up'state'
up'stream'
up'surge' *n.*

up•surge' -surged',
  -surg'ing
up'sweep'
up'swept'
up'swing'
up'take'
up'tick'
up'tight' *also* up tight
up'-to-date'
up'town'
up'trend'
up'turn'
up'ward *also* up'-
  wards
up'wind'
u•rae'us
u•ra'ni•um
U'ra•nus
ur'ban *(of a city)*
ur•bane' *(suave)*
ur'ban•ist
ur'ban•ite'
ur•ban'i•ty
ur•ban•i•za'tion
ur•ban•ize', -ized',
  -iz'ing
ur'chin
u•re'a
u•re'mi•a
u•re'ter
u•re'thra *pl.* -thras *or*
  -thrae
u•re'thral
urge, urged, urg'ing
ur'gen•cy
ur'gent
u'ric

u'ri•nal
u'ri•nal'y•sis
u'ri•nar'y
u'ri•nate', -nat'ed,
  -nat'ing
u'rine
urn *(vase)*
  ♦*earn*
Ur'sa Major
Ursa Minor
ur'sine'
us
us'a•ble *also* use'-
  a•ble
us'age
use *(to employ),* used,
  us'ing
  ♦*yews*
use'ful
use'less
us'er
ush'er
u'su•al
u'su•fruct'
u'su•rer
u•su'ri•ous
u'surp'
u'sur•pa'tion
u'su•ry
u•ten'sil
u'ter•ine
u'ter•us
u•til'i•tar'i•an
u•til'i•tar'i•an•ism
u•til'i•ty
u'til•i•za'tion
u'til•ize', -ized', -iz'-

ing
ut′most′
u•to′pi•a
u•to′pi•an
ut′ter
ut′ter•ance
ut′ter•most′
U′-turn′
u′vu•la
u′vu•lar
ux•o′ri•al
ux•o′ri•ous

V

va′can•cy
va′cant
va′cate′, -cat′ed, -cat′-
  ing
va•ca′tion
vac′ci•nate′, -nat′ed,
  -nat′ing
vac′ci•na′tion
vac′ci•na′tor
vac′cine′
vac′il•late′, -lat′ed,
  -lat′ing
vac′il•la′tion
vac′il•la′tor
va•cu′i•ty
vac′u•ole′
vac′u•ous
vac′u•um *pl.* -u•ums
  or -u•a
vac′u•um-packed′
va′dc mc′cum *pl.* va′-
  de me′cums

vag′a•bond′
va′gar•y
va•gi′na *pl.* -nas *or*
  -nae
vag′i•nal
va′gran•cy
va′grant
vague, vagu′er, vagu′-
  est
vain *(unsuccessful,*
  conceited)
  ♦*vane, vein*
vain•glo′ri•ous
vain′glo′ry
val′ance *(drapery)*
  ♦*valence*
vale *(valley)*
  ♦*veil*
val′e•dic′tion
val′e•dic•to′ri•an
val′e•dic′to•ry
va′lence *(capacity to*
  combine), also va′-
  len•cy
  ♦*valance*
val′en•tine′
va•le′ri•an
val′et
val′e•tu′di•nar′i•an
val′e•tu′di•nar′-
  i•an•ism
Val•hal′la
val′iant
val′id
val′i•date′, -dat′ed,
  -dat′ing
val′i•da′tion

va•lid′i•ty
va•lise′
Val•kyr′ie
val′ley *pl.* -leys
val′or
val′or•ous
val′u•a•ble
val′u•a′tion
val′u•a′tor
val′ue, -ued, -u•ing
val′ue-add′ed tax
valve
val′vu•lar
va•moose′, -moosed′,
  -moos′ing
vamp
vam′pire′
vam′pir•ism
van
va•na′di•um
van′dal *(defacer)*
Van′dal *(tribesman)*
van′dal•ism
van′dal•ize′, -ized′,
  -iz′ing
Van•dyke′
vane *(wind indicator)*
  ♦*vain, vein*
van′guard′
va•nil′la
va•nil′lin
van′ish
van′i•ty
van′quish
van′tage
vap′id
va•pid′i•ty

va'por
va'por•iz'a•ble
va'por•i•za'tion
va'por•ize', -ized',
 -iz'ing
va'por•ous
va'por•ware'
va•que'ro *pl.* -ros
var'i•a•bil'i•ty
var'i•a•ble
var'i•ance
var'i•ant
var'i•a'tion
var'i•col'ored
var'i•cose'
var'i•cos'i•ty
var'ied
var'i•e•gate', -gat'ed,
 -gat'ing
var'i•e•ga'tion
va•ri'e•ty
var'i•ous
var'let
var'mint
var'nish
var'si•ty
var'y *(to change)*, -ied,
 -y•ing
 ♦*very*
vas'cu•lar
vase
va•sec'to•my
Vas'e•line'®
vas'so•con•stric'-
 tion
vas'so•con•stric'tor
vas'so•dil'a•ta'tion

also va'so•di•la'tion
va'so•di•la'tor
vas'o•mo'tor
vas'sal
vas'sal•age
vast
vat
Vat'i•can
vaude'ville
vaude'vil'lian
vault'ing
vaunt'ed
veal
vec'tor
vec•to'ri•al
Ve'da
Ve•dan'ta
veep
veer
Ve'ga
veg'e•ta•ble
veg'e•tal
veg'e•tar'i•an
veg'e•tar'i•an•ism
veg'e•tate', -tat'ed,
 -tat'ing
veg'e•ta'tion
veg'e•ta•tive *also*
 veg'e•tive
ve'he•mence *also* ve'-
 he•men•cy
ve'he•ment
ve'hi•cle
ve•hic'u•lar
veil *(covering)*
 ♦*vale*
vein *(vessel, strip,*

 crack)
 ♦*vain, vane*
ve'lar
Vel'cro®
veldt *also* veld
vel•le'i•ty
vel'lum *(parchment)*
 ♦*velum*
ve•loc'i•pede'
ve•loc'i•ty
ve•lour' *pl.* -lours', *or*
 ve•lours'
ve'lum *(membrane)*,
 pl. -la
 ♦*vellum*
vel'vet
vel'vet•een'
vel'vet•y
ve'na ca'va *pl.* ve'-
 nae' ca'vae'
ve'nal *(open to brib-*
 ery)
 ♦*venial*
ve•nal'i•ty
ve•na'tion
vend•ee'
vend'er *also* ven'dor
ven•det'ta
vend'i•ble *also* vend'-
 a•ble
vend'ing machine
ve•neer'
ven'er•a•bil'i•ty
ven'er•a•ble
ven'er•ate', -at'ed,
 -at'ing
ven'er•a'tion

ven'er•a'tor
ve•ne're•al
Ve•ne'tian blind
　also ve•ne'tian blind
venge'ance
venge'ful
ve'ni•al *(minor)*
　♦*venal*
ve'ni•al'i•ty
ve•ni're
ven'i•son
ven'om
ven'om•ous
ve'nous
vent
ven'ti•late', -lat'ed,
　-lat'ing
ven'ti•la'tion
ven'ti•la'tor
ven'tral
ven'tri•cle
ven'tri•cose *also* ven'-
　tri•cous
ven'tri•cos'i•ty
ven•tric'u•lar
ven•tril'o•quism
　also ven•tril'o•quy
ven•tril'o•quist
ven•tril'o•quis'tic
ven•tril'o•quize',
　-quized', -quiz'ing
ven'ture, -tured, -tur-
　ing
ven'ture•some
ven'tur•ous
ven'ue
Ve'nus

Ve•nu'sian
Ve'nus's-fly'trap'
ve•ra'cious *(truthful)*
　♦*voracious*
ve•rac'i•ty
ve•ran'dah *or* ve-
　ran'da
verb
ver'bal
ver'bal•ism
ver'bal•ist
ver'bal•i•za'tion
ver'bal•ize', -ized',
　-iz'ing
ver•ba'tim
ver•be'na
ver'bi•age
ver•bose'
ver•bos'i•ty
ver'dan•cy
ver'dant
ver'dict
ver'di•gris
ver'dure
verge, verged, verg-
　ing
verg'er
ver'i•fi'a•ble
ver'i•fi•ca'tion
ver'i•fi'er
ver'i•fy', -fied', -fy'-
　ing
ver'i•ly
ver'i•si•mil'i•tude'
ver'i•ta•ble
ver•i'ty
ver'meil

ver'mi•cel'li
ver'mi•cide'
ver•mic'u•lar
ver•mic'u•lite'
ver'mi•form'
ver'mi•fuge'
ver•mil'ion *also* ver-
　mil'lion
ver'min *pl.* -min
ver'min•ous
Ver•mont'er
ver'mouth'
ver•nac'u•lar
ver'nal
ver'ni•er
ve•ron'i•ca
ver'sa•tile
ver'sa•til'i•ty
verse
versed
ver'si•cle
ver'si•fi•ca'tion
ver'si•fi'er
ver'si•fy', -fied', -fy'-
　ing
ver'sion
ver'so *pl.* -sos
ver'sus
ver'te•bra *pl.* -brae *or*
　-bras
ver'te•bral
ver'te•brate'
ver'tex' *pl.* -tex'es *or*
　-ti•ces'
ver'ti•cal
ver'ti•cal'i•ty
ver•tig'i•nous

ver'ti•go' *pl.* -goes' or -gos'
verve
ver'y *(extremely)*
♦*vary*
ves'i•cant
ves'i•cate' -cat'ed, -cat'ing
ves'i•cle
ve•sic'u•lar
ves'per *(bell)*
Ves'per *(star)*
ves'pers *also* Ves'pers
ves'sel
ves'tal
vest'ed
ves•tib'u•lar
ves'ti•bule'
ves'tige
ves•tig'i•al
vest'ment
vest'-pock'et *adj.*
ves'try
ves'try•man
ves'ture
vetch
vet'er•an
Vet'er•ans Day
vet'er•i•nar'i•an
vet'er•i•nar'y
ve'to *pl.* -toes
ve'to, -toed, -to•ing
vex•a'tion
vex•a'tious
vexed
vi'a
vi•a•bil'i•ty

vi'a•ble
vi'a•duct'
vi'al *(container), also* phi'al
♦*vile, viol*
vi'and
vi•at'i•cum *pl.* -ca or -cums
vibes
vi'bran•cy
vi'brant
vi'bra•phone'
vi'bra•phon'ist
vi'brate', -brat'ed, -brat'ing
vi•bra'tion
vi•bra'to *pl.* -tos
vi'bra'tor
vi'bra•to'ry
vi•bur'num
vic'ar
vic'ar•age
vi•car'i•ous
vice *(evil, deputy)*
♦*vise*
vice-pres'i•den•cy
vice-pres'i•den'tial
vice•re'gal
vice'roy'
vice'roy'al•ty
vi'ce ver'sa
vi'chys•soise'
Vi'chy water
vic'i•nage
vi•cin'i•ty
vi'cious
vi'cious•ness

vi•cis'si•tude'
vic'tim
vic'tim•i•za'tion
vic'tim•ize', -ized', -iz'ing
vic'tim•iz'er
vic'tor
vic•to'ri•a
Vic•to'ri•an
vic•to'ri•ous
vic'to•ry
vict'ual
vi•cu'ña *also* vi•cu'-na
vi'de
vi•del'i•cet
vid'e•o'
vid'e•og'ra•phy
vid'e•o•phile'
vie, vied, vy'ing
Vi'en•nese' *pl.* -nese'
Vi•et'cong' *pl.* -cong', *also* Vi•et' Cong'
Vi•et'minh' *pl.* -minh', *also* Vi•et' Minh'
Vi•et'nam•ese' *pl.* -ese'
view
view'er
view'er•ship'
view'point'
vi•ges'i•mal
vig'il
vig'i•lance
vig'i•lant

vig'i•lan'te

vi•gnette', -gnet'ted,
  gnet'ting

vig'or

vig'or•ish

vig'or•ous

Vi'king

vile *(hateful)*, vil'er,
  vil'est
  ♦*vial, viol*

vil'i•fi•ca'tion

vil'i•fy', -fied', -fy'ing

vil'la

vil'lage

vil'lag•er

vil'lain *(scoundrel)*
  ♦*villein*

vil'lain•ous

vil'lain•y

vil'la•nelle'

vil'lein *(serf)*
  ♦*villain*

vil'lein•age

vim

vin'ai•grette'

vin'ci•ble

vin'cu•lum *pl.* -lums
  or -la

vin'di•cate', -cat'ed,
  -cat'ing

vin'di•ca'tion

vin'di•ca'tor

vin•dic'tive

vin'e•gar

vin'e•gar•y

vine'yard

vin'i•cul'ture

vin' or•di•naire' *pl.*
  vins' or•di•naires'

vi'nous

vin'tage

vint'ner

vi'nyl

vi'ol *(instrument)*
  ♦*vial, vile*

vi•o'la

vi'o•la•bil'i•ty

vi'o•la•ble

vi'o•late', -lat'ed,
  -lat'ing

vi'o•la'tion

vi'o•la'tive

vi'o•la'tor

vi'o•lence

vi'o•lent

vi'o•let

vi'o•lin'

vi'o•lin'ist

vi•o'list

vi'o•lon•cel'list

vi'o•lon•cel'lo *pl.*
  -los

vi'per

vi'per•ous

vi•ra'go -goes *or* -gos

vi'ral

vir'e•o' *pl.* -os'

vir'gin

vir'gin•al

Vir•gin'ian

vir•gin'i•ty

Vir'go

vir'gule

vir'ile

vi•ril'i•ty

vi•rol'o•gist

vi•rol'o•gy

vir'tu *(fine arts)*, *also*
  ver'tu
  ♦*virtue*

vir'tu•al

vir'tu•al•ly

vir'tue *(goodness)*
  ♦*virtu*

vir'tu•o'sic

vir'tu•os'i•ty

vir'tu•o'so *pl.* -sos *or*
  -si

vir'tu•ous

vi'ru•cide'

vir'u•lence

vir'u•lent

vi'rus *pl.* -rus•es

vi'sa

vis'age

vis-à-vis' *pl.* vis'-à-
  vis'

vis'cer•a

vis'cer•al

vis'cid

vis•cid'i•ty

vis'cose'

vis•cos'i•ty

vis'count'

vis'cous *(thick)*
  ♦*viscus*

vise *(clamp)*, *also* vice

Vish'nu

vis'i•bil'i•ty

vis'i•blc

Vis'i•goth'

vi'sion
vi'sion•ar'y
vis'it
vis'i•tant
vis'i•ta'tion
vis'i•tor
vi'sor *also* vi'zor
vis'ta
vis'u•al
vis'u•al•i•za'tion
vis'u•al•ize', -ized', -iz'ing
vi'tal
vi•tal'i•ty
vi'tal•i•za'tion
vi'tal•ize', -ized', -iz'ing
vi'ta•min
vi'ti•ate', -at'ed, -at'ing
vi'ti•a'tion
vi'ti•a'tor
vit'i•cul'ture
vit'i•cul'tur•ist
vit're•ous
vit'ri•fi•a•bil'i•ty
vit'ri•fi'a•ble
vit'ri•fi•ca'tion
vit'ri•fy', -fied', -fy'ing
vit'ri•ol'
vit'ri•ol'ic
vi•tu'per•ate', -at'ed, -at'ing
vi•tu'per•a'tion
vi•tu'per•a•tive
vi•tu'per•a'tor

vi•va'cious
vi•vac'i•ty
vi'va vo'ce
vive
viv'id
viv'i•fi•ca'tion
viv'i•fy', -fied', -fy'ing
viv'i•par'i•ty
vi•vip'a•rous
viv'i•sect'
viv'i•sec'tion
viv'i•sec'tor
vix'en
viz'ard
vi•zier' *also* vi•zir'
vo•cab'u•lar'y
vo'cal
vo•cal'ic
vo'cal•ist
vo'cal•i•za'tion
vo'cal•ize', -ized', -iz'ing
vo•ca'tion
vo•ca'tion•al
voc'a•tive
vo•cif'er•ate', -at'ed, -at'ing
vo•cif'er•a'tion
vo•cif'er•a'tor
vo•cif'er•ous
vod'ka
vogue
voice, voiced, voic'ing
voice'less
voice'-o'ver
voice'print'

void
void'a•ble
voi•là'
voile
vo'lant
vol'a•tile
vol'a•til'i•ty
vol'a•til•i•za'tion
vol'a•til•ize', -ized', -iz'ing
vol'a•tiz'a•ble
vol•can'ic
vol•ca'no *pl.* -noes *or* -nos
vole
vo•li'tion
vol'ley *pl.* -leys
vol'ley•ball'
volt'age
vol•ta'ic
vol•tam'e•ter
volt'am'me'ter
volt'-am'pere'
volt'me'ter
vol'u•bil'i•ty
vol'u•ble
vol'ume
vol'u•met'ric
vo•lu'mi•nous
vol'un•tar'y
vol'un•teer'
vo•lup'tu•ar'y
vo•lup'tu•ous
vo•lute'
vol'vox'
vom'it
voo'doo *pl.* -doos

voo'doo•ism
vo•ra'cious *(greedy)*
♦*veracious*
vo•ra'ci•ty
vor'tex *pl.* -tex•es *or*
-ti•ces'
vor'ti•cel'la
vot'a•ble *also* vote'-
a•ble
vo'ta•ry
vote, vot'ed, vot'ing
vo'tive
vouch'er
vouch'safe', -safed',
-saf'ing
vow
vow'el
vox pop'u•li'
voy'age, -aged, -ag-
ing
voy'ag•er *(traveler)*
vo•ya•geur' *(boat-
man, guide), pl.*
-geurs
vo•yeur'
vo•yeur'ism
vo'yeur•is'tic
Vul'can
vul'ca•nite'
vul'can•i•za'tion
vul'can•ize', -ized',
-iz'ing
vul'gar
vul'gar'i•an
vul'gar•ism
vul'gar'i•ty
vul'gar•i•za'tion

vul'gar•ize', -ized',
-iz'ing
vul'gate' *(speech)*
Vul'gate' *(Bible)*
vul'ner•a•bil'i•ty
vul'ner•a•ble
vul'pine
vul'ture
vul'va *pl.* -vae
vy'ing

W

wack'y *also* whack'y
wad, wad'ded, wad'-
ding
wad'dle, -dled, -dling
wade *(to walk in wa-
ter)*, wad'ed, wad'ing
♦*weighed*
wa'di *pl.* -dis, *also* wa'-
dy
wa'fer
waf'fle, -fled, -fling
waft
wag, wagged, wag'ging
wage, waged, wag'ing
wa'ger
wag'gish
wag'gle, -gled, -gling
Wag•ne'ri•an
wag'on
wag'on•ette'
waif
wail *(cry)*
♦*wale, whale*
wain *(wagon)*

♦*wane*
wain'scot, -scot•ed *or*
-scot•ted, -scot•ing
or -scot•ting
waist *(middle)*
♦*waste*
waist'band'
waist'coat
waist'line'
wait *(delay)*
♦*weight*
wait'er
wait'ress
waive *(to give up)*,
waived, waiv'ing
♦*wave*
waiv'er *(relinquish-
ment)*
♦*waver*
wake, woke *or* waked,
waked *or* wok'en,
wak'ing
wake'ful
wak'en
Wal'dorf' salad
wale *(to mark with
ridges)*, waled, wal'-
ing
♦*wail, whale*
walk'a•way'
walk'ie-talk'ie
walk'-in' *adj. & n.*
walk'-on' *n.*
walk'-out' *n.*
walk'-through' *n.*
walk'up' *n., also*
walk'-up'

wal'la•by
wall'board'
wal'let
wall'eye'
wall'eyed'
wall'flow'er
Wal•loon'
wal'lop
wal'lop•ing
wal'low
wall'pa'per
wall'-to-wall' *adj.*
wal'nut'
wal'rus *pl.* -rus *or*
 -rus•es
waltz
wam'pum
wan, wan'ner, wan'-
 nest
wand
wan'der
wan'der•lust'
wane *(to decrease)*,
 waned, wan'ing
 ♦*wain*
wan'gle, -gled, -gling
want *(lack)*
 ♦*wont*
want'ing
wan'ton
wap'i•ti *pl.* -ti *or* -tis
war, warred, war'ring
war'ble, -bled, -bling
war'den
ward'er
ward'robe'
ward'room'

ward'ship'
ware *(articles)*
 ♦*wear, where*
ware'house'
war'fare'
war'head'
war'-horse' *also* war
 horse
war'like'
war'lock'
war'lord'
warm'-blood'ed
warm'-heart'ed
war'mon'ger
warmth
warm'-up' *n.*
warn'ing
warp
war'path'
war'plane'
war'rant
war'ran•tor
war'ran•ty
war'ren
war'ri•or
war'ship'
wart
war'time'
war'y
wash'a•ble
wash'-and-wear'
wash'board'
wash'bowl'
wash'cloth'
wash'day'
washed'-out' *adj.*
washed'-up' *adj.*

wash'er
wash'er•wom'an
wash'ing
Wash'ing•to'ni•an
wash'out' *n.*
wash'room'
wash'stand'
wash'tub'
wasp'ish
wasp'waist'ed
was'sail
Was'ser•mann test
wast'age
waste *(to squander)*,
 wast'ed, wast'ing
 ♦*waist*
waste'bas'ket
waste'ful
waste'land'
wast'rel
watch'band'
watch'dog'
watch'ful
watch'mak'er
watch'man
watch'tow'er
watch'word'
wa'ter
wa'ter•borne'
wa'ter-col'or *adj.*
wa'ter-cool'
wa'ter•course'
wa'ter•cress'
wa'ter•fall'
wa'ter•fowl', *pl.*
 -fowl' *or* -fowls'
wa'ter•front'

Wa'ter•gate'
wa'ter•less
wa'ter-log', -logged',
  -log'ging
Wa'ter•loo'
wa'ter•mark'
wa'ter•mel'on
wa'ter•pow'er
wa'ter•proof'
wa'ter-re•pel'lent
wa'ter-re•sis'tant
wa'ter•shed'
wa'ter•side'
wa'ter-ski', -skied',
  -ski'ing
wa'ter-ski' *pl.* -skis'
  or -ski'
wa'ter-ski'er
wa'ter•spout'
wa'ter•tight'
wa'ter•way'
wa'ter•works'
wa'ter•y
watt
watt'age
watt'-hour'
wat'tle
wave *(water)*
  ♦*waive*
wave *(to flutter),*
  waved, wav'ing
  ♦*waive*
wave'band'
wave'length'
wav'er *(one that
  waves)*
  ♦*waiver*

wa'ver *(to sway)*
  ♦*waiver*
wax
wax'en
wax'wing'
wax'work'
wax'y
wa'y
way *(course)*
  ♦*weigh, whey*
way'bill'
way'far'er
way'far'ing
way'lay', -laid', -lay-
  ing
way'-out' *adj.*
way'side'
way'ward
we *pron.*
  ♦*wee*
weak *(feeble)*
  ♦*week*
weak'en
weak'fish' *pl.* -fish' *or*
  -fish'es
weak'ling
weak'ly *(sickly)*
  ♦*weekly*
weak'-mind'ed
weak'ness
weal *(prosperity, welt)*
  ♦*we'll, wheal, wheel*
wealth'y
wean
weap'on
weap'on•ry
wear *(to have on,*

damage, rub away),
  wore, worn, wear'-
  ing
  ♦*ware, where*
wear'a•ble
wea'ri•some
wea'ry, -ried, -ry•ing
wea'sel
weath'er *(climate)*
  ♦*wether, whether*
weath'er-beat'en
weath'er•board'
weath'er-bound'
weath'er•cast'
weath'er•cock'
weath'cred
weath'er•ing
weath'er•man'
weath'er•proof'
weath'er-strip',
  -stripped', -strip'-
  ping
weave *(to interlace),*
  wove, wov'en, weav'-
  ing
  ♦*we've*
weav'er•bird'
web, webbed, web'-
  bing
web'-foot'ed
wed, wed'ded, wed *or*
  wed'ded, wed'ding
wedge, wedged, wedg'-
  ing
wedg'ie
wed'lock'
Wednes'day

wee *(tiny)*, we′er, we′-
est
♦*we*
weed *(plant)*
♦*we'd*
weed′y
week *(seven days)*
♦*weak*
week′day′
week′end′
week′end′er
week′long′
week′ly *(once a week)*
♦*weakly*
wee′nie
weep, wept, weep′ing
weep′y
wee′vil
weft
weigh *(to determine
weight)*
♦*way, whey*
weigh′-in′ *n.*
weight *(measure of
heaviness)*
♦*wait*
weight′less
weight′lift′ing
weight′y
weir *(dam)*
♦*we're*
weird′ness
weird′o *pl.* -oes
wel′come, -comed,
-com•ing
weld
wel′fare′

wel′kin
well *(satisfactorily)*,
bet′ter, best
well *(shaft)*
we'll *contraction*
♦*weal, wheal, wheel*
well′-bal′anced
well′-be′ing
well′-born′
well′-bred′
well′-dis•posed′
well′-done′
well′-fed′
well′-fixed′
well′-found′ed
well′-groomed′
well′-ground′ed
well′-known′
well′-man′nered
well′-mean′ing
well′-meant′
well′ness
well′-nigh′
well′-off′
well′-read′
well′spring′
well-thought′-of′
well′-timed′
well′-to-do′
well′-turned′
well′-wish′er
well′-worn′
Wels′bach′ burner
welsh *(to swindle)*,
also welch
Welsh *(of Wales)*
Welsh′man

Welsh rab′bit *also*
Welsh rare′bit
wel′ter
wel′ter•weight′
welt′ing
wen *(cyst)*
♦*when*
wench
wend
we're *contraction*
♦*weir*
were′wolf′
wes′kit
west′bound′
west′er•ly
west′ern
west′ern•er
west′ern•ize′, -ized′,
-iz′ing
west′ern•most′
West In′di•an
west′-north′west′
west′-south′west′
West Vir•gin′ian
west′ward *also* west′-
wards
wet *(damp)*, wet′ter,
wet′test
♦*whet*
wet *(to dampen)*, wet′-
ted, wet′ting
♦*whet*
wet′back′
weth′er *(sheep)*
♦*weather, whether*
wet′land′
we've *contraction*

◆*weave*
whack
whale *(mammal)*
  ◆*wail, wale*
whale′boat′
whale′bone′
whal′er
whal′ing
wham, whammed,
  wham′ming
wham′my
wharf *pl.* wharves *or*
  wharfs
wharf ′age
what•ev′er
what′not′
what′so•ev′er
wheal *(swelling)*
  ◆*weal, we'll, wheel*
wheat′en
whee′dle, -dled,
  -dling
wheel *(disk)*
  ◆*weal, we'll, wheal*
wheel′bar′row
wheel′chair′
wheeled
wheel′er-deal′er
wheel′wright′
wheeze, wheezed,
  wheez′ing
wheez′y
whelk
whelm
whelp
when *(at what time)*
  ◆*wen*

whence′so•ev′er
when•ev′er
when′so•ev′er
where *(at what place)*
  ◆*ware, wear*
where′a•bouts′
where•as′
where•at′
where•by′
where′fore′
where′from′
where•in′
where•of ′
where•on′
where′so•ev′er
where•to′
wherc′up•on′
wher•ev′er
where′with′
where′with•al′
wher′ry
whet *(to sharpen)*,
  whet′ted, whet′ting
  ◆*wet*
wheth′er *(if)*
  ◆*weather, wether*
whet′stone′
whey *(part of milk)*
  ◆*way, weigh*
whey′ey
which *pron.*
  ◆*witch*
which•ev′er
whiff
whif ′fle•tree
Whig
while *(period of time)*

◆*wile*
while *(to spend idly)*,
  whiled, whil′ing
  ◆*wile*
whi′lom
whilst
whim
whim′per
whim′si•cal
whim′si•cal′i•ty
whim′sy *also* whim′-
  sey *pl.* -seys
whine *(to complain)*,
  whined, whin′ing
  ◆*wine*
whin′ny, -nied, -ny-
  ing
whin′y
whip, whipped *or*
  whipt, whip′ping
whip′cord′
whip′lash′
whip′per•snap′per
whip′pet
whip′poor•will′ *also*
  whip′-poor-will′
whip′saw′
whir, whirred, whir′-
  ring
whirl′i•gig′
whirl′pool′
whirl′wind′
whirl′y•bird′
whisk′broom′
whisk′er
whis′key *pl.* -keys
whis′per

whist
whis'tle, -tled, -tling
whis'tle-stop',
  -stopped', -stop'ping
whit *(particle)*
  ♦*wit*
white, whit'er, whit'-
  est
white, whit'ed, whit'-
  ing
white'cap'
white'-col'lar *adj.*
white'-faced'
white'fish' *pl.* -fish'
  or -fish'es
white'-hot'
whit'en
white'ness
white'out' *n.*
white'-tailed' deer
white'wall'
white'wash'
whith'er *(where)*
  ♦*wither*
whit'ish
whit'low
Whit'sun•day
whit'tle, -tled, -tling
whiz, whizzed, whiz'-
  zing, *also* whizz
who•dun'it
who•ev'er
whole *(complete)*
  ♦*hole*
whole'heart'ed
whole'sale', -saled',
  -sal'ing

whole'sal'er
whole'some
whole'-wheat'
whol'ly *(totally)*
  ♦*holy*
whom•ev'er
whom'so•ev'er
whoop *(cough)*
  ♦*hoop*
whoop'ee
whoop'ing cough
whooping crane
whoops
whoosh
whop, whopped,
  whop'ping
whop'per
whorl
who's *contraction*
whose *pron.*
who'so
who'so•ev'er
why *pl.* whys
wick
wick'ed
wick'er
wick'er•work'
wick'et
wick'i•up'
wide, wid'er, wid'est
wide'-an'gle lens
wide'-a•wake'
wide'-bod'ied
wide'-eyed'
wid'en
wide'-o'pen
wide'spread'

wid'geon *pl.* -geon *or*
  -geons
widg'et
wid'ow
wid'ow•er
wid'ow•hood'
width
wield'a•ble
wie'ner
Wie'ner schnit'zel
wie'ner•wurst'
wife *pl.* wives
wig, wigged, wig'ging
wig'gle, -gled, -gling
wig'wag', -wagged',
  -wag'ging
wig'wam'
wild'cat'
wild'cat'ter
wil'de•beest'
wil'der•ness
wild'-eyed'
wild'fire'
wild'flow'er
wild'fowl' *pl.* -fowl'
  or -fowls'
wild'-goose' chase
wild'life'
wile *(to entice)*, wiled,
  wil'ing
  ♦*while*
will *(volition)*
will *auxiliary, past
  tense* would
willed
will'ful *also* wil'ful
will'ing

will'-o'-the-wisp'
wil'low
wil'low•y
wil'ly-nil'ly
wilt
wi'ly
wim'ple
win, won, win'ning
wince, winced, winc'-
  ing
winch
wind *(air)*
wind *(to wrap
  around)*, wound,
  wind'ing
wind'bag'
wind'-blown'
wind'break'
Wind'break'er®
wind'-chill' factor
wind'ed
wind'fall'
wind'flow'er
wind'jam'mer
wind'lass
wind'mill'
win'dow
win'dow-dress'er
win'dow-dress'ing
win'dow•pane'
win'dow-shop',
  -shopped', -shop'-
  ping
win'dow•sill'
wind'pipe'
wind'row'
wind'shield'

wind'sock'
Wind'sor tie
wind'storm'
wind'swept'
wind'-up' *n. & adj.*
wind'ward
wind'y
wine *(fermented juice)*
  ♦*whine*
wine'glass'
win'er•y
Wine'sap'
wine'skin'
wing'ding'
winged
wing'span'
wing'spread'
wink
win'kle
win'ner
win'ning
win'now
win'some
win'ter
win'ter•green'
win'ter•ize', -ized',
  -iz'ing
win'ter•time'
win'try *also* win'ter•y
wipe, wiped, wip'ing
wipe'out' *n.*
wire, wired, wir'ing
wire'-haired'
wire'less
wire'pull'er
wire'pull'ing
wire'tap', -tapped',

-tap'ping
wir'ing
wir'y
wis'dom
wise, wis'er, wis'est
wise'a'cre
wise'crack'
wish'bone'
wish'ful
wish'y-wash'y
wisp'y
wis•ter'i•a *also* wis-
  tar'i•a
wist'ful
wit *(intelligence, hu-
  mor)*
  ♦*whit*
witch *(hag)*
  ♦*which*
witch'craft'
with•al'
with•draw', -drew',
  -drawn', -draw'ing
with•draw'al
withe
with'er *(to dry up)*
  ♦*whither*
with'ers
with•hold', -held',
  -hold'ing
with•in'
with'-it' *adj.*
with•out'
with•stand', -stood',
  -stand'ing
wit'less
wit'ness

wit'ti•cism

wit'ty

wiz'ard

wiz'ard•ry

wiz'ened

woad

wob'ble, -bled, -bling

wob'bly

woe'be•gone'

woe'ful

wok

wolf *pl.* wolves

wolf 'hound'

wolf 'ram

wol'ver•ine'

wom'an *pl.* wom'en

wom'an•hood'

wom'an•ish

wom'an•ize' -ized',
   -iz'ing

wom'an•kind'

womb

wom'bat'

wom'en•folk'

won'der

won'der•ful

won'der•land'

won'der•ment

won'der•work'er

won'drous

wont *(custom)*
   ♦*want*

wont'ed *(usual)*
   ♦*wanted*

won ton

woo

wood *(lumber)*

♦*would*

wood'bine'

wood'carv'ing

wood'chuck'

wood'cock' *pl.* -cock'
   or -cocks'

wood'craft'

wood'cut'

wood'cut'ter

wood'ed

wood'en

wood'land

wood'peck'er

wood'pile'

wood'shed'

woods'man

wood'wind'

wood'work'

wood'y

woof 'er

wool'en *also* wool'len

wool'gath'er•ing

wool'ly *also* wool'y

wooz'y

Worces'ter•shire

word'age

word'book'

word'ing

word'less

word proc'ess•ing

word proc'es•sor

word'y

work'a•ble

work'a•day'

work'a•hol'ic

work'bench'

work'book'

work'box'

work'day'

work'er

work'horse'

work'house'

work'ing-class' *adj.*

work'ing•man'

work'load'

work'man

work'man•like' *also*
   work'man•ly

work'man•ship'

work'place'

work'out' *n.*

work'room'

work'shop'

work'ta'ble

work'week'

world'ly

world'ly-wise'

world'-shak'ing

world'wide'

worm'-eat'en

worm'hole'

worm'wood'

worn'-out' *adj.*

wor'ri•some

wor'ry, -ried, -ry•ing

wor'ry•wart'

worse

wors'en

wor'ship, -shiped *or*
   -shipped, -ship•ing
   or -ship•ping

wor'ship•er *or* wor'-
   ship•per

wor'ship•ful

worst *(most inferior)*
♦*wurst*
wor'sted
worth'less
worth'while'
wor'thy
would *auxiliary*
♦*wood*
would'-be'
wound
wow
wrack *(to ruin)*
♦*rack*
wraith *(ghost)*
♦*wrath*
wran'gle, -gled, -gling
wran'gler
wrap *(to enclose)*,
wrapped *or* wrapt,
wrap'ping
♦*rap*
wrap'a•round'
wrap'per
wrap'-up' *n.*
wrath *(anger)*
♦*wraith*
wreak *(to punish)*
♦*reek*
wreath *pl.* wreaths
wreathe, wreathed,
wreath'ing, wreathes
wreck *(to destroy)*
♦*reck*
wreck'age
wren
wrench
wrest *(to obtain by*

force)
♦*rest*
wres'tle, -tled, -tling
wretch *(miserable per-*
son)
♦*retch*
wretch'ed
wrig'gle, -gled, -gling
wring *(to squeeze)*,
wrung, wring'ing
♦*ring*
wring'er
wrin'kle, -kled, -kling
wrist'band'
writ *(order)*
write *(to compose)*,
wrote, writ'ten, writ'-
ing
♦*right, rite*
write'-in' *n.*
write'-off' *n.*
writ'er
write'-up' *n.*
writhe, writhed,
writh'ing
writ'ing
wrong'do'er
wrong'do'ing
wrong'-head'ed
wrought
wry *(crooked)*, wri'er
or wry'er, wri'est *or*
wry'est
♦*rye*
wun'der•kind' *pl.*
-kinds' *or* -kind'er

wurst *(sausage)*
♦*worst*

X

x'-ax'is *pl.* -es
X'-chro'mo•some'
xe'non'
xen'o•phile'
xe•noph'i•lous
xen'o•phobe'
xen'o•pho'bi•a
xen'o•pho'bic
xe•rog'ra•pher
xer'o•graph'ic
xe•rog'ra•phy
Xer'ox®
X'mas
x'-ra'di•a'tion
X'-rat'ed
x'-ray' *also* X'-ray'
xy'lem
xy'lo•phone'
xy'lo•phon'ist

Y

yacht'ing
yachts'man
ya'hoo *pl.* -hoos
Yah'weh *also* Yah'-
veh
yak *(animal)*
yak *(to talk)*, yakked,
yak'king
ya•ku•za' *pl. n.*
yam

yam'mer
yank (to pull)
Yank (Yankee)
Yan'kee
yap, yapped, yap'ping
yard'age
yard'arm'
yard'mas'ter
yard'stick'
yar'mul•ke also yar'-
   mel•ke
yarn
yar'row
yaw
yawl
yawn'ing
yawp also yaup
yaws
y'-ax'is pl. -es
Y'-chro'mo•some'
ye
yea
yeah
year'book'
year'ling
year'long'
year'ly
yearn'ing
year'-round' adj.
yeast'y
yell'ing
yel'low
yel'low•ham'mer
yel'low•legs' pl. -legs'
yellow pages or
   Yellow Pages
yel'low•tail'

yelp
yen
yen'ta
yeo'man
yeo'man•ry
yes pl. yes'es
yes, yessed, yes'sing
ye•shi'va or ye•shi'-
   vah
yes'ter•day'
yes'ter•year'
yet
yet'i pl. -is
yew (tree)
   ♦ewe, you
Yid'dish
yield'ing
yip, yipped, yip'ping
yip'pee
yo'del, -deled or
   -delled, -del•ing or
   -del•ling
yo'ga
yo'gi pl. -gis
yo'gurt also yo'ghurt
yoke (to join), yoked,
   yok'ing
   ♦yolk
yo'kel
yolk (yellow of an egg)
   ♦yoke
Yom Kip'pur
yon'der
yoo'-hoo'
yore
York'shire' pudding
you pron.

   ♦ewe, yew
you'll contraction
   ♦Yule
young'ster
your possessive
you're contraction
yours
your•self' pl. -selves'
youth pl. youths
youth'ful
yowl
yo'-yo' pl. -yos'
yt•ter'bic
yt•ter'bi•um
yt'tric
yt'tri•um
yuc•ca
Yu'go•slav' or Yu'-
   go•sla'vi•an
Yule (Christmas)
   ♦you'll
Yule'tide'
Yu'man
yum'my
yup'pie
yurt

Z

za'ba•glio'ne
za'ny
zap, zapped, zap'ping
zeal'ot
zeal'ous
ze'bra
ze'bu
zed

ze'nith
zeph'yr
zep'pe•lin *also* Zep'-
  pe•lin
ze'ro *pl.* -ros *or* -roes
ze'ro, -roed, -ro•ing
zest'ful
Zeus
zig'gu•rat'
zig'zag', -zagged',
  -zag'ging
zil'lion
Zim•bab'we•an *also*
  Zim•bab'wi•an
zinc
zin'fan•del' *also* Zin'-
  fan•del'
zing'er
zin'ni•a
Zi'on *also* Si'on
Zi'on•ism
Zi'on•ist
zip, zipped, zip'ping

Zip Code *also* zip
  code, ZIP Code
zip'per
zip'py
zir'con'
zir•co'ni•um
zith'er *also* zith'ern
zo'di•ac
zo•di'a•cal
zom'bie *also* zom'bi
  pl. -bis
zo'nal *also* zo'na•ry
zone, zoned, zon'ing
zonked
zoo *pl.* zoos
zo'o•ge•o•graph'ic
  also zo'o•ge-
  o•graph'i•cal
zo'o•ge•og'ra•phy
zo'o•graph'ic *also*
  zo'o•graph'ic•al
zo•og'ra•phy
zo'oid'

zo•oid'al
zoo'keep'er
zo'o•log'i•cal *also*
  zo'o•log'ic
zo•ol'o•gist
zo•ol'o•gy
zoom
zo'o•phyte'
zo'o•spore'
Zou•ave'
zuc•chi'ni *pl.* -ni
zwie'back'
zy'go•mat'ic
zy'go•spore'
zy'gote'
zy•got'ic
zy'mase'
zy'mo•gen
zy'mo•gen'ic *also*
  zy•mog'e•nous
zy•mol'o•gy
zy'mur•gy
zyz'zy•va

Guide to Plurals

1. The plural of most nouns is formed by adding -s to the singular: *arm, arms; chief, chiefs; doll, dolls; epoch, epochs; jaw, jaws; log, logs; skate, skates; George, Georges;* the *Walkers;* the *Romanos.*

2. a. Common nouns ending in **ch** *(soft)*, **sh, s, ss, x,** or **zz** usually form their plurals by adding -es: *church, churches; slash, slashes; gas, gasses; class, classes; fox, foxes; buzz, buzzes.*
b. Proper nouns of this type always add -es: *Charles, Charleses;* the *Keaches;* the *Joneses;* the *Coxes.*

3. a. Common nouns ending in **y** preceded by a vowel usually form their plurals by adding -s: *bay, bays; guy, guys; key, keys; toy, toys.*
b. Common nouns ending in **y** preceded by a consonant or by **qu** change the **y** to **i** and add -es: *baby, babies; city, cities; faculty, faculties; soliloquy, soliloquies.*
c. Proper nouns ending in **y** form their plurals regularly, and do not change the **y** to **i** as common nouns do: the two *Kathys;* the *Connallys;* the two *Kansas Citys.* Exceptions: the *Alleghenies,* the *Ptolemies,* the *Rockies;* the *Two Sicilies.*

4. Most nouns ending in **f, ff,** or **fe** form their plurals regularly by adding -s to the singular: *clef, clefs; sheriff, sheriffs; fife, fifes.* However, some nouns ending in **f** or **fe** change the **f** or **fe** to **v** and add -es: *calf, calves; half, halves; loaf, loaves; self, selves; thief, thieves; wife, wives; wolf, wolves.*

Note: *Scarf, staff,* and *wharf* have two plural forms: *scarfs* or *scarves; staffs* or *staves; wharves* or *wharfs.* Sometimes different forms have different meanings, as in the case of *staffs* (members of an organization) and *staves* (long poles), or in the case of *beeves* (animals) and *beefs* (complaints).

5. a. Nouns ending in **o** preceded by a vowel form their plurals by adding -s to the singular: *cameo, cameos; duo, duos; studio, studios; zoo, zoos.*

b. Most nouns ending in **o** preceded by a consonant usually add -es: *echo, echoes; hero, heroes; tomato, tomatoes.*

Note: There are many exceptions to this rule since the consonant or cluster of consonants preceding the **o** does not determine whether the plural will add -s or -es: *alto, altos; ego, egos; piano, pianos; poncho, ponchos; silo, silos.*

c. Some nouns ending in **o** preceded by a consonant have two plural forms. In the following examples the preferred form is given first: *buffaloes* or *buffalos; cargoes* or *cargos; halos* or *haloes; zeros* or *zeroes.*

6. Most nouns ending in **i** form their plurals by adding -s: *alibi, alibis; rabbi, rabbis; ski, skis.*

Note: A few nouns add either -s or -es: *alkalis* or *alkalies; taxis* or *taxies.*

7. a. A few nouns undergo a change in the stem exhibiting a different medial vowel: *foot, feet; goose, geese; louse, lice; man, men; mouse, mice; tooth, teeth; woman, women.*

Note: Compounds in which one of these nouns is the final element form their plurals in the same way: *clubfoot, clubfeet; mailman, mailmen; dormouse, dormice; bucktooth, buckteeth; Englishwoman, Englishwomen;* but, *mongoose, mongooses.* Many words ending in **-man** are not compounds: *German, talisman, ottoman,* etc. These words form their plurals by adding -s: *Germans, talismans, ottomans.*

b. Only three nouns have plurals ending in **-en:** *ox, oxen; child, children; brother, brothers* (of the same parents), or *brethren* (a fellow member of a society, order, etc.).

8. Many nouns derived from a foreign language retain their foreign plurals, for example:

From Latin: alumna, alumnae; alumnus, alumni; bacillus, bacilli; genus, genera; series, series; species, species.

From Greek: analysis, analyses; basis, bases; crisis, crises; criterion, criteria or criterions; phenomenon, phenomena or phenomenons.

From French: adieu, adieux or adieus; beau, beaux or beaus; madame, mesdames.

Others: paparazzo, papparazzi (Italian); cherub, cherubim (Hebrew).

Many words of this class also have a regular -s or -es English plural that is often preferred; however, a foreign plural often signals a difference in meaning, for example: antenna, antennas (radio antennas) or antennae (the antennae of an insect).

9. a. Compounds written as a single word form their plurals like any other word of the same ending: clothesbrush, clothesbrushes; dishcloth, dishcloths; housewife, housewives; mailman, mailmen; manhunt, manhunts.

b. In rare cases both parts of the compound are made plural: manservant, menservants.

c. Compounds ending in -ful normally form their plurals by adding -s at the end: cupful, cupfuls; handful, handfuls; tablespoonful, tablespoonfuls.

d. Compound words, written with or without a hyphen, that consist of a noun followed by an adjective or other qualifying expression form their plurals by making the same change in the noun as when the noun stands alone: aide-de-camp, aides-de-camp; attorney-general, attorneys-general; court-martial, courts-martial; daughter-in-law, daughters-in-law; hanger-on, hangers-on; heir apparent, heirs apparent.

10. Some nouns, mainly names of birds, fishes, and mammals, have the same form in the plural as in the singular: deer,

grouse, moose, swine, trout. But some of these words, as well
as a few others that ordinarily have no plural, such as *coffee,
flour, wheat,* have a normal plural form different from the
singular to denote different varieties or species or kinds. In
such cases the unchanged plural denotes that the idea is collective or is the form commonly used in the language of
sportsmen: *fish, fish* or *fishes; trout, trout* or *trouts.*

11. **a.** Many names of tribes, peoples, etc., have the same form
    in the plural as in the singular: *Iroquois; Sioux.*
    b. Similarly certain names of peoples, city inhabitants, etc.,
    ending in **-ese** have the same form in the plural as in the sin-
    gular: *Cantonese, Milanese, Portuguese, Siamese.*

12. Nouns ending in **-ics** are construed as singular when the
    word denotes a subject or a scientific study or treatise. They
    are construed as plural when the word denotes matters of
    practice, activities, or qualities.
    Mathematics is his chief interest but *The mathematics of the
    tax proposal were all wrong.*
    "Strategy wins wars, tactics wins battles" but *The union's tac-
    tics were discrediting the industry.*
    Acoustics is a difficult subject for the layman but *The acous-
    tics of this room are excellent.*

13. Some nouns are rarely or never construed as singular: *cattle,
    clothes, scissors, pants, trousers.*

14. **a.** Plurals of letters, symbols, and numbers, and abbrevia-
    tions are normally formed by adding an apostrophe and **s**
    (**'s**): *A's; ABC's; 2's; -'s; GI's; +'s*
    b. The plural of a word regarded as a word is indicated by an
    apostrophe and an **s** (**'s**): no *if's, and's,* or *but's.*
    Note: All entries in *The Word Book* will show plurals
    wherever needed.

Guide to Spelling

The complexities and frustrating inconsistencies of modern English spelling have been produced by a variety of causes. Three major factors have been: (1) The lack of consistency shown by older scribers, printers, and writers, who did not always spell the same sound in the same way, or, for that matter, the same word in the same way. (2) The extensive sound shifts that took place after the spelling of English became fairly well established about the year 1500, shortly after the introduction of printing. (3) The fact that the standard alphabet of twenty-six characters adopted by printers and writers did not provide one character, and one only, for each of the forty or more separate sounds in the English language.

Moreover, since the English vocabulary contains thousands of words borrowed from foreign languages, and in some cases these borrowings have retained their original spelling and pronunciation, it is difficult to formulate a set of rules that will cover the spelling of all English words. Many spelling difficulties arise in connection with suffixes, and the seven basic rules given here are intended as an aid in learning and understanding the correct spelling of a large number of English words.

SEVEN BASIC RULES OF SPELLING

First rule: *Adding a suffix to a one-syllable word.* Words of one syllable that end in a single consonant preceded by a single vowel double the final consonant before a suffix beginning with a vowel:

bag + -age	= baggage		red + -er	= redder
hop + -er	= hopper		run + -ing	= running
hot + -est	= hottest		stop + -ed	= stopped

Exceptions: bus, buses or *busses, busing* or *bussing;* derivatives of the word *gas (gasses* or *gases, gassing, gassy,* but *gasoline, gasiform, gasify).*

Note: This rule does not apply if a word ends with two or more consonants or if it ends with one consonant preceded by two or more vowels instead of one:

debt	+	-or	=	debtor	mail	+	-ed	=	mailed
lick	+	-ing	=	licking	sweet	+	-est	=	sweetest

Second rule: *Adding a suffix to a word with two or more syllables.* Words of two or more syllables that have the accent on the last syllable and end in a single consonant preceded by a single vowel double the final consonant before a suffix beginning with a vowel:

admit + -ed = admitted   control + -er   = controller
confer + -ing = conferring   regret   + -able = regrettable

Exceptions: (a) *chagrin, chagrined; transfer, transferable, transference,* but *transferred, transferring.*
(b) When the accent shifts to the first syllable of the word after the suffix is added, the final consonant is not doubled: *prefer + -ence = preference; refer + -ence = reference*

Note: This rule does not apply:

(1) If the word ends with two consonants or if the final consonant is preceded by more than one vowel:

perform + -ance = performance
repeal   + -ing = repealing

(2) If the word is accented on any syllable except the last:

benefit + -ed = benefited   kidnap + -er = kidnaper

Exceptions: Some words like *cobweb, handicap, outfit,* follow the models of *web, cap, fit,* even though these words may not be true compounds. A few others ending in **g** double the final **g** so that it will not be pronounced like **j**: *humbug, humbugged; zigzag, zigzagged.*

Third rule: *Adding a suffix beginning with a vowel to a word ending in a silent e.* Words ending with a silent **e** usually drop the **e** before a suffix beginning with a vowel:

agitate	+ -ion	= agitation	glide	+ -ing = gliding
force	+ -ible	= forcible	operate	+ -or = operator
route	+ -ed	= routed	trifle	+ -er = trifler

Exceptions: Here the exceptions are many:
(a) Many words of this type have alternative forms. In *The Word Book III* the preferred form is always shown first.

blue	+ -ish	= bluish *or* blueish
move	+ -able	= movable *or* moveable

Note: In certain cases, alternative forms have different meanings. Thus: *line + -age = linage* or *lineage* (number of lines), but *lineage* (the only form for "ancestry").

(b) Words ending in **ce** or **ge** keep the **e** before the suffixes **-able** and **-ous.**

advantage	+ -ous	= advantageous
change	+ -able	= changeable
trace	+ -able	= traceable

(c) Words ending in a silent **e** keep the **e** if the word could be mistaken for another word:

dye + -ing = dyeing   singe + -ing = singeing

(d) If the word ends in **ie,** the **e** is dropped and the **i** changed to **y** before the suffix **-ing.** A word ending in **i** remains unchanged before **-ing:**

die + -ing = dying   ski + -ing = skiing

(e) *Mile* and *acre* do not drop the **e** before the suffix **-age.** Thus, *mileage* and *acreage.*

Fourth rule: *Adding a suffix with a consonant to a word ending in a silent e.* Words ending with a silent **e** generally retain the **e** before a suffix that begins with a consonant, such as **-ful, -less, -ment, -ness, -some, -ty:**

plate	+ -ful	= plateful
shoe	+ -less	= shoeless
arrange	+ -ment	= arrangement
white	+ -ness	= whiteness
awe	+ -some	= awesome
nice	+ -ty	= nicety

Exceptions: There are many exceptions to this rule. Some of the most common are: *abridge, abridgment; acknowledge, acknowledgment; argue, argument; awe, awful; due, duly; judge, judgment; nine, ninth; true, truly; whole, wholly; wise, wisdom.*

Fifth rule: *Adding a suffix to a word ending in y.*
1. Words ending in **y** preceded by a consonant generally change the **y** to **i** before the addition of a suffix, except a suffix that begins with an **i:**

accompany	+ -ment	= accompaniment
beauty	+ -ful	= beautiful
reply	+ -ing	= replying

Note: (1) Adjectives of one syllable ending in **y** usually retain the **y** when a suffix is added: *sly, slyly; shy, shyness.* But, *dry, drier, driest, dryly* or *drily, dryness.*

(2) The **y** is retained in derivatives of *baby, city* and *lady* and before the suffixes **-ship** and **-like:** *babyhood, citylike, cityward, ladyship, ladylike.*

(3) Some words drop the final **y** before the addition of the suffix **-eous:** *beauty + eous = beauteous.*

2. Words ending in **y** preceded by a vowel usually retain the **y** before a suffix:

buy + -er = buyer   key + -less = keyless

Exceptions: day, daily; gay, gaily, gaiety.

Sixth rule: *Adding a suffix to a word ending in c.* Words ending in **c** almost always have the letter **k** inserted after the **c** when a suffix beginning with **e, i,** or **y** is added. This is done so that the letter **c** will not be pronounced like **s.**

panic + -y = panicky   picnic + -er = picnicker

Seventh rule: *The problem of "ie" or "ei."*

1. When the two letters have a long **e** sound (as in *feet*):
(a) **I** comes before **e,** except after **c:** *believe, grieve, niece, siege, shield, mischievous.*
Exceptions: either, leisure, neither, plebeian, seize, sheik.
(b) After **c, e** comes before **i:** *ceiling, conceit, deceive, perceive, receive, receipt.*
Exceptions: ancient, financier, specie.

2. **E** comes before **i** when **ei** has the sound **a** (as in *cake*), **e** (as in *pet*), **i** (as in *fit*), or **i** (as in *mine*): *Fahrenheit, foreign, forfeit, height, neighbor, sleight, sovereign, surfeit.*
Exceptions: friend, handkerchief, mischief, sieve.

Note: Many words spelled with **ie** or **ei** present no difficulties because the vowels are pronounced separately: *deity, piety, science.* For other exceptions to the rules outlined above, *The Word Book III* or *The American Heritage Dictionary, Second College Edition* will help you spell the word correctly.

Abbreviations

A 1. ammeter. **2.** Also **a., A.** acre. **3.** ampere. **4.** area.

a. 1. acceleration. **2.** adjective. **3.** answer. **4.** Also **A.** are (measurement).

A. 1. alto **2.** America; American.

A.A. Associate in Arts.

A.B. Bachelor of Arts.

abbr., abbrev. abbreviation.

abr. 1. abridge. **2.** abridgment.

acad. 1. academic. **2.** academy.

acct. account.

ack. 1. acknowledge. **2.** acknowledgment.

ACLU American Civil Liberties Union.

A.D. anno Domini (usually small capitals A.D.).

add. 1. addition. **2.** additional. **3.** address.

adj. 1. adjacent. **2.** adjective. **3.** adjourned. **4.** adjunct.

ad loc. to (or at) the place (Latin *ad locum*).

admin. administration.

adv. 1. adverb. **2.** adverbial.

adv., advt. advertisement.

A.F., AF 1. air force.

2. Anglo-French. **3.** audio frequency.

AFL-CIO, A.F.L.-C.I.O. American Federation of Labor and Congress of Industrial Organizations.

agr. 1. agriculture. **2.** agricultural.

agt. 1. agent. **2.** agreement.

AIDS acquired immune deficiency syndrome.

AK Alaska (with Zip Code).

Alta. Alberta.

Am., Amer. 1. America. **2.** American.

a.m. Also **A.M.** ante meridiem (usually small capitals A.M.).

amt. amount.

anal. 1. analogy. **2.** analysis. **3.** analytic.

ans. answer.

approx. 1. approximate. **2.** approximately.

appt. 1. appoint. **2.** appointed.

Apr. April.

AR 1. account receivable. **2.** Arkansas (with Zip Code).

art. article.

ASCII American Standard Code for Information Interchange.

ASPCA American Society for the Prevention of Cruelty to Animals.

assoc. 1. associate. **2.** Also **assn.** association.

asst. assistant.

ATM automated teller machine.

attn. attention.

atty., at., att. attorney.

Aug. August.

av., ave., avenue.

avg., av. average.

AZ Arizona (with Zip Code).

b, B. 1. base. **2.** bay. **3.** book.

B. 1. bachelor. **2.** Baume scale. **3.** British. **4.** Bible.

B.A. Bachelor of Arts.

bal. balance.

bar. 1. barometer. **2.** barometric. **3.** barrel.

B.B.A. Bachelor of Business Administration.

BBC British Broadcasting Corporation.

B.C. 1. before Christ (usually small capitals B.C.). **2.** British Columbia.

bd. 1. board. **2.** bond. **3.** bookbinding. **4.** bound.

B.D. 1. bank draft. **2.** bills discounted.

bdl. bundle.

B/E. 1. bill of entry. **2.** bill of exchange.

bet. between.

bf, bf., b.f. boldface.

B/F *Accounting.* brought forward.

bg. bag.

Bib. 1. Bible. **2.** Biblical.

bibliog. 1. bibliographer. **2.** bibliography.

biog. 1. biographer. **2.** biographical. **3.** biography.

biol. 1. biological. **2.** biologist. **3.** biology.

bk. 1. bank. **2.** book.

bkg. banking.

bkpg. bookkeeping.

bkpt. bankrupt.

bl. 1. barrel. **2.** black. **3.** blue.

B/L bill of lading.

bldg. building.

blk. 1. black. **2.** block. **3.** bulk.

blvd. boulevard.

b.o. 1. box office. **2.** branch office. **3.** buyer's option.

B/P bills payable.

br. 1. branch. **2.** brief. **3.** bronze. **4.** brother. **5.** brown.

B.S. 1. Bachelor of Science. **2.** balance sheet. **3.** bill of sale.

bu. 1. Also **Bur.** bureau. **2.** bushel.

bull. bulletin.

bus. business.

bx. box.

c 1. carat. **2.** centi-. **3.** cubic.

C 1. Celsius. **2.** centigrade.

c., C. 1. cape. **2.** cent. **3.** century. **4.** Also **chap.** chapter. **5.** Also **ca** circa. **6.** copy. **7.** copyright.

CA California (with Zip Code).

CAD Computer-aided design.

cal. 1. calendar. **2.** caliber.

CAM Computer-aided manufacturing.

canc. cancel.

C.B.D. cash before delivery.

cc cubic centimeter.

cc. chapters.

c.c., C.C. carbon copy.

c.d. cash discount

CD 1. Also **C/D** certificate of deposit. **2.** compact disk.

C.D. civil defense.

Cdr., Cmdr., Comdr. commander.

CD/ROM compact disk/read-only memory.

CEO chief executive officer.

cert. 1. certificate. **2.** certification. **3.** certified.

cf., cp. compare.

c.f.i., C.F.I. cost, freight, and insurance.

CFO chief financial officer.

char. charter.

chg. charge.

cit. 1. citation. **2.** cited. **3.** citizen.

C.J. 1. chief justice. **2.** corpus juris.

ck. check.

cl. 1. class. **2.** classification. **3.** clause. **4.** clearance. **5.** Also **clk.** clerk.

cm. centimeter.

cml. commercial.

C/N credit note.

CO Colorado (with Zip Code).

co. 1. Also **Co.** company. **2.** county.

c.o. 1. Also **c/o** care of. **2.** *Accounting.* carried over. **3.** cash order.

COD, C.O.D. 1. cash on delivery. **2.** collect on delivery.

col. 1. collect. **2.** collected. **3.** collector. **4.** college. **5.** collegiate. **6.** column.

COM computer output microfilm.

Com. 1. commission. **2.** commissioner.

comm. 1. commission. **2.** commissioner. **3.** commerce. **4.** communication.

con. 1. *Law:* conclusion. **2.** consolidate. **3.** consolidated.

conj. conjunction.

cons. 1. consignment. **2.** construction. **3.** constitution.

Const. 1. constable. **2.** constitution.

cont. 1. contents. **2.** continue. **3.** continued. **4.** control.

contr. contract.

COO chief operating officer.

coop. cooperative.

corp. corporation.

cos., c.o.s. cash on shipment.

C.P.A. certified public accountant.

cpd. compound.

CPI consumer price index.

CPR cardiopulmonary resuscitation.

CPU central processing unit.

cr. credit.

CRT cathode-ray tube.

CST, C.S.T. Central Standard Time.

CT Connecticut (with Zip Code).

CT, C.T. Central Time.

ct. 1. Also **c., C.,** cent. **2.** court.

ctn. carton.

ctr. center.

cu. Also **c** cubic.

cur. currency.

c.w.o. 1. cash with order. **2.** chief warrant officer.

cwt. hundredweight.

CZ Canal Zone (with Zip Code).

d. 1. date. **2.** daughter. **3.** day. **4.** died. **5.** Also **D.** dose.

D. 1. December. **2.** Also **D.** democrat; democratic. **3.** doctor (in academic degrees).

D.A. district attorney.

DASD direct access storage device.

dB decibel.

D.B. daybook.

d.b.a. doing business as.

dbl. double.

DC District of Columbia (with Zip Code).

D.D.S. Doctor of Dental Science.

DE Delaware (with Zip Code).

deb. debenture.

dec. 1. deceased. **2.** decrease.

Dec. December.

def. 1. definite. **2.** definition.

deg, deg. degree (thermometric).

del. 1. delegate. **2.** delegation. **3.** delete.

Dem. Democrat.

dep. 1. depart. **2.** departure. **3.** deposit. **4.** deputy.

dept. department.

dia. diameter.

dim. dimension.

dir. director.

disc. discount.

div. 1. divided. **2.** division. **3.** dividend.

dlvy. delivery.

do. ditto.

DOB date of birth.

dol. dollar.

DOS disk operating system.

doz. Also **dz.** dozen.

DP data processing.

dr. 1. debit. **2.** debtor.

DST, D.S.T. daylight-saving time.

dup. duplicate.

dz. Also **doz.** dozen.

e. 1. electron. **2.** Also **E, e., E.,** east; eastern.

E Earth.

E. 1. Also **e.,** engineer; engineering. **2.** Also **E** English.

ea. each.

econ. 1. economics. **2.** economist. **3.** economy.

ed. 1. edition. **2.** editor.

EDT, E.D.T. Eastern Daylight Time.

educ. 1. education. **2.** educational.

EEC European Economic Community.

e.g. for example (Latin *exempli gratia*).

elec. 1. electric. **2.** electrical. **3.** electricity.

enc., encl. 1. enclosed. **2.** enclosure.

eng., engr. Also **e., E.,** engineer.

EPA Environmental Protection Agency.

eq. 1. equal. **2.** equation. **3.** equivalent.

equip. equipment.

ERA 1. *Baseball.* earned run average. **2.** Equal Rights Amendment.

ESL English as a second language.
esp. especially.
Esq. Esquire (title).
est. 1. established. **2.** *Law.* estate. **3.** estimate.
EST, E.S.T. Eastern Standard Time.
ET, E.T. Eastern Time.
et al. and others (Latin *et alii*).
etc. and so forth (Latin *et cetera*).
Eur. 1. Europe. **2.** European.
ex. 1. example. **2.** Also **exch.** exchange. **3.** Also **exam.** examination.
exec. 1. executive. **2.** executor.
exp. 1. expenses. **2.** export. **3.** express.

F, Fahr. Fahrenheit.
f. 1. Also **f, F., F** female. **2.** Also **F.** folio.
F.B. freight bill.
FBI, F.B.I. Federal Bureau of Investigation.
FDA Food and Drug Administration.
Feb. February.
fed. 1. federal. **2.** federated. **3.** federation.
fem. feminine.
FICA Federal Insurance Contributions Act.
FL Florida (with Zip Code).
fl oz fluid ounce.

fm frequency modulation.
F.O.B., f.o.b. free on board.
fol. 1. folio. **2.** following.
fpm, f.p.m. feet per minute.
fr. 1. franc. **2.** from. **3.** Also **freq.** frequently.
Fri. Friday.
frt. freight.
ft foot.
FTC Federal Trade Commission.
fut. future.
fwd. forward.
FYI for your information.

g 1. gravity. **2.** gram.
GA Georgia (with Zip Code).
gal. gallon.
GAW guaranteed annual wage.
gds. goods.
gen., genl. general.
geog. 1. geographer. **2.** geographic. **3.** geography.
geol. 1. geologic. **2.** geologist. **3.** geology.
geom. 1. geometric. **2.** geometry.
gm gram.
GNP gross national product.
gov., Gov. governor.
govt. government.
G.P. general practitioner.
gr. 1. grade. **2.** gross. **3.** group.

grad. 1. graduate. **2.** graduated.
GU Guam (with Zip Code).
guar., gtd. guaranteed.

h hour.
h. Also **H.,** height.
ha hectare.
hdqrs. headquarters.
hf high frequency.
HI Hawaii (with Zip Code).
HMO health maintenance organization.
Hon. 1. Honorable (title). **2.** Also **hon.** honorary.
hor. horizontal.
hosp. hospital.
hp horsepower.
hr hour.
h.s., H.S. high school.
ht height.
HUD, H.U.D. Housing and Urban Development.
hyp., hypoth. hypothesis.
Hz hertz.

i., I., 1. island. **2.** isle.
IA Iowa (with Zip Code).
ib., ibid. in the same place (Latin *ibidem*).
ID Idaho (with Zip Code).
I.D. 1. identification. **2.** intelligence department.
i.e. that is (Latin *id est*).
IF, i.f. intermediate frequency.

IL Illinois (with Zip Code).
IN Indiana (with Zip Code).
in. inch.
inc. 1. income. **2.** Also **Inc.** incorporated. **3.** increase.
ins. inspector.
inst. 1. instant. **2.** institute. **3.** institution. **4.** instrument.
int. 1. interest. **2.** interior. **3.** interval. **4.** international.
interj. interjection.
intr. *Grammar.* intransitive.
inv. 1. invention. **2.** invoice.
IQ, I.Q. intelligence quotient.
IRA 1. Individual Retirement Account. **2.** Also **I.R.A.** Irish Republican Army.
IRS Internal Revenue Service.
Is., is. island.
ital. italic.

J joule.
J. 1. journal. **2.** judge. **3.** justice.
J.A. 1. joint account. **2.** judge advocate.
Jan. January.
jct., junc. junction.
J.D. Doctor of Laws.
jour. 1. journal. **2.** journalist. **3.** journeyman.
J.P. justice of the peace.
jr., Jr. junior.

k 1. karat. **2.** kilo.
K 1. Kelvin (temperature unit). **2.** Kelvin (temperature scale).
kc kilocycle.
kg kilogram.
km kilometer.
KS Kansas (with Zip Code).
kW kilowatt.
KY Kentucky (with Zip Code).

l liter.
l. 1. Also **L.** lake. **2.** left. **3.** length. **4.** line.
LA Louisiana (with Zip Code).
lab. laboratory.
LAN local area network.
lat. latitude.
Lat. Also **L.** Latin.
lb pound.
LBO leveraged buyout.
l.c. lower-case.
L/C letter of credit.
l.c.d. lowest common denominator.
leg., legis. 1. legislation. **2.** legislative. **3.** legislature.
lf 1. *Printing.* lightface. **2.** low frequency.
lg., lge. large.
lib. 1. liberal. **2.** librarian. **3.** library.
LISP list processing.
lit. 1. literary. **2.** literature.
LL.B. Bachelor of Laws.
LL.D. Doctor of Laws.

loc. cit. in the place cited (Latin *loco citato*).
log logarithm.
long. longitude.
ltd., Ltd. limited.

m 1. Also **M, m., M.** male; medium. **2.** meter.
m. mile.
MA Massachusetts (with Zip Code).
M.A. Master of Arts.
Man. Manitoba.
Mar. March.
masc. masculine.
math. 1. mathematical. **2.** mathematician. **3.** mathematics.
max. maximum.
M.B.A. Master of Business Administration.
Mc megacycle.
m.c. master of ceremonies.
MD Maryland (with Zip Code).
M.D. Doctor of Medicine.
mdse. merchandise.
ME Maine (with Zip Code).
M.E. 1. mechanical engineer. **2.** mechanical engineering. **3.** Middle English.
meas. 1. measurable. **2.** measure.
mech. 1. mechanical. **2.** mechanics. **3.** mechanism.

med. 1. medical. **2.** medieval. **3.** medium.

M.Ed. Master of Education.

mem. 1. member. **2.** memoir. **3.** memorandum. **4.** memorial.

Messrs. 1. Messieurs. **2.** Plural of **Mr.**

mfg. 1. manufacture. **2.** manufactured. **3.** manufacturing.

mfr. 1. manufacture. **2.** manufacturer.

MI Michigan (with Zip Code).

mi. 1. mile. **2.** mill (monetary unit).

min minute (unit of time).

min. minimum.

misc. miscellaneous.

mkt. market.

ml milliliter.

mm millimeter.

MN Minnesota (with Zip Code).

MO Missouri (with Zip Code).

mo. month.

m.o., M.O. 1. mail order. **2.** medical officer. **3.** money order.

mol. 1. molecular. **2.** molecule.

mon. monetary.

Mon. Monday.

mpg, m.p.g. miles per gallon.

mph, m.p.h. miles per hour.

Mr. Mister.

Mrs. mistress.

ms 1. manuscript. **2.** millisecond.

MS 1. manuscript. **2.** Mississippi (with Zip Code). **3.** multiple sclerosis.

Ms., Ms Title of courtesy for a woman.

msg. message.

MST, M.S.T. Mountain Standard Time.

MT Montana (with Zip Code).

mt., Mt. 1. mount. **2.** mountain.

m.t., M.T. metric ton.

MT, M.T. Mountain Time.

mtg. 1. meeting. **2.** Also **mtge.** mortgage.

mtn. mountain.

mun. 1. municipal. **2.** municipality.

mus. 1. museum. **2.** music. **3.** musical. **4.** musician.

MVP most valuable player.

N Also **n, N., n.** north; northern.

n. 1. net. **2.** noun. **3.** number.

N. 1. Norse. **2.** November.

N.A. North America.

NAACP, N.A.A.C.P. National Association for the Advancement of Colored People.

NASA National Aeronautics and Space Administration.

nat. 1. Also **natl.** national. **2.** native. **3.** natural.

NATO North Atlantic Treaty Organization.

nav. 1. naval. **2.** navigation.

n.b. note carefully (Latin *nota bene*).

N.B. New Brunswick.

NBA 1. National Basketball Association. **2.** National Boxing Association.

NC North Carolina (with Zip Code).

NCO noncommissioned officer.

ND North Dakota (with Zip Code).

NE 1. Nebraska (with Zip Code). **2.** northeast.

N.E. New England.

neg. negative.

NFL National Football League.

Nfld. Newfoundland.

NH New Hampshire (with Zip Code).

NHL National Hockey League.

NJ New Jersey (with Zip Code).

NM New Mexico (with Zip Code).

no., No. 1. north. **2.** northern. **3.** number.

nos., Nos. numbers.

Nov. November.

NOW National Organization for Women.

N.P. notary public.

N.S. Nova Scotia.

NV Nevada (with Zip Code).
NW northwest.
N.W.T. Northwest Territories.
NY New York (with Zip Code).

O 1. Also **O.** ocean. **2.** Also **O.** order.
obj. 1. *Grammar.* object; objective. **2.** objection.
obs. 1. obscure. **2.** observation. **3.** Also **Obs.** observatory. **4.** obsolete.
Oct. October.
O.D. 1. Doctor of Optometry. **2.** overdraft. **3.** overdrawn.
OEM original equipment manufacturer.
OH Ohio (with Zip Code).
OK Oklahoma (with Zip Code).
Ont. Ontario.
OPEC Organization of Petroleum Exporting Countries.
OR Oregon (with Zip Code).
org. 1. organic. **2.** organization. **3.** organized.
o.s., o/s out of stock.
OTB off-track betting.
oz ounce.

p. 1. page. **2.** participle. **3.** per. **4.** pint. **5.** population. **6.** Also **P.** president.

PA 1. Pennsylvania (with Zip Code). **2.** public-address system.
P.A. 1. Also **P/A** power of attorney. **2.** press agent. **3.** prosecuting attorney.
Pac. Pacific.
par. 1. paragraph. **2.** parallel. **3.** parenthesis. **4.** parish.
pat. patent.
P.A.Y.E. 1. pay as you earn. **2.** pay as you enter.
payt. Also **p.t.** payment.
P.B. 1. passbook. **2.** prayer book.
PBS Public Broadcasting System.
p.c. Also **pct.** per cent.
PC personal computer.
p/c, P/C 1. Also **p.c.** petty cash. **2.** prices current.
pd. paid.
P.E.I. Prince Edward Island.
pf. preferred.
Pfc, Pfc. private first class.
phar., Phar., pharm., Pharm., 1. pharmaceutical. **2.** pharmacist. **3.** pharmacy.
phi., philos. 1. philosopher. **2.** philosophical. **3.** philosophy.
phr. phrase.
pk. 1. pack. **2.** park. **3.** peak. **4.** Also **pk** peck.
pkg., pkge. package.

pl. 1. platform. **2.** platoon. **3.** plural.
plf. plaintiff.
pm., prem. premium.
p.m. 1. post mortem. **2.** Also **P.M.** post-mortem examination. **3.** Also **P.M.** post meridiem (usually small capitals P.M.).
P.M. 1. past master. **2.** Also **PM** postmaster. **3.** prime minister. **4.** provost marshal.
P.M.G. postmaster general.
p.n., P/N promissory note.
P.O. 1. Personnel Officer. **2.** Also **p.o.** petty officer; post office. **3.** postal order.
P.O.E. port of entry.
poet. 1. poetic. **2.** poetical. **3.** poetry.
pol. 1. Also **polit.** political. **2.** politician. **3.** Also **polit.** politics.
pos. 1. position. **2.** positive.
poss. 1. possession. **2.** possessive. **3.** possible. **4.** possibly.
pot. potential.
POW, P.O.W. prisoner of war.
pp. 1. pages. **2.** past participle.
p.p., P.P. 1. parcel post. **2.** parish priest. **3.** past participle. **4.** postpaid.

ppd. 1. postpaid. **2.** prepaid.

PR. 1. Also **P.R.** public relations. **2.** Puerto Rico (with Zip Code).

pr. 1. pair. **2.** present. **3.** price. **4.** printing. **5.** pronoun.

Pr. 1. priest. **2.** prince.

pref. 1. preface. **2.** prefatory. **3.** preference. **4.** preferred. **5.** prefix.

prep. 1. preparation. **2.** preparatory. **3.** prepare. **4.** preposition.

pres. 1. present (time). **2.** Also **Pres.** president.

prim. 1. primary. **2.** primitive.

prin. 1. principal. **2.** principle.

prob. 1. probable. **2.** probably. **3.** problem.

prof., Prof. professor.

pron. 1. pronominal. **2.** pronoun. **3.** pronounced. **4.** pronunciation.

prop. 1. proper. **2.** properly. **3.** property. **4.** proposition. **5.** proprietary. **6.** proprietor.

pro tem., p.t. for the time being; temporarily (Latin *pro tempore*).

P.S. 1. Police Sergeant. **2.** postscript. **3.** public school.

PST, P.S.T. Pacific Standard Time.

pt. 1. part. **2.** pint. **3.** point. **4.** port.

PT, P.T. Pacific Time.

P.T. physical therapy.

PTA, P.T.A. Parent-Teachers Association.

ptg. printing.

pub. 1. public. **2.** publication. **3.** published. **4.** publisher.

pvt. Also **Pvt.** private.

q. 1. Also **qt.** quart. **2.** Also **qu., ques.** question.

qr. 1. quarter. **2.** quarterly.

qt. 1. quantity. **2.** Also **q.** quart.

quad. 1. quadrangle. **2.** quadrant. **3.** quadrilateral.

Que. Quebec.

ques. Also **q., qu.** question.

quot. quotation.

r 1. Also **R** radius. **2.** *Electricity.* Also **R** resistance.

r. 1. Also **R.** railroad; railway. **2.** range. **3.** rare. **4.** retired. **5.** Also **R.** right. **6.** Also **R.** river. **7.** Also **R.** road. **8.** rod (unit of length). **9.** Also **R.** rouble.

R. 1. rabbi. **2.** rector. **3.** Republican (party). **4.** royal.

R & D research and development.

RAM random access memory.

rd. 1. road. **2.** round.

RD, R.D. rural delivery.

RDA recommended daily allowance.

re concerning; in reference to; in the case of.

R.E. real estate.

rec. 1. receipt. **2.** recipe. **3.** record. **4.** recording. **5.** recreation.

recd. received.

ref. 1. reference. **2.** referred. **3.** refining. **4.** reformation. **5.** reformed. **6.** refunding.

reg. 1. Also **Regt.** regent. **2.** regiment. **3.** region. **4.** Also **regd.** register; registered. **5.** registrar. **6.** registry. **7.** regular. **8.** regularly. **9.** regulation. **10.** regulator.

rep. 1. repair. **2.** Also **rpt.** report. **3.** reporter. **4.** Also **Rep.** representative. **5.** reprint. **6.** Also **Rep.** republic.

Rep. Republican (party).

req. 1. require. **2.** required. **3.** requisition.

rev. 1. revenue. **2.** reverse. **3.** reversed. **4.** review. **5.** reviewed.

6. revise. 7. revision. 8. revolution. 9. revolving.

RF radio frequency.

RFD, R.F.D. rural free delivery.

RI Rhode Island (with Zip Code).

rm. 1. ream. **2.** room.

RN, R.N. registered nurse.

ROM read-only memory.

ROTC Reserve Officers' Training Corps.

r.p.m. revolutions per minute.

R.R. 1. Also **RR** railroad. **2.** Also **RT. Rev.** Right Reverend (title). **3.** rural route.

r.s.v.p., R.S.V.P. please reply.

s 1. second. **2.** Also **S, s., S.** south; southern. **3.** stere.

s. 1. son. **2.** substantive. **3.** shilling.

S. 1. Saturday. **2.** school. **3.** sea. **4.** September. **5.** Sunday.

S.A. 1. South Africa. **2.** South America.

SALT Strategic Arms Limitations Talks.

Sask. Saskatchewan.

Sat. Saturday.

S.B. Bachelor of Science.

SC 1. Security Council (United Nations). **2.** South Car-

olina (with Zip Code).

sc. 1. scene. **2.** scruple (weight). **3.** scilicet.

s.c. *Printing.* small capitals.

S.C. Supreme Court.

sch. school.

sci. 1. science. **2.** scientific.

SD South Dakota (with Zip Code).

S.D. special delivery.

SDI Strategic Defense Initative.

SE 1. southeast. **2.** southeastern.

sec. 1. Also **secy.** secretary. **2.** sector. **3.** second.

SEC Securities and Exchange Commission.

sen., Sen. 1. senate. **2.** senator. **3.** Also **sr.** senior.

Sept. September.

seq. 1. sequel. **2.** the following (Latin *sequens*).

ser. 1. serial. **2.** series. **3.** sermon.

serv. service.

sgd. signed.

sgt. sergeant.

sh. 1. Also **shr.** share (capital stock). **2.** sheet. **3.** shilling.

shpt. shipment.

shtg. shortage.

sic thus; so.

sig. 1. signal. **2.** signature.

sing. singular.

sm. small.

so. 1. south. **2.** southern.

s.o. 1. seller's option. **2.** strikeout.

soc. 1. socialist. **2.** society.

soln solution.

SOP standard operating procedure.

soph. sophomore.

SOS 1. international distress signal. **2.** Any call or signal for help.

sp. 1. special. **2.** species. **3.** spelling.

SPCA Society for the Prevention of Cruelty to Animals.

SPF sun protection factor.

Sr. 1. senior (after surname). **2.** sister (religious).

S.R.O. standing room only.

st. 1. stanza. **2.** state. **3.** Also **St.** statute. **4.** stet. **5.** stitch. **6.** stone. **7.** Also **St.** street. **8.** strophe.

St. 1. saint. **2.** strait.

sta. 1. station. **2.** stationary.

std. standard.

stk. stock.

sub. 1. Also **subs.** subscription. **2.** Also **subst.** substitute. **3.** suburb. **4.** suburban.

subj. 1. subject. **2.** subjective. **3.** subjunctive.

suff. 1. sufficient. **2.** Also **suf.** suffix.

Sun. Sunday.
sup. 1. above (Latin *supra*). **2.** Also **super.** superior. **3.** *Grammar.* Also **superl.** superlative. **4.** supplement. **5.** supply.
supt., Supt. Also **super.** superintendent.
surg. 1. surgeon. **2.** surgery. **3.** surgical.
SW southwest.
sym. 1. symbol. **2.** symphony.
syn. 1. synonymous. **2.** synonym. **3.** synonymy.

t 1. ton. **2.** troy.
T temperature.
t. 1. teaspoon. **2.** *Grammar.* tense. **3.** Also **T.** time. **4.** *Grammar.* transitive.
T. 1. tablespoon. **2.** territory. **3.** Testament. **4.** transit.
TA teaching assistant.
t.b. trial balance.
tbs., tbsp. tablespoon.
TCAM telecommunications access method.
tech. technical.
technol. 1. technological. **2.** technology.
TEFL teaching English as a foreign language.
tel. 1. telegram. **2.** telegraph. **3.** telephone.

temp. 1. in the time of (Latin *tempore*). **2.** temperature. **3.** temporary.
Thurs. Thursday.
tkt. ticket.
TM trademark.
TN Tennessee (with Zip Code).
tn. 1. town. **2.** train.
tnpk. turnpike.
t.o. turnover.
trans. 1. transaction. **2.** *Grammar,* transitive. **3.** translated. **4.** translation. **5.** translator. **6.** Also **transp.** transportation.
treas. 1. treasurer. **2.** treasury.
Tues. Tuesday.
TV television.
TX Texas (with Zip Code).

U. 1. university. **2.** upper.
uhf ultra high frequency.
UN United Nations.
UNESCO United Nations Educational, Scientific, and Cultural Organization.
UNICEF United Nations International Children's Emergency Fund.
univ. 1. universal. **2.** Also **Univ.** university.
USA, U.S.A. 1. United States Army.

2. United States of America.
UT Utah (with Zip Code).
UV ultraviolet.

V 1. *Physics.* velocity. **2.** *Electricity.* volt. **3.** volume.
v. 1. verb. **2.** verse. **3.** version. **4.** Also **vs.** versus. **5.** vide. **6.** voice. **7.** volume (book). **8.** vowel.
V. 1. Also **v.** vice (in titles). **2.** village.
VA 1. Also **V.A.** Veterans' Administration. **2.** Virginia (with Zip Code).
var. 1. variable. **2.** variant. **3.** variation. **4.** variety. **5.** various.
VAT value-added tax.
VCR video cassette recorder.
VD venereal disease.
VDT visual display terminal.
VFW Veterans of Foreign Wars.
vhf, VHF very high frequency.
VI Virgin Islands (with Zip Code).
VIP *Informal.* very important person.
VISTA Volunteers in Service to America.
vol. 1. volume. **2.** volunteer.
V.P. Vice President.

VT Vermont (with Zip Code).
v.v. vice versa.

w 1. width. **2.** Also **W, w., W.** west; western.
W 1. *Electricity.* watt. **2.** *Physics.* Also **w** work.
w. 1. week. **2.** width. **3.** wife. **4.** with.
W. Wednesday.
WA Washington (with Zip Code).
Wed. Wednesday.
WHO World Health Organization.
whse., whs. warehouse.
whsle. wholesale.
WI Wisconsin (with Zip Code).

w.i. when issued (financial stock).
wk. 1. weak. **2.** week. **3.** work.
wkly. weekly.
w.o.c. without compensation.
wt. weight.
WV West Virginia (with Zip Code).
WY Wyoming (with Zip Code).

x symbol for an unknown or unnamed factor, thing, or person.
XL extra large.
Xmas *Informal.* Christmas.

y ordinate.
y. year.
YMCA Young Men's Christian Assocation.
yr. 1. year. **2.** younger. **3.** your.
Y.T. Yukon Territory.
YWCA Young Women's Christian Association.

Z 1. atomic number. **2.** *Electricity.* impedance.
z. 1. zero. **2.** zone.
zool. 1. zoological. **2.** zoology.
ZPG zero population growth.